# Psychoneuroimmunology

## THIRD EDITION

## Volume 2

Edited by

**Robert Ader**

*Department of Psychiatry*
*Center for Psychoneuroimmunology Research*
*University of Rochester Medical Center*
*Rochester, New York*

**David L. Felten**

*Center for Neuroimmunology*
*Loma Linda University School of Medicine*
*Loma Linda, California*

**Nicholas Cohen**

*Department of Microbiology and Immunology*
*Center for Psychoneuroimmunology Research*
*University of Rochester Medical Center*
*Rochester, New York*

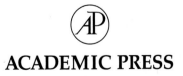

## ACADEMIC PRESS

A Harcourt Science and Technology Company

San Diego   San Francisco   New York   Boston   London   Sydney   Tokyo

Academic Press
*A Harcourt Science and Technology Company*
525 B Street, Suite 1900, San Diego, California 92101-4495, USA
http://www.academicpress.com

Academic Press
Harcourt Place, 32 Jamestown Road, London NW1 7BY, UK
http://www.academicpress.com

Library of Congress Catalog Card Number: 00-102888

International Standard Book Number: 0-12-044314-7 (Set)
International Standard Book Number: 0-12-044315-5 Volume 1
International Standard Book Number: 0-12-044316-3 Volume 2

PRINTED IN THE UNITED STATES OF AMERICA
00  01  02  03  04  05  WP  9  8  7  6  5  4  3  2  1

*For Gayle,*
        *Deb,*
        *Janet,*
        *Rini, and*
        *Leslie;*

                *Mary,*
                        *Mike,*
                        *Matt, and*
                        *Brannon;*

                                *Inike,*
                                        *Jamie,*
                                        *Jessica,*
                                        *Mischa, and*
                                        *Mark*

# Contents

# VOLUME 1

# BEHAVIORAL EFFECTS ON IMMUNITY

# 29

# Conditioning and Immunity

ROBERT ADER, NICHOLAS COHEN

## I. INTRODUCTION

Learning, a primary function of brain activity, is the primary means by which higher organisms adapt to their environment. Thus, a dramatic illustration of the role of the nervous system in the modulation of immunity is provided by several demonstrations that immune responses can be modified by learning, i.e., classical conditioning (Ader & Cohen, 1991). As frequently happens, clinical observations antedate experimental research and such is the case for conditioned immune reactions. In 1896, Mackenzie described his use of an artificial rose to induce a "so-called 'rose cold'" in an allergic patient. He also reported that, in 1557, "...Amatus Lusitanus related the case of a Dominican monk, who, whenever he perceived the odor of roses *or saw them at a distance*, was immediately seized with syncope and fell unconscious to the ground." (Mackenzie 1896, p. 51, italics added). Hill (1930), too, reported that the mere picture of a hay field was sufficient to provoke an attack of hay fever in very sensitive subjects. The literature contains other vignettes that describe what appear to be conditioned allergic responses and these

receive some experimental confirmation from clinical studies in humans (Dekker, Pelser, & Groen, 1957; Khan, 1977) and animals (Ottenberg, Stein, Lewis, & Hamilton, 1958). Exposure to symbolic, nonallergenic stimuli (conditioned stimuli) previously associated with allergens (unconditioned stimuli) can elicit asthmatic symptoms in some subjects.

The classical (Pavlovian) conditioning of non-immunologically specific host defense mechanisms and antigen-specific immune responses was first studied by Russian scientists in the 1920s and adhered to the principles and procedures of the day (e.g., Metal'nikov & Chorine, 1926, 1928). The classic example of Pavlovian conditioning is the salivation of dogs in response to a formerly neutral *conditioned* stimulus (CS) such as a tone that has, in the past, been repeatedly paired with food in the mouth, the *unconditioned* stimulus (UCS) for salivation. Similarly, after multiple pairings of a neutral CS and an injection of antigen, the UCS, exposure to the CS, alone, was purported to effect conditioned increases in nonspecific defense responses and, in some cases, conditioned increases in antibody production. Conversely, repeated injections of immunologically neutral material suppressed the response to the subsequent presentation of an antigenic stimulus. More recent observations have been made of an attenuated immune response when animals (Moynihan, Koota, Brenner, Cohen, & Ader, 1989; Shaskin & Lovett, 1981) or humans (Smith & McDaniels, 1983) are injected with antigen under circumstances that had been associated repeatedly with the injection of immunologically neutral material.

Most of these early Russian studies were inadequately described and poorly designed. They constituted little more than preliminary observations. Nevertheless, the studies of nonspecific cellular events (e.g., changes in leukocyte number, phagocytosis, inflammatory responses), in particular, were consistent and suggested that conditioning could, indeed, modulate host defenses. Early English language reviews of these Russian studies (Hull, 1934; Kopeloff, 1941), however, attracted little attention. The most detailed review of these early studies was provided by Ader (1981). In the present chapter, we will provide a brief review of modern studies on the conditioned modulation of immune function, concentrating on studies published since our review of this topic in the Second edition of *Psychoneuroimmunology* (Ader, Felten, & Cohen, 1991).

To provide some overall perspective on experimental strategies, Table I defines the major treatment groups that are used in studies of the conditioned modulation of immune responses. All these groups may not be necessary in all experiments (and, in fact, cannot be included in some experiments), but most of these groups are critical in one or another stage of most research programs.

Group CS is the primary experimental group. These are a subgroup of conditioned animals that, at the time of testing for conditioned responses, are reexposed to the CS previously paired with the UCS (e.g., an immunomodulating drug, an endogenous immunomodulating agent, an antigen).

Identically treated conditioned animals that are not reexposed to the CS at the time of testing (Group CSo) serve as a control for any direct or indirect immunomodulating effects of the conditioning procedures, per se, and as a control for the residual effects of the UCS. In the absence of a CSo group, one cannot be certain that some component of either the CS, the UCS, or some combination thereof did not have long-term, sensitization effects (Domjan & Burkhard, 1986) that could influence one or another immune response.

Another critical control group is composed of animals that, at the time of testing, are reexposed to the UCS (Group UCS). This is the "positive" control group that defines the effects unconditionally elicited by the UCS and, additionally, serves as a procedural check on the immunological assays being conducted. Ideally, Group UCS would also experience the conditioning procedures and would be reexposed to the UCS at the same time that Group CS is reexposed to the CS. A Group UCS that is exposed to the UCS at any other time may more accurately satisfy the definition of a nonconditioned group.

There are several nonconditioned control groups that have been used in examining the conditioned modulation of immunity. The most appropriate group of nonconditioned animals (Group NC) in a situation in which there is only a single (or just a few) conditioning trial(s) is a group that is exposed to the CS and to the UCS, but in an unpaired or noncontingent manner, such that the number of exposures to the CS and the UCS is the same for all groups. Group NC (like Group CS) is also reexposed to the CS at the time of testing to be certain that, for these animals, the immunologically neutral CS has, in fact, remained neutral. In the absence of this NC group, one cannot be certain that the response in Group CS reflects conditioning or that the difference between a Group CS and a Group CSo, for example, represents a conditioned response in one or the other of these groups or conditioned responses of different magnitudes in both groups. A nonconditioned group that does not experience noncontingent CS–UCS presentations or is not reexposed to the CS at the time of testing (and, thus, receives fewer exposures to the CS and/or the UCS than Group CS) will be referred to here as Group [NC].

## TABLE I  Treatment Conditions

| Group | PRE | Treatment | Sub-group | Test trial(s) | Rationale |
|-------|-----|-----------|-----------|---------------|-----------|
| Cond. | None | CS + UCS | CS | CS + Sal | Experimental group: conditioning effects |
|       | None |          | CSo | $H_2O$ | Control: effects of conditioning, per se; residual effects of CS + UCS |
|       | CS   |          | CSp | CS + Sal | Control: effects of CS preexposure (attenuation of CR) |
|       | None |          | UCS | $H_2O$ + UCS | Unconditioned effects |
| Noncond. | None | CS ≠ UCS | NC | CS | Control: noncontingent CS–UCS pairing; nonassociative factors; residual effects of UCS |
| Placebo | None | CS + Sal | P | CS + Sal | Control: residual effects of CS and handling, injections, etc. |

Note. CS, conditioned stimulus; CSo, no conditioned stimulus; UCS, unconditioned stimulus; +, paired; ≠, unpaired; Sal, saline.

Still another control group consists of animals that are exposed to the CS (as often as Group CS) but are never exposed to the UCS. Instead, they are treated with an immunologically neutral stimulus or placebo (the "negative" control) and will be referred to as Group P.

Unfortunately, all studies on the classical conditioning of immunologic effects do not use all the necessary control groups or treat the several control groups in the most appropriate manner. Such omissions should influence one's interpretation of any observed differences but should be considered in relation to other information that may be available, such as the demonstrated effects of experimental extinction. Repeated exposures to the CS that are not followed (reinforced) by the UCS should diminish and eventually extinguish the conditioned response. Preexposure to the CS interferes with the acquisition of conditioned responses (Lubow, 1973). Therefore, the addition of a Group CSp that is exposed to the CS before it is paired with the UCS should attenuate the conditioned response and thus furnish additional evidence of the effects of associative processes. (If a CSp group is used, the remaining groups should, at the same time(s) be exposed to an irrelevant stimulus.) Also, there are circumstances in which it is not possible to impose certain control conditions. One cannot, for example, administer immunomodulating agents to conscious human patients in the absence of conditioned stimuli. However, there are still other experimental strategies (e.g., discriminative conditioning protocols) that can be used to validate conditioning effects.

## II. CONDITIONED IMMUNOSUPPRESSION

Modern studies of conditioned alterations of immune responses were initiated by Ader and Cohen (1975), who used an especially powerful, one-trial passive avoidance conditioning paradigm known as taste aversion learning (Garcia & Koelling, 1967). Consumption of a novel, distinctively flavored drinking solution, the CS, is paired with a stimulus that unconditionally elicits some noxious internal effects, the UCS. Animals reexposed to a novel, distinctively flavored drinking solution previously paired with the noxious internal effects unconditionally elicited by lithium chloride or cyclophosphamide (or any number of other drugs) will avoid drinking the CS solution when it is subsequently offered. Exposure to the novel drinking solution before conditioning trials begin will interfere with acquisition of the conditioned taste

aversion, and repeatedly exposing conditioned animals to the CS in the absence of the UCS will lead to extinction of the conditioned response.

## A. Conditioned Immunopharmacolgic Effects

In the initial study of conditioned immunosuppression, Ader and Cohen (1975) paired saccharin-flavored water, the CS, with an intraperitoneal (ip) injection of cyclophosphamide (CY), an immunosuppressive UCS that also produces a transient gastrointestinal upset. Nonconditioned animals were injected with CY after drinking plain water (saccharin was provided at some other time in subsequent experiments), and a placebo group was injected with saline following consumption of plain water or saccharin. Subsequently, (3 days later in this first experiment), all animals were injected with antigen (sheep red blood cells, SRBC) and, at that same time (and/or 3 days after immunization), the several groups were treated as follows:

One group of conditioned animals (Group CS) was reexposed to the saccharin solution and injected with saline instead of CY; a second conditioned group (Group CSo) was not reexposed to the CS but furnished with plain water to control for the effects of conditioning, per se, and any residual effects of CY; and a third group of conditioned animals (Group UCS) was provided with plain water and injected with CY to define the unconditioned effects of the drug. The nonconditioned animals (Group NC) that received CY but not saccharin were, at the time of immunization and/or 3 days later, exposed to the saccharin drinking solution. Placebo-treated animals (Group P) were also provided with saccharin.

As expected, conditioned animals showed an aversion to the saccharin solution previously paired with CY. Also, conditioned animals that were reexposed to the CS showed an attenuated anti-SRBC serum antibody response compared to nonconditioned animals that were exposed to saccharin and conditioned animals that were not reexposed to the CS. These results, immediately verified in other laboratories (Rogers, Reich, Strom, & Carpenter, 1976; Wayner, Flannery, & Singer, 1978), have been taken as evidence for behaviorally conditioned suppression of immune function.

When last reviewed (Ader & Cohen, 1991), there was already an extensive literature documenting the conditioned modulation of non-immunologically- specific host defense reactions (e.g., Hiramoto, Hiramoto, Solvason, & Ghanta, 1987; Kusnecov, Husband, & King, 1988; Lysle, Cunnick, Fowler, &

Rabin, 1988; Neveu, Dantzer, & LeMoal, 1986; O'Reilly & Exon, 1986), the acquisition and/or the extinction of the conditioned suppression of antibody production (e.g., Ader, Cohen, & Bovbjerg, 1982; Bovbjerg, Kim, Siskind, & Weksler, 1987; Gorczynski, 1987a, 1991a; Gorczynski & Kennedy, 1984), and the acquisition and/or extinction of the conditioned suppression of cell-mediated immune responses (e.g., Bovbjerg, Ader, & Cohen, 1982, 1984). A considerably smaller literature dealt the conditioned enhancement of immunologic reactivity (e.g., Bovbjerg, Cohen, & Ader, 1987a; Gorczynski, Macrae, & Kennedy, 1982; MacQueen, Marshall, Perdue, Siegel, & Bienenstock, 1989).

Many of these studies used the taste aversion conditioning model and immunopharmacologic agents as UCSs, and while the phenomenon is not restricted to conditioned immunopharmacologic effects, there have been important additions to the literature using these procedures. For example, Morato, Gerbase-DeLima, and Gorczynski (1996) examined such conditioning in the context of mucosal immunity and T to B-cell collaboration. Splenic or Peyer's patch T cells from mice that had been immunized orally (with either SRBC or keyhole limpet hemocyanin) were cocultured with primed splenic B cells and antigen, and the numbers of specific IgM and IgA antibody forming cells were determined in vitro. Fewer IgM and IgG antibody forming cells were detected in cultures that contained T cells from conditioned mice (pairing of CY with chocolate milk) that had been reexposed to the CS than were present in cultures in which T cells were from either conditioned animals that had not been reexposed to the CS or nonconditioned mice. Levels of antigen-stimulated IL-2 and IL-4 from Peyer's patch T cells were also reduced in the conditioned group relative to the aforementioned controls.

One of the early questions about conditioning concerned the possibility that there are populations of lymphocytes that might be especially sensitive to the changes induced by conditioning and, thus, responsible for the conditioned changes in immune function. The conditioned suppression of lymphoproliferative responses in animals, for example, has been found in response to T-cell mitogens but not (or less reliably) in response to B-cell mitogens (Kusnecov et al., 1988; Lysle, Cunnick, Kucinski, Fowler, & Rabin, 1990a; Neveu et al., 1986). The results of adoptive transfer experiments (Gorczynski, 1987b) also suggest that the effects of conditioning might operate primarily through an effect on T cells. The transfer of splenocytes from conditioned or unconditioned mice into irradiated conditioned or unconditioned mice

that were or were not exposed to the CS resulted in increases or decreases in the production of anti-SRBC IgG depending upon the source of the donor cells and the treatment condition of the recipient. The separate transfer of T-cell- and B-cell-enriched splenocytes suggested that the conditioning effects derived from the adoptively transferred T cells (see also Gorczynski, 1991b).

In this regard, only a few studies on conditioning have examined the response to T-cell-independent antigens. Cohen, Ader, Green, and Bovbjerg (1979) observed a conditioned suppression of the response to immunization with the hapten, 2,4,6-trinitrophenol (TNP) coupled to the T-independent carrier, lipopolysaccharide (LPS), a type 1 thymus independent antigen (Mosier & Subbarao, 1982). Wayner and her colleagues (1978), however, did not find conditioned immunosuppression using the thymus-independent antigen, *Brucella abortus*. Although considered a type 1 antigen, there is a literature suggesting that *B. abortus* behaves like a type 2 thymus- independent immunogen (Boswell, Nerenberg, Scheer, & Singer, 1980), resembling pneumoccocal polysaccharide rather than LPS in its actions. Similarly, Schulze, Benson, Paule, and Roberts (1988) were able to demonstrate conditioned immunosuppression using SRBC, but they were unable to observe a conditioned suppression of the antibody response to pneumococcal polysaccharide, a type 2 T-cell- independent immunogen.

That the nature of the antigen determines whether the immune responses it evokes can be modulated by conditioning is evidenced by other recent data reported by Morato, Gerbase-DeLima, and Gorczynski (1997). Bacterial LPS stimulates murine B cells without the involvement of macrophages or T cells (Andersson & Blomgren, 1971; Jacobs & Morrison, 1975). Thus, using the same procedures previously used to demonstrate conditioned suppression of antibody and cytokine production in mice orally immunized with SRBC (Morato et al., 1996), Morato and his colleagues (1997) next studied the effects of conditioning with cyclophosphamide on the response to orally ingested LPS. Mice were conditioned by pairing saccharin consumption with an ip injection of CY. Two weeks later, these animals were divided into subgroups that were or were not reexposed to the CS and then given LPS and an ip injection of vehicle. Nonconditioned groups were exposed to saccharin and then treated with LPS. Conditioned animals received a second reexposure to the CS 3 days later and were sacrificed 3 days after that. There was a dramatic suppression of anti-LPS IgM production in the spleens of conditioned mice that were reexposed to the CS compared to each of the control groups that did not differ from each other. The conditioned suppression of T-independent antibody responses confirmed the findings of Cohen et al. (1979) and indicates that conditioning may influence B cells and is not necessarily confined to T cells as previously hypothesized (Gorczynski, 1987b, 1991).

The immunosuppressive effects of CY can also be used to condition a suppression of cell-mediated immunity. When splenic leukocytes from inbred Lewis strain rats are injected into a hind footpad of hybrid (Lewis × Brown Norwegian)F1 rats, the grafted cells see the host as "foreign" and a local inflammatory reaction, the graft-versus-host (GvH) response, ensues. The GvH response can be measured by weighing the popliteal lymph node draining the injection site. Although a single, low-dose injection of CY is only moderately effective, multiple low-dose injections of CY will suppress this GvH response. Bovbjerg et al., (1982) asked if reexposures to a CS previously paired with CY in conjunction with a single, low-dose injection of CY would suppress the GvH response. That is, rather than expect a symbolic stimulus to suppress immunity by itself, they asked if a CS presented in conjunction with a minimally effective UCS would be more effective than either stimulus alone.

In the studies by Bovbjerg and colleagues (1982, 1984), then, (Lewis × Norwegian)F1 rats were first conditioned by pairing saccharin consumption and CY. Seven weeks later, experimental and control groups were injected with splenic leukocytes from Lewis strain donors. On the day of grafting and on the succeeding 2 days, they were reexposed to the CS; on the day after grafting, they were also injected with a low dose of CY. The single low-dose injection of CY *plus* reexposure to the CS significantly suppressed the GvH response relative to nonconditioned animals that were initially given noncontingent CS and UCS exposures and conditioned animals that received the low dose of CY but was not reexposed to the CS. There was no difference between conditioned animals given a single, low-dose injection of CY in conjunction with reexposures to the CS and a UCS group that received three low-dose injections of CY (Bovbjerg et al., 1982). Unreinforced exposures to the CS introduced during the 7-week interval between conditioning and induction of the GvH response resulted in extinction of the conditioned behavioral and immunosuppressive responses.

Roudebush and Bryant (1991) studied the conditioned immunosuppression of a delayed-type hypersensitivity (DTH) reaction, another cell-mediated immune response. The primary purpose of this study was to directly address the possibility that condition-

ally suppressed T-cell-mediated responses might be the result of elevated adrenocortical steroid levels. Mice were conditioned by pairing the taste of saccharin with an injection of CY. On the conditioning day, mice were also sensitized by the topical application of picryl chloride to a shaved section of the abdomen. Three days later, when animals were challenged with footpad injections of picryl chloride, conditioned and nonconditioned mice were or were not reexposed to saccharin. Footpad swelling was measured the next day. Group CS showed a conditioned taste aversion to saccharin and a suppressed DTH response. However, there were no differences between conditioned and nonconditioned animals at any of the several sample times that followed reexposure to plain water or saccharin, respectively. In another experiment using dexamethasone instead of CY as the UCS, reexposure to the CS induced an aversion to saccharin but there was no conditioned immunosuppressive response.

Lesions in the insular cortex region of the neocortex disrupt the acquisition and retention of conditioned taste aversions (Garcia, Lasiter, Bermúdez-Rattoni, & Deems, 1985). Thus, Ramírez-Amaya et al. (1996) inquired into the effects of insular cortex (IC) lesions on acquisition of conditioned immunosuppressive responses. Insular cortex and parietal cortex lesions were made by bilateral microinjections of N-methyl-D-aspartate (NMDA) several days before the rats were conditioned by the pairing of a saccharin drinking solution and an injection of CY. Three weeks later, lesioned and sham-treated animals were immunized with either SRBC or ovalbumin (OVA) and experimental animals were reexposed to the CS. Lesions in the insular cortex but not the parietal cortex blocked the acquisition of a conditioned aversion to the CS solution and the conditioned suppression of antibody production to both antigens. IC lesions did not, however, influence the humoral immune response of normal (placebo-treated) animals or animals immunosuppressed by CY.

Because of the functional relationships between the IC and the amygdala, a second study (Ramírez-Amaya, Alvarez-Borda, & Bermúdez-Rattoni, 1998) examined the effects of NMDA-induced IC and amygdala lesions made before or after acquisition of the CY-induced conditioned responses. Again, IC lesions disrupted the acquisition and the expression of the conditioned taste aversion and the immunosuppressive response to OVA. Lesions in the amygdala interfered with acquisition of the conditioned immunosuppressive response but had no effect on the performance of the learned response. Amygdala lesions also had no effect on the acquisition or expression of the conditioned taste aversion. These are not nonspecific effects because neither lesion influenced the immune response in normal animals and amygdala lesions did not alter the sensory systems necessary for taste aversion learning.

It appears from these studies that the integrity of the insular cortex is essential for whatever neural mechanisms underlie the acquisition of an association between a gustatory CS and the effects of cyclophosphamide—in much the same way, perhaps, that the insular cortex is critical for the learning of other taste aversions and avoidance responses (e.g., Bermúdez-Rattoni & McGaugh,1991; Garcia et al., 1985). The involvement of the IC in the conditioning of immunosuppression, the authors suggest, is achieved through its connections with the hypothalamus and/or the autonomic nervous system. Because lesions in the amygdala affect the acquisition of a conditioned immune response but not the conditioned taste aversion, the authors hypothesize that the amygdala provides the feedback from the immune system to the central nervous system (CNS) that is required for the associations that are responsible for conditioned changes in immune function—or, at least, conditioned changes in antibody production. It will be of interest to determine if the same structures subserve conditioned alterations of cell-mediated immunity.

It is not necessary to use cytotoxic agents that unconditionally suppress immune function in order to condition an immunosuppressive response. Other drugs (e.g., psychotropic drugs) induce a variety of psychophysiological changes—including changes in immunocompetence. Morphine, for example, has immunological consequences (e.g., Lysle, Coussons, Watts, Bennett, & Dykstra, 1993) and can be used as a UCS to condition changes in immune function. Coussons, Dykstra, and Lysle (1992) observed a decrease in mitogen responsiveness and nature killer (NK)-cell activity when rats that experienced 2, 4, 8, or 16 daily trials on which a sc injection of morphine (15 mg/kg) was paired with a 1-h exposure to a distinctive environment (CS) were later reexposed to the CS. In a second experiment using the same conditioning procedures, they observed a decrease in the blastogenic response of splenic and blood lymphocytes to both T- and B-cell mitogens, a decrease in NK-cell activity, and a decrease in IL-2 production in conditioned rats reexposed to the CS compared to that seen in conditioned animals that were not reexposed to the CS—and nonconditioned and placebo-treated animals that were returned to the distinctive environment. Rats develop a preference for environments in which they have received morphine (Carr, Fibinger, & Phillips, 1989; Eikelboom &

Stewart, 1979; Schwarz & Cunningham, 1990; Stefurak, Martin, & Van der Kooy, 1990). These data, then, provide additional evidence that aversive conditioning is not necessary in order to observe conditioned immunosuppressive responses.

As elaborated in earlier chapters of this book, primary and secondary lymphoid tissues are sympathetically innervated and there are adrenergic receptors on lymphocytes. Such data provide grounds for expecting that catecholamines might have a direct effect on immune function and, since morphine increases plasma levels of catecholamines, Coussons-Read, Dykstra, and Lysle (1994a) explored the role of $\beta$-adrenergic receptor activity in the acquisition and expression of morphine-induced conditioned alterations of immune function. In their first experiment, nalodol, a peripheral $\beta$-adrenergic receptor antagonist, was given to rats 15 min before each of two trials on which morphine was paired with a 1-h exposure to a distinctive cage environment. Twelve days later, half the animals were reexposed to the CS and half remained undisturbed. Nalodol had no effect on conditioned immunosuppressive responses at any of the doses used. When introduced after conditioning but before testing, nalodol, at the higher or highest doses, blocked the effects of conditioning on lymphoproliferation and IL-2 production by splenocytes but had no effect on the conditioned suppression of NK-cell activity. The latter finding is consistent with the report that $\beta$-adrenergic antagonists have no effect on the unconditioned decrease in NK-cell activity induced by morphine (Fecho, Dykstra, & Lysle, 1993). It is also of interest that, in contrast to the effects of morphine on lymphoproliferation and interferon (IFN)-$\gamma$ production, prior exposure to morphine results in tolerance to morphine's suppressive effect on NK-cell activity (West, Lysle, & Dykstra (1997).

Observations such as these (e.g., Luecken & Lysle, 1992), demonstrating that different lymphocyte populations are differentially sensitive to $\beta$-adrenergic stimulation, are important for the study of the mechanisms underlying conditioned immunologic effects. Coussons-Read and her colleagues make a case for the possibility that centrally acting catecholamines may still play a role in the conditioned suppression of NK-cell activity. The central depletion of catecholamines does appear to abrogate a conditioned enhancement of NK-cell activity (Hiramoto, Solvason, Ghanta, Lorden, & Hiramoto, 1990). More generally, though, such findings undermine any expectation that a single mechanism could account for the diverse effects of conditioning. If, based on other data from the authors' laboratory (Fecho et al.,

1993), we infer that nalodol given before conditioning blocked some or all of the immunological effects of morphine, then the observation of a conditioned response suggests that the CS–UCS association is being made centrally and that different mechanisms are involved in the development as opposed to the expression of conditioned immune changes.

Coussons-Read, Dykstra, and Lysle (1994b) also examined the role of opioid receptors in the conditioning of morphine-induced immune alterations. Using the same behavioral conditions, naltrexone injected before conditioning prevented acquisition of the conditioned suppression of splenic lymphoproliferation, NK-cell activity, and IL-2 production. Naltrexone injected before testing blocked the expression of conditioned alterations in lymphoproliferative responses, attenuated the suppression of NK-cell activity only at the highest dose of drug, and had no effect on IL-2 production. Thus, these data show that an opioid receptor antagonist can attenuate the response to a CS paired with morphine under conditions in which morphine is a positive reinforcer (Mucha, Van der Kooy, O'Shaughnessey, & Bucenieks, 1982) as well as attenuate the response to electric shocks, a noxious stimulus (Lysle, Luecken, & Maslonek, 1992a), or a morphine-induced conditioned taste aversion (LeBlanc & Cappell, 1975). Apparently, the noxious or so-called stressful nature of the UCS is not a critical factor. It is also clear from these data that the development and expression of conditioned changes in immune function depend upon the parameter of immune function being examined and that different pathways support the development and expression of conditioned alterations of different immune responses. Apropos of one potential pathway, these authors note the analogous observation that chemically induced peripheral sympathectomy suppresses concanavalin A (ConA) -induced lymphoproliferation but has no effect on IL-2 production (Madden et al., 1994).

## B. Conditioned Stress Effects

Conditioned immunomodulatory effects can also be obtained without using immunomodulatory drugs. Sato, Flood, and Makinodan (1984), for example, delayed the recovery of a humoral immune response in irradiated mice that were reexposed to the complex of CSs previously paired with electric shock stimulation. Other stressors have also been effective UCSs for the conditioning of alterations of lymphoproliferative and antibody responses in mice (Drugan et al., 1986; Gorczynski & Kennedy, 1984; Zalcman, Richter, &

Anisman, 1989). The most extensive series of studies demonstrating that cues associated with the immunosuppressive effects of stress can, through conditioning, assume immunosuppressive properties were conducted by Lysle and his colleagues (Luecken & Lysle, 1992; Lysle et al., 1988, 1990a, 1992a; Lysle & Maslonek, 1991; Lysle, Cunnick, & Maslonek, 1991; Perez & Lysle, 1995, 1997).

These investigators first characterized the conditioned suppression of lymphoproliferative responses in rats reexposed to cues previously paired with stressful stimulation (Lysle et al., 1988). On 2 successive days, experimental animals were placed into a novel chamber for 40 min and subjected to a series of conditioning trials involving paired presentations of an auditory or visual CS and electric footshocks. Six days later, these conditioned animals were returned to the experimental chambers and reexposed to the CS. Compared to animals in Group NC, Group CS showed decreased proliferative responses to Con A and phytohemagglutinin (PHA), two T-cell mitogens. Unreinforced exposures to the CS during the interval between conditioning and testing resulted in experimental extinction (actually, a reduction but not complete elimination of the conditioned responses), and preexposure to the CS attenuated the conditioned immunosuppressive responses. These additional observations support the proposition that the observed suppression of lymphoproliferative responses was the result of associative learning.

In further characterizing the conditioned responses of male, Lewis strain rats (Lysle, Cunnick & Rabin, 1990b Lysle & Maslonek, 1991), these investigators again observed a conditioned suppression of lymphoproliferative responses to Con A, PHA, and lipopolysaccharide (LPS), a B-cell mitogen. The magnitude of the suppression depended upon the immune compartment from which the cells were obtained and, as previously noted (Zalcman et al., 1989), the interval between conditioning and testing. Splenic lymphocytes from conditioned rats reexposed to the CS were suppressed in their response to both T- and B-cell mitogens; whole blood lymphocytes showed the depressed responsiveness to Con A and PHA, but not to LPS; and no conditioned response was observed in cells obtained from mesenteric lymph nodes. In addition, there was a conditioned suppression of splenic NK-cell activity.

Using female, Sprague–Dawley rats and a longer interval between conditioning and testing, Shanks, Kusnecov, Pezzone, Berkun, and Rabin (1997) observed an enhanced PHA-stimulated production of IL-2 and LPS-stimulated production of IL-1 in splenocytes from conditioned animals reexposed to the CS. This level of variability is not surprising considering the strain differences in different dimensions of immunologic reactivity described by Shurin, Kusnecov, Riechman, and Rabin (1995). Shanks and colleagues (1997) and others (Zhou, Kusnecov, Shurin, DePaoli, & Rabin, 1993) also found an elevation in plasma IL-6 levels when rats were returned to the environment in which they had been given electric footshocks. The enhanced levels of IL-6 were viewed as a product of the neuroendocrine response to the stressful experience rather than being of immune origin since there was, if anything, a decreased production of IL-6 in cultures of splenic and peripheral blood mononuclear cells.

Several lines of evidence—the sympathetic innervation of lymphoid tissues, the effects of catecholamines and adrenocortical steroids on immune function, and the effects of $\beta$-adrenergic and opioid antagonists on the stress-induced suppression of immunologic reactivity—suggested that catecholamines and/or endogenous opioids might be pathways through which conditioned stress effects were realized. Thus, Lysle and his colleagues (1991) examined the effects of a nonselective $\beta$-adrenergic receptor antagonist, propranolol, on the conditioned suppression of mitogen responsiveness. Animals were conditioned, as described above, and injected with varying doses of propranolol before being divided into groups that were or were not reexposed to the CS. Propranolol blocked the conditioned suppression of the splenic lymphoproliferative responses to T- and B-cell mitogens of conditioned rats that were reexposed to the CS. Propranol did not affect adrenocortical activity; plasma corticosterone levels were elevated in all animals reexposed to the shock chamber, but only the animals injected with saline rather than propranolol showed the conditioned immunosuppression.

When administered 30 min before each of the two conditioning sessions, propranolol had no effect on the subsequent expression of the conditioned response, even though we can assume that propranolol blocked the unconditioned effects of the electric shock stimulation (Cunnick, Lysle, Kucinski, & Rabin, 1990). Like the effects of nadolol on morphine-induced conditioned immune responses (Coussons-Read et al., 1994a), such results may be an example of conditioning that is not dependent on the peripheral expression of the conditioned change in immunologic reactivity during the course of training. It is possible, however, that conditioned behavioral, affective, and/or neuroendocrine responses elicited by reexposure to the CS constitute unconditioned stimuli for changes in some aspects of immune function.

Using selective $\beta$-adrenergic receptor antagonists and an expanded battery of immune measures, Luecken and Lysle (1992) found that treatment with $\beta_1$- and $\beta_2$-receptor antagonists before reexposing conditioned animals to the CS yielded similar results: an attenuation of the conditioned suppression of lymphoproliferative responses of splenic T cells and of IFN-$\gamma$ production and no effects on the conditioned suppression of the response to LPS, splenic NK-cell activity, or IL-2 production. It is of additional interest that $\beta$-adrenergic receptor antagonists, which blocked the unconditioned effects of electric shock on the mitogen responsiveness of splenic but not peripheral blood lymphocytes (Cunnick et al., 1990), also failed to interfere with the shock-induced conditioned suppression of whole blood lymphoproliferative responses. Based on this series of experiments, it would appear that the release of catecholamines is instrumental for the conditioned suppression of some immune responses. Along similar lines, Exton et al., (1998), using cyclosporin A (CsA) as the UCS, reported that surgical denervation of the spleen abrogated the conditioned suppression of lymphoproliferation and of IL-2 and IFN-$\gamma$ production without influencing the unconditioned effects of CsA— and without affecting the acquisition of a conditioned taste aversion.

In an attempt to identify those brain areas that might be involved in unconditioned and conditioned changes in immune function, Pezzone, Lee, Hoffman, and Rabin (1992) measured the immunocytochemical localization of c-Fos in the rat forebrain in response to a series of electric shocks or an auditory cue previously paired with electric shocks. c-Fos, the product of a nuclear protooncogene that effectively "marks" stimulated neurons, was expressed in cells of the paraventricular nucleus of the hypothalamus (some of which contain corticotropin-releasing hormone (CRH)) and other hypothalamic areas related to autonomic function in conditioned animals reexposed to the CS. CS exposure also induced c-Fos immunoreactivity in noradrenergic neurons in several brainstem areas (Pezzone, Lee, Hoffman, Pezzone, & Rabin, 1993), which is consonant with the findings of Lysle and his colleagues described above.

There is also evidence that central opioid activity mediates the conditioning of some stress-induced conditioned immune changes (Lysle et al., 1992a). When administered before reexposing conditioned animals to the CS, naltrexone, a centrally and peripherally acting opiate receptor antagonist, caused a dose-dependent attenuation of the CS-induced suppression of splenic lymphocytes to mitogen stimulation and of NK-cell activity. Methyl-naltrexone, a quaternary form of naltrexone that does not cross the blood–brain barrier, did not interfere with expression of a conditioned suppression of mitogen responsiveness or NK-cell activity. Thus, it would appear that the conditioned immunosuppressive responses were mediated by the central action of endogenous opioids. Perez and Lysle (1997) further refined the involvement of opioid function by demonstrating that the central blocking of the selective $\mu$-opioid receptor was responsible for the observed interference with the conditioned immunosuppression of lymphoproliferative responses, NK-cell activity, and IFN-$\gamma$ production.

The results of these explorations of potential mediators of conditioned changes in immunologic reactivity are summarized in Table II. They clearly indicate that multiple mechanisms are involved. It would appear that interference with the release of catecholamines or the central action of endogenous opioids are equally effective (and may interact) in attenuating lymphoproliferative responses to T-cell mitogens. Nitric oxide production by macrophages has been proposed as a link in the chain that connects opioid and catecholaminergic responses to the conditioned suppression of lymphoproliferation (Coussons-Read, Maslonek, Fecho, Perez, & Lysle, 1994). In the case of NK-cell activity, however, different mechanisms would seem to be involved. The potential involvement of central opioid effects (conditioned or otherwise) would have to be transmitted to peripheral immune cells through a pathway other than the release of catecholamines since $\beta$-adrenergic receptor antagonists do not affect the conditioned suppression of NK-cell activity. Also, since it would appear that the central actions of the opioid receptor antagonist, naltrexone, are able to block the conditioned suppression of NK-cell activity (Coussons-Read et al., 1994b; Lysle et al., 1992a), the conditioned enhancement of NK-cell activity (Solvason, Hiramoto, & Ghanta, 1989), and a specific cytotoxic lymphocyte response (Hiramato et al., 1993), we infer that naltrexone is acting on neural pathways involved in associative processes rather than on a CNS pathway that directly influences lymphocyte function.

Corticotropin-releasing hormone may have some additional mediational role. As noted above, in response to a CS associated with electric shocks, c-Fos was expressed in some hypothalamic neurons containing CRH (Pezzone et al., 1992). Also, the intraventricular administration of $\alpha$-helical CRH$_{(9-41)}$, a CRH-selective receptor antagonist, before reexposing conditioned animals to the CS, blocked the conditioned suppression of NK-cell activity while

having no effect on the conditioned suppression of mitogen responsiveness, IL-2 or IFN-$\gamma$ production, or the increase in plasma levels of corticosterone (Perez & Lysle, 1995).

These observations, incidentally, are quite consistent with the differential effects of naltrexone on the immunosuppressive effects unconditionally elicited by electric shock stimulation. The suppression of NK-cell activity induced by electric shock could be prevented by preshock treatment with naltrexone, whereas naltrexone had no impact on the stressor-induced suppression of lymphoproliferation (Cunnick, Lysle, Armfield, & Rabin, 1988). There is a seeming inconsistency in these several observations in that the electric shock-induced suppression of NK cell function but not lymphoproliferation was blocked by naltrexone while naltrexone was effective in attenuating the *conditioned* suppression of both NK-cell activity and lymphoproliferative responses. These differences might be dose or timing effects; they might also indicate, again, that conditioned and unconditioned alterations in immunologic reactivity are mediated by somewhat different neural–immune pathways.

## C. Dissociation of Conditioned Immune Responses from Behavioral and Adrenocortical Responses

Although it is not necessary to use pharmacologic agents with aversive properties (e.g., Coussons-Read et al., 1994a,b), conditioned changes in immune function have most frequently been studied in the context of a conditioned taste aversion and, most frequently, using UCSs with noxious physiologic effects. Even if one excludes studies in which antigen has served as the UCS, inducing a conditioned enhancement of immunologic reactivity in the absence of an aversive response (e.g., Alvarez-Borda, Ramírez-Amaya, Pérez-Montfort, & Bermúdez-Rattoni, 1995), the available literature reveals no consistent relationship between conditioned behavioral and immune responses:

- Taste aversions can be expressed without concomitant changes in immune function (Ader & Cohen, 1975; Gorczynski, 1991b; Neveu, Crestani, & LeMoal, 1987; Roudebush & Bryant, 1991)
- Conditioned changes in immune function occur in the absence of conditioned taste aversions (Ader, Grota, & Cohen, 1987; Klosterhalfen & Klosterhalfen, 1990; Neveu et al., 1986)
- There are differences in the rate of acquisition or extinction of conditioned behavioral and immune

**TABLE II  Effects of Neurochemical Interventions on the Expression of Conditioned Immune Responses[a]**

| Agent | Action | US[b] | Splenic lymphocyte response to:[c] | | | | Splenic NK cell activity | CTL | IL-2 | IFN-γ | Cort[d] | Source |
|---|---|---|---|---|---|---|---|---|---|---|---|---|
| | | | ConA | PHA | LPS | PMA | | | | | | |
| Naltrexone (sc) | Central/peripheral opioid receptor antagonist | Stress | ↓[e] | ↓ | ↓ | ↓ | ↓ | | | | | Lysle et al., 1992 |
| N-methylnaltrexone (sc) | Peripheral opioid receptor antagonist | | 0 | | 0 | 0 | 0 | | | | | |
| Naltrexone (sc) | Central/peripheral opioid receptor antagonist | Morphine | ↓ | | ↓ | | ↓ | | 0 | | | Coussons-Read et al., 1994a |
| Naltrexone (sc) | | Poly I:C | | | | | ↓ | | | | | Solvason et al., 1989 |
| Naltrexone methobromide (sc) | Peripheral opioid receptor antagonist | | | | | | 0 | | | | | |
| Naltrexone methobromide (sc) | | Allogeneic cells | | | | | | 0 | | | | Hiramoto et al., 1993 |
| Naltrexone (icv) | Central/peripheral opioid receptor antagonist | Stress | ↓ | | ↓ | | ↓ | | | ↓ | | Perez & Lysle, 1997 |
| Naloxazine (icv) | Selective μ1-opioid receptor antagonisit | | ↓ | | ↓ | 0 | ↓ | | | ↓ | | |
| Naloxazine (sc) | | | 0 | | 0 | | 0 | | | 0 | | |
| Nor-binaltorphi-mine (icv) | κ-opioid receptor antagonist | | 0 | | 0 | | 0 | | | 0 | | |
| Naltrindole (sc) | δ-opioid receptor | | | | ↓ | | 0 | | | 0 | | |
| Propranolol (sc) | β-Adrenergic receptor antagonist | Stress | ↓ | ↓ | ↓ | | 0 | | | | 0 | Lysle et al., 1991 |
| Nadolol (sc) | β-Adrenergic receptor antagonist | Morphine | ↓ | ↓ | ↓ | | 0 | | ↓ | | | Coussons-Read et al., 1994b |
| Atenolol (sc) | β1-Adrenergic receptor antagonist | Stress | ↓ | ↓ | 0 | ↓ | 0 | | 0 | ↓ | | Luecken & Lysle, 1992 |
| ICI 118,551 (sc) | β2-Adrenergic receptor antagonist | | ↓ | ↓ | 0 | ↓ | 0 | | 0 | | | |
| Reserpine (ip) | Depletion of central/peripheral catecholamines | Poly(I:C) | | | | | ↓ | | | ↓ | | Hiramoto et al., 1990 |
| 6-OHDA (ip) | Peripheral sympathectomy | | | | | | 0 | | | | | |
| α-helical CRH(9-41)(icv) | CRH-Selective receptor antagonist | Stress | 0 | 0 | 0 | 0 | ↓ | | 0 | 0 | 0 | Perez & Lysle, 1995 |

[a]Interventions were introduced after conditioning and before testing for the conditioned response.
[b]Unconditioned stimulus for suppression (stress, morphine) or enhancement (Poly(I:C), allogeneic cells) of immunologic reactivity.
[c]Con A, concanavalin A; PHA, phytohemagglutanin; LPS, lipopolysaccharide; PMA, ionomycin/phorbol-myristate-acetate.
[d]Corticosterone.
[e]Attenuation or block of conditioned response; 0, no effect on conditioned response.

responses (Bovbjerg et al., 1984; Gorczynski & Kennedy, 1984; Klosterhalfen & Klosterhalfen, 1987; Kusnecov et al., 1988; Schulze et al., 1988; Wayner et al., 1978)

- Several investigators infer or document the lack of a correlation between conditioned behavioral and immune responses (Ader & Cohen, 1975; Bovbjerg et al., 1987b, 1990; Gorczynski, 1987a; Krank & MacQueen, 1988; Rogers et al., 1976; Solvason, Ghanta, & Hiramoto, 1988)
- Mice selectively bred for differences in open-field activity also differed in their expression of a conditioned suppression of antibody production but did not differ in taste aversion learning performance (Gorczynski & Kennedy, 1987); and, on still another level of analysis,
- Surgical or neurochemical interventions can differentially affect the expression of conditioned behavioral and immune responses (Exton et al., 1998; Gorczynski & Holmes, 1989).

These and other current data (Lennartz & Weinberger, 1992) suggest that multiple and independent processes are involved in the acquisition of conditioned behavioral and physiological responses.

Because of the conditioned taste aversion model, the use of UCSs with noxious physiologic effects, and the pervasive generalization that "stress" effects are, primarily, adrenocortical effects, it has been suggested that conditioned immunosuppressive responses are mediated by stress-induced (or conditioned) elevations of glucocorticoids. This hypothesis provided a ready "explanation" of an observation for which no other explanation existed. Adrenocortical steroids do have immunomodulating effects, and the exogenous administration of corticosteroids is, in general, immunosuppressive. However, the vast majority of the literature either fails to support or, with few exceptions, is inconsistent with the hypothesis that conditioned changes in immune function are mediated by increased adrenocortical activity. This research, reviewed elsewhere (Ader, 1987; Ader & Cohen, 1991, 1993), demonstrates that conditioned suppression and enhancement of antibody- and cell-mediated immune responses occur in the absence of or with equivalent changes in corticosterone levels in experimental and control groups. Recent studies confirm these observations.

With respect to stressor-induced conditioned responses, for example, propranolol blocked the suppression of splenic lymphoproliferative responses without affecting plasma levels of corticosterone (Lysle et al., 1991); a CRH receptor antagonist blocked the conditioned suppression of NK cell activity but

had no effect on the elevated plasma corticosterone levels (Perez & Lysle, 1995); and strain differences in conditioned alterations of immunologic reactivity among rats were not paralleled by differences in adrenocortical reactivity (Shurin et al., 1995). Roudebush & Bryant (1991) found a CY-induced conditioned suppression of a DTH response but no differences in the corticosterone responses of experimental and control groups, and Exton and his associates (1998) reported a cyclosporin A-induced conditioned suppression of lymphoproliferation and cytokine production in the absence of CS-induced differences in corticosterone secretion. In humans, an epinephrine-induced conditioned increase in NK-cell activity occurred in the absence of cortisol elevations (Kirschbaum et al., 1992).

Although the available data are inconsistent with the notion that conditioned alterations of immunity are mediated simply by nonspecific (stressor-induced) changes in circulating adrenocortical steroids, there are a variety of other hormones and neurotransmitters capable of providing the signaling to lymphocytes that form part of the pathway through which conditioning is able to suppress or enhance immune responses. Thus, the possibility that endocrine responses are being conditioned along with behavioral and immune changes should be examined more extensively to provide additional clues about the nature of the relationship between neuroendocrine activity and immune function.

## III. CONDITIONED IMMUNOENHANCEMENT

Until recently, relatively few studies had addressed the conditioned enhancement of immunologic reactivity. One early study took advantage of the differential effects of CY on different T-cell subsets. Depending on concentration and timing, CY can suppress an initial DTH response and enhance the response to subsequent antigenic challenges (Bovbjerg, Cohen, & Ader, 1986; Turk & Parker, 1982). When sensitized animals, previously conditioned by pairing saccharin and CY, were reexposed to the CS before an initial challenge, there was no evidence of conditioned immunosuppression. How-ever, reexposure to the CS enhanced DTH in response to two subsequent challenges compared to the DTH response in control groups with an identical drug history (Bovbjerg et al., 1987a). This conditioned enhancement of a DTH response may actually represent a conditioned immunosuppressive effect since CY may be depressing suppressor cell function (Gill & Lieu, 1978; Mitsuoka, Morikawa, Baba, & Harada, 1979). Using levamisole as the UCS, Husband, King, and Brown (1986/87) reported a conditioned increase in the T-helper: T-suppressor subset ratio that also appeared to be the result of a selective depletion of cytotoxic/suppressor T cells.

Most studies of conditioned immunoenhancement have used UCSs that more directly enhance antigen-specific and nonspecific responses.

## A. Natural Killer Cell Activity

Polyinosinic:polycytidylic acid (poly(I:C)) elicits an interferon response which, in turn, stimulates natural killer cell activity. Hiramoto and his colleagues have published an extensive series of studies in which reexposure to an odor previously paired with poly(I:C) is associated with an increase in NK-cell activity. In the basic experimental paradigm, group-housed mice are placed into an experimental cage in which they are exposed to the odor released by heated camphor for a period of 1 h. Immediately thereafter, the mice are injected with 20 µg poly(I:C). Some days later, these animals (Group CS) are reexposed on one or more occasions to the odor of camphor alone, or to the odor of camphor plus the injection of a suboptimal dose of poly(I:C) (1 µg). Blood samples are subsequently obtained for the assay of NK-cell activity. Control groups consist of similarly treated mice that are not reexposed to the camphor odor before sampling for NK-cell activity (Group CSo) and/or mice that receive only the injection of poly(I:C) on the treatment day but are later exposed to the odor of camphor, a Group [NC], and mice that are never exposed to either camphor odor or poly(I:C). The elevation in NK-cell activity observed in Group CS compared to that seen in one or more control groups is taken as evidence of a conditioned response, and such an elevation in NK-cell activity has been observed on many occasions. The studies that include most of the relevant control groups (e.g., Ghanta 1987a; Solvason, Ghanta, Lorden, Soong & Hiramoto, 1991a) would appear to demonstrate a conditioned enhancement of NK cell activity. However, the variable inclusion of different control groups in different studies and findings that are inconsistent with what is known about classical conditioning raise concerns about the variables that might be responsible for these data.

The study by Solvason and colleagues (1991a) on the conditioned augmentation of NK-cell activity, for example, is one of the very few studies using poly(I:C) as the unconditioned stimulus in which most of the relevant control groups are present. In this particular experiment, however, there was no control (placebo) group that was exposed to the odor of camphor, injected with saline, and subsequently reexposed to camphor. More directly relevant, perhaps, there were no nonconditioned animals that received the same number of camphor exposures as the "conditioned and reexposed to camphor" group. The need for such groups is evidenced by the fact that mice that received three exposures to camphor had the highest NK cell activity, mice that received two exposures to camphor had the next highest levels, and animals that had only one exposure to camphor had still lower levels which were, in turn, higher than the levels in mice that were never exposed to the odor of camphor. Thus, the immunologic effects of repeatedly confining mice to an inescapable environment permeated with the odor of heated camphor for 1 h cannot be ruled out as a factor contributing to the observed effects. Certainly, as hypothesized, Group CS should show the highest NK cell activity, but there is no reason to expect any consistent difference among the control groups that were injected with poly(I:C). As it happens, though, the elevation in NK-cell activity has been a function of the number of exposures to the odor of camphor in every such study involving multiple control groups (Hiramoto et al., 1992; Solvason et al., 1988; Solvason, Ghanta, Soong, & Hiramoto, 1991b; Solvason, Ghanta, Soong, Rogers, Hsueh, Hiramoto, & Hiramoto, 1992). The potential problem was recognized early on using a different CS (Solvason et al., 1988), but has not been addressed in designing the studies using camphor as a CS.

In support of the proposition that the elevation in NK cell activity is a conditioned response, Solvason and his colleagues (1991a) also examined the stimulus specificity of the conditioned response. Using the same basic conditioning procedures, one group of animals was exposed to poly(I:C) following exposure to the odor of camphor and a second group was exposed to poly(I:C) following a 1-h exposure to the odor of citronella. On two subsequent occasions, half of each group was reexposed to camphor and half was reexposed to citronella. An elevation in NK-cell activity in response to a 1-µg dose of poly(I:C) was observed only among mice reexposed to the odor previously paired with poly(I:C). Unfortunately, this experiment included none of the control groups that would be required to support the conclusion that these were conditioned responses that showed stimulus specificity as opposed, for example, to the possibility that the observed levels of NK-cell activity in all groups were conditioned responses of different magnitudes.

The purported conditioning of enhanced NK-cell activity using poly(I:C) as the UCS generated a series of experiments which, despite major variations of some of the variables that are known to influence learned responses, yielded remarkably consistent results. CS–UCS intervals of 1–2 days which have never before been observed—even for the conditioning of avoidance responses (taste aversions) critical to the immediate health of the animal—have been reported to be as effective in conditioning enhanced NK-cell activity as a CS–UCS interval of 1–5 minutes (Hiramoto et al., 1992; Solvason et al., 1992). The authors are aware of the extensive literature describing an inverse relationship between the length of the CS–UCS interval and the magnitude or probability of observing a conditioned response (Rescorla, 1988). They interpret the greatly attenuated conditioned response observed after a 4-day CS–UCS interval as evidence of such a gradient. The failure to discriminate between intervals as disparate as a few minutes versus 48 h necessarily raises questions about whether the elevation in NK-cell activity can be attributed to conditioning or some other component(s) of the experimental procedures that need to be addressed. "Conditioned" immunoenhancement has even been used to describe results obtained when the UCS does not or is not reported to elicit an observable unconditioned response under the conditions used in the experiment (Solvason et al., 1988; Solvason, Ghanta, Soong & Hiramoto, 1991b). Conversely, conditioning has not been observed under experimental circumstances referred to as a backward conditioning control procedure (Demissie, Rogers, Hiramoto, Ghanta, & Hiramoto, 1995) but which these (e.g., Ghanta et al., 1987a,b) and other investigators (e.g., Coussons-Read et al., 1992) used to obtain conditioned responses. Although the authors claim that animals in the backward conditioning group were not conditioned, there were no nonconditioned groups to determine if the observed NK-cell activity represented a conditioned response or a control level of activity.

Procedural and analytical issues aside, the failure to include appropriate control groups, the observation of effects that are of approximately the same magnitude irrespective of the CS, the UCS, or the CS–UCS interval, and the absence of any systematic data that address the role of associative factors such as the effects of varying the number of conditioning trials, preexposure to the CS or the UCS, or experimental extinction make the results of these studies susceptible to alternative interpretations. For example, the absence of a conditioned group that is not reexposed to the CS becomes all the more problematic

in view of results obtained by Gee and Johnson (1994). In several independent experiments, these investigators found that NK-cell activity was greater in conditioned mice that were returned to the experimental apparatus in which they had been exposed to the odor of camphor (Group CSo) than in conditioned animals that were reexposed to the full CS (Group CS). In another population, there were no differences in NK-cell activity between Groups CS and CSo (Gee, Thiele, & Johnson, 1994). These experiments address the omission of the CSo control group in many of the studies conducted by Hiramoto and his colleagues, but they do not resolve the issue of whether these are conditioning effects because the studies by Gee and his colleagues did not include nonconditioned animals. We cannot determine, then, whether either or both Groups CS and CSo were showing conditioned responses.

Because poly(I:C) induces interferon-$\beta$ (IFN-$\beta$) production, it was hypothesized (Solvason et al., 1988) that IFN-$\beta$ might be the critical signal in inducing the (putative) conditioned enhancement of NK-cell activity using poly(I:C) as the UCS. Using a combination of the taste of saccharin and an injection of LiCl as the compound CS, IFN-$\alpha$ and -$\beta$ elevated NK-cell activity in animals that were exposed only to these UCSs, but only IFN-$\beta$ was an effective UCS for inducing a conditioned elevation in NK-cell activity. Using a 1-h exposure to camphor as the CS paired with IFN-$\beta$, there was a subsequent increase in NK-cell activity in response to the CS alone. It is not clear, however, that the observed effect was due to conditioning since IFN-$\beta$, itself, did not elicit an observable unconditioned elevation in NK-cell activity. In a second study (Solvason et al., 1991b), 100 IU IFN-$\beta$ injected into the cisterna magna was paired with the odor of camphor. In this experiment, the evidence for conditioning was subverted by the fact that there was no discernable unconditioned effect of IFN-$\beta$ injected into the cisterna magna and there were no conditioned animals that were not reexposed to the CS to determine the effects of conditioning with this new UCS.

To be sure, an attempt was made (Solvason et al., 1991b) to define the unconditioned effects of cisterna magna IFN-$\beta$ by comparing the effects of injecting anesthetized animals with IFN-$\beta$ (200 IU/mouse) or sterile saline on the response to a suboptimal dose of poly(I:C) injected immediately thereafter. While it is reported that IFN-$\beta$ was then able to increase NK-cell activity, the dose of IFN-$\beta$ was twice as high as that used in the conditioning experiment and the circumstances under which IFN-$\beta$ was administered were totally different. Thus, these results were consistent with the earlier data (Solvason et al., 1988) indicating that peripheral IFN-$\beta$, in the doses used in the conditioning experiment, was not an effective UCS for the activation of NK-cell activity. The interferon-inducing properties of poly(I:C) may be related to the elevation of NK-cell activity in conditioned animals, but this series of experiments does not establish that relationship.

Pursuing this line of research with camphor and poly(I:C) activation of NK cells, Hsueh, Tyring, Hiramoto, and Ghanta (1994) measured changes in IFN messenger RNA in spleen cells by Northern blotting. In contrast to what might be expected based on the above findings, IFN-$\alpha$ (but not IFN-$\beta$) gene expression was higher in conditioned than in non-conditioned animals. There were no differences in plasma levels of $\beta$-endorphin, but animals in Group CS had the highest ACTH levels. Also, there was a correlation of .99 between ACTH level and NK-cell activity, but it is not clear how this was derived since these samples were obtained from different animals. The authors concluded that IFN-$\alpha$ and ACTH were conditioned along with an elevation in NK-cell activity but, again, the control groups required for such a conclusion were not included in this study. Previously, Ghanta and her associates (1987b) had reported that they were unable to detect a conditioned elevation in IFN levels in the serum of conditioned mice.

There can be no doubt that the manipulations introduced by Hiramoto and his colleagues result in an increase in NK cell activity. Our criticisms of these studies, enabled by the sheer number of experiments, highlight the difficulties in selecting control groups and in designing studies of conditioning. They should not be taken as evidence that the observed changes in NK- cell activity are not conditioned responses; they mean that, in the absence of certain kinds of data and in the face of some contradictory and some anomalous findings, we cannot be sure that they are. Thus, to proceed with studies that attempt to identify the pathways involved on the presumption rather than the demonstration that these are conditioned responses could seriously confound and misdirect future research.

## B. Antigen as Unconditioned Stimulus

An antigen is, by definition, an unconditioned stimulus for activation of the immune system, and antigens have been used for the study of the conditioned enhancement of immune as opposed to immunopharmacologic responses. In the first modern study of this sort, Gorczynski et al. (1982) measured the precursors of cytotoxic T lymphocytes (CTLp) reacting against an alloantigen. CBA mice were repeatedly grafted with skin from C57BL/6J mice. The procedure, which involved shaving, anesthetizing, grafting, and bandaging the mice (the compound CS), was repeated three times at 40-day intervals. On the fourth (test) trial, all groups received sham grafts; that is, the mice were reexposed to the stimulus conditions associated with grafting in the absence of the immunogenic stimulus. Conditioned mice displayed an increase in CTLp in response to the CS.

Only about half the conditioned mice in each of the several replications of this experiment showed the enhanced immune response. Those that did respond were divided into subgroups that were given two additional conditioning trials or two extinction trials (unreinforced exposures to the compound CS). All of the mice that had additional training showed the conditioned increase in CTLp, whereas none of the "responder" mice that experienced extinction trials showed the conditioned change in immunologic reactivity. These results affirm the proposition that the increase in CTLp was the result of associative processes.

In a reasonably well controlled study, Hiramato and his colleagues (1993) exposed BALB/c mice to the odor of camphor for 1 h and then injected them ip with C57BL/6 spleen cells. An [NC] group received only the injection of allogeneic cells. In response to the number of allogeneic cells injected, there was a specific cytotoxic T-lymphocyte (CTL) response that peaked 4 days after immunization and was already declining by 6 days postimmunization. Therefore, to determine if conditioning could evoke a CTL response (or, more precisely, retard the waning of the CTL response), the animals were manipulated 6 days after immunization. Half the conditioned and nonconditioned animals were reexposed to the camphor odor and half remained unmanipulated. On the following day the CTL response to the allogeneic cells was measured. CTL activity was significantly greater in conditioned animals reexposed to the CS than in any of the comparison groups.

In an incompletely controlled followup experiment, half the conditioned and nonconditioned BALB/c mice injected with C57BL/6 spleen cells on Day 0 were subsequently injected with naltrexone and half were injected with saline 10 min before being reexposed to the camphor odor. The CTL response measured the following day was attenuated by naltrexone. Conditioned mice injected with saline and reexposed to the CS showed a higher level of CTL activity than the other groups that did not differ significantly from one another. This experiment was followed by one in which the CTL response was compared in conditioned and nonconditioned animals, all of which were injected with quaternary naltrexone. The level of CTL activity was, again, greater in the conditioned than in the nonconditioned animals, implicating central opioid receptor mechanisms in the mediation of the observed effects.

Continuing with this line of inquiry (Demissie, Rogers, Hiramoto, Ghanta, & Hiramoto, 1996), lipopolysaccharide or IL-1 were used as UCSs in an attempt to condition elevations in NK-cell activity. In the case of LPS, mice were exposed to the odor of camphor for 1 h and then injected with 10 or 50 μg LPS. On day 2, conditioned animals were reexposed to the camphor odor and injected with 1 μg of poly(I:C) to activate NK cells and, on day 3, NK-cell activity was assessed. Although the 10-μg dose of LPS produced greater NK-cell activity than the 50-μg dose, only the 50-μg dose of LPS resulted in an elevation in NK-cell activity in conditioned relative to nonconditioned animals. The data on LPS as a UCS for an increase in NK-cell activity remain incomplete, though, because there was no CSo group to determine the effects of conditioning, per se, with this new CS–UCS combination.

In the experiment with IL-1α, conditioned mice were first exposed to the odor of camphor after which they were anesthetized before IL-1α was injected into the cisterna magna. Two days later, conditioned animals were reexposed to the camphor odor and injected with the suboptimal dose of poly(I:C). NK-cell activity was measured on day 3. In this experiment, there was a group of conditioned animals that was not reexposed to the CS on day 2 and a group of nonconditioned animals that received only IL-1α on the conditioning day and the camphor odor on day 2. There was also a backward conditioning group that received IL-1α on the conditioning day and the odor of camphor on day 1; i.e, this group might also be described as a nonconditioned group that experienced the CS and the UCS in a noncontingent manner. Irrespective of label, this group received the same number of exposures to the camphor odor as the critical experimental group and is therefore a more appropriate comparison group than the group labeled as "nonconditioned." The results showed that animals reexposed to the CS had higher NK-cell activity than animals in any of the comparison groups. Whatever the specific pathways, these results provide evidence of the potential for CNS involvement in the in vivo regulation of NK-cell activity.

Using a discriminative conditioning procedure, Russell et al., (1984) gave sensitized guinea pigs weekly trials on which an olfactory CS+ was paired with bovine serum albumin; a second odor, the CS–, was paired with saline. On test trials, reexposure to the CS+, alone, resulted in a release of histamine, a nonspecific mediator of allergic reactions. The response to the CS– did not differ from the pretraining baseline level. Unreinforced presentations of the CS+ resulted in extinction of the conditioned histamine release (Dark, Peeke, Ellman, & Salfi, 1987) and, although there was a differential histamine response to the CS+ and CS–, there was no difference in the adrenocortical response to the previously reinforced and unreinforced odor cues (Peeke, Elman, Dark, Salfi, & Reus,1987).

Histamine is released from a variety of cells throughout the body. Therefore, MacQueen and her colleagues (1989) measured rat mast cell protease II (RCMP II), an enzyme found only in thymus-dependent mast cells in the mucosal lamina propria of the intestine and lung. Sensitized rats were given three trials on which they were exposed to audio-visual cues paired with a subcutaneous injection of egg albumin. Relative to a pretest baseline, conditioned animals reexposed to the CS showed an elevation of RMCP II equivalent to the elevation shown by animals injected with egg albumin on the test trial—and significantly greater than that shown by nonconditioned animals that experienced unpaired CS and UCS presentations. These results provide compelling evidence for the conditioning of a specific mediator of mucosal mast cell function.

Using essentially the same basic protocol that had proven effective in conditioning immunosuppression, Ader, Kelly, Moynihan, Grota, and Cohen (1993) paired a gustatory CS with a low dose of antigen, keyhole limpet hemocyanin (KLH), on as many as five trials, each of which was separated by a 3- to 4-week interval. The pairing of a neutral stimulus with antigen did not induce a conditioned taste aversion. In a manner analogous to the use of a subthreshold dose of CY to increase the visibility of a conditioned immunosuppressive response (Bovbjerg et al., 1982, 1984)—a technique also used by Hiramoto and his colleagues to increase the magnitude of a poly(I:CV)-induced conditioned increase in NK-cell activity-half the animals in all groups were given a low-dose, "booster" injection of KLH on the test trial. In the absence of the "boost," antibody titers remained low and there were no discernable effects of conditioning. Using the booster injection of antigen, however, there was clear evidence of a conditioned enhancement of antibody production (Figure 1). Anti-KLH antibody titers in conditioned animals reexposed to the CS did not differ from the levels in conditioned animals that were again injected with the dose of KLH used on

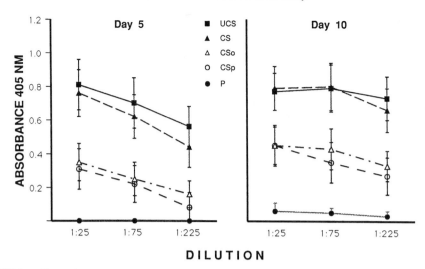

**FIGURE 1**   Effects of conditioning on the enhancement of anti-KLH IgG antibody production in response to a low-dose booster injection of KLH. CS, conditioned mice reexposed to the CS at the time of challenge; CSo, conditioned mice not reexposed to the CS; CSp, conditioned mice preexposed to the CS; P, placebo-treated (nonimmunized) mice; UCS, conditioned mice injected with the full dose of KLH on the test day. Reprinted from Ader et al. (1993) with permission of Academic Press.

conditioning trials. In addition, Group CS showed a significant enhancement of antibody production compared to conditioned animals that were not reexposed to the CS. As predicted, the conditioning effect was obviated by exposing conditioned animals to the CS before the initiation of conditioning trials, providing further evidence that the observed effects were the result of associative processes.

Since neither the CS nor the booster dose of antigen was sufficient, by itself, to evoke a robust antibody response in conditioned animals, Ader and his colleagues (1993) speculated that the conditioned enhancement of antibody production required two signals: a neural or neuroendocrine response elicited by reexposure to the CS, and a signal from within the immune system recognizing the booster immunization. This analysis was consistent with the argument that only such a juxtaposition of signals could enable CNS-derived information to influence an immune response (Roszman & Carlson, 1991). In the case of conditioning using an antigen as the UCS, the response being measured—the response elicited by reexposure to the CS—is a secondary response and, as such, is predicated upon information existing within the immune system. Whether memory cells can sufficiently represent the signals required of the immune system in this proposed two-signal model or whether the expression of a conditioned enhancement of immunity is limited to the potentiation of the response to otherwise ineffective or subthreshold antigenic stimuli remains to be seen. For whatever (procedural?) reason(s), a low-dose booster injection

of antigen was required to detect the effects of conditioning in this study. This was not a prerequisite for the ostensible conditioned enhancement of antibody production reported by Russian investigators beginning in the 1920s (Ader, 1981).

At a meeting of the Australian Behavioural Immunology Group, Husband, Lin, Madsen, and King (1993) reported a conditioned enhancement of antibody production following a single conditioning trial. After consuming a saccharin-flavored drinking solution, rats were injected with a protein antigen, ovalbumin (OVA), emulsified in Freund's complete adjuvant. A conditioned group was injected ip with OVA immediately after drinking saccharin and, 14 days later, given access to bottles containing saccharin or plain tap water; an [NC] group was immunized with OVA after drinking plain water and subsequently provided with plain water rather than the CS solution; and a placebo-treated group was injected with saline after drinking a saccharin solution and later provided with saccharin or plain water. Four days later, the animals were sacrificed.

Anti-OVA antibody titers were higher after CS reexposure in the conditioned rats than in the nonconditioned animals that were simply exposed to plain water. Similarly, the in vitro proliferative response of spleen cells cultured with OVA were higher in conditioned than in nonconditioned and placebo-treated animals. The groups did not differ in proliferative responses to mitogenic stimulation. Also, there was no relationship between corticosterone levels sampled at the time of sacrifice and anti-OVA antibody titers or the magnitude of the behavioral aversion to saccharin in conditioned rats (induced, perhaps, by the Freund's adjuvant). While suggestive, the absence of appropriate control conditions—a conditioned group that was not reexposed to the CS and/or a nonconditioned group that was exposed to saccharin—makes it difficult to attribute the observed differences to conditioning.

Alvarez-Borda and his associates (1995) conducted a well controlled study documenting a conditioned enhancement of antibody production using the protein antigen, hen egg-white lysozyme, as the UCS. Individually caged rats were maintained under a restricted drinking schedule and manipulated during the dark phase of a reversed light–dark schedule. Conditioned animals were injected with 0.5 mg of hen egg lysozyme (HEL) following consumption of a saccharin-flavored drinking solution. Twenty-five days after immunization, when the primary anti-HEL antibody response was no longer detectable, these animals were reexposed to saccharin and blood samples were collected 4, 8, 12, and 16 days later. Control groups in this study included conditioned animals that were not reexposed to the CS, nonconditioned animals that were immunized after drinking plain water and given saccharin on the test trial, and a UCS group that was immunized on the training day and immunized again on the test day to define the normal secondary response to HEL.

As can be seen in Figure 2, conditioned animals that were reexposed to the CS had higher anti-HEL IgM and IgG antibody titers than conditioned animals that were not reexposed to the CS or nonconditioned animals that were exposed to the saccharin solution. It should be noted that these dramatic effects were observed in response to a nonaversive stimulus (the one-trial pairing of saccharin consumption with an injection of HEL did not induce an aversion to saccharin)—and in the absence of a low-dose booster injection of antigen. Our laboratory has successfully replicated these findings (unpublished observations), although the differences were not as large as those reported by Alvarez-Borda and his colleagues (1995).

Having demonstrated that the insular cortex and amygdala are involved in the acquisition of a conditioned immunosuppressive response, Ramírez-Amaya and Bermúdez-Rattoni (1998) examined the effects of brain lesions on the conditioning of immunoenhancement. Bilateral lesions were placed in the IC, the amygdala, and the dorsal hippocampus of rats with NMDA several days before conditioning. Lesioned animals and sham-operated controls were exposed to a saccharin-flavored drinking solution or to the odor of almond while drinking plain water

and immediately thereafter immunized with HEL. Twenty-five days later, when the primary response was no longer detectable, conditioned and nonconditioned animals (except for a CSo group) were reexposed to the CS. The results obtained from sham-operated animals repeated their earlier findings (Alvarez-Borda et al., 1995): there were no conditioned taste aversions, but there was an enhancement of anti-HEL IgG production in Group CS compared with Group CSo and nonconditioned rats exposed to either the saccharin flavor the or almond odor.

Lesions did not affect normal immune responses, but NMDA-induced lesions in the IC and amygdala, but not the hippocampus, obviated the acquisition of an enhanced antibody production in response to the gustatory and the olfactory CSs. As in the case of the conditioned suppression of antibody production, the insular cortex and amygdala are involved in the conditioned enhancement of antibody production. By virtue of the nature of their connections to other brain areas involved with immune responses and with neuroendocrine and autonomic nervous system functions, the authors posit, again, that the insular cortex is critical to the mechanisms underlying the association of stimuli responsible for the conditioning while the role of the amygdala is to provide the feedback information from the immune system that enables the conditioned alteration of immune responses. Ramírez-Amaya and Bermúdez-Rattoni note that the insular cortex and the amygdala, among other brain areas, show changes in c-Fos expression in association with an immunologic challenge (Elmquist, Scammell, Jacobsen, & Saper, 1996; Tkacs, Li, & Strack, 1997). Also, a recent study has shown that peripheral chemical sympathectomy with 6-OHDA results in CNS activation as reflected by c-Fos expression in several regions including the amygdala (Callahan, Moynihan, & Piekut, 1998). In light of the results described by Pezzone and his colleagues (1992, 1993) on c-Fos expression elicited by conditioned as well as unconditioned stressful stimuli, it might be of particular interest to determine if c-Fos expression in the insular cortex and/or the amygdala could be elicited by reexposing animals to a CS previously paired with antigen.

Some studies (Krank & MacQueen, 1988; MacQueen & Siegel, 1989) have obtained results interpreted to reflect the conditioned enhancement of immune responses. Actually, these are studies in which there were no observable conditioned effects. For theoretical reasons, these studies in which CY was paired with environmental and/or gustatory stimuli were conducted with the expectation of observing compensatory conditioning (a conditioned response

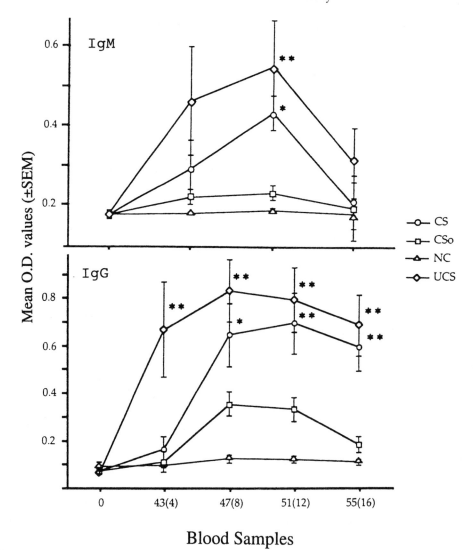

**FIGURE 2**   Effects of conditioning on the enhancement of anti-HEL IgM and IgG production by conditioned rats that were (CS) or were not (CSo) reexposed to the CS, nonconditioned animals (NC), and animals injected with HEL (UCS) on the test day. Reconfigured and reprinted from Alvarez-Borda et al. (1995) with permission of the authors and Academic Press.

opposite in direction to the unconditioned response). The failure to discriminate between the antibody responses of experimental and control groups permits one to hypothesize the operation of compensatory conditioning. The investigators acknowledge, however, that they obtained no direct evidence of a conditioned enhancement of immune function.

In the absence of any recent data, the best evidence for the possibility of compensatory conditioning of host defense reactions comes from studies on the role of conditioning in the development of pharmacological tolerance to repeated injections of poly(I:C) (Dyck, Greenberg, & Osachuk, 1986; Dyck, Driedger, Nemeth, Osachuk, & Greenberg, 1987). Four weekly injections of poly(I:C) resulted in a diminution of the NK response to an injection of poly(I:C) administered

8 weeks later. In keeping with a conditioning analysis of the development of tolerance to some other pharmacologic agents (Siegel, 1983), tolerance to the enhancing effects of poly(I:C) on NK cell activity was abrogated by unreinforced exposures to the CS (weekly extinction trials) imposed after conditioning and by preexposure to the CS before the imposition of conditioning trials. Also, tolerance was attenuated when poly(I:C) was injected in the absence of the environmental cues previously paired with injections of the drug. Tolerance was retained when animals conditioned with an olfactory CS received extinction trials with a different (visual and auditory) stimulus.

Thus, the data obtained by Dyck and his colleagues (1986, 1987) implicate conditioning processes in the development of tolerance to an immunomodulating agent in much the same way as it has been found to influence the development of tolerance to some other pharmacologic substances (Siegel, 1983). Whether this tolerance derives from the development of compensatory responses, however, remains an open question. There are experimental conditions under which some drugs, morphine (e.g., Siegel, 1976), for example, induce compensatory (hyperalgesic) responses; under other circumstances, however, compensatory responses are not observed (e.g., Shapiro, Dudek, & Rosellini, 1983; Tiffany, Petrie, Baker, & Dahl, 1983). Insofar as immune responses are concerned, the data remain sparse, but, as discussed above, Coussons-Read and her colleagues (1992) found a mimicking suppression not an enhancement of lymphoproliferative responses, NK-cell activity, and cytokine production in response to a CS previously associated with injections of morphine.

Although somewhat tangential to the focus of the present discussion, it is worth noting that immunogenic stimuli that induce behavioral and physiological changes can be used as UCSs for the conditioning of these responses. Parenteral administration of LPS, for example, unconditionally elicits a variety of immunologically relevant changes including the production of the proinflammatory cytokine, IL-1. IL-1 is a pleiotropic cytokine that can activate the HPA axis resulting in production of glucocorticoids. Pairing IL-1 with environmental cues in a taste aversion or odor conditioning protocol can result in a conditioned corticosterone response (Dyck et al., 1990; Janz et al., 1996). LPS can also cause plasma hypoferremia; altered levels of iron can be conditioned by associating LPS with saccharin (Exton, Bull, King, & Husband, 1995). LPS, or more precisely, the cytokines it elicits, also induces behavioral changes that include increased body temperature and anorexia, and both of these behavioral manifestations of IL-1-associated sickness behavior have been conditioned in rats by pairing LPS with saccharin (Bull, Exton, & Husband, 1994; Exton, Bull, & King, 1995; Exton et al., 1995; Exton, Lightfoot, Stanton, Bull, King, & Husband, 1995; Hiramoto, Ghanta, Rogers, & Hiramoto, 1991).

## IV. CONDITIONING IN HUMAN SUBJECTS

There are a few experimental studies that describe conditioned alterations of immunologic reactivity in human subjects. In one of the earliest of these (Ikemi & Nakagawa, 1962), four subjects were painted with a methylene blue solution containing the extract of a Japanese lacquer tree which unconditionally induces eczema. After several CS–UCS pairings, the CS alone was able to elicit a skin reaction in all the subjects. In the study by Smith and McDaniels (1983), subjects volunteered for tuberculin skin testing six times at monthly intervals. In a counterbalanced manner, tuberculin obtained from a green vial was applied to one arm and saline drawn from a red vial was applied to the other. On the test day, the contents of the colored vials were reversed. Saline administered to the arm previously treated with tuberculin did not elicit a delayed type hypersensitivity reaction, but the erythema and induration elicited by tuberculin in the arm previously injected with saline was significantly reduced. The latter observation is remarkably similar to some earlier work from the Soviet Union (Ader, 1981) and to the results of more recent studies (Moynihan et al., 1989); the failure to elicit a DTH response in the absence of antigen, however, contrasts with the results described in the early Russian studies.

As previously noted (Bovbjerg et al., 1982, 1984), the combination of a CS for immunosuppression and a low dose of cyclophosphamide depressed a GvH response more than the low dose of CY or the CS was able to accomplish alone. Also, only when combined with a low-dose booster injection of KLH was it possible to observe an enhancement of anti-KLH antibody production in response to a CS previously paired with KLH (Ader et al., 1993). In an analogous manner, the use of a subthreshold level of antigenic stimulation (which may be a necessary but not sufficient stimulus) in conjunction with reexposure to CSs might enable the observation of conditioned enhancement of a delayed type hypersensitivity reaction. In especially sensitive individuals, a CS might prove to be sufficient by itself.

Booth, Petrie, and Brook (1995) crafted a very carefully executed study that followed an experimental protocol similar to the one used by Smith and McDaniels (1983). Colored vials and tags clearly identified the arm to which coded allergens were to be applied. In this instance, a titration schedule for elicitation of an immediate hypersensitivity reaction was determined for and applied to each individual subject. After a series of daily trials, the contents of the visually coded vials were reversed (e.g., the arm receiving allergen now received saline) and, after two such test trials, reversed again. The measurement of weal size, titration gradient, or titration endpoint revealed no consistent changes in response that could reflect conditioning.

A group of investigators in Trier, Germany, obtained preliminary evidence of conditioned increases in NK-cell activity in human subjects. A group of investigators in Utrecht, The Netherlands, however, were unable to repeat these findings. Communication between these groups resulted in the all-too-rare publication of a single paper describing both sets of data (Kirschbaum et al., 1992). In the Trier study, volunteer subjects received four trials on which the CS (a sweet candy) was immediately followed by a sc injection of 0.2 mg epinephrine, which unconditionally elevates NK-cell activity. Control subjects were injected with saline after eating the candy. On the fifth day, both groups were given the candy and injected with saline. After the four CS–UCS presentations, exposure to the CS alone was sufficient to elevate NK-cell activity although there was no rise in plasma epinephrine or changes in cortisol levels. Placebo-treated subjects showed no change in NK-cell activity. Under very similar experimental conditions, these results could not be repeated by investigators in Utrecht. One might even speculate that the conditioning protocol in Utrecht, for some undetected reason, gave rise to a conditioned compensatory response.

Two possible reasons for the disparity were discussed. One difference in the experimental protocols was the amount of information given to subjects. In contrast to the Trier group, researchers in Utrecht were required to inform their subjects that they were being injected with epinephrine and what side-effects might be expected. A second, related suggestion concerns the cultural differences between the two populations. While there were no problems attracting subjects in Trier, even without telling them about the substance with which they were to be injected, "...Dutch subjects in general tend to be very critical of experiments in which they participate." Thus, differences in expectations, attitudes, compliance, and, perhaps, other cultural factors may have influenced the results. One might have hypothesized, for example, that expectations based on the known effects of epinephrine would have favored a positive response in the Dutch sample, which was not the case. On the other hand, confirmed expectations about the effects of epinephrine and its side effects on the conditioning trials may have made the eventual substitution of a saline injection immediately recognizable.

Despite the unexplained differences, the Trier group pursued this line of research. In a second study (Buske-Kirschbaum, Kirschbaum, Stierle, Lehnert, & Hellhammer, 1992), conditioned subjects reexposed to the CS and injected with saline instead of epinephrine showed an elevation in NK-cell activity relative to placebo-treated subjects and a nonconditioned group previously exposed to the CS and UCS in an unpaired manner. In still another study using a discriminative conditioning protocol (Buske-Kirschbaum, Kirschbaum, Stierle, Jabaij, & Hellhammer, 1994), support for the conditioned enhancement of NK cell function was evidenced by an elevated response to a CS+ (a stimulus previously paired with epinephrine) as distinct from a CS− (a stimulus that had not been paired with the UCS).

Studies of conditioned immunosuppression in humans have taken advantage of clinical situations such as the natural circumstances surrounding the chemotherapy of cancer patients. The findings are not consistent and these studies have inherent design problems. It is not possible, for example, to create conditions for a noncontingent presentation of the cues associated with chemotherapy and the chemotherapy, itself. Even so, the data are of some interest because apparent conditioning effects are already evident in cancer patients who display nausea and vomiting in the presence of cues associated with their chemotherapy such as the odors of the clinic, the nurse, and the hospital itself (Andrykowski, Redd, & Hatfield, 1985; Andrykowski et al., 1988; Andrykowski & Redd 1987; Carey & Burish, 1988; Morrow & Dobkin, 1988; Redd, Andresen, & Minagawa, 1982). These are commonly viewed as conditioned responses. Since chemotherapy suppresses the immune system in addition to causing nausea, Bovbjerg and his associates (1990) examined the possibility that chemotherapy patients might show conditioned immunosuppression as well as conditioned nausea and vomiting.

Women receiving chemotherapy for ovarian cancer were sampled at home 3–8 days before their scheduled chemotherapy session and again in the hospital, on the day of chemotherapy. They found no differences in NK cell activity or in lymphocyte counts or lymphocyte subset numbers, but the lymphoproliferative response to the T-cell mitogens, Con A, and PHA, were significantly lower in the hospital just before chemotherapy than they were at home. There was no evidence, however, that the decreased mitogen responsiveness was related to anticipatory nausea or to increased anxiety in the hospital. To some extent, these findings are consistent with the experimental data on conditioned immunosuppression. However— and recognizing the major differences in the population and in experimental conditions—a conceptually similar study by Fredrikson, Fürst, Lekander, Rotstein, and Blomgren (1993) failed to confirm these observations.

In multiple sclerosis patients undergoing monthly immunosuppressive drug treatment, Giang et al., (1996) paired cyclophosphamide with a distinctively flavored drinking solution. After five or six such treatments, patients were given a sham trial (the CS plus an ineffective dose of 10 mg CY). Eight of the 10 patients showed a peripheral leukopenia in response to the sham trial. One of the two patients that did not show evidence of conditioning was found to have had a prior course of cyclophosphamide therapy and the other volunteered that the CS solution tasted like ouzo, which the patient happened to like. Preexposure to either the CS (Lubow, 1973) or the UCS (Randich & LoLordo, 1979) tends to interfere with the acquisition of conditioned responses.

Positive results were obtained in a study by Gauci, Husband, Saxarra, and King (1994), who attempted to condition nasal tryptase release in patients with a history of perennial allergic rhinitis. Mast cell tryptase, a specific marker of mucosal mast cell degranulation, is released in response to allergenic stimulation. Conditioned subjects drank a novel tasting and smelling blue solution and were immediately given an intranasal challenge with house dust mite allergen. Two days later, conditioned patients were reexposed to the CS and challenged with normal saline. A placebo group that originally received the distinctive solution and a challenge with saline were again stimulated with the drinking solution and saline. A third group received only the allergen on the conditioning day and only saline on the test day; they never experienced the novel CS. Nasal washings with normal saline were performed before and 15 min after the challenge on both days. The subjects also completed a subjective symptom scale, rating the severity of their nasal symptoms before and after the challenge. The pre–post change in mast cell tryptase release was significantly greater in the conditioned subjects reexposed to the CS than in either of the other two groups. There were no corresponding differences, however, in the change in symptom severity. The results provide presumptive evidence of conditioning. Assuming that the distinctive drinking solution was the most salient cue, such studies would be more definitive if they included conditioned subjects who were not reexposed to the CS and if nonconditioned subjects were exposed to the CS and UCS in a noncontingent manner and were exposed to the CS on the day of testing.

In a recent study by Longo et al., (1999), an attempt was made to condition immune responses using recombinant interferon-$\gamma$ (rhIFN-$\gamma$) as the UCS. The primary outcome measures were serum concentrations of quinolinic acid (QUIN) and neopterin, two nonspecific markers of immunologic activity, and the expression of Fc receptors (CD64) on monocytes, each of which is transiently produced by rhIFN-$\gamma$. Volunteer subjects in a CS Group were provided with a distinctively flavored drinking solution 4 days per week for 4 weeks. The CS was followed by a sc injection of rhIFN-$\gamma$ on the 4 days during week 1, on 3 of the days during week 2, and on 2 of the 4 days during week 3. Only the CS was presented on week 4. A placebo-treated group was exposed to the same gustatory stimulus followed by an injection of saline according to the same schedule, and a UCS group was not exposed to the CS solution but was injected with rhIFN-$\gamma$ on the same schedule as subjects in the experimental group.

Placebo-treated subjects showed no change in any measure of immunologic reactivity at any time during the experiment. Groups CS and UCS, which received the same amount of rhIFN-$\gamma$ throughout the study, showed the expected rise in QUIN values at the end of the first and second weeks. At the end of week 3, however (when both groups had received only two injections of rhIFN-$\gamma$), subjects that also received the CS solution had higher QUIN values than subjects that received only the two rhIFN-$\gamma$ injections. Reexposure to the CS had delayed the decay in the response to the decline in the cumulative amount of rhIFN-$\gamma$. The authors took care to note that the difference was probably due to half the subjects in Group CS who showed exaggerated responses to the CS. The neopterin data and the expression of CD64 on rhIFN-$\gamma$-activated monocytes were consistent with the QUIN results, but were even smaller in magnitude and, again, could have been attributable to the dramatic responses of just a few subjects in the experimental group. As these investigators point out (and as it turned out), the design of this study did not enable the direct observation of a CS-induced elevation in QUIN or neopterin levels. Nevertheless, these preliminary observations suggest that it may well be possible to demonstrate a cytokine-induced conditioned enhancement of immunologic reactivity in human subjects.

## V. BIOLOGICAL SIGNIFICANCE OF CONDITIONED CHANGES IN IMMUNE FUNCTION

The effects of conditioning in suppressing or enhancing immune responses have not been large. They have, however, been consistent and independently reproducible. Thus, the question arises: do behaviorally induced alterations of immunity have any biological or clinical significance? With respect to conditioning, there are now several illustrations of the potential clinical significance of such processes. One demonstration comes from a study of lupus-prone mice.

Female, (NZBxNZW)F1 mice spontaneously develop an autoimmune disease similar to systemic lupus erythematosus (SLE) in man. These animals, then, constitute a model of disease in which immunosuppression is in the biological interests of the organism. Ader and Cohen (1982) hypothesized that, based on the ability to condition immunosuppressive responses, the substitution of CSs for active immunosuppressive drug would have a salutary effect on the course of the autoimmune disease in conditioned relative to nonconditioned animals treated with the same amount of drug. Over a period of 2 months, lupus-prone mice received weekly injections of CY that were or were not paired with the taste of saccharin. For the experimental group, CSs (saccharin plus an ip injection of saline) were substituted for half the weekly treatments with active immunosuppressive drug. Nonconditioned animals that received half the cumulative amount of CY received by the animals treated weekly did not differ from mice that received no CY at all. However, as hypothesized, the onset of proteinuria and mortality was significantly delayed in conditioned animals compared to that seen in nonconditioned animals treated with the same amount of drug; i.e., the onset of autoimmune disease in these genetically susceptible mice was delayed using a cumulative dose of active drug that was not, by itself, sufficient to alter progression of the autoimmune disorder. Furthermore, in lupus-prone mice that previously received weekly treatments with CY paired with the taste of saccharin, reexposure to saccharin after active drug treatment was discontinued prolonged survival relative to similarly conditioned animals that received neither active drug nor saccharin (Ader, 1985). Besides their substantiation of the biological impact of conditioned alterations of immune function, these data indicate that there would be some heuristic value in viewing some pharmacotherapeutic protocols as a series of conditioning trials and suggest that conditioning operations might be engaged to reduce the amount of drug required in the treatment of chronic disease. These issues are discussed in detail elsewhere (Ader, 1985, 1997).

Consensual validity for these observations comes from a study in which reexposure to a CS previously paired with poly(I:C) resulted in decreased NK-cell activity (Gorczynski & Kennedy, 1984), rather than the increased NK-cell activity reported by others in other experimental situations (e.g., Solvason et al., 1988). The mice that showed the immunosuppressive response also showed a decreased survival to an adoptively transferred NK-sensitive tumor (the YAC-1 lymphoma). No such effects were seen using an NK-resistant tumor. In another study (Gorczynski, Kennedy, & Ciampi, 1985), mice that had been conditioned by pairing saccharin consumption with CY were subsequently challenged with a syngeneic plasmacytoma. Conditioned mice that were reexposed to the CS showed an accelerated mortality rate compared to conditioned animals that were not reexposed to the CS and nonconditioned and placebo-treated groups.

Using an NK-resistant, transplanted MOPC 104 E myeloma, Ghanta, Hiramoto, Solvason, and Spector (1987a) claim that reexposure to a CS previously paired with poly(I:C) can reverse the growth of the tumor and enhance survival in BALB/c mice. Conditioned mice were exposed to the odor of camphor for 4 h on each of 10 trials given at 3-day intervals. They were then inoculated with tumor cells and reexposed to the camphor for 4 h every 3 days thereafter. A second group of conditioned animals was not reexposed to the CS following transplantation of the tumor. A third group received only the poly(I:C) before transplantation and was subsequently exposed to camphor plus injections of poly(I:C), and another group received no treatment at any time. There were no overall differences among the several groups. There were two "outlier" mice in the conditioned group reexposed to the CS that did not die; the median survival time for the remaining animals in the CS group, however, was essentially identical to that of the other groups—including those that actually received poly(I:C) every 3 days throughout the study.

At a subsequent meeting, Ghanta, Miura, Hiramoto, and Hiramoto (1988) presented additional data on the susceptibility of BALB/c mice to the NK-resistant, MOPC 104 E plasmacytoma. Again, the odor of camphor was paired with an injection of poly(I:C) 10 times at 3-day intervals. Twenty-four hours later the mice were injected with tumor cells and the next day (and every 3 days thereafter), some conditioned animals were reexposed to the odor of camphor while others remained undisturbed. The results suggested that there was a slower mortality rate among the animals reexposed to the CS. However, there were no nonconditioned groups or a concurrent control group to define the unconditioned effects of poly(I:C) on tumor growth and mortality, so the findings can not yet be attributed to conditioning. These investigators report other successful attempts to use conditioning to influence the response to tumors (e.g., Ghanta, Hiramoto, Solvason, Soong, & Hiramoto, 1990), but, however provocative, problems with design and data analyses preclude any conclusions about the biologic impact or clinical significance of conditioned alterations of immune function based on these results.

Blom, Tamarkin, Shiber, and Nelson (1995) paired saccharin consumption with CY on a single trial and then reexposed conditioned mice to the CS when they were subsequently injected with the chemical carcinogen, 9,10-dimethylbenanthracene (DMBA). Some conditioned mice were reexposed to the CS a second time, 3 days after the injection of DMBA. There was no CSo group, but this study did include an NC group that was exposed to the CS and UCS in a noncontingent manner and later reexposed to saccharin and a placebo-treated group that was also reexposed to saccharin when they were injected with DMBA (and again 3 days later). In the first experiment, the critical comparisons indicated that a greater percentage of the twice-reexposed CS group had verified tumors than the nonconditioned (noncontingent) animals that were also reexposed to the CS on two occasions. In a second experiment, the CS group had a greater percentage of animals with tumors than the NC group that did not experience the noncontingent CS–UCS presentation, but they did not differ from an NC group that did experience the noncontingent CS–UCS presentation. The results, then, are less than definitive, but consistent with previous findings (Gorczynski et al., 1985).

There are several animal models of arthritis that are demonstrably sensitive to the manipulation of psychosocial and stressful life events (see Rogers et al., this volume). They are also sensitive to conditioned immunosuppressive responses. Klosterhalfen and Klosterhalfen (1983) initially found that reexposure to a CS paired with CY prevented the spread of an inflammatory reaction from a paw that had been injected with Freund's complete adjuvant to a contralateral, noninjected paw. Expressing some concern for the potentially confounding aversive properties of CY, they studied the effects of a conditioned immunosuppressive response on adjuvant-induced arthritis using cyclosporine A as the UCS (Klosterhalfen & Klosterhalfen, 1990). While a high dose of CsA (150 mg/kg) paired with a taste stimulus will induce avoidance behavior (Neveu et al., 1987), a low dose of CsA (20 mg/kg) will not necessarily do so. In this discriminative conditioning study, then, a CS+ preceded an ip injection of 20 mg/kg CsA, and another distinctive taste stimulus, the CS−, was not associated with CsA. Rats were first given a subplantar injection of Freund's adjuvant. Conditioning trials began 1 week later. On alternating days, the animals were exposed to the CS+ plus an injection of CsA or the CS−, alone. After 14 days of discriminative conditioning trials and a 3-day interval, each of these

groups was exposed to either the CS+ or the CS− alone on each of three test trials administered every other day. There was no apparent taste aversion among animals treated with CsA. However, the degree of foot pad swelling after reexposure to the CS+ was significantly reduced relative to that seen in animals exposed to the CS−.

When arthritis was induced after acquisition of the discrimination between stimuli that were and were not associated with CsA, paw swelling was again reduced in the animals reexposed to the CS+ compared to those reexposed to the CS−. Similar results were obtained when adjuvant-induced arthritis was introduced after rats had received a 12-day series of electric footshocks in a distinctive environment (Lysle, Luecken, & Maslonek, 1992b). Reexposure to the distinctive environment on days 12, 14, and 16 reduced the severity of disease relative to animals that were reexposed to the CS 0, 2, and 4 days after receiving adjuvant, and compared to conditioned animals that were not reexposed to the CS or nonconditioned animals.

In an earlier study (Sato et al., 1984), mice were exposed to low-dose X-irradiation after a series of conditioning trials which paired the sound of a buzzer with inescapable footshocks. After irradiation, some mice were reexposed to the CS and others were not. In the absence of irradiation, there were no group differences in antibody production in response to an injection of SRBC. In irradiated animals, however, there was an attenuated antibody response among animals that were reexposed to the CS compared to conditioned animals that were not reexposed to the CS and nonconditioned animals. Although we are not here dealing with a direct measure of pathology, the reexposure of immunocompromised animals to environmental cues associated with stressful experiences delayed the recovery of immune function.

Acquired resistance to *Leishmania* parasites depends on T-cell immunity in which IFN-γ plays a significant role. CBA mice that produce primarily a pattern of Th-1 cytokines (including IFN-γ and IL-2) in response to infection are more resistant to the parasite than BALB/c mice that respond to infection with a more predominant Th-2 pattern of cytokine production (e.g., IL-4). Also, young mice preferentially produce Th-1 type cytokines and old mice preferentially produce Th-2 type cytokines. Gorczynski (1996) confirmed the predictions that young mice would be more resistant than old mice and that CBA mice would be more resistant than BALB/c mice to infection with *Leishmania major* and that the differences in susceptibility were paralleled by differences in the patterns of IL-2 and IL-4 that were produced in response to the infection.

Gorczynski (1996) then proceeded to determine if a stressor-induced conditioned immunosuppressive state would affect the response to *L. major*. Young (8 weeks) and old (≥75 weeks) CBA mice were exposed to a "rotational stress" on three occasions and subsequently infected with the parasite. Every 4 days thereafter, half the animals were reexposed to the environment in which the stressful experience had occurred. Neither lesion size nor cytokine production discriminated between the CS and CSo groups in the "old" population. Among the young animals, however, conditioned animals that were reexposed to the CS following infection were more susceptible than conditioned animals that were not reexposed to the CS. In a separate population rechallenged with antigen in vitro, IL-4 production exceeded IL-2 production in the more susceptible conditioned/reexposed group, while the reverse was true for the conditioned/nonreexposed group. When susceptible BALB/c mice were made resistant to the parasitic infection by a series of preimmunization injections of irradiated *L. major*, reexposure of conditioned animals to the CS suppressed the acquired immunity to the infection. While these dramatic results appear to reflect the effects of associative processes, the absence of a control group that experienced the repeated (and, for them, presumably neutral) postinfection stimulation experienced by conditioned animals precludes any definitive conclusions on this issue.

Transplantation models offer another dramatic illustration of the impact of conditioned immunosuppressive responses. Normally, A/J recipient mice will reject skin grafts from BALB/c or C57BL/6 donors

within 2 weeks. Injecting a low dose of CY on the day of grafting or a pretransplantation transfusion of donor blood, however, prolongs graft survival. Based on these data, Gorczynski (1990) paired saccharin consumption and CY and then reexposed conditioned A/J mice to the CS alone on the day of grafting and at 5-day intervals thereafter. As can be seen in Figure 3, whether or not the recipients received transfusions of donor blood, survival of the skin allograft was extended in conditioned mice reexposed to the CS relative to that seen in the several control groups. Similar results were obtained by Grochowicz et al., (1991) and by Exton and his associates (1998). In the first of these studies (Figure 4A), the nonconditioned groups were not reexposed to the gustatory CS but, in the second study (Figure 4B) the NC group did experience noncontingent CS–UCS training trials. Also, there was no CSo group in either study, but the other control groups suggest that there are no residual effects of either the CS or the UCS. Both studies found that the survival of a heterotopic heart transplant was prolonged when recipient mice were reexposed to a CS previously paired with cyclosporin A.

Finally, as a direct extension of the animal research on conditioning in lupus-prone mice, a conditioning protocol was superimposed on the regimen of chemotherapy prescribed for a child with systemic lupus erythematosus (Olness & Ader, 1992). In this single case study, a combined gustatory and olfactory CS was administered with the infusion of cytoxan. During the course of the 12 monthly treatment sessions, the patient received only half the amount of cytoxan she would normally have received; half the treatment sessions consisted of CS exposures and

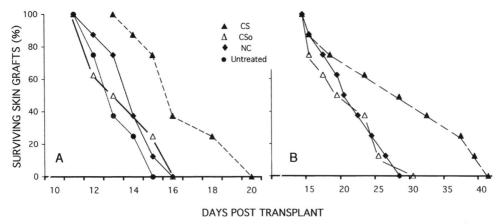

**FIGURE 3** Effects of conditioning on the survival of BALB/c skin grafts in untreated A/J mice (A) and in A/J mice that were pretransfused with BALB/c blood (B). CS, conditioned mice reexposed to the CS; CSo, conditioned mice not reexposed to the CS; NC, nonconditioned mice; and untreated animals. Redrawn from Gorczynski (1990) and reprinted with permission of the author and Academic Press.

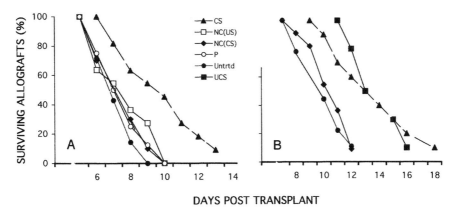

**FIGURE 4** Effects of conditioning on the survival of Lewis strain cardiac allografts in DA strain rats reported by Grochowicz et al. (1991) (A) and Exton et al. (1998) (B). CS, conditioned animals reexposed to the CS; NC, nonconditioned groups; UCS, animals that received repeated injections of cyclosporine, the unconditioned stimulus; and placebo (P) and untreated control groups. Drawn or redrawn with permission of the authors and of Academic Press and Elsevier Science B.V.

vehicle infusions. There are few definitive conclusions that can be drawn from a single case study, but the patient improved clinically and continued to do well for several years.

Other preliminary but provocative data come from a study of asthmatic children on Coche Island, Venezuela (Castes, Palenque, Canelones, Hagel, & Lynch, 1998). For a conditioned group, β2 agonist bronchodilator inhalation (salbutamol) was paired with the odor of vanilla twice a day for 15 days. Control groups received only the bronchodilator or unpaired exposures to the vanilla odor. Pulmonary function was significantly increased in the conditioned children following a test trial with the odor alone. The authors also reported that, in children accustomed to inhaler therapy, a placebo inhaler produced a significant increase in pulmonary function.

In these several studies, then, the pairing of an immunologically neutral stimulus, the CS, with an immunomodulating agent or the immunologic effects of a stressful experience enabled reexposure to the CS to evoke responses that influenced immunocompetence or the progression of a pathophysiologic process and, ultimately, the survival of the organism. As such, these studies, hint at the potential clinical significance and therapeutic potential of conditioned alterations in immune function.

## VI. SUMMARY

Even if there are methodological issues that remain to be resolved and even if every study does not contain every control group, the available evidence leaves little doubt that learning processes contribute to the development and expression of immunoregulatory function. The acquisition and extinction of the conditioned suppression or enhancement of nonspecific and antigen-specific antibody- and cell-mediated immune responses have been documented under a variety of experimental circumstances. Much of the original evidence was generated using a taste aversion conditioning model. It is now clear, however, that the phenomenon is not confined to conditioned immunopharmacologic responses or to any single conditioning model or procedure. The effects of aversive and nonaversive immunopharmacologic agents and the immunologic effects of stress have been conditioned and influence both B and T cells. More to the issue of conditioned *immune* responses, conditioning effects have also been observed using a variety of antigens as unconditioned stimuli. Conversely, and in keeping with the bidirectional nature of the relationship between the nervous and immune systems, immunogenic stimuli are capable of serving as unconditioned stimuli for the conditioning of other psychophysiological responses.

Most of the conditioning work has been based on one-trial taste aversion conditioning or situations involving relatively few conditioning trials. Considering the nature of immune responses, the ability to observe conditioning effects after a single CS–UCS trial has its virtues; it also has its limitations, and the "optimal" experimental circumstances for the elaboration of conditioning effects may not yet have been identified. For example, experimental and clinical studies in immunology typically immunize with suprathreshold levels of antigenic stimulation calculated to induce an "optimal" response. However, that "optimal" (frequently, "maximal") response may not provide the latitude to observe the effects of behavioral interventions. Systematic studies of the kinetics of the response to varying concentrations of different antigenic stimuli that are used as UCSs or as the vehicle for assessing antigen-specific responses are needed in order to design studies that have the potential to reveal the true magnitude and extent of the effects of conditioning (and other behavioral interventions).

Conditioning studies that permit the parametric variation of other relevant variables (e.g., number of conditioning trials) also need to be explored in an attempt to magnify conditioned immunologic effects, better define conditioning effects (e.g., resistance to extinction, retention), and determine if the functional relationships that obtain in the conditioning of immunologic reactivity are the same as those that characterize other conditioned (physiologic) responses. In the case of immunopharmacologic UCSs, the ability to use multiple conditioning trials might enable more comprehensive analyses of the circumstances under which compensatory immune responses might occur. Multiple trial paradigms would also permit assessment of the extent to which tolerance to immunopharmacologic agents (like the tolerance to some other drugs) can be attributed to conditioning processes.

The neural or neuroendocrine mechanisms underlying the behavioral modulation of immune responses have not yet been identified. The notion that there might be some direct relationship between conditioned behavioral and immunologic responses or that conditioning effects are a consequence of stress-induced elevations of glucocorticoids is not supported by the existing literature. As described throughout this volume, the sympathetic innervation of lymphoid organs, the ability of lymphocytes to receive and generate neuroendocrine signals, and the ability of the nervous system to produce and to receive cytokine signals provide myriad pathways through which learning processes could modulate antigen-specific and nonspecific immune defenses and be modified by the activity of the immune system. It is clear from the data accumulated thus far that different immunologic and neuroendocrine mechanisms are involved in mediating the effects of different behavioral interventions on different immune responses measured in different compartments of the immune system.

If we are not yet able to specify the mechanisms underlying the functional relationships between the nervous system and the immune system illustrated by the conditioned modulation of different immune responses, neither can we specify the functional significance of the neuroanatomical, neurochemical, and neuroendocrine connections between the brain and the immune system. Research conducted during the past decade has, however, begun to address these issues. Adrenocortical steroids, opioids and catecholamines, acting singly or in tandem, have been offered as mediators of conditioned alterations of immunity. One or another of these systems has been implicated in the mediation of some conditioning effects observed under some experimental conditions. This latter summation is not a "hedge"; it is simply an acknowledgment that different conditioning circumstances, particularly, different unconditioned stimuli, elicit different patterns of autonomic and neuroendocrine responses that define the environment within which immunologic processes and the response to immunologic signals take place. To add to these interactions, the biologic impact of conditioned (or stress-induced or environmentally determined) alterations of immune function will depend upon the immunologic status of the host. The effects of conditioned immunosuppressive responses in lupus-prone mice and in animals bearing an NK-sensitive tumor would be one example; the effects of conditioning in young and old animals would be another.

These host characteristics are not complications; they are opportunities. Individual differences, gender differences, age differences, strain differences, and species differences in behavioral and physiologic (including immunologic) function permit one to identify and focus on empirically derived candidates for the mediation of behaviorally- induced changes in immune function. Thus, rather than a discrete but intrusive intervention that can and often does induce multiple physiological changes, sometimes in an artificial or nonphysiological manner, one could take advantage of the neuroendocrine and immunologic differences between young and old animals or the difference in the pattern of cytokine responses that characterize different strains of animals to identify processes that could be involved in mediating conditioned and other behaviorally induced changes in immune function.

Not infrequently, one stimulus (e.g., an UCS) is substituted for another with the implicit assumption that, if the outcome is the same, the two stimuli are equivalent and, further, that the substituted stimulus "explains" the action of the original stimulus. Similarly, the fact that some agonistic or antagonistic neurochemical or pharmacologic intervention can block or mimic the immunologic effects of reexposure to a CS or stressful stimulation is not nearly enough information to constitute an explanation of the behaviorally induced effects. It suggests only that such a pathway is one (of perhaps several) means by which such an effect could occur. Even that conclusion depends on whether or not other behavioral, neuroendocrine, or immune responses are similarly affected. Also, in attempting to discover how conditioning processes are able to modulate immune processes, it is necessary to distinguish between: (a) the effects of some intervention (e.g., brain lesions, receptor agonists and antagonists) on the acquisition of a conditioned response, i.e., the neural events that mediate associative processes, and (b) the effects of interventions that influence pathways between the nervous system and the immune system that could support the acquisition and expression of conditioned changes in immune responses, per se.

Some neural or neuroendocrine intervention studies can be difficult to interpret. Using receptor-blocking agents, for example, a central receptor antagonist can be administered before conditioning or after conditioning but before testing for the conditioned response. Interventions introduced before conditioning address the associative processes involved in the acquisition of a conditioned response. The results would be instructive if there are differential effects on different parameters of humoral and/or cell-mediated immune responses and/or there are different effects on behavioral or neuroendocrine and immune responses. The results would also be instructive if the intervention had no effect on conditioning. If all conditioned responses are blocked (or if there is only a single measure of immunity and that response is blocked), no conclusion about the role of the interrupted circuitry in the conditioning of an alteration of immunity (as distinct from any other conditioned response) would be possible; all learning may have been affected.

Similarly, if a blocking agent or brain lesion introduced after conditioning interferes with the expression of a conditioned change in immune function, such results bear on relevant CNS–immune system interactions only if there are other immune responses that are not affected or if other conditioned (behavioral or neuroendocrine) responses remain intact. Again, if the only immune response being measured is blocked, it is not possible to identify the circuitry involved as having a mediational role, a permissive effect, or some general effect on the expression of conditioned responses.

Research conducted over the past several years has also provided a glimpse of some of the clinical implications of conditioned immunologic effects. Consistent with a voluminous experimental literature on psychosomatic relationships, susceptibility to naturally occurring or experimentally induced disease states can be altered if animals are exposed to cues associated with specific immunomodulating substances or environmental circumstances. One of the most direct and immediate extrapolations from these data would be the application of conditioning principles in the design of pharmacotherapeutic protocols calculated to reduce the cumulative amount of immunomodulating drugs required to maintain some physiologic (immunologic) state within homeostatic bounds. These observations and the hypotheses they generate reinforce the expectation that an elaboration of the conditions under which and the mechanisms through which conditioning and other psychosocial circumstances can alter immune function could have important clinical and therapeutic ramifications.

## Acknowledgments

Preparation of this chapter was supported by a Research Scientist Award (K05 MH06318) to R.A. from the National Institute of Mental Health.

## References

Ader, R. (1981). A historical account of conditioned immunobiologic responses. In R. Ader (Ed.), *Psychoneuroimmunology* (pp. 321–352). New York: Academic Press.

Ader, R. (1985). Conditioned immunopharmacologic effects in animals: Implications for a conditioning model of pharmacotherapy. In L. White, B. Tursky, & G. Schwartz (Eds.), *Placebo: Theory, research, and mechanisms* (pp. 306–323). New York: Guilford.

Ader, R. (1987). Conditioned immune responses: Adrenocortical influences. *Progress in Brain Research, 72,* 79–90.

Ader, R. (1997). The role of conditioning in pharmacotherapy. In A. Harrington (Ed.), *The placebo: An interdisciplinary exploration* (pp. 138–165). Cambridge: Harvard University Press.

Ader, R., & Cohen, N. (1975). Behaviorally conditioned immunosuppression. *Psychosomatic Medicine, 37,* 333–340.

Ader, R., & Cohen, N. (1982). Behaviorally conditioned immunosuppression and murine systemic lupus erythematosus. *Science, 215,* 1534–1536.

Ader, R., & Cohen, N. (1991). The influence of conditioning on immune responses. In R. Ader, D. L. Felten, & N. Cohen (Eds.), *Psychoneuroimmunology,* (2nd ed.) (pp. 611–646). New York: Academic Press.

Ader, R., & Cohen, N. (1993). Psychoneuroimmunology: Conditioning and stress. *Annual Review of Psychology, 44,* 53–85.

Ader, R., Cohen, N., & Bovbjerg, D. (1982). Conditioned suppression of humoral immunity in the rat. *Journal of Comparative and Physiological Psychology, 96,* 517–521.

Ader, R., Felten, D. L., & Cohen, N. (1991). *Psychoneuroimmunology,* (2nd ed.). New York: Academic Press.

Ader, R., Grota, L. J., & Cohen, N. (1987). Conditioning phenomena and immune function. *Annals of the New York Academy of Sciences, 496,* 532–544.

Ader, R., Kelly, K., Moynihan, J. A., Grota, L. J., & Cohen, N. (1993). Conditioned enhancement of antibody production using antigen as the unconditioned stimulus. *Brain, Behavior, and Immunity, 7,* 334–343.

Alvarez-Borda, B., Ramírez-Amaya, V., Pérez-Montfort, R., & Bermúdez-Rattoni, F. (1995). Enhancement of antibody production by a learning paradigm. *Neurobiology of Learning and Memory, 64,* 103–105.

Andersson, B., & Blomgren, H. (1971). Evidence for thymus-independent humoral antibody production in mice against polyvinylpyrrolidone and *E. coli.* lipopolysaccharide. *Cellular Immunology, 2,* 411.

Andrykowski, M. A., Jacobsen, P. B., Marks, E., Gorfinkle, K., Hakes, T. B., Kaufman, R. I., Currie, V. E., Holland, J. C., & Redd, W. H. (1988). Prevalence, predictors and course of anticipatory nausea in women receiving adjuvant chemotherapy for breast cancer. *Cancer, 62,* 2607–2613.

Andrykowski, M. A., & Redd, W. H. (1987). Longitudinal analysis of the development of anticipatory nausea. *Journal of Consulting and Clinical Psychology, 55,* 36–41.

Andrykowski, M., Redd, W. H., & Hatfield, A. (1985). The development of anticipatory nausea: A prospective analysis. *Journal of Consulting and Clinical Psychology, 53,* 447–454.

Bermúdez-Rattoni, F., & McGaugh, J. L. (1991). Insular cortex and amygdala lesions differentially affect acquisition of inhibitory avoidance and conditioned taste aversion. *Brain Research, 549,* 165–170.

Blom, J. M. C., Tamarkin, L., Shiber, J. R., & Nelson, R. J. (1995). Learned immunosuppression is associated with an increased risk of chemically-induced tumors. *Neuroimmunomodulation, 2,* 92–99.

Booth, R. J., Petrie, K. J., & Brook, R. J. (1995). Conditioning allergic skin responses in humans: A controlled study. *Psychosomatic Medicine, 57,* 492-495.

Boswell, H. S., Nerenberg, M. I., Scher, I., & Singer, A. (1980). Role of accessory cells in B cell activation. III. Cellular analysis of primary immune response deficits in CBA/N mice: Presence of an accessory cell-B cell interaction defect. *Journal of Experimental Medicine, 152,* 1194–1209.

Bovbjerg, D., Ader, R., & Cohen, N. (1982). Behaviorally conditioned suppression of a graft-vs-host response. *Proceedings of the National Academy of Sciences, USA, 79,* 583–585.

Bovbjerg, D., Ader, R., & Cohen, N. (1984). Acquisition and extinction of conditioned suppression of a graft-vs-host response in the rat. *Journal of Immunology, 132,* 111–113.

Bovbjerg, D., Ader, R., & Cohen, N. (1986). Long-lasting enhancement of the delayed-type hypersensitivity response to heterologous erythrocytes in mice after a single injection of cyclophosphamide. *Clinical and Experimental Immunology, 66,* 539–550.

Bovbjerg, D., Cohen, N., & Ader, R. (1987). Behaviorally conditioned enhancement of delayed-type hypersensitivity in the mouse. *Brain, Behavior and Immunity, 1,* 64–71.

Bovbjerg, D., Kim, Y. T., Siskind, G. W., & Weksler, M. E. (1987). Conditioned suppression of plaque-forming cell response with cyclophosphamide. *Annals of the New York Academy of Sciences, 496,* 588–594.

Bovbjerg, D. H., Redd, W. H., Maier, L. A., Holland, J. C., Lesko, L. M., Niedzwiecki, D., Rubin, S. C., & Hakes T. B. (1990). Anticipatory immune suppression and nausea in women receiving cyclic chemotherapy for ovarian cancer. *Journal of Consulting and Clinical Psychology, 58,* 153–157.

Bull, D. F., Exton, M. S., & Husband, A. J. (1994). The acute phase immune response: Lipopolysaccharide-induced fever and sleep alterations are not simultaneously conditionable in the rat during the inactive (light) phase. *Physiology and Behavior, 56,* 143–149.

Buske-Kirschbaum, A., Kirschbaum, C., Stierle, H., Jabaij, L., & Hellhammer, D. (1994). Conditioned manipulation of natural

killer (NK) cells in humans using a discriminative learning protocol. *Biological Psychology, 38,* 143–155.

Buske-Kirschbaum, A., Kirschbaum, C., Stierle, H., Lehnert, H., & Hellhammer, D. (1992). Conditioned increase of natural killer cell activity (NKCA) in humans. *Psychosomatic Medicine, 54,* 123–132.

Callahan, T. A., Moynihan, J. A., & Piekut,, D. T. (1998). Central nervous system activation following peripheral chemical sympathectomy: Implications for neural-immune interactions. *Brain, Behavior, and Immunity, 12,* 230–241.

Carey, M. P., & Burish, T. G. (1988). Etiology and treatment of the psychological side effects associated with cancer chemotherapy: A critical review and discussion. *Psychological Bulletin, 104,* 307–325.

Carr, G., Fibinger, H. C., & Phillips, A. G. (1989). Conditioned place preference as a measure of drug reward. In J. M. Lieberman & S. J. Cooper (Eds.), *The neuropharmacological basis of reward* (pp. 264–319). Oxford: Clarendon Press.

Castes, M., Palenque, M., Canelones, P., Hagel, I., & Lynch, N. (1998). Classic conditioning and placebo effects in the bronchodilator response of asthmatic children. *Neuroimmunomodulation, 5,* 70.

Cohen, N., Ader, R., Green, N., & Bovbjerg, D. (1979). Conditioned suppression of a thymus independent antibody response *Psychosomatic Medicine, 41,* 487–491.

Coussons, M. E., Dykstra, L. A., & Lysle, D. T. (1992). Pavlovian conditioning of morphine-induced alterations of immune status. *Journal of Neuroimmunology, 39,* 219–230.

Coussons-Read, M. E., Dykstra, L. A., & Lysle, D. T. (1994a). Pavlovian conditioning of morphine-induced alterations of immune status: Evidence for peripheral β-adrenergic receptor involvement. *Brain, Behavior, and Immunity, 8,* 204–217.

Coussons-Read, M. E., Dykstra, L. A., & Lysle, D. T. (1994b). Pavlovian conditioning of morphine-induced alterations of immune status: Evidence for opioid receptor involvement. *Journal of Neuroimmunology, 55,* 135–142.

Coussons, M. E., Maslonek, K. A., Fecho, K., Perez, L., & Lysle, D. T. (1994). Evidence for the involvement of macrophage-derived nitric oxide in the modulation of immune status by a conditioned aversive stimulus. *Journal of Neuroimmunology, 50,* 51–58.

Cunnick, J. E., Lysle, D. T., Armfield, A., & Rabin, B. S. (1988). Shock-induced modulation of lymphocyte responsiveness and natural killer activity: Differential mechanisms of induction. *Brain, Behavior, and Immunity, 2,* 102–113.

Cunnick, J. E., Lysle, D. T., Kucinski, B. J., & Rabin, B. (1990). Evidence that shock-induced suppression is mediated by adrenal hormones and peripheral β-adrenergic receptors *Pharmacology, Biochemistry, and Behavior, 36,* 645–651.

Dark, K., Peeke, H. V. S., Ellman, G., & Salfi, M. (1987). Behaviorally conditioned histamine release. *Annals of the New York Academy of Sciences, 496,* 578–582.

Dekker, E, Pelser, H. E., & Groen, J. (1957). Conditioning as a cause of asthmatic attacks: A laboratory study. *Journal of Psychosomatic Research, 2,* 97–108.

Demissie, S., Rogers, C. F., Hiramoto, N. S, Ghanta, V. K., & Hiramoto, R. N. (1995). Arecoline a muscarinic cholinergic agent conditions central pathways that modulate natural killer cell activity. *Journal of Neuroimmunology, 59,* 57–63.

Demissie, S., Rogers, C. F., Hiramoto, N. S, Ghanta, V. K., & Hiramoto, R. N. (1996). Lipopolysaccharide and IL-1 activate CNS pathways as measured by NK cell activity. *Physiology and Behavior, 59,* 499–504.

Domjan, M., & Burkhard, B. (1986). *The principles of learning and behavior* (2nd ed.) Brooks/Cole: Belmont, CA.

Drugan, R. C., Mandler, R., Crawley, J. N., Skolnick, P., Barker, J. L., Novotny, B., Paul, S. M., & Weber, R. J. (1986). Conditioned fear induced rapid immunosuppression in the rat. *Neuroscience Abstracts, 12,* 337.

Dyck, D. G., Driedger, S. M., Nemeth, R., Osachuk, T. A. G., & Greenberg, A. H. (1987). Conditioned tolerance to drug-induced (Poly I:C) natural killer cell activation: Effects of drug-dosage and context-specificity parameters. *Brain, Behavior, and Immunity, 1,* 251–266.

Dyck, D. G., Greenberg, A. H., & Osachuk, T. (1986). Tolerance to drug-induced (Poly I:C) natural killer (NK) cell activation: Congruence with a Pavlovian conditioning model. *Journal of Experimental Psychology: Animal Behavior Processes, 12,* 25–31.

Dyck, D., Janz, L., Osachuk, T. A. G., Falk, J., Labinsky, J., & Greenberg, A. H. (1990). The Pavlovian conditioning of IL-1-induced glucocorticoid secretion. *Brain, Behavior, and Immunity, 4,* 93–104.

Eikelboom, R., & Stewart, J. (1979). Conditioned temperature effects using morphine as the unconditioned stimulus. *Psychopharmacology, 61,* 31–38.

Elmquist, J. K., Scammell, T. E., Jacobsen, C. D., & Saper, C. B. (1996). Distribution of Fos-like immunoreactivity in the rat brain following intravenous lipopolysaccharide administration. *Journal of Comparative Neurology, 371,* 85–103.

Exton, M. S., Bull, D. F., & King, M. G. (1995). Behavioral conditioning of endotoxin-induced anorexia. *Physiology and Behavior, 57,* 401–405.

Exton, M. S., Bull, D. F., King, M. G., & Husband, A. J. (1995). Behavioral conditioning of endotoxin-induced plasma iron alterations. *Pharmacology, Biochemistry, and Behavior, 50,* 675–679.

Exton, M. S., Lightfoot, J. B., Stanton, M. W., Bull, D. F., King, M. G., & Husband, A. J. (1995). Behaviorally conditioned anorexia: Role of gastric emptying and prostaglandins *Physiology and Behavior, 58,* 471–476.

Exton, M. S., von Hörsten, S. B., Schult, M., Vöge, J., Strubel, T., Donath, S., Steinmüller, C., Seeliger, H., Nagel, E., Westermann, J., & Schedlowski, M. (1998). Behaviourally conditioned immunosuppression using cyclosporin A: Central nervous system reduces IL-2 production via splenic innervation. *Journal of Neuroimmunology, 88,* 182–191.

Fecho, K., Dykstra, L. A., & Lysle, D. T. (1993). Evidence for beta adrenergic receptor involvement in the immunomodulatory effects of morphine. *Journal of Pharmacology and Experimental Therapeutics, 265,* 1079–1087.

Fredrikson, M., Fürst, C. J., Lekander, M., Rotstein, S., & Blomgren, H. (1993). Trait anxiety and anticipatory immune reactions in women receiving adjuvant chemotherapy for breast cancer. *Brain, Behavior and Immunity, 7,* 79–90.

Garcia, J., & Koelling, R. A. (1967). The relationship of cue to consequence in avoidance learning. *Psychonomic Science, 4,* 123–124.

Garcia, J., Lasiter, P. S., Bermúdez-Rattoni, F., & Deems, D. A. (1985). A general theory of aversion learning. *Annals of the New York Academy of Sciences, 443,* 8–21.

Gauci, M., Husband, A. J., Saxarra, H., & King, M. G. (1994). Pavlovian conditioning of nasal tryptase release in human subjects with allergic rhinitis. *Physiology and Behavior, 55,* 823–825.

Gee, A. L., & Johnson, D. R. (1994). Behaviorally conditioned modulation of natural killer cell activity: Effects of preconditioning manual restraint and apparatus exposure. *International Journal of Neuroscience, 77,* 139–152.

Gee, A. L., Thiele, G. M., & Johnson, D. R. (1994). Behaviorally conditioned modulation of natural killer cell activity: Enhancement of baseline and activated natural killer cell activity. *International Journal of Neuroscience, 77,* 127–137.

Ghanta, V. K., Hiramoto, N. S., Solvason, H. B., Soong, S.-J., & Hiramoto, R. N. (1990). Conditioning: A new approach to immunotherapy. *Cancer Research, 50,* 4295–4299.

Ghanta, V., Hiramoto, R. N., Solvason, B., & Spector, N. H. (1987a). Influence of conditioned natural immunity on tumor growth. *Annals of the New York Academy of Sciences, 496,* 637–646.

Ghanta, V. K., Hiramoto, N. S., Solvason, H. B., Tyring, S. K., Spector, N. H., & Hiramoto, R. N. (1987b). Conditioned enhancement of natural killer cell activity, but not interferon, with camphor or saccharin-LiCl conditioned stimulus. *Journal of Neuroscience Research, 18,* 10–15.

Ghanta, V. K., Miura, T., Hiramoto, N. S., & Hiramoto, R. N. (1988). Augmentation of natural immunity and regulation of tumor growth by conditioning. *Annals of the New York Academy of Sciences, 521,* 29–42.

Giang, D. W., Goodman, A. D., Schiffer, R. B., Mattson, D. H., Petrie, M., Cohen, N., & Ader, R. (1996). Conditioning of cyclophosphamide-induced leukopenia in humans. *Journal of Neuropsychiatry and Clinical Neuroscience, 8,* 194–201.

Gill, H. K., & Liew, F. Y. (1978). Regulation of delayed-type hypersensitivity. III. Effects of cyclophosphamide on the suppressor cells for delayed-type hypersensitivity to sheep erythrocytes in mice. *European Journal of Immunology, 8,* 172–176.

Gorczynski, R. M. (1987a). Conditioned enhancement of natural killer cell activity, but not interferon, with camphor or saccharin-LiCl conditioned stimulus. *Journal of Neuroscience Research, 18,* 10–15.

Gorczynski, R. M. (1987b). Analysis of lymphocytes in, and host environment of, mice showing conditioned immunosuppression to cyclophosphamide. *Brain, Behavior, and Immunity, 1,* 21–35.

Gorczynski. R. M. (1990). Conditioned enhancement of skin allografts in mice. *Brain, Behavior, and Immunity, 4,* 85–92.

Gorczynski, R. M. (1991a). Toward an understanding of the mechanisms of classical conditioning of antibody responses. *Journal of Gerontology, 46,* P152–P156.

Gorczynski, R. M. (1991b). Conditioned immunosuppression: Analysis of lymphocytes and host environment of young and aged mice. In R. Ader, D. L. Felten, & N. Cohen (Eds.), *Psychoneuroimmunology* (2nd ed.) (pp. 647–662). New York: Academic Press.

Gorczynski, R. M. (1996). Conditioned immunity to *L. Major* in young and aged mice. In H. Friedman, T. W. Klein, & Friedman, A. L. (Eds.), Psychoneuroimmunology, stress, and infection (pp. 137–151). CRC Press: Boca Raton, FL.

Gorczynski, R. M., & Holmes, W. (1989). Neuroleptic and antidepressant drug treatment abolishes conditioned immunosuppression in mice. *Brain, Behavior and Immunity, 3,* 312–319.

Gorczynski, R. M., & Kennedy, M. (1984). Associative learning and regulation of immune responses. *Progress in Neuropsychopharmacology and Biological Psychiatry, 8,* 593–600.

Gorczynski, R. M., & Kennedy, M. (1987). Behavioral trait associated with conditioned immunity. *Brain, Behavior and Immunity, 1,* 72–80.

Gorczynski, R. M., Kennedy, M., & Ciampi A. (1985). Cimetidine reverses tumor growth enhancement of plasmacytoma tumors in mice demonstrating conditioned immunosuppression. *Journal of Immunology, 134,* 4261–4264.

Gorczynski, R. M., Macrae, S., & Kennedy, M. (1982). Conditioned immune response associated with allogeneic skin grafts in mice. *Journal of Immunology, 129,* 704–709.

Grochowicz, P., Schedlowski, M., Husband, A. J., King, M. G., Hibberd, A. D., & Bowen, K. M. (1991). Behavioral conditioning prolongs heart allograft survival in rats. *Brain, Behavior and Immunity, 5,* 349–356.

Hill, L. E. (1930). *Philosophy of a Biologist.* London: Arnold.

Hiramoto, R. N., Ghanta, V. K., Lorden, J. F., Solvason, H. B., Soong, S.-J., Rogers, C. F., Hsueh, C.-M., & Hiramoto, N. S. (1992). Conditioning of enhanced natural killer cell activity: Effects of changing interstimulus intervals and evidence for long-delayed learning. *Progress in NeuroEndocrinImmunology, 5,* 13–20.

Hiramoto, R. N., Ghanta, V. K., Rogers, C. F., & Hiramoto, N. S. (1991). Conditioning the elevation of body temperature, a host defense reflex response. *Life Sciences, 49,* 903–909.

Hiramoto, R., Hiramoto, N. S., Solvason, H. B., & Ghanta, V. K. (1987). Regulation of natural immunity (NK) activity by conditioning. *Annals of the New York Academy of Sciences, 496,* 545–552.

Hiramato, R. N., Hsueh, C.-M., Rogers, C. F., Demissie, S., Hiramoto, N. S., Soong, S.-J., & Ghanta, V. K. (1993). Conditioning of the allogeneic cytotoxic lymphocyte response. *Pharmacology, Biochemistry, and Behavior, 44,* 275–280.

Hiramoto, R., Solvason, B., Ghanta, V., Lorden, J., & Hiramoto, N. (1990). Effect of reserpine on retention of the conditioned NK cell response. *Pharmacology, Biochemistry, and Behavior, 36,* 51–56.

Hsueh, C.-M., Tyring, S. K., Hiramoto, R. N., & Ghanta, V. K. (1994). Efferent signal(s) responsible for the conditioned augmentation of natural killer cell activity. *Neuroimmunomodulation, 1,* 74–81.

Hull, C. L. (1934). The factor of conditioned reflex. In C. Murchison (Ed.), *A handbook of general experimental psychology.* Worcester: Clark University.

Husband, A. J., King, M. G., & Brown, R. (1986/87). Behaviorally conditioned modification of T cell subset ratios in rats. *Immunology Letters, 14,* 91–94.

Husband, A. J., Lin, W., Madsen, G., & King, M. G. (1993). A conditioning model for immunostimulation: Enhancement of the antibody response to ovalbumin by behavioral conditioning in rats. In A. J. Husband (Ed.), *Psychoimmunology: CNS–immune interactions* (pp. 139–147). CRC Press: Boca Raton, FL.

Ikemi, Y., & Nakagawa, S. (1962). A psychosomatic study of contagious dermatitis. *Kyushu Journal of Medicine/Science, 13,* 335–350.

Jacobs, D. M., & Morrison, D.C. (1975). Stimulation of a T-independent primary anti-hapten response in vitro by TNP-lipopolysaccharide (TNP-LPS). *Journal of Immunology, 114,* 360–364.

Janz, L. J., Green-Johnson, J., Murray, L., Vriend, C. Y., Nance, D. M., Greenberg, A. H., & Dyck, D. G. (1996). Pavlovian conditioning of LPS-induced responses: Effects on corticosterone, splenic norepinephrine, and IL-2 production. *Physiology and Behavior, 59,* 1103–1109.

Khan, A. U. (1977). Effectiveness of biofeedback and counter-conditioning in the treatment of bronchial asthma. *Journal of Psychosomatic Research, 21,* 97–104.

Kirschbaum, C., Jabaij, L., Buske-Kirschbaum, A., Hennig, J., Blom, M., Dorst, K., Bauch, J., DiPauli, R., Schmitz, G., Ballieux, R., & Hellhammer, D. (1992). Conditioning of drug-induced immunomodulation in human volunteers: A European collaborative study. *British Journal of Clinical Psychology, 31,* 459–472.

Klosterhalfen, S., & Klosterhalfen, W. (1987). Classically conditioned cyclophosphamide effects on white blood cell counts in rats. *Annals of the New York Academy of Sciences, 496,* 569–577.

Klosterhalfen, S., & Klosterhalfen, W. (1990). Conditioned cyclosporine effects but not conditioned taste aversion in immunized rats. *Behavioral Neuroscience, 104,* 716–724.

Klosterhalfen, W., & Klosterhalfen, S. (1983). Pavlovian conditioning of immunosuppression modifies adjuvant arthritis in rats. *Behavioral Neurosciences, 97*(4), 663–666.

Kopeloff, N. (1941). *Bacteriology in Neuropsychiatry.* Springfield: Charles C. Thomas.

Krank, M. D., & MacQueen, G. M. (1988). Conditioned compensatory responses elicited by environmental signals for cyclophosphamide-induced suppression of antibody production in mice. *Psychobiology, 16,* 229–235.

Kusnecov, A. V., Husband, A. J., & King, M. G. (1988). Behaviorally conditioned suppression of mitogen-induced proliferation and immunoglobulin production: Effect of time span between conditioning and reexposure to the conditioned stimulus. *Brain, Behavior and Immunity, 2,* 198–211.

LeBlanc, A. E., & Cappell, H. (1975). Antagonism of morphine-induced aversive conditioning by naloxone. *Pharmacology, Biochemistry, and Behavior, 3,* 185–188.

Lennartz, R. C., & Weinberger, N. M. (1992). Analysis of response systems in Pavlovian conditioning reveals rapidly versus slowly acquired conditioned responses: Support for two factors, implications for behavior and neurobiology. *Psychobiology, 20,* 93–119.

Longo, D. L., Duffey, P. L., Kopp, W. C., Heyes, M. P., Alvord, W. G., Sharfman, W. H., Schmidt, P. J., Rubinow, D. R., & Rosenstein, D. L. (1999). Conditioned immune response to interferon-γ in humans. *Clinical Immunology* (in press).

Lubow, R. E. (1973). Latent inhibition. *Psychological Review, 79,* 398–407.

Luecken, L. J., & Lysle, D. T. (1992). Evidence for the involvement of beta-adrenergic receptors in conditioned immunomodulation. *Journal of Neuroimmunology, 38,* 209–220.

Lysle, D. T., Coussons, M. E., Watts, V. J., Bennett, E. H., & Dykstra, L. A. (1993). Morphine-induced alterations of immune status: Dose-dependency, compartment specificity, and antagonism by naltrexone. *Journal of Pharmacology and Experimental Therapeutics, 265,* 1071–1078.

Lysle, D. T., Cunnick, J. E., Fowler, H., & Rabin, B. (1988). Pavlovian conditioning of shock-induced suppression of lymphocyte reactivity: Acquisition, extinction, and preexposure effects. *Life Sciences, 42,* 185–2194.

Lysle, D. T., Cunnick, J. E., Kucinski, B. J., Fowler, H., & Rabin, B. S. (1990a). Characterization of immune alterations induced by a conditioned aversive stimulus. *Psychobiology, 18,* 220–226.

Lysle, D. T., Cunnick, J. E., & Maslonek, K. A. (1991). Pharmacological manipulation of immune alterations induced by an aversive conditioned stimulus: Evidence for β-adrenergic receptor-mediated Pavlovian conditioning process. *Behavioral Neuroscience, 105,* 443–449.

Lysle, D. T., Cunnick, J. E., & Rabin, B. S. (1990b). Stressor-induced alteration of lymphocyte proliferation in mice: Evidence for enhancement of mitogen responsiveness. *Brain, Behavior, and Immunity, 4,* 269–277.

Lysle, D. T., Luecken, L. J., & Maslonek, K. A. (1992a). Modulation of immune function by a conditioned aversive stimulus: Evidence for the involvement of endogenous opioids *Brain, Behavior, and Immunity, 6*(2), 179–188.

Lysle, D. T., Luecken, L. J., & Maslonek, K. A. (1992b). Suppression of the development of adjuvant arthritis by a conditioned aversive stimulus. *Brain, Behavior and Immunity, 6,* 64–73.

Lysle, D. T., & Maslonek, K. A. (1991). Immune alterations induced by a conditioned aversive stimulus: Evidence for a time-dependent effect. *Psychobiology, 19,* 339–344.

Mackenzie, J. N. (1896). The production of the so-called "rose cold" by means of an artificial rose. *American Journal of Medical Science, 91,* 45–57.

MacQueen, G. M., & Siegel, S. (1989). Conditional immunomodulation following training with cyclophosphamide. *Behavioral Neurosciences, 103,* 638–647.

MacQueen, G. M., Marshall, J., Perdue, M., Siegel, S., & Bienenstock, J. (1989). Pavlovian conditioning of rat mucosal mast cells to secrete rat mast cell protease II. *Science, 243,* 83–85.

Madden, K. S., Moynihan, J. A., Brenner, G. J., Felten, S. Y., Felten, D. L., & Livnat, S. (1994). Sympathetic nervous system modulation of the immune system. III. Alterations in T and B cell proliferation and differentiation *in vitro* following chemical sympathectomy. *Journal of Neuroimmunology, 49,* 77–87.

Metal'nikov, S., & Chorine, V. (1926). Rôle des réflexes conditionnels dans l'immunité. *Annals L'Institute Pasteur, 40,* 893–900.

Metal'nikov S., & Chorine, V. (1928). Rôle des réflexes conditionnels dans la formation des anticorps. *Comptes Rendus des Seances de la Societe de Biologie et de Ses Filiales, 102,* 133–134.

Mitsuoka, A., Morikawa, S., Baba, M., & Harada, T. (1979). Cyclophosphamide eliminates suppressor T cells in age-associated central regulation of delayed hypersensitivity in mice. *Journal of Experimental Medicine, 149,* 1018–1028.

Morato, E. F., Gerbase-DeLima, M., & Gorczynski, R. M. (1996). Conditioned immunosuppression in orally immunized mice. *Brain, Behavior and Immunity, 10,* 44–54.

Morato, E. F., Gerbase-DeLima, M., & Gorczynski, R. M. (1997). Conditioned immunosuppression of lipopolysaccharide-induced antibody response of orally immunized mice. *Brain, Behavior, and Immunity, 11,* 133–139.

Morrow, G. R., & Dobkin, P. L. (1988). Anticipatory nausea and vomiting in cancer patients undergoing chemotherapy treatment: Prevalence, etiology and behavioral interventions. *Clinical Psychology, Review, 8,* 517–556.

Mosier, D. E., & Subbarao, B. (1982). Thymus-independent antigens: Complexity of B lymphocyte activation revealed. *Immunology Today, 3,* 217–222.

Moynihan, J., Koota, D., Brenner, G., Cohen, N., & Ader, R. (1989). Repeated intraperitoneal injections of saline attenuate the antibody response to a subsequent intraperitoneal injection of antigen. *Brain, Behavior and Immunity, 3(1),* 90–96.

Mucha, R. F., van der Kooy, D., O'Shaughnessey, M., & Bucenieks, P. (1982). Drug reinforcement studies by the use of place conditioning in rat. *Brain Research, 243,* 91–105.

Neveu, P. J., Crestani, F., & LeMoal, M. (1987). Conditioned immunosuppression: A new methodological approach. *Annals of the New York Academy of Sciences, 496,* 595–601.

Neveu, P. J., Dantzer, R., & Le Moal, M. (1986). Behaviorally conditioned suppression of mitogen-induced lymphoproliferation and antibody production in mice. *Neuroscience Letters, 65,* 293–298.

Olness, K., & Ader, R. (1992). Conditioning as an adjunct in the pharmacotherapy of lupus erythematosus: A case report. *Journal of Developmental and Behavioral Pediatrics, 13,* 124–125.

O'Reilly, C. A., & Exon, J. H. (1986). Cyclophosphamide-conditioned suppression of the natural killer cell response in rats. *Physiology and Behavior, 37,* 759–764.

Ottenberg, P., Stein, M., Lewis, J., & Hamilton, C. (1958). Learned asthma in the guinea pig. *Psychosomatic Medicine, 20,* 395–400.

Pavlov, I. P. (1928). *Lectures on conditioned reflexes.* New York: Liveright.

Peeke, H. V. S., Ellman, G., Dark, K., Salfi, M., & Reus, V. I. (1987). Cortisol and behaviorally conditioned histamine release. *Annals of the New York Academy of Sciences, 496,* 583–587.

Perez, L., & Lysle, D. T. (1995). Corticotropin-releasing hormone is involved in conditioned stimulus-induced reduction of natural killer cell activity but not in conditioned alterations in cytokine production or proliferation responses. *Journal of Neuroimmunology, 63,* 1–8.

Perez, L., & Lysele, D. T. (1997). Conditioned immunomodulation: Investigations of the role of endogenous activity at $\mu$, $\kappa$, and $\delta$ opioid receptor subtypes. *Journal of Neuroimmunology, 79,* 101–112.

Pezzone, M. A., Lee, W-S., Hoffman, G. E., Pezzone, K. M., & Rabin, B. S. (1993). Activation of brainstem catecholaminergic neurons by conditioned and unconditioned aversive stimuli as revealed by c-Fos immunoreactivity. *Brain Research, 608,* 310-318.

Pezzone, M. A., Lee, W-S., Hoffman, G. E., & Rabin, B. S. (1992). Induction of c-Fos immunoreactivity in the rat forebrain by conditioned and unconditioned aversive stimuli. *Brain Research, 597,* 41–50.

Ramírez-Amaya, V., Alvarez-Borda, B., & Bermúdez-Rattoni, F. (1998). Differential effects of NMDA-induced lesions into the insular cortex and amygdala on the acquisition and evocation of conditioned immunosuppression. *Brain, Behavior, and Immunity, 12,* 149–160.

Ramírez-Amaya, V., Alvarez-Borda, B., Ormsby, C. E., Martínez, R. D., Pérez-Montfort, R., & Bermúdez-Rattoni, F. (1996). Insular cortex lesions impair the acquisition of conditioned immunosuppression. *Brain, Behavior, and Immunity, 10,* 103–114.

Ramírez-Amaya, V., & Bermúdez-Rattoni, F. (1998). Conditioned enhancement of antibody production is disrupted by insular cortex and amygdala but not hippocampal lesions. *Brain, Behavior, and Immunity, 13,* 46–60.

Randich, A., & LoLordo, V. M. (1979). Associative and non-associative theories of the UCS preexposure phenomenon: Implications for Pavlovian conditioning. *Psychological Bulletin, 86,* 523–548.

Redd, W. H., Andresen, G. V., & Minagawa, R. (1982). Hypnotic control of anticipatory nausea in patients undergoing cancer chemotherapy. *Journal of Consulting and Clinical Psychology, 50,* 12–19.

Rescorla, R. (1988). Behavioral studies of Pavlovian conditioning. *Annual Review of Neuroscience, 11,* 329–334.

Rogers, M. P., Reich, P., Strom, T. B., & Carpenter, C. B. (1976). Behaviorally conditioned immunosuppression: Replication of a recent study. *Psychosomatic Medicine, 38,* 447–452.

Roszman, T., & Carlson, S. (1991). Neural-immune interactions: Circuits and networks. *Progress in Neuroendocrinimmunology, 4,* 69–78.

Roudebush, R. E., & Bryant, H. U. (1991). Conditioned immunosuppression of a murine delayed type hypersensitivity response: Dissociation from corticosterone elevation. *Brain, Behavior, and Immunity, 5,* 308–317.

Russell, M., Dark, K. A., Cummins, R. W., Ellman, G., Callaway, E., & Peeke, H. V. S. (1984). Learned histamine release. *Science, 225,* 733–734.

Sato, K., Flood, J. F., & Makinodan, T. (1984). Influence of conditioned psychological stress on immunological recovery in mice exposed to low-dose x-irradiation. *Radiation Research, 98,* 381–388.

Schulze, G. E., Benson, R. W., Paule, M. G., & Roberts, D. W. (1988). Behaviorally conditioned suppression of murine T-cell dependent but not T-cell independent antibody responses. *Pharmacology, Biochemistry and Behavior, 30,* 859–865.

Schwarz, K. S., & Cunningham, C. L. (1990). Conditioned stimulus control of morphine hypothermia. *Psychopharmacology, 101,* 77–84.

Shand, F. L., & Liew, F. Y. (1980). Differential sensitivity to cyclophosphamide of helper T cells for humoral response and suppressor T cells for delayed-type hypersensitivity. *European Journal of Immunology, 10,* 480–483.

Shanks, N., Kusnecov, A., Pezzone, M., Berkun, J., & Rabin, B. S. (1997). Lactation alters the effects of conditioned stress on immune function. *American Journal of Physiology, 272,* R16–25.

Shapiro,N. R., Dudek, B. C., & Rosellini, R. A. (1983). The role of associative factors in tolerance to the hypothermic effects of morphine in mice. *Pharmacology, Biochemistry, and Behavior, 19,* 327–333.

Shaskin, E. G., & Lovett, E. J., III (1981). Effects of halperidol, a dopamine receptor antagonist, on a delayed-type hpersensitivity reaction to 1-chloro,-2,4-dinitrobenzene in mice. *Research Communications in Psychology, Psychiatry, and Biology, 5,* 241–254.

Shurin, M. R., Kusnecov, A. W., Riechman, S. E., & Rabin, B. S. (1995). Effect of a conditioned aversive stimulus on the immune response in three strains of rats. *Psychoneuroendocrinology, 20,* 837–849.

Siegel, S. (1976). Morphine analgesia tolerance: Its situation specificity supports a Pavlovian model. *Science, 193,* 323–325.

Siegel, S. (1983). Classical conditioning, drug tolerance, and drug dependence. In Y. Israel, F. B. Gaser, H. Kalant, R. E. Popham, W. Schmidt, & R. G. Smart (Eds.), *Research advances in alcohol and drug problems* (pp. 207–246). New York: Plenum.

Smith, G. R., & McDaniels, S. M. (1983). Psychologically mediated effect on the delayed hypersensitivity reaction to tuberculin in humans. *Psychosomatic Medicine, 45,* 65–70.

Solvason, H. B., Ghanta, V. K., & Hiramoto, R. N. (1988). Conditioned augmentation of natural killer cell activity: Independence from nociceptive effects and dependence on interferon-β. *Journal of Immunology, 140,* 661–665.

Solvason, H. B., Ghanta, V. K., Lorden, J. F., Soong, S.-J., & Hiramoto, R. N. (1991a). A behavioral augmentation of natural immunity: Odor specificity supports a Pavlovian conditioning model. *International Journal of Neuroscience, 61,* 277–288.

Solvason, H. B., Ghanta, V. K., Soong, S.-J., & Hiramoto, R. N. (1991b). Interferon interaction with the CNS is required for the conditioning of the NK cell response. *Progress in Neuroendocrinimmunology, 4,* 258–264.

Solvason, H. B., Ghanta, V. K., Soong, S.-J., Rogers, C. F., Hsueh, C.-M., Hiramoto, N. S., & Hiramoto, R. N. (1992). A simple, single-trial learning paradigm for conditioned increase in natural killer cell activity. *Proceedings of the Society for Experimental Biology and Medicine, 199,* 199–203.

Solvason, H. B., Hiramoto, R. N., & Ghanta, V. K. (1989). Naltrexone blocks the expression of the conditioned elevation of natural killer cell activity in BALB/c mice. *Brain, Behavior and Immunity, 3,* 247–262.

Stefurak, T. L., Martin, G., & Van der Kooy, D. (1990). The representation in memory of morphine's unconditioned motivational effects depends on the nature of the conditioned stimulus. *Psychobiology, 18,* 435–442.

Tiffany, S. T., Petrie, E. C., Baker, T. B., & Dahl, J. (1983). Conditioned morphine tolerance in the rat: Absence of a compensatory response and cross-tolerance with stress. *Behavioral Neuroscience, 97,* 335–353.

Tkacs, N. C., Li, J. H., & Strack, A. M. (1997). Central amygdala Fos expression during hypotensive or febril non-hypotensive endotoxemia in conscious rats. *Journal of Comparative Neurology, 379,* 592-602.

Turk, J. L., & Parker, D. (1982). The effect of cyclophosphamide on immunological control mechanisms. *Immunology Reviews, &,* 99–113.

Wayner, E. A., Flannery, G. R., & Singer, G. (1978). The effects of taste aversion conditioning on the primary antibody response to sheep red blood cells and *Brucella abortus* in the albino rat. *Physiology and Behavior, 21,* 995–1000.

West, J. P. Lysle, D. T., & Dykstra, L. A. (1997). Tolerance development to morphine-induced alterations of immune status. *Drug and Alcohol Dependence, 46,* 147–157.

Zalcman, S., Richter, M., & Anisman, H. (1989). Alterations of immune functioning following exposure to stressor-related cues. *Brain, Behavior, and Immunity, 3,* 99–109.

Zhou, D. A., Kusnecov, A., Shurin, M. R., DePaoli, M., & Rabin, B. S. (1993). Exposure to physiological and psychological stressors elevates plasma interleukin 6: Relationship to the activation of hypothalamic-pituitary-adrenal axis. *Endocrinology, 133,* 2523–2530.

# 30

# From Psychoneuroimmunology to Ecological Immunology: Life History Strategies and Immunity Trade-offs

C. J. BARNARD, J. M. BEHNKE

I. OPTIMIZING IMMUNE RESPONSIVENESS
II. IMMUNITY TRADE-OFFS
III. IMPLICATIONS OF ADAPTIVE IMMUNITY
TRADE-OFFS

Bidirectional interactions between immune function and the central nervous system (CNS) are wellestablished (e.g., Ader, Felten, & Cohen, 1991; Khansari, Murgo, & Faith, 1990; Maier & Watkins, 1998; Maier, Watkins, & Fleshner, 1994; Rook & Zumia, 1997) and provide plausible mechanisms by which psychological state and behavior can influence immune function and vice versa (the field of psychoneuroimmunology (Ader et al., 1991; Maier et al., 1994; Maier & Watkins, 1998)). While mechanisms (particularly stress-related hormonal) and metabolic pathways underlying the interrelationships have been elucidated over the years (see Ader et al., 1991; Maier et al., 1994 for reviews), their functional and evolutionary significance have only recently begun to be considered (Folstad & Karter, 1992; Maier et al., 1994; Sheldon & Verhulst, 1996). Functional considerations have come to the fore for two reasons. First, the emerging intricacy of the bidirectional interaction and its mediators beg the question as to why the system is designed the way it is—why should stress, for instance, reduce immunocompetence, and why is immune challenge often associated with downregulated locomotory and maintenance behaviors and increased sleep? Interpretations here center on the adaptive redistribution of limited resources in the face of immune challenge and new metabolic demands (Maier et al., 1994; Maier & Watkins, 1998). Second, interest among evolutionary biologists in the role of parasites and disease in the evolution of elaborate secondary sexual characters (SSCs) (Hamilton & Zuk, 1982; Read, 1990) has recently focused on the immunomodulatory effects of steroid hormones, particularly androgens and glucocorticoids, involved in the development of some SSCs and competitive behaviors (Folstad & Karter, 1992; Siva-Jothy, 1995; Owens & Short, 1995; Wedekind & Folstad, 1994; Sheldon & Verhulst, 1996; Hillgarth & Wingfield, 1997). Elaborate SSCs may thus be sustainable only at some cost to immune function, and, since reduced immunocompetence is likely to lead to higher parasite burdens which impair SSCs, only competent individuals (that can tolerate parasite burdens or resist infection despite high steroid levels) can afford the androgen levels necessary to develop sexual signals fully; thus elaborate SSCs become honest indicators of mate quality in terms of freedom from parasites (the 'immunocompetence handicap' hypothesis (IHH) (Folstad & Karter, 1992)).

While their starting points are very different, these two directions of thought converge on the same

35

central issue, that immune function may be subject to adaptive trade-offs between competing demands; in the first case, a switch of resources from other activities into the immune response in the face of a threatening challenge, in the other an adaptive switch away from the immune system (Wedekind & Folstad, 1994), or an incidental cost of inducing appropriate metabolic pathways, to invest in developments with high short-term reproductive benefits. Such trade-offs are part of the animal's adaptive life history strategy (relative investment in growth, survival, and reproduction) and reflect choices that maximize transmission of the alleles coding for them to the next generation. Immune responses contribute to reproductive success via survival. Investment in immunity, and therefore decisions relating to potential immunomodulators, will thus be determined by the extent to which the reproductive benefits of its survival-enhancing effects outweigh those of shorter-term, but potentially life-threatening, reproductive bonanzas. From this point of view, we can consider any action—physiological, behavioral, developmental—that impacts on immune function and is instigated or suppressed in that light, as an immunomodulator, and seek evidence for its adaptive regulation, as we should seek evidence for adaptive regulation of immune responses themselves. In this chapter, we review the arguments and evidence for the adaptive regulation of immune responses and immunomodulators and consider their functional significance in the context of individual life history strategies (the field of *ecological immunology* (Sheldon & Verhulst, 1996)). Before we do that, however, we consider the general implications of a life history approach for immunity trade-offs in more detail.

## I. OPTIMIZING IMMUNE RESPONSIVENESS

As Sheldon and Verhulst (1996) have pointed out, a feature shared by all classes of immune function, whether the antigen-specific, cell-mediated responses of vertebrates, the simpler humoral and cell-mediated responses of invertebrates, barrier mechanisms, or behaviors that reduce exposure to or the severity of infections, is the demand for resources the animal could have used for some other function. Resource costs may be either direct (e.g., energy costs of mounting cell-mediated responses, fever, etc. (Keymer & Read, 1991; Maier et al., 1994; Sheldon & Verhulst, 1996)) or indirect (e.g., associations between poor nutrition and disease (Keymer & Read, 1991; Lochmiller, Vestey, & Boren., 1993)). The metabolic,

and therefore reproductive, cost of mounting an immune response must be outweighed by the reproductive cost of sustaining an infection unchallenged. On this basis, Behnke, Barnard and Wakelin (1992) introduced the notion of optimal parasite regulation using a simple graphical model in which the strength of the expected immune response depended on the potential reproductive impact of the infection on the host. The crucial point about the optimal immune response model is the explicit acknowledgment that reproductive priorities will vary between hosts on the basis of life history considerations: age, sex, reproductive status, competitive ability, migratory phase, risk of predation, risk of infecting kin, to mention obvious ones. Variation in life history strategies within host populations is thus likely to be at least as important as other key factors, such as the metabolic cost of immunity and the life cycle and virulence of infective agents, in determining exposure to infection and immune responses among hosts and thereby distributions of prevalence and intensity of infection across host populations.

While there is accumulating evidence for immunity trade-offs with other components of life history (e.g. Apanius, 1994; Barnard, Behnke, & Sewell, 1996a,b; Demas & Nelson, 1996; Festa-Bianchet, 1989; Gustafsson, Nordling, Andersson, Sheldon, & Qvarnstrom, 1994; Norris, Anwar, & Read, 1994; Richner, Christe, & Oppliger, 1995; Saino & Moller, 1996; Smith et al., 1996), it is necessary to be clear as to what is expected in such trade-offs. There are two considerations: first, the conditions per se under which we should expect trade-offs between immune function and other components of life history and, second, the effects of life history strategy on the tendency to show expected trade-offs under any given set of conditions.

## II. IMMUNITY TRADE-OFFS

Immune function is a vital component of survivorship for most animal species. In general, therefore, we should expect animals to attach a high priority to maintaining immunocompetence. However, if the immune system competes for resources with other activities important for survival and reproduction, investment in immunity must be prioritized. This is illustrated schematically in Figure 1. The $x$-axis characterizes the immune status of the animal from intense immune activity under challenge at one extreme to a state of immunodepression at the other. The $y$-axis plots changes in other important activities that impact on immunity (immunomodulators); these

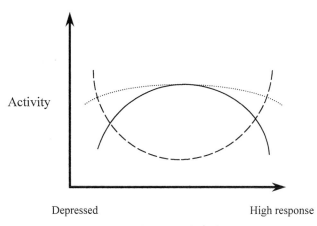

Activity

Depressed　　　　　　　　　　High response

Immune function

**FIGURE 1** Relationships between potentially immunodepressive activities and imposition or demand on the immune system expected under conditions of adaptive immunity trade-off (see text). The x-axis ranges from acute immunodepression to high demand for response. Under conditions of immunodepression or high demand, further immunodepressive activities (e. g., steroid hormone secretion, aggressive behavior—see text) are expected to be downregulated (solid curve), with the converse holding for activities that conserve metabolic resources or enhance immunity (dashed curve). If short-term reproductive opportunities are increased, however, it may be worth reducing the degree of downregulation of immunodepressants in order to capitalize on them (dotted line).

could be energy-demanding behaviors such as aggression or copulatory activity, steroid hormone levels that reduce immune responsiveness, or any of several other factors. Our expectation would be that activities with a depressing effect on immune function would be downregulated, and those with an enhancing effect (e.g., through releasing resources) would be upregulated, in situations where antigen challenge increased the demand for immune response. However, since the risk of infection is likely to be an ever-present one in the real world, we should expect animals to maintain a minimum level of responsiveness even in the absence of a challenge. Thus we should expect similar modulation of activities under conditions of immunodepression. The idea that a base level of immune responsiveness ultimately acts as a constraint on other activities is at the core of the IHH (Folstad & Karter, 1992), but the IHH is merely a special case (relating to constraints on sexually selected signals) of the general principle; we should expect to see evidence of such constraints wherever activities impinge on responsiveness. More importantly for our present purposes, the constraining effects of both extremes of immune status in Figure 1 provide the most fertile ground for seeking adaptive differences in modulation between individuals with different life history priorities, since it is here that

decisions have to be made about conserving or sacrificing immune responsiveness. Since the reproductive value of conserving immunity is only as great as its contribution to reproductive output relative to other courses of action, short-term reproductive opportunities may tempt other priorities and reduce modulation (dashed lines in Fig. 1). However, the attractiveness of the alternatives is likely to depend at least partly on the ability of the animal to invest in them. Trading off immunity against aggressive competition for mating opportunities, for instance, will be adaptive only if sufficient energy reserves are available to maintain aggression and the likelihood of success and avoiding serious injury is great enough. Such trade-offs are intuitively more likely among robust, high-ranking individuals than among less competitive, weaker individuals. We might thus expect immunity trade-offs to vary with physical condition, social status or other indices of competitive ability (and thereby resource availability) and so with life history strategies placing different emphasis on short-term competitiveness. Is there any evidence for these kinds of constraints on immunomodulatory activities and adaptive individual variation in modulation?

## A. Social Rank and Immunity Trade-offs in Mice

While life history trade-offs may vary more or less continuously within a population, they can frequently be characterized in terms of adaptive suites and thus more discrete categories of life history strategy (Arak, 1984; Bass, 1996; Hutchings & Myers, 1996; Rohwer & Ewald, 1981). Social rank classifications are a good example. Rank classifications are usually based on measures of competitive ability, but are often associated with differences in several other important life history traits, such a growth and body size, disease resistance, and reproductive status (Freeland, 1981; Komers, Pelabon, & Stenstrom, 1997; Meikle, Drickamer, Vessey, Arthur, & Rosenthal, 1996; Schur, 1987). In a recent series of studies, Barnard, Behnke, and co-workers have shown that male mice (*Mus musculus*) of the outbred CFLP strain can be classified into two discrete rank categories ("high" and "low" rankers) based on the relative amount of aggression initiated and received and that ranks are associated with different strategies of immunity modulation and susceptibilty to experimental infections (Barnard, Behnke, & Sewell, 1994; Barnard et al., 1996a,b; Barnard, Behnke, Gage, Brown, & Smithhurst, 1997a,b, 1998a,b; Smith et al., 1996). Moreover, the fact that these differences precede the emergence of clear rank categories in random groups (and the development of rank is influenced by maternal condition (Barnard et al., 1998b)) suggests deeper differences in life history strategies between individuals than of responses to current aggression (see below). Other recent evidence, from relationships between nerve growth factor secretion, corticosterone, mast cell responses, and aggressive behavior, also suggests that rank categories in mice are associated with different strategies of immune response (e.g., Bigi, Huber, DeAcetis, Alleva, & Dixon, 1994; Aloe et al., 1995).

## B. Modulation under Conditions of Immune Challenge

As Maier and colleagues (1994) have pointed out, the clearest basis for arguing that the immune system competes for metabolic resources with other physiological and behavioral systems derives from the stress-response-like consequences of immune activation. Studies have long indicated increased autonomic nervous system activity and serum concentrations of pituitary-adrenal "stress" hormones during immune responses to antigen (Besedovsky, Sorkin, Keller, & Muller, 1975), implying a peripheral physiological equivalent to a classical stress response. Indeed, the pituitary-adrenal response is activated by the same mechanisms that trigger their response to classical environmental stressors — induction of the paraventricular nucleus of the hypothalamus to release corticotropin-releasing factor and thus stimulate secretion of glucocorticoid (stress) hormones from the adrenal glands (Maier et al., 1994), a chain of events mediated by cytokines released by cells of the immune system during immune response (Berkenbosch, Oers, Rey, Tilders, & Besedovsky, 1987). The use of harmless antigen (rather than pathogens) to stimulate immune responses confirmed that it was the immune response per se that was responsible for triggering the physiological stress response. Significantly, however, immune responses have been shown to be associated with behavioral changes, particularly increased somnolence and a reduction in activity, social and sexual interaction, exploration of novel objects, and food and water intake, that imply a redirection of energy away from muscular activity and mimic changes that often follow a period of "fight–flight"-inducing stress (Maier et al., 1994). All these stress-like changes can be induced by the administration of interleukin (IL)-1 or substances that stimulate immune cells to secrete IL-1 and other cytokines (Cirulli, DeAcetis, & Alleva, 1998; Dantzer, Bluthe, Kent, & Goodall, 1993) that

may be instrumental in coordinating behavioral and other (e.g., slowed digestion, hyperalgesia) changes via cells of the immune system and CNS (Maier et al., 1994). The obvious functional interpretation of the changes is that redirected energy can be made available for the clonal expansion of T and B cells, inflammation, fever, and other energy-demanding components of the immune response, and attention is focused (via hyperalgesia) on sites of injury, infection, or other distress (Maier et al., 1994). Conversely, it makes functional sense at times of acute danger or conflict to direct resources into muscular activity and analgesia to facilitate aggressive or escape responses and reduce distraction by injuries (Kelly, 1986; Maier et al., 1994). Thus, changing priorities can, in principle, dictate shifts in the pattern of energy investment between behavior and other responses and the immune system. As Maier and his associates (1994) point out, glucocorticoid hormones, which modulate immunity in several ways (Wilckens & de Rijk, 1997), including downregulating inflammatory responses in the later stages, provide a convincing potential mechanism for mediating such shifts in resource allocation between immune function and behavior. The characteristic (indeed, commonly accepted diagnostic) elevation in glucocorticoid levels during stress responses may thus (at least partly) reflect such immunity trade-offs. A similar argument can be made for the immunomodulatory effects of other steroid hormones, such as testosterone (Alexander & Stimson, 1988; Grossman, 1985; Grossman & Roselle, 1986; Roberts, Satoskar, & Alexander, 1996), in which downregulation of some aspects of immunity may reflect adaptive shifts of resources away from the immune system into, in the case of testosterone, elaborate sexual signals and competitive behavior (Mooradian, Morley, & Korenman, 1987; Penn & Potts, 1998; Wedekind & Folstad 1994; though see Folstad & Skarstein, 1997; Hillgarth, Ramenofsky, & Wingfield, 1997, for an alternative view of the origin of the immunodepressive effects of testosterone).

The above argues at a general level for adaptive trade-offs between immune function and other systems competing for metabolic resources. As we have already intimated, however, individuals are likely to vary in the trade-offs they show depending on the relative reproductive advantage of investing in immunity rather than other competing systems, variation that ultimately reflects differences in life history strategy. In particular, we might expect individuals of high competitive ability, that are able to take advantage of short-term mating opportunities, to be more likely to invest in energy-demanding social and sexual activities at the expense of immune responses. Some evidence in this direction comes from our studies of laboratory mice.

Barnard and co-workers (1998a) infected male CFLP mice in single-sex groups with the trichostrongyloid nematode *Heligmosomoides polygyrus*. Overall, high rankers (males with a disproportionately high attack rate and high attack initiation:receipt ratios within their group) showed reduced immune responsiveness compared with low rankers, the difference between ranks being accountable in terms the interrelationship between aggression, plasma corticosterone concentration, peripheral immune responsiveness (measured as hemagglutination titer to sheep red blood cells (SRBCs)), and resistance to *H. polygyrus* among high rankers. Among high ranking males, aggressive behavior following infection correlated positively with corticosterone concentration and negatively with hemagglutination titer to SRBCs and resistance to *H. polygyrus*. These relationships compounded a tendency for high rankers to maintain corticosterone levels during the infection, when corticosterone concentrations dropped among low rankers and uninfected controls. Partial regression analyses revealed that the change in corticosterone levels during the period of infection was the best hormone-measure predictor of eventual worm burden, a relationship in keeping with the impact of glucocorticoids on the secretion of Th2 cytokines (Padgett, Sheridan, & Loria, 1995; Rook & Zumia, 1997) and depression of the Th2 arm of the immune response considered to be vital in resistance to helminth infections (Behnke & Parish, 1979; Else & Grencis, 1991; Finkelman et al., 1997; Finkelman & Urban 1992; Quinnell, Behnke, & Keymer, 1991; Wakelin & Selby, 1974). The results are thus consistent with our expectation that individuals of greater competitive ability will be more likely to trade off immune responsiveness under conditions of antigenic challenge.

The important point to stress about Barnard and co-workers (1998a) results is that it was the *change* in corticosterone concentration over the period of infection, rather than differences in absolute concentration generally, that accounted for the difference in resistance to *H. polygyrus* between high- and low-ranking males. The conclusion that this reflected a tendency for high competitive ability males to trade off worm burden against short-term investment in aggressive competition is strengthened by the fact that the negative relationship between corticosterone concentration and resistance among high rankers emerged as a specific component effect within a multivariate analysis, an analysis that controlled for differences in absolute corticosterone concentration and the concentration of potentially immunodepressive testosterone that have been associated with rank differences in immune responsiveness and infection in other studies (e.g. Barnard et al., 1994, 1996a,b; Brain & Nowell, 1970; Chapman, Dejardins, & Bronson 1969; Vessey, 1964). The association between corticosterone and immunodepression in circumstances of social stress has usually arisen among low rankers (e.g., Beden & Brain, 1985; Leshner & Politch, 1979; Maestripieri, Desimone, Aloe, & Alleva, 1990; Vessey, 1964), presumably trading off potential immune responsiveness to a future challenge against the present priority for escaping attack. The question, of course, remains as to whether the apparent tendency for high rankers to trade off resistance to helminth infection in Barnard and co-workers (1998a) study reflects a sacrifice of future survivorship in favor of short-term competitiveness or an ability of higher quality individuals to withstand greater parasite burdens at little cost to survivorship. We shall say more about this later. However, this distinction does not alter the putative role of corticosterone in shifting resources between inflammatory immune responses and other systems among high rankers. The more widely reported, corticosterone-induced immunodepression among socially stressed subordinate mice appears to reflect a similar role of corticosterone but in the context of a simple trade-off of survival risks.

## C. Modulation under Conditions of Immunodepression

Modulation of potential immunodepressants at the other extreme of the $x$-axis in Figure 1 reflects choices about the maintenance of immune responsiveness in the event of a challenge at some point in the future. Since infection with some kind of agent is an ongoing risk for most animals, maintaining a minimum base level of responsiveness is likely to be a constraint on competing avenues of resource investment. As discussed above, interest here has focused particularly on the modulation of sex steroids, especially testosterone, which serve a number of important metabolic functions, but also have direct and indirect influences on the immune system (see Folstad & Karter, 1992). The evolution of SSCs as honest sexual signals may be one manifestation of immunity trade-offs involving androgens (but see Owens & Short, 1996), but other recent work suggests that such trade-offs may be a more fundamental feature of physiological and behavioral decision making. Again, male laboratory mice provide a good example.

In a series of studies, Barnard and colleagues (1993, 1994, 1996a,b) exposed male CFLP mice to varying conditions of social stress in randomly constituted single sex groups. Plasma concentrations of testosterone, corticosterone, and total IgG were measured before and after periods of social grouping and mice were finally subjected to an experimental infection of *Babesia microti*, a piroplasmid protozoan infecting the erythrocytes of its vertebrate host (Clark & Howell, 1990, Cox & Young, 1969). The time course of *B. microti* infection allows a number of measures of the host's ability to respond immunologically to the parasite, the main ones being the magnitude of the peak of infection (percentage cells infected, usually peaking around 8–10 days post infection) and the time to clear the infection (usually around 17–22 days post infection). The social rank of males during the random grouping phase was calculated on the basis of attacks initiated and received, as in Barnard and co-workers' (1998a) study above, and allowed comparisons of hormone levels, immunocompetence, responses to infection and interrelationships between the three in males of different competitive life history strategy.

Of particular interest were the relationships between aggressive behavior, changing testosterone, corticosterone, and IgG levels during the period of grouping, and their impact on later resistance to *B. microti*. Several lines of evidence point to an immunodepressive effect of androgens and glucocorticoids in the context of intraerythrocytic protozoan parasites, including *B. microti* (Benten, Bettenhauser, Wunderlich, Van Vliet, & Mossmann, 1991; Davies, 1998; Hughes, 1998; Schmitt-Wrede et al., 1991; Wunderlich, Marinovski, Benten, Schmitte-Wrede, & Mossmann, 1992). Many more indicate that immunodepressive effects of both groups of hormones are associated with aggression and social stress (see Broom & Johnson, 1993). One expectation, therefore, was that testosterone would be modulated in relation to current immunocompetence, of which total IgG was a peripheral bystander measure (Davies (1998) has since demonstrated that total IgG correlates well with the production of *B. microti*-specific antibody during infection), and the level of corticosterone, a stress-associated immunodepressant. However, on the basis of differences in competitive life history strategy, we might expect such modulation to be more apparent among high-ranking, rather than low-ranking, males. In addition, if modulating testosterone influences resistance, we should expect an effect of testosterone on resistance to be more apparent in individuals that fail to modulate. Both expectations have been borne out in a series of studies in our laboratory (Barnard et al., 1994, 1996a,b, 1998a,b; Smith et al., 1996).

## 1. Social Rank and Modulation of Testosterone

Barnard and colleagues (1994, 1996a) found that an independent effect of change in testosterone concentration over the period of random grouping on subsequent resistance to *B. microti* was confined to high-ranking males. When relationships between changing hormone and total IgG concentrations were partialled out, it emerged that high rankers tended to decouple changes in testosterone from those in total IgG whereas low rankers showed significant positive correlations between the two (Barnard et al., 1996a). High rankers subsequently showed a significant negative effect of testosterone concentration on resistance to *B. microti*, an effect absent among low rankers (Barnard et al., 1994, 1996a). However, while high rankers appeared to decouple changes in testosterone and IgG, both rank categories showed some evidence of downregulating testosterone as corticosterone concentration increased (Barnard et al., 1994, 1996a). It is important to stress here that absolute testosterone concentration did not differ between rank categories; the effect of testosterone on resistance appeared to be due entirely to the tendency or otherwise to modulate levels relative to current immunocompetence. While aggression resulted in increased levels of corticosterone and reduced IgG concentration and resistance to *B. microti*, these relationships were restricted to low ranking males when ranks were analyzed separately. However, in both studies, it was high rankers that experienced the greatest reduction in immunocompetence over the period of grouping. These results therefore suggest that high ranking males, by decoupling testosterone secretion from current immunocompetence at a time when they appear to be immunocompromised, actively trade off future survival against the presumed competitive and reproductive benefits of maintaining testosterone levels.

The role of modulation in these rank differences in resistance has received further support from recent experiments in which hormone levels were manipulated experimentally (Davies, 1998). Administration of testosterone and glucocorticoids accelerated the time course and increased the peak of *B. microti* infection, as expected from previous work with *Babesia* and other blood-borne protozoan infections (e.g., Hussein, 1984; Wunderlich et al., 1991, 1992). If modulation of testosterone, rather than absolute serum concentration, is what determines the hormone-related resistance to *B. microti*, however, our prediction would be that increasing testosterone levels experimentally, and thus overriding any tendency to modulate, would reduce resistance among low rankers, but not among high rankers. The prediction was borne out by Davies's results: time to reach peak infection and the magnitude of the peak were significantly increased in testosterone-treated low rankers compared with vehicle controls, while there was no significant difference in the time course of infection among high rankers.

Interestingly, mice that turned out to be high rankers in the Barnard and co-workers' randomly constituted groups showed a tendency to enter their groups with higher testosterone and corticosterone, but lower IgG, levels than eventual low rankers (Barnard et al., 1993, 1994, 1996a), implying preexisting differences in their natal litters. A later study in our laboratory (Barnard et al., 1998b) has shown that the rank difference in testosterone modulation referred to above is present in natal litters, with eventual high rankers lacking the correlation between testosterone levels and IgG shown by eventual low rankers, but in the absence of any polarized aggressive social relationships. These early differences may have their origin in the effects of maternal condition on suckling and weight gain, or in its effects on the prenatal environment (Barker, 1995). Extensive work in humans and rodents (Barker, 1995; Phillips, 1996; Rao, 1996) has identified a crucial role of nutritional constraints and other mother/fetus conflicts (Haig, 1993) in utero in determining a suite of life history attributes in resultant offspring, including patterns of growth and organ development, immune function, menopause, and longevity (via susceptibility to adult disease such as cardiovascular disease, hypertension, and adult-onset diabetes) (Barker, 1995, 1996; Cresswell et al., 1997; Hales, 1997; Langley-Evans, 1997). These differences are underpinned by various endocrine changes involving many different hormones, but particularly glucocorticoids, insulin, and growth hormone (Barker, 1995; Phillips, 1996; Rohner-Jeanrenaud & Jeanrenaud, 1997). Such fundamental shifts in development and metabolism, mediated by maternal condition, could account for the early differences in life history trade-offs in CFLP rank categories prior to the aggressive social environment in which rank is normally expressed.

## 2. Constraints on Immunity Trade-offs

While these results support the idea of life history-dependent immunity trade-offs, there is likely to be a limit to the benefits of discounting future survivorship. If immunocompetence becomes severely de-pressed it may pay all individuals to downregulate potentially immunodepressive activities and physiological responses, regardless of their short-term payoffs in other contexts. Both correlational evidence and evidence from experimental manipulation of immunocompetence among laboratory mice lend support to this expectation.

Correlational evidence emerges from hormonal responses of animals at times of increased social stress, such as on first introduction into an unfamiliar group or maintenance in environments that encourage aggressive interaction. Comparisons of pregrouping and immediately postgrouping testosterone levels among male CFLP mice consistently show a precipitate drop in hormone concentration when individuals are introduced into new groups (Barnard et al., 1996a,b; 1997a,b) and the frequency of aggressive encounters is high (Barnard et al., 1993, 1996a; see also Poole & Morgan, 1973). In some cases the marked decline removed preexisting differences in testosterone concentration between high and low ranking males (Barnard et al., 1996a), which then decayed back toward pregrouping levels in relation to apparent peripheral immune responsiveness (low rankers) or independently of immune responsiveness (high rankers) with the consequences for resistance discussed earlier. However, whether or not a rank difference in testosterone modulation emerges depends on the degree of social stress in the group environment. One potential, if somewhat counterintuitive, source of increased social stress is so-called environmental enrichment.

Environmental enrichment has been an important element in the drive to improve the welfare of captive animals, including standard laboratory species (Chamove, 1989; Markowitz, 1982). In caged environments, this often means the provision of objects that create spatial heterogeneity or opportunities for different activities, shelter, and so on (Chamove, 1989). Such initiatives can have unexpected results, however. In laboratory mice, the addition of various objects, such as bricks, flowerpots, and labyrinths, to cages can result in increased aggression and plasma corticosterone concentrations (Barnard et al., 1996b; Brain, 1988; Haemisch & Gartner, 1994; McGregor & Ayling, 1990), probably because they provide defendable resources for dominants (Hurst, 1987, 1990).

Barnard and co-workers (1996b) equipped the unfurnished cages used in some of their earlier studies (Barnard et al., 1993, 1994) with shelving and nestboxes to act as refuges where mice could escape or avoid aggressive encounters. The rest of the experimental design repeated that of Barnard et al. (1994). In comparison with the earlier experiment, mice in the furnished cages showed significantly elevated aggression and reduced subsequent resistance to *B. microti*. Moreover, both total IgG concentration and resistance to *B. microti* decreased as the number of attacks received by mice increased, implying that it was the change in the aggressiveness of the social environment that was instrumental in the reduction in immunocompetence and resistance. From a welfare perspective, it is interesting to note that, when time spent on the shelves or in the nestboxes was partialled out of the analyses, their use showed a significant enhancing effect on both IgG levels and resistance to *B. microti* (Barnard et al., 1996b). The availability of the refuges thus appeared to offset to some extent their negative effects on overall social stress within the furnished cage environment. The crucial point in terms of the adaptive modulation hypothesis, however, was the lack of any hormone-related reduction in resistance. In part this appeared to be due to a general downregulation of testosterone and corticosterone levels in comparison with mice in the unfurnished cages, but it also appeared to be due to the fact that *both* rank categories now showed significant positive correlations between change in testosterone concentration and levels of total IgG. Among low rankers there was a similar correlation between corticosterone and IgG concentrations, the only study of ours to date in which there has been evidence for the modulation of corticosterone levels in relation to immunocompetence (see Smith et al., 1996, for some discussion of this). The conclusion from this seems to be that, when environmental stressors depress immunity, other potential immunodepressants become more tightly regulated, despite their important role in various functional systems, so as to reduce further impact on the animal's immune capability.

This conclusion is reinforced by a very different study in which singly housed male mice were exposed to the odors of unfamiliar males and/or females (Smith et al., 1996). In Smith and colleagues' (1996) study, male mice, previously identified as high or low rankers within small, randomly constituted groups were presented with the substrate odors of unfamiliar individuals in their home cage, assayed for changing hormone and IgG concentrations during the period of exposure, then infected with *B. microti*. Exposure to odors resulted in a marked decrease in IgG levels relative to that seen in clean sawdust controls, with levels being reduced most when male and female odors were presented together. As in our experiment with *H. polygyrus* (Barnard et al., 1998a), previously high ranking males showed a severer infection than previous low rankers, and infections

among high rankers were severest after they had been presented with male and female odors combined. However, when relationships between resistance and hormone concentrations were analyzed, resistance related to corticosterone concentration but not testosterone. Reduced resistance across ranks and odor treatments was associated with elevated corticosterone relative to pretreatment concentrations and posttreatment corticosterone concentrations were higher among previous high rankers and among high rankers when female odors (especially when combined with those of a male) had been presented. Importantly, as in all our other experiments, corticosterone showed no evidence of being modulated with respect to IgG concentration. Testosterone concentration, on the other hand, showed a significant positive correlation with IgG concentration across both rank categories. Once again, therefore, the absence of an independent effect of testosterone on resistance to *B. microti* was associated with a tendency to modulate levels of the hormone in relation to current immunocompetence.

The correlational evidence is thus in keeping with the idea of constraints on adaptive immunity trade-offs. If this conclusion is robust, however, we should be able to manipulate the tendency to modulate potential immunodepressants by reducing immunocompetence experimentally. We tested this by temporarily depressing immunocompetence with antithymocyte serum (ATS) (Barnard et al., 1997a). ATS treatment was selected because it acts primarily on T lymphocytes that are essential for efficient antibody responses and cell-mediated immunity and because it is relatively innocuous in other respects, without the general side-effects of other forms of immunodepressive therapy (e.g., cytotoxic drugs, whole-body irradiation, ablation of lymphoid tissue) (see references in Barnard et al., 1997a). In addition, there are known feedback mechanisms mediating the secretion of sex steroids in relation to immunocompetence via the thymus (Alexander & Stimson, 1988; Grossman, 1985). Our expectation from the adaptive immunity trade-off hypothesis was that ATS-treated mice would show a downregulation of testosterone and aggressive and other energy-consuming behaviors commensurate with the degree of immunodepression experienced. From our previous results, however, we did not expect to see a reduction in corticosterone concentration.

Male CFLP mice were observed in small groups prior to separation and treatment with ATS or naive rabbit serum (NRS) control, then reallocated to their pretreatment groups for further observation. Blood samples for hormone and IgG concentrations were taken at the beginning and end of the two periods of grouping, and, terminal blood samples were assayed for SRBC haemagglutination titers. Following treatment, ATS-treated animals showed an absence of detectable antibody response to SRBCs and a pronounced reduction in IgG concentration compared with NRS controls. The change in IgG was reflected in a simultaneous decline in testosterone. However, when relationships were partialled out, the decline in testosterone among ATS males correlated with a reduction in thymus weight rather than IgG concentration, supporting the idea of thymus-mediated regulation of testosterone secretion. As expected, there was no associated change in corticosterone concentration.

The downregulation of testosterone among ATS animals was accompanied by a reduction in the amount of aggression and general activity relative to both pretreatment levels and NRS controls, the reduction being particularly striking because overall activity, and especially aggression, are usually greatly increased when groups are first introduced or reconstituted after a period of separation (Barnard et al., 1993; Poole & Morgan, 1973). Time spent sleeping, however, was maintained among ATS mice but fell sharply among controls. The fact that the reduction in aggression correlated with that in IgG concentration across both ATS mice and controls strengthened the conclusion that the treatment effect was the result of increased immunodepression among ATS mice. Relationships between immunocompetence measures and sleep were confined to ATS animals and involved thymus weight rather than IgG. Interestingly, neither the changes in activity and aggression nor those in sleep (or other behaviors) correlated with testosterone concentration. The recurrent finding in our experiments that aggressive (and other) behavior show little correlation with testosterone suggests that hormonal and behavioral changes are independent responses to immunodepression.

Of course, if the modulation of hormones and behavior by immunodepressed ATS males reflected an adaptive trade-off between survival and reproduction, an increased reproductive incentive might be expected to reduce their tendency to modulate. Barnard and co-workers (1997b) repeated the ATS experiment, but this time introduced the substrate odors of females into the males' cages during the posttreatment phase. Under these conditions, ATS-treated males failed to show any of the behavioral changes observed in our experiment (Barnard et al.,1997a). Indeed, there was a significant increase in aggression and general locomotory activity, and a reduction in sleep, during the posttreatment phase

relative to pretreatment levels with no difference between ATS-treated and control mice. There was also an increase in mounting behavior in both ATS and control mice, a behavior which was shown very infrequently and with little change from pre- to posttreatment phases in the previous experiment. The presence of female cues to some extent therefore appeared to override the downregulation of active behaviors in immunodepressed males.

## III. IMPLICATIONS OF ADAPTIVE IMMUNITY TRADE-OFFS

The idea of adaptive immunity trade-offs clearly has implications for the way we think about how other species prioritize health and well-being in the context of life history strategy. In this review, we have discussed experimental evidence for immunity-driven trade-offs in behavior and hormone secretion that is in keeping with this view and imply a fundamental role of immune status in time budgeting and behavioral priorities. However, the implications of such trade-offs extend well beyond these individual-level issues to affect our view of a number of important areas relating to immune function. We shall briefly discuss just two.

### A. Sterilizing Immunity

As Behnke and colleagues (1992) noted, trade-offs between life history components and the need to respond to different challenges is likely to affect the assessment of vaccination programs in which sterilizing immunity is the yardstick of success. Sterilizing immunity, however, may be a vain objective because the natural immune response on which the vaccines depend may not be designed to produce such an absolute outcome. Indeed the scarcity of sterilizing immunity among host species in nature suggests that it is rarely favored by natural selection. The likely reason, of course, is that sterilizing immunity is a naïve expectation. It ignores both the cost of elimination to the host and the fact that the cost of infection, and thus the benefit of attacking the parasite, may not be a simple linear function of parasite burden. If we consider the cost of infection by a given parasite to be a reduced probability of the host reproducing due to loss of metabolic resources and parasite-induced pathology, it is reasonable to suppose that, in many cases, the cost will be an accelerating curvilinear function of parasite burden (Behnke et al., 1992). Increases in burden when the overall burden is low make little difference to the host's reproductive potential. As burden increases, however, additional increments are likely to be very detrimental. Cost functions of this form mean that a law of diminishing returns is likely to operate on the benefits of attacking the parasite. At high burdens, when the cost of infection is high, the benefit of a given reduction in burden is correspondingly high, so the slope of the benefit curve is initially steep. As the burden, and thus the cost to the host, decreases, the benefit accruing from the same degree of reduction also decreases and the slope of the benefit curve begins to decline. Of course, several factors may affect the form of the cost and benefit curves, for instance cross-regulatory effects of responding to one infection on the potential to respond to another may reduce the optimal degree of clearance still further. Conversely, while incomplete elimination may be the optimal response in these terms, such a strategy leaves a residual infection which may be transmissible to other potential hosts. If vulnerable hosts include relatives of the infected individual, inclusive fitness (Hamilton, 1964) benefits may accrue from reduction beyond the individual host's optimum. On top of these considerations, the ongoing modulation of immune responsiveness discussed above introduces further life history factors into optimal response strategies.

## B. Animal Welfare

Adaptive immunity trade-offs also have implications for clinical indicators of welfare. We have briefly discussed hormone modulation in the context of environmental enrichment, but immunity trade-offs have far wider implications for the assessment of welfare.

The scientific study of animal, including human, welfare has generated a welter of complex, equivocal, and often contradictory results (e.g., Barnard & Hurst, 1996; Broom & Johnson, 1993; Dawkins, 1990; Fraser, 1993; Mendl, 1991; Rushen, 1986), many relying on clinical measures of ill health and impaired well-being such as immunodepression, disease, injury, and physiological stress responses (see Broom & Johnson, 1993; Mason & Mendl, 1993; Barnard, & Hurst, 1996). While some solutions to the confusion have been suggested, these have usually relied on more sophisticated versions of, or greater control over, traditional welfare yardsticks (Mason & Mendl, 1993). However, Barnard & Hurst (1996) have argued that the difficulties arise because of questionable assumptions in the definition and measurement of welfare, in particular the measurement of suffering and the presumed importance of the physical well-being of the individual. They contend that welfare can be interpreted only in terms of what natural selection has designed organisms to do and how circumstances impinge on their ability to do it. Organisms are designed for self-expenditure in that resources and survivorship are spent in the pursuit of reproduction. The relative importance of self-preservation and survival varies, as we have argued above, with their contribution to reproductive success and therefore with life history strategy. As a result, the clinical and other measures of well-being currently accepted as indicating poor welfare cannot be so interpreted without appreciating the functional significance of the apparent impairment (a parallel line of reasoning underpins the field of Darwinian medicine (Nesse & Williams, 1994)). The traditional notions of coping and stress imply homeostatic maintenance of the individual. While a degree of self-preservation is likely to be important in any life history strategy, other considerations may conflict with it in the pursuit of reproductive success; physical injury, immunodepression, or even death may be adaptive trade-offs built into the decision making machinery of the organism. Our own preoccupation with welfare and well-being can be seen as an anthropomorphism based on our relative longevity and lengthy period of parental care, life history characteristics that place a high premium on survival as a route to reproductive opportunity. Generalizing this to other species in the absence of appropriate life history considerations has little a priori validity.

## Acknowledgments

We thank Jane Sewell, Alex Gage, Ian Davies, Charlotte Nevison, Frances Smith, Hazel Brown, Jill Brown, David Fox, Jim Reader, Faisal Wahid, Lisa Truslove, Jane Hurst, Francis Gilbert, Derek Wakelin, David Pritchard, Mike Doenhoff , Padraic Fallon, and several anonymous referees for help, advice, discussion, and comment. Sadly, we also record our thanks for the last time to our technician Peter Smithurst who died on September 15, 1998, after a short illness.

## References

Ader, R., Felten, D. L., & Cohen, N. (Eds.) (1991). *Psychoneuroimmunology* (2nd ed.). New York, Academic Press.

Alexander, J., & Stimson, W. H. (1988). Sex hormones and the course of parasitic infection. *Parasitology Today, 4,* 189–193.

Aloe, L, Musi, B., Micera, A., Santucci, D., Tirassa, P., & Alleva, E. (1995). NGF antibody production as a result of repeated psychosocial stress in adult mice. Neuroscience Research Communications, *16,* 19–28.

Apanius, V. (1994). Reproductive effort and parasite resistance: Evidence for an energetically based trade-off. *Journal of Ornithology, 135,* 404.

Arak, A. (1984). Sneaky breeders. In C. J. Barnard (Ed.), *Producers and scroungers: Strategies of exploitation and parasitism* (pp. 154–194). New York: Chapman & Hall.

Barker, D. J. P. (1995). The foetal and infant origins of disease. *European Journal of Clinical Investigation, 25*, 457–463.

Barker, D. J. P. (1996). The foetal origins of hypertension. *Journal of Hypertension, 14*, S117–S120.

Barnard, C. J., Behnke, J. M., & Sewell, J. (1993). Social behavior, stress and susceptibility to infection in house mice (*Mus musculus*): Effects of duration of grouping and aggressive behavior prior to infection on susceptibility to *Babesia microti*. *Parasitology, 107*, 183–192.

Barnard, C. J., Behnke, J. M., & Sewell, J. (1994). Social behavior and susceptibility to infection in house mice (*Mus musculus*): Effects of group size, aggressive behavior and status-related hormonal responses prior to infection on resistance to *Babesia microti*. *Parasitology, 108*, 487–496.

Barnard, C. J., Behnke, J. M., & Sewell, J. (1996a). Social status and resistance to disease in house mice (*Mus musculus*): Status-related modulation of hormonal responses in relation to immunity costs in different social and physical environments. *Ethology, 102*, 63–84.

Barnard, C. J., Behnke, J. M., & Sewell, J. (1996b). Environmental enrichment, immunocompetence and resistance to *Babesia microti* in male laboratory mice. Physiology and Behavior, *60*, 1223–1231.

Barnard, C. J., Behnke, J. M., Gage, A. R., Brown, H., & Smithurst, P. R. (1997a). Modulation of behavior and testosterone concentration in immunodepressed male laboratory mice (*Mus musculus*). *Physiology and Behavior, 61*, 907–917.

Barnard, C. J., Behnke, J. M., Gage, A. R., Brown, H., & Smithurst, P. R. (1997b) Immunity costs and behavioral modulation in male laboratory mice (*Mus musculus*) exposed to the odour of females. *Physiology and Behavior, 62*, 857–866.

Barnard, C. J., Behnke, J. M., Gage, A. R., Brown, H., & Smithurst, P. R. (1998a). The role of parasite-induced immunodepression, rank and social environment in the modulation of behavior and hormone concentration in male laboratory mice (*Mus musculus*). *Proceedings of the Royal Society of London Series B, 265*, 693–701.

Barnard, C. J., Behnke, J. M., Gage, A. R., Brown, H., & Smithurst, P. R. (1998b). Maternal effects on the development of social rank and immunity trade-offs in male laboratory mice (*Mus musculus*). *Proceedings of the Royal Society of London, Series B, 265*, 2087–2093.

Barnard, C. J., & Hurst, J. L. (1996). Welfare by design: The natural selection of welfare criteria. *Animal Welfare, 5*, 405–433.

Beden, S. N., & Brain, P. F. (1985) Effects of attack-related stress on the primary immune response to sheep red blood cells in castrated mice. *IRCS Medical Science, 12*, 675.

Behnke, J. M., Barnard, C. J., & Wakelin, D. (1992). Understanding chronic nematode infections: Evolutionary considerations, current hypotheses and the way forward. *International Journal of Parasitology, 22*, 861–907.

Behnke, J. M., & Parish, H. A. (1979). *Nematospiroides dubius*: Arrested development of larvae in immune mice. *Experimental Parasitology, 47*, 116–127.

Benten, W. P. M., Bettenhauser, U., Wunderlich, F., Van Vliet, F., & Mossman, H. (1991). Testosterone-induced abrogation of self-healing of *Plasmodium chabaudi* malaria in B10 mice: mediation by spleen cells. *Infection and Immunity, 59*, 4486–4490.

Berkenbosch, F., Oers, J. van, Rey, A. del, Tilders, F., & Besedovsky, H. (1987). Corticotropin-releasing factor-producing neurons in the rat activated by interleukin-1. *Science, 238*, 524–526.

Besedovsky, H. O., Sorkin, E., Keller, M., & Muller, J. (1975). Changes in blood hormone levels during immune response. *Proceedings of the Society for Experimental Biology and Medicicine, 150*, 466–470.

Bigi, S., Huber, C., DeAcetis, L., Alleva, E., & Dixon, A. K. (1994). Removal of the submaxillary salivary glands first increases then abolishes the agonistic response of male mice in social encounters. *Physiology and Behavior, 55*, 13–19.

Brain, P. F. (1988). Social stress in laboratory mouse colonies. In Universities' Federation for Animal Welfare (Ed.), *Laboratory animal welfare research: Rodents* (pp. 49–61). Potters Bar, Universities' Federation for Animal Welfare.

Brain, P. F., & Nowell, N. W. (1970). The effects of differential grouping on endocrine function of mature albino mice. *Physiology and Behavior, 5*, 907–910.

Broom, D. M., & Johnson, K. (1993). *Stress and animal welfare.* London: Chapman & Hall.

Chamove, A. S. (1989). Environmental enrichment: A review. *Animal Technology, 40*, 155–178.

Chapman, V. M., Desjardins, C., & Bronson, F. H. (1969). Social rank in male mice and adrenocortical response to open field exposure. *Proceedings of the Society for Experimental Biology and Medicine, 130*, 624–627.

Cirulli, F, DeAcetis, L., & Alleva, E. (1998). Behavioral effects of peripheral interleukin-1 administration in adult CD-1 mice: Specific inhibition of the offensive components of intermale agonistic behavior. *Brain Research, 791*, 308–312.

Clark, I. A., & Nowell, M. J. (1990). Protozoan parasites of erythrocytes and macrophages. In J. M. Behnke (Ed.), *Parasites, immunity and pathology: The consequences of parasitic infection in mammals* (pp. 146–168). London: Taylor & Francis.

Cox, F. E. G., & Young, A. S. (1969). Acquired immunity to *Babesia microti* and *Babesia rodhaini* in mice. *Parasitology, 75*, 189–196,

Cresswell, J. L., Egger, P., Fall, C. H. D., Osmond, C., Fraser, R. B., & Barker, D. J. P. (1997). Is the age of menopause determined in utero? *Early Human Development, 49*, 143–148.

Dantzer, R., Bluthe, R. M., Kent, S., & Goodall, G. (1993). Behavioral effects of cytokines: An insight into mechanisms of sickness behavior. In D. B. DeSouza (Ed.), *Neurobiology of cytokines* (pp. 130–151). Academic Press: San Diego.

Davies, I. B. (1998). *The effects of hormone treatment on social status-related differences in infection with Babesia microti in adult male CFLP mice.* Unpublished Ph. D. thesis, University. of Nottingham, UK.

Dawkins, M. S. (1990). From an animal's point of view: Motivation, fitness and animal welfare. *Behavior and Brain Science, 20*, 200–225.

Demas, G. E., & Nelson, R. J. (1996). Photoperiod and temperature interact to affect immune parameters in adult deer mice (*Peromyscus maniculatus*). *Journal of Biological Rhythms, 11*, 94–102.

Else, K. J., & Grencis, R. K. (1991). Helper T-cell subsets in mouse trichuriasis. Parasitology Today, *7*, 313–316.

Festa-Bianchet (1989). Individual differences, parasites, and the costs of reproduction in birds. *Philosophical Transactions of the Royal Society of London B, 346*, 323–331.

Finkelman, F. D., Shea-Donaghue, T., Goldhill, J., Sullivan, C. A., Morris, S. C., Madden, K. B., Gause, W. C., & Urban, J. F., Jr. (1997). Cytokine regulation of host defense against parasitic gastrointestinal nematodes: lessons from studies with rodent models. *Annual Review of Immunology , 15*, 505–533.

Finkelman, F. D., & Urban, J. F., Jr. (1992). Cytokines: making the right choice. Parasitology Today, *8*, 311–313.

Folstad, I., & Karter, A. J. (1992). Parasites, bright males and the immunocompetence handicap. *American Naturalist, 139*, 603–622.

Folstad, I., & Skarstein, F. (1997). Is male germ line control creating avenues for female choice? *Behavioral Ecology, 8*, 109–111.

Fraser, D. (1993). Assessing animal well-being: Common sense, uncommon science. In *Food animal well-being* (pp. 37–54). West

Lafayette: Purdue University Office of Agricultural Research Programs.

Freeland, W. J. (1981). Parasitism and behavioral dominance among male mice. *Science, 213,* 461–462.

Grossman, C. J. (1985). Interactions between the gonadal steroids and the immune system. Science, *227,* 257–261.

Grossman, C. J., & Roselle, G. A. (1986). The control of immune response by endocrine factors and the clinical significance of such regulation. *Progress in Clinical Biochemistry and Medicine, 4,* 9–56.

Gustafsson, L., Nordling, D., Andersson, M. S., Sheldon, B. C., & Qvarnstrom, A. (1994). Infectious diseases, reproductive effort and the cost of reproduction in birds. Philosophical Transactions of the Royal Society B, *260,* 323–331.

Haemisch, A., & Gartner, K. (1994) The cage design affects intermale aggression in small groups of male laboratory mice: Strain specific consequences of social organization, and endocrine activations, in two inbred strains (DBA/2J and CBA/J). *Journal of Experimental Animal Science, 36,* 101–116.

Hales, C. N. (1997). Metabolic consequences of intrauterine growth retardation. *Acta Paediatrica, 86,* 184–187.

Hamilton, W. D. (1964). The genetical evoluton of social behavior I, II. *Journal of Theoretical Biology, 7,* 1–52.

Hamilton, W. D., & Zuk, M. (1982). Heritable true fitness and bright birds: A role for parasites? *Science, 218,* 384–387.

Hillgarth, N., & Wingfield, J. C. (1997). Testosterone and immuno-suppression in vertebrates: Implications for parasite–mediated sexual selection. In N. E. Beckage (Ed.), *Parasites and pathogens; Effects on host hormones and behavior* (pp. 143–155). London: Chapman and Hall.

Hillgarth, N., Ramenofsky, M., & Wingfield, J. (1997). Testosterone and sexual selection. Behavioral Ecology, *8,* 108–109.

Hughes, V. L. (1998) *The effect of testosterone on parasitic infections in rodents, with respect to disease transmission by ticks.* Unpublished D. Phil thesis, University of Oxford, UK.

Hurst, J. L. (1987) Behavioral variation in wild house mice (*Mus domesticus* Rutty): A quantitative assessment of female social organization. *Animal Behavior, 35,* 1846–1857.

Hurst, J. L. (1990). Urine marking in population of wild house mice (*Mus domesticus* Rutty). I. Communication between males. *Animal Behavior, 40,* 209–222.

Hussein, H. S. (1984). *Babesia hylomysci* and *Babesia microti*: Dexamethasone treatment of infected mice. *Experimental Parasitology, 57,* 165–171.

Hutchings, J. A., & Myers, R. A. (1994). The evolution of alternative mating strategies in variable Environments. *Evolutionary Ecology, 8,* 256–268.

Kelly, D. D. (1986). Stress-induced analgesia. *Annals of the New York Academy of Science, 467,* 426–445.

Keymer, A. E., & Read, A. F. (1991). Behavioral ecology: The impact of parasitism. In C. A. Toft, A. Aeschlimann, & L. Bolis (Eds.), *Parasite–host associations: Coexistence or conflict?* (pp. 37–61), Oxford: Oxford University Press.

Khansari, D. N., Murgo, A. J., & Faith, R. E. (1990). Effects of stress on the immune system. *Immunology Today, 11,* 170–175.

Komers, P. E., Pelabon, C., & Stenstrom, D. (1997). Age at first reproduction in male fallow deer: Age-specific versus dominance-specific behaviors. *Behavioral Ecology, 8,* 456–462.

Langley-Evans, S. (1997). Fetal programming of immune function and respiratory disease. *Clinical Experimental Allergy, 27,* 1377–1379.

Leshner, A. I., & Politch, J. A. (1979). Hormonal control of submissiveness in mice: Irrelevance of the androgens and relevance of the pituitary-adrenal hormones. *Physiology and Behavior, 22,* 531–534.

Lochmiller, R. L., Vestey, M. R., & Boren, J. C. (1993). Relationship between protein nutritional status and immunocompetence in northern bobwhite chicks. *Auk, 110,* 503–510.

Maestripieri, D., Desimone, R., Aloe, L., & Alleva, E. (1990). Social status and nerve growth factor serum level affect agonistic encounters in mice. *Physiology and Behavior, 47,* 161–164.

Maier, S. F., & Watkins, L. R. (1998). Cytokines for psychologists: Implications of bidirectional immune-to-brain communication for understanding behavior, mood, and cognition. *Psychological Reviews, 105,* 83–107.

Maier, S. F., Watkins, L. R., & Fleshner, M. (1994). Psychoneuroimmunology: The interface between behavior, brain and immunology. *American Psychologist, 49,* 1004–1017.

Markowitz, H. (1982) *Behavioral enrichment in the Zoo.* New York, van Nostrand.

Mason, G., & Mendl, M. (1993). Why is there no simple way of measuring animal welfare? *Animal Welfare, 2,* 301–319.

McGregor, P. K., & Ayling, S. J. (1990). Varied cages result in more aggression in male CFLP mice. *Applied Animal Behavior Science, 26,* 277–281.

Meikle, D. B., Drickamer, L. C., Vessey, S. H., Arthur, R. D., & Rosenthal, T. L. (1996). Dominance rank and parental investment in swine (*Sus scrofa domesticus*). *Ethology, 102,* 969–978.

Mendl, M. (1991). Some problems with the concept of a cut-off point for determining when an animal's welfare is at risk. *Applied Animal Behavior Science, 31,* 139–146.

Mooradian, A. D., Morley, J. E., & Korenman, S. G. (1987). Biological action of androgens. *Endocrine Review, 8,* 1–28.

Nesse, R. M., & Williams, G. C. (1994). *Why we get sick: The new science of Darwinian Medicine.* New York, Random House.

Norris, K., Anwar, M., & Read, A. F. (1994). Reproductive effort influences the prevalence of haematozoan parasites in great tits. *Journal of Animal Ecology, 63,* 601–610.

Owens, I. P. F., & Short, R. V. (1995). Hormonal basis of sexual dimorphism in birds: implications for new theories about sexual selection. *Trends in Ecology & Evolution, 10,* 44–47.

Padgett, D. A., Sheridan, J. F., & Loria, R. (1995). Steroid hormone regulation of a polyclonal Th2 immune response. *Annals of the New York Academy of Science, 774,* 323–325.

Penn, D., & Potts, W. K. (1998). Chemical signals and parasite-mediated sexual selection. *Trends in Ecology and Evolution, 13,* 391–396.

Poole, T. R., & Morgan, H. D. R. (1973). Differences in aggressive behavior between male mice (*Mus musculus* L.) in colonies of different sizes. *Animal Behavior, 21,* 788–795.

Quinnell, R. J., Behnke, J. M., & Keymer, A. E. (1991). Host specificity of and cross-immunity between two strains of *Heligmosomoides polygrus*. *Parasitology, 102,* 419–427.

Read, A. F. (1990). Parasites and the evolution of host sexual behavior. In C. J. Barnard & J. M. Behnke (Eds.), *Parasitism and host behavior*. London: Taylor & Francis.

Richner, H., Christe, P., & Oppliger, A. (1995). Paternal investment affects prevalence of malaria. *Proceedings of the National Academy of Sciences USA, 92,* 1192–1194.

Roberts, C. W., Satoskar, A., & Alexander, J. (1996). Sex steroids, pregnancy-associated hormones and immunity to parasitic infections. *Parasitology Today, 12,* 382–388.

Rohner-Jeanrenaud, F., & Jeanrenaud, B. (1997). Central nervous system and body weight regulation. *Annals of Developmental Endocrinology, 58,* 137–142.

Rohwer, S., & Ewald, P. (1981). The cost of dominance and advantage of subordination in a badge signalling system. *Evolution 35,* 441–454.

Rook, G. A. W., & Zumia, A. (1997). Gulf War syndrome: Is it due to a systemic shift in cytokine balance towards a Th2 profile? *Lancet, 349*, 1831–1833.

Rushen, J. (1986). Some problems with the physiological concept of stress. *Australian Veterinary Journal, 63*, 359–361.

Saino, N., & Moller, A. . P. (1996). Sexual ornamentation and immunocompetence in the barn swallow. *Behavioral Ecology, 7*, 227–232.

Schmitt-Wrede, H. P., Fiebig, S., Wunderlich, F., Benten, W. P. M., Bettenhauser, U., Beden, K., & Mossmann, H. (1991). Testosterone-induced susceptibility to *Plasmodium chabaudi* malaria: Variant protein expression in functionally changed spenic non-T cells. *Molecular and Cellular Endocrinolody, 76*, 207–214.

Schur, B. (1987). Social structure and plasma corticosterone level in female albino mice. *Physiology and Behavior, 40*, 698–693.

Sheldon, B. C., & Verhulst, S. (1996). Ecological immunology: Costly parasite defences and trade-offs in evolutionary ecology. *Trends in Ecology and Evolution, 11*, 317–321.

Siva-Jothy, M. T. (1995). Immunocompetence: Conspicuous by its absence. *Trends in Ecology and Evolution, 10*, 205.

Vessey, S. H. (1964). Effects of grouping on levels of circulating antibodies in mice. *Proceedings of the Society for Experimental Biology and Medicine, 115*, 252–255.

Wakelin, D., & Selby, G. R. (1974). The induction of immunological tolerance to the parasitic nematode *Trichuris muris* is cortisone-treated mice. *Immunology, 26*, 1–10.

Wedekind, C., & Folstad, I. (1994). Adaptive or nonadaptive immunosuppression by sex hormones? *American Naturalist, 143*, 936–938.

Wilckens, T., & Rijk, R. de (1997). Glucocorticoids and immune function: unknown dimensions and new frontiers. *Immunology Today, 18*, 418–424.

Wunderlich, F., Benten, W. P. M., Bettenhauser, U., Schmitte-Wrede, H., & Mossmann, H. Testosterone unresponsiveness of existing immunity against *Plasmodium chabaudi*. *Parasite Immunology, 14*, 307–320.

Wunderlich, F., Marinovski, P., Benten, W. P. M., Schmitte-Wrede, H., & Mossmann, H. Testosterone and other gonadal factor(s) restrict the efficacy of genes controlling resistance to *Plasmodium chabaudi* malaria. *Parasite Immunology, 13*, 357–367.

# 31

# Fetal Alcohol Syndrome and Immunity

ANNA N. TAYLOR, FRANCESCO CHIAPPELLI, RAZ YIRMIYA

## I. INTRODUCTION

The characteristic features of the fetal alcohol syndrome (FAS), first described three decades ago, include cranio-facial dysmorphologies, growth retardation, mental retardation, cognitive, psychosocial and behavioral problems, altered motor performance and impaired communication skills (Abel, 1996; Gottesfeld & Abel, 1991; Hanson, Jones, & Smith, 1976; Jones & Smith, 1973; Jones, Smith, Streissguth, & Myrianthopoulos, 1974; Jones, Smith, Ulleland, & Streissguth, 1973; Lemoine, Harosseau, Borteryu, & Menuet, 1968).

Children exposed to alcohol in utero also exhibit serious impairments in both cellular and humoral immunity (Chiappelli & Taylor, 1995; Gottesfeld & Abel, 1991). One of the early descriptions of these impairments (Johnson, Knight, Harmer, & Steele, 1981) compared a group of 13 children with the FAS with control subjects. Signs of immune pathology were found in the FAS group, including a 36% decrease in the number of circulating E-rosette forming lymphocytes (i.e., CD2+ T cells), a 40–50% decrease in mitogen-induced proliferative responses of T and B lymphocytes, a blunted delayed hypersensitivity response, decreased counts of eosinophils and neutrophils, and decreased immunoglobulin (Ig)

levels (Johnson et al., 1981). Furthermore, infants diagnosed with congenital thymic aplasia (DiGeorge Syndrome), which is associated with various morpho- and immunopathological dysfunctions, including impaired T-cell-mediated responses and increased susceptibility to infections, were found to be born to women who had a history of chronic alcohol consumption during pregnancy (Amman, Wara, Cowan, Barrett, & Stiehm, 1982). The impairments in immune functions following fetal alcohol exposure (FAE) may be responsible for the increased morbidity from infections associated with this syndrome. Indeed, children with FAS show a predisposition for viral, bacterial, and fungal infections, including upper respiratory and urinary tract infections, recurrent otitis media, sepsis, acute gastroenteritis, and pneumonia caused by *Mycobacterium tuberculosis* (Amman et al., 1982; Church & Gerkin, 1988; Johnson et al., 1981). FAE-induced suppression of cellular immunity may also contribute to the increased incidence of malignancies (particularly of embryonic origin) observed in children with FAS (Chiappelli & Taylor, 1995; Gottesfeld & Abel, 1991).

The development of animal models of the FAS is valuable and necessary because histories of FAE in human subjects are often imprecise and incomplete (Calvani et al., 1985; Chiappelli et al., 1993; Giberson & Weinberg, 1992; Gottesfeld & Abel, 1991; Hanson et al., 1976; Johnson et al., 1981; Nelson & Taylor, 1987; Yirmiya, Pilati, Chiappelli, & Taylor 1993; Yirmiya, Tio, & Taylor, 1996). Animal models provide precise and controlled patterns of prenatal alcohol exposure crucial for the characterization of alcohol teratogenicity. The rat and the mouse are particularly convenient models that have been extensively studied to characterize the mechanisms of fetal alcohol toxicity to neural, endocrine, and immune development. Studies using murine and rodent models of the less severe manifestations of FAE have shown serious disturbances in the development of central and peripheral systems, including the regulation of the neuroendocrine and immune systems. In particular, these studies clearly demonstrated that exposure to alcohol in utero leads to a profound derangement of the immunophysiological system that involves the hypothalamo-pituitary-adrenal (HPA) axis and cell-mediated immunity (CMI) (Chiappelli et al., 1993; Clarren et al., 1990; Giberson & Weinberg, 1992; Gottesfeld, Christie, Felten, & LeGrue, 1990; Lee, Imaki, Vale, & Rivier, 1990; Nelson & Taylor, 1987; Watson & Gottesfeld, 1993; West, 1986; Yirmiya et al., 1993, 1996).

Alcohol has primary metabolites that have documented immunotoxicity. In addition, alcohol may have direct toxic effects upon cells of the central nervous system (CNS), upon endocrine cells, and upon immune cells (Braun, Pearce, & Peterson, 1995; Chiappelli, Kung, Stefanini, & Foschi, 1998). Pathological sequelae of alcohol abuse and alcoholism (e.g., liver pathology, malnutrition) produce significant deleterious neuroendocrine-immunoregulatory outcomes. These issues, however, will not be addressed here.

This chapter reviews the current knowledge of the effects of FAE on immune functions and their interactions with the neural and neuroendocrine systems, with emphasis on central and peripheral outcomes of the HPA-CMI axis in animal models. Specifically, this chapter discusses murine and rodent models of FAE in the context of peripheral measures of immune surveillance, of the febrile and behavioral responsiveness to immune challenges, and of central and peripheral neuroendocrine dysregulation, which may partly account for the immunological and neuroimmune impairments.

## II. FAE AND IMMUNE SURVEILLANCE

Immune surveillance refers to the complex set of events mediated by cells and soluble factors of the immune system that work in concert to provide the host with the necessary resistance against viruses, bacteria, fungi, and foreign bodies (for review, Chiappelli et al., 1998; Huston, 1997; Roitt, Brostoff, & Male, 1989). The immune system has two broad functional divisions, based on whether or not recognition of the infectious agent is directed by the major histocompatibility complex (MHC). The innate immune system is MHC-unrestricted, and represents the initial line of defense of the host. It consists primarily of monocytes/macrophages and other antigen-presenting cells, and natural killer (NK) cells, which act in MHC-unrestricted cytotoxicity. By definition, NK cells are neither T nor B cells; indeed, their developmental lineage is somewhere between the myeloid and the lymphoid lineages. They are closer to the lymphoid cells in general morphology and in plastic nonadherence properties, but they do not carry the T-cell marker, CD3, nor the B-cell marker, CD20. NK cells do not mature in the thymus, nor do they secrete immunoglobulins. The NK-cell population, while CD3−, CD16+, CD56+, and expressing other NK-specific markers, is morphologically similar to large granular lymphocytes, which are CD3+ CD8+ cells, i.e., activated and mature cytotoxic T lymphocytes. The large granular morphology of NK cells has led to the loose nomenclature of NK/LGL. The antigen-dependent immune system is MHC-restricted, and represents the adaptive resistance of the host to a pathogen. It consists primarily of T and B lymphocytes. Humoral immunity is brought about by antibodies produced by B cells; cellular immunity is brought about by T-cell-initiated and T-cell-driven events (e.g., lymphokine production, delayed hypersensitivity reaction, MHC-restricted cytotoxicity). These two intertwined branches of the immune system interact and communicate via cytokines, growth factors produced by the diverse immune cell populations. MHC-unrestricted responses form the first barrier to invading pathogens. Sustained immunity toward a given pathogen is directed and maintained by MHC-restricted processes, which therefore are critical to effective immune surveillance (for review, Chiappelli et al., 1998; Roitt et al., 1989).

Immune surveillance occurs through the concerted action of several intertwined pathways, which do not usually take place in the circulating blood lymphocytes, but in secondary lymphoid organs (e.g., spleen, lymph nodes) and body surfaces, including the oral and the intestinal mucosa. These mucosa represent the first line of defense against the cytopathic and physiopathic effects of ingested alcohol. Immune cells migrate from immune organs to other sites, and it is in that process of transit that they are found in peripheral blood. Therefore it is critical to interpret cellular immune data in the context of the site within which the immune cells were collected, as well as other temporal and experimental conditions. At any given site, immune cells represent a rather narrow window of the immune system (for review, Chiappelli, 1991; Chiappelli et al., 1998; Huston, 1997; Roitt et al., 1989).

## A. FAE Alters Immunity at the Feto-Placental Interface

From the ontogenetic perspective, FAE is detrimental because it alters the maternal immune competence during pregnancy, including cellular immune events that help prevent the rejection of the fetus. Particularly in the vicinity of the feto-placental interface, one finds maternal immune response bias toward antibody production and away from cell-mediated responses. Mounting evidence suggests that this change in maternal immunity is critical for successful pregnancy and may be mediated by a localized shift in the cytokine milieu. The fetal–maternal relationship is bidirectional. As the feto-placental unit affects the regulation of the maternal pattern of cellular immune response, it is also likely that the mother's immune responses direct the development of the fetus' immune system (Wegmann, Lin, Guilbert, & Mosmann, 1993). The maternal–fetal interface is rich in TH2-type cytokines (i.e., interleukin (IL)-3, IL-4, IL-5), which play a crucial role in the maturation and clonal expansion of antibody-producing B-cell populations. By contrast, the feto-placental unit is generally low in TH1 cytokines (i.e., IL-2, interferon-$\gamma$ (IFN)), which favor immune cytotoxicity and graft rejection (Lin, Mosmann, Guilbert, Tuntipopipat, & Wegmann, 1993; Wegmann et al., 1993). Activation of the naive helper T cells initiates their process of maturation to either of these two polarized terminal stages, in which the cells produce either one or the other pattern of cytokines (for review, Romagnani, 1996). Because alcohol blunts helper T-cell activation and maturation under experimental conditions (for review, Chiappelli et al., 1998), FAE could alter patterns of cytokine production by altering the regulation of the process of naive helper T-cell activation and maturation. These lines of evidence converge to suggest that FAE may significantly alter the early development of the immune system. For example, maternal alcohol consumption could result in altered patterns of cytokines at the feto-placental interface, thus contributing to the increased risk of spontaneous abortions and premature births by alcoholic mothers (i.e., immune rejection of the fetus). This hypothesis, supported in part by recent observations made from cord blood samples of a cohort of 2631 infants, which indicated that alcohol consumption by the mothers during pregnancy was associated with significant alterations in IgE concentrations (Bjerke, Hedegaard, Henriksen, Nielsen, & Schiotz, 1994), remains to be tested experimentally.

## B. FAE Disturbs Lactational Immunity

The transfer of immunity via lactation also plays an important role in providing early protection to the neonate. To test the hypothesis that maternal exposure to ethanol results in an altered transfer of immunity to the neonate by milk against the intestinal parasite *Trichinella spiralis*, a rat model of FAE was established. Cytokine production by mammary milk leukocytes stimulated either by the T-cell mitogen concanavalin A (Con A) or by the Gram-negative bacterial cell wall lipopolysaccharide (LPS) was tested. Findings showed significantly decreased production of IL-6 and tumor necrosis factor-$\alpha$ (TNF-$\alpha$), and increased production of IL-2 (Na & Seelig, 1994). Further studies involving the same model of in vivo infection established that the immune response of rat pups to *T. spiralis* was diminished following maternal consumption of ethanol. Taken together, these data confirmed that FAE pups show depressed immune capacity, which involves altered development of T- and B-cell-mediated reactions. These data also confirmed that FAE affects cytokine production systemically, that is by blood leukocytes, as well as locally (Seelig, Steven, & Stewart, 1996).

These results led to the question of whether the effects of FAE on immune surveillance were attributable to lactation alone, or could evolve from events that occur in utero. To begin to test this issue, the effect of fostering was examined experimentally. The outcomes of surrogate fostering were found to vary with age and to have differential long-term effects on female and male FAE offspring. In this model, litters were fostered at birth to surrogate untreated dams who had given birth within the same 12-h period or were reared by their biological mothers, and their splenic leukocytes examined for expression of differentiation antigens. At 15 days, fostered FAE animals showed reduced percentages of CD4+, CD45RA+, and CD5+ cells compared to fostered control rats. At 60 days of age, fostered FAE females showed a higher percentage of CD4+ and of CD45RA+ splenocytes than fostered control females. Nonfostered animals showed no FAE effects on the expression of these differentiation antigens (Giberson & Weinberg, 1997). Indeed, fostering at birth has differential effects on splenic lymphocyte populations in FAE animals, and these effects interact with the actions of FAE. It appears that fostering at birth may further exacerbate the effects of in utero and/or lactational ethanol exposure.

Alcohol consumption during pregnancy alters certain key cellular immune components. A recent study compared the distribution of lymphocytes, the production of cytokines by lymphocytes, and the level of IgA and IgG in breast milk and in peripheral blood of 10 women who reported to be moderate to heavy drinkers and in 10 nondrinkers at 3 days post partum. Since drinkers also most often smoke, nondrinker control women were assigned to either a smoker control group or a nonsmoker control group. The milk and serum from the alcohol-consuming group contained a statistically elevated amount of IL-8 and IL-6 as compared with milk from nonsmoker controls, but not the smoker control group. Blood from the alcohol-consuming women also had a statistically elevated level of IL-8 when compared to that from both smoker and nonsmoker control groups. The total number of white blood cells was statistically higher in milk from the alcohol-consuming group than the milk of either the smoker or the nonsmoker groups. These differences were attributable to IL-8-mediated migration of polymorphonuclear cells, but most likely not of cells of the lymphoid or the myeloid lineages. The observed alterations could not be attributed solely to the consumption of alcohol during pregnancy, as smoking was revealed to be a significant confounding variable (Na, Daniels, & Seelig, 1997).

The relevance of these findings, in particular, to the present public health threat of the transmission of the human immunodeficiency virus by women who abuse alcohol during pregnancy and lactation remains to be tested. Nevertheless, emerging research appears to support this contention (Spencer et al., 1997).

## C.  FAE and Cell-Mediated Immunity

Evidence from in vivo and in vitro studies indicates that FAE is associated with a selective impairment of cell-mediated immune function, including primarily T-cell-mediated responses. Responses mediated by NK cells, by myeloid cells, and by B cells appear to be only selectively affected by FAE (Gottesfeld & Ullrich, 1995; Wolcott, Jennings, & Chervenak, 1995).

### 1.  FAE Retards Development of the Thymus and the Spleen

T-cell progenitor cells migrate from the bone marrow as preprothymocytes and are directed toward the thymus for positive and negative selection maturational sequences. The thymus is critical for the development of immune competence. Its ontogenesis is determined by a series of precisely timed events during which the pharyngeal pouch endoderm interacts with embryonic connective tissue and migrating blood-borne lymphoid stem cells. The portion of the neural crest associated with the developing hindbrain migrates ventrolaterally through the branchial arches and is to become the mesenchyme that will form the layers around the epithelial primordia of the thymus. Experimental alterations of this sequence of events, or ablation of the cranial neural crest before its migration to the nascent thymus results in delayed, aborted, or abnormal thymic ontogenesis and in aberrant development of immune competence (for review, Bockman & Kirby, 1985; Chiappelli et al., 1993). From a neuroendocrinimmune perspective, the development of the thymus is intertwined with the regulation of gonadal, adrenocortical, pituitary, and other hormones. Indeed, the HPA–thymus interaction (Hall, O'Grady, & Farah, 1991; Revskoy, Halasz, & Redei, 1997) and the deleterious effects of FAE on HPA ontogenesis (see below) predict that substantial damaging effects of FAE on thymic ontogenesis should be expected. Nevertheless, and despite our understanding of the teratogenic effects of FAE upon the neuroendocrine system (see below), research to date has not yet tested experimentally whether or not FAE significantly alters specific events of thymic histologic ontogeny.

What is known today about the teratogenicity of FAE upon thymic ontogeny is complex and multifaceted. Studies involving a murine model (C57BL/6 mice fed 4.8% (w/v) ethanol for up to 2 weeks before and throughout pregnancy), for example, show, upon histological examination, that the cortico-medullary junction (which normally appears at 17–19 days of fetal life in the mouse as the thymus becomes functionally mature) is all but absent in FAE mice. The absence of this landmark of thymic development suggests that FAE may lead to a retardation of thymic ontogeny (Ewald & Walden, 1988). Three lines of evidence support this hypothesis: (1) A positive linear relationship was obtained between fetal weight and thymocyte number in 18-day-old fetal mice. FAE animals were clustered in the lower left quadrant, but control animals were found in the upper ranges of thymocyte number and fetal weight. (2) Immature thymocytes are generally enlarged and reduce their size as they traverse the thymus and acquire signs of thymocyte maturity. By flow cytometric forward scatter analysis, thymocytes from FAE fetuses appeared generally enlarged, compared to thymocytes from control cohorts. (3) FAE produces changes in the normal development of T-cell marker expression. The murine pan-thymocyte and pan-T-lymphocyte marker, Thy-1, is acquired early during thymic ontogeny and thymocyte maturation. This membrane antigen, a 18 to 25-kDa glycoprotein of the Ig superfamily, is associated with the phosphatidylinositol transmembrane signaling system and is expressed in cerebellar and brain stem neurons as well as thymocytes and T lymphocytes (Greene et al., 1987). Committed T-cell precursors from the murine hematopoietic fetal liver—where toxic alcohol metabolites are presumably produced in FAE animals—initially migrate to the thymic primordia by day 10–11 of gestation. These enlarged basophilic cells engage in active differentiation and maturation within the thymus, and express Thy-1 by day 15 (Pardoll, Fowlkes, Lechler, Germain, & Schwartz, 1987). By day 16 of gestation, thymocytes acquire Lyt-2. The appearance of L3T4 generally does not occur before day 17. By day 18–19 of fetal life, murine fetal thymocytes generally express the Lyt-2 and L3T4 antigens in a proportion similar to that found in adult mice. Helper T-cell activity is conferred to the L3T4+/Lyt-2− subpopulation, and cytotoxic/suppressor T-cell activity resides in the L3T4−/Lyt-2+ thymocyte subpopulation in mature normal mice. Double negative populations are immature and remain in the thymus. By single color fluorescence flow cytometry measurements, the proportion of Thy-1+ fetal murine thymocytes was not different in FAE vs. control animals, but the proportions of L3T4+ and Lyt-2+ thymocytes were two to three fold reduced in FAE animals compared to controls (Ewald & Walden, 1988).

In more recent studies designed to determine whether ethanol allows escape of potentially autoreactive T-cell clones from negative selection, ethanol was fed to sublethally irradiated, young adult C57BR mice during the time of thymic and splenic repopulation as a new model of human third trimester FAE. T-cell populations were monitored by flow cytometry. Findings established that there was no discernible effect of ethanol exposure during thymic and splenic repopulation on the expression of $V\beta17\alpha$ on thymocytes and splenic T lymphocytes, indicating that prenatal ethanol does not appear to affect negative selection (Livant, Welles, & Ewald, 1997).

Murine splenocyte development appears normal up to day 17 of gestation in mice exposed to 25% ethanol-derived calories (EDC) during fetal development. This period of time corresponds to the events leading to the invasion of the splenic environment by lymphoid cells capable of differentiation along the B lineage pathway. Thereafter, however, flow cytometric analyses showed that B-cell developmental patterns were altered, i.e., whereas B-cell precursor and early intermediates were equally present in the spleens of FAE and control fetuses, the more mature progenitor B cells were significantly decreased in FAE animals (Biber, Moscatello, Dempsey, Chervenak, & Wolcott, 1998).

A related murine model (20% EDC during pregnancy and/or lactation) demonstrated that the population of immune cells in the spleen of 21-day-old offspring was significantly altered by FAE. The number of CD4+ or CD8+ T splenocytes expressing the marker Thy1.2 and the number of splenocytes expressing the IgG receptor (B cells) were significantly reduced in FAE animals and in animals exposed to ethanol prior to weaning (Giberson & Blakley, 1994).

The generation of functionally competent T cells from thymocyte precursors involves several finely regulated processes modulated in part by the interaction between thymocytes and the thymic epithelium (Singer, 1990), as well as the intrathymic environment determined in part by secreted cytokines (Carding, Hayday, & Bottomly, 1991; Montgomery & Dallman, 1991; Street & Mosmann, 1991). In addition, different subpopulations of thymocytes are characterized biochemically by the expression of distinct isozymes of protein kinase C, and maturation of thymocytes seems linked to the sequential expression and deexpression of these isozymes (for review, Chiappelli et al., 1993). Similar cellular interactions occur in the spleen and other lymphoid organs. The putative effects of FAE on the thymic and splenic epithelia and on thymocyte and splenocyte cellular and molecular biology must be addressed in future research to understand fully the mechanisms of action of FAE upon those immune compartments.

## 2. FAE Generally Impairs T-Cell Proliferative Responses

From the functional standpoint, the proliferative response of thymic, splenic, lymph node, or blood lymphocytes to mitogen stimulation is generally lower in FAE animals than in control cohorts. Seminal studies have used the male offspring of Sprague-Dawley rats, intubated daily with 6 g/kg ethanol from 2 weeks before mating until delivery, to measure the response of splenocytes at 7, 11, and 18 months of postnatal life. No differences in proliferation were obtained between FAE and control animals when the B-cell mitogen, lipopolysaccharide (LPS), was used. Stimulation with the T-cell mitogen, Con A, led to a suppression of the proliferative response that was greatest at 7 months (5% of control), less pronounced at 11 months (40% of control), and all but abolished at 18 months (90–100% of control) (Monjan & Mandell, 1980). Moreover, the proliferative response to Con A of splenocytes and thymocytes obtained from 21-day-old offspring from Sprague–Dawley rats treated with ethanol (35% EDC) during the last week of gestation was suppressed eight-fold in splenocytes and two-fold in thymocytes compared to controls (Redei, Clark, & McGivern, 1989). Neuro-endocrine assessments revealed correlated HPA dys-regulation in FAE animals (elevated hypothalamic adrenocorticotrophin (ACTH), but decreased hypo-thalamic CRF and pituitary ACTH compared to con-trol animals at day 1 postnatally) (see below) (Redei et al., 1989).

Studies to-date have used the male progeny primarily to avoid the complexities associated with the possible neuroimmune outcomes derived from the neuroendocrine fluctuations of the estrous cycle. Despite putative neuroimmune sexual dimorphic characteristics (Grossman, 1990), studies designed to characterize the outcome of FAE on immune surveil-lance mechanisms in females remain sparse to date. In general, however, data indicate that alterations in T-cell responsiveness due to FAE are primarily evident in males (Weinberg & Jerrells, 1991).

We have shown, in our laboratory, an eightfold age-dependent increase in response by thymocytes to Con A by postnatal day 44 in male FAE rats (35% EDC in a liquid diet, during the last 2 weeks of gestation). The response of stimulated thymocytes tended to normalize by young adulthood (day 72, Fig. 1) (Wong et al., 1992). We have also noted a 2-fold decrease in response by splenocytes of FAE animals about day 44. Stimulated thymocytes from FAE rats were less responsive to further stimulation with crude Con A

supernatant compared to normal rats at day 44, as were stimulated splenocytes. Maximal suppression of the proliferative response of splenocytes to Con A occurred at 3–5 months, and the response failed to normalize in adult animals (Figure 1) (Norman, Chang, Castle, van Zuylen, & Taylor, 1989; Norman, Chang, Wong, Branch, Castle, & Taylor, 1991). We also noted that splenocytes from these animals were significantly less responsive to further stimulation with crude Con A supernatant or with human recombinant IL-2, compared to controls, following prestimulation with ConA. This loss of responsive-ness was age-dependent (Norman et al., 1989, 1991). Flow cytometric analyses of splenocyte populations confirmed the data by others (see above) that showed that FAE alters the proportion of T- cell subsets that home to the spleen, and that these alterations may be sustained into adulthood (Chang, Yamaguchi, Yeh, Taylor, & Norman, 1994).

By contrast, a combined prenatal–postnatal expo-sure to ethanol was found to alter the proliferative response of splenic T cells up to 4 weeks postnatally in mice. These differences were all but abrogated by 12 weeks. The number of splenic and thymic T cells were not significantly altered (Basham, Whitmore, Adcock, & Basta, 1998).

Our studies further showed that the diminished T-cell proliferation in young adult FAE rats was due to a decreased responsiveness to IL-2. Impaired produc-

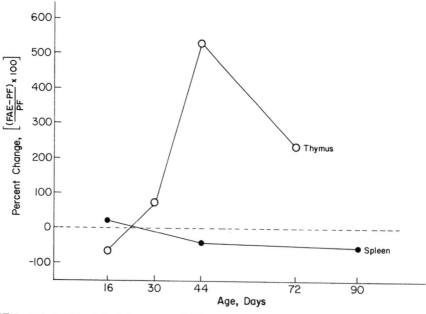

**FIGURE 1**   Effects of fetal alcohol exposure (FAE) on Con A (0.5 µg/mL) mitogenesis in thymocytes and splenocytes between postnatal day 16 and postnatal day 90. Data are expressed as the percentage change in the mitogenic response obtained with cells from FAE rats compared to the response of cells from pair-fed (PF) control rats. (Data based on Norman et al., 1991 and Wong et al., 1992.)

tion of IL-2 or expression of IL-2 receptor was excluded based on our data, as was the putative presence of an excessive suppressor T-cell activity. We also showed that the increase in intracellular calcium induced by Con A in T cells from FAE rats was not changed compared to cells obtained from control animals. The results of IL-2-binding studies established that the $K_d$ values and the number of both high- and low-affinity IL-2 receptor binding sites on the T cells of FAE rats were comparable to those of pair-, or chow-fed control rats. Indeed, our data clearly determined that the amount of the internalized IL-2 was significantly reduced in T cells from FAE rats, and that the half-time for dissociation of IL-2 from the receptors in the T cells of FAE rats was greater than that of the control rats. These results suggested that FAE suppresses T-cell proliferation by interfering with events following the interaction between IL-2 and its receptor (Chang et al., 1994).

Progression of peripheral immune cells toward maturation and memory requires initial sine qua non interactions between cytokines and their receptors. In the instance of T cells, the premier interaction is that which we showed to be altered in FAE animals: the interaction between IL-2 and its receptor. Should the immune cell "read" an inappropriate interaction, or inappropriate steps thereafter, then the cell engages in the pathway leading to spontaneous cell death, or apoptosis. To a certain degree, cell proliferation and apoptosis seem to concur since some modulators of cell proliferation can also trigger the onset of apoptosis or can repress it. Representatives of a group of positive regulators of both processes have been found among cellular as well as viral proteins, such as c-*myc* (Evan et al., 1992), c-*fos* (Preston et al., 1996), cyclin D1 (Kranenburg, van der Eb, & Zantema, 1996; Sofer-Levi & Resnitzky, 1996), cyclin A (Hoang et al., 1994), E2F (Qin, Livingston, Kaelin, & Adams, 1994; Shan & Lee, 1994), and viral oncogenes (Howes et al., 1994). Conversely, the retinoblastoma protein, pRb, is a candidate with growth-suppressive properties and protective properties against apoptosis. The pathway of association of pRb with the transcription factor, E2F, may be important in inducing apoptosis. Indeed, pRb and its related pocket proteins such as p107 and p130 block G1/S transition in a variety of cell types by binding and thereby sequestering E2F, which is essential for entering S phase (Ewen, 1994). The activity of pRb is regulated by the cyclin-dependent kinases (CDK)-4, CDK-6, and CDK-2 complexed with specific regulatory subunits of cyclins D and E, respectively, during late G1 (Yamato et al., 1997). They inactivate pRb by phosphorylating it at multiple tyrosine residue sites. Hyperphosphorylated pRb

releases the transcription factor E2F in late G1 phase, allowing cells to enter S phase (Liu, Dawes, Lu, Shubeita, & Zhu, 1997). Negative regulation of CDK complexes is mediated via inhibitor peptides, such as p21$^{cip1/waf1}$ and p27$^{kip1}$ (Marches, Scheuermann, & Uhr, 1998). It is critical to characterize the effects of FAE upon these molecular immune mechanisms, and upon neuroendocrine–immune interactive pathways, to elucidate further the cellular immune events impaired by FAE and to determine whether FAE preferentially induces T cells to engage in apoptosis rather than maturation.

### 3. FAE Affects T-Cell Maturation

The maturation of T cells is characterized by marked changes in naive T cells phenotypically as well as functionally. Phenotypically, naive T cells lose the A (human) or the C (rodent) restriction fragment of CD45, the common leukocyte antigen, and acquire the 0 fragment. Functionally, naive T cells acquire the capability of producing cytokines, and eventually establish a TH1 or a TH2 pattern of cytokines, which plays a pivotal role in determining immune surveillance in vivo (for review, Chiappelli et al., 1998; Romagnani, 1996).

In our studies on the phenotypic maturation of thymocytes in male FAE rats, we examined the proportion of CD4+ and CD8+ thymocytes that express or are devoid of the maturational markers, the alpha/beta configuration of the T-cell receptor (TcR) and CD45RC (Taylor, Tio, & Chiappelli, 1999). We noted significant age-dependent effects on the numbers of total double positive CD4-TcR and CD8-TcR or CD45RC thymocytes and significantly lower numbers of total CD4+ and CD8+ cells in FAE than in control rats at 20, 28, 35, and 48 days of age, a finding consistent with the significantly lower total number of thymocytes in FAE than in control rats throughout this period. The developmental patterns for both markers were similar in FAE and control groups, in both the rising (days 20–28) and the declining (days 35–48) phases. However, on day 35, FAE rats had significantly lower numbers of double positive CD8-TcR and -CD45RC cells than control rats. It therefore appears that FAE tends to accelerate the decline of double positive CD8-TcR and CD8-CD45RC cells. The contribution of this phenotypic change to the thymic functional alterations induced by FAE remains to be determined.

### 4. FAE and Monocyte/Macrophage Function

We have begun to monitor the effects of FAE upon monocyte/macrophage function. In a first set of studies, we chose a design that involved the in vivo priming of the peripheral myeloid populations with a low dose of LPS (5 μg/kg), considered to be suboptimal from the perspective of mounting detectable levels of circulating monokines. An hour and a half after priming, we monitored the production of immunoreactive TNF-$\alpha$ in response to a further in vitro challenge of peripheral blood mononuclear cells with LPS (2.5 μg/mL). We showed that the response to the LPS pathogen in vitro after priming was significantly blunted in male FAE rats compared with that seen in control male animals. FAE female rats, either intact or ovariectomized (OVX), failed to show significant differences in the priming response, compared with the respective control female animals. Furthermore, there was no correlation between plasma corticosterone levels and TNF-$\alpha$ production after priming in any of the groups (Chiappelli et al., 1997). These results support the putative role of gonadal hormones in the neuroendocrine modulation of macrophage responses (Grossman, 1990) and provide another demonstration of the previously cited observation that fetal alcohol-induced alterations in cellular immune responses are most often detected in male, rather than in female, FAE rats (Weinberg & Jerrells, 1991; Redei, Halasz, Prystowsky, & Aird, 1993).

### 5. FAE and B-Cell Responses and Antibody Production

The development of immunity to an antigenic challenge, such as with keyhole limpet hemocyanin (KLH), reflects the integrated action of those immune processes normally invoked during the host response to antigenic challenge, including T/B-cell interactions leading to B-cell activation, Ig production, and isotype switching. Antibody secretion and isotype switching depend upon certain cytokines produced by TH1 cells (e.g., IL-2, IFN) and TH2 cells (e.g., IL-4, IL-5), as discussed above. The patterns of generation and interaction of TH1 and TH2 cells and T-cell cytokine production that occur in response to an antigenic challenge are modulated by the regulatory influences on gene expression exerted by glucocorticoids and androgens (Daynes & Araneo, 1989; Purkerson & Isakson, 1992). Thus, it is reasonable to expect that physiologic alterations capable of enhancing the output of glucocorticoids, such as stress or ethanol, would repress immune responses that depend upon IL-2 or IFN for optimal expression while augmenting those that are driven by IL-4 and IL-5.

To study the integrated immune response of FAE subjects, we have begun to assess T-cell-dependent responses in vivo with the T-dependent antigen, KLH. At 7, 14, and 21 days after immunization with KLH, production of the immunoglobulins, IgM and IgG, was determined by an enzyme-linked immunosorbent assay (ELISA) (Laudenslager et al., 1988), modified in our laboratory. We found no effects of FAE on IgM production in either males or females. In contrast, IgG production was suppressed after a high dose of KLH (250 μg/kg) in male FAE rats while it was enhanced in response to a low dose (10 μg/kg) in FAE females. Interestingly, maternal pair-feeding also enhanced the IgG response of female offspring. Given that IgM production was unaffected by FAE, it appears that FAE affects the switch from IgM to IgG production in response to KLH and that this is another gender-specific effect of FAE (Taylor, Tio, Pilati, Tritt, & Chiappelli, 1995). Cytokine production by lymphocytes in KLH-challenged FAE and control rats remains to be characterized.

## III. FAE AND NEUROIMMUNE INTERACTIONS

Considerable evidence now exists for bidirectional communication between the immune system and the central nervous system (CNS), such that the immune system can signal the brain to initiate physiological and behavioral processes that promote recovery following infection (reviewed in Besedovsky & Del Rey, 1996; Maier & Watkins, 1998). Infection characteristically elicits fever and a series of systemic and behavioral responses that collectively have been termed "sickness behavior" (Hart, 1988; Kent, Bluthe, Kelley, & Dantzer, 1992). The fever and its nonthermal correlates (i.e., behavioral responses such as anorexia and immobility, metabolic responses such as hepatic synthesis of acute-phase proteins and other chemical changes detectable in blood, neuroendocrine responses such as activation of glucocorticoid release, and immune responses such as activation of lymphocytes) represent a primary host defense response to infection (Blatteis, 1988; Kluger, 1991; Kent et al., 1992). Cytokines, released from antigen-activated immune cells, play a key role as regulators of the host defense response by providing bidirectional signals to the immune system and to the CNS (Besedovsky & Del Rey, 1996). Accumulating evidence, as reviewed below, indicates that FAE affects both directions of this communication, i.e., CNS to immune and immune to CNS signaling. Indeed, impairment of this cytokine-mediated reciprocal communication between the immune and the nervous systems may be an important risk factor for increased susceptibility to infection and altered immune competence of children exposed to alcohol in utero.

## A. FAE Alters the Communication from the CNS to the Immune System

The CNS controls peripheral organs such as those of the immune system by two major outflow systems, i.e., the autonomic nervous system and the neuroendocrine system. In the following sections we discuss evidence for the effects of FAE on CNS signaling to the immune system via these outflow systems.

### 1. FAE and Autonomic Innervation of Lymphoid Organs

Sympathetic innervation of lymphoid organs, e.g., thymus and spleen, has been shown to play an important role in regulating immune responses (Felten et al., 1987). Although the effects of prenatal alcohol exposure per se on the development of sympathetic innervation of lymphoid organs during gestation have not been studied, the developmental pattern of autonomic innervation of the thymus provides some indications as to possible periods of vulnerability. Both myelinated and unmyelinated fibers of the autonomic nervous system are known to innervate the thymus (Bulloch, Cullen, Schwartz, & Longo, 1987). Acetylcholinesterase-positive fibers innervate the murine thymic cortex and the corticomedullary junction as early as gestational day 18. This pattern of innervation is similar to that seen in fully developed mature murine thymus. Perivascular catecholaminergic innervation of the thymus is also evident at gestational day 18. In mature murine thymus, catecholaminergic innervation is both perivascular and nonperivascular, particularly within the cortical area. This pattern of innervation is apparent only within the third week of postnatal life in the mouse. The hypothesis that catecholaminergic innervation of the thymus modulates the regulation of the influx/efflux of lymphocytes from the blood stream through the thymic tissue, while innervation by cholinergic fibers is critical to the maturation and differentiation of the thymus, as originally proposed (Bulloch et al., 1987), still requires testing, particularly within the context of FAE.

Biochemical evidence confirms the existence of adrenergic receptors early in thymic development. At gestational day 18, the level of $\beta$-adrenergic receptors in fetal thymus is comparable to that found in adult thymus, as determined by binding studies with the potent $\beta$-adrenergic antagonist, dihydroalprenolol (Singh, Millson, Smith, & Owen, 1979). The immuno-

functional relevance of lymphocytic adrenergic receptors is suggested by studies such as those demonstrating an enhancement of expression of the activation marker, Tac (CD25, low molecular weight $\alpha$ subunit of the IL-2 receptor), by human lymphocytes after treatment with the $\beta$-adrenoreceptor antagonist, propanolol ($10^{-6}$ M) (Malec & Novak, 1988).

The spleen, as does the thymus, receives rich noradrenergic innervation. In the rat, noradrenergic nerve fibers are present in the white pulp of the spleen at birth. Innervation is evident among surface IgM-positive B lymphocytes at the outer border of the periarteriolar lymphatic sheath, distally from the central artery. Noradrenergic innervation develops steadily in the first 3 to 4 weeks of life (Ackerman, Felten, Bellinger, & Felten, 1987; Ackerman, Felten, Dijkstra, Livnat, & Felten, 1989). A selective age-related loss of sympathetic noradrenergic nerve endings from the spleen and other lymphoid organs occurs in the rodent, whereas the nerve fiber density rises dramatically in the thymus. Decreased splenic noradrenergic innervation in aging rodents has been attributed to cumulative oxidative metabolic autodestruction of nerve terminals by high concentrations of norepinephrine released during specific time periods of immunologic reactivity, which can be prevented by L-deprenyl (Madden, Thyagarajan, & Felten, 1998).

It has been reported that FAE leads to a selective developmental delay of sympathetic innervation of the thymus and spleen but not the heart (Gottesfeld et al., 1990). The young adult (5–10 weeks of age) progeny of C57BL/6J mice born from dams exposed to ethanol (25% EDC) throughout gestation exhibited decreased in vivo measures of cell-mediated immunity (e.g., contact hypersensitivity, local graft vs. host response), and altered synaptic transmission in noradrenergic fibers of lymphoid organs—that is, a rise in splenic and thymic, but not cardiac, norepinephrine turnover, a drop in the norepinephrine content, and a drop in $\beta$-adrenergic receptor number, but a retention of the "sympatolymphoid" noradrenergic system of innervation of the spleen (Gottesfeld et al., 1990). Chronic, but not acute, treatments with nerve growth factor reversed the FAE-related deficits in splenic norepinephrine concentrations as well as in pineal N-acetyltransferase activity in a time- and age-dependent manner (Gottesfeld, Simpson, Yuwiler, & Perez-Polo, 1996). The splenic neural response (i.e., norepinephrine turnover) to immune signals, such as endotoxin and IL-1$\beta$ is blunted in FAE cohorts (Gottesfeld, Simpson, & Maier, 1997). Taken together, these findings have led to the hypothesis that, because the sympathetic outflow to lymphoid organs is considered an important immune modulator, the anomalous neural response to immune signals may partly account for the impaired cellular immunity and, thus, for the increased susceptibility to infections associated with FAE (Gottesfeld et al., 1997).

## 2. FAE and Immune Responsiveness to Stress

One of the hallmarks of FAE in adult rodent models is enhanced HPA responsiveness to certain physical and pharmacological stressors, including ethanol, morphine, LPS, and IL-$1\beta$ (Lee & Rivier, 1996; Nelson et al., 1986; Taylor, Branch, Liu, & Kokka, 1982; Taylor, Branch, van Zuylen, & Redei, 1988; Taylor et al., 1981; Weinberg, 1989). Maternal drinking during pregnancy has also been found to be associated with higher poststress cortisol levels in infants (Jacobson, Jacobson, Bihun, Chiodo, & Sokol, 1993). In view of the role of the neuroendocrine outflow pathway in CNS–immune system communication (Besedovsky & Del Rey, 1996; Maier & Watkins, 1998) and the stress hyperresponsiveness associated with FAE, it is of interest to assess the effect of stress upon immune surveillance in FAE subjects.

### a. FAE and Cold Stress

To study the possible interactive effects of FAE and exposure to cold stress, differential vulnerability to this challenge was assessed in 5 to 6-month-old female and male offspring (Giberson et al., 1997). The stimulation of splenocytes by Con A and by the B-cell mitogen, pokeweed mitogen (PWM), was significantly increased in stressed female FAE rats compared to control females 1 day following the cold stress, but not prior to the stress paradigm or after 3 days of stress. Lymphocyte proliferation was unaffected before or after cold stress in male FAE rats. These findings appeared not to be correlated with HPA responses, since after cold stress for 1 or 3 days, females, regardless of prenatal treatment, and only FAE males had significantly elevated basal plasma corticosterone levels. These findings implicate the involvement of gonadal hormones in the stress-induced lymphocyte response since only FAE females responded to cold stress. These findings also indicate that the interactive effects of FAE and cold stress may result in enhanced rather than suppressed immune responsiveness in the female progeny 24 h following the stress (Giberson et al., 1997).

Indeed, these results complement an earlier report that showed that adult stressed FAE males (3-week chronic intermittent, variety of stressors to prevent habituation) had a greater reduction in the number of pan-T cells in the thymus, but, by contrast, showed an increased expression of peripheral blood pan-T antigen, compared to controls. Stressed FAE animals also showed reduced numbers of peripheral blood CD4+ T cells compared to nonstressed FAE males. These effects were noted preferentially in FAE males rather than females (Giberson & Weinberg, 1995).

### b. FAE and Food Restriction

We have examined the effects of restriction of food availability, a reliable stress model for studying neuroendocrine–immune interactions since it leads to significant HPA activation to which rats do not habituate (Amkraut, Solomon, Kasper, & Purdue, 1972; Gallo & Weinberg, 1981; Gilman-Sachs, Kim, Pollard, & Snyder, 1991; Meites, 1990). We monitored the phenotypic maturation of thymocytes in FAE male and female rats at 30–35 days of age. We observed that food restriction induced significant changes in body weight, thymus weight-to-body weight ratio, adrenal weight-to-body weight ratio, plasma corticosterone levels, as well as thymocyte number and the percentage and absolute number of CD4+ and CD8+ thymocytes that express CD45RC; however, FAE and control male and female rats were equally affected. These results indicate that food restriction is an example of a stressful stimulus that is too stringent to permit any distinction between FAE and control rats of prepubertal age (Taylor, Tio, & Chiappelli, 1995).

### c. FAE and Alcohol Ingestion

Alcohol consumption, in and of itself, is a significant stressor, i.e., an effective stimulus for activation of the HPA axis. Therefore, it is of interest to establish the effects of alcohol consumption upon immune surveillance in FAE subjects. In one study (Halasz, Aird, Li, Prystowsky, & Redei, 1993), prolonged ethanol exposure activated the HPA axis and suppressed T-cell function. FAE led to a specific HPA-related vulnerability in males to the effects of ethanol in adulthood, i.e., FAE decreased anterior pituitary pro-opiomelanocortin (POMC) mRNA levels and increased glucocorticoid receptor (GR) mRNA levels in males, while in FAE females, GR mRNA levels were decreased. There were no differences in hypothalamic corticotropin releasing factor (CRF) mRNA and GR mRNA levels between the prenatal treatment groups, nor was there a significant difference in Con A-stimulated lymphocyte proliferation between FAE and PF males. In contrast, FAE females showed Con A-stimulated lymphocyte proliferation significantly higher than those of PF females. This finding of an enhanced Con A-stimulated lymphocyte proliferative response is reminiscent of the cold stress results in FAE females, summarized above.

A recent study (Jerrells & Weinberg, 1998) confirmed that long-term consumption of ethanol diets in adulthood produced significant immunosuppressive effects on T-cell responses to Con A, LPS, and IL-2 in both males and females. In this study, however, FAE did not further aggravate the immunosuppressive effects of chronic alcohol exposure in either males or females.

Whether FAE effects on lymphocyte trafficking, and consequent expression of adhesion molecules and homing receptors, may be responsible for the observed stress-induced outcomes remains to be determined.

## B.  FAE Alters the Communication from the Immune System to the CNS

During infection, the initial host defense response is elicited by bacterial endotoxin or other pathogen products which stimulate macrophages and monocytes to release cytokines, such as IL-$1\beta$, TNF-$\alpha$, and IL-6, into the circulation to mediate the activation of and interactions among various components of the immune system (Kundel & Remik, 1992). The release of cytokines by cells of the immune system provides a sensory-like signal to the nervous system, alerting it to pathogen-induced immune activation (Maier & Watkins, 1998; Schobitz, De Kloet, & Holsboer, 1994). It is currently postulated that cytokines produced in the periphery by macrophages in response to LPS induce the production of IL-$1\beta$ within the brain, as reflected by increased brain IL-$1\beta$ immunoreactivity (Van Dam, Bauer, Tilders, & Berkenbosch, 1995), bioactivity (Quan, Sundar, & Weiss, 1994), and mRNA (Laye et al., 1995). The effect of LPS on brain IL-$1\beta$ is mediated by the vagus nerve since severing the vagus prevents the induction of brain IL-$1\beta$ following intraperitoneal (ip) administration of LPS (Laye et al., 1995; Watkins, Maier, & Goehler, 1995).

Cytokines in general, and IL-$1\beta$ in particular, affect neural, neuroendocrine, and behavioral function via specific receptors located throughout the CNS (Maier & Watkins, 1998; Rothwell, 1991; Schobitz et al., 1994). The interaction of IL-$1\beta$ with its receptors, particularly within the hypothalamus, produces an increase in body temperature by raising the thermoregulatory set point (Kluger, 1991; Rothwell, 1993). Also acting at the hypothalamic level, these cytokines exert potent effects on the hypothalamo-pituitary axis, generally activating the HPA axis, but with varying species-dependent effects on the other neuroendocrine axes

(Besedovsky & Del Rey, 1996; McCann, Rettori, Milenkovic, Jurcovicova, & Gonzalez, 1990; Schobitz et al., 1994). During infections, these cytokines also facilitate behavioral patterns which promote conservation of heat and body resources, while inhibiting goal-directed behavior (Yirmiya, 1996, 1997; Maier & Watkins, 1998). Following administration of IL-$1\beta$, motor activity is retarded (Avitsur, Donchin, Cohen, & Yirmiya, 1995; Otterness, Seymour, Golden, Reynolds, & Daumy, 1988), slow-wave sleep is increased (Krueger, Walter, Dinarello, Wolff, & Chedid, 1984), and marked suppression of food ingestion (Mrosovsky, Molony, Conn, & Kluger, 1989), exploratory behavior (Dunn, Antoon, & Chapman, 1991), social activity (Crestani, Seguy, & Dantzer, 1991), and sexual behavior (Avitsur, Pollak, & Yirmiya, 1997; Yirmiya, Avitsur, Donchin, & Cohen, 1995) are observed.

### 1.  FAE and Cytokines

Consumption of alcohol by adult rats, as well as exposure of immune cells to alcohol in vitro, alters the induction and release of several cytokines, particularly TNF-$\alpha$. Alterations in TNF-$\alpha$ production, for example, have been reported in patients with alcoholic hepatitis and cirrhosis (Khoruts, Stahnke, McClain, Logan & Allen, 1991; McClain & Cohen, 1989; Muzes et al., 1989). Moreover, TNF-$\alpha$ secretion by macrophages taken from healthy human volunteers was suppressed by exposure to alcohol in vitro (Bermundez, Wu, Marinelli, & Young, 1991). In experimental animals, both acute (Nelson, Bagby, Bainton, & Summer, 1989; Nelson, Bagby, & Summer, 1989) and chronic (Chen, Huang, Watzl, & Watson, 1993; Na & Seelig, 1994; Nanji, Hossein Sadrzadeh, Thomas, & Yamanaka, 1994; Wang, Huang, & Watson, 1994; Wang & Watson, 1994) alcohol administration significantly decreased spontaneous and mitogen-stimulated secretion of TNF-$\alpha$.

In view of the immune consequences of FAE, and the marked effects of alcohol on cytokine secretion in adult animals, we examined the effects of FAE on LPS-induced secretion of TNF-$\alpha$ (Yirmiya, Chiappelli, Tio, Tritt, & Taylor, 1998) and several other cytokines, i.e., IL-$1\beta$ IL-6, and IL-10 in blood (Taylor, Tio, & Yirmiya, 1999). TNF-$\alpha$ secretion was maximal within 2 h after LPS (Yirmiya et al., 1996) as was that of IL-10, while secretion of IL-$1\beta$ was maximal at 4 h and that of IL-6 was higher at 2 and 4 h than at 6 h. FAE did not affect either the pattern or amount of cytokine secretion in blood in males. Blood levels of LPS-induced TNF-$\alpha$ were also unaffected in FAE females. In contrast, blood levels of LPS-induced TNF-$\alpha$ were significantly reduced by FAE in OVX females compared to that seen in controls, an effect that was not reversed by long-term estradiol replacement (Yirmiya et al., 1998). The particular sensitivity of FAE rats to ovariectomy in this in vivo paradigm (in contrast to the in vitro priming experiment reported above) may be related to the known dysregulation of gonadotropin releasing hormone expression and luteinizing hormone secretory patterns in these rats (Handa, McGivern, Noble, & Gorski, 1985; Wilson, Marshall, Bollnow, McGivern, & Handa, 1995).

Peripheral administration of LPS has been shown to induce IL-1$\beta$ production in the brain, as reflected by increased brain IL-1$\beta$ immunoreactivity (Hagan, Poole, & Bristow, 1993; Hillhouse & Mosley, 1993; Nguyen et al., 1998; Van Dam et al., 1995), bioactivity (Laye et al., 1995), and mRNA and gene expression (Goujon et al., 1995; Laye et al., 1995). These studies indicate that in addition to the hippocampus and brain stem, the hypothalamus is a particularly rich source of IL-1$\beta$, which is detectable at 2 or more h following injection of LPS systemically. We assessed LPS-induced IL-1$\beta$ secretion in the brain in two studies. In the first, normal (N) 60-day-old male rats, offspring of dams fed a liquid diet supplemented with ethanol (FAE) and pair-fed control offspring (PF) were injected with LPS (50–1000 µg/kg, ip). At 4–6 h after LPS injection, brains were removed, dissected and the hypothalamic, hippocampal, and brain-stem regions were excised and frozen. Tissue homogenates were prepared in radioimmunoprecipitation assay (RIPA) buffer supplemented with phosphatase and protease inhibitors (usually 1:1, wet weight:volume), separated in a standard denaturing SDS-$\beta$-mercaptoethanol Tris-glycine buffer, 10–20% gradient polyacrylamide gel with a 4% stacking gel, and analyzed by Western blot. A prestained SDS–PAGE low-range

reference standard (Bio-Rad) was added to the gel. Following transfer, the nitrocellulose membranes were incubated with rabbit anti-rat IL-1$\beta$ (Cytokine Sciences) and rabbit anti-rat actin as control, and the gels were stained with goat anti-rabbit horseradish peroxidase. The developed membranes were photographed and scanned. Band intensities were assessed with the Photoshop (ADOBE) computer software, and expressed as the difference between the band intensity and background. This value was then expressed as the percentage of the actin control band and of that obtained for the corresponding band on the molecular weight standard lane.

As shown in Figure 2, all animals tested in the three groups at 6 h after 1.0 mg/kg LPS exhibited only one band slightly above the band corresponding to actin, that is, at a molecular weight corresponding to that of the IL-1$\beta$ pro-form (Dinarello, 1996). The lower doses and shorter time points tested resulted in no detectable product with the anti-rat IL-1$\beta$ antibody used. The detected pro-IL-1$\beta$ band was not a contaminant or an artifact produced by the anti-actin antibody since it could be detected equally well in the absence or the presence of anti-actin antibody. In all experiments performed, pro-IL-1$\beta$ was mainly expressed in hypothalamic extracts with less expression in hippocampus and brain stem. Individual differences in pro-IL-1$\beta$ band intensity can be observed, as noted in Figure 2. Computerized analysis of the intensity of the pro-IL-1$\beta$ band in the hippocampus, brain stem, and hypothalamus lane on a gray scale produced a reliable quantification of the band standardized for its own background, for its corresponding actin band, and for the proximal molecular weight standard on the gel (actin, approx. 43 kDa molecular weight, comigrates with the ovalbumin 45 to 46-kDa standard). This operation permitted the

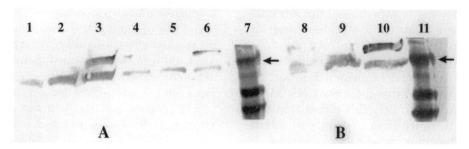

**FIGURE 2**　Effects of fetal alcohol exposure (FAE) on production of proIL-1$\beta$ in hippocampus, brain stem, and hypothalamus 6 h after ip LPS (1 mg/kg). The figure presents Western blots of two independent gels (A and B) immunostained with polyclonal rabbit anti-actin antibody (arrow) and polyclonal rabbit anti-rat IL-1$\beta$ antibody. Tissue homogenates from one representative pair-fed (lanes 1–3), FAE (lanes 4–6), and normal animal (lanes 8–10) are shown. Hippocampus homogenates are shown in lanes 1, 4, and 8; brain stem homogenates are shown in lanes 2, 5, and 9; hypothalamus homogenates are shown in lanes 3, 6, and 10. Low molecular weight standards are given in lanes 7 and 11.

**TABLE I** Pro-IL-1β Band Intensities across Animals and Experiments Presented as Percentage of Standard Band Intensity on Computerized Gray Scale

| Group | Brain region | | |
| | Hippocampus | Brain stem | Hypothalamus |
| --- | --- | --- | --- |
| Normal | $29.0+0^a$ (1)[b] | 19.0+0 (1) | 44.8+18.0 (4) |
| Pair fed | 27.3+8.1 (4) | 38.8+11.8 (4) | 183.2+34.3 (5) |
| FAE | 30.6+8.1 (5) | 21.3+11.3(4) | 126.8+33.4 (6) |

Note. FAE, fetal alcohol exposure.
[a]Data expressed as mean+SEM of band intensity as percent of the intensity of the control band.
[b]Number of animals tested.

compilation of summary statistics across gels and across experiments (Table I) and indicated that while there were no significant differences among the FAE, PF, and N groups in terms of pro-IL-1β detected in hippocampus and brain stem, there was significantly more pro-IL-1β in hypothalami of PF than N rats. FAE hypothalami showed a similar trend.

Using a highly sensitive rat IL-1β ELISA kit (R & D Systems, Minneapolis MN) (cf. Nguyen et al., 1998), we found that FAE altered the kinetics of LPS-induced hypothalamic IL-1β production, i.e., at 2 h, but not at 4 and 6 h following LPS administration, hypothalamic content of IL-1β was significantly lower in FAE than in normal rats (Taylor, Tio, & Yirmiya, 1999). The significance of this reduction in hypothalamic IL-1β, albeit short-lived, to neuroimmune function in FAE is discussed below.

## C. FAE, Fever, and Sickness Behavior

Fever is a component of the acute-phase response elicited by infectious agents and serves to enhance host defense responses to infection. Indeed, it has been documented that elevated body temperature reduces the morbidity and mortality caused by a variety of pathogens (Kluger, 1991; Moltz, 1993). Whereas IL-1β is regarded as the major endogenous pyrogen, IL-6 and, to a lesser extent, TNF-α also produce fever.

### 1. LPS, IL-1β, Fever, and Sickness Behavior

FAE has been shown to affect neuroimmune interactions, including the febrile response to LPS. We have reported that FAE rats manifest markedly decreased LPS-induced fever (i.e., they require a higher dose than control rats to show any LPS-induced hyperthermia, and even with the higher LPS

dose, they manifest a weaker hyperthermia, which declines faster than that in control animals) (Yirmiya et al., 1993). LPS-induced fever is at least partly mediated by the endogenous release of IL-1β. Administration of IL-1β antiserum suppresses the fever (Long, Otterness, Kunkel, Vandar, & Kluger, 1990) and the increase in thermogenic and metabolic responses (Rothwell, 1993) induced by LPS. Similarly, administration of the human IL-1β receptor antagonist also partially suppresses LPS-induced fever in rats (Smith & Kluger, 1992). These findings suggest that the reduced LPS-induced fever in FAE rats may result from an impairment in the response to IL-1β. We assessed this hypothesis by examining the effects of IL-1β on body temperature as well as on other behavioral and neuroendocrine parameters, including motor activity, ingestive behavior, and pituitary-adrenal activation in FAE and control rats (Yirmiya et al., 1996). Transmitters for continuous biotelemetric recording of body temperature and motor activity were implanted ip in FAE, PF, and N 60-day-old male rats.

In one experiment, FAE, PF, and N rats were injected with either saline (Sal) or IL-1β (2 μg/kg, ip) during the light period and body temperature and activity levels were recorded continuously for 8 h. Baseline body temperature and activity levels were not different among the groups. Rats in all groups responded with an initial transient increase in body temperature, attributable to the stress of the injection protocol (Figure 3). IL-1β-injected rats began to develop fever at 100 min after the injection, which subsided around 420 min postinjection. IL-1β-induced fever was significantly lower in FAE rats than in N and PF rats (Figure 3).

In order to characterize the effects of FAE on aspects of sickness behavior, in another experiment rats were administered either IL-1β (10 μg/kg, ip) or Sal immediately prior to the onset of the dark period, and body temperature, activity, and 24-h food and water consumption were monitored. Under these conditions, IL-1β produced a biphasic effect on body temperature, resulting in an initial hypothermia (at 90–150 min) followed by a longer-lasting hyperthermia (at 240–420 min). There were no differential effects of FAE on the extent and duration of the hypothermia. During the second phase, fever in the FAE rats was significantly lower than in the PF rats, but comparable to fever in the N rats. IL-1β significantly reduced motor activity during both the hypothermic and hyperthermic phases. This effect was similar in all prenatal treatment groups. IL-1β also significantly suppressed 24-h food consumption in N and PF rats and water consumption in PF rats,

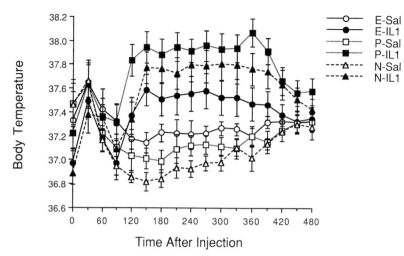

**FIGURE 3**   Effects of fetal alcohol exposure (FAE) on IL-1β-induced alterations in body temperature during the light phase of the circadian cycle. Mean (±SEM) body temperature (°C) in rats exposed prenatally to ethanol (E), pair-feeding (P), or normal diet (N). Male rats within each of the prenatal treatment groups were injected with either IL-1β (2 μg/kg, ip) or saline (Sal) at the beginning of the light period and body temperature was recorded continuously by a biotelemetric system for 8 h (from Yirmiya et al., 1996).

but it did not affect food and water consumption in FAE rats.

Overall these findings are consistent with many other studies demonstrating similar IL-1β-induced sickness behavior symptoms (Rothwell, 1991; Kent et al., 1992). The effects of IL-1β on motor activity were observed only during the dark period, probably because activity during the light phase is already very low, creating a floor effect. Interestingly, suppression of motor activity was observed during both the hypothermic and hyperthermic responses to IL-1β, indicating that this behavioral effect of IL-1β is not secondary to IL-1β's effect on body temperature. Together, these findings indicate that exposure to ethanol in utero produces impairments in mechanisms that mediate the effects of IL-1β on the febrile response (particularly during the light period) and ingestive behavior, but not on motor activity (cf. Table II).

The blunting effect of FAE on the febrile response following ip administration of LPS or IL-1β may reflect a decrease in the production of brain IL-1β and/or alterations in neurochemical signaling mechanisms, which are affected by brain IL-1β. Having observed an alteration in the production kinetics of IL-1β in FAE rats (as described above), it was of interest to determine whether intracerebroventricular (icv) administration of IL-1β could bypass this FAE-related impairment and produce a normal febrile response. Infusion of IL-1β (20 ng/rat) via an icv cannula produced characteristic febrile responses (cf. Figure 3) in N and PF 60-day-old male rats. However,

the febrile response of FAE rats was significantly blunted (Taylor et al., 1999) (cf. Table II). These results indicate that FAE has a direct effect on central mechanisms which mediate the pyrogenic effects of IL-1β. In contrast, there were no differential effects of FAE on icv IL-1β-induced ingestive behavior, although food and water consumption and body weight were significantly reduced in the 24-h period after icv IL-1β in all groups.

Having found that the febrile response to icv IL-1 was blunted in FAE rats, it was of interest to ascertain whether this was indicative of a general impairment of thermoregulatory effector mechanisms in FAE rats, which mediate the febrile response. Our recent results with icv administration of PGE₂, which bypasses the IL-1β signal and produces fever by acting directly on temperature-sensitive neurons in the hypothalamus (Scammell, Elmquist, Griffin, & Saper, 1996; Sehic & Blatteis, 1996), indicated that FAE rats have a normal febrile response to exogenously administered PGE₂ (Taylor et al., 1999) (cf. Table II). Taken together, these results strongly implicate a FAE-induced impairment in one or more of the central neurochemical signaling mechanisms for the febrile response, perhaps PGE₂ itself.

### 2. Mechanisms for the Effects of FAE on Fever

Although numerous mechanisms have been proposed to mediate the febrile effects of IL-1β (see Kluger, Bartfai, & Dinarello, 1998), this discussion will focus on several thermoregulatory mechanisms which

**TABLE II   Comparison of LPS- and IL-1β-Induced Fever and Sickness Behavior in FAE and Control Rats**

| Treatment | Effects in control rats | Effects in FAE rats |
|---|---|---|
| LPS (ip) | | |
| Males | Fever | Blunting of the febrile response |
| IL-1β (ip, light period) | | |
| Males | Fever | Blunting of the febrile response |
| Males | Fever | Fever |
| (offspring of adrenalectomized dams) | | |
| Females | Fever | Blunting of the febrile response |
| IL-1β (ip, dark period) | | |
| Males | Hypothermia followed by fever | Blunting of the febrile response (compared to pair-fed) |
| | Anorexia | Blunting of anorexia |
| | Reduced locomotion | Reduced locomotion |
| Females | Hypothermia followed by fever | Enhanced hypothermia and blunting of the febrile response |
| IL-1β (icv, light period) | | |
| Males | Fever | Blunting of the febrile response |
| | Anorexia | Anorexia |
| PGE₂ | | |
| Males | Fever | Fever |

Note. LPS, lipopolysaccharide; IL, interleukin.

are known to be affected by exposure to alcohol in utero and thus may be involved in the effects of FAE on fever production.

### a. HPA Hormones

Glucocorticoids are potent inhibitors of many actions of IL-1β, either directly by blocking its synthesis or secondarily by blocking its effects, e.g., on fever and thermogenesis. IL-1β-induced fever was almost completely prevented by preadministration of the synthetic glucocorticoid, dexamethasone (Carey et al., 1990). This effect of glucocorticoids is at least partly mediated by the release of lipocortin-1, which acts as an endogenous inhibitor of the pyrogenic and thermogenic responses to IL-1β (Carey et al., 1990), probably by interfering with the thermogenic effects of CRF (Strijbos, Hardwick, Relton, Carey, & Rothwell, 1992). Moreover, alterations in the concentration and/or sensitivity to glucocorticoids, which increase the release of endogenous lipocortin-1, may be responsible for the impaired IL-1β-induced febrile response of aging mice (Strijbos, Hardwick, Relton, Carey, & Rothwell, 1993). Consistent with these findings, we found that male PF rats, which showed significantly lower levels of IL-1β-induced corticosterone secretion, also showed significantly elevated IL-1β-induced fever compared to FAE rats when IL-1β was administered at the onset of the dark period

(Yirmiya et al., 1996). Although IL-1β-induced corticosterone secretion was not differentially affected by FAE in male rats (Yirmiya et al., 1996, 1998), hypothalamic glucocorticoid receptor expression has been shown to be increased in adult FAE progeny (Redei et al., 1993) and the resulting augmented sensitivity to normal corticoid levels could contribute to their decreased febrile response.

CRF has been shown to be involved in several components of the febrile response, including stimulation of sympathetic outflow, thermogenesis, and activity of brown adipose tissue (BAT) (Rothwell, 1993). These effects are probably independent of the role of CRF in activation of the HPA axis, which actually inhibits IL-1β-induced fever (see above). Administration of exogenous IL-1β-induces the release of hypothalamic CRF, which mediates the effects of IL-1β on fever and thermogenesis. For example, icv administration of a CRF receptor antagonist or neutralizing antibody to CRF inhibits the febrile and thermogenic responses to IL-1β (Strijbos et al., 1992). FAE has been shown to alter hypothalamic CRF levels, although the results of such studies are not consistent, showing either an increase (Lee et al., 1990; Redei et al., 1993) or no change (Lee and Rivier, 1993) in CRF mRNA levels. On the other hand, CRF content in the median eminence is decreased in FAE rats (Lee & Rivier, 1994). If the latter finding represents a decrease of CRF content in nerve terminals of the median eminence of FAE rats, particularly during the light period of the circadian cycle, a reduced thermogenic response to IL-1$\beta$ could be expected following FAE, consistent with the results reported above.

### b. Gonadal Hormones

Female rats exhibit less LPS-induced fever than male rats (Murakami & Ono, 1987) and less IL-1$\beta$-induced fever (Taylor et al., 1998b). Moreover, castrated male rats have lower febrile responses than intact male rats, and androgenization of females by injection of testosterone (T) on the first postnatal day produces a male-like febrile response in adult females (Murakami & Ono, 1987).

Similarly, FAE-induced alterations in perinatal T levels may contribute to the gender differences in neuroimmune and neuroendocrine function repeatedly alluded to above. For example, male neonates exposed to alcohol in utero do not exhibit the normal preparturition T surge (McGivern, Raum, Salido, & Redei, 1988; Revskoy et al., 1997) and their plasma levels of T are significantly depressed from control levels on the day of birth (Rudeen, 1988). Consistent with these findings, FAE feminizes physiological and behavioral systems in male rats (McGivern et al., 1984), and the size of the sexually dimorphic nucleus of the preoptic hypothalamus (Barron, Tieman, & Riley, 1988; Ahmed, Shryne, Gorski, Branch, & Taylor, 1991). Serum T levels as well as testis, prostate, and seminal vesicle weights were significantly reduced in 55-day-old FAE rats compared to control rats (Udani, Parker, Gavaler, & Van Thiel, 1985). These findings suggest the testable hypothesis that the blunted febrile response in FAE males may result from a FAE-induced feminization of this response.

Whereas the daytime IL-1$\beta$-induced febrile response of females is less robust than that of males, the response in FAE (and PF) females is blunted, as it is in males (Taylor et al., 1998b). Furthermore, in females, blunting of the febrile response appears to be mediated by gonadal hormones as OVX normalized this response. OVX reversal of FAE's blunting of fever in the light phase may be due to specific alterations in cytokine production in OVX-FAE females given that OVX was found to inhibit LPS-induced TNF-$\alpha$ (i.e., a known cryogen (Kluger, 1991)) production in FAE females, but not in PF and N controls (Yirmiya et al., 1998). When IL-1$\beta$ was administered just prior to the dark phase, females, like males, as reported above, showed a biphasic temperature response, i.e., hypothermia followed by hyperthermia. In contrast to males, FAE females showed significantly lower responses than PF or N controls during both phases of

the response. Also, in contrast to males, there was no differential effect of FAE on IL-1$\beta$-induced anorexia. Interestingly, in the dark period, OVX did not affect the differential febrile responses of FAE females, suggesting that the effects of FAE on fever in females are mediated by different mechanisms at different phases of the diurnal cycle. The mechanisms for these gender differences in the effects of FAE on the IL-1$\beta$-induced temperature response are currently under investigation.

### c. Nitric Oxide (NO)

In addition to its myriad functions in the inflammatory process, NO may act as an endogenous antipyretic factor (Gourine, 1995). In fetal guinea pigs chronic maternal administration of ethanol decreased hippocampal NO synthase (NOS) activity (Kimura, Parr, & Brien, 1996). In contrast, blockade of NO synthesis with L$_w$nitro-L-arginine methylester (L-NAME) reversed the blunted ACTH response to iv administration of IL-1$\beta$ in weanling male FAE rats (Lee & Rivier, 1994). The latter finding suggests that endogenous NO levels may be increased by prenatal ethanol exposure and interfere with the release of CRF from the median eminence (Lee & Rivier, 1994). Indeed, it has recently been demonstrated that in response to LPS, FAE rats have substantially higher plasma levels of the NO metabolites, nitrite and nitrate, as well as higher splenic inducible NOS immunoreactivity than control rats (Gottesfeld, 1998; Gottesfeld, Maier, Mailman, Lai, & Weisbrodt, 1998). Taken together, these findings suggest that increased NO levels in FAE rats may also be involved in the reduced febrile response to LPS and IL-1$\beta$.

### d. Peripheral Mechanisms

The febrile response to IL-1$\beta$ depends to a large extent on activation of the sympathetic nervous system (SNS), which induces thermogenesis in BAT (Rothwell, 1993). FAE has been found to markedly alter the development of the SNS innervation of the heart (Thadani & Wells, 1984), thymus, and spleen (Gottesfeld et al., 1990), as reviewed above, and BAT (Zimmerberg, Carson, Kaplan, Zuniga, & True, 1993). Norepinephrine concentration in BAT was significantly lower in 5-day-old FAE rats and significantly higher in 20-day-old FAE rats compared to control rats, suggesting a delay in the development of SNS innervation, followed by a compensatory overactivation (Zimmerberg et al., 1993). The number of $\beta$1-adrenoreceptor binding sites in BAT was also increased in FAE rats (Zimmerberg, Smith, Weider, & Teitler, 1995). The significance of the latter finding is not clear, since norepinephrine-stimulated thermogenic responses in BAT are mediated primarily by $\beta3$-adrenoreceptors (Arch, 1989). Taken together, however, these findings suggest that alterations in SNS activation of BAT may be involved in the reduced febrile response of FAE.

## D. LPS, IL-1$\beta$, and Activation of the HPA Axis

In weanling FAE rats, the release of ACTH and $\beta$-endorphin following administration of IL-1$\beta$ was found to be attenuated (Lee & Rivier, 1993, 1994). Furthermore, the ACTH response could be stored by inhibition of NO synthesis (Lee & Rivier, 1994). It should be noted, however, that attenuation of the IL-1-induced ACTH response appeared to be transitory because in young adult rats, ACTH release was enhanced following LPS or IL-1$\beta$ (Lee & Rivier, 1996). Indeed, an age-dependent transition in FAE rats from suppressed stress-induced HPA responsiveness in the preweaning period to enhanced HPA responsiveness in adulthood has been documented (Taylor, Branch, Nelson, Lane, & Poland, 1986; Angelogianni & Gianoulakis, 1989; Weinberg, 1992).

In adult rats, we have reported that LPS-induced corticosterone secretion at 60 min post-LPS was significantly higher in FAE and PF compared to N females, while there were no differences among the male groups (Yirmiya et al., 1998). At 2 h after ip administration of IL-1$\beta$, we found similarly elevated levels of plasma ACTH in all adult male rats, irrespective of prenatal treatment (Yirmiya et al., 1996). (This is in contrast to the enhanced ACTH release of adult FAE rats reported at 30 min after IL-1$\beta$ (Lee & Rivier, 1996).) Furthermore, at 2 h after IL-1$\beta$, the corticosterone response was significantly lower in the PF males than in either the FAE or the N male offspring. Taken together with our finding higher levels of LPS-induced pro-IL-1$\beta$ expression in PF males, as described above, these results indicate that the pair-feeding paradigm constitutes an experimental manipulation, which may have effects on mechanisms that are not altered by FAE. The facts that pair-feeding is associated with caloric restriction and that pair-fed animals usually consume most of their food during the first few hours after diet is presented suggest that pair-feeding constitutes a prenatal stress paradigm. Indeed, pair-feeding was found to activate the HPA axis of both the dam and her offspring (Weinberg & Gallo, 1982), which may have long-lasting consequences for the HPA responsiveness of the adult offspring.

Differential regulation of the HPA axis may not only be involved in FAE-induced impairment of neuroimmune interactions in the mature offspring, but may in part underlie the effects of alcohol in the prenatal period. Previous work by ourselves and other investigators has demonstrated that maternal adrenalectomy can prevent various postnatal effects of FAE, such as growth retardation (Tritt, Tio, Brammer, & Taylor, 1993), HPA hyperresponsiveness to stress (Lee et al., 1990), and suppression of certain cellular immune functions such as mitogen-stimulated splenocyte proliferation, as described above (Redei et al., 1993). Moreover, we recently found that maternal adrenalectomy also normalized the blunted IL-1$\beta$-induced febrile response in adult male FAE rats (Taylor, Tio, Tritt, & Yirmiya, 1998a) (cf. Table II). These diverse effects of maternal alcohol consumption may well reflect a long-term effect of the increased plasma corticosterone levels that occur in alcohol-consuming dams (Tritt et al., 1993; Weinberg & Bezio, 1987). However, as corticosteroid replacement to adrenalectomized dams did not restore the effects of FAE on HPA activity in 21-day old offspring (Lee & Rivier, 1992), other factors may be involved. Indeed, recent data indicate that prenatal alcohol exposure and maternal adrenalectomy interact to produce sexually dimorphic effects on the expression of two glucocorticoid-regulated genes, hypothalamic CRF and anterior pituitary POMC, during the first 3 weeks postnatally (Aird, Halasz, & Redei, 1997).

## IV. SUMMARY

Human and animal studies have established that FAE is associated with significant impairments in cellular immune functions which may be responsible for increased susceptibility of the neonate to infection and malignancies. Human and animal studies concur in two fundamental observations: first, the immune defects associated with FAE appear to be principally of the cellular immune component and thus driven to affect primarily T-cell-mediated immune events; and secondly, these dysfunctions do not seem to diminish with increasing age of the child or offspring. These observations have profound clinical implications in that they suggest that FAE may lead to grave impairments in those aspects of the immune system that are most crucial for initiating, regulating, and sustaining immune competence against minor as well as lethal infectious agents, and against malignancies.

Animal studies have established the serious effects of FAE upon neuroimmune interactions which mediate many of the host's defense responses to infection. Specifically, FAE is now known to blunt CNS-mediated responses to immune signals such as LPS and IL-1$\beta$, including sympathetic outflow to the spleen, thermoregulatory and neuroendocrine processes, and sickness behavior. The deleterious effects of FAE on neuroimmune interactions may involve impairments in the regulation of central cytokine production, and/or alterations in neuroendocrine and neurochemical mediators of the acute-phase response. Based on our demonstration that blunting of the febrile response was also observed after central administration of IL-1$\beta$ in FAE rats and the evidence that central infusion of IL-1$\beta$ has been shown to suppress peripheral cellular immune responses (Sundar et al., 1989; Hodgson, Yirmiya, & Taylor, 1998), it appears evident that the immunophysiological disturbances associated with FAE may in part reflect a direct effect of FAE on the communication between the CNS and peripheral immune organs.

## Acknowledgments

We are grateful to Delia L. Tio, Michelle Kung, and Ngy S. Heng for their expert assistance in our studies. Our work reported herein was supported by grants from the NIH (AA 09850), the Department of Veterans Affairs Medical Research Service, and by the United States–Israel Binational Science Foundation (94-00062 and 97-00204).

## References

Abel, E. L. (Ed.) (1996). *Fetal alcohol syndrome*. Boca Raton; FL: CRC Press.

Ackerman, K. D., Felten, S. Y., Bellinger, D. L., & Felten, D. L. (1987). Noradrenergic sympathetic innervation of the spleen, III. Development of innervation in the rat spleen. *Journal of Neuroscience Research, 18*, 49–54.

Ackerman, K. D., Felten, S. Y., Dijkstra, C. D., Livnat, S., & Felten, D. L. (1989). Parallel development of noradrenergic innervation and cellular compartmentation in the rat spleen. *Experimental Neurology, 103*, 239–255.

Ahmed, I. J., Shryne, J. E., Gorski, R. A., Branch, B. J., & Taylor, A. N. (1991). Prenatal ethanol and the prepubertal sexually dimorphic nucleus of the preoptic area. *Physiolology and Behavior, 49*, 427–432.

Aird, F., Halasz, I., & Redei, E. (1997). Ontogeny of hypothalamic corticotropin-releasing factor and anterior pituitary pro-opio-melanocortin expression in male and female offspring of alcohol-exposed and adrenalectomized dams. *Alcoholism: Clinical and Experimental Research, 21*, 1560–1566.

Amkraut, A. A., Solomon, G. F., Kasper, P., & Purdue, A. (1972). Stress and hormonal intervention in the graft-versus-host response. *Advances in Experimental Biology, 23*, 667–674.

Amman, A. J., Wara, D. W., Cowan, M. J., Barrett, D. J., & Stiehm, R. (1982). The DiGeorge syndrome and the fetal alcohol syndrome. *American Journal of Diseases in Childhood, 136*, 906–908.

Angelogianni, P., & Gianoulakis, C. (1989). Prenatal exposure to ethanol alters the ontogeny of the beta-endorphin response to stress. *Alcoholism: Clinical and Experimental Research, 13*, 564–571.

Arch, J. R. C. (1989). The brown adipocyte $\beta$-adrenoreceptor. *Proceedings of the Nutritional Society, 48*, 215–223.

Avitsur, R., Donchin, O., Cohen, E., & Yirmiya, R. (1995). Differential effects of IL-1$\beta$ on the activity of male and female rats in the open field test. *Brain Behavior and Immunity, 9*, 234–241.

Avitsur, R., Pollak, Y., & Yirmiya, R. (1997). Different receptor mechanisms mediate the effects of endotoxin and interleukin-1 on female sexual behavior. *Brain Research, 772*, 149–161.

Barron, S., Tieman, S. B., & Riley, E. P. (1988). Effects of prenatal alcohol exposure on the sexually dimorphic nucleus of the preoptic area of the hypothalamus in male and female rata. *Alcoholism: Clinical and Experimental Research, 12*, 59–64.

Basham, K. B., Whitmore, S. P., Adcock, A. F., & Basta, P. V. (1998). Chronic and acute prenatal and postnatal ethanol exposure on lymphocyte subsets from offspring thymic, splenic and interstinal intraepithelial sources. *Alcoholism: Clinical and Experimental Research, 22*, 1501–1508.

Bermundez, L. E., Wu, M., Martinelli, J., & Young, L. S. (1991). Ethanol affects release of TNF and GM-CSF and membrane expression of TNF receptors by human macrophages. *Lymphokine Cytokine Research, 10*, 413–419.

Besedovsky, H. O., & Del Rey, A. (1996). Immune-neuro-endocrine interactions: Facts and hypotheses. *Endocrine Reviews, 17*, 64–102.

Biber, K. L., Moscatello, K. M., Dempsey, D. C., Chervenak, R., & Wolcott, R. M. (1998). Effects of in utero alcohol exposure on B-cell development in the murine fetal liver. *Alcoholism: Clinical and Experimental Research, 22*, 1706–1712.

Bjerke, T., Hedegaard, M., Henriksen, T. B., Nielsen, B. W., & Schiotz, P. O. (1994). Several genetic and environmental factors influence cord blood IgE concentration. *Pediatric Allergy Immunology, 5*, 88–94.

Blatteis, C. M. (1988) Neural mechanisms in the pyrogenic and acute-phase responses to interleukin-1. *International Journal of Neuroscience, 38*, 223–232.

Bockman, D. E., & Kirby, M. L. (1985). Neural crest interactions in the development of the immune system. *Journal of Immunology, 135*, 766s–768s.

Braun, K. P., Pearce, R. B., & Peterson, C. M. (1995). Acetaldehyde-serum protein adducts inhibit interleukin-2 secretion in concanavalin A-stimulated murine splenocytes: A potential common pathway for ethanol-induced immunomodulation. *Alcoholism: Clinical and Experimental Research, 19*, 345–349.

Bulloch, K., Cullen, M. R., Schwartz, R. H., & Longo, D. L. (1987). Development of innervation within syngeneic thymus tissue transplanted under the kidney capsule of the nude mouse: A light and ultrastructural microscope study. *Journal of Neuroscience Research, 18*, 16–27.

Calvani, M., Ghirelli, D., Calvani, M., Fortuna, C., Lalli, F., & Marcolini, P. (1985). La sindrome feto-alcolica: Follow-up clinico-metabolico-immunitario di 14 casi. *Minerva Pediatrica, 37*, 77–88.

Carding, S. R., Hayday, A. C., & Bottomly, K. (1991). Cytokines in T cell development. *Immunology Today, 12*, 239–245.

Carey, F., Forder, R., Edge, M. D., Greene, A. R., Horan, M. A., Strijbos, P. J. L. M., & Rothwell, N. J. (1990). Lipocortin-1 fragment modifies pyrogenic actions of cytokines in rats. *American Journal of Physiolology, 259*, R266–R269.

Chang, M. P., Yamaguchi, D. T., Yeh, M., Taylor, A. N., & Norman, D. C. (1994). Mechanism of the impaired T-cell proliferation in adult rats exposed to alcohol in utero. *International Journal of Immunopharmacology, 16*, 345–357.

Chen, G. J., Huang, D. S., Watzl, B., & Watson, R. R. (1993). Ethanol modulation of tumor necrosis factor and gamma interferon production by murine splenocytes and macrophages. *Life Sciences, 52*, 1319–1326.

Chiappelli, F. (1991). Neuroimmunological perspectives on lymphocyte homing and adhesion. *International Journal Immunopathology and Pharmacology, 4*, 115–121.

Chiappelli, F., Kung, M. A., Stefanini, G. F., & Foschi, F. G. (1998). Alcohol and immune function. In M. E. Gershwin, B. German & C. L. Keen (Eds.), *Nutrition and immunology: Principles and practice*, (Chap. 23). Totawa, New Jersey: Humana Press.

Chiappelli, F., Kung, M. A., Tio, D. L., Tritt, S. H., Yirmiya, R., & Taylor, A. N. (1997). Fetal alcohol exposure augments the blunting of tumor necrosis factor production in vitro resulting from in vivo priming with lipopolysaccharide in young adult male but not female rats. *Alcoholism: Clinical and Experimental Research, 21*, 1542–1546.

Chiappelli, F., & Taylor, A. N. (1995). The fetal alcohol syndrome and fetal alcohol effects on immune competence. *Alcohol and Alcoholism, 30*, 259–263.

Chiappelli, F., Wong, C. M. K., Yirmiya, R., Norman, D. C., Chang, M.-P., & Taylor, A. N. (1993). Fetal alcohol exposure (FAE) and neuroimmune surveillance. In R. Yirmiya & A. N. Taylor (Eds.), *Alcohol, immunity and cancer* (pp. 141–156). Boca Raton, FL: CRC Press.

Church, M., & Gerkin, K. P. (1988). Hearing disorders in children with fetal alcohol syndrome: Findings from case reports. *Journal of Pediatrics, 82*, 147–154.

Clarren, S. K., Astley, S. J., Bowden, D. M., Lai, H., Milam, A. H., Rudeen, P. K., & Shoemaker, W. J. (1990). Neuroanatomic and neurobiochemical abnormalities in non-human primate infants exposed to weekly doses of ethanol during gestation. *Alcoholism: Clinical Experimental Research, 14*, 674–683.

Crestini, F., Seguy, F., & Dantzer, R. (1991). Behavioral effects of peripherally injected interleukin-1: Role of prostaglandins. *Brain Research, 542*, 330–335.

Daynes, R. A., & Araneo, B. A. (1989). Contrasting effects of glucocorticoids on the capacity of T cells to produce the growth factors interleukin 2 and interleukin 4. *European Journal of Immunology, 19*, 2319–2325.

Dinarello C. A. (1996). Biologic basis for interleukin-1 in disease. *Blood, 87*, 2095–2147.

Dunn A. J., Antoon, M., & Chapman, Y. (1991). Reduction of exploratory behavior by intraperitoneal injection of interleukin-1 involves brain corticotropin releasing factor. *Brain Research Bulletin, 2*, 539–542.

Evan, G. I., Wyllie, A. H., Gilbert, C. S., Littlewood, T. D., Land, H., Brooks, M., Waters, C. M., Penn, L. Z., & Hancock, D. C. (1992). Induction of apoptosis in fibroblasts by c-myc protein. *Cell, 69*, 119–128.

Ewald, S. J., and Walden, S. M. (1988). Flow cytometric and histological analysis of mouse thymus in fetal alcohol syndrome. *Journal of Leukocyte Biology, 44*, 434–440.

Ewen, M. E. (1994). The cell cycle and the retinoblastoma protein family. *Cancer and Metastasis Reviews, 13*, 45–66.

Felten, D. L. K., Felten, S. Y., Bellinger, D. L., Carlson, S. L., Ackerman, K. D., Madden, K. S., Olschowska, J. A., & Livnat, S. (1987). Noradrendergic sympathetic neural interactions with the immune system: Structure and function. *Immunology Reviews, 100*, 225–260.

Gallo, P. V., & Weinberg, J. (1981). Corticosterone rhythmicity in the rat: Interactive effects of dietary restriction and schedule of feeding. *Journal of Nutrition, 111*, 208–218.

Giberson, P. K., & Blakley, B. R. (1994). Effect of postnatal ethanol exposure on expression of differentiation antigens of murine splenic lymphocytes. *Alcoholism: Clinical and Experimental Research, 18*, 21–28.

Giberson, P. K., Kim, C. K., Hutchison, S., Yu, W., Junker, A., & Weinberg, J. (1997). The effect of cold stress on lymphocyte proliferation in fetal ethanol-exposed rats. *Alcoholism: Clinical and Experimental Research, 21*, 1440–1447.

Giberson, P. K., & Weinberg, J. (1992). Fetal alcohol syndrome and functioning of the immune system. *Alcohol World, 16*, 29–39.

Giberson, P. K., & Weinberg, J. (1995). Effects of prenatal ethanol exposure and stress in adulthood on lymphocyte populations in rats. *Alcoholism: Clinical and Experimental Research, 19*, 1286–1294.

Giberson, P. K., & Weinberg, J. (1997). Effect of surrogate fostering on splenic lymphocytes in fetal ethanol exposed rats. *Alcoholism: Clinical and Experimental Research, 21*, 44–55.

Gilman-Sachs, A., Kim, Y. B., Pollard, M., & Snyder, D. L. (1991). Influence of aging, environmental antigens and dietary restriction on expression of lymphocyte subsets in germ-free conventional Lobund-Wistar rats. *Journal of Gerontology, 46*, B101–B106.

Gottesfeld, Z. (1998). Sympathetic neural response to immune signals involves nitric oxide: Effects of expsoure to alcohol in utero. *Alcohol, 16*, 177–181.

Gottesfeld, Z., & Abel, E. L. (1991). Maternal and paternal use: Effects on the immune system of the offspring. *Life Sciences, 48*, 1–8.

Gottesfeld, Z., Christie, R., Felten, D. L., & LeGrue, S. J. (1990). Prenatal ethanol exposure alters immune capacity and noradrenergic synaptic transmission in lymphoid organs of the adult mouse. *Neuroscience, 35*, 85–94.

Gottesfeld, A., Maier, M., Mailman, D., Lai, M., & Weisbrodt, N. W. (1998). Splenic sympathetic response to endotoxin is blunted in the fetal alcohol-exposed rat: Role of nitric oxide. *Alcohol, 16*, 19–24.

Gottesfeld, Z., Simpson, S., & Maier, M. (1997). Exposure to alcohol in utero blunts splenic sympathetic neural response to endotoxin and interleukin-1beta in the rat. *Journal of Neuroimmunology, 78*, 180–183.

Gottesfeld, Z., Simpson, S., Yuwiler, A., & Perez-Polo, J. R. (1996). Effects of nerve growth factor on splenic norepinephrine and pineal N-acetyl-transferase in neonate rats exposed to alcohol in utero: Neuroimmune correlates. *International Journal of Developmental Neuroscience, 14*, 655–662.

Gottesfeld, Z., & Ullrich, S. E. (1995). Prenatal alcohol exposure selectively suppresses cell-mediated but not humoral immune responsiveness. *International Journal of Immunopharmacology, 17*, 247–254.

Goujon, E., Parnet, P., Laye, S., Combe, C., Kelley, K. W., & Dantzer, R. (1995). Stress downregulates lipopolysaccharide-induced expression of proinflammatory cytokines in the spleen, pituitary, and brain of mice. *Brain Behavior and Immunity, 9*, 292–303.

Gourine A. V. (1995). Pharmacological evidence that nitric oxide can act as an endogenous antipyretic factor in endotoxin-induced fever in rabbits. *General Pharmacology, 26*, 835–841.

Greene, M. I., Kokai, Y., Gaulton, G. N., Powell, M. B., Geller, H., & Cohen, J. A. (1987). Receptor systems in tissues of the nervous system. *Immunology Reviews, 100*, 153–184.

Grossman, C. S. (1990). Are the underlying immune–neuroendocrine interactions responsible for immunological sexual dimorphism? *Progress in NeuroEndocrineImmunology, 3*, 75–81.

Hagan, P., Poole, S., & Bristow, A. F. (1993). Endotoxin-stimulated production of rat hypothalamic interleukin-1$\beta$ in vivo and in vitro, measured by specific immunoradiometric assay. *Journal of Molecular Endocrinology, 11*, 31–36.

Halasz, I., Aird, F., Lifang, L., Prystowsky, M. B., & Redei, E. (1993). Sexually dimorphic effects of alcohol exposure in utero on neuroendocrine and immune functions in chronic alcohol-exposed adult rats. *Molecular and Cellular Neuroscience, 4,* 343–353.

Hall, N. R. S., O'Grady, M. P., & Farah, J. M. (1991). Thymic hormones and immune function: Mediation via neuroendocrine circuits. In R. Ader, D. L. Felten & N. Cohen (Eds.), *Psychoneuroimmunology* (2nd ed.) (pp. 515–528). San Diego: Academic Press.

Handa, R. J., McGivern, R. F., Noble, E. S., & Gorski, R. A. (1985). Exposure to alcohol in utero alters the adult patterns of luteinizing hormone secretion in male and female rats. *Life Sciences, 37,* 1683–1690.

Hanson, J. W., Jones, K. L., & Smith, D. W. (1976). Fetal alcohol syndrome—Experience with 41 patients. *Journal of the American Medical Association, 235,* 1458–1460.

Hart, B. L. (1988). Biological basis of the behavior of sick animals. *Neuroscience and Biobehavioral Reviews, 12,* 123–137.

Hillhouse, E. W., & Mosley, K. (1993). Peripheral endotoxin induces hypothalamic immunoreactive interleukin-1$\beta$ in the rat. *British Journal of Pharmacology, 109,* 289–290.

Hoang, A. T., Cohen, K. J., Barrett, J. F., Bergstrom, D. A., & Dang, C. V. (1994). Participation of cyclin A in Myc-induced apoptosis. *Proceedings of the National Academy of Science, USA, 91,* 6875–6879.

Hodgson, D. M., Yirmiya, R., & Taylor, A. N. (1998). Intracerebral HIV glycoprotein (gp120) enhances tumor metastasis via centrally released interleukin-1. *Brain Research, 781,* 244–251.

Howes, K. A., Ransom, N., Papermaster, D. S., Lasudry, J. G., Albert, D. M., & Windle, J. J. (1994). Apoptosis or retinoblastoma: Alternative fates of photoreceptors expressing the HPV-16 E7 gene in the presence or absence of p53. *Genes and Development, 8,* 1300–1310.

Huston, D. P. (1997). The biology of the immune system. *Journal of the American Medical Association, 278,* 1804–1814.

Jacobson, S. W., Jacobson, J. L., Bihun, J. T., Chiodo, L., & Sokol, R. J. (1993). Effects of prenatal alcohol exposure on poststress cortisol levels in infants. *Alcoholism: Clinical and Experimental Research, 17,* 456.

Jerrells, T. R., & Weinberg, J. (1998). Influence of ethanol consumption on immune competence of adult animals exposed to ethanol in utero. *Alcoholism: Clinical and Experimental Research, 22,* 391–400.

Johnson, S., Knight, R., Harmer, D. J., & Steele, R. W. (1981). Immune deficiency in fetal alcohol syndrome. *Pediatrics Research, 15,* 908–911.

Jones, K. L., & Smith, D. W. (1973). Recognition of the fetal alcohol syndrome in early infancy. *Lancet, 2,* 999–1001.

Jones, K. L., Smith, D. W., Streissguth, A. P., & Myrianthopoulos, N. C. (1974). Outcome in offspring of chronic alcoholic women. *Lancet, 1,* 1076–1078.

Jones, K. L., Smith, D. W., Ulleland, C. N., & Streissguth, A. P. (1973). Pattern of malformation in offspring of chronic alcoholic mothers. *Lancet, 1,* 1267–1271.

Kent, S., Bluthe, R., Kelley, K. W., & Dantzer, R. (1992). Sickness behavior as a new target for drug development. *Trends in Pharmacological Science, 13,* 24–28.

Khoruts, A., Stahnke, L., McClain, C. J., Logan, G., & Allen, J. I. (1991). Circulating tumor necrosis factor, interleukin-1 and interleukin-6 concentrations in chronic alcoholic patients. *Hepatology, 13,* 267–276.

Kimura K. A., Parr, A. M., & Brien, J. F. (1996). Effect of chronic maternal ethanol administration on nitric oxide synthase activity in the hippocampus of the mature fetal guinea pig. *Alcoholism: Clinical and Experimental Research, 20,* 1–6.

Kluger, M. J. (1991). Fever: Role of pyrogens and cryogens. *Physiological Reviews, 71,* 93–127.

Kluger, J. J., Bartfai, T., & Dinarello, C. A. (Eds.) (1998). Molecular mechanisms of fever. *Annals of the New York Academy of Science, 856.*

Kranenburg, O., van der Eb, A. J., & Zantema, A. (1996). Cyclin D1 is an essential mediator of apoptotic neuronal cell death. *Embo Journal, 15,* 46–54.

Krueger, J. M., Walter, J., Dinarello, C. A., Wolff, S. M., & Chedid, L. (1984). Sleep promoting effects of endogenous pyrogen (interleukin-1). *American Journal of Physiology, 246,* R994–R999.

Kundel, S. L., & Remik, D. G. (1992). *Cytokines in health and disease.* New York: Dekker.

Laudenslager, M. L., Fleshner, M., Hofstadter, P., Held, P. E., Simons, L., & Maier, S. F. (1988). Suppression of specific antibody production by inescapable shock: Stability under varying conditions. *Brain, Behavior and Immunity, 2,* 92–101.

Laye, S., Bluthe, R.-M., Kent, S., Comb, C., Medina, C., Parnet, P., Kelley, K., & Dantzer, R. (1995). Subdiaphragmatic vagotomy blocks induction of IL-1b mRNA in mice brain in response to peripheral LPS. *American Journal of Physiology, 268,* R1327–R1331.

Lee, S., & Rivier, C. (1993). Prenatal alcohol exposure blunts interleukin-1-induced ACTH and B-endorphin secretion by immature rats. *Alcoholism: Clinical and Experimental Research, 17,* 940–945.

Lee, S., & Rivier, C. (1994). Prenatal alcohol exposure alters the hypothalamic-pituitary-adrenal axis response of immature offspring to interleukin-1: Is nitric oxide involved? *Alcoholism: Clinical and Experimental Research, 18,* 1242–1247.

Lee, S., & Rivier, C. (1996). Gender differences in the effect of prenatal alcohol exposure on the hypothalamic-pituitary-adrenal axis response to immune signals. *Psychoneuroendocrinology, 21,* 145–155.

Lee, S. Y., Imaki, T., Vale, W., & Rivier, C. (1990). Effects of prenatal exposure to alcohol on the activity of hypothalamic-pituitary-adrenal axis of the offspring: Importance of the time of exposure to ethanol and possible modulating mechanisms. *Molecular and Cellular Neuroscience, 1,* 168–177.

Lemoine, P., Harosseau, H., Borteryu, J. P., & Menuet, J.-C. (1968). Les enfants de parents alcooliques: Anomalies observées à propos de 127 cas. *Ouest Médical, 21,* 476–482.

Lin, H., Mosmann, T. R., Guilbert, L., Tuntipopipat, S., & Wegmann, T. G. (1993). Synthesis of T helper 2-type cytokines at the maternal-fetal interface. *Journal of Immunology, 151,* 4562–4573.

Liu, Q., Dawes, N. J., Lu, Y., Shubeita, H. S., & Zhu, H. (1997). $\beta$-Adrenergic stimulation induces phosphorylation of retinoblastoma protein in neonatal rat ventricular myocytes. *Biochemical Journal, 327,* 305–309.

Livant, E. J., Welles, E. G., & Ewald, S. J. (1997). Chronic ethanol exposure alters leukocyte subsets in repopulating spleens, but does not alter negative selection in thymuses of sublethally irradiated mice. *Alcoholism: Clinical and Experimental Research, 21,* 1520–1529.

Long, N. D., Otterness, I., Kunkel, S. L., Vandar, A. J., & Kluger, M. J. (1990). Roles of interleukin-1$\beta$ and tumor necrosis factor in lipopolysaccharide fever in rats. *American Journal of Physiology, 259,* R724–R728.

Madden, K. S., Thyagarajan, S., & Felten, D. L. (1998). Alterations in sympathetic noradrenergic innervation in lymphoid organs with age. *Annals of the New York Academy of Science, 840,* 262–268.

Maier, S. F., & Watkins, L. R. (1998). Cytokines for psychologists: Implications of bi-directional immune-to-brain communication for understanding behavior, mood, and cognition. *Psychological Review, 105,* 83–107.

Malec, P., & Nowak, Z. (1988). Propanolol enhances in vitro interleukin-2 receptor expression on human lymphocytes. *Immunology Letters, 17,* 319–321.

Marches, R., Scheuermann, R. H., & Uhr, J. W. (1998). Cancer dormancy: Role of cyclin-dependent kinase inhibitors in induction of cell cycle arrest mediated via membrane IgM. *Cancer Research, 58,* 691–697.

McCann, S. M., Rettori, V., Milenkovic, L., Jurcovicova, J., & Gonzalez, M. C. (1990). Role of monokines in control of anterior pituitary hormone release. In J. C. Porter & D. Jezova (Eds.), *Circulating regulatory factors and neuroendocrine function* (pp. 315–329). New York: Plenum.

McClain, C. J., & Cohen, D. A. (1989). Increased tumor necrosis factor production by monocytes in alcoholic hepatitis. *Hepatology, 9,* 349–351.

McGivern, R. F., Clancy, A. N., Hill, M. A., & Noble, E. P. (1984). Prenatal alcohol exposure alters adult expression of sexually dimorphic behavior in the rat. *Science, 224,* 896.

McGivern, R. F., Raum, W. J., Salido, E., & Redei, E. (1988). Lack of prenatal testosterone surge in fetal rats exposed to alcohol: Alterations in testicular morphology and physiology. *Alcoholism: Clinical and Experimental Research, 12,* 243–247.

Meites, J. (1990). Aging: Hypothalamic catecholamines, neuroendocrine–immune interactions, and dietary restriction. *Neuroendocrine and Dietary Influences, 195,* 304–310.

Moltz, H. (1993). Fever: Causes and consequences. *Neuroscience and Biobehavioral Reviews, 17,* 237–269.

Monjan, A. A., & Mandell, W. (1980). Fetal alcohol and immunity: Depression of mitogen-induced lymphocyte blastogenesis. *Neurobehavioral Toxicology, 2,* 213–220.

Montgomery, R. A., & Dallman, M. J. (1991). Analysis of cytokine gene expression during fetal thymic ontogeny using the polymerase chain reaction. *Journal of Immunology, 147,* 554–560.

Mrosovsky, N., Molony, L. A., Conn, C. A., & Kluger, M. J. (1989). Anorexic effects of interleukin-1 in the rat. *American Journal of Physiology, 257,* R1315–R1321.

Murakami, N., & Ono, T. (1987). Sex-related differences in fever development of rats. *American Journal of Physiology, 252,* R284–R289.

Muzes, G., Deak, G., Lang, G., Gonzalez-Cabello, R., Gergely, P., & Feher, J. (1989). Depressed monocyte production of interleukin-1 and tumor necrosis factor-alpha in patients with alcoholic liver cirrhosis. Liver, 9, 302–306.

Na, H. R., & Seelig, L. L., Jr. (1994). Effect of maternal ethanol consumption on in vitro tumor necrosis factor, interleukin-6 and interleukin-2 production by rat milk and blood leukocytes. *Alcoholism: Clinical and Experimental Research*, 18, 398–402.

Na, H. R., Daniels, L. C., & Seelig, L. L., Jr. (1997). Preliminary study of how alcohol consumption during pregnancy affects immune components in breast milk and blood of postpartum women. *Alcohol and Alcoholism, 32,* 581–589.

Nair, M. P., Kronfol, Z. A., Greden, J. F., Chadha, K. C., Dumaswala, U. J., Sweet, A. M., & Schwartz, S. A. (1994). Selective inhibition by alcohol and cortisol of natural killer cell activity of lymphocytes from cord blood. *Progress in NeuroPsychopharmacology & Biological Psychiatry, 18,* 1293–1305.

Nanji, A. A., Hossein Sadrzadeh, S. M., Thomas, P., & Yamanka, T. (1994). Ethanol-induced suppression of interleukin-1 activity: Reversal by a quinone derivative. *Biochemical Pharmacology, 47,* 925–928.

Nelson, L. R., & Taylor, A. N. (1987). Long-term behavioral and neuroendocrine effects of prenatal alcohol exposure. In M. C. Braude & A. M. Zimmerman (Eds.), *Genetic and perinatal effects of abused substances* (pp. 177–203). Orlando: Academic Press.

Nelson, L. R., Taylor, A. N., Lewis, J. E., Poland, R. E., Redei, E., & Branch, B. J. (1986). Pituitary-adrenal responses to morphine and footshock stress are enhanced following prenatal alcohol exposure. *Alcoholism: Clinical and Experimental Research, 10,* 397–402.

Nelson, S., Bagby, G., & Summer, W. R. (1989). Alcohol suppresses lipopolysaccharide-induced tumor necrosis factor activity in serum and lung. *Life Sciences, 44,* 673–676.

Nelson, S., Bagby, G. J., Bainton, B. G., & Summer, W. R. (1989). The effects of acute and chronic alcoholism on tumor necrosis factor and the inflammatory responses. *Journal of Infectious Diseases, 160,* 422–429.

Nguyen, K. T., Deak, T., Owens, S. M., Kohno, T., Fleshner, M., Watkins, L. R., & Maier, S. F. (1998). Exposure to acute stress induces brain interleukin-1$\beta$ protein in the rat. *Journal of Neuroscience, 18,* 2239–2246.

Norman, D. C., Chang, M.-P., Castle, S. C., van Zuylen, J. E., & Taylor, A. N. (1989). Diminished proliferative response of Con-A blast Cells to interleukin-2 in adult rats exposed to ethanol in utero.*Alcoholism: Clinical and Experimental Research, 13,* 69–72.

Norman, D. C., Chang, M.-P., Wong, C. M. K., Branch, B. J., Castle, S., & Taylor, A. N. (1991). Changes with age in the proliferative response of splenic T cells from rats exposed to ethanol in utero. *Alcoholism: Clinical and Experimental Research, 15,* 428–32.

Otterness, I. G., Seymour, P. A., Golden, H. W., Reynolds, J. A., & Daumy, G. O. (1988). The effects of continuous administration of murine interleukin-1 alpha in the rat. *Physiology and Behavior, 43,* 797–804.

Pardoll, D. M., Fowlkes, B. J., Lechler, R. I., Germain, R. N., & Schwartz, R. H. (1987). Early genetic events in T cell development analyzed by in situ hydridization. *Journal of Experimental Medicine, 165,* 1624–1638.

Preston, G. A., Lyon, T. T., Yin, Y., Lang, J. E., Solomon, G., Annab, L., Srinivasan, D. G., Alcorta, D. A., & Barrett, J. C. (1996). Induction of apoptosis by c-Fos protein. *Molecular and Cellular Biology, 16,* 211–218.

Purkerson, J., & Isakson, P. (1992). A two-signal model for regulation of immunoglobulin isotype switching. *FASEB Journal, 6,* 3245–3252.

Qin, X. Q., Livingston, D. M., Kaelin, W. G., Jr. & Adams, P. D. (1994). Deregulated transcription factor E2F-1 expression leads to S-phase entry and p53-mediated apoptosis. *Proceedings of the National Academy of Science, USA, 91,* 10918–10922.

Quan, N., Sundar, S. K., & Weiss, J. M. (1994). Induction of interleukin-1 in various brain regions after peripheral and central injections of lipopolysaccharide. *Journal of Neuroimmunology, 49,* 125–134.

Redei, E., Clark, W., & McGivern, R. F. (1989). Alterations in immune responsiveness, ACTH and CRF content of brains in animals exposed to alcohol during the last week of gestation. *Alcoholism: Clinical and Experimental Research, 13,* 439–443.

Redei, E., Halasz, I., Li, L., Prystowsky, M. B., & Aird, F. (1993). Maternal adrenalectomy alters the immune and endocrine functions of fetal alcohol-exposed male offspring. *Endocrinology, 133,* 452–460.

Revskoy, S., Halasz, I., & Redei, E. (1997). Corticotropin-releasing hormone and proopiomelanocortin gene expression is altered selectively in the male rat fetal thymus by maternal alcohol consumption. *Endocrinology, 138,* 389–396.

Roitt, I., Brostoff, J., & Male, D. (1989). *Immunology* (2nd ed.). London: Gower Medical.

Romagnani, S. (1996). Development of Th 1- or Th 2-dominated immune responses: What about the polarizing signal. *International Journal of Clinical Laboratory Research, 26,* 83–98.

Rothwell, N. J. (1991). Functions and mechanisms of interleukin 1 in the brain. *Trends in Pharmacological Science, 12,* 430–436.

Rothwell, N. J. (1993). Cytokines and thermogenesis. *International Journal of Obesity, 17*, S98–S101.

Rudeen, P. I. (1988). Fetal ethanol exposure in the rat: A mechanism for brain defects. In K. Kuriyama, A. Takada, & H. Ishii (Eds.), *Biomedical and social aspects of alcohol and alcoholism* (pp. 859–862). Amsterdam: Elsevier Scientific.

Scammell, T. E., Elmquist, J. K., Griffin, J. D., & Saper, C. B. (1996). Ventromedial preoptic prostaglandin E2 activates fever-producing autonomic pathways. *Journal of Neuroscience, 16*, 6246–6254.

Schobitz, B., De Kloet, E. R., & Holsboer, F. (1994). Gene expression and function of interleukin 1, interleukin 6 and tumor necrosis factor in the brain. *Progress in Neurobiology, 44*, 397–432.

Seelig, L. L. Jr., Steven, W. M., & Stewart, G. L. (1996). Effects of maternal ethanol consumption on the subsequent development of immunity to Trichinella spiralis in rat neonates. *Alcoholism: Clinical and Experimental Research, 20*, 514–522.

Sehic, E., & Blatteis, C. M. (1996). Blockade of lipopolysaccharide-induced fever by subdiaphragmatic vagotomy in guinea pigs. *Brain Research, 726*, 160–166.

Shan, B., & Lee, W. H. (1994). Deregulated expression of E2F-1 induces S-phase entry and leads to apoptosis. *Molecular and Cellular Biology, 14*, 8166–8173.

Singer, K. H. (1990). Interactions between epithelial cells and T lymphocytes: Role of adhesion molecules. *Journal of Leukocyte Biology, 48*, 367–374.

Singh, U., Millson, D. S., Smith, P. A., & Owen, J. J. T. (1979). Identification of beta-adrenoreceptors during thymocyte ontogeny in mice. *European Journal of Immunology, 9*, 31–35.

Smith, B. K., & Kluger, J. J. (1992). Human IL-1 receptor antagonist partially suppresses LPS fever but not plasma levels of IL-6 in Fischer rats. *American Journal of Physiology, 263*, R653–R655.

Sofer-Levi, Y., & Resnitzky, D. (1996). Apoptosis induced by ectopic expression of cyclin D1 but not cyclin E. *Oncogene, 13*, 2431–2437.

Spencer, J. D., Ladd, N., Beeby, P. J., Collins, E., Saunders, J. B., McCaughan, G. W., & Cossart, Y. E. (1997). Transmission of hepatitis C virus to infants of human immunodeficiency virus-negative intravenous drug-abusing mothers: Rate of infection and assessment of risk factors for transmission. *Journal of Viral Hepatitis, 4*, 395–409.

Street, N. E., & Mosmann, T. R. (1991). Functional diversity of T lymphocytes due to secretion of different cytokine patterns. *FASEB Journal, 5*, 171–177.

Strijbos, P. J., Hardwick, A. J., Relton, J. K., Carey, F., & Rothwell, N. J. (1992). Inhibition of central actions of cytokines on fever and thermogenesis by lipocortin-1 involves CRF. *American Journal of Physiology, 263*, E632–E636.

Strijbos, P. J. L. M., Hardwick, A. J., Relton, J. K., Carey, F., & Rothwell, N. J. (1993). Inhibition of central actions of cytokines on fever and thermogenesis by lipocortin-1 involves CRF. *American Journal of Physiology, 265*, E289–E297.

Sundar, S. K., Becker, K. J., Cierpal, M. A., Carpenter, M. D., Rankin, L. A., Fleener, S. L., Ritchie, J. C., Simson, P. E., & Weiss, J. M. (1989). Intracerebroventricular infusion of interleukin 1 rapidly decreases peripheral cellular immune responses. *Proceedings of the National Academy of Science, USA, 86*, 6398–6402.

Taylor, A. N., Branch, B. J., Liu, S. H., & Kokka, N. (1982). Long-term effects of fetal alcohol exposure on pituitary-adrenal response to stress. *Pharmacology Biochemistry and Behavior, 16*, 585–589.

Taylor, A. N., Branch, B. J., Liu, S., Weichman, A. F., Hill, M. A., & Kokka, N. (1981). Fetal exposure to ethanol enhances pituitary-adrenal and temperature responses to ethanol in adult rats. *Alcoholism: Clinical and Experimental Research, 5*, 237–246.

Taylor, A. N., Branch, B. J., Nelson, L. R., Lane, L. A., & Poland, R. E. (1986). Prenatal ethanol and ontogeny of pituitary-adrenal responses to ethanol and morphine. *Alcohol, 3*, 255–259.

Taylor, A. N., Branch, B. J., van Zuylen, J. E., & Redei, E. (1988). Maternal alcohol consumption and stress responsiveness in offspring. Mechanisms of physical and emotional stress. *Advances in Experimental Medicine and Biology, 245*, 311–317.

Taylor, A. N., Tio, D. L., & Chiappelli, F. (1995). Fetal alcohol and thymocyte phenotypes in offspring: Response to food deprivation. *Alcoholism: Clinical and Experimental Research, 19*, 545–550.

Taylor, A. N., Tio, D. L., & Chiappelli, F. (1999). Thymocyte development in male fetal alcohol-exposed rats. *Alcoholism: Clinical and Experimental Research, 23*, 465–470.

Taylor, A. N., Tio, D. L., Pilati, M. L., Tritt, S. H., & Chiappelli, F. (1995). Sexually dimorphic effects of fetal alcohol exposure (FAE) on plasma antibody production. *Alcoholism: Clinical and Experimental Research, 19*, 20A.

Taylor, A. N., Tio, D. L., Tritt, S. H., & Yirmiya, R. (1998a). Attenuation of interleukin-1$\beta$-induced fever in fetal alcohol-exposed rats is prevented by maternal adrenalectomy. *Abstracts of the Society for Neuroscience, 24*, 47.

Taylor, A. N., Tio, D. L., & Yirmiya, R. (1998b). Fetal alcohol exposure (FAE) and ovariectomy interact to affect febrile and hypothermic responses to interleukin-1B (IL-1). *Alcoholism: Clinical and Experimental Research, 22*, 27A.

Taylor, A. N., Tio, D. L., & Yirmiya, R. (1999). Fetal alcohol exposure attenuates interleukin-1$\beta$-induced fever: Neuroimmune mechanisms. *Journal of Neuroimmunology, 99*, 44–52.

Thadani, P. V., & Wells, M. R. (1984). Histoflourescence evaluation of sympathetic nerve fibers in hearts of developing rats exposed to ethanol during gestation. *Neuropharmacol, 23*, 1075–1079.

Tritt, S. H., Tio, D. L., Brammer, G., & Taylor, A. N. (1993). Adrenalectomy but not adrenal demedullation during pregnancy prevents the growth retarding effects of fetal alcohol exposure. *Alcoholism: Clinical and Experimental Research, 17*, 1281–1289.

Udani, M., Parker, S., Gavaler, J., & Van Thiel, D. H. (1985). Effects of in utero exposure to alcohol upon male rats. *Alcoholism: Clinical and Experimental Research, 9*, 355–359.

Van Dam, A.-M., Bauer, J., Tilders, F. J., & Berkenbosch, F. (1995). Endotoxin-induced appearance of immunoreactive interleukin-1 beta in ramified microglia in rat brain: A light and electron microscopic study. *Neuroscience, 65*, 815–828.

Wang, Y., Huang, D. S., & Watson, R. R. (1994). Dietary vitamin E modulation of cytokine production by slpenocytes and thymocytes from alcohol-fed mice. *Alcoholism: Clinical and Experimental Research, 18*, 355–362.

Wang, Y., & Watson, R. R. (1994). Chronic ethanol consumption prior to retrovirus infection alters cytokine production by thymocytes during murine AIDS. *Alcohol 11*, 361–365.

Watkins, L. R., Maier, S. F., & Goehler, L. E. (1995). Cytokine-to-brain communication: A review and analysis of alternative mechanisms. *Life Sciences, 57*, 1011–1026.

Watson, R. R., & Gottesfeld, Z. (1993). Neuroimmune effects of alcohol and its role in AIDS. *Advances in Neuroimmunology, 3*, 151–162.

Wegmann, T. G., Lin, H., Guilbert, L., & Mosmann, T. R. (1993). Bidirectional interactions in the maternal-fetal relationship: Is successful pregnancy a Th2 phenomenon? *Immunology Today, 14*, 353–356.

Weinberg, J. (1989). Hyperresponsiveness to stress: Differential effect of prenatal ethanol in male and female. *Alcoholism: Clinical and Experimental Research, 12*, 647–652.

Weinberg, J. (1992). Prenatal ethanol exposure alters adrenocortical response to predictable and unpredictable stressors. *Alcohol, 9,* 427–432.

Weinberg, J., & Bezio, S. (1987). Alcohol-induced changes in pituitary-adrenal activity during pregnancy. *Alcoholism: Clinical and Experimental Research, 11,* 274–280.

Weinberg, J., & Gallo, P. V. (1982). Prenatal ethanol exposure: Pituitary-adrenal activity in pregnant dams and offspring. Neurobehavioral Toxicology and Teratology, 4, 515–520.

Weinberg, J., & Jerrells, T. R. (1991). Suppression of immune responsiveness: Sex differences in prenatal ethanol effects. *Alcoholism: Clinical and Experimental Research, 15,* 525–531.

West, J. R. (Ed.) (1986) *Alcohol and brain development.* New York: Oxford Press.

Wilson, M. E., Marshall, M. T., Bollnow, M. R., McGivern, R. F., & Handa, R. J. (1995). Gonadotropin-releasing hormone mRNA and gonadotropin β-subunit mRNA expression in the adult female rat exposed to ethanol in utero. *Alcoholism: Clilnical and Experimental Research, 19,* 1211–1218.

Wolcott, R. M., Jennings, S. R., & Chervenak, R. (1995). In utero exposure to ethanol affects postnatal development of T- and B-lymphocytes, but not natural killer cells. *Alcoholism: Clinical and Experimental Research, 19,* 170–176.

Wong, C. M. K., Chiappelli, F., Norman, D. C., Chang, M.-P., Cooper, E. L., Branch, B. J. & Taylor, A. N. (1992). Prenatal exposure to alcohol enhances thymocyte mitogenic responses postnatally. *International Journal Immunopharmacology, 14,* 303–309.

Yamato, K., Koseki, T., Ohguchi, M., Kizaki, M., Ikeda, Y., & Nishihara, T. (1997). Activin A induction of cell-cycle arrest involves modulation of cyclin D2 and p21CIP1/WAF1 in plasmacytic cells. *Molecular Endocrinology, 11,* 1044–1052.

Yirmiya, R. (1996). Endotoxin produces a depressive-like episode in rats. *Brain Research, 711,* 163–174.

Yirmiya, R. (1997). Behavioral and psychological effects of immune activation: Implication for "depression due to a general medical condition." *Current Opinions in Psychiatry, 10,* 470–476.

Yirmiya, R., Avitsur, R., Donchin, O., & Cohen, R. (1995). Interleukin-1 inhibits sexual behavior in female but not in male rats. *Brain, Behavior and Immunity, 9,* 220–233.

Yirmiya, R., Chiappelli, F., Tio, D. L., Tritt, S. H., & Taylor, A. N. (1998). Effect of fetal alcohol exposure and pair feeding on lipopolysaccharide-induced secretion of TNFalpha and corticosterone. *Alcohol, 15,* 327–335.

Yirmiya, R., Pilati, M. L., Chiappelli, F., & Taylor, A. N. (1993). Fetal-alcohol exposure attenuates LPS-induced fever in rats. *Alcoholism: Experimental and Clinical Research, 17,* 906–910.

Yirmiya, R., Tio, D. L., & Taylor, A. N. (1996). Effects of fetal alcohol exposure on fever, sickness behavior, and pituitary-adrenal activation induced by interleukin-1 beta in young adult rats. *Brain, Behavior and Immunity, 10,* 205–220.

Zimmerberg, B., Carson, E. A., Kaplan, L. J., Zuniga, J. A., & True, R. C. (1993). Role of noradrenergic innervation of brown adipose tissue in thermoregulatory deficits following prenatal alcohol exposure. *Alcoholism: Clinical and Experimental Research, 17,* 418–422.

Zimmerberg, B., Smith, C. D., Weider, J. M., & Teitler, M. (1995). The development of β₁-adrenoreceptors in brown adipose tissue following prenatal alcohol exposure. *Alcohol, 12,* 71–77.

# 32

# Effects of Early Rearing Experiences and Social Interactions on Immune Function in Nonhuman Primates

JULIE M. WORLEIN, MARK L. LAUDENSLAGER

## I. VALIDITY OF NONHUMAN PRIMATE MODELS

Animal models allow control of extraneous, confounding variables to a degree that is not possible with human subjects. The use of animal models also allows the researcher to perform experimental manipulations that may not be possible in humans. An animal model should meet several commonly accepted criteria, including similarities in etiology, pathophysiology, phenomenology, and effective treatments (physiological, pharmacological, or behavioral) for amelioration of negative outcomes to the targeted human condition (McKinney & Bunney, 1969). Nonhuman primates have been used extensively as models for human conditions such as grief and bereavement, affiliative and agonistic social interactions, and early development and aging, as they fulfill many of these criteria. Monkeys develop more rapidly

than human children, reaching adulthood in 3 to 4 years, and thus are particularly useful in studies of development and the influence of early experience on later outcomes.

Probably the most important features of nonhuman primate models are their close parallels to the social relationships characteristic of the human species (see for example, Hinde, 1983). Like humans, most nonhuman primates have an extended, dependent infancy and live in large, complex social organizations where they form strong and long-lasting social bonds. This is especially true of rhesus, pigtailed, bonnet, and cynomolgus macaques, the species most commonly used in psychoneuroimmunological research. It is therefore not surprising that interactions with conspecifics play a key role in modulating both behavior and physiology from birth to senescence, particularly during times of challenge. The present chapter will focus on the role of these social interactions in modulating aspects of immune regulation as they have been studied in nonhuman primates.

## II. EFFECTS OF EARLY EXPERIENCE ON IMMUNE RESPONSES

### A. Maternal Rearing

Infant monkeys spend most of their time in physical contact with their mothers for the first few months of life and during that time are totally dependent on her as a source of food, warmth, and protection. The mother also has a role in regulating infant physiology (Hofer, 1994). An extensive literature on rodents has elucidated the various aspects of tactile, olfactory, and nutritive interactions of the mother on the body temperature, blood pressure, heart rate and activity levels of her infants (Hofer, 1994). Monkey mothers also influence both body temperature and activity in their infants. Infants that are hand reared in a nursery show lower nighttime body temperatures, different diurnal temperature patterns, and more variability in body temperature than mother-reared infants (Lubach, Kittrell, & Coe, 1992). However, the disrupted circadian temperature changes that typically occur when an infant monkey is separated briefly from its mother are *not* reversed if the infant is adopted by a conspecific female (Reite, Seiler, & Short, 1978). The role of the mother as a zeitgeber for circadian processes in young macaques seems to be unique to the infant's mother and evidently cannot be fulfilled by others in the social group.

During infancy the mother monkey carries the infant, grooms it, occasionally punishes it, and often restricts its early attempts at independence. Thus, the first social experience that an infant encounters is with its mother. It has been hypothesized that these first mother–infant interactions form the basis of subsequent social interactions and patterns of coping with stressors (Coe, Wiener, & Levine, 1983). Several lines of evidence indicate that patterns of maternal behavior have considerable impact on the behavioral development of infants. Vervet monkey juveniles whose mothers had been more protective and restrictive during their infancy showed less interest in the external environment and took longer to enter a novel environment than juveniles whose mothers had not been overprotective (Fairbanks & McGuire, 1988). Early brief maternal separation experiences seem to be associated with delayed weaning and increased maternal restriction in offspring as old as 15 months (Laudenslager, unpublished observations). At 18 months of age, these offspring also appear timid in a novel setting and fail to habituate in comparison with normally reared controls (Laudenslager, unpublished observations). Bonnet macaque mothers, which normally are unrestrictive in the care of their young, become quite restrictive after being subjected to the stress of varied foraging demands (Boccia, Reite, & Laudenslager, 1991). This change in parenting produces tension in the mother–infant relationship, with negative consequences for the infant. Such infants show signs of less secure attachment to their mothers,

lower frequencies of breaking contact, lower levels of affiliative social behaviors including play and social subordination, and more distress during brief maternal separation (Andrews & Rosenblum, 1991, 1993, 1994a, 1994b; Boccia et al., 1991). Rhesus macaque infants whose mothers are inattentive or rejecting react most adversely when the mother–infant social bond is disrupted through separation (Hinde & Spencer-Booth, 1971; Kraemer, Ebert, Schmidt, & McKinney, 1991). This is also true for human infants: if the mother is inconsistent, unresponsive, or rejecting, her infant is more likely to evince an insecure attachment (Ainsworth, Blehar, Waters, & Wall, 1978) and be more disturbed by separation (Rutter, 1979). What is not known, at present, is whether these individual differences in maternal behavior have a long-term impact on immune responses in their offspring. However, given the far-reaching effects on behavioral responses, it would be surprising if this were not the case. Thus, the influence of individual differences in maternal parenting style on development of the immune system in infants is an important issue for future study.

## B. Nursery Rearing

Monkey infants that are hand reared by humans in a nursery environment and thus do not experience interactions with their mother and/or peers have different behavioral and immune profiles than infants that are reared by their mothers in a social group. Early studies by Harry Harlow and his colleagues demonstrated that rearing infant rhesus macaques without maternal or peer interactions (isolation rearing) had devastating effects on their behavioral repertoires. Isolation rearing for 6 or 12 months created animals that, as juveniles, showed exaggerated fearfulness, little or no play, and inappropriate aggressive behavior. These animals were sexually incompetent as adults, and females, if they became pregnant, showed cruel or indifferent maternal behavior toward their infants (Harlow & Harlow, 1969). Isolation-reared animals also showed differences in physiological profiles, including autonomic nervous system imbalances as measured by evoked heart rate responses to a loud auditory stimulus (Martin, Sackett, Gunderson, & Goodlin-Jones, 1988), lower levels of cerebrospinal norepinephrine (Kraemer, Ebert, Schmidt, & McKinney, 1989), and basal plasma cortisol levels nearly twice as high as those of mother-reared infants (Sackett, Bowman, Meyer, Tripp, & Grady, 1973). Given the breadth of the behavioral and physiological consequences of isolation rearing, it is not surprising that isolation-reared animals also had different immunological profiles. As adults, isolation-reared rhesus macaques had a lower ratio of helper to suppressor T cells, an increased proportion of natural killer cells, and a decreased survival rate compared with non-isolation-reared infants (Gluck et al., 1989). Taken together, these studies clearly indicate that early interactions with mother and peers are necessary for normal behavioral and physiological development, including immunocompetence.

Rearing environments in which infant monkeys are hand-reared by humans in a nursery but routinely socialized with peers also have a long-lasting impact on immune development even though this form of rearing produces few, if any, behavioral anomalies (Worlein & Sackett, 1997). Such nursery-reared (NR) rhesus macaques had significantly higher lymphocyte responses to mitogen stimulation at 5–8 months of age than did infants that were reared by their mothers. Although levels were still elevated 1.5 years later, by 2.5 years of age only responses to concanavalin A (Con A) were still significantly elevated; responses to phytohemagglutinin (PHA) and pokeweed mitogen (PWM) had returned to normal ranges (Coe, Lubach, Ershler, & Klopp, 1989). The NR infants also had a significantly higher ratio of CD4+ (T-helper) to CD8+ (T-cytotoxic/suppressor) cells at 6, 12, 18, and 24 months of age and consistently lower natural cytotoxicity than infants that had been reared with their mothers (Lubach, Coe, & Ershler, 1995). Young monkeys that were left with their mothers and weaned at 6 months of age (early weaning) had mitogen stimulation profiles that were intermediate between the profiles of NR infants and those of monkeys that were reared with their mothers until they were more than 1 year old, the age at which macaques are normally weaned from their mothers under free-ranging conditions (Coe et al., 1989). Nursery rearing also affects other physiological set points. NR infants reared with cloth surrogates or in continuous housing with peers showed lower basal cortisol levels at 14, 30, and 60 days of age than did mother-reared infants (Shannon, Champoux, & Suomi, 1998).

Although some of these effects on immune profiles are undoubtedly due to the psychological and physiological impact of rearing without regulatory input from the mother, NR infants differ from mother-reared infants in a number of other ways. NR infants that received human infant formula were larger and heavier than mother-reared infants (Coe, Lubach, Schneider, Dierschke, & Ershler, 1992). They also experienced more gastrointestinal infections than infants raised with their mothers (Coe, 1993), possibly because they are exposed to a different range of infectious agents owing to their close exposure to humans during rearing. Although there is no doubt that this form of early rearing can have long-term effects on immune profiles in macaques, the functional significance of these differences is not entirely clear. For example, in vivo antibody responses to vaccination with three different antigens were no different in NR than in mother-reared infants (Coe, Lubach, Schneider, Dierschke, & Ershler, 1992). Studies that relate nursery rearing to subsequent morbidity and mortality are necessary to truly assess the significance, if any, of immune differences seen in these infants.

## C. Disruption of the Mother–Infant Bond

Even at a time when the infant is physiologically able to live independently of its mother, disruption of this social bond can produce dramatic changes in behavior and physiology, including immunomodulation. Maternal separation has been conceptualized as a nonhuman primate model of human loss, bereavement, and depression (Kaufman & Rosenblum, 1967a,b; McKinney & Bunney, 1969; Reite & Boccia, 1994). A number of studies have investigated acute and chronic behavioral and physiological impacts of maternal separation on young nonhuman primates (Mineka & Suomi, 1978). The studies have involved a variety of separation experiences, but most separations occurred when the infants were 4 to 7 months of age. In some experimental paradigms the mother–infant dyads were socially housed and the mother was removed from the social group for a period of time and then returned to the group. In other designs the infants were removed from the social group and placed in novel housing without their mothers. In some cases singly housed mother–infant dyads have been separated. Finally, other studies have investigated the impact of naturally occurring separations, such as those during mating season when the infant is about 6 months old. As a general rule, more unfamiliar separation environments and greater social isolation during separation are associated with greater behavioral and physiological effects. As will be discussed later, the presence of positive social support (social affiliation) has considerable utility in ameliorating the effects of all types of social disturbance, including separation.

The behavioral response to maternal separation has been characterized as a two-step process that begins with an initial agitation (protest) phase followed by a despair or depression phase similar to that seen in human children separated from their parents for prolonged periods of time (Bowlby, 1973; Kaufman & Rosenblum, 1967a,b; Mineka & Suomi, 1978; Reite, Short, Seiler, & Pauley, 1981). The agitation phase generally lasts 24 to 48 h. The young monkey vocalizes frequently and increases its vigilance, activity, and locomotion during this phase. Under free-ranging conditions, these behaviors would be instrumental in reuniting the isolated infant with the mother (Bowlby, 1973). After the initial agitation period, the monkey withdraws. Activity and vocalization decline and the young monkey may assume a withdrawn, huddled posture. Social interactions and play behavior decline and ingestive behaviors increase (Laudenslager, Held, Boccia, Reite, & Cohen, 1990).

These behavioral changes are accompanied by dysregulation in a number of physiological systems, including the immune system. The initial agitation phase is associated with increased heart rate and body temperature. The subsequent depression phase is characterized by altered sleep patterns (decreased total sleep, increased REM latency, reduced number of REM periods, and more frequent arousals), lower heart rate and body temperature, cardiac arrhythmia, and changes in circadian rhythms of heart rate and body temperature (Reite et al., 1981). There are also multiple indications of hypothalamo-pituitary activation (Levine & Wiener, 1988), including increased plasma cortisol and growth hormone (Laudenslager et al., 1995) and prolactin (Laudenslager, unpublished observations). Changes in central nervous system biogenic amines and peripheral sympathetic activity have also been reported (Kraemer et al., 1991). The magnitude of these physiological changes is related to a number of factors such as the species under investigation, presence of conspecifics, and ability to have visual and tactile contact with the mother. Physiological changes in the separated infant often covary with the magnitude of behaviors that reflect distress. Elevation in plasma cortisol during the first week after separation is positively correlated with vocalization and time spent in a withdrawn posture and negatively correlated with play and physical proximity to others (Laudenslager et al., 1995).

These physiological alterations are exactly the changes expected to affect the regulation of the immune response. Thus it is not surprising that immunomodulation also occurs following maternal separation in nonhuman primates. These alterations are evident in a wide variety of immunological systems. Bonnet macaque infants that were separated from both their mothers and their social group showed reduced lymphocyte activation in response to both Con A and PHA (Laudenslager, Reite, &

Harbeck, 1982). Squirrel monkey infants that were separated from their mothers had an increase in hemolytic complement activity evident 24 h after separation and still apparent 2 weeks later (Coe, Rosenberg, & Levine, 1988a). The primary antibody response to a bacteriophage was also lower in both squirrel monkey and rhesus macaque infants following maternal separation, although decreases were not as great in the rhesus infants. A dramatic increase in macrophage chemiluminescence by zymosan-stimulated macrophages was seen following a 24-h separation of singly housed squirrel monkey mother–infant dyads. This effect was present in both mother and infant and lingered for 2 weeks after the dyads were reunited (Coe, Rosenberg, & Levine, 1988b). Infant squirrel monkeys that were separated from their mothers and housed individually in a novel separation cage showed a significant decrease in total plasma IgG levels. Interestingly, infants separated from their mothers and left in their home cage with three or four familiar peers showed no decrease in plasma nonspecific IgG levels. Both groups did, however, show a reduction in the C4 complement protein (Coe, Cassayre, Levine, & Rosenberg, 1988). Squirrel monkeys that were separated from their mothers and housed in a single cage showed a decrease in natural cytotoxicity 1 and 3 days after separation. However, levels of cytolytic activity returned to baseline in most groups by 7 days postseparation (Coe & Erickson, 1997).

Although maternal separation can reliably elicit changes in behavioral and physiological systems, nearly every study has shown that the magnitudes of the responses are extremely variable among individuals. In a study of behavior and immune responses, two species of macaque were housed in social groups with their mothers and age-matched controls (Laudenslager et al., 1990). When the mothers were removed from the group, lymphocyte activation declined in some, but not all, subjects. The effects were limited to the young monkeys that exhibited the greatest behavioral distress after maternal separation. Monkeys that vocalized the most on the first day of separation and spent the greatest amount of time in huddled, withdrawn postures were the most likely to show indications of immunomodulation. This relation between behavioral and physiological indices of stress also occurs in free-ranging infant macaques. Rhesus macaque females typically resume mating activity when their infants are 5–8 months old, before completion of weaning. This is distressing for the infant because the mother is frequently out of sight and often rejects and punishes the infant as she develops consortships with males. However, the response to this experience is quite variable among the infants. Antibody levels after immunization with tetanus toxoid at 1 year of age were related to behavioral responses that an infant had shown during its mother's mating activity; infants that exhibited high levels of distress had lower antibody levels to immunization (Laudenslager, Rasmussen, Berman, Suomi, & Berger, 1993). Therefore, not all monkeys are affected equally by disruption of the mother–infant relationship. An important area for continued investigation is determination of the sources of these individual differences in response and identification of individuals that are most vulnerable to social separation experiences. Variations in response could be due to the prior mother–infant relationship, maternal dominance status, infant gender, infant parity, the availability of social support during these experiences, and inherent behavioral and/or physiological reactivity, to name only a few.

Some experimental attention has been given to several of these factors. As discussed previously, the prior mother–infant relationship is known to impact behavioral responses. This relationship may be an important predictor of subsequent response to social stressors such as maternal separation and deserves further experimental attention. Autonomic indicators of physiological reactivity, such as resting heart rate, may serve as useful predictors of risk for problematic behavioral and physiological stress responses. Pigtailed macaques whose baseline heart rates were above the median heart rate also had higher rates of vocalization (indicative of agitation) after maternal separation at 6 months and spent more time in slouched postures (indicative of depression) than did infants whose heart rates were below the median (Boccia, Laudenslager, & Reite, 1994). Higher heart rates may reflect more reactive physiological and behavioral patterns in these monkeys. The obvious prediction is that monkeys with higher heart rates at baseline would also show greater immunological and endocrinological responses to separation. Human children with more reactive response patterns are at greater risk for immunological disease such as allergic disorders (Kagan, Snidman, Julia-Sellers, & Johnson, 1991). Studies have also demonstrated that humans with high cardiac sympathetic reactivity also have high hypothalamo-pituitary-adrenal (HPA) reactivity and immune modulation during stress (Cacioppo, 1994). However, adolescents with atopic illness have a blunted response to socially stressful situations (Buske-Kirschbaum et al., 1998). This blunted HPA response in adolescents with allergic disorders bears a strong similarity to the blunted HPA response observed in strains of rats at greater risk for auto-

immune illness (Sternberg, 1995). Given the inherent variability in the response of monkeys to maternal and other forms of social separation (Lewis, McKinney, Young, & Kraemer, 1976), intrinsic differences in biological reactivity, as reflected by these autonomic parameters, may act as important markers for individuals at greater risk for untoward responses to social stressors.

Other studies indicate that certain behavioral styles in monkeys are related to viral antibody titers to cytomegalovirus (Laudenslager et al., in press). Young, free-ranging rhesus macaques characterized as irritable, active, aggressive, and excitable had significantly higher titers to cytomegalovirus than monkeys scoring low on these scales. None of the immune parameters were related to gender or maternal dominance status.

Species differences in response to maternal separation have also been reported. These variations appear to be mediated by the availability of social support for separated infants and are related to differences in maternal behavior and social organization between the two species studied (pigtailed and bonnet macaques). Pigtailed macaque mothers are quite restrictive in the care of their infants, preventing other members of the social group from interacting with their offspring. Socially housed adult females of this species usually maintain spatial separation from each other rather than sitting in close proximity (Boccia, Laudenslager, & Reite, 1988; Kaufman & Rosenblum, 1966). As a result, their infants seldom interact with adults other than their mothers. During an experimental separation, when a mother is removed from the social group, the young monkey is therefore unlikely to find other individuals willing to provide either protection or social interaction. Often when the infant attempts to interact with other adults, it is punished or chased away. The resulting behavioral and physiological responses to maternal separation in pigtailed macaques can be quite profound (although as discussed previously responses are quite variable). However, if the infant succeeds in receiving positive social support from other members of the group, the negative effects of maternal separation can be lessened. Greater contact with other members of the social group has been shown to reduce the magnitude of heart rate changes following maternal separation in pigtailed macaques (Caine & Reite, 1981).

Bonnet macaques display a far less restrictive pattern of maternal care and much greater interaction with other individuals in the social group. Females and infants typically sit in close proximity in small clusters. Bonnet macaque infants, therefore, have the opportunity to participate in a number of social interactions and form a familiarity with many members of their natal group. If a mother is removed from the social group, her offspring has alternate adults with which it can interact. These alternative caregivers hold the infants on their ventral surfaces, groom them, and provide protection. As a result, behavioral and physiological disturbances evinced by separation are more transient in bonnet macaques than in pigtailed macaques (Laudenslager et al., 1990).

The importance of the availability of these alternative caregivers during separation was further delineated in a subsequent set of studies. Bonnet macaque infants separated from their mothers in the presence of a preferred peer partner showed no changes in natural cytotoxicity. However, when infants were separated from their mothers in the absence of a preferred peer partner, cytotoxicity toward tumor targets declined as rapidly as 2 h after separation, although it returned to baseline after 1 week (Boccia et al., 1997). A similar pattern of changes was shown in proliferative responses to Con A and PWM. Interestingly, monkeys that were separated from their mothers without the presence of preferred peer partners, had developed significant interactions with the less preferred older peers by the end of the week of separation. This was coincident with the time that immune parameters returned to baseline. The magnitude of immunological changes was related to the allomaternal and affiliative behaviors that the young monkey experienced during the separation period. The more social affiliation a monkey experienced, the higher the cytotoxicity of peripheral blood lymphocytes toward tumor cells. The presence of these affiliative or allomaternal behaviors in nonhuman primates models similar influences of social support in humans. Certainly the presence of social support reduces the negative consequences of stressors on health in humans. Such support is particularly important in recovery from serious illnesses of many etiologies (Cohen, 1988) and minor illnesses such as the common cold (Cohen, Doyle, Skoner, Rabin, & Gwaltney, 1997).

## D.  Disruption of Bonds in Peer Reared Infants

Nursery reared infants are sometimes housed with peers during infancy. This type of continuous exposure to peers during development produces individuals with impaired behavioral repertoires compared with mother-reared infants and NR infants that are housed singly and socialized daily (Ruppenthal, Walker, & Sackett, 1991; Worlein &

Sackett, 1997). Peer-reared animals do form attachment bonds with each other and experimental separation of these infants has been shown to alter behavioral and physiological responses. However, these alterations are somewhat different from those seen during maternal separation. Infants that do not experience multiple separations typically show fewer and less profound behavioral and physiological effects than infants separated from their mothers (Mineka & Suomi, 1978). Peer-separated infants usually show only the agitation phase of the separation response, characterized by more activity and vocalization, and higher heart rate and body temperature (Boccia, Reite, Kaemingk, Held, & Laudenslager, 1989), although despair responses have been reported in some paradigms involving multiple separations from peers (Suomi, Harlow, & Domek, 1970). Separation of peer-reared infants also resulted in modest effects on mitogen-stimulated lymphocyte activation during a 2-week separation of 6-month-old pair-reared macaques (Reite, Harbeck, & Hoffman, 1981). Proliferative response to PHA and Con A was decreased when the monkeys were separated, and returned to baseline when they were reunited. In a larger study consisting of eight pairs of infants, decreased lymphocyte proliferation in response to PWM was observed in the second week of separation (Boccia et al., 1989). Peer-reared infants subjected to 4 weeks of repeated social separation showed a small but statistically significant decrease in total IgG levels following separation (Scanlan, Coe, Latts, & Suomi, 1987). An obvious obstacle inherent to in vitro stimulation studies and enumerative procedures is the lack of clear implications for in vivo immune function (Maier & Laudenslager, 1988) and, more specifically, health in general (Cohen, Doyle, & Skoner, 1999).

## E.  Long-Term Effects of Social Separation

Early social separation experiences, even if brief, can have long-term behavioral and immunological consequences. A single 2-week maternal separation occurring at 6 months of age (followed by reunion with the mother) affects subsequent behavioral responses to novelty in juvenile and adult monkeys (Capitanio et al., 1988; Capitanio & Reite, 1984). These monkeys are timid in new situations, taking longer to explore novel objects or obtain preferred fruit under conditions of novelty. They have smaller social networks and fewer grooming partners as adults than conspecifics that did not undergo maternal separation. Infant pigtailed macaques that had experienced a single 10-day maternal separation when they were

4–7 months old were significantly less sociable as juveniles than animals that had not undergone a separation (Caine, Earle, & Reite, 1983).

Immunologically, adult monkeys that have had early experiences with brief social separation have lower mitogen activation of lymphocytes than do adults that have not experienced these events (Coe et al., 1992; Laudenslager, Capitanio, & Reite, 1985). In contrast, the influence of similar experiences on natural cytotoxicity is quite different. Under resting, nonchallenged conditions, lymphocytes from adult monkeys separated at 6 months for 2 weeks and subsequently reunited showed *greater* lysis of tumor targets than lymphocytes compared to control animals (Laudenslager, Berger, Boccia, & Reite, 1996).

It is possible that differences seen in individuals that have undergone a maternal separation may be partly mediated through long-term changes in the mother-infant relationship following reunion. We have noted that pigtailed macaque mothers that have been separated briefly from their infants tend to be more attentive and restrictive when they are reunited and wean the infants at a later age than mothers whose infants had not been separated. Mothers of previously separated infants also maintain greater control over their infants' physical proximity when observed at 15 months of age (Laudenslager, unpublished observations). The preceding observations are reminiscent of data showing that rat pups that experienced early handling were more responsive to antigenic challenge as adults (Solomon, Levine, & Kraft, 1968). It turns out that handled pups received increased grooming from the mother after return to the nest (Smotherman, Brown, & Levine, 1977). The changes in behavioral and physiological regulation in rats following early handling may therefore have been attributable to differential reactions of the mother to the pups that were handled. Increased maternal care has been shown to affect the nature of HPA responses to stressors (Liu et al., 1997). Therefore, a part of the long-term differences observed in monkeys that experienced early separation may be related to long-term alterations in the mother–infant relationship after reunion.

## F. Disease Risk and Early Rearing

If one is to implicate early experience as a significant factor affecting health and well-being, then one must identify associations of negative early experiences with disease course. For example, stressful early experiences in nonhuman primates have been shown to alter the course of simian immunodeficiency virus (SIV). Animals that were peer reared after undergoing a permanent separation from their mothers at 3–7 months of age had shorter latencies to leukopenia and lymphopenia after inoculation with SIV as adults (Capitanio & Lerche, 1991). Thus, early experience not only affects immunomodulation but also impacts disease course in immune related illness.

## III. EFFECTS OF SOCIAL INTERACTION ON IMMUNE FUNCTION IN JUVENILES AND ADULTS

### A. Disruption of Social Bonds at Later Ages

Nonhuman primates form strong and enduring bonds with conspecifics resulting in complex social interactions and social organization. Just as separation from the mother in infancy results in dysregulation in a variety of behavioral and physiological systems, disruption of social bonds results in behavioral changes and immunomodulation in older animals. Trapping and 24-h social isolation of free-ranging juvenile rhesus macaques resulted in lower natural cytotoxicity and lower percentages of CD2+ and CD8+ lymphocytes (Laudenslager et al., in press). The magnitude of these changes was not associated with gender or maternal social rank. Experimentally removing juvenile rhesus macaques from their natal social groups and housing them in peer groups produced marked changes in behavioral and immune parameters as well as an increase in cortisol (Gordon et al., 1992; Gust et al., 1992). Similar to young monkeys separated from their mothers, juveniles that were separated from their natal groups exhibited less play and more coo vocalizations (a separation distress call) than control juveniles that remained in their social groups. Separated juveniles also showed a rise in cortisol on the day of separation. Although cortisol levels returned to baseline by 3–4 weeks, separated individuals showed continued reductions in peripheral blood CD4+ and CD8+ cells for up to 11 weeks after separation. It is likely that separation also produced dysregulation in other physiological systems, since weight gain in separated subjects was one-third of that exhibited by controls. These observations indicate that adaptation to social separation and/or rehousing is a prolonged process, a consideration that should be noted by investigators who are using these highly social animals in studies of infectious diseases and of immune and endocrine function.

Adult female rhesus macaques separated from their social group and housed either alone or with a preferred companion underwent changes similar to those seen in juveniles, namely, an increase in plasma cortisol concentrations, a decrease in CD4+ and CD8+ populations, and an increase in coo vocalizations. As noted with separated bonnet macaque infants (Boccia et al., 1997), the presence of social support in the form of a preferred companion modulated these changes and was associated with a quicker return to baseline levels (Gust, Gordon, Brodie, & McClure, 1994). However, there were large individual differences in the degree to which the companion modulated the stress-associated changes in lymphocyte subsets.

Although separation from social partners resulted in immunomodulation for both male and female juveniles and for adult females, effects were somewhat different for adult male rhesus macaques. Removal from their social group had no effect on cortisol, absolute number of CD4+ and CD8+ or CD20+, or absolute number of white blood cells (Gust, Gordon & Hambright, 1993). These differences in immunomodulation probably reflect different life histories of male and female macaques. Females remain in the social group in which they are born and maintain strong social bonds with maternal kin, whereas males emigrate to other troops as young adults. Therefore adult males appear to be more physiologically adapted to separation from familiar conspecifics than females.

## B. Disease Risk and Social Separations

Immunomodulation associated with separations seems to result in increased morbidity and mortality. Capitanio and Lerche (1998) found that in rhesus macaques, housing relocations and social separations occurring in the 90-day period before inoculation with SIV and 30 days after were associated with decreased survival. Thus, social separation is associated with greater health risk in adult monkeys.

## C. Formation of Social Groups

Immune functioning is affected not only by social separation but by any situation that increases social conflict among animals. Macaques form linear dominance hierarchies. In undisturbed groups of animals this hierarchy is extremely stable. Females remain in their natal social group and acquire the dominance rank that their mothers hold. Attainment of dominance status is somewhat different for males because they leave their natal group and emigrate to other groups as young adults. The dominance status of adult males is positively correlated with their age and the amount of time they have spent in residence in a particular social group. When unfamiliar animals are experimentally placed together in a common housing area they must establish a new social structure and dominance hierarchy. This results in increased levels of aggression that typically diminish after a short period of time as a dominance hierarchy is established and social alliances are formed. Groups of unfamiliar female rhesus macaques had increased levels of cortisol and decreased numbers of lymphocytes in plasma 24 h after their groups were formed (Gust et al., 1991). These decreases were longer lasting in females that attained low social rank. Lymphocyte levels returned to baseline by 8 days after group formation in females that attained high rank, whereas lymphopenia was still apparent 9 weeks later in females that attained low rank. Although decreases in lymphocytes were not highly correlated with amounts of aggression received, they were associated with grooming, an important affiliative behavior. Higher ranking individuals received more social support in the form of grooming and also recovered from the adverse immunological effects of group formation more rapidly. Social grooming in macaques is an important means of establishing social relationships and modulating autonomic function. The elevation in heart rate, which occurs after an agonistic encounter, decreases most rapidly if a monkey receives grooming from the other monkey involved in the encounter (Boccia, Reite, & Laudenslager, 1989).

## D. Reintroduction of Individuals into Familiar Social Groups

Formation of groups of unfamiliar individuals is not the only experimental manipulation that can result in increased levels of aggression in macaques. Return of individuals to a familiar group also results in increased aggression directed toward the familiar intruder. When familiar adult male rhesus macaques were released into a familiar group after a 1-year absence, they received threats from the majority of the resident group members. These males showed significant increases in cortisol and significant decreases in absolute numbers of CD4+ and CD8+ lymphocytes. Changes in physiological parameters were significantly correlated with the amount of aggression that the monkeys received. Individuals that received more aggression showed a greater increase in cortisol and a greater decrease in T lymphocytes (Gust et al., 1993).

A similar pattern of behavioral and physiological responses was seen in juvenile animals that were returned to their social group after shorter absences (11–18 weeks) (Gordon & Gust, 1993). After their return to the social group, the animals experienced aggression and showed significantly higher levels of cortisol and significant reductions in CD4+ and CD8+ lymphocytes. There were also significant correlations between the increase in cortisol and decrease in T cell subsets within subjects as well as significant correlations between aggression and T-cell subsets and cortisol. The immune changes in this study were related to cortisol, which increased in response to aggression received.

## E. Constantly Changing Social Conditions

Experimentally induced social instability in the form of continuous group reorganizations has been shown to negatively impact both behavior and physiology. In a study of the cardiovascular and immune consequences of long-term exposure to unstable social conditions, cynomolgus macaque males were subjected to monthly reorganizations of their social groups. After 26 months of social instability the subjects showed lower responses to mitogen stimulation than monkeys that were housed in stable social groups. Immunomodulation was correlated with behaviors exhibited by individuals. Subjects that were more affiliative and less aggressive showed higher levels of lymphocyte response to Con A and PHA at the end of the study. Natural cytotoxicity was positively correlated with higher levels of affiliation even in the more aggressive males. Interestingly, even in the stable social groups, animals that showed more affiliative behavior had higher levels of Con A mitogenesis (Cohen, Kaplan, Cunnick, Manuck, & Rabin, 1992; Kaplan et al., 1991). It is possible that behaviors such as social grooming, an integral component of affiliation, served to modulate the physiological changes that occurred during these reorganizations. The functional significance of these differences has not yet been fully explored. Surprisingly, the primary IgG response to tetanus toxoid immunization was higher in subordinate animals (those receiving more aggression) at the beginning of the 26-month study (Cunnick et al., 1991). When secondary response to tetanus toxoid was measured 9 months later, animals that had undergone repeated social reorganization had a greater IgG response regardless of rank. These observations emphasize the need for immune panels that include measures of in vivo immune function (Maier & Laudenslager, 1988) so that the functional significance of these changes can be ascertained.

Male cynomolgus monkeys that underwent reorganization of their social groups four times over a period of 5 months also had increased lymphocyte counts and decreased lymphocyte proliferation. These effects were especially prevalent in individuals that showed high levels of fear. As with the previously described longer study, a functional measure of immune competence (antibodies to herpes B virus) was not negatively affected by the stressor (Line et al., 1996). However, a more recent study indicates that social instability can have considerable impact on the course of disease. Animals that were socialized for 100 min daily in stable social groups survived longer after inoculation with SIV than did animals whose social groups were reorganized daily (Capitanio, Mendoza, Lerche, & Mason, 1998). A very important aspect of these findings was that early in the study animals that received social threats (aggression) had higher levels of SIV viral RNA in plasma and animals that engaged in affiliative behaviors had lower levels of viral RNA regardless of social condition. This indicates that the nature of social interactions (affiliative versus aggressive) can also influence disease course, regardless of social condition.

## F. Competition for Restricted Resources

Another situation that increases social conflict in nonhuman primates and results in immunomodulation is competition for a restricted resource. Significant changes in in vitro immune parameters have been observed under these conditions. When groups of macaques were prevented from access to water for 18–24 h, the animals displayed increased agonistic behavior and competition for the water spout when access was restored. Although linear dominance hierarchies existed in these groups, there was no relation between dominance status and the immune parameters measured. Behavioral and immunological changes did, however, vary according to species (Boccia, Laudenslager, Broussard, & Hijazi, 1992). There were clear differences between pigtailed and bonnet macaques in immune and endocrine measures, both at baseline (before experimental manipulation) and in response to experimental manipulation. At baseline, pigtailed macaques showed lower lymphocyte activation in response to mitogens, higher natural cytotoxicity, lower percentages of lymphocytes and higher percentages of segmented neutrophils in plasma, and lower total white blood counts than did bonnet macaques. After the experimental manipulation, only pigtailed macaques showed an immunological change, that is, significantly increased natural cytotoxicity and decreased proliferative responses to mitogens compared with baseline values. These changes may be related to the fact that agonistic behaviors were consistently higher in pigtailed macaques. Although, as noted before, immune measures were not directly influenced by the dominance status of the individual, there was a relation between the number of times a given individual was displaced from the water spout during the test and the proportion of change in responses to PHA and Con A. Animals that received more displacements also showed a greater decrease in mitogen stimulation.

## G. Aggression under Free-Ranging Conditions

Physiological correlates of increased aggression are not unique to laboratory settings. Increased rates of aggression have also been associated with altered numbers of lymphocytes and higher levels of cortisol in baboons in free-ranging situations. When an extremely aggressive adult male baboon joined a troop of baboons, the troop experienced increased levels of aggression, mostly instigated by the immigrating male and disproportionately aimed at females (Alberts, Sapolsky, & Altmann, 1992). Physiological profiles of troop members taken 2 weeks later showed that levels of cortisol were higher than before the male joined the troop, and these levels were significantly higher in animals that were the focus of his aggressive behavior. Interestingly, even the immigrating male had high levels of cortisol. Mean numbers of lymphocytes in blood of resident troop members were lower after the male's immigration and negatively correlated with plasma cortisol.

## IV. SOCIAL INTERACTION AND IMMUNE FUNCTIONING IN AGING MACAQUES

Although frequent and intense social interactions are extremely important in regulating behavioral and physiological systems in developing and adult monkeys, the consequences of these interactions seem to change during senescence. Macaques can live to be over 30 years of age, with females exhibiting signs of menopause at about 25 years of age. Since younger monkeys have been shown to benefit from social housing in a laboratory setting, it was thought that older animals might also benefit from increased social interactions. Behavioral observations seemed to indicate that social housing does indeed enhance the well-being of older animals (Coe, Ershler, Champoux, & Olson, 1992). Aged rhesus macaques that were housed with one or more juveniles were more active than their counterparts that were housed alone or with one other aged individual. However, the immunological data presented a different picture. Socially housed aged individuals exhibited decreases in lymphocyte proliferation and natural cytotoxicity. It is therefore apparent that unregulated social interaction was very stressful for older animals. However, housing the older monkey in a cage that allowed it to control the social access of a single juvenile alleviated these effects. Under these conditions, lymphocyte proliferation and natural cytotoxicity were not depressed. Thus, the value of social interaction is not constant but actually changes quite significantly as an individual reaches senescence.

As monkeys age they show signs of decreased immune functioning, including significantly lower proliferative responses to mitogens, lower natural cytotoxicity than in younger animals (Ershler et al., 1988) and lower antibody responses to tetanus vaccine. Under free-ranging conditions, old macaques (>25 years of age) engage in fewer social interactions than younger individuals (Worlein, unpublished observations). It is possible that decreased social interactions result in less exposure to transmittable diseases and thus may actually increase longevity in aged animals, which are no longer as able to mount an effective immune response as when they were younger.

## V. SUMMARY

It is abundantly clear that early experience profoundly affects subsequent behavioral and physiological development in nonhuman primates. Factors encountered by the developing organism, including maternal care and stressors, have the ability to permanently alter behavioral and physiological set points. Absence of mother and/or peers, and stressors such as social separation, are known to be associated with long-term alterations in behavior and physiology. Maternal parenting style is known to alter behavioral repertoires in infants. To date, however, very little is known about the effect of maternal parenting style and other social situations on physiological development in nonhuman primates.

Monkeys (and humans) show a great degree of variability in both behavioral and physiological responses to stressful situations. Studies in nonhuman primates indicate that behavioral and physiological distress are closely coupled. For example, individuals who show the greatest behavioral response to maternal separation also are the most likely to show immunomodulation. Although there are probably a variety of factors that influence these responses, mother–infant interactions and inherent behavioral/

physiological reactivity appear to be two especially promising avenues of future research.

Social instability, whether naturally occurring or experimentally induced, results in immunomodulation. The nature of social interactions with conspecifics during these periods of stress can have significant impact on the physiological effects of the stressor. Animals that receive and engage in aggressive behavior tend to experience exacerbated physiological effects of stress, whereas animals that engage in affiliative behaviors and receive social support show diminished physiological effects of the stressor. Grooming is an important component of affiliative social interactions between nonhuman primates with heart rate falling as low during social grooming as it does during sleep. Grooming is used for reconciliation among nonhuman primates following agonistic encounters. In adult monkeys the elevation in heart rate associated with agonistic encounters or fighting declines most rapidly when an individual receives social grooming. Social grooming may also alter sympathetic activity in other autonomically regulated systems and perhaps influence immunoregulatory processes to reduce the impact of the stressor. The link between social affiliation and diminished changes in immune responses under social stressors is not surprising in light of these observations.

## Acknowledgments

Preparation of this chapter was supported in part by USPHS Grant MH37373 (M.L.L.). The authors are grateful to Lisa Aimes and Kate Elias, Washington Regional Primate Research Center, for their editorial assistance.

## References

Ainsworth, M. D. S., Blehar, M. C., Waters, E., & Wall, S. (1978). *Patterns of attachment: a psychological study of the strange situation.* Hillsdale, NJ: Erlbaum.

Alberts, S. C., Sapolsky, R. M., & Altmann, J. (1992). Behavioral, endocrine, and immunological correlates of immigration by an aggressive male into a natural primate group. *Hormones and Behavior, 26,* 167–178.

Andrews, M. W., & Rosenblum, L. A. (1991). Attachment in monkey infants raised in variable- and low-demand environments. *Child Development, 62,* 686–693.

Andrews, M. W., & Rosenblum, L. A. (1993). Assessment of attachment in differentially reared infant monkeys (*Macaca radiata*): Response to separation and a novel environment. *Journal of Comparative Psychology, 107,* 84–90.

Andrews, M. W., & Rosenblum, L. A. (1994a). Influences of environmental demand on maternal behavior and infant development. *Acta Paediatrica, Supplement, 397,* 57–63.

Andrews, M. W., & Rosenblum, L. A. (1994b). The development of affiliative and agonistic social patterns in differentially reared monkeys. *Child Development, 65,* 1398–1404.

Boccia, M. L., Laudenslager, M. L., Broussard, C. L., & Hijazi, A. S. (1992). Immune responses following competitive water tests in two species of macaques. *Brain, Behavior and Immunity, 6,* 201–213.

Boccia, M. L., Laudenslager, M. L., & Reite, M. L. (1988). Spatial distribution of food and dominance related behavior in Bonnet macaques. *American Journal of Primatology, 16,* 123–130.

Boccia, M. L., Laudenslager, M. L., & Reite, M. L. (1994). Intrinsic and extrinsic factors affect infant responses to maternal separation. *Psychiatry, 57,* 43–49.

Boccia, M. L., Reite, M., Kaemingk, K., Held, P., & Laudenslager, M. (1989). Behavioral and autonomic responses to peer separation in pigtail macaque monkey infants, *Developmental Psychobiology, 22,* 447–461.

Boccia, M. L., Reite, M. L., & Laudenslager, M. L. (1989). On the physiology of grooming in pigtail macaques. *Physiology and Behavior, 45,* 667–670.

Boccia, M. L., Reite, M. L., & Laudenslager, M. L. (1991). Early social environment may alter the development of attachment and social support: Two case reports. *Infant Behavior and Development, 14,* 253–260.

Boccia, M. L., Scanlan, J. L., Laudenslager, M. L., Berger, C. L., Hijazi, A. S., & Reite, M. L. (1997). Juvenile friends, behavior, and immune responses to separation in bonnet macaque infants. *Physiology and Behavior, 61,* 191–198.

Bowlby, J. (1973). *Attachment and loss. II. Separation: Anxiety and anger.* New York: Basic Books.

Buske-Kirschbaum, A., Jobst, S., Psych, D., Wustmans, A., Kirschbaum, C., Rauh, W., & Hellhammer, D. (1998). Attenuated free cortisol response to psychosocial stress in children with atopic dermatitis. *Psychosomatic Medicine, 59,* 419–426.

Cacioppo, J. T. (1994). Social neuroscience: Autonomic, neuroendocrine, and immune responses to stress. *Psychophysiology, 31,* 113–128.

Caine, N. G., Earle, H., & Reite, M. (1983). Personality traits of adolescent pig-tailed monkeys (*Macaca nemestrina*): An analysis of social rank and early separation experience. *American Journal of Primatology, 4,* 253–260.

Caine, N., & Reite, M. (1981). The effect of peer contact upon physiological response to maternal separation. *American Journal of Primatology, 1,* 271–276.

Capitanio, J. P., & Lerche, N. W. (1991). Psychosocial factors and disease progression in simian AIDS: A preliminary report. *AIDS, 5,* 1103–1106.

Capitanio, J. P., & Lerche, N. W. (1998). Social separation, housing relocation, and survival in simian AIDS: A retrospective analysis. *Psychosomatic Medicine, 60,* 235–244.

Capitanio, J. P., Mendoza, S. P., Lerche, N. W., & Mason, W. A. (1998). Social stress results in altered glucocorticoid regulation and shorter survival in simian acquired immune deficiency syndrome. *Proceedings of the National Academy of Sciences of the United States of America, 95,* 4714–4719.

Capitanio, J. P., Rasmussen, K. L. R., Snyder, D. S., Laudenslager, M. L., & Reite, M. L. (1988). Long-term follow-up of previously separated pigtail macaques: Group and individual differences in response to novel situations. *Journal of Child Psychology and Psychiatry and Allied Disciplines, 27,* 531–538.

Capitanio, J. P., & Reite, M. L. (1984). The roles of early separation experience and prior familiarity in the social relations of pigtail macaques: A descriptive multivariate study. *Primates, 25,* 475–484.

Coe, C. L. (1993). Psychosocial factors and immunity in nonhuman primates: A review. *Psychosomatic Medicine, 55,* 298–308.

Coe, C. L., Cassayre, P., Levine, S., & Rosenberg, L. T. (1988). Effects of age, sex, and psychological disturbance on immunoglobulin levels in the squirrel monkey. *Developmental Psychobiology, 21*(2), 161–175.

Coe, C. L., & Erickson, C. M. (1997). Stress decreases lymphocyte cytolytic activity in the young monkey even after blockade of steroid and opiate hormone receptors. *Developmental Psychobiology, 30*, 1–10.

Coe, C. L., Ershler, W. B., Champoux, M., & Olson, J. (1992). Psychosocial factors and immune senescence in the aged primate. *Annals of the New York Academy of Sciences, 650*, 276–282.

Coe, C. L., Lubach, G. R., Ershler, W. B., & Klopp, R. G. (1989). Influence of early rearing on lymphocyte proliferation responses in juvenile rhesus monkeys. *Brain Behavior and Immunity, 3*, 47–60.

Coe, C. L., Lubach, G. R., Schneider, M. L., Dierschke, D. J., & Ershler, W. B. (1992). Early rearing conditions alter immune responses in the developing infant primate. *Pediatrics, 90*, 505–509.

Coe, C. L., Rosenberg, L. T., & Levine, S. (1988a). Prolonged effect of psychological disturbance on macrophage chemiluminescence in the squirrel monkey. *Brain Behavior and Immunity, 2*, 151–160.

Coe, C. L., Rosenberg, L. T., & Levine, S. (1988b). Effect of maternal separation on the complement system and antibody responses in infant primates. *International Journal of Neuroscience, 40*, 289–302.

Coe, C. L., Wiener, S. G., & Levine, S. (1983). Psychoendocrine responses of mother and infant monkeys to disturbance and separation. In *Symbiosis in parent–offspring interactions* (pp. 189–214). New York: Plenum.

Cohen, S. (1988). Psychosocial models of the role of social support in the etiology of physical disease. *Health Psychology, 7*, 269–297.

Cohen, S., Doyle, W. J., & Skoner, D. P. (1999). Psychological stress, cytokine production, and severity of upper respiratory illness. *Psychosomatic Medicine, 61*, 175–180.

Cohen, S., Doyle, W. J., Skoner, D. P., Rabin, B. S., & Gwaltney, J. M. (1997). Social ties and susceptibility to the common cold. *Journal of the American Medical Association, 277*, 1940–1944.

Cohen, S., Kaplan, J. R., Cunnick, J. E., Manuck, S. B., & Rabin, B. S. (1992). Chronic social stress, affiliation and cellular immune response in nonhuman primates. *Psychological Science, 3*, 301–304.

Cunnick, J. E., Cohen, S., Rabin, B. S., Carpenter, A. B., Manuck, S. B., & Kaplan, J. R. (1991). Alterations in specific antibody production due to rank and social instability. *Brain Behavior and Immunity, 5*, 357–369.

Ershler, W. B., Coe, C. L., Gravenstein, S., Schultz, K. T., Klopp, R. G., Meyer, M., & Houser, W. D. (1988). Aging and immunity in nonhuman primates. I. Effects of age and gender on cellular immune function in rhesus monkeys *(Macaca mulatta). American Journal of Primatology, 15*, 181–188.

Fairbanks, L. A., & McGuire, M. T. (1988). Long-term effects of early mothering behavior on responsiveness to the environment in vervet monkeys. *Developmental Psychobiology, 21*, 711–724.

Gluck, J. P., Ozer, H. Hensley, L. L., Beauchamp, A., Mailman, R. B., & Lewis, M. H. (1989). Early isolation in rhesus monkeys: Longterm effects on survival and cell mediated immunity. *Society of Neuroscience Abstracts, 15*, 197.

Gordon, T. P., & Gust, D. A. (1993). Return of juvenile rhesus monkeys (Macaca mulatta) to the natal social group following an 18 week separation. *Aggressive Behavior, 19*, 231–239.

Gordon, T. P., Gust, D. A., Wilson, M. E., Ahmed-Ansari, A., Brodie, A. R., & McClure, H. M. (1992). Social separation and reunion affects immune system in juvenile rhesus monkeys. *Physiology and Behavior, 51*, 467–472.

Gust, D. A., Gordon, T. P., Brodie, A. R., & McClure, H. M. (1994). Effect of a preferred companion in modulating stress in adult female rhesus monkeys. *Physiology and Behavior, 55*, 681–684.

Gust, D. A., Gordon, T. P., & Hambright, M. K. (1993). Response to removal from and return to a social group in adult male rhesus monkeys. *Physiology and Behavior, 53*, 599–602.

Gust, D. A., Gordon, T. P., Wilson, M. E., Brodie, A. R., Ahmed-Ansari, A., & McClure, H. M. (1991). Formation of a new social group of unfamiliar female rhesus monkeys affects the immune and pituitary adrenocortical systems. *Brain Behavior and Immunity, 5*, 296–307.

Gust, D. A., Gordon, T. P., Wilson, M. E., Brodie, A. R., Ahmed-Ansari, A., & McClure, H. M. (1992). Removal from natal social group to peer housing affects cortisol levels and absolute numbers of T-cell subsets in juvenile rhesus monkeys. *Brain Behavior and Immunity, 6*, 189–199.

Harlow, H. F., & Harlow, M. K. (1969). Effects of various mother-infant relationships on rhesus monkey behaviors. In B.M. Foss (Ed.), *Determinants of infant behaviour* (Vol. 4, pp. 15–36). London: Methuen.

Hinde, R. A. (Ed.) (1983). *Primate social relationships: An integrated approach.* Suderland, MA: Sinauer Associates.

Hinde, R. A., & Spencer-Booth, Y. (1971). Effects of brief separation from mother on rhesus monkeys. *Science, 173*, 111–118.

Hofer, M. A. (1994). Early relationships as regulators of infant physiology and behavior. *Acta Pediactrica Scandanavia, 397*, 9–18.

Kagan, J., Snidman, N., Julia-Sellers, J., & Johnson, M. O. (1991). Temperament and allergic symptoms. *Psychosomatic Medicine, 53*, 332–340.

Kaplan, J. R., Heise, E. R., Manuck, S. B., Shively, C. A., Cohen, S., Rabin, B. S., & Kasprowicz, A. L. (1991). The relationship of agonistic and affiliative behavior patterns to cellular immune function among cynomolgus monkeys *(Macaca fascicularis)* living in unstable social groups. *American Journal of Primatology, 25*, 157–173.

Kaufman, I. C., & Rosenblum, L. (1966). A behavioral taxonomy for *Macaca nemestrina* and *Macaca radiata*: Based on longitudinal observation of family groups in the laboratory. *Primates, 7*, 206–258.

Kaufman, I. C., & Rosenblum, L. A. (1967a). Depression in infant monkeys separated from their mothers. *Science, 155*, 1030–1031.

Kaufman, I. C., & Rosenblum, L. A., (1967b). The reactions to separation in infant monkeys: Anaclitic depression and conservation-withdrawal. *Psychosomatic Medicine, 29*, 648–675.

Kraemer, G. W., Ebert, M. H., Schmidt, D. E., & McKinney, W. T. (1989). A longitudinal study of the effect of different social rearing conditions on cerebrospinal fluid norepinephrine and biogenic amine metabolites in rhesus monkeys. *Neuropsychopharmacology, 2*(3), 175–189.

Kraemer, G. W., Ebert, M. H., Schmidt, D. E., & McKinney, W. T. (1991). Strangers in a strange land: A psychobiological study of infant monkeys before and after separation from real or inanimate mothers. *Child Development, 62*, 548–566.

Laudenslager, M. L., Berger, C. L., Boccia, M. L., & Reite, M. L. (1996). Natural cytotoxicity toward K562 cells by macaque lymphocytes from infancy through puberty: Effects of early social challenge. *Brain Behavior and Immunity, 10*, 275–287.

Laudenslager, M. L., Boccia, M. L., Berger, C. L., Gennaro-Ruggles, M. M., McFerran, B., & Reite, M. L. (1995). Total cortisol, free cortisol, and growth hormone associated with brief social separation experiences in young macaques. *Developmental Psychobiology, 28*, 199–212.

Laudenslager, M., Capitanio, J. P., & Reite, M. (1985). Possible effects of early separation experiences on subsequent immune function in adult macaque monkeys. *American Journal of Psychiatry, 142,* 862–864.

Laudenslager, M. L., Held, P. E., Boccia, M. L., Reite, M. L., & Cohen, J. J. (1990). Behavioral and immunological consequences of brief mother-infant separation: A species comparison. *Developmental Psychobiology, 23,* 247–264.

Laudenslager, M. L., Rasmussen, K. L. R., Berman, C. M., Suomi, S. J., & Berger, C. L. (1993). Specific antibody levels in free-ranging rhesus monkeys: Relationships to plasma hormones, cardiac parameters, and early behavior. *Developmental Psychobiology, 26,* 407–420.

Laudenslager, M. L., Rasmussen, K. L. R., Berman, C. M., Lilly, A. A., Shelton, S. E., Kalin, N. H., & Suomi, S. J. (1999). A preliminary description of free-ranging rhesus monkeys' responses to brief capture experiences: Behavioral, endocrine and immune relationships. *Brain, Behavior, and Immunity, 13,* 124–137.

Laudenslager, M. L., Reite, M., & Harbeck, R. J. (1982). Suppressed immune response in infant monkeys associated with maternal separation. *Behavioral and Neural Biology, 36,* 40–48.

Levine, S., & Wiener, S. G. (1988). Psychoendocrine aspects of mother-infant relationships in nonhuman primates. *Psychoneuroendocrinology, 13,* 143–154.

Lewis, J. K., McKinney, W. T., Young, L. D., & Kraemer, G. W. (1976). Mother-infant separation in rhesus monkeys as a model of human depression. A reconsideration. *Archives of General Psychiatry, 33,* 699–705.

Line, S. W., Kaplan, J. R., Heise, E. R., Hilliard, J. K., Cohen, S., Rabin, B. S., & Manuck, S. B. (1996). Effects of social reorganization on cellular immunity in male cynomolgus monkeys. *American Journal of Primatology, 39,* 235–249.

Liu, D., Diorio, J., Tannenbaum, B., Caldji, C., Francis, D., Freedman, A., Sharma, S., Pearson, D., Plotsky, P.M., & Meaney, M. J. (1997). Maternal care, hippocampal glucocorticoid receptors, and hypothalamic-pituitary-adrenal responses to stress. *Science, 277,* 1659–1662.

Lubach, G. R., Coe, C. L., & Ershler, W. B. (1995). Effects of early rearing environment on immune responses of infant rhesus monkeys. *Brain, Behavior, and Immunity, 9,* 31–46.

Lubach, G. R., Kittrell, E. M., & Coe, C. L. (1992). Maternal influences on body temperature in the infant primate. *Physiology and Behavior, 51,* 987–994.

Maier, S., & Laudenslager, M. (1988). Commentary: Inescapable shock, shock controllability and mitogen stimulated lymphocyte proliferation. *Brain Behavior, and Immunity, 2,* 87–91.

Martin, R. E., Sackett, G. P., Gunderson, V. M., & Goodlin-Jones, B. L. (1988). Auditory evoked heart rate responses in pigtailed macaques (*Macaca nemestrina*) raised in isolation. *Developmental Psychobiology, 21*(3), 251–260.

McKinney, W. T., Jr., & Bunney, W. E., Jr. (1969). Animal model of depression. I. Review of evidence: Implications for research. *Archives of General Psychiatry, 21,* 240–248.

Mineka, S., & Suomi, S. J. (1978). Social separation in monkeys. *Psychological Bulletin, 85,* 1376–1400.

Reite, M. L., & Boccia, M. L. (1994). Physiological aspects of adult attachment. In M. B. Speling & W. H. Berman (Eds.), *Attachment in adults: Clinical and developmental perspectives.* (pp. 98–127). New York: Guilford Press.

Reite, M., Harbeck, R., & Hoffman, A. (1981). Altered cellular immune response following peer separation. *Life Sciences, 29,* 1333–1136.

Reite, M., Seiler, C., & Short, R. (1978). Loss of your mother is more than loss of a mother. *American Journal of Psychiatry, 135,* 370–371.

Reite, M., Short, R., Seiler, C., & Pauley, J. D. (1981). Attachment, loss and depression. *Journal of Child Psychology and Psychiatry, 22,* 141–169.

Ruppenthal, G. C., Walker, C. G., & Sackett, G. P. (1991). Rearing infant monkeys (*Macaca nemestrina*) in pairs produces deficient social development compared with rearing in single cages. *American Journal of Primatology, 25,* 103–113.

Rutter, M. (1979). Maternal deprivation, 1972–1978: New findings, new concepts, new approaches. *Child Development, 50,* 283–305.

Sackett, G. P., Bowman, R. E., Meyer, J. S., Tripp, R. L., & Grady, S. S. (1973). Adrenocortical and behavioral reactions by differentially raised rhesus monkeys. *Physiological Psychology, 1,* 209–212.

Scanlan, J. M., Coe, C. L., Latts, A., & Suomi, S. J. (1987). Effects of age, rearing, and separation stress on immunoglobulin levels in rhesus monkeys. *American Journal of Primatology, 13,* 11–22.

Shannon, C., Champoux, M., & Suomi, S. J. (1998). Rearing condition and plasma cortisol in rhesus monkey infants. *American Journal of Primatology, 46,* 311–321.

Smotherman, W. P., Brown, C. P., & Levine, S. (1977). Maternal responsiveness following differential pup treatment and mother-pup interactions. *Hormones and Behavior, 8,* 242–253.

Solomon, G. F., Levine, S., & Kraft, J. K. (1968). Early experience and immunity. *Nature, 220,* 821–822.

Sternberg, E. M. (1995). Neuroendocrine factors in susceptibility to inflammatory disease: Focus on the hypothalamic-pituitary-adrenal axis. *Hormone Research, 43,* 159–161.

Suomi, S. J., Harlow, H. F., & Domek, C. J. (1970). Effect of repetitive infant–infant separation of young monkeys. *Journal of Abnormal Psychology, 76,* 161–172.

Worlein, J. M., & Sackett, G. P. (1997). Social development in nursery-reared pigtailed macaques (*Macaca nemestrina*). *American Journal of Primatology, 41,* 23–35.

# Individual Difference Factors in Psychoneuroimmunology

SUZANNE C. SEGERSTROM, MARGARET E. KEMENY,
MARK L. LAUDENSLAGER

## I. INTRODUCTION

The role of individual difference factors in psychoneuroimmunology (PNI) is an important area of inquiry. Does the relationship between stressor exposure and immune change depend on the nature of the individual's response to the stressor? What are the key domains of individual differences that have physiological relevance? Do certain stable characteristics of the organism play a key role in shaping immune responses? The vast majority of studies of behavior and immune processes in humans and other animals focus on the impact of the environment, particularly stressors. These studies have generated clear evidence that exposure to stressors can impact a variety of immune parameters measured in peripheral blood and lymphoid organs (see chapters by Biondi, Rabin, & Kusnecov, and Kiecolt-Glaser, this volume). However, inspection of the raw data in these studies suggests that effects of stressors are not uniform across individuals, even when the specific nature of the stressor and other contextual factors are kept relatively constant across exposures (e.g., in human experimental studies with tight control over laboratory conditions and in carefully controlled animal studies). Some individuals show particular immunologic changes with exposure to a particular stressor, while others do not, and when changes are apparent, the magnitude and even direction of these changes vary across individuals. It seems likely that host differences play a role in determining the nature of physiological changes following stressor exposure.

There are a variety of individual difference factors that may govern the immunologic response to stressful situations, as well as exerting an ongoing influence on physiology. This chapter will review studies of stable individual difference factors (e.g., *traits*) and their relationship to immune system functioning in humans and animals, both within and outside the context of stressor exposure. Stable individual difference factors exert an organizing influence on behavior and physiology, including responses to stressors (Mendoza & Mason, 1989), and may therefore influence the immune system. Observations of vertebrates from fish to humans reveal individual differences: In rodents, a particular stressor can provoke freezing, defeat postures, aggressive behavior, or no response. In humans, responses can include changes in behavior, affective responses such as anxiety, fear, depression, sadness, or a combination thereof, as well as an infinite array of cognitions. Furthermore, the specific nature of these responses may affect physiological consequences. For example, pleasant and unpleasant affective states, as well as different unpleasant affective states (e.g., sadness and disgust), show different patterns of brain activity as measured by electroencephalogram (EEG) or positron emission tomographic (PET) measurements of regional blood flow (Heller, Nitschke, Etienne, & Miller, 1997; Lane et al., 1997; Lane, Reiman, Ahern, Schwartz, & Davidson, 1997). There is also some evidence for different patterns of change in the autonomic nervous system during different emotional states (Ekman, Levenson, & Friesen, 1983; Levenson, 1992). Behavioral and psychological states, therefore, potentially mediate the effects of stable individual differences on the immune system. Throughout the chapter, we will examine these potential mediators of individual differences and include relevant evidence linking them to the immune system.

Despite the possibility that individual differences can account for additional variance in psychoneuroimmunology studies, there are a relatively small number of studies of stable individual difference factors and the immune system. We will review these studies and consider behavioral and psychological states that might mediate the effects of these individual difference factors. They are organized into three areas: affective characteristics, social characteristics, and cognitive characteristics.

## II. MODELS OF INDIVIDUAL DIFFERENCES

### A. Genetics

At the core of the investigation of individual differences, particularly in nonhuman animals, rests the role of each individual's genetic background in directing individual phenotypes. Tools provided by quantitative methods of behavioral genetics have permitted questions to be posed that no longer focus on sole contributions of environmental or genetic factors to individual differences but allow for the estimation of the interactions of these factors in determining differences (Plomin, DeFries, & McClearn, 1990). Selective breeding and knockout and transgenic approaches for identifying genetic contributions to mechanisms of control of immune regulation (Paul, 1998) and behavioral differences (Plomin et al., 1990) are important approaches in this endeavor. A recent report suggests that there are often uncontrolled environmental variables present in behavioral

genetic research that unwittingly confound the role of small genetic contributions (Crabbe, Wahlstrom, & Dudek, 1999). When the same strains of mice were tested in three laboratories under rigorously controlled conditions, there were significant differences in behavior across laboratories. Presumed contributing factors included time of testing, specific experimenter, and shipping variables. It was concluded when studying mutant mice strains that the role of large genotypic effects would not be influenced by these factors whereas smaller effect sizes are quite likely to be affected. With these caveats in mind, the use of behavioral genetic technologies has been advocated in the study of individual differences in PNI (see Bonneau, Moremede, Vogler, McClearn, & Jones, 1998). Sophisticated analytic techniques such as quantitative trait loci linkage studies permit identification of both genetic and environmental contributions for complex behavioral phenotypes (Cardon, 1995).

Two approaches to genetic individual differences dominate the animal PNI literature. Initial investigations focused on genetic differences between strains and the behavioral and immune concomitants. For example, strain differences in the reactivity of the hypothalamio-pituitary-adrenal (HPA) axis in Lewis and Fischer rats have been closely associated with differences in reactivity to acute stressors such as open field exposure (Sternberg, 1995). These differences co-vary with susceptibility to experimentally induced rheumatoid arthritis (RA) and encephalomyelitis (EAE) (Mason, 1991; Sternberg, 1995). Lewis rats that show reduced activity in an open field and lower HPA activity are far more susceptible to these induced phenomena. It is generally thought that the lower activity of the HPA axis noted in the Lewis strain is responsible for an overreaction of the immune system to the eliciting antigens for EAE (myelin basic protein) and RA (Streptococcal cell walls).

However, this characterization of trait differences in murine models has moved from a focus on between-species or -strain differences to within-strain differences. For example, the outbred Wistar rat shows a wide range of variation in a number of behavioral and neurobiological parameters (Cools, Brachten, Heeren, Willemen, & Ellenbroek, 1990). Based on their behavioral response to the dopaminergic agonist, apomorphine, an unselected population of Wistar rats can be characterized into two distinctly different populations with regard to endocrine, immune, and behavior characteristics (Cools, Rots, Ellenbroek, & deKloet, 1993). Apomorphine susceptible (APO-SUS) Wistar rats are more resistant to EAE, having greater HPA axis reactivity than the apomorphine unsusceptible (APO-UN) rats (Kavelaars, Heijnen, Ellenbroek, van Loveren, & Cools, 1997). Similar observations were made with regard to adjuvant-induced arthritis in this outbred strain (van de Langerijt, van Lent, Hermus, Sweep, Cools, & Van den Berg, 1994). The preceding observations are consistent with *between*-strain comparison of Lewis and Fischer rats (Sternberg , 1995). However, HPA reactivity is a necessary condition for greater EAE susceptibility. Initial observations of wild-type rats (*Rattus norvegicus*) indicates that although short attack latency toward an intruder is correlated with greater resistance to EAE, attack latency is not correlated with HPA activation or EAE resistance (Kavelaars, Heijnen, Tennekes, Briggink, & Koolhaas, 1999).

## B. Personality

In humans, PNI research necessarily focuses on stable individual differences unrelated to strain, though many may have a genetic component. The term *personality* encompasses most of these stable individual differences. *Trait* may be used to indicate continuous variables or dimensions on which people differ (e.g., conscientiousness), while *type* indicates a discontinuous or categorical description of personality (e.g., Type A). In addition, some individual differences are more narrowly defined: *temperament* is a stable individual difference which is present in early life and which results from inherited physiological processes (Kagan, 1994; Kagan & Snidman, 1991). Personality differs from other individual differences such as mood and coping primarily by being stable over long periods of time, even a lifetime. That is, most people show stable predispositions over time to feel, think, behave, or relate to others in particular ways when presented with similar situations, though the evidence for cross-situational consistency is weaker (Mischel & Shoda, 1995).

Several theoretical models for the effects of human individual differences on the immune system are possible (Segerstrom, in press). The first such model would propose tonic effects: Personality is associated with differences in the immune system on an ongoing basis. This model enjoys some support, as illustrated below by the empirical literature. There is, however, reason to believe that other models are equally, if not more, promising. For example, psychological and behavioral effects of personality, including those which could affect the immune system, are more pronounced when both personality and the environment are taken into effect (Bowers, 1973; Mischel &

Shoda, 1995), suggesting that immune effects would also be more evident in a more complex model.

Personality research has identified a number of such models which could apply to individual difference effects on the immune system. For example, models of the relationship between personality and psychopathology include the *predisposition* model, in which personality is a risk factor for pathology, the *pathoplastic* model, in which personality and psychopathology mutually affect each other's presentation, and the *common cause model*, in which the two share a single etiology (Klein, Wonderlich, & Shea, 1993; Widiger, Verheul, & van den Brink, 1999). Some of these personality models have already been applied to the immune system. For example, the predisposition model describes how personality affects stressor-related immune change (e.g., a personality dimension is a "risk factor" for stressor-related immune change). Such a model fits evidence that individual differences such as optimism, hostility, and worry predict the magnitude of immune responses to stressors. In the common cause model, personality traits which are driven by elevated autonomic reactivity, such as inhibited temperament and extraversion, are associated with immune system differences also associated with autonomic activity. While the pathoplastic model has not been applied to the relationship between personality and the immune system, such a model is possible, for example, if the inflammation associated with rheumatoid arthritis were thought to both affect and be affected by personality.

Finally, personality is a multidimensional construct, and there are probably an infinite number of personality dimensions along which people could be characterized. Much research in personality now employs five dimensions which are thought to subsume most of the variance in personality. These dimensions are neuroticism (predisposition to negative affect and impulsiveness), extraversion (lively sociability and positive affect), openness to experience (appreciation of and desire for new experiences), conscientiousness (carefulness and dependability), and agreeableness (warmth and cooperativeness) (Digman, 1990). While only a few psychoneuroimmunology studies have employed these dimensions, their use has the distinct advantage of linking PNI studies with other personality research (e.g., investigations of the heritability of personality; e.g., Jang, Livesley, & Vernon, 1996; Jang, McCare, Angleitner, Riemann, & Livesley, 1998). Furthermore, some personality dimensions already important in PNI correspond to these factors. For example, hostility is the inverse of agreeableness (Digman, 1990; Friedman, Tucker, & Reise, 1995; Watson & Clark, 1992).

The use of the five-factor model of personality should not be used indiscriminately, however. First, as Smith and Williams (1992) warned, "Much of behavioral medicine is atheoretical. The unsophisticated adoption of a powerful descriptive taxonomy [the five-factor model] presents the risk of making it even more atheoretical" (p. 412). Second, the five factors are necessarily broad characterizations of personality. Only some facets of each dimension may be physiologically significant. For example, agreeableness subsumes hostility, trait anger, anger dyscontrol, and anger-out (Friedman et al., 1995). Distinct effects of these facets could be obscured if agreeableness were the only personality measure used. Third, when the combination of environment and personality is considered, personality measures that are specific to the environment may be more powerful predictors than the more general five factors (for some examples of specificity, see Reed, Kemeny, Taylor, Wang, & Visscher, 1994; Segerstrom, Taylor, Kemeny, & Fahey, 1998; Strauman, Lemieux, & Coe, 1993).

Few of the studies below have employed the five-factor model; therefore, we have imposed a different structure on the research linking stable individual differences to the immune system. We consider individual differences related to affect first, followed by individual differences related to social behavior and relationships and, finally, cognitive representations of self and future. It should be noted that many individual difference constructs could fit into more than one category. For example, while inhibited temperament primarily involves differences in social behavior, it also has elements of emotionality, particularly increased fearfulness, and may be relevant to cognitive representations of how one will be perceived by others (rejection sensitivity; Cole, Kemeny, & Taylor, 1997).

## III. INDIVIDUAL DIFFERENCES RELATED TO AFFECT

### A. The Nature of Affect

Individual differences in affect and affect regulation include the degree to which individuals are predisposed to negative and positive emotions and moods and how they experience or express their emotions and moods. Animal models of emotionality are somewhat limited in that emotional states must be inferred from the animal's behavioral responses, as Blanchard described for a rodent's behavioral response reflecting fear to a threatening stimulus

(Blanchard, Flannelly, & Blanchard, 1986). Within a species or strain, there are considerable individual differences in the manner that a rodent might respond in an open field (freezing versus exploration) or to auditory stimuli (small versus large startle responses). These differences are associated with significant neurochemical and endocrine differences (Cools et al., 1990). Not surprisingly, behavioral differences are associated with significant differences in a rodent's immune response associated with a variety of stressors (auditory stressor: Irwin, Segal, Hauger, & Smith, 1989; social interaction: Kavalaars, Heijnen, Tenbekes, Bruggink, & Koolhas, in press).

In humans, affective experience is distinguished in at least two ways: emotion versus mood and positive versus negative valence. Emotions are thought to be universal, intensely felt states which last seconds to minutes and are associated with distinct facial expressions, behavioral predispositions, and possibly patterns of autonomic arousal (Ekman, 1994; Ekman et al., 1983; Levenson, 1992). Researchers differ in their assessment of the number of basic emotions, but often identify fear, sadness, anger, surprise, and disgust. Moods, on the other hand, are less intense, may be a blend of different feelings (e.g., anxiety and depression), last longer periods of time, and do not have the universal qualities of emotion (e.g., distinct facial expressions; Ekman, 1994). With regard to valence, some evidence suggests that positive and negative affect are not two ends of a bipolar dimension, but rather two separate dimensions. That is, the degree to which people report positive mood is often orthogonal to the degree to which they report negative mood (see Stone, (1995), for a discussion of dimensional models of mood). This may be due to the different relationships of mood states to personality dimensions (e.g., negative affect with neuroticism and positive affect with extraversion), different neurological substrates of negative and positive affect, or both.

### B. Emotionality and Immune Function in Animal Strains

As noted above, Lewis and Fischer rats differ in their reactivity to acute stressors such as the open field task, with Lewis rats showing less activity in the open field. Lewis rats have also been categorized as low stress responders on the basis of their reduced plasma corticosterone output in response to stressors; Fischer rats, conversely, have higher corticosterone levels in response to stressors and so may be categorized as a high-stress-responder strain. Low-stress-responder strains such as Lewis are more susceptible to experimentally induced autoimmune disease (Mason, 1991; Sternberg, 1995). Greater stress or fearfulness in the experimental situation is inferred from increases in adrenal output (since with animals models one can never know what the animal is "thinking"). In addition, a number of interindividual behavioral differences can model fearfulness. For example, when introduced into the territory of resident rats, the intruder may assume postures indicative of submissiveness to the residents. Rats showing these defeated postures are more likely to have an attenuated specific antibody response to benign protein antigen challenge (Fleshner, Laudenslager, Simons, & Maier, 1989), increased retention of exogenously administered tumors (Stefanski & Ben-Eliyahu, 1996), and reduced concanaralin A (Con A) lymphocyte activation and fewer CD4 and CD8 cells (Stefanski, 1998). Thus, animals exposed to the same experimental conditions will express responses to the stressor or social situation that vary in important ways for determining immune responses. Can one predict outcome based on any behavioral indices prior to stressor exposure? The approach of identifying specific behavioral and physiological differences prior to stressor exposure has not been used for predicting individual differences in immune response following stressor exposure. However, using a multivariate strategy in a different disease model, the level of gastric ulceration following stressor exposure, Overmier, Murison, and Johnsen (1997) determined if there were preexisting behavioral and physiological factors that were predictive of outcome. The tasks used to determine the individual differences were based on several accepted behavioral measures of "emotionality" (Archer, 1973), including open field exploration, open field defecation, body weight, defensive burying, response to a bitter solution, and stereotypical responses to apomorphine, a dopamine agonist (Overmier et al., 1997). Interestingly, none of the behavioral factors predicted gastric ulceration. However, apomorphine sensitivity alone was highly correlated with risk for gastric ulceration, accounting for 25% of the variance (see also Cools et al., 1990). Apomorphine sensitivity has also been critical in prediction of responses to EAE in other rodent models (Kavallars et al., 1997). How preexisting individual differences in behavior relate to immune responses during stressor exposure in animal models has not been well documented at present. However, Sandi, Borrell, and Guaza (1992a,b) have found that exploratory responses in a novel environment are associated with immune responses noted during stressor exposure. Rats showing the

greatest exploration showed the least reduction in immune parameters associated with the stressor. The presence of stable individual differences in rodent models has not been tested directly, although one might infer that they exist, based on studies such as that by Sandi and colleagues (1992a,b), in which behavior in one situation predicts reaction, including immune reactions, in another (cf. Capitanio, 1999).

Strain differences in emotional reactivity in mice have been noted as well (Royce, Carran, & Howarth, 1970). Strain differences contribute significantly to the impact of stressor exposure (restraint) on the manifestation of experimentally induced influenza virus immune mediated lung pathophysiology in mice (Hermann, Tovar, Beck, Allen, & Sheridan, 1993). During social confrontations, the DBA strain, in comparison to the C57Bl/6 and C3H/HeN strains, was more likely to show escape behavior and postural defeat. Not surprisingly, when compared to C57BL/6 and C3H/HeN strains, the inflammatory response of the lung to the influenza virus was suppressed most by restraint in DBA/2 mice. The DBA/2 mice also showed enhanced survival after infection and a greater corticosterone response to the restraint. Treatment with a glucocorticoid antagonist, RU486, was associated with increased lung pathophysiology (Hermann, Becks, & Sheridan, 1995). It was argued that the activation of the HPA axis in the mouse model is essential for terminating the inflammatory response in the lungs (Sheridan, 1998) in much the way that the HPA has been implicated in strain differences in susceptibility to EAE in the rat model (Sternberg, 1995). Variations in HPA reactivity may play a role in individual differences in immune/behavior relationships, but this may not be a necessary condition (Kavelaars et al., 1999).

To what degree do these potential links between emotional behavior and immune responsiveness reflect shared or linked genes? Mice bred for high and low responsiveness to antigenic challenge with keyhole limpet hemocyanin (KLH) show individual differences in behavior (Vidal & Rama, 1994). However, behavioral patterns (open field [activity level, rearing, and defecation], aversion to light, and responses to handling) were statistically independent of the antibody response. Individual differences in behavior of these mice did not seem to be set by the genes controlling immune regulation. Although a particular pattern of behavioral differences might covary consistently with specific immune patterns, they are not necessarily controlled by the same gene but may indeed reflect linked gene loci.

## C. Trait Negative and Positive Affect

There are stable individual differences in the degree to which people report positive and negative moods (McCrae, 1993). These differences are referred to as positive and negative affectivity (Watson & Clark, 1984) and are important elements of the major personality dimensions of extraversion and neuroticism (Costa & McCrae, 1980; Watson & Clark, 1992). On the positive affectivity side, Miller, Cohen, Rabin, Skoner and Doyle (1999) found that extraversion was associated with lower blood pressure, epinephrine, norepinephrine, and natural killer cell cytotoxicity (NKCC) in 276 healthy adults. Despite the reduction in cellular immunity implied by lower NKCC, extraversion was associated with a decreased likelihood of developing clinical cold symptoms after controlled exposure to rhinovirus (Cohen et al., 1997). It is possible that the relationship between extraversion and the immune system is due to extraversion's positive affectivity facet. However, extraversion contains other facets such as sociability and social dominance (McCrae & Costa, 1987), and it may be these factors that are driving the relationship with the immune system (see below). Furthermore, a common cause model involving autonomic differences is also possible. Eysenck (1967) proposed that higher sympathetic nervous system arousal in introverts caused their more withdrawn behavior as they attempted to avoid overarousal. The lower sympathetic arousal in extroverts might also cause the immune difference observed in these individuals, to wit, lower NKCC.

Neuroticism and negative affectivity were not related to either tonic physiology (including NKCC; Miller et al., 1999) or rhinovirus immunity (Cohen, Doyle, Skoner, Rabin, & Gwaltney, 1997; Cohen et al., 1997). Investigators often find that neuroticism is not related to physiological outcomes but, instead, is a strong predictor of symptom reports (see, e.g., Cohen et al., 1995; Costa & McCrae, 1987; Watson & Pennebaker, 1989). However, in a number of studies, state negative affect was associated with lower functional immune measures and reduced resistance to rhinovirus (Cohen et al., 1995; Stone, Cox, Valdimarsdotti, Jandort, & Neale, 1987; Stone et al., 1994; Zorrilla, Redei, & DeRubeis, 1994). To the degree that negative affectivity leads to state negative affect, the immune system can be affected by the former (Cohen et al., 1995). One problem is that if state negative affect is assessed on only one occasion, the error with regard to negative affectivity is large. On any given occasion, state affect will be a product not only of affectivity but also factors specific to that occasion such as interactions with other people, daily life events, or even weather. Over a series of occasions, however, the effects of affectivity on state affect are more clearly seen (Epstein, 1979). Studies which repeatedly measure state affect, immune parameters, and immunity will be stronger tests of the associations between negative, as well as positive, affectivity and the immune system.

## D. Other Contributors to Affective Experience

### 1. Cerebral Lateralization

Affective dispositions have neurophysiological correlates. Using recordings of brain electrical activity from the scalp, Davidson (1998) has demonstrated that there are stable individual differences in prefrontal activation asymmetry and that individuals with greater relative right prefrontal activation report less positive and more negative trait affect and more behavioral inhibition than those with greater left prefrontal activation. These individuals also respond more strongly to negative affective challenges (see Davidson, 1998). Greater relative right-sided prefrontal activation in Rhesus monkeys has been associated with higher basal levels of cortisol (Kalin, Larson, Shelton, & Davidson, 1998), a finding consistent with increased emotionality in the monkey. Interestingly, freezing behaviors, indicative of fear in nonhuman primates as well, are present early in development and may set developmental markers for later individual differences in adult behavior (Kalin & Shelton, 1998).

In terms of the immune system, female college students with greater right prefrontal activation had lower NK-cell activity levels than left-activated participants (Kang et al., 1991). These associations at baseline were confirmed in a subsequent study (Davidson, Coe, Dolski, & Donzella, 1999). In addition, individuals with greater right prefrontal activation showed a greater decrease in NKCC after exams and a smaller increase in NKCC after exposure to a positive film. Thus, this neurophysiological trait may influence both basal as well as stressor-induced immune changes.

### 2. Worry

People differ in the degree to which they worry, that is, they anticipate and imagine potential future negative events. At mild or moderate levels, people report that worry facilitates problem-solving (Davey, 1994); however, for others, worry is uncontrollable and unproductive and may consume most of their waking hours. Reports of such pathological worry are stable, at least over periods of weeks or months (Molina & Borkovec, 1994).

Higher levels of worry have been associated with autonomic dysregulation, particularly tonic withdrawal of parasympathetic tone (Thayer, Friedman, & Borkovec, 1996) and lack of heart rate and skin conductance responses to acute stressors (Borkovec & Hu, 1990; Borkovec, Lyonfields, Wiser, & Deihl, 1993; Lader & Wing, 1964; Lyonfields, Borkovec, & Thayer, 1995; Hoehn-Saric, McLeod, & Zimmerli, 1989). Autonomic dysregulation would be expected to dysregulate the natural killer (NK) cell response to stress; acute autonomic activation is ordinarily associated with an increase in the percentage of natural killer (NK) cells (e.g., Gerritsen, Heijnen, Wiegant, Bermond, & Frijda, 1996; Kiecolt-Glaser, Cacioppo, Malarkey, & Glaser, 1992; Uchino, Cacioppo, Malarkey, & Glaser, 1995). Segerstrom, Glover, Craske, and Fahey (1999) exposed seven participants with high levels of trait worry and eight individuals with normal levels of trait worry to a phobic stimulus (spider or snake) for five min, to which both groups responded with increases in heart rate and skin conductance. However, only the normal worry group had an increase in the percentage of natural killer cells in peripheral blood. The high worry group, despite normal autonomic responses elicited by a high level of fear, failed to show an immunologic response.

A chronic stressor, the aftermath of the 1994 Northridge, California, earthquake, also interacted with worry to predict changes in the immune system (Segerstrom, Solomon, Kemeny, & Fahey, 1998). Forty-seven employees of a hospital near the earthquake's epicenter were divided into high and low trait worriers based on a median split. Two weeks after the earthquake, the high worriers had 25% fewer natural killer cells in peripheral blood compared with preearthquake controls, while the low worriers had 9% fewer. A significant difference between high and low worriers persisted over 4 months after the earthquake. While worry has been associated with more intrusive thoughts, anxious mood, and sleep disturbance, these did not mediate the effect of worry on the immune system in this sample. Furthermore, while worry and negative affectivity overlap significantly, the associations with worry were independent of negative affectivity.

Worry, therefore, has been associated with a lack of immune system response to acute stressors and autonomic activation and an overresponse to chronic stressors. It is possible that worry dysregulates the interaction between the autonomic and immune systems (Segerstrom et al., 1999).

## 3. Repressive Style

It is important to consider individual differences in the degree to which people experience or inhibit their affective responses. Individuals with a repressive style appear to minimize or inhibit negative emotional responses (Jamner, Schwartz, & Leigh, 1988; Barger, Kircher, & Croyle, 1997) which may be an automatic method of affect regulation. For example, individuals with a repressive style report low levels of anxiety but demonstrate high behavioral and physiological indications of distress, such as autonomic reactivity, during a laboratory stressor (Weinberger, Schwartz, & Davidson, 1979). When survivors of a major fire followed by significant flooding within 1 month were characterized as repressors or nonrepressors, these categories were associated with the identification of different circadian cortisol patterns the following year. Repressors showed a flattened diurnal decline in salivary cortisol and higher mean cortisol levels than nonrepressors, indicating dysregulation of cortisol secretion. Furthermore, the flattened decline in salivary cortisol was also associated with greater intrusive memories of the fire and flooding (Laudenslager, Benight, Harper, & Goldstein, 1999). Disrupted circadian cortisol patterns are very likely to have negative impacts on immunoregulation in general (see Munck & Guyre, 1991).

Consistent with the evidence for autonomic and neuroendocrine dysregulation, repressors also show evidence of immune dysregulation. Repressors have higher antibody titers to latent Epstein–Barr virus (EBV), indicating poorer cellular control over the virus. Esterling, Antoni, Kumar, and Schneiderman (1990) had 80 undergraduate students complete measures of repressive personality and write a letter describing a highly stressful event. Higher emotional expression in the letter was associated with lower antibody titers after writing only in students who did not have repressive personality traits. Students with repressive personality traits had higher antibody titers regardless of the emotionality of their letters. In a second study, tonic associations between repression and EBV antibody titers were investigated in sample of 54 undergraduate students. Defensiveness, as measured by a social desirability scale, was associated with higher antibody titers (Esterling, Antoni, Kumar, & Schneiderman, 1993). Jamner et al. (1988) found that defensiveness was also associated with lower monocyte and eosinophil counts in 312 patients at a behavioral medicine clinic, a relationship which they proposed to result from higher levels of endogenous opiates associated with repressive and defensive coping. Finally, Shea,

Burton, and Girgis (1993) found that both repression and extreme anxiety were associated with lower numbers of T cells in 48 female undergraduate students.

### 4. Alexithymia

Alexithymia is a construct related to repression which implies deficits in the processing of emotions. Characteristics associated with alexithymia include difficulty identifying and describing affective experiences, difficulty distinguishing between emotional and physiological arousal, and a paucity of fantasies (Taylor, Bagby, & Parker, 1991). Support for a possible neurophysiological substrate of alexithymia comes from the work of Lane and colleagues who have shown that level of "emotional awareness" is correlated with level of neuronal activity in certain brain regions, specifically the anterior cingulate cortex (Lane et al., 1998). These regions may be more involved in response to emotion cues in individuals better at detecting complex cues.

Two studies of alexithymia and lymphocyte cell subsets included 65 women with cervical dysplasia and 103 women without dysplasia. Among women without dysplasia, alexithymic and not alexithymic women had equal numbers of cells in 15 cell subsets in one study and alexithymic women had only fewer CD2+ cells in the other; among women with dysplasia, those who were also alexithymic had lower numbers of CD2+ and CD3+ cells in both studies (Todarello et al., 1994, 1997).

### E. Potential Psychological Mechanisms

What psychological mechanisms might explain the associations between trait negative and positive affect, individual differences in affect regulation, and the immune system? First among the potential psychological mediators is the experience of state positive and negative affect. In addition, emotional processing and disclosure are also potentially important.

State negative affect includes the experience of moods such as anxiety, depression, and hostility. Such moods have been associated with lower functional and in vivo immune parameters, as well as differences in lymphocyte subsets and cytokine production (Connor & Leonard, 1998; Herbert & Cohen, 1993; LaVia et al., 1996; Stone et al., 1987, 1994; Zorrilla et al., 1994). For example, major depression has been found to be associated with a decrease in the proliferative response to mitogens across a number of studies as well as an increase in the production of interleukins-1, -2, and -6 (see Herbert & Cohen, 1993; Maes et al.,

1995; Seidel et al., 1995, 1996). However, the direction of causality in these relationships remains unclear especially given recent rodent studies suggesting that cytokines can influence psychological states (Maier & Watkins, 1998). Some evidence suggests that positive moods may be associated with higher values on functional and in vivo immune assays, although there are only a few studies in this area (Stone et al., 1987, 1994). Short, intense emotional responses induced in a laboratory can also result in immunologic alterations. Futterman, Kemeny, Shapiro, and Fahey (1994) used improvisational monologues to induce emotions in method-trained actors. After 25 min of involvement in these monologues, NK-cell number and NKCC were increased in those involved in positive emotion induction as well as in those involved in negative emotion induction. In contrast, proliferative response to high-dose PHA increased during positive emotions and decreased during negative emotions. These immune changes returned to baseline following a 20-min neutral period.

The immune correlates of individual differences in other affective constructs (e.g., repressive style, worry, alexithymia) may be due to the behavioral, affective, and cognitive processes involved with the inhibition of affect. At one level, the simple act of inhibition may have physiological effects. Gross and Levenson (1993) found increased skin conductance levels (indicating sympathetic nervous system activation) in students asked to suppress facial expressions while watching emotional movie clips. Furthermore, inhibition may prevent processing of emotional information. A number of investigators have found physiological effects of disclosing traumatic experiences. Changes include decreases in skin conductance levels (Pennebaker, Hughes, & O'Heeron, 1987), decreases in EBV antibody titers (Esterling et al., 1994; Lutgendorf, Antoni, Kumar, & Schneiderman, 1994), higher proliferative responses to Con A (Pennebaker, Kiecolt-Glaser, & Glaser, 1988), and higher antibody levels after hepatitis B vaccination (Petrie, Booth, Pennebaker, Davison, & Thomas, 1995) as well as reduced health center visits over a 6-month follow-up period (Pennebaker & Beall, 1986). There is some indication that the positive effects of disclosure are due to increases in emotional processing, since the effects were linked to greater evidence of negative emotion and cognitive insight and understanding of the problem during the disclosure task (e.g., Esterling et al., 1994). Thus, individual differences in the tendency to inhibit emotional experience may interfere with the ability to successfully process stressful or traumatic experiences. Both the experience of negative emotion and its processing may be necessary; Foa and Kozac (1986) propose that the complete activation of negative emotion permits its processing and change (cf. Lang, 1977).

## IV. INDIVIDUAL DIFFERENCES RELATED TO SOCIAL RELATIONSHIPS

### A. Types and Qualities of Social Relationships

Individual differences with relevance to social relationships include status in hierarchical social structures, preference for social activity, and cognitive predispositions to perceive others, for example, as threatening or malicious. Social relationships are not unidimensional; they may be assessed in terms of both quantity and quality. The term *social support* is often applied to human social relationships. This term implies both that social relationships exist and that they are supportive, but these two dimensions are not redundant, as social relationships can sometimes be negative. Therefore, the number of social relationships (i.e., social network size) is a quantitative measure of the number of contacts an individual has within a fixed period of time (e.g., every 2 weeks). The quality of social relationships (i.e., social support) is a qualitative measure in which an individual is asked to make a subjective judgment about the quality of relationships and his or her satisfaction with those relationships (see, e.g., Sarason, Levine, Basham, & Sarason, 1983).

### B. Aggression, Sociability, and Social Perception

In mice, individual differences are evident in an animal's predisposition to aggress. Selective breeding of outbred mice produced two lines with distinctly different levels of aggression by the fourth generation, a highly aggressive group (NC900) and a nonaggressive group (NC100) (Gariepy, Hood, & Cairnset, 1988). Continued selective breeding lowered the probability of aggression in the NC100 line but led to little increase in aggression in the NC900 line (Gariepy et al, 1988). In an elegant series of studies, Petitto and colleagues (Petitto, et al., 1993; Petitto, Lysle, Gariepy, & Lewis, 1994) found that the low aggressive group (NC100) compared to the high aggressive group (NC900) had increased tumor growth in response to 3-methylcholanthrene and lower overall lysis of YAK-1 targets. Furthermore, in vitro measures of cellular immunity (responses to

T- and B- cell mitogens and IL-2 and IFN-$\gamma$ production) were lower in the low aggressive group (NC100) than in the high aggressive group (NC900) (Petitto et al., 1994). The low aggressive group, defined as "socially inhibited" by Petitto, was no different in response to either tactile stimuli or performance on an elevated "plus" maze (a behavioral measure of anxiety) compared to the high aggressive line.

Is the phenotypic expression of these immune parameters a function of differences in behavioral aggression or is it independent of the behavioral manifestation of aggression? Aggression in these lines is a function of the postweaning isolation rearing condition. Single housing immediately postweaning is associated with increased aggression in the NC900 line, whereas social housing postweaning is less likely to result in the observed differences in aggression. These observations are clearly in support of the recent observations of Crabb, Wahlsten and Dudek (1999) regarding small effect size observed in behavioral genetics and the extent to which housing differences can influence outcomes. If socially and nonsocially housed mice from both lines were compared, the differences in cellular responses (mitogen activation and cytokine production) and NK activity between the high and low aggressive lines remain (Petitto et al., 1994). These data suggest that the differences were more likely attributable to genetic (e.g., linked gene loci) and not experiential factors. These investigators addressed the specifics of the housing condition (same line versus mixed lines), gender (e.g., females fail to show differences except postpartum), and social hierarchy influences in another series of studies (Petitto et al., 1999). The differences in NK activity between the aggressive and nonaggressive lines were not affected by housing experience, social rank, or gender, each of which can modify aggressive behavior. Thus, the association of these behavioral and immune traits could simply be a fortuitous association or related to linkages of genes contributing to these characteristics. A clarification of the relationships between behavior and immune responses would require crossing the two lines and determining if the behavioral patterns and NK activity cosegregate in the F2 generation (Crabbe, Phillips, Kosobud, & Belknap, 1990). This approach was followed by Vidal and Rama (1994) in mice bred for high and low antibody responses. The behavioral traits reflecting emotionality that co-varied with antibody responses (e.g., the low responsiveness mice were more emotional) were independent of the antibody response in the F2 generation. Care must be taken in concluding that behavior–immune relationships observed in selective breeding studies are necessarily based on shared genes.

Human personality dimensions related to aggressiveness, sociability, and social perception include extraversion and agreeableness or, conversely, hostility. Extraversion implies a preference for social activity as well as more positive mood. As noted above, extraversion has been related to lower tonic physiological arousal and NKCC and better immunity against rhinovirus (Miller et al., 1999; Cohen et al., 1997). However, it is not clear which facet of extraversion—positive affectivity or sociability—is associated with these physiological changes, or whether lower arousal is a common cause of both extraversion and immune differences. A sociability interpretation is supported by findings that extraverts are more likely to seek social support, and social support is generally associated with higher functional immune measures (Uchino et al., 1996).

However, it is important to note that preference for social activity and seeking social support does not guarantee positive or supportive responses. In addition to the quantity of social relationships, the quality of behavior within relationships may have immunologic concomitants or sequelae. Agreeableness versus antagonism or hostility is a personality dimension which predicts the quality of behavior within social relationships. Hostility is characterized by perceptions that others are likely to mistreat, provoke, or frustrate; suspiciousness and mistrust; and easily aroused anger (Smith, 1992) and may lead to hostile interpersonal behavior such as criticism and disapproval. On the other hand, agreeable individuals are described as warm, generous, cooperative, and trusting (McCrae & Costa, 1987, 1991). On a tonic basis, more agreeableness and less antagonism and hostility was associated with lower blood pressure and serum epinephrine, but not immune differences, in 287 healthy adults (Miller et al., 1999). The immune associations with agreeableness–hostility were evident during acute stressors in three studies: In each, hostility was associated with more pronounced changes in the NK-cell subset. In the first study, 46 male subjects were asked to talk to a confederate about either a stressful event that they had personally experienced (self-disclosure) or a hypothetical situation occurring to another person (nondisclosure). Only hostile subjects who were also in the self-disclosure condition showed an increase in NKCC (Christensen et al., 1996). In the second, 104 subjects (69% male) were asked to present a 3-min speech to a video camera defending themselves against a shoplifting charge. Hostility was associated with larger increases in the number of CD57+ cells in peripheral blood during the task (Mills, Dimsdale, Nelesen, & Dillon, 1996). In the third, 41 married couples were asked to discuss a topic about which they disagreed. Hostile husbands who expressed anger during the discussion showed a large increase in NKCC, while wives' hostility and anger did not predict immune changes (Miller, Dopp, Myers, Felten, & Fahey, 1999). Hostility, therefore, appears to be associated with increased NK reactivity to interpersonal communication tasks which may involve cognitive structures involving mistrust, anger, or both. Furthermore, men appear to be more prone to these effects than women.

## C. Social Inhibition

Inhibition is a temperamental quality evident by a few months of age. Inhibited infants show accelerated heart rate responses to sour tastes, reflecting sympathetic reactivity, and increased muscle tension, motor activity, and crying in response to novel events, reflecting a low threshold to novel events in the limbic system. As inhibited children get older, they tend toward shyness, emotional restraint, and timidity when encountering novel people, which are potent social stimuli (Kagan & Snidman, 1991). There is some evidence that this trait, which is at least partially heritable (Robinson, Kagan, Reznick, & Corley, 1992), is associated with physical characteristics such as facial width (Arcus & Kagan, 1995) and blue eyes, as well as differences in immunologically mediated diseases. In particular, first- and second-degree relatives of inhibited children were more likely to have hay fever (Kagan, Snidman, Julia-Sellers, & Johnson, 1991). Cole, Kemeny, Weitzman, Schoen, and Anton (1999) examined social inhibition and delayed type hypersensitivity (DTH) responses in a predominantly female group of 36 functional bowel disease and fibromyalgia patients. Patients underwent a 5-week psychosocial intervention which involved discussing their psychological state, behavior, and physical health with a clinician, with additional focus on either health education or controlling inflammatory processes through hypnosis. Tetanus toxoid was injected intradermally and DTH responses quantitated at baseline, 4 weeks, and 6 weeks. Hypersensitivity reactions increased in size over the intervention period in more socially inhibited patients, who were presumably more affected by the social demands of participation.

Social inhibition has also been examined in the context of homosexual identity. Cole and his colleagues have examined the health consequences of concealing one's identity from others (i.e., being "in the closet"). In 222 HIV seronegative gay men, concealment was associated with increased risk of infectious disease and cancer, particularly skin cancer (Cole, Kemeny, Taylor, & Visscher, 1996). In HIV seropositive gay men, concealment was associated with accelerated disease course, including CD4 T-cell decline, time to AIDS diagnosis, and time to death (Cole, Kemeny, Taylor, Vescher, & Fahey, 1996). A construct related to social inhibition, rejection sensitivity, reflects the expectation that one will be perceived negatively by others. Rejection sensitivity was a significant predictor of CD4 decline, AIDS onset and death over a 9-year follow-up period (Cole, Kemeny, & Taylor, 1997). Furthermore, there was an interaction between concealment and rejection sensitivity: The less rejection sensitive a man was, the more negative the health effects of concealment. Therefore, inhibition in those not dispositionally predisposed to do so may have particularly negative effects.

## D. Social Confrontation and Dominance

Genetic breeding studies in mice have focused on particular behavioral tendencies as discriminating characteristics and then assessed basal immune parameters in the absence of behavioral challenge that brings out these differences. A contrasting approach has examined the nature of the behavioral response (defeat or attack) to a social challenge such as territorial intrusion or social group rearrangement and related that to concurrent immune parameters measured *at the time of social challenge*. For example, Fleshner et al. (1988) noted that repeated experiences with territorial intrusion in the rat was associated with reduced specific antibody levels to KLH inoculated at the time of intrusion. Individual differences in reduction in specific antibody level were related to the amount of time the intruders spent in defeat postures, accounting for practically 50% of the variance in antibody level. Thus, intruders falling *below* the median of time spent in defeat postures (e.g., exposure of vulnerable body region and other species-typical defeat behaviors) have significantly higher antibody titers toward KLH than those *above* the median ("defeated").

Individual differences in behavioral responses to social confrontation also affect another in vivo response, the clearance of tumor cells from the lung (Stefanski & Ben-Eliyahu, 1996). Male Fischer 344 rats, injected with mammary tumor cells, were exposed to 6 h of social confrontation with a pair of resident Long–Evans rats. The tumor line chosen is characterized by the fact that metastases appear only in the lung and is to a great extent controlled by the activity of NK cells. Twenty-four hours following the con-

frontation, lung retention of tumor cells was quantified (Ben-Eliyahu & Page, 1992). Compared to controls not experiencing social confrontation, the intruders had significantly higher levels of lung retention of tumors. Tumor retention in intruders was directly related to defensive postures, number of attacks received, and number of bites received. Thus, the nature of in vivo responses (antibody level or tumor metastases) was significantly related to individual differences in behaviors occurring at the time of the challenge.

Social confrontation also affects trafficking patterns in the peripheral blood of the intruder rats in a time-dependent manner (Stefanski, Solomon, Kling, Thomas, & Plaeger, 1996) that is also affected by individual differences in their response to the confrontation (Stefanski, 1998). The number of total WBCs was unaffected after 2 h, increased after 6 h., and decreased after 48 h of social confrontation. The numbers of CD8+ cells were decreased at 2 and 48 h and numbers of CD4+ cells were decreased only at 48 h. The number of CD4+ cells (CD4+/CD45RC−/CD90−) was below baseline at all time points. These effects appear to be selective to trafficking of mature, activated T helper cells from peripheral blood to other sites. When the behavioral response of the intruder was characterized by the presence (submissive) or absence (subdominant) of defeat behavior, significant differences are observed between groups. Basal immune parameters were not different between submissive and subdominant rats. However, after 7 days of social confrontation, the percentage of helper and cytotoxic T cells was significantly decreased and B cells increased in the submissive intruders. As lymphocytopenia was greatest in the subdominant rats, subdominant intruders showed a larger decrease in number of helper T cells and B cells relative to control or submissive rats. Indeed, characterization of individual differences in the behavioral response of intruder rats predicted trafficking patterns in much the same way that characterizing defeat accounted for 50% of the variance in specific antibody levels in intruder rats (Fleshner et al., 1988).

Dominance ranks within nonhuman primate social groups provide order to complex primate societies. A number of implications including priority of access to preferred resources are associated with dominance status (Bernstein, 1981). High rank generally predicts better quality of life even under plentiful conditions (Sapolsky, 1990). Dominance status carries with it a number of physiological correlates including differential hormone levels between high and low ranking members of the group and different patterns of hormonal responses following challenge (Sapolsky,

1993). For example, resting cortisol levels of male baboons are related to unstable relationships only with lower ranking males and are also related to the social stability of the individual (e.g., whether the male's rank is rising or falling; Sapolsky, 1992; Sapolsky, Alberts, & Altmann, 1997; Virgin & Sapolsky, 1997). As seen under stable conditions in rat models of aggression (Stefanski, 1998), there are few differences between high and low ranking female pigtail and bonnet macaques in stable conspecific social groups (Boccia, Laudenslager, Broussard, & Hijazi, 1992). However, if competition is exaggerated by limiting access to a resource (e.g., colony water supply), the species showing greater conflict (pigtail macaques) during testing had increased natural cytotoxic activity and reduced lymphocyte activation. Levels of conflict noted during these tests were directly related to changes in the immune parameters measured with the greatest aggression received by lower ranking members of the group. Thus immune modulation is not only related to social rank but its relative direction during encounters.

Heart rate regulation (e.g., relative levels of sympathetic and parasympathetic tone) has been linked to individual differences in risk for a number of medical disorders in human populations (Jemerin & Boyce, 1990; Kagan, 1994) or immune changes following a laboratory stressor (Cacioppo, Maclarkey, Kiecolt-Glaser, Uchino, Sgoutas-Emich, Sheridan, Berntson, & Glaser, 1995). Resting heart rate is also useful in predicting individual differences in behavioral responses to social separation in nonhuman primates (Boccia, Laudenslager, & Reite, 1995). Monkeys can be characterized as reactors and nonreactors based on heart rate while experiencing a threatening stimulus (Bowers, Crocket, & Bowden, 1998). Many of the individual differences in biological reactivity change little over time and the underlying biochemical differences seem to be subject to genetic influences in nonhuman primates (see, e.g., Higley et al., 1993). However, resting heart rate is inversely related to relative dominance status (Kaplan, Manuck, & Gatsonis, 1990) and shifts with changes in dominance status much like hormone patterns (Sapolsky, 1993; Virgin & Sapolsky, 1997). There are considerable individual differences in cardiovascular and behavioral reactivity even between closely related species (Clarke, Mason, & Mendoza, 1994; Clarke, Mason, & Moberg, 1988). Unfortunately, individual differences in immunologic reactivity in nonhuman primates has not achieved the same level of empirical study.

The role of dominance status and behavioral interactions in predicting individual differences in hormone and immune (both in vitro and in vivo) responses during reorganization of stable nonhuman primate groups or introduction of a monkey into a new social group has been assessed (see Worlein & Laudenslager, this volume, for a review). In this paradigm, group membership is periodically changed and new dominance relationships must be reestablished within the new group. Specific antibody responses to antigenic challenge with tetanus toxoid and resistance to viral challenge have been followed in conjunction with these manipulations and related to individual differences in dominance status (high versus low) ranking, preexisting behavioral traits, and behavior noted during the reorganization process. Cunnick et al. (1991) noted that there was no effect of a single social reorganization on specific antibody responses in macaques. However, subordinate monkeys demonstrated a higher specific antibody response to immunization with tetanus toxoid. When the monkeys were subjected to either repeated reorganizations (unstable condition) or no reorganization (stable condition), secondary response to tetanus toxoid were higher under the unstable social group conditions without an influence of social status. Thus the response to tetanus toxoid is counterintuitive; that is, the chronic social stress of lower dominance status or a chronic stressor of repeated social reorganization was associated with elevated specific antibody responses. It is unlikely that the mediator of these differences in antibody responses is due entirely to altered glucocorticoid regulation. Under the acute condition, subordinate monkeys have higher plasma cortisol levels (Sapolsky, 1993; Virgin & Sapolsky, 1997) and single social group reorganizations are associated with a rise in plasma cortisol (Gust et al., 1991). During chronic reorganizations, basal plasma cortisol levels are lower and the monkeys hypersuppress to dexamethasone challenge (Capitanio, Mendoza, Lerche, & Mason, 1998). In a similar manner, repeated social reorganizations did not affect monkeys experimentally challenged with an upper respiratory virus (Cohen et al., 1997). However, independent of the reorganization, subordinate monkeys had a greater risk for viral infection. The increased risk for infection with the virus was not accounted for by lower body weight, elevated cortisol, or less aggressive behavior in the subordinate monkeys.

Simian immunodeficiency virus (SIV)-infected macaques experiencing repeated social reorganizations have higher concentrations of SIV viral RNA (indicative of a greater viral load) in their plasma than monkeys housed under stable conditions (Capitanio et al., 1998). Monkeys that received more threats had higher SIV RNA and lower SIV-specific antibodies. Similar to the observations of Cunnick and colleagues (1992), monkeys housed under unstable conditions had elevated plasma antibodies to tetanus toxoid immunization (Capitanio et al., 1998). Furthermore, individual differences in behavioral traits observed 1.5 years prior to inoculation with SIV account for variations in the initial response to the virus (Capitanio, Mendoza, & Baroncelli, 1999). The initial response (rise in serum antibody titers and decline SIV RNA) is predictive of long-term outcome following infection with SIV (Baroncelli et al., 1997). Monkeys high in sociability (the tendency to engage in positive affiliative social interactions) had lower viral loads and higher antibody titers during the initial weeks following inoculation with SIV. Importantly, these traits are stable over time and predict behavioral responses to social manipulations (Capitanio, 1999). In nonhuman primates, these behavioral characteristics or temperaments have been linked to age, sex, and social rank (Clarke & Boinski, 1995).

Social dominance may also be immunologically relevant in humans. Though we know of no direct evidence involving the immune system, other evidence points to effects of social dominance on health and hormone levels. A study of social dominance in a group of 750 men linked a competitive, dominating speech style to an increased risk of mortality (standardized relative risk = 1.6 after controlling for traditional risk factors such as smoking, cholesterol, and blood pressure) (Houston, Babyak, Chesney, Black, & Ragland, 1997). As in other primate and rodent species, increased social dominance may be related to increased testosterone in humans. This has been shown in male chess players, whose testosterone levels rise after winning tournaments; testosterone also rises before competitions (Mazur, Booth, & Dabbs, 1992).

### E. Potential Psychological Mechanisms

As noted, social support—both the presence of social relationships and support provided therein—is a probable mediator of many socially relevant individual differences, including hostility, extraversion, and social inhibition. For example, hostile individuals may demonstrate immunologic and health impairment in part because their behavioral characteristics interfere with supportive relationships. The quality and quantity of social support has been linked to both immune parameters and immunologically relevant diseases. For example, a greater number of social relationships was related to better protection

against common cold viruses (Cohen et al., 1997), and, in general, more social support is related to higher functional immune measures (Uchino et al., 1996). However, social relationships are not uniformly positive. For example, while spouses often provide an important source of social support for each other, hostile interactions in married couples were associated with lower functional immune measures (Kiecolt-Glaser et al., 1993).

## V. COGNITIVE REPRESENTATIONS OF SELF AND FUTURE

### A. Types of Cognitive Representation

People vary in the ways in which they typically think about themselves and the world around them, and there are several conceptualizations of the nature of these important cognitive representations. These conceptualizations, including self-representations, attributional style, and optimism, are reviewed separately below, but they have some characteristics in common. First, many of them have an element of beliefs about the future. For some constructs, this future focus is explicit, as in optimism. For other constructs, the focus is indirect, but still important. For example, results from self research suggest that the cognitive representation of what one is likely to be like in the future has a more profound influence on self-esteem and mood than the representation of what one is like now (Markus & Nurius, 1986). Second, there is evidence that these cognitive representations are stable. For example, while self-representations can be primed or inhibited by the environment (including the internal or affective environments), and therefore are somewhat changeable, a core self-representation also exists that is stable and reflects those factors which are essential to the identification or definition of the self (Markus & Nurius, 1986). As another example, attributional style shows stability over periods of over 50 years (Burns & Seligman, 1989).

### B. Representations of Self: Self-Discrepancy Theory

Self theory posits that cognitive representations of the self have potent effects on motivation and mood. For example, representations of likely future selves are strongly related to current self-esteem and hopelessness, and discrepancies between actual and ideal self-representations lead to negative moods such as dejection, disappointment, and dissatisfaction (Higgins, 1987; Markus & Nurius, 1986).

To test whether self-discrepancy could have physiological consequences, Strauman, Lemieux, and Coe (1993) recruited groups of dysphoric but not anxious ($n = 10$), anxious but not dysphoric ($n = 8$), and neither anxious nor dysphoric ($n = 20$) adults (primarily students). As predicted by self-discrepancy theory (Higgins, 1987), dysphoric participants' "actual self" was most different from their "ideal self" representation, and anxious participants' "actual self" was most different from their representation of what they thought their parents would like them to be ("ought self"). Furthermore, after priming self-representations, the anxious group showed the lowest NKCC ($M = 23.9$ lytic units [LU]), followed by the dysphoric group (32.1 LU) and the control group (69.3 LU). The authors posited that self-discrepancies are associated with lower NKCC and that the effect of self-discrepancy on NKCC is mediated by anxiety and dysphoria.

## C. Representations of Causes: Attributional Style

Attribution theory focuses on the perceived causes of events, which are evaluated along three dimensions: internal/external, stable/unstable, and global/specific (Abramson, Seligman, & Teasdale, 1978). A stable predisposition to attribute negative events to internal, stable, and global causes is known as pessimistic attributional or explanatory style (Burns & Seligman, 1989). Pessimistic attributions ("I am a stupid person") are associated with lower self-esteem and more hopelessness than optimistic attributions ("The referee had a bad day").

Two studies have examined the immune correlates of pessimistic attributional style. Kamen-Siegel, Rodin, Seligman, and Dwyer (1991) coded attributional style explanatory from a series of interviews with 8 elderly men and 18 elderly women. These individuals also had blood drawn for measurement of T-cell subsets and the proliferative response to PHA. Pessimistic attributional style was associated cross-sectionally with a lower CD4/CD8 T-cell ratio and low-dose (.05 mg/mL) PHA proliferation. Segerstrom and her colleagues (Segerstrom, Taylor, Kemeny, Reed, & Visscher, 1996) coded attributional style from interviews with 86 HIV seropositive gay men, using the following attributional dimensions: internal-behavioral (what the participant does or did), internal-characterological (what the participant is or was), external, general (stable + global), and controllable. Only the internal-characterological dimension for

negative events predicted CD4 T-cell slope over the subsequent 18 months: The more the participant tended to explain negative events with internal-characterological causes, the more rapidly CD4 cells declined.

As attributional style has a long history of association with the initiation and promotion of depression, both of these studies examined negative mood (e.g., depression) and health behavior (e.g., alcohol intake) as potential mediators of the relationship between attributional style and immune parameters. Neither found such a relationship.

## D. Representations of the Future

Optimism has been operationalized as positive outcome expectancies. Dispositionally, optimism is reflected in such statements as "In uncertain times, I usually expect the best." (Scheier, Carver, & Bridges, 1994). Optimism may also be operationalized as expectancies in a more specific domain such as academic achievement or health. Positive expectancies are thought to be beneficial in maintaining motivation during setbacks and minimizing defeat-related emotions (Scheier & Carver, 1992). Dispositional optimism has been found to be associated with positive health outcomes (see Scheier & Carver, 1992, for review) such as reduced complications during and faster recovery from coronary artery bypass surgery (Scheier et al., 1989). However, some studies have found no health correlates of dispositional optimism (e.g., Reed, Kemeny, Taylor, Wang, & Visscher, 1994; Reed, Kemeny, Taylor, & Visscher, 1998; Segerstrom et al., 1998).

In one study measuring dispositional optimism and immune responses, optimism buffered the effects of acute life stress on specific lymphocyte subsets. However, optimists were more vulnerable to stress-related immune changes, including a decrease in NK-cell activity, if the stressful experiences persisted (Cohen et al., 1999). Thus, the effects of dispositional optimism may depend on stressor parameters, such as chronicity. In a related experimental study, more dispositionally optimistic participants showed the greatest decrease in NK cell activity after exposure to an uncontrollable laboratory stressor of 20 min duration; however, the effects did not continue once the stressor was over (Sieber, Rodin, Larson, Ortega, & Cummings, 1992). A slightly different version of pessimism, "premorbid pessimism" (which consists of a stable predisposition to see life as a succession of problems and misfortunes) was associated with immune differences among HIV seropositive women: NKCC and CD8+ T-cell percentages were lower in women who were higher in premorbid pessimism. However, the interaction between stressful life events and pessimism was not tested (Byrnes et al., 1998).

## E. Potential Psychological Mechanisms

### 1. Mood

The effects of these various cognitive styles on immune parameters may be mediated by moods that are consistent with these styles. For example, as noted above, self-discrepancies are associated with negative mood, pessimistic attributional style has long been associated with depression, and optimism is associated with a reduction in defeat-related emotion and mood. However, attempts to find affective mediators of these cognitive states have not always met with success (see, e.g., Segerstrom et al., 1998), raising the possibility that certain cognitive states may have physiological correlates that cannot be explained fully by differences in affect (see Kemeny & Gruenewald (2000) for a more extensive discussion of this issue).

### 2. Situation-Specific Expectancies

Effects of dispositional optimism on the immune system and health may be mediated by the positive situation-specific expectancies that they engender. Dispositionally optimistic individuals are more likely to have positive expectancies for a variety of situations. A number of studies have demonstrated beneficial health and immunologic correlates of positive situation-specific expectancies and, conversely, detrimental correlates of negative expectancies. Three studies of health-specific expectancies have been conducted in HIV positive individuals. In the first study, Reed and colleagues (1994) found that negative HIV-specific expectations among men with AIDS predicted a shorter survival time, controlling for medication regimen, health behaviors, health and immune status at the time of assessment of expectations, and other possible confounds. The shortest survival time was observed in the men with high levels of negative expectancies about future health in combination with an AIDS-related bereavement over the past year. In a second study, this group (Reed et al., 1999) studied CDC Stage A (asymptomatic) HIV positive men. They found that negative expectations about future health in combination with an AIDS-related bereavement predicted an increased likelihood of the development of HIV-related symptoms over the next 2.5 to 3.5 years. In a final study, 128 HIV positive men who were either highly optimistic or highly pessimistic about their future health were selected, stratified on CD4 T-cell count at baseline.

Negative HIV-specific expectancies plus exposure to a bereavement event predicted a number of immunologic indicators of HIV progression over a 2- to 3-year follow-up period, including a more rapid loss of CD4 T cells and more deficient proliferative response to mitogens as well as more evidence of immune activation (both in the serum and expressed on the surface of lymphocyte subsets; Kemeny, Reed, Taylor, Visscher, & Fahey, 1999). In a sample of healthy law students, Segerstrom et al. (1998) found that situation-specific optimism (in this case, optimism about succeeding in law school) predicted higher CD4 T-cell levels and higher NK-cell activity during the stress of first semester law school. It is interesting that *dispositional* optimism was not a significant predictor of outcomes in any of these studies while *situation-specific* optimism was. Also, these relationships were not due to more global psychological states such as depression, social isolation, and negative affectivity.

### 3. Perceived Control

Certain cognitive styles may have physiological correlates because they increase or decrease perceptions of control. For example, pessimistic attributional style is thought to lead to a perception that stressors are uncontrollable events, resulting in helplessness (Abramson et al., 1978). In addition, pessimism can be accompanied by a sense of helplessness. An experimental study, mentioned above, found that exposure to an uncontrollable stressor for 20 min resulted in a decrease in NKCC while exposure to a controllable version of the stressor did not. A stressor condition that gave subjects the *perception* that they had control over the stressor, when in fact they did not, had no effect on NKCC (Sieber et al., 1992). While the stressor exposure across conditions was the same, apparently perceptions of control buffered the effects of the stressor on the immune parameters measured. In addition, animal models have documented physiological, including immune, alterations using the learned helplessness paradigm, at the center of which lies uncontrollable stressors (Laudenslager, Ryan, Drugan, Hyson, & Maier, 1983; Maier & Laudenslager, 1988; Peterson, Maier, & Seligman, 1993; Sandi, Borrell, & Guaza, 1992b).

### 4. Finding Meaning

Dispositionally optimistic individuals may show beneficial outcomes because they are more likely to show other positive cognitive changes following a stressful situation. For example, optimists are more likely to find meaning in a stressful circumstance such as bereavement (Davis, Nolen-Hoeksema, & Larson,

1998). Finding meaning, in turn, may lead to resilience to stressors (Davis et al., 1998). One study found that bereaved HIV positive individuals who found meaning in the loss showed greater CD4 T-cell stability and lower mortality rates over a 9-year follow-up period, controlling for confounding factors and other psychological states such as depression (Bower, Kemeny, Taylor & Fahey, 1998).

### 5. Self-Evaluative States

In addition to the stable cognitive conceptualizations of self reviewed above, there are also fluctuating, state constructs regarding the self. Some evidence suggests that these constructs have physiological correlates and may mediate the immunologic correlates of self-related traits (e.g., self-discrepancy, internal-characterological attributions). For example, low self-esteem predicted a failure to show habituation of adrenocortical responses to repeated psychological stress (Kirschbaum et al., 1995). In addition, the self-reproach aspect of a depression inventory predicted CD4 decline in a sample of HIV positive men, while depressed mood did not (Kemeny & Dean, 1995).

## VI. CONCLUSION

Individual differences play an essential role in promoting or compromising health from variability in major histocompatibility complex, to patient compliance, to individual responses to medications, and, probably, brain–behavior–immune relationships (Cohen, 1999; Scheier & Bridges, 1995). However, this is an understudied topic of investigation. An almost exclusive focus on stressor exposure has excluded examination of the correlates of the organism's response to the stressor. The studies reviewed in this chapter suggest that stable individual difference factors may in fact play a role in modifying the physiological responses to stressors. Unfortunately, in most cases there are few studies—if not a single study—focusing on a given trait characteristic. Also, most studies examine only a limited number of immune parameters, thereby reducing the range of possible associations.

Some themes emerge from the studies of stable individual difference factors. A variety of negative traits were associated with lower levels of NK cells and NKCC, including worry, self-discrepancy, and right prefrontal activation, which is observed in individuals with high levels of negative affect and behavioral inhibition. However, hostile individuals were more likely to show *increased* NKCC under stressful laboratory conditions when compared to less hostile individuals. These opposing findings mirror the stress literature, in which naturalistic and usually more persistent stressors are associated with decreased NK-cell activity while acute laboratory stressors are associated with increased NK values. Thus, certain traits may amplify the stress response and its neurophysiological and immunologic effects.

It is also possible that traits show immunologic associations similar to those seen during stressors, but outside the context of a stressful encounter. For example, socially inhibited individuals may have physiological patterns consistent with stress exposure under a variety of stressful and nonstressful conditions. Repressive style, pessimistic explanatory style, and social inhibition have been associated with immune function decrements or immune changes known to confer increased disease risk (i.e., CD4 decline among HIV positive individuals) on an ongoing basis. On the other hand, positive traits such as agreeableness and dispositional optimism did not have consistent or interpretable relationships to immune parameters. It is possible that negative traits elicit similar physiological patterns as psychological stressors do, except that they are steady, internal rather than intermittent, external stimuli, creating a more constant demand on physiological systems. The effects of positive traits are less clear, as they have been the focus of less research; positive traits appear to mitigate against effects of some stressors, but their ongoing effects are less clear.

In a large number of studies, depression has been associated with functional decrements such as decreased NK-cell activity and proliferative capacity, coupled with increased evidence of immune activation. The largest body of evidence in this area comes from studies of individuals with extremely depressed mood accompanied by cognitive and somatic symptoms such as loss of energy and excessive self-blame; that is, a major depressive episode. Traits related to these depressive symptoms, such as negative future expectancies, pessimistic attributional style, and negative representations of the self, have been shown in multiple studies to be associated with immune alterations, including CD4 decline in HIV positive individuals and decreased NK-cell activity in healthy individuals. Animal and human studies suggest that perceived lack of control or learned helplessness is associated with immune and other physiological alterations. In animal models, defeat responses to aggressive encounters correlated with a number of immunologic changes. All of these constructs—negative cognitive representations, helplessness, and

**TABLE I**  **Summary of Studies of Stable Individual Difference Factors and the Immune System**

| Factor | Findings | No. of studies | Sample | Stressor |
|---|---|---|---|---|
| **Affective characteristics** | | | | |
| Extraversion | ↓ NKCA | 1 | Healthy humans | None |
| Neuroticism | —NKCA | 1 | Healthy humans | |
| Worry | —%NK | 1 | Healthy humans | Experimental |
| | ↓ %NK | 1 | Healthy humans | Naturalistic |
| Repressive style | ↑ AB to EBV | 2 | Healthy humans | |
| | ↓ Monos, eosinos | 1 | Clinic patients | |
| | ↓ T cells | 1 | Healthy humans | |
| Alexythymia | ↓ CD2, CD3 | 1 | Women with dysplasia | |
| Right prefrontal activation | ↓NKCA | 2 | Healthy humans | |
| | ↓NKCA | 1 | Healthy humans | Experimental |
| **Social characteristics** | | | | |
| NC900 mice | ↑ Prolif. to mitogen, cytokine production, NKCA | 1 | Mice | |
| Bred for aggressiveness | | | | |
| Agreeableness | —NKCA | 1 | Healthy humans | |
| Hostility | ↑NKCA | 3 | Healthy males | Experimental |
| Social inhibition | ↑ DTH | 1 | Fibromyalgia, irritable bowel syndrome | Naturalistic |
| | ↑ CD4 decline | 1 | HIV+ men | |
| Conflict | ↑ NKCA; ↓ activation | 1 | Female macaques | Naturalistic |
| Subordinates | ↑ AB to tetanus | 1 | Macaques | |
| Sociability | ↓ SIV viral load; | | | |
| | ↑ AB to SIV | 1 | SIV+ macaques | |
| **Cognitive characteristics** | | | | |
| Self-discrepancy | ↓ NKCA | 1 | Healthy humans | Experimental |
| Pessimistic attributional style | ↓ CD4/CD8, | | | |
| | Prolif. to mitogen | 1 | Healthy humans | |
| | ↑ CD4 decline | 1 | HIV+ men | |
| Dispositional optimism | ↓ NKCA | 1 | Healthy humans | Naturalistic |
| | ↓ NKCA | 1 | HIV+ women | |
| | ↓ CD3+ CD8+ | 1 | Healthy humans | Experimental |
| | ↓ NKCA | | | |

Note. NKCA, natural killer cell cytotoxicity; NK, natural killer cells; AB to EBV, antibody to the Epstein–Barr Virus; monos, Eosinos, monocytes, eosinophils; prolif. to mitogen; proliferation to mitogenic stimulation; DTH, delayed type hypersensitivity response.

defeat—resemble aspects of major depressive episodes. Notably, many of the human studies have controlled for depressed mood and found that individual differences predicted immune parameters above and beyond mood. These results might suggest that the cognitive and behavioral—rather than affective—characteristics of major depression, as well as the traits that reflect them, are physiologically potent. However, the physiological mechanisms explaining most of the findings regarding these traits are not yet clear.

The role of individual difference factors in psychoneuroimmunology deserves increased attention. Clearly, examining individual difference factors in studies of naturalistic and laboratory stressors will improve our ability to understand behavior–immune relationships. Examining the physiological correlates of stable individual difference factors under basal conditions as well as provocation would be a useful addition to the literature. Finally, at the present time, the animal literature is superior to the human literature in that the constructs under investigation are limited in number; the diversity of traits examined in the human literature makes drawing conclusions across studies difficult (see Table I for a summary of findings). Effort to duplicate both trait and immune measures across studies will help this literature coalesce into the substantive and substantial research domain that it deserves to be.

## Acknowledgments

This chapter was supported by a Summer Faculty Research Fellowship from the University of Kentucky, NIMH Research Scientist Development Award (MH00820), and NIMH Grant MH37373.

# References

Abramson, L. Y., Seligman, M. E. P., & Teasdale, J. D. (1978). Learned helplessness in humans: Critique and reformulation. *Journal of Abnormal Psychology, 87*, 49–74.

Archer, J. (1973). Tests for emotionality in rats and mice: A review. *Animal Behavior, 21*, 205–235.

Arcus, D., & Kagan, J. (1995). Temperament and craniofacial variation in the first two years. *Child Development, 66*, 1529–1540.

Barger, S. D., Kircher, J. C., & Croyle, R. T. (1997). The effects of social context and defensiveness on the physiological responses of repressive copers. *Journal of personality and Social Psychology, 73*, 1118–1128.

Baroncelli, S., Barry, P., Capitanio, J. P., Lerche, N. W., Otyula, M., & Mendoza, S. P. (1997). Cytomegalovirus and simian immuno-deficiency virus coinfection: Longitudinal study of antibody responses and disease progression. *Journal of Acquired Immune Deficiency Syndrome and Human Retroviruses, 15*, 5–15.

Ben-Eliyahu, S., & Page, G. G. (1992). The *in vivo* assessment of natural killer cell activity in the rat. *Progress in NeuroEndocrinImmunology, 5*, 199–214.

Bernstein, I. S. (1981). Dominance: The baby and the bathwater. *Behavioral and Brain Sciences, 4*, 419–457.

Blanchard, R. J., Flannnelly, K. J., & Blanchard, D. C. (1986). Defensive behaviors of laboratory and wild Rattus norvegicus. *Journal of comparative Psychology, 100*, 100–107.

Boccia, M. L., Laudenslager, M. L., & Reite, M. L. (1995). Individual differences in macaques' responses to stressors based on social and physiological factors: Implications for primate welfare and research outcomes. *Laboratory Animal, 29*, 250–257.

Boccia, M. L., Laudenslager, M. L., Broussard, C. L., & Hijazi, A. S. (1992). Immune response following competitive water tests in two species of macaques. *Brain, Behavior, and Immunity, 6*, 201–213.

Bonneau, R. H., Mormede, P., Vogler, G. P., McClearn, G. E., & Jones, B. C. (1998). A genetic basis for neuroendocrine-immune interactions. *Brain, Behavior, and Immunity, 12*, 83–89.

Borkovec, T. D., & Hu, S. (1990). The effect of worry on cardiovascular response to phobic imagery. *Behaviour Research and Therapy, 28*, 69–73.

Borkovec, T. D., Lyonfields, J. D., Wiser, S. L., & Deihl, L. (1993). The role of worrisome thinking in the suppression of the cardiovascular response to phobic imagery. *Behaviour Research and Therapy, 31*, 321–324.

Bower, J., Kemeny, M. E., Taylor, S. E., & Fahey, J. L. (1998). Cognitive processing, discovery of meaning, CD4 decline, and AIDS-related mortality among bereaved HIV seropositive men. *Journal of Consulting and Clinical Psychology, 66*, (6), 979–986.

Bowers, C. L., Crockett, C. M., & Bowden, D. M. (1998). Differences in stress reactivity of laboratory macaques measured by heart period and respiratory sinus arrhythmia. *American Journal of Primatology, 45*, 245–261.

Bowers, K. S. (1973). Situationism in psychology: An analysis and a critique. *Psychological Review, 80*, 307–336.

Burns, M. O., & Seligman, M. E. P. (1989). Explanatory style across the life span: Evidence for stability over 52 years. *Journal of Personality and Social Psychology, 56*, 471–477.

Byrnes, D. M., Antoni, M. H., Goodkin, K., Efantis-Potter, J., Asthana, D., Simon, T., Munajj, J., Ironson, G., & Fletcher, M. A. (1998). Stressful events, pessimism, natural killer cell cytotoxicity, and cytotoxic/suppressor T cells in HIV+ Black women at risk for cervical cancer. *Psychosomatic Medicine, 60*, 714–722.

Cacioppo, J. T., Malarkey, W. B., Kiecolt-Glaser, J. K., Uchino, B. N., Sgoutas-Emich, S. A., Sheridan, J. F., Berntson, G. G., & Glaser, R. (1996). Heterogeneity in neuroendocrine and immune responses to brief psychological stressors as a function of autonomic cardiac activation. *Psychosomatic Medicine, 57*, 154–164.

Capitanio, J. P. (in press). Personality dimensions in adult male rhesus macaques: Predictions of behaviors across time and situations. *American Journal of Primatology*.

Capitanio, J. P., Mendoza, S. P., & Baroncelli, S. (1999). The relationship of personality dimension sin adult male rhesus macaques to progression of simian immunodeficiency virus disease. *Brain, Behavior, and Immunity, 13*, 138–154.

Capitanio, J. P., Mendoza, S. P., Lerche, N. W., & Mason, W. A. (1998). Social stress results in altered glucocorticoid regulation and shorter survival in simian acquired immune deficiency syndrome. *Proceedings of the National Academy of Sciences, 95*, 4714–4719.

Cardon, L. R. (1995). Quantitative trait loci: Mapping genes for complex traits. In J. R. Turner, L. R. Cardon, & J. R. Hewitt (Eds.), *Behavioral genetic approaches in behavioral medicine* (pp. 237–250). New York: Plenum.

Christensen, A. J., Edwards, D. L., Wiebe, J. S., Benotsch, E. G., McKelvey, L., Andrews, M., & Lubaroff, D. M. (1996). Effect of verbal self-disclosure on natural killer cell activity: Moderating influence of cynical hostility. *Psychosomatic Medicine, 58*, 150–155.

Clarke, A. S., & Boinski, S. (1995). Temperament nonhuman primates. *American Journal of Primatology, 37*, 103–125.

Clarke, A. S., Mason, W. A., & Mendoza, S. P. (1994). Heart rate patterns under stress in three species of macaques. *American Journal of Primatology, 33*, 133–148.

Clarke, A. S., Mason, W. A., & Moberg, G. P. (1988). Differential behavioral and adrenocortical responses to stress among three macaque species. *American Journal of Primatology, 14*, 37–52.

Cohen, F., Kearney, K., Zegans, L., Kemeny, M. E., Neuhaus, J., & Stites, D. (1999). Differential immune system changes with acute and persistent stress for optimists vs. pessimists. *Brain, Behavior, and Immunity, 13*, 155–174.

Cohen, J. J. (1999). Individual variability and imunity. *Brain, Behavior, and Immunity, 13*, 76–79.

Cohen, S., Doyle, W. J., Skoner, D. P., Fireman, P., Gwaltney, J. M., & Newson, J. T. (1995). State and trait negative affect as predictors of objective and subjective symptoms of respiratory viral infections. *Journal of Personality and Social Psychology, 68*, 159–169.

Cohen, S., Doyle, W. J., Skoner, D. P., Rabin, B. S., & Gwaltney, J. M. (1997). Social ties and susceptibility to the common cold. *JAMA, 277*, 1940–1944.

Cohen, S., Line, S., Manuck, S. B., Rabin, B. S., Heise, E. R., & Kaplan, J. R. (1997). Chronic social stress, social status, and susceptibility to upper respiratory infections in nonhuman primates. *Psychosomatic Medicine, 59*, 213–221.

Cole, S. W., Kemeny, M. E., & Taylor, S. E. (1997). Social identity and physical health: Accelerated HIV progression in rejection-sensitive gay men. *Journal of Personality and Social Psychology, 72*, 320–335.

Cole, S. W., Kemeny, M. E., Taylor, S. E., & Visscher, B. R. (1996). Elevated physical health risk among gay men who conceal their homosexual identity. *Health Psychology, 15*, 243–251.

Cole, S.W., Kemeny, M.E., Taylor, S.E., & Visscher, B.R. (1997). Social identity and physical health: Accelerated HIV progression in rejection-sensitive gay men. *Journal of Personality and Social Psychology, 72*, 320–335.

Cole, S. W., Kemeny, M. E., Taylor, S. E., Visscher, B. R., & Fahey, J. L. (1996). Accelerated course of human immunodeficiency virus infection in gay men who conceal their homosexual identity. *Psychosomatic Medicine, 58*, 219–231.

Cole, S. W., Kemeny, M. E., Weitzman, O. B., & Anton, P. (1999). Socially inhibited individuals show heightened DTH response during intense social engagement. *Brain, Behavior, & Immunity, 13*, 187–200.

Cole, S. W., Kemeny, M. E., Weitzman, O. B., Schoen, M., & Anton, P. A. (1999). Socially inhibited individuals show heightened DTH response during intense social engagement. *Brain Behavior and Immunity, 13*, 187–200.

Connor, T. J., & Leonard, B. E. (1998). Depression, stress, and immunological activation: The role of cytokines in depressive disorders. *Life Sciences, 62*, 583–606.

Cools, A. R., Brachten, R., Heerren, D., Willemen, A., & Ellenbroek, B. (1990). Search after neurobiological profile of individual-specific features of Wistar rats. *Brain Research Bulletin, 24*, 49–69.

Cools, A. R., Ros, N. Y., Ellenbroek, B., & deKloet, E. R. (1993). Bimodal shape of individual variation in behavior of Wistar rats: The overall outcome of a fundamentally different make-up and reactivity of the brain, the endocrinological, and the immunological system. *Neuropsychobiology, 28*, 100–105.

Costa, P. T., & McCrae, R. R. (1980). Influence of extraversion and neuroticism on subjective well-being: Happy and unhappy people. *Journal of Personality and Social Psychology, 38*, 668–678.

Crabbe, J. C., Phillips, J. J., Kosobud, A., & Belknap, J. K. (1990). Estimation of genetic correlations: Interpretation of experiments using selectively bred and inbred animals. *Alcoholism: Clinical and Experimental Research, 14*, 141–151.

Crabbe, J. C., Wahlsten, D., & Dudek, B. C. (1999). Genetics of mouse behavior: Interactions with the laboratory environment. *Science, 284*, 1670–1672.

Cunnick, J. E., Cohen, S., Rabin, B. S., Carpenter, A. B., Manuck, S. B., & Kaplan, J. R. (1991). Alteration in specific antibody production due to rank and social instability. *Brain Behavior, and Immunity, 5*, 357–369.

Davey, G. C. L. (1994). Pathological worrying as exacerbated problem-solving. In G. C. L. Davey & F. Tallis (Eds.), *Worrying: Perspectives on theory, assessment, and treatment*. New York: Wiley.

Davidson, R. J. (1998). Affective style and affective disorders. Perspectives from affective neuroscience. *Cognition and Emotion, 12*, 307–330.

Davidson, R. J., Coe, C. C., Dolski, I., & Donzella, B. (1999). Individual differences in prefrontal activation asymmetry predict natural killer cell activity at rest and in response to challenge. *Brain, Behavior, and Immunity, 13*, 93–108.

Davis, C. G., Nolen-Hoeksema, S., & Larson, J. (1998). Making sense of loss and benefiting from the experience: Two construals of meaning. *Journal of Personality and Social Psychology, 75*, 561–574.

Digman, J. M. (1990). Personality structure: Emergence of the five-factor model. *Annual Review of Psychology, 41*, 417–440.

Ekman, P., Levenson, R. W., & Friesen, W. V. (1983). Autonomic nervous system activity distinguishes among emotions. *Science, 4616*, 1208–1210.

Ekman, P. (1994). Moods, emotions, and traits. In R.J. Davidson, P. Ekman, and K. Scherer (Eds.), *The nature of emotion: Fundamental questions* (pp. 56–58). New York: Oxford Univ. Press.

Epstein, S. (1979). The stability of behavior. I. On predicting most of the people much of the time. *Journal of Personality and Social Psychology, 37*, 1097–1126

Esterling, B. A., Antoni, M. H., Fletcher, M. A., Margulies, S., & Schneiderman, N (1994). Emotional disclosure through writing or speaking modulates latent Epstein–Barr virus antibody titers. *Journal of Consulting and Clinical Psychology, 62*, 130–140.

Esterling, B. A., Antoni, M. H., Kumar, M., & Schneiderman, N. (1990). Emotional repression, stress disclosure responses, and Epstein–Barr viral capsid antigen titers. *Psychosomatic Medicine, 52*, 397–410.

Esterling, B. A., Antoni, M. H., Kumar, M., & Schneiderman, N. (1993). Defensiveness, trait anxiety, and Epstein–Barr capsid antigen antibody titers in healthy college students. *Health Psychology, 12*, 132–139.

Eysenck, H. J. (1967). *The biological basis of personality*. Springfield, IL: Thomas.

Fleshner, M., Laudenslager, M. L., Simons, L., & Maier, S. F. (1989). Reduced serum antibodies associated with social defeat in rats. *Physiology and Behavior, 45*, 1183–1187.

Foa, E. B., & Kozac, M. J. (1986). Emotional processing of fear: Exposure to corrective information. *Psychological Bulletin, 99*, 20–35.

Friedman, H. S., Tucker, J. S., & Reise, S. P. (1995). Personality dimensions and measures potentially relevant to health: A focus on hostility. *Annals of Behavioral Medicine, 17*, 245–251.

Futterman, A. D., Kemeny, M. E., Shapiro, D., & Fahey, J. L. (1994). Immunological and physiological changes associated with induced positive and negative mood. *Psychosomatic Medicine, 56*, 499–511.

Gariepy, J. L., Hood, K. E. & Cairns, R. B. (1988). A developmental-genetic analysis of aggressive behavior in mice: III. Behavioral mediation by heightened reactivity or increased immobility. *Journal of Comparative Psychology, 102*, 392–399.

Gerritsen, W., Heijnen, C. J., Wiegant, V. M., Bermond, B., & Frijda N. H. (1996). Experimental social fear: Immunological, hormonal, and autonomic concomitants. *Psychosomatic Medicine, 58*, 273–286.

Gross, J. J., & Levenson, R. W. (1993) Emotional suppression: Physiology, self-report, and expressive behavior. *Journal of Personality and Social Psychology, 64*, 970–986.

Gust, D. A., Gordon, T. P., Wilson, M. E., Ahmed-Ansari, A., Brodie, A. R., & McClure, H.M. (1991). Formation of new social group of unfamiliar female rhesus monkeys affects the immune and pituitary adrenocortical systems. *Brain, Behavior, and Immunity, 5*, 296–307.

Heller, W., Nitschke, J. B., Etienne, M. A., & Miller, G. A. (1997). Patterns of regional brain activity differentiate different types of anxiety. *Journal of Abnormal Psychology, 106*, 376–385.

Herbert, T. B., & Cohen, S. (1993). Depression and immunity: A meta-analytic review. *Psychological Bulletin, 113*, 472–486.

Hermann, G., Beck, M. F., & Sheridan, J. F. (1995). Stress-induced glucocorticoid response modulates mononuclear cell trafficking during an experimental influenza viral infection. *Journal of Neuroimmunology, 56*, 179–186.

Hermann, G., Tovar, C. A., Beck, M. F., Allen, C., & Sheridan, J. F. (1993). Restrain stress differentially affects the pathogenesis of an experimental influenza viral infection in three inbred strains of mice. *Journal of Neuroimmunology, 47*, 83–94.

Higgins, E. T. (1987). Self-discrepancy: A theory relating self and affect. *Psychological Review, 94*, 319–340.

Higley, J. D., Thompson, W. W., Champoux, M., Goldman, D., Hasert, M. F., Kraemer, G. W., Scanlan, J. M., Suomi, S. J., & Linnoila, M. (1993). Patterns and maternal genetic and environmental contributions to cerebrospinal fluid monoamine metabolites in rhesus monkeys (*Macaca mulatta*). *Archives of General Psychiatry, 50*, 615–623.

Hoehn-Saric, R., McLeod, D. R., & Zimmerli, W. D. (1989). Somatic manifestations in women with generalized anxiety disorder: Psychophysiological responses to psychological stress. *Archives of General Psychiatry, 46*, 1113–1119.

Houston, B. K., Babyak, M. A., Chesney, M. A., Black, G., & Ragland, D. R. (1997). Social dominance and 22-year all-cause mortality in men. *Psychosomatic Medicine, 59*, 5–12.

Irwin, M. R., Segal, D. S., Hauger, R. L., & Smith, T. L. (1989). Individual behavioral and neuroendocrine differences in responsiveness to audiogenic stress. *Pharmacology, Biochemistry, and Behavior, 32*, 913–917.

Jamner, L. D., Schwartz, G. E., & Leigh, H. (1988). The relationship between repressive and defensive coping style and monocyte, eosinophil, and serum glucose levels: Support for the opioid peptide hypothesis of repression. *Psychosomatic Medicine, 50*, 567–575.

Jang, K. L., Livesley, W. J., & Vernon, P. A. (1996). Heritability of the Big Five personality dimensions and their facets: A twin study. *Journal of Personality, 64*, 577–617.

Jang, K. L., McCrae, R. R., Angleitner, A., Riemann, R., & Livesley, W. J. (1998). heritability of facet-level traits in a cross-cultural twin sample: Support for a hierarchical model of personality. *Journal of Personality and Social Psychology, 74*, 1556–1565.

Jemerin, J. M. & Boyce, W. T. (1990). Psychobiological difference in childhood stress response. II. Cardiovascular markers of vulnerability. *Developmental and Behavioral Pediatrics, 11*, 140–150.

Kagan, J. (1994). *Galen's prophecy: Temperament in human nature.* New York: Basic Books.

Kagan, J., & Snidman, N. (1991). Temperamental factors in human development. *American Psychologist, 46*, 856–862.

Kagan, J., Snidman, N., Julia-Sellers, M., & Johnson, M.O. (1991). Temperament and allergic symptoms. *Psychosomatic Medicine, 53*, 332–340.

Kalin, N. H., Larson, C., Shelton S. E., & Davidson, R. J., (1998). Asymmetric frontal brain activity cortisol, and behavior associated with fearful temperament in Rhesus monkeys. *Behavioral Neuroscience, 112*, 286–292.

Kalin, N. H., & Shelton, S. E. (1998). Ontogeny and stability of separation and threat-induced defensive behaviors in rhesus monkeys during the first year of life. *American Journal of Primatology, 44*, 125–135.

Kamen-Siegel, L., Rodin, J., Seligman, M. E. P., & Dwyer, J. (1991). Explanatory style and cell-mediated immunity in elderly men and women. *Health Psychology, 10*, 229–235.

Kang, D. H., Davidson, R. J., Coe, C. L. Wheeler, R. W., Tomarken, A. J., & Ershler, W. B. (1991). Frontal brain asymmetry and immune function. *Behavioral Neuroscience, 105*, 860–869.

Kaplan, J. R., Manuck, S. B., & Gatsonis, C. (1990). Heart rate and social status among cynomolgus monkeys (*Macaca fascicularis*) housed in disrupted social groupings. *American Journal of Primatology, 21*, 175–187.

Kavelaars, A., Heijnen, C.J., Ellenbroek, B., vanLoeveren, H., Cools, A.R. (1997). Apomorphine-susceptible and apomorphine-unsusceptible Wistar rats differ in their susceptibility to inflammatory and infectious diseases: A study on rats with group-specific differences in structure and reactivity of hypothalamic-pituitary-adrenal axis. *Journal of Neuroscience, 17*, 2580–2584.

Kavelaars, A., Heijnen, C. J., Tenbekes, R., Bruggink, J. E., & Koolhas, J. M. (1999). Individual behavioral characteristics of wild type rats predict susceptibility to experimental autoimmune encephalomyelitis. *Brain, Behavior, and Immunity, 13*, 279–286.

Kemeny, M., Reed, G., Taylor, S., Visscher, B., & Fahey, J.L. (1999). *Negative HIV-specific expectancies predict immunologic evidence of HIV progression.* Submitted.

Kemeny, M. E., & Dean, L. (1995). Effects of AIDS-related bereavement on HIV progression among gay men in New York City. *AIDS Education and Prevention, 7*, 36–47.

Kemeny, M. E., & Gruenewald, T. L. (2000). Affect, cognition, the immune system and health. In Mayer, E.A. & Saper, C. (Eds.) *The biological basis for mind body interactions. Progress in brain research series* (pp. 291–308). Amsterdam: Elsevier Science.

Kiecolt-Glaser, J. K., Cacioppo, J. T., Malarkey, W. B., & Glaser, R. (1992). Acute psychological stressors and short-term immune changes: What, why, for whom, and to what extent? *Psychosomatic Medicine, 54*, 680–685.

Kiecolt-Glaser, J. K., Malarkey, W. B., Chee, M. A., Newton, T., Cacioppo, J. T., Mao, H. Y., & Glaser, R. (1993). Negative behavior during marital conflict is associated with immunological down-regulation. *Psychosomatic Medicine, 55*, 395–409.

Kirschbaum, C., Prussner, J. C., Stone, A. A., Federenko, I., Gaab, J., Lintz, D., Schommer, N., & Hellhammer, D. H. (1995). Persistent high cortisol responses to repeated psychological stress in a subpopulation of healthy men. *Psychosomatic Medicine, 57*, 468–474.

Klein, M. H., Wonderlich, S., & Shea, M. T. (1993). Models of relationships between personality and depression: Toward a framework for theory and research. In M. H. Klein, D. K. Kupfer, & M. T. Shea (Eds.), *Personality and depression* (pp. 1–54). New York: Guilford.

Lader, M. H., & Wing, L. (1964). Habituation of the psycho-galvanic reflex in patient with anxiety states and in normal subjects. *Journal of Neurology, Neurosurgery, and Psychiatry, 27*, 210–218.

Lane, R .D., Reiman, E. M., Ahern, G. L., Schwartz, G. E., & Davidson, R. J. (1997). Neuroanatomical correlates of happiness, sadness, and disgust. *American Journal of Psychiatry, 154*, 926–933.

Lane, R. D., Reiman, E. M., Axelrod, B., Yun, L., Holmes, A., & Schwartz, G. E. (1999). Neural correlates of levels of emotional awareness: Evidence of an interaction between emotion and attention in the anterior cingulate cortex. *Journal of Cognitive Neuroscience, 10*, 525–535.

Lane, R. D., Reiman, E. M., Bradley, M. M., Lang, P. J., Ahern, G. L. Davidson, R. J., & Schwartz, G. E. (1997). Neuroanatomical correlates of pleasant and unpleasant emotion. *Neuropsychologica, 35*, 1437–1444.

Lang, P. J. (1977). Imagery in therapy: An information processing analysis of fear. *Behavior Therapy, 8*, 862–886.

Laudenslager, M. L., Benight, C., Harper, M., & Goldstein, M. (1999). Long-term individual differences in the salivary cortisol diurnal decline following a series of natural disasters. *Neuroimmunomodulation, 6*, 231. [abstract]

Laudenslager, M. L., Ryan, S. M., Drugan, R. C., Hyson, R. L., & Maier, S. F. (1983). Coping and immunosuppression: Inescapable but not escapable shock suppresses lymphocyte proliferation. *Science, 221*, 568–570.

LaVia, M. F., Munro, I., Lydiard, R. B., Workman, E. W., Hubbard, J. R., Michel, Y., & Paulling, E. (1996). The influence of stress intrusion on immunodepression in generalized anxiety disorder patients and controls. *Psychosomatic Medicine, 58*, 138–142.

Levenson, R. W. (1992). Autonomic nervous system differences among emotions. *Psychological Science, 3*, 23–27.

Lutgendorf, S. K., Antoni, M. H., Kumar, M., & Schneiderman, N. (1994). Changes in cognitive coping strategies predict EBV-antibody titre change following a stressor disclosure induction. *Journal of Psychosomatic Research, 38*, 63–78.

Lyonfields, J. D., Borkovec, T. D., & Thayer, J. F. (1995). Vagal tone in generalized anxiety disorder and the effects of aversive imagery and worrisome thinking. *Behavior Therapy, 26*, 457–466.

Maes, M., Meltzer, H. Y., Bosmans, E., Bergmans, R., Vandoolaeghe, E., Ranjan, R., & Desnyder, R. (1995). Increased plasma concentrations of interleukin-6, soluble interleukin-6, soluble interleukin-2 and transferrin receptor in major depression. *Journal of Affective Disorders, 34*, 301–309.

Maier, S.F., & Laudenslager, M.L. (1988). Inescapable shock, shock controllability, and mitogen stimulated lymphocyte proliferation. *Brain, Behavior, and Immunity, 2*, 87–91.

Maier, S. F., & Watkins, L. R. (1998). Cytokines for psychologists: Implications of bidirectional immune-to-brain communication for understanding behavior, mood, and cognition. *Psychological Review, 105,* 83–107.

Markus, H., & Nurius, P. (1986). Possible selves. *American Psychologist, 41,* 954–969.

Mason, D. (1991). Genetic variation in the stress response: Susceptibility to experimental allergic encephalomyelitis and implications for human inflammatory disease. *Immunology Today, 12,* 57–60.

Mazur, A., Booth, A., & Dabbs, J. M. (1992). Testosterone and chess competition. *Social Psychology Quarterly, 55,* 70–77.

McCrae, R. R. (1993). Moderated analyses of longitudinal personality stability. *Journal of Personality and Social Psychology, 65,* 577–585.

McCrae, R. R., & Costa, P. T. (1987). Validation of the five-factor model of personality across instruments and observers. *Journal of Personality and Social Psychology, 52,* 81–90.

McCrae, R. R., & Costa, P. T. (1991). Adding *Liebe und Arbeit*: The full five-factor model and well-being. *Personality and Social Psychology Bulletin, 17,* 227–232.

Mendoza, S. P., & Mason, W. A. (1989). Primate relationships: Social dispositions and physiological responses. In P. K. Seth & S. Seth (Eds.), *Perspectives in primate biology* (Vol. 2, pp. 129–143). New Delhi: Today's & Tomorrow's Printers.

Miller, G. E., Cohen, S., Rabin, B. S., Skoner, D. P., & Doyle, W. J. (1999). Personality and tonic cardiovascular, neuroendocrine, and immune function. *Brain, Behavior, and Immunity, 13,* 109–123.

Miller, G. E., Dopp, J. M., Myers, H. F., Felten, S. Y., & Fahey, J. L. (1999). Psychosocial predictors of natural killer cell mobilization during marital conflict. *Health Psychology, 18,* 262–271.

Mills, P. J., Dimsdale, J. E., Nelesen, R. A., & Dillon, E. (1996). Psychologic characteristics associated with acute stressor-induced leukocyte subset redistribution. *Journal of Psychosomatic Research, 40,* 417–423.

Mischel, W., & Shoda, Y. (1995). A cognitive-affective system theory of personality: Reconceptualizing situations, dispositions, dynamics, and invariance in personality structure. *Psychological Review, 102,* 246–268.

Molina, S., & Borkovec, T. D. (1994). The Penn State Worry Questionaire: Psychometric properties and associated characteristics. In Davey, G. C. L. & Tallis, F. (Eds.) *Worrying: Perspectives on theory, assessment, and treatment.* New York: Wiley.

Munck, A., & Guyre, P. M. (1991). Glucocorticoids and immune function. In R. Ader, D. Felten, & N. Cohen (Eds.), *Psychoneuroimmunology* (pp. 447–474). San Diego: Academic Press.

Overmier, J. B., Murison, R., & Johnsen, T. B. (1997). Prediction of individual variability to stress-induced gastric ulceration in rats: A factor analysis of selected behavioral and biological indices. *Physiology and Behavior, 61,* 555–562.

Paul, W. E. (1998). *Fundamental immunology* (4th ed.), Philadelphia: Lippincott Raven.

Pennebaker, J. K., Kiecolt-Glaser, J. K., & Glaser, R. (1988). Disclosure of traumas and immune function: Health implications for psychotherapy. *Journal of Consulting and Clinical Psychology, 56,* 239–245.

Pennebaker, J. W., & Beall, S. K. (1986). Confronting a traumatic event: Toward an understanding of inhibition and disease. *Journal of Abnormal Psychology, 95,* 274–281.

Pennebaker, J. W., Hughes, C. F., & O'Heeron, R. C. (1987). The psychophysiology of confession: Linking inhibitory and psychosomatic processes. *Journal of Personality and Social Psychology, 58,* 528–537.

Peterson, C., Maier, S. F., & Seligman, M. E. P. (1993). *Learned helplessness: A theory for the age of personal control.* New York: Oxford University Press.

Petitto, J. M., Lysle, D. T., Gariepy, J., Clubb, P. H., Cairns, R.L., & Lewis, M.H. (1993). Genetic differences in social behavior: Relation to natural killer cell function and susceptibility to tumor development. *Neuropsychopharmacology, 8,* 35–43.

Petitto, J. M., Lysle, D. T., Gariepy, J., & Lewis, M. H. (1994). Association of genetic differences in social behavior and cellular immune responsiveness: Effects of social experience. *Brain Behavior, and Immunity, 8,* 111–123.

Petrie, K. J., Booth, R. J., Pennebaker, J. W., Davison, K. P., & Thomas, M. G. (1995). Disclosure of trauma and immune response to a hepatitis B vaccination program. *Journal of Consulting and Clinical Psychology, 63,* 787–792.

Petitto, J. M., Gariepy, J., Gendreau, P. L., Rodriguiz, R., Lewis, M. H., & Lyle, D. T. (1999). Differences in NK function in mice bred for high and low aggression: Genetic linkage between complex behavioral and immunological traits? *Brain, Behavior, and Immunity, 13,* 175–186.

Pettito, J. M., McIntyre, T. D., McRae, B. L., Skolnick, P., & Arora, P. K. (1990). Differential immune responsiveness in mouse line selectively bred for high and low sensitivity to ethanol. *Brain, Behavior, and Immunity, 4,* 39–49.

Plomin, R., DeFries, J. G., & McClearn, G. E. (1990). *Behavioral genetics: A primer* (2nd ed.). New York: Freeman.

Plomin, R., DeFries, J. C., McClearn, G. E., & Rutter, M. (1997). *Behavioral genetics* (3rd ed.). New York: Freeman.

Reed, G., Kemeny, M. E., Taylor, S. E., & Visscher, B. (1999). Negative HIV-specific expectancies and AIDS-related bereavement as predictors of symptom onset in asymptomatic HIV seropositive gay men. *Health Psychology. 18,* 354–363.

Reed, G. M., Kemeny, M. E., Taylor, S. E., Wang, H.-Y., & Visscher, B. R. (1994). Realistic acceptance as a predictor of decreased survival time in gay men with AIDS. *Health Psychology, 13,* 299–307.

Robinson, J. L., Kagan, J., Reznick, J. S., & Corley, R. (1992). The heritability of inhibited and uninhibited behavior: A twin study. *Developmental Psychology, 28,* 1030–1037.

Roths, J. B., Foxworth, W. B., McArthur, M. J., Montgomery, C. A., & Kier, A. B. (1999). Spontaneous and engineered mutant mice as models for experimental and comparative pathology: History, comparison, and developmental technology. *Laboratory Animal Science, 49,* 12–34.

Royce, J. R., Carran, A., & Horwarth, E. (1970). Factor analysis of emotionality in ten inbred strains of mice. *Multivariate Behavioral Research, 5,* 19–48.

Sandi, C., Borrell, J., & Guaza, C. (1992a). Behavioral factors in stress-induced immunomodulation. *Behavioral Brain Research, 48,* 95–98.

Sandi, C., Borrell, J., & Guaza, C. (1992b). Behavioral, neuroendocrine, and immunological outcomes of escapable and inescapable shocks. *Physiology and Behavior, 51,* 651–656.

Sapolsky, R. M. (1992). Cortisol concentrations and the social significance of rank instability among wild baboons. *Psychoneuroendocrinology, 17,* 701–709.

Sapolsky, R. M. (1993). Endocrinology alfresco: Psychoneuroendocrine studies of wild baboons. *Recent Progress in Hormone Research, 48,* 437–468.

Sapolsky, R. M., Alberts, S. C., & Altmann, J. (1997). Hypercortisolism associated with social subordinance or social isolation among wild baboons. *Archives of General Psychiatry, 54,* 1137–1143.

Sapolsky, R. M. (1990). Adrenocortical function, social rank, and personality among the wild baboons. *Biological Psychiatry, 28,* 862–878.

Sarason, I. G., Levine, H. M., Basham, R. B., & Sarason, B.R. (1983). Assessing social support: The Social Support Questionnaire. *Journal of Personality and Social Psychology, 44,* 127–139.

Scheier, M. F., & Bridges, M. W. (1995). Person variables and health: Personality predispositions and acute psychological states and shared determinants for disease. *Psychosomatic Medicine, 57,* 255–268.

Scheier, M. F., & Carver, C. S. (1992). Effects of optimism on psychological and physical well-being: Theoretical overview and empirical update. *Cognitive Therapy and Research, 16,* 201–228.

Scheier, M. F., Carver, S. C., & Bridges, M. W. (1994). Distinguishing optimism from neuroticism (and trait anxiety, self-mastery, and self-esteem): A reevaluation of the Life Orientation Test. *Journal of Personality and Social Psychology, 67,* 1063–1078.

Scheier, M. F., Matthews, K. A., Owens, J. F., Magovern, G. J. Sr., Lefebvre, R. C., Abbott, R. A., & Carver, C. S. (1989). Dispositional optimism and recovery from coronary artery bypass surgery: The beneficial effects on physical and psychological well-being. *Journal of Personality and Social Psychology, 57,* 1024–1040.

Segerstrom, S. C. (in press). Personality and the immune system: Models, methods, and mechanisms. *Annals of Behavioral Medicine.*

Segerstrom, S. C., Glover, D. A., Craske, M. G., & Fahey, J. L. (1999). Worry affects the immune response to phobic fear. *Brain, Behavior, and Immunity, 13,* 80–92.

Segerstrom, S. C., Solomon, G. F., Kemeny, M. E., & Fahey, J. L. (1998). Relationship of worry to immune sequelae of the Northridge earthquake. *Journal of Behavioral Medicine, 21,* 433–450.

Segerstrom, S. C., Taylor, S. E., Kemeny, M. E., & Fahey, J. L. (1998). Optimism is associated with mood, coping, and immune change in response to stress. *Journal of Personality and Social Psychology, 74,* 1646–1655.

Segerstrom, S. C., Taylor, S. E., Kemeny, M. E., Reed, G. R., & Visscher, B. R. (1996). Causal attributions predict rate of immune decline in HIV-seropositive gay men. *Health Psychology, 15,* 485–493.

Seidel, A., Arolt, V., Hunstiger, M., Rink, L., Behnisch, A., & Kirchner, H. (1995). Cytokine production and serum proteins in depression. *Scandinavian Journal of Immunology, 41,* 534–538.

Seidel, A., Arolt, V., Hunstiger, M., Rink, L., Behnisch, A., & Kirchner, H. (1996). Increased CD56+ natural killer cells and related cytokines in major depression. *Clinical Immunology and Immunopathology, 78,* 83–85.

Shea, J. D. C., Burton, R., & Girgis, A. (1993). Negative affect, absorption, and immunity. *Physiology and Behavior, 53,* 449–457.

Sheridan, J. F. (1998). Stress-induced modulation of anti-viral immunity. *Brain, Behavior, and Immunity, 12,* 1–6.

Sieber, W. J., Rodin, J., Larson, L., Ortega, S., & Cummings, N. (1992). Modulation of human natural killer cell activity by exposure to uncontrollable stress. *Brain, Behavior, and Immunity, 6,* 141–156.

Smith, T. W. (1992). Hostility and health: Current status of a psychosomatic hypothesis. *Health Psychology, 11,* 139–150.

Smith, T. W., & Williams, P. G. (1992). Personality and health: Advantages and limitations of the five-factor model. *Journal of Personality, 60,* 395–423.

Stefanski, V. (1998). Social stress in loser rats: Opposite immunological effects in submissive and subdominant males. *Physiology and Behavior, 63,* 605–613.

Stefanski, V. & Ben-Eliyahu, S. (1996). Social confrontation and tumor metastasis in rates: Defeat and b-adrenergic mechanisms. *Physiology and Behavior, 60, 277–282.*

Stefanski, V., Solomon, G. F., Kling, A. S., Thomas, J., & Plaeger, S. (1996). Impact of social confrontation on rat CD4 T cells bearing different CD45R isoforms. *Brain, Behavior, and immunity, 10,* 364–379.

Sternberg, E. M. (1995). Neuroendocrine factors in susceptibility to inflammatory disease: focus on the hypothalamic-pituitary-adrenal axis. *Hormone Research, 43,* 159–161.

Stone, A. A. (1995). Measurement of affective response. In S. Cohen, R. C. Kessler, & L. U. Gordon (Eds.), *Measuring stress: A guide for health and social scientists* (pp. 148–171). New York: Oxford University Press.

Stone, A. A., Cox, D. S., Valdimarsdottir, H., Jandorf, L., & Neale, J. M. (1987). Evidence that secretory IgA antibody is associated with daily mood. *Journal of Personality and Social Psychology, 52,* 988–993.

Stone, A. A., Neale, J. M., Cox, D. S., Napoli, A., Valdimarsdottir, H., & Kennedy-Moore, E. (1994). Daily events are associated with a secretory immune response to an oral antigen in men. *Health Psychology, 13,* 440–446.

Strauman, T. J., Lemieux, A. M., & Coe, C. L. (1993). Self-discrepancy and natural killer cell activity: Immunological consequences of negative self-evaluation. *Journal of Personality and Social Psychology, 64,* 1042–1052.

Taylor, G. J., Bagby, R. M., & Parker, J. D. A. (1991). The alexithymia construct: A potential paradigm for psychosomatic medicine. *Psychosomatics, 32,* 153–164.

Thayer, J. F., Friedman, B. H., & Borkovec, T. D. (1996). Autonomic characteristics of generalized anxiety disorder and worry. *Biological Psychiatry, 39,* 255–266.

Todarello, O., Casamassima, A., Daniele, S., Marinaccio, M., Fanciullo, F., Valentino, L., Tedesco, N., Wiesel, S., Simone, G., & Marinaccio, L. (1997). Alexithymia, immunity, and cervical intraepithelial neoplasia: Replication. *Psychotherapy and Psychosomatics, 66,* 208–213.

Todarello, O., Casamassima, A., Marinaccio, M., La Pesa, M.W., Caradonna, L., Valentino, L., & Marinaccio, L. (1994). Alexithymia, immunity, and cervical intraepithelial neoplasia: A pilot study. *Psychotherapy and Psychosomatics, 61,* 199–204.

Uchino, B. N., Cacioppo, J. T., Malarkey, W., & Glaser, R. (1995). Individual differences in cardiac sympathetic control predict endocrine and immune responses to acute psychological stress. *Journal of Personality and Social Psychology, 69,* 736–743.

Uchino, B. N., Cacioppo, J. Y., & Kiecolt-Glaser, J. K. (1996). The relationship between social support and physiological processes: A review with emphasis on underlying mechanisms and implications for health. *Psychological Bulletin, 119,* 488–531.

Van de Langerijt, A. G., Van Lent, P. L., Hermus, A. R., Sweep, C. G., Cools, A. R., & Van den Berg, W. B. (1994). Susceptibility to adjuvant arthritis: Relative importance of adrenal activity and bacterial flora. *Journal of Clinical Investigation, 97,* 33–38.

Vidal, J., & Rama, R. (1994). Association of the antibody response to hemocyanin with behavior in mice bred for high or low antibody responsiveness. *Behavioral Neuroscience, 108,* 1172–1178.

Virgin, C. E., & Sapolsky, R. M. (1997). Styles of male social behavior and their endocrine correlates among low-ranking baboons. *American Journal of Primatology, 42,* 25–39.

Watson, D., & Clark, L. A. (1984). Negative affectivity: The disposition to experience aversive emotional states. *Psychological Bulletin, 96,* 465–490.

Watson, D., & Clark, L. A. (1992). On traits and temperament: General and specific factors of emotional experience and their relation to the five-factor model. *Journal of Personality, 60,* 441–476.

Watson, D., & Pennebaker, J. W. (1989). Health complaints, stress, and distress: Exploring the central role of negative affectivity. *Psychological Review, 96,* 234–254.

Weinberger, D. A., Schwartz, G. E., & Davidson, R. J. (1979). Low-anxious, high-anxious, and repressive coping styles: Psychometric patterns and behavioral and physiological responses to stress. *Journal of Abnormal Psychology, 88,* 369–380.

Widiger, T. A., Verheul, R., & van den Brink, W. (1999). Personality and psychopathology. In L. A. Pervin & O. P. John (Eds.), *Handbook of personality: Theory and research.* New York: Guilford.

Worlein, J., & Laudenslager, M. L. (in press). Effects of early rearing experiences and social interactions on immune function in nonhuman primates. In R. Ader, D. Felten, & N. Cohen (Eds.), *Psychoneuroimmunology* (3rd ed.). New York: Academic Press.

Zorrilla, E. P., Redei, E., & DeRubeis, R. J. (1994). Reduced cytokine levels and T-cell function in healthy males: Relation to individual differences in subclinical anxiety. *Brain, Behavior, and Immunity, 8,* 293–312.

# 34

# Pain and Immune Function

HALINA MACHELSKA, SHAABAN A. MOUSA, CHRISTOPH STEIN

## I. INTRODUCTION

A communication between the nervous and immune systems can be brought about by the release of compounds from immunocompetent cells and their action upon neurons and/or vice versa. Such interactions have been described in both the central (see, e.g., Reichlin, Maier & Nance and Dunn, Dantzer, & McGeer, this volume) and the peripheral nervous systems. This chapter will focus on the peripheral nervous system–immune system communication. The novel concept that there is an interrelation between peripheral sensory nerves and immune cells has been proposed by a number of authors, based mostly on microanatomical findings in inflammatory processes (reviewed in Weihe et al., 1990). Similar to the situation in the central nervous system, mutual interactions may take place; i.e., substances released from peripheral nerves may act on immune cells and/ or vice versa. Effects resulting from these interactions include immunomodulatory, pro- or anti-inflammatory, hyperalgesic (i.e., enhancing pain), or analgesic (i.e., inhibiting pain) phenomena. This chapter is divided into two main parts, the first covers substances released from peripheral neurons; the second covers substances derived from immune cells. The focus will be on functional studies that examine the

cross-talk between cells of the immune system and peripheral sensory nerves and the role of this communication in pain.

## II. NEURON-DERIVED SUBSTANCES

### A. Substance P

Substance P (SP) is one of the best characterized neurogenic mediators of immune hyperactivity. SP is contained in dorsal root ganglion neurons and is released from their peripheral and central terminals (Yaksh, 1988; Zhang, Mi, & Qiao, 1994). SP is capable of modulating immune functions via multiple signaling pathways. One pathway is the neurokinin-1 (NK-1) receptor, which is well-characterized in the nervous system. These receptors have been demonstrated on T and B lymphocytes by cell sorting, radioligand-binding, and immunohistochemical techniques (Bost & Pascual, 1992; Goode et al., 1998; McGillis, Mitsuhashi, & Payan, 1990). Moreover, messenger ribonucleic acid (mRNA) encoding the NK-1 receptor is constitutively expressed in mast cell lines (Ansel, Brown, Payan, & Brown, 1993), in T and B lymphocytes (Bost & Pascual 1992; McCormack, Hart, & Ganea, 1996), and in macrophages (Bost, Breeding, & Pascual, 1992). Sequencing of polymerase chain reaction fragments from purified T lymphocytes showed complete identity to the brain NK-1 receptor sequence (McCormack et al., 1996). This was also demonstrated by radioreceptor binding assays and determining the gene encoding the NK-1 receptor

(Bost et al., 1992; Bost & Pascual 1992). SP can also activate monocytes and B lymphocytes via a non-neurokinin SP receptor, whose stimulation leads to activation of mitogen-activated protein kinase, an important second messenger in the cascade leading to cytokine production by monocytes. Finally, SP can activate G proteins and calcium influx into T cells, followed by an increase in proliferation of these cells in a receptor-independent manner (Kavelaars, Jeurissen, & Heijnen, 1994).

The majority of studies indicate that the effects of SP on cell-mediated immunity are stimulatory. SP can activate mononuclear and polymorphonuclear cells, leading to proliferation, immunoglobulin synthesis and secretion, chemotaxis, lysosomal enzyme release, and phagocytosis (Bost & Pascual, 1992; Kavelaars et al., 1994; McGillis, Organist, & Payan, 1987). Also, SP can modulate the production and secretion of several cytokines from immune-competent cells. Thus, SP has been found to induce mRNA for tumor necrosis factor (TNF)-$\alpha$ and stimulate TNF-$\alpha$ secretion in mast cell lines or peritoneal mast cells in rodents (Ansel et al., 1993; Cocchiara, Bongiovanni, Albeggiani, Azzolina, & Geraci, 1997). SP analogs induce TNF secretion also from human blood monocytes and macrophages, and secretion is inhibited by NK-1 receptor antagonists (Ho et al., 1998). Other cytokines like interleukin (IL)-1 and IL-2, as well as histamine and serotonin, are released by SP from neutrophils, macrophages, or mast cells, respectively (Heller et al., 1994; Lotz, Vaughan, & Carson, 1988). Furthermore, treatments which increase SP concentrations in the periphery increase the number of immunoglobulin-secreting B cells and NK-1 receptor antagonists or depletion of SP-containing neurons reduces the organism's ability to synthesize immunoglobulins (Bost & Pascual, 1992). Mechanisms involved in these responses may include mobilization of intracellular $Ca^{2+}$, stimulation of $Cl^-$ currents and changes in the cell surface expression of cell adhesion molecules and cytokine receptors (Kavelaars et al., 1994; Lambert et al., 1998). Studies suggest that these modulatory effects of SP are important in human inflammatory diseases such as rheumatoid arthritis (McGillis et al., 1990; Walker, Wilson, Binder, Scott, & Carmody, 1997). In addition, SP immunoreactivity has been detected in human peripheral leukocytes, which can represent an additional source of tachykinins in inflamed tissue. This can provide a nonneurogenic tachykininergic contribution to the local inflammatory process (De Giorgio, Tazzari, Barbara, Stanghellini, & Corinaldesi, 1998). This, however, needs to be further examined.

## B. Calcitonin Gene-Related Peptide (CGRP)

Similar to SP, CGRP is contained and released from primary afferent nerves (Zhang et al., 1994). It has also been found in nerve endings within lymphoid organs (Wang, Fiscus, Yang, & Mathews, 1995). Specific CGRP receptors are present on T and B lymphocytes and on a macrophage-like cell line (Abello, Kaiserlian, Cuber, Revillard, & Chayvialle, 1991; Wang et al., 1995). CGRP can modulate mitogenic responses in human peripheral blood mononuclear cells (Casini, Geppetti, Maggi, & Surrenti, 1989) and can inhibit the production of $H_2O_2$ (Nong, Titus, Ribeiro, & Remold, 1989). In T cells, CGRP inhibits the production of IL-2, TNF-$\alpha$ and interferon-$\gamma$ (Wang, Millet, Bottomly, & Vignery, 1992). In human epidermis, CGRP-containing nerve fibers are intimately associated with Langerhans cells and can inhibit their antigen-presenting functions (Hosoi et al., 1993). These findings suggest an inhibitory role of CGRP on cellular immune functions. Anatomical studies have shown a close relationship between mast cells and CGRP-containing enteric nerves (Stead et al., 1987) and between various immunocytes and CGRP-immunoreactive cutaneous nerves under inflammatory conditions (Hassan, Przewlocki, Herz, & Stein, 1992; Przewlocki, Hassan, Lason, Herz, & Stein, 1992). Additionally, CGRP immunoreactivity has been found in extracts of rat lymphocytes from thymus and mesenteric lymph nodes (Xing, Guo, Tang, Tang, & Wang, 1998). However, the functional significance of CGRP derived from immune cells has not been studied in detail.

## C. Opioids

Three families of opioid peptides are well characterized in the central nervous and neuroendocrine systems. Each family derives from a distinct gene and precursor protein, namely proopiomelanocortin (POMC), proenkephalin (PENK), and prodynorphin. Appropriate processing yields their respective major representative opioid peptides $\beta$-endorphin (END), enkephalin (ENK), and dynorphin (DYN). Each peptide exhibits different affinities and selectivities for the three opioid receptor types, $\mu$ (END, ENK), $\delta$ (ENK, END), and $\kappa$ (DYN) (Höllt, 1986). Recently, two additional endogenous opioid peptides have been isolated from bovine brain: endomorphin-1 and endomorphin-2 (Zadina, Hackler, & Kastin, 1997); their precursors are not known yet. Both peptides are considered $\mu$-receptor ligands, having the highest selectivity and affinity for these receptors of any endogenous substance described so far (Zadina et al.,

1997). Opioid peptides have been found in sensory ganglia (ENK, DYN) (Pohl et al., 1997; Przewlocki, Gramsch, Pasi, & Herz, 1983) and in peripheral terminals of sensory nerves (DYN) (Hassan et al., 1992). Also, END and endomorphin-2 have been detected in cultured human and rat spinal ganglion neurons (Kim, Kim, & Kito, 1984; Martin-Schild, Zadina, Geral, Vigh, & Kastin, 1997).

Opioid receptors and the expression of opioid receptor transcripts have been conclusively demonstrated in immune cells (Gaveriaux et al., 1995; Hassan et al., 1993; Sharp et al., 1998). Opioids can modulate lymphoproliferation, chemotaxis, superoxide and cytokine production, and mast cell degranulation (Bryant & Holaday, 1993; Pacifici et al., 1994; Panerai & Sacerdote, 1997). These immunomodulatory actions can be stimulatory as well as inhibitory (Heijnen, Kavelaars, & Ballieux, 1991; Panerai & Sacerdote, 1997) and have been ascribed to the activation of opioid receptors (Sharp et al., 1998). Although these findings signal the potential for interactions between nociceptor-derived opioid peptides and their receptors on immune cells, direct functional evidence for a role in pain perception is lacking at this time.

### D. Other Neurotransmitters

Other neurotransmitters implicated in the mediation of nociception and/or inflammation in the periphery include acetylcholine (ACh), vasoactive intestinal peptide (VIP), and noradrenaline. Choline acetyltansferase (ChAT), an enzyme synthetizing ACh, has been immunohistochemically detected in small diameter sensory neurons in rat dorsal root ganglia (Sann, McCarthy, Mader, & Schemann, 1995). ACh and ChAT mRNA have also been detected in thymic, splenic and peripheral blood T and B lymphocytes (Rinner, Kawashima, & Schauenstein, 1998), suggesting that ACh is produced, and possibly released, from immune cells. Muscarinic cholinergic receptors have been found in peripheral blood lymphocytes (Bronzetti et al., 1996).

VIP is present in small diameter sensory neurons in dorsal root ganglia and is upregulated after sciatic nerve transection (Verge, Richardson, Wiesenfeld-Hallin, & Hökfelt, 1995). It is also produced in primary and secondary lymphoid organs. Mast cells, macrophages, and B and T cells recognize and respond to VIP in patterns that are controlled by the relative levels of expression of VIP receptors. Activation of VIP receptors alters human T-cell chemotaxis, expression of matrix metalloproteinases, proliferation, and cytokine production (for review see

Goetzl et al., 1998). The involvement of immune cell-derived ACh and VIP in pain modulation remains to be evaluated.

There is good evidence for noradrenergic sympathetic innervation of primary and secondary lymphoid organs. In addition to the presence of $\alpha$- and $\beta$-adrenergic receptors on different types of immunocompetent cells, histological studies have demonstrated direct contact between tyrosine hydroxylase-positive nerve terminals and lymphocytes in the spleen and thymus. The exposure of lymphocytes and macrophages to adrenergic agonists in vitro modulates cytokine production, antibody secretion, and proliferation. In vivo, surgical or chemical sympathectomy is known to alter immune responses in rodents. Moreover, in animal models of autoimmune disease, sympathetic innervation is reduced prior to the onset of disease symptoms, and chemical sympathectomy can exacerbate inflammatory disease severity (for review see Hori, Katafuchi, Take, Shimizu, & Niijama, 1995; Madden, Sanders, & Felten, 1995). The role of postganglionic sympathetic neurons and their transmitters in opioid mechanisms of pain control is currently under investigation. Preliminary experiments suggest that adrenergic agonists can release opioid peptides from immune cells and that these opioids interact with peripheral opioid receptors to inhibit inflammatory pain (Zhou, Zhang, & Stein, 1997).

## III. IMMUNE CELL-DERIVED SUBSTANCES

### A. Opioids

Interactions between immune-derived opioid peptides and sensory nerves can result in the inhibition of pain. This notion has emerged during studies on peripheral antinociceptive actions of opioids, which are particularly prominent in painful (hyperalgesic) inflammatory conditions (Barber & Gottschlich, 1992; Stein, 1993). Opioid receptors are present on peripheral sensory nerves and are upregulated during the development of inflammation. Their endogenous ligands, opioid peptides, are synthesized in circulating immune cells which migrate preferentially to injured sites (Figure 1). In response to stressful stimuli or to releasing agents (e.g., corticotropin releasing factor, cytokines), these immunocytes can secrete opioids to activate peripheral opioid receptors and to produce analgesia by inhibiting either the excitability of these nerves or the release of excitatory, proinflammatory neuropeptides. This concept shall be outlined in detail below.

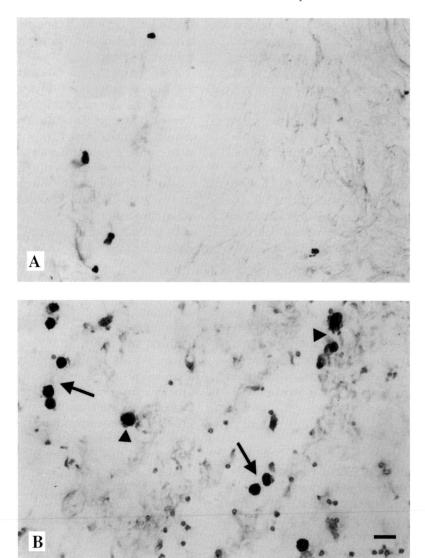

**FIGURE 1**   Immunostaining of $\beta$-endorphin in subcutaneous tissue of (A) noninflamed and (B) Freund's complete adjuvant inflamed rat paws. Photomicrographs demonstrate staining with antibody against $\beta$-endorphin performed at 4 days after induction of inflammation. Cells staining for $\beta$-endorphin include macrophages (arrow heads) and lymphocytes (arrows). Bar, 10 μm.

### 1. Peripheral Opioid Receptors

Anatomical and molecular studies have shown that all three opioid receptors ($\mu$, $\delta$, and $\kappa$) are expressed within sensory neurons. They have been found on cell bodies in the dorsal root ganglia (Ji et al., 1995; Mansour, Fox, Akil, & Watson, 1995; Zhang, Schäfer, Elde, & Stein, 1998) and on central (LaMotte, Pert, & Snyder, 1976) and peripheral terminals of primary afferent neurons in animals (Coggeshall, Zhou, & Carlton, 1997; Hassan et al., 1993; Stein et al., 1990b) and in humans (Stein et al., 1996). Saturation and competition experiments indicate that the pharmacological characteristics of these receptors are very similar to those in the brain. In vivo experiments have shown that the peripheral antinociceptive effects of $\mu$-, $\delta$- and $\kappa$-selective agonists are abolished by pretreatment with capsaicin, a neurotoxin selective for primary afferent neurons (Zhou, Zhang, Stein, & Schäfer, 1998).

After the induction of peripheral inflammation, the axonal transport of opioid receptors in fibers of the sciatic nerve is greatly enhanced. Subsequently, the density of opioid receptors on cutaneous nerve fibers in the inflamed tissue increases and this increase is abolished by ligating the sciatic nerve (Hassan et al., 1993). These findings demonstrate that inflammation enhances the peripherally directed axonal transport of opioid receptors, which leads to an increase in their number (upregulation) on peripheral nerve terminals. In addition, preexistent, but possibly inactive, neuronal opioid receptors may undergo changes owing to the specific milieu (e.g., low pH) of inflamed tissue and thus be rendered active. Indeed, low pH increases opioid agonist efficacy in vitro by altering the interaction of opioid receptors with G proteins in neuronal membranes (reviewed in Stein et al., 1997). Furthermore, inflammation entails a disruption of the perineurium (a normally rather impermeable barrier sheath encasing peripheral nerve fibers) and increases the number of peripheral sensory nerve terminals in inflamed tissue, a phenomenon known as "sprouting" (Antonijevic, Mousa, Schäfer, & Stein, 1995).

Activation of these opioid receptors results in potent peripherally mediated analgesia, particularly in inflamed subcutaneous tissue, viscera, and joints (reviewed in Stein, 1993). Opioid-mediated central side-effects can be excluded by using compounds that do not cross the blood-brain barrier (Barber & Gottschlich, 1997) or by the local application of small, systemically inactive doses of agents (Stein, 1993). Rigorous criteria such as reversibility by standard opioid antagonists (e.g., naloxone), dose-dependency, and stereospecificity have been applied to demonstrate the opioid receptor-specificity of these peripheral effects. Comparing agonists with differing affinities for the three types of opioid receptors ($\mu$, $\delta$, and $\kappa$) has shown that ligands with a preference for $\mu$ receptors are generally most potent, but $\delta$ and $\kappa$ ligands are active as well. Considering the different characteristics of the various inflammatory models, it is conceivable that, depending on the nature and stage of the inflammatory reaction, different types of local opioid receptors become active. Thus, depending on the particular circumstances, all three receptor types can be present and functionally active in peripheral tissues (for details, see Stein, 1993).

Apart from primary afferent neurons, it has been suggested that opioid receptors are also located on sympathetic postganglionic neuron (SPN) terminals and that they may contribute to peripheral opioid antinociception in bradykinin hyperalgesia (Taiwo & Levine, 1991). However, there are reports arguing against the involvement of sympathetic neurons in this model, and studies attempting the direct demonstration of opioid receptor mRNA in sympathetic ganglia have produced negative results (see references in Zhou et al., 1998). Moreover, recent studies using chemical sympathectomy with 6-hydroxydopamine have shown that peripheral antinociception mediated by $\mu$-, $\delta$- and $\kappa$-opioid receptors is indepen-dent of SPN in Freund's adjuvant inflammation (Zhou et al., 1998).

## 2. Opioid Peptides in Cells of the Immune System

Opioid peptides and their precursors are present in immune cells. Pro-opiomelanocortin (POMC)-derived peptides have been highly conserved during evolution (Ottaviani, Franchini, & Franceschi, 1997). Their presence and production were first reported in human lymphocytes by Blalock and Smith (for review, see Blalock, 1994). Since then, POMC-related opioid peptides have been found in immune cells of many vertebrates and nonvertebrates (reviewed in Blalock, 1994; Ottaviani et al., 1997; Panerai & Sacerdote, 1997). To determine whether these leukocytes actually synthesize POMC, rather than simply absorbing related peptides from plasma, mRNA encoding POMC was sought and demonstrated in many of these studies (reviewed in Ottaviani et al., 1997; Panerai & Sacerdote, 1997). In spite of the initial notion that only truncated forms of POMC mRNA are present in immune cells (Panerai & Sacerdote, 1997; Sharp & Yaksh, 1997), recently, full-length POMC mRNA identical in sequence to that isolated from the pituitary gland has been demonstrated in rat mononuclear leukocytes. This POMC transcript is spliced in the same way as the pituitary transcript and consequently contains the sequence for the signal peptide. The 31-kDa POMC protein is also proteolytically processed in a way consistent with the pituitary gland (Lyons & Blalock, 1997).

Proenkephalin (PENK)-derived opioid peptides have also been detected in human and rodent immune cells (in normal lymphocytes, in activated T lymphocytes, and in macrophages) (reviewed in Weisinger, 1995). Upon in vitro stimulation or under pathological conditions, these cells express enhanced levels of PENK mRNA, probably as a result of the induction of transcription factors (e.g., NF-$\kappa$B) and the subsequent activation of the preproenkephalin promoter. In subpopulations of these cells, this mRNA is highly homologous to brain PENK mRNA. It is abundant and apparently translated since immunoreactive ENK is present and/or released (Weisinger, 1995). The appropriate enzymes necessary for post-translational processing of both POMC and PENK have also been identified in immune cells (Vindrola, Mayer, Citera, Spitzer, & Espinoza, 1994).

Immune cell-derived opioid peptides apparently play a substantial role in modulation of inflammatory pain (Stein, 1995). Persistent inflammation is a pathophysiological in vivo stimulus for the immune system and represents a condition that is closer to the clinical setting than some of the early in vitro studies. In a rat model of unilateral localized paw inflammation, mRNAs encoding POMC and PENK and their respective opioid peptide products, END and ENK, are found predominantly within inflamed tissue (Przewlocki et al., 1992) (Figure 1). Histomorphological (Stein et al., 1990) (Figure 1) and double-staining procedures (Przewlocki et al., 1992; Cabot et al., 1997) have identified the opioid-containing cells as T and B lymphocytes as well as monocytes and macrophages. Small amounts of DYN are also detectable by immunocytochemistry (Hassan et al., 1992). Thus, a growing body of evidence indicates that both POMC- and PENK-derived opioid peptides are produced by and stored in immune cells.

### 3. Interaction of Immune-Derived Opioids with Peripheral Opioid Receptors

Recent studies investigating the production, release, and antinociceptive effects of lymphocyte-derived END in relation to cell trafficking have suggested that circulating END-producing lymphocytes home to inflamed tissue where they secrete the opioid to inhibit pain. Afterward, depleted of the peptide, they travel to the regional lymph nodes (Cabot et al., 1997). This migratory pattern is reminiscent of memory type T cells. The trafficking of those cells is not random but they are specifically directed to sites of antigenic or microbial invasion (e.g., inflammatory lesions of the skin) (Butcher & Picker, 1996). Consistent with this notion, END was indeed found mostly in memory-type T cells (Cabot et al., 1997). These findings suggest that local signals not only stimulate the synthesis of opioid peptides in different types of resident inflammatory cells but also attract opioid-containing cells from the circulation to the site of tissue injury to reduce pain.

What are the mechanisms underlying the migration of opioid-containing immunocytes to inflamed tissue? Extensive studies during the past 10 years revealed that extravasation of immune cells is a multistep process involving the sequential activation of various adhesion molecules located on immune cells and vascular endothelium. Initially, the circulating leukocytes are captured and roll on the endothelial cells of vessels, a process mediated by selectins present on leukocytes (L-selectin) and endothelial cells (P- and E-selectin) and their carbohydrate ligands. The rolling leukocytes can then be activated by chemoattractants and this leads to upregulation and increased avidity of integrins, which mediate the firm adhesion of leukocytes to endothelial cells by binding to their immunolgobulin ligands. Finally, the leukocytes transmigrate through the endothelial wall and are directed to the sites of inflammation. Interruption of the leukocyte-endothelial cell cascade (e.g., by monoclonal antibodies against adhesion molecules or by blocking agents like polysaccharides) has been found to block immune cell extravasation (for review see Butcher & Picker, 1996; Springer, 1994). Recently, it has been shown that this treatment can influence endogenous pain control in inflammation. Pretreatment of rats with a selectin blocker (fucoidin) (Ley, Linnemann, Meinen, Stoolman, & Gaehtgens, 1993) abolishes peripheral opioid analgesia. This results from a blockade of the infiltration of END-containing immunocytes and the consequent decrease of the END content in the inflamed tissue (Machelska, Cabot, Mousa, Zhang, & Stein, 1998). These findings indicate that the immune system uses mechanisms of cell migration not only to fight pathogens but also to control pain within injured tissue. Thus, pain may be exacerbated by measures inhibiting the immigration of opioid-producing cells or, conversely, analgesia may be conveyed by adhesive interactions that recruit those cells to injured tissue.

Once opioid-containing immune cells reach the site of inflammation, they have to secrete opioids to produce pain relief. Endogenous opioid peptides are released by different kinds of stress. Following cold water swim, nociceptive thresholds increase selectively in inflamed tissue and this effect is blocked by peripherally acting opioid antagonists (Parsons, Czlonkowski, Stein, & Herz, 1990; Stein, Gramsch, & Herz, 1990a; Stein et al., 1990b). Moreover, this effect is abolished by antibodies against opioid peptides, by immunosuppression, and by blocking the extravasation of opioid-containing immune cells (Machelska et al., 1998; Przewlocki et al., 1992; Stein et al., 1990a,b). Together, these findings suggest that peripheral opioid receptors can mediate local antinociception following their activation by opioids released from immune cells during stress. Studies have supported this notion by the direct demonstration of opioid peptide release within subcutaneous tissue following a noxious thermal stimulus (Yonehara, Takiuchi, Imai, & Inoki, 1993).

The exact mechanisms and stimuli triggering opioid secretion within inflamed tissue are currently under investigation. Corticotropin releasing factor (CRF) is a major physiological secretagogue for opioid peptides in the pituitary. Its releasing effects are potentiated by IL-1$\beta$, and cytokines can stimulate END release directly. Receptors for each of these agents are present on immune cells and are upregulated within inflamed tissue (reviewed in Schäfer,

Mousa, & Stein, 1997). In vivo, the local application of small, systemically inactive doses of CRF, IL-1, and other cytokines produces potent antinociceptive effects in inflamed, but not in noninflamed tissue (Schäfer, Carter, & Stein, 1994; Schäfer et al., 1997). These effects are reversible by immunosuppression, by passive immunization with antibodies against opioid peptides and by opioid antagonists. Furthermore, short-term incubation with CRF or IL-1 can release END in immune cell suspensions prepared from lymph nodes in vitro (Cabot et al., 1997). This release is specific to CRF and IL-1 receptors, is calcium-dependent, and is mimicked by elevated extracellular concentrations of potassium. This is consistent with a regulated pathway of release from secretory vesicles, as in neurons and endocrine cells (Cabot et al., 1997). In summary, these findings indicate that CRF and cytokines can cause secretion of opioids from immune cells, which subsequently activate opioid receptors on sensory nerves to inhibit pain. The most important endogenous secretagogue appears to be locally produced CRF, because endogenous analgesia in inflamed tissue is abolished when the synthesis of CRF in inflamed tissue is inhibited by antisense oligodeoxynucleotides or when antagonists and antibodies against CRF are administered locally (Schäfer et al., 1996).

Opioids produce antinociception by several mechanisms. They increase potassium and decrease calcium currents in the soma of dorsal root ganglion sensory neurons through interactions with G proteins ($G_i$ and/or $G_o$). Recently, the inhibition of a tetrodotoxin-resistant sodium current by a $\mu$-opioid agonist was also described (Gold & Levine, 1996). Provided that these events are similar throughout the neuron, they may underlay the following observations. Opioids attenuate the excitability of the peripheral nociceptive terminal and the propagation of action potentials. Similar to their effects at the soma and at central terminals, opioids inhibit the (calcium-dependent) release of excitatory proinflammatory compounds (e.g., SP) from peripheral sensory nerve endings. In addition, morphine has been shown to inhibit the antidromic vasodilatation evoked by stimulation of C fibers. These mechanisms may also account for opioid anti-inflammatory and antiarthritic actions (reviewed in Stein et al., 1997).

### 4. Clinical Implications

Peripheral opioid interactions with nociceptors are of clinical relevance. A sizeable body of literature demonstrates the analgesic efficacy of exogenous opioids outside the central nervous system (reviewed in Stein, 1993, 1995). To test opioid analgesic actions in the vicinity of peripheral sensory nerve terminals, several controlled studies have examined the intraarticular application of small, systemically inactive doses of morphine in knee surgery or chronic arthritis (Likar et al., 1997; Stein et al., 1997). The majority of these trials have reported significant analgesic effects. Opioid receptors are present on peripheral terminals of nerve fibers in human synovia (Stein et al., 1996). The fact that intraarticular naloxone antagonizes locally applied morphine indicates that these receptors are capable of mediating analgesia in humans (Stein, Comisel, Haimerl, Yassouridis, Lehrberger, Herz, & Peter, 1991).

To search for the endogenous ligands, inflamed synovial tissue from patients undergoing arthroscopic knee surgery was examined. Opioid peptides were found in synovial lining cells and in lymphocytes, macrophages and mast cells. The prevailing peptides were END and ME, while only minor amounts of DYN were detectable (Stein et al., 1993). The interaction of synovial opioids with peripheral opioid receptors was examined in patients undergoing knee surgery. Blocking of intraarticular opioid receptors by the local administration of the antagonist naloxone resulted in significantly increased postoperative pain. This pain-enhancing effect was demonstrated by subjective measures as well as by increased supplemental analgesic requirements (Stein, Hassan, Lehrberger, Giefing, & Yassouridis, 1993). Taken together, these findings suggest that in a stressful (e.g., postoperative) situation, opioids are tonically released from inflamed tissue and activate peripheral opioid receptors to attenuate clinical pain.

Importantly, these endogenous opioids do not interfere with exogenous morphine; i.e., intraarticular morphine is an equally potent analgesic in patients with and without opioid-producing inflammatory synovial cells (Stein et al., 1996). This suggests that, in contrast to the rapid development of tolerance in the central nervous system, the immune cell-derived opioids do not produce cross-tolerance to morphine at the level of peripheral opioid receptors. This finding is at variance with some animal experiments that have used exogenous agonists to produce tolerance of peripheral opioid receptors (see references in Stein et al., 1996). Importantly, however, in these studies normal animals *without inflammation* were pretreated with repeated opioid injections to induce tolerance. Since the number, affinity and coupling efficacy of opioid receptors appear to be markedly enhanced under inflammatory conditions (Hassan et al., 1993; Stein et al., 1997), these studies do not permit conclusions regarding tolerance in the clinical situation. Indeed, earlier studies have suggested that tolerance to peripheral opioid antinociception does not occur when the opioid pretreatment is performed in presence of brief, transient inflammatory stimuli (Ferreira, Lorenzetti, & Rae, 1984). These considerations raise questions whether tolerance development is different at central versus peripheral opioid receptors and in inflamed versus noninflamed tissue. Clarification of these issues is important for the treatment of chronic pain in arthritis and other inflammatory conditions with peripherally acting opioids.

## B. Nerve Growth Factor (NGF)

NGF is the prototype of neurotrophic factors critical for the development and maintenance of specific peripheral and central neuronal populations (Eide, Lowenstein, & Reichardt, 1993). NGF accumulates in inflammatory sites or exudates caused by various noxious stimuli (Aloe, Tuveri, Carcassi, & Levi-Montalcini, 1992). T lymphoctytes and mast cells have been shown to synthesize, store, and release NGF (Ehrhard, Erb, Graumann, & Otten, 1993; Leon et al., 1994). Receptors for NGF are expressed by dorsal root ganglion (DRG) sensory neurons (Barrett, Georgiou, Reid, Bartlett, & Leung, 1998; Farinas, Wilkinson, Backus, Reichardt, & Patapoutian, 1998; Meakin, & Shooter 1992). NGF is thought to bind to its receptor on nerve terminals and to be transported retrogradely together with its receptor to the cell body. Neurochemical studies have suggested an interaction of NGF with primary afferent neurons innervating inflamed tissue. NGF upregulates the synthesis and content of SP and CGRP in DRG and sciatic nerves (Donaldson, Harmar, Mcqueen, & Seckl, 1992; Donnerer, Schuligoi, & Stein, 1992; Schuliogoi & Amann, 1998; Vedder, Affolter, & Otten, 1993). Moreover, the axonal transport of both peptides toward the periphery is induced by NGF (Donnerer et al., 1992). The elevated levels of neuropeptides likely result in their increased release from peripheral (Donnerer et al., 1992) and/or central (Garry & Hargreaves 1992) terminals. Since SP and CGRP are commonly considered excitatory and/or proinflammatory neuropeptides, these investigations suggest that NGF plays a role in sustaining pain and inflammation. In addition, NGF can influence immune cell function. Receptors for NGF have been demonstrated on human B lymphocytes, and NGF enhances proliferation of these cells (Melamed et al., 1996). NGF also stimulates phagocytosis, parasite killing, and IL-1 production by murine peritoneal macrophages (Susaki et al., 1996). Finally, NGF-induced accumulation of neutrophils has been held responsible for hyperalgesia induced by intraplantar injection of NGF into the rat paw (Bennett, al-Rashed, Hoult, & Brian, 1998).

## C. Cytokines

A few studies have suggested an interaction of cytokines and nociceptors. IL-6-deficient mice have a lower response threshold to noxious stimulation and under inflammatory conditions they develop less hyperalgesia and exhibit less plasma extravasation (Xu et al., 1997). Electrophysiological studies show that TNF-$\alpha$ increases the responses of isolated sensory neurons grown in culture (Nicol, Lopshire, & Pafford, 1997). The injection of IL-1 into noninflamed tissue has been shown to cause hyperalgesia, which was presumed to result from prostaglandin release (Ferreira, Lorenzetti, Bristow, & Poole, 1988). Macrophage-derived IL-1 enhances NGF synthesis in Schwann cells and other nonneuronal cells of the sciatic nerve after nerve lesion (Lindholm, Heumann, Meyer, & Thoenen, 1987) and IL-1 may be produced and released from nonneuronal cells residing in the damaged nerve (Rotshenker, Aamar, & Barak, 1992). None of these studies, however, have shown direct interactions between immune cell-derived cytokines and nociceptors.

## IV. CONCLUSIONS

At this time, the most extensively studied compounds mediating direct interactions between nociceptors and immunocytes are SP and opioids. SP is the prototype of a neuropeptide released from sensory neurons and its actions upon immune cells appear to be largely stimulatory. Some studies have suggested that the effects of SP are of importance in human diseases such as rheumatoid arthritis and inflammatory bowel disease. A large number of experimental and clinical trials have demonstrated interactions of exogenous and immune cell-derived endogenous opioids with nociceptors, resulting in the inhibition of inflammatory pain. These findings have stimulated research into novel routes of opioid administration and into production, release, and pharmacokinetics of opioids in inflamed tissue. Clinical studies have already shown promising results, suggesting that peripheral opioid neuro-immune interactions provide a novel perspective for pain management and for the treatment of chronic inflammatory conditions.

# References

Abello, J., Kaiserlian, D., Cuber, J. C., Revillard, J. P., & Chayvialle, J. A. (1991). Characterization of calcitonin gene-related peptide receptors and adenylate cyclase response in the murine macrophage cell line P388 D1. *Neuropeptides, 19*, 43–49.

Aloe, L., Tuveri, M. A., Carcassi, U., & Levi-Montalcini, R. (1992). Nerve growth factor in the synovial fluid of patients with chronic arthritis. *Arthritis and Rheumatism, 35*, 351–355.

Ansel, J. C., Brown, J. R., Payan, D. G., & Brown, M. A. (1993). Substance P selectively activates TNF-α gene expression in murine mast cells. *Journal of Immunology, 150*, 4478–4485.

Antonijevic, I., Mousa, S. A., Schäfer, M., & Stein, C. (1995). Perineurial defect and peripheral opioid analgesia in inflammation. *The Journal of Neuroscience, 15*(1), 165–172.

Barber, A., & Gottschlich, R. (1992). Opioid agonists and antagonists: An evaluation of their peripheral actions in inflammation. *Medicinal Research Reviews, 12*, 525–562.

Barber, A., & Gottschlich, R. (1997). Central and peripheral nervous system. Novel developments with selective, non-peptidic kappa-opioid receptor agonists. Experimental Opinion in Investigation of Drugs, 6, 1351–1368.

Barrett, G. L., Georgiou, A., Reid, K., Bartlett, P. F., & Leung, D. (1998). Rescue of dorsal root sensory neurons by nerve growth factor and neurotrophin-3, but not brain-derived neurotrophic factor or neurotrophin-4, is dependent on the level of the p75 neurotrophin receptor. *Neuroscience, 85*(4), 1321–1328.

Bennett, G., al-Rashed, S., Hoult, J. R. S., & Brian, S. D. (1998). Nerve growth factor induced hyperalgesia in the rat hind paw is dependent on circulating neutrophils. *Pain, 77*, 315–322.

Blalock, J. E. (1994). The syntax of immune-neuroendocrine communication. *Immunology Today, 15*, 504–511.

Bost, K. L., Breeding, S. A., & Pascual, D. W. (1992). Modulation of the mRNAs encoding substance P and its receptor in rat macrophages by LPS. *Regional Immunology, 4*, 105–112.

Bost, K. L., & Pascual, D. W. (1992). Substance P: A late acting B lymphocyte differentiation cofactor. *American Journal of Physiology, 262*, C537–C545.

Bronzetti, E., Adani, O., Amenta, F., Felici, L., Mannino, F., & Ricci, A. (1996). Muscarinic cholinergic receptor subtypes in human peripheral blood lymphocytes. Neuroscience Letters, 208(3), 211–215.

Bryant, H. U., & Holaday, J. W. (1993). Opioids in immunologic processes. In A. Herz (Ed.), *Opioids II* (pp. 551–570). Berlin: Springer-Verlag.

Butcher, E. C., & Picker, L. J. (1996). Lymphocyte homing homeostasis. *Science, 272*, 60–66.

Cabot, P. J., Carter, L., Gaiddon, C., Zhang, Q., Schäfer, M,. Loeffler, J. P., & Stein, C. (1997). Immune cell-derived β-endorphin: Production, release and control of inflammatory pain in rats. *Journal of Clinical Investigation, 100*, 142–148.

Casini, A., Geppetti, P., Maggi, C. A., & Surrenti, C. (1989). Effects of calcitonin gene-related peptide (CGRP), neurokinin A and neurokinin A (4-10) on the mitogenic response of human peripheral blood mononuclear cells. *Naunyn Schmiedeberg's Archives of Pharmacology, 339*, 354–358.

Cocchiara, R., Bongiovanni, A., Albeggiani, G., Azzolina, A., & Geraci, D. (1997). Substance P selectively activates TNF-α mRNA in rat uterine immune cells: A neuroimmune link. *Neuroreport, 8*(13), 2961–2964.

Coggeshall, R. E., Zhou, S., & Carlton, S. M. (1997). Opioid receptors on peripheral sensory axons. *Brain Research, 764*, 126-132.

De Giorgio, R., Tazzari, P. L., Barbara, G., Stanghellin, V., & Corinaldesi, R. (1998). Detection of substance P immunoreactivity in human peripheral leukocytes. *Journal of Neuroimmunology, 82*(2), 175–181.

Donaldson, L. F., Harmar, A. J., Mcqueen, D. S., & Seckl, J. R. (1992). Increased expression of preprotachykinin, calcitonin gene-related peptide, but not vasoactive intestinal peptide messenger RNA in dorsal root ganglia during the development of adjuvant monoarthritis in the rat. *Molecular Brain Research, 16*, 143–149.

Donnerer, J., Schuligoi, R., & Stein, C. (1992). Increased content and transport of substance P and calcitonin gene-related peptide in sensory nerves innervating inflamed tissue: evidence for a regulatory function of nerve growth factor in vivo. *Neuroscience, 49*, 693–698.

Ehrhard, P. B., Erb, P., Graumann, U., & Otten, U. (1993). Expression of nerve growth factor and nerve growth factor receptor tyrosine kinase Trk in activated CD4-positive T-cell clones. *Proceedings of the National Academy of Sciences, USA, 90*, 10984–10988.

Eide, F. F., Lowenstein, D. H., & Reichardt, L. F. (1993). Neurotrophins and their receptors—Current concepts and implications for neurologic disease. *Experimental Neurolology, 121*, 200–214.

Farinas, I., Wilkinson, G. A., Backus, C., Reichardt, L. F., & Patapoutian, A. (1998). Characterization of neurotrophin and Trk receptor functions in developing sensory ganglia: Direct NT-3 activation of TrkB neurons in vivo. *Neuron, 21*(2), 325–334.

Ferreira, S. H., Lorenzetti, B. B., Bristow, A. F., & Poole, S. (1988). Interleukin-1 beta as a potent hyperalgesic agent antagonized by a tripeptide analogue. *Nature, 334*, 698–700.

Ferreira, S. H., Lorenzetti, B. B., & Rae, G. A. (1984). Is methyl-nalorphinium the prototype of an ideal peripheral analgesic. *European Journal of Pharmacology, 99*, 23–29.

Garry, M. G., & Hargreaves, K. M. (1992). Enhanced release of immunoreactive CGRP and substance P from spinal dorsal horn slices occurs during carrageenan inflammation. *Brain Research, 582*, 139–142.

Gaveriaux, C., Peluso, J., Simonin, F., Laforet, J., & Kieffer, B. (1995). Identification of kappa- and delta-opioid receptor transcripts in immune cells. *FEBS Letters, 369*, 272–276.

Goetzl, E. J., Pankhaniya, R. R., Gaufo, G. O., Mu, Y., Xia, M., & Sreedharan, S. P. (1998). Selectivity of effects of vasoactive intestinal peptide on macrophages and lymphocytes in compartmental immune responses. *Annals of the New York Academy of Sciences, 840*, 540–550.

Goode, T., O'Connell, J., Sternini, C., Anton, P., Wong, H., O'Sullivan, G. C., Collins, J. K., & Shanahan, F. (1998). Substance P (neurokinin-1) receptor is a marker of human mucosal but not peripheral mononuclear cells: Molecular quantitation and localization. *Journal of Immunology, 161*(5), 2232–2240.

Hassan, A. H. S., Ableitner, A., Stein, C., & Herz. A. (1993). Inflammation of the rat paw enhances axonal transport of opioid receptors in the sciatic nerve and increases their density in the inflamed tissue. *Neuroscience, 55*, 185–195.

Hassan, A. H. S., Przewlocki, R., Herz, A., & Stein, C. (1992). Dynorphin, a preferential ligand for kappa-opioid receptors, is present in nerve fibers and immune cells within inflamed tissue of the rat. *Neuroscience Letters, 140*, 85–88.

Heller, P. H., Green, P. G., Tanner, K. D., Miao, F. J.-P., & Levine, J. D. (1994). Peripheral neural contributions to inflammation. In K. L. Fields & J. C. Liebeskind (Eds.), *Progress in Pain Research and Management* (pp. 31–42). Seattle: IASP Press.

Heijnen, C. J., Kavelaars, A., & Ballieux, R. E. (1991). Beta-endorphin: Cytokine and neuropeptide. *Immunological Review, 119*, 41–63.

Ho, W. Z., Stavropoulos, G., Lai, J. P., Hu, B, F., Magafa, V., Anagnostides, S., & Douglas, S. D. (1998). Substance P C-terminal octapeptide analogues augment tumor necrosis factor-$\alpha$ release by human blood monocytes and macrophages. *Journal of Neuroimmunology, 82*(2), 126–132.

Höllt, V. (1986). Opioid peptide processing and receptor selectivity. *Annual Review of Pharmacology and Toxicology, 26*, 59–77.

Hori, T., Katafuchi, T., Take, S., Shimizu, N., & Niijama, A. (1995). The autonomic nervous system as a communication channel between the brain and the immune system. *Neuroimmunomodulation, 2*(4), 203–215.

Hosoi, J., Murphy, G. F., Egan, C. L., Lerner, E. A., Grabbe, S., Asahina, A., & Granstein, R. D. (1993). Regulation of Langerhans cell function by nerves containing calcitonin gene-related peptide. *Nature, 363*, 159–163.

Ji, R.-R., Zhang, Q., Law, P.-Y., Low, H. H., Elde, R., & Hökfelt, T. (1995). Expression of mu-, delta-, and kappa-opioid receptor-like immunoreactivities in rat dorsal root ganglia after carrageenan-induced inflammation. *Journal of Neuroscience, 15*, 8156–8166.

Kavelaars, A., Jeurissen, F., & Heijnen, C. J. (1994). Substance P receptors and signal transduction in leukocytes. *Immunomethods, 5*(1), 41–48.

Kim, J. H., Kim, S. U., & Kito, S. (1984). Immunocytochemical demonstration of beta-endorphin and beta-lipotropin in cultured human spinal ganglion neurons. *Brain Research, 304*, 192–196.

Lambert, N., Lescoulie, P. L., Yassine-Diab, B., Enault, G., Mazieres, B., De Preval, C., & Cantagrel, A. (1998). Substance P enhances cytokine-induced vascular cell adhesion molecule-1 (VACAM-1) expression on cultured rheumatoid fibroblast-like synoviocytes. *Clinical and Experimental Immunology, 113*(2), 269–175.

LaMotte, C., Pert, C. B., & Snyder, S. H. (1976). Opiate receptor binding in primate spinal cord: Distribution and changes after dorsal root section. *Brain Research, 112*, 407–412.

Leon, A., Buriani, A., Dal Toso, R., Fabris, M., Romanello, S., Aloe, L., & Levi-Montalcini, R. (1994). Mast cells synthesize, store, and release nerve growth factor. *Proceedings of the National Academy of Sciences, USA, 91*, 3739–3743.

Ley, K., Linnemann, G., Meinen, M., Stoolman, L. M., & Gaehtgens, P. (1993). Fucoidin, but not polyphosphomannan PPME, inhibits leukocyte rolling in venules of the rat mesentery. *Blood, 81*, 177–185.

Likar, R., Schäfer, M., Paulak, F., Sittl, R., Pipam, W., Schalk, H., Geissler, D., & Bernatzky, G. (1997). Intraarticular morphine analgesia in chronic pain patients with osteoarthritis. *Anesthesia and Analgesia, 84*(6), 1313–1317.

Lindholm, D., Heumann, R., Meyer, M., & Thoenen, H. (1987). Interleukin-1 regulates synthesis of nerve growth factor in non-neuronal cells of rat sciatic nerve. *Nature, 330*, 658–659.

Lotz, M., Vaughan, J. H., & Carson, D. (1988). Effects of neuropeptides on prduction of inflammatory cytokines by human monocytes. *Science, 241*, 1218–1221.

Lyons, P. D., & Blalock, J. E. (1997). Pro-opioimelanocortin gene expression and protein processing in rat mononuclear leukocytes. *Journal of Neuroimmunology, 78*, 47–56.

Machelska, H., Cabot, P. J., Mousa, S. A., Zhang, Q., & Stein, C. (1998). Pain control in inflammation governed by selectins. *Nature Medicine, 4*, 1425–1428.

Madden, K. S., Sanders, V. M., & Felten, D. L. (1995). Catecholamine influences and sympathetic neural modulation of immune responsiveness. *Annual Review of Pharmacology and Toxicology, 35*, 417–448.

Mansour, A., Fox, C. A., Akil, H., & Watson, S. J. (1995). Opioid-receptor mRNA expression in the rat CNS: Anatomical and functional implications. *Trends in Neurosciences, 18*, 22–29.

Martin-Schild, S., Zadina, J. E., Geral, A. A., Vigh, S., & Kastin, A. J. (1997). Localization of endomorphin-2-like immunoreactivity in the rat medulla and spinal cord. *Peptides, 18*, 1641–1649.

McCormack, R. J., Hart, R. P., & Ganea, D. (1996). Expression of NK-1 receptor mRNA in murine T lymphocytes. *Neuroimmunomodulation, 3*(1), 35–46.

McGillis, J. P., Mitsuhashi, M., & Payan, D. G. (1990). Immunomodulation by tachykinin neuropeptides. *Annals of the New York Acadademy of Sciences, 594*, 85–94.

McGillis, J. P., Organist, M. L., & Payan, D. G. (1987). Substance P and immunoregulation. *Federation Proceedings, 46*, 196–199.

Meakin, S. O., & Shooter, E. M. (1992). The nerve growth family of receptors. *Trends in Neurosciences, 15*, 323–331.

Melamed, I., Kelleher, C. A., Franklin, R. A., Brodie, C., Hempstead, B., Kaplan, D., & Gelfand, E. W. (1996). Nerve growth factor signal transduction in human B lymphocytes is mediated by gp140trk. *European Journal of Immunology, 26*(9), 1985–1992.

Nicol, G. D., Lopshire, J. C., & Pafford, C. M. (1997). Tumor necrosis factor enhances the capsaicin sensitivity of rat sensory neurons. *Journal of Neuroscience, 17*(3), 975–982.

Nong, Y. H., Titus, R. G., Ribeiro, J. M., & Remold, H. G. (1989). Peptides encoded by the calcitonin gene inhibit macrophage function. *Journal of Immunology, 143*, 45–49.

Ottaviani, E., Franchini, A., & Franceschi, C. (1997). Pro-opiomelanocortin-derived peptides, cytokines, and nitric oxide in immune responses and stress: An evolutionary approach. *International Review of Cytology, 170*, 79–141.

Pacifici, R., Patrini, G., Venier, I., Parolaro, D., Zuccaro, P., & Gori, E. (1994). Effect of morphine and methadone acute treatment on immunological activity in mice:pharmacokinetic and pharmacodynamic correlates. *Journal of Pharmacology and Experimental Therapeutics, 269*(3), 1112–1116

Panerai, A. E., & Sacerdote, P. (1997). Beta-endorphin in the immune system: a role at last? *Immunology Today, 18*, 317–319.

Parsons, C. G., Czlonkowski, A., Stein, C., & Herz, A. (1990). Peripheral opioid receptors mediating antinociception in inflammation. Activation by endogenous opioids and role of the pituitary-adrenal axis. *Pain, 41*, 81–93.

Pohl, M., Ballet, S., Collin, E., Mauborgne, A., Bourgoin, S., Benoliel, J. J., Hamon, M., & Cesselin, F. (1997). Enkephalinergic and dynorphinergic neurons in the spinal cord and dorsal root ganglia of the polyarthritic rat—In vivo release and cDNA hybridization studies. *Brain Research, 749*, 18–28.

Przewlocki, R., Gramsch, C., Pasi, A., & Herz, A. (1983). Characterization and localization of immunoreactive dynorphin, alpha-neoendorphin, met-enkephalin and substance P in human spinal cord. *Brain Research, 280*, 95–103.

Przewlocki, R., Hassan, A. H. S., Lason, W., Epplen, C., Herz, A., & Stein, C. (1992). Gene expression and localization of opioid peptides in immune cells of inflamed tissue. Functional role in antinociception. *Neuroscience, 48*, 491–500.

Rinner, I., Kawashima K., & Schauenstein, K. (1998). Rat lymphocytes produce and secrecte acetylcholine independent of differentiation and activation. *Journal of Neuroimmunology, 81*(1–29), 31–37.

Rotshenker, S., Aamar, S., & Barak, V. (1992). Interleukin-1 activity in lesioned peripheral nerve. *Journal of Neuroimmunology, 39*, 75–80.

Sann, H., McCarthy, P. W., Mader M., & Schemann, M. (1995). Choline acetyltransferase-like immunoreactivity in small diameter neurons of the rat dorsal root ganglion. *Neuroscience Letters, 198*(1), 17–20.

Schäfer, M., Carter, L., & Stein, C. (1994). Interleukin-1 beta and corticotropin-releasing-factor inhibit pain by releasing opioids from immune cells in inflamed tissue. *Proceedings of the National Academy of Sciences, USA, 91*, 4219–4223.

Schäfer, M., Mousa, S. A., & Stein, C. (1997). Corticotropin-releasing factor in antinociception and inflammation. *European Journal of Pharmacology, 323*, 1–10

Schäfer, M., Mousa, S. A., Zhang, Q., Carter, L., & Stein, C. (1996). Expression of corticotropin-releasing factor in inflamed tissue is required for intrinsic peripheral opioid analgesia. *Proceedings of the National Academy of Sciences, USA, 93*, 6096–6100.

Schuligoi, R., & Amann, R. (1998). Differential effects of treatment with nerve growth factor on thermal nociception and on calcitonin gene-related peptide content of primary afferent neurons in the rat. *Neuroscience Letters, 252*(2), 147–149.

Sharp, B. M., Roy, S., & Bidlack, J. M. (1998). Evidence for opioid receptors on cells involved in host defense and the immune system. *Journal of Neuroimmunology, 83*, 45–56.

Sharp, B., & Yaksh, T. (1997). Pain killers of the immune system. T lymphocyte produce opioid immunopeptides that control pain at sites of inflammation. *Nature of Medicine, 3*, 831–832.

Springer, T. A. (1994). Traffic signals for lymphocyte recirculation and leukocyte emigration: The multistep paradigm. *Cell, 76*, 301–314.

Stead, R. H., Tomioka, M., Quinonez, G., Simon, G. T., Felten, S.Y., & Bienenstock, J. (1987). Intestinal mucosal mast cells in normal and nematode-infected rat intestines are in intimate contact with peptidergic nerves. *Proceedings of the National Academy of Sciences, USA, 84*, 2975–2979.

Stein, C. (1993). Peripheral mechanisms of opioid analgesia. *Anesthesia and Analgesia, 76*, 182–191.

Stein, C. (1995). The control of pain in peripheral tissue by opioids. *New England Journal of Medicine, 332*, 1685–1690.

Stein, C., Comisel, K., Haimerl, E., Yassouridis, A., Lehrberger, K., Herz, A., & Peter, K. (1991). Analgesic effect of intraarticular morphine after arthroscopic knee surgery. *New England Journal of Medicine, 325*, 1123–1126.

Stein, C., Gramsch, C., & Herz, A. (1990a). Intrinsic mechanisms of antinociception in inflammation. Local opioid receptors and beta-endorphin. *Journal of Neuroscience, 10*, 1292–1298.

Stein, C., Hassan, A. H. S., Lehrberger, K., Giefing, J., & Yassouridis, A. (1993). Local analgesic effect of endogenous opioid peptides. *Lancet, 342*, 321–324.

Stein, C., Hassan, A. H. S., Przewlocki, R., Gramsch, C., Peter, K., & Herz, A. (1990b). Opioids from immunocytes interact with receptors on sensory nerves to inhibit nociception in inflammation. *Proceedings of the National Academy of Sciences, USA, 87*, 5935–5939.

Stein, C., Pflüger, M., Yassouridis, A., Hoelzl, J., Lehrberger, K., Welte, C., & Hassan, A H. S. (1996). No tolerance to peripheral morphine analgesia in presence of opioid expression in inflamed synovia. *Journal of Clinical Investigation, 98*, 793–799.

Stein, C., Schäfer, M., Cabot, P. J., Carter, L., Zhang, Q., Zhou, L., & Gasior, M. (1997). Peripheral opioid analgesia. *Pain Reviews, 4*, 171–185.

Susaki, Y., Shimizu, S., Katakura, K., Watanabem, N., Kawamoto, K., Matsumoto, M., Tsudzuki, M., Furusaka, T., Kitamura, Y., & Matsuda, H. (1996). Functional properties of murine macrophages promoted by nerve growth factor. *Blood, 88*(12), 4630–4637.

Taiwo, Y. O., & Levine, J. D. (1991). Kappa- and delta-opioids block sympathetically dependent hyperalgesia. *Journal of Neuroscience, 11*, 928–932.

Vedder, H., Affolter, H. U., & Otten, U. (1993). Nerve growth factor (NGF) regulates tachykinin gene expression and biosynthesis in rat sensory neurons during early postnatal development. *Neuropeptides, 24*(6), 351–357.

Verge, V. M., Richardson, P. M., Wiesenfeld-Hallin, Z., & Hökfelt, T. (1995). Differential influence of nerve growth factor on neuropeptide expression in vivo: A novel role in peptide suppression in adult sensory neurons. *Journal of Neuroscience, 15*(3 Pt), 2081–2096.

Vindrola, O., Mayer, A. M. S., Citera, G., Spitzer, J. A., & Espinoza, L. R. (1994). Prohormone convertases PC2 and PC3 in rat neutrophils and macrophages. *Neuropeptides, 27*, 235–244.

Walker, J. S., Wilson, J. L., Binder, W., Scott, C., & Carmody, J. J. (1997). The anti-inflammatory effects of opioids: their possible relevance to the pathophysiology and treatment of rheumatoid arthritis. *Rheumatoid Arthritis, 1*(6), 291–299.

Wang, X., Fiscus, R. R., Yang, L., & Mathews, H. L. (1995). Suppression of the functional activity of IL-2-activated lymphocytes by CGRP. *Cell Immunology, 162*(1), 105–113.

Wang, F., Millet, I., Bottomly, K., & Vignery, A. (1992). Calcitonin gene-related peptide inhibits interleukin 2 production by murine T lymphocytes. *Journal of Biological Chemistry, 267*, 21052–21057.

Weihe, E., Büchler, M., Müller, S., Friess, H., Zentel, H. J., & Yanaihara, N. (1990). Peptidergic innervation in chronic pancreatitis. In H. G. Beger, M. Büchler, H. Ditschuneit, & P. Malfertheiner (Eds.), *Chronic pancreatitis* (pp. 83–105). Berlin Heidelberg: Springer.

Weisinger, G. (1995). The transcriptional regulation of the preproenkephalin gene. *Journal of Biochememistry, 307*, 617–629.

Xing, L., Guo, J., Tang, J., Tang, Y., & Wang, X. (1998). Morphological evidence for the location of calcitonin gene-related peptide (CGRP) immunoreactivity in rat lymphocytes. *Cell Vision, 5*(1), 8–12.

Xu, X. J., Hao, J. X., Andell-Jonsson, S., Poli, V., Bartfai, T., & Wiesenfeld-Hallin, Z. (1997). Nociceptive responses in interleukin-6-deficient mice to peripheral inflammation and peripheral nerve section. *Cytokine, 9*(12), 1028–1033.

Yaksh, T. L. (1988). Substance P release from knee afferent terminals: modulation by opioids. *Brain Research, 458*, 319–324.

Yonehara, N., Takiuchi, S., Imai, Y., & Inoki, R. (1993). Opioid peptide release evoked by noxious stimulation of the hind instep of rats. *Regulatory Peptides, 48*, 365–372.

Zadina, J. E., Hackler, L., Ge, L-J., & Kastin, A. J. (1997). A potent and selective endogenous agonist for the i-opiate receptor. *Nature, 386*, 499–502.

Zhang, R. X., Mi, Z. P., & Qiao, J. T. (1994). Changes of spinal substance P, calcitonin gene-related peptide, somatostatin, Met-enkephalin and neurotensin in rats in response to formalin-induced pain. *Regulatory Peptides, 51*(1), 25–32.

Zhou, L., Zhang, Q., & Stein, C. (1997). Role of sympathetic postganglionic neurons in endogenous peripheral opioid analgesia. *Society of Neuroscience Abstract, 23*(2), 2042.

Zhou, L., Zhang, Q., Stein, C., & Schäfer, M. (1998). Contribution of opioid receptors on primary afferent versus sympathetic neurons to peripheral opioid analgesia. *Journal of Pharmacology and Experimental Therapeutics, 261*, 1–7.

# 35

# Immune Responses to Acute Exercise: Hemodynamic, Hormonal, and Cytokine Influences

LAURIE HOFFMAN-GOETZ, BENTE K. PEDERSEN

## I. INTRODUCTION

Exercise and physical activity are important human behaviors that influence the immune system. Some of the immunological effects reflect the dynamic physical nature of the cardiovascular response to exercise involving recirculation, shear forces, and plasma volume shifts. This category of effects might include redistribution of lymphocytes as a result of splanchnic contraction with exercise. Some immunological effects are due to the metabolic demands and oxygen uptake resulting from work. This category of effects might include the generation of oxygen free radicals, such as superoxide anion, due to increased ventilation as well as cellular respiration. Some immunological effects are related to skeletal muscle trauma and induction of the inflammatory response. Other immunological effects of exercise might reflect the action of stress hormones, such as corticosteroids, inducing programmed cell death or apoptosis in lymphoid tissues. Still other immunological effects concomitant with exercise are due to the actions of cytokine regulatory signals. This chapter briefly describes the range of innate and acquired immune responses to an acute exercise bout. Although humans usually engage in repeated physical activity, rather than in an isolated and novel exposure, most of the research in exercise immunology has focused on exercise as a reproducible and highly quantifiable model of acute stress (Hoffman-Goetz & Pedersen, 1994).

## II. IMMUNOLOGICAL RESPONSE TO ACUTE EXERCISE

### A. Innate Immune Responses

Neutrophils, mononuclear phagocytes, and natural killer (NK) cells are primary effector cells mediating the innate or nonspecific host defense response to diverse physical and psychological stimuli. While nonspecific host defense responses are involved in various inflammatory conditions, these highly stereotyped responses also occur following an episode of acute exercise stress.

Neutrophils, which contribute approximately half of the total circulating leukocyte pool, demonstrate a prolonged neutrocytosis following acute long-term exercise (McCarthy & Dale, 1988). Although the phenomenon of neutrocytosis with exercise has been described, the underlying mechanisms have not been clearly identified. Some data to suggest that the neutrocytosis may reflect changes in the expression of intercellular adhesion molecules (ICAMs), leading to selective demargination from tissue compartments or the extravasation of neutrophils into damaged tissues. Smith and colleagues (1996) reported that the expression of CD11b on the surface of neutrophils was increased in response to acute submaximal exercise. Kurokawa, Shinkai, Torii, Hino, and Shek (1995) in contrast found no change in the granulocyte expression of either CD11a or CD11b after exercise. In an older study, Lewicki, Tchorzewski, Denys, Kowalska, and Golinska (1987) showed that neutrophil adherence (reflecting ICAM expression) was reduced following a single maximal physical exercise bout relative to preexercise function.

The effect of exercise on the function of neutrophils depends on the type and duration of exercise, and the neutrophil parameter in question. Several independent laboratories have shown that extreme exercise (either prolonged or of very high intensity) reduces respiratory oxidative burst activity of neutrophils but does not affect chemotaxis and phagolysosomal degranulation (Dziedziak, 1990; Rodriguez, Barriga & De La Feunte, 1991; Smith, McKenzie, Telford, & Weidemann, 1992; Smith, Telford, Mason, & Weidemann, 1990). In contrast, exercise of moderate intensity and short duration is associated with increases in oxidative burst activity in vivo but not in vitro. In response to graded cycle ergometry exercise (10 min at 45%, 5 min at 60 and 75% maximal oxygen uptake), plasma myeloperoxidase (MPO) concentration was markedly elevated, suggestive of a spillover from neutrophils following activation (Pincemail et al., 1990). Macha and colleagues (Macha, Shlafer, & Kluger, 1990) found that exercise at 50% of maximal capacity for 1 h was associated with a diminished capacity for hydrogen peroxide generation by human neutrophils after PMA stimulation in vitro.

Blood monocytes and tissue macrophages have been the focus of many studies using an acute exercise model. In the postexercise period the number of monocytes in the circulation increases. Early studies suggested that a single exhaustive running-exercise bout in humans (Fehr, Lötzerich, & Michna, 1989) and swimming bout in rodents (Voronina & Mayanskii, 1987) increased macrophage phagocytic index. Interestingly, the enhanced phagocytic index varied by tissue compartment. For peritoneal macrophages, the capacity to phagocytose met acrylate granules did

not differ between exercised and control mice and rats; in alveolar macrophages, both the capacity to phagocytose met acrylate and free radical generation (as measured by nitroblue tetrazolium dye reduction) were higher in exercise relative to control mice and rats. Two recent studies (Kohut et al., 1998; Wong, Thompson, Thong, & Thornton,1990) failed to confirm higher alveolar macrophage responses (chemiluminescence and antiviral functions) following strenuous exercise. De La Fuente, Martin, and Ortega (1990) and Ortega, Collazos, Barriga, and De La Feunte (1992) reported enhanced engulfment and phagocytosis of *Candida albicans* by peritoneal macrophages obtained from exercise subjects relative to preexercise values. These studies suggest that although local paracrine influences may modify macrophage responses to exercise stress, further studies are necessary to resolve the magnitude and repeatability of these tissue differences.

Natural killer cells are a population of CD3 negative lymphoid cells that express characteristic surface cell markers or epitopes (CD16 and CD56 in humans; pan NK, NK1.1, and asialo GM$_1$ in mice) and which mediate non-MHC-restricted cytotoxicity reactions against viruses and tumors. A functionally related group of cells are LAK cells (lymphokine activated killer) generated in vitro from NK cells following incubation with interferon-$\alpha$ and interleukin-2 (Ortaldo et al., 1983; O'Shea & Ortaldo, 1992). The effects of single bouts of exercise, of varying types, durations, and intensities, on NK cell numbers and functions have been well documented over the past 10 years. Using flow cytometric methods, numerous studies demonstrate a marked increase in the percentage of NK cells following a single bout of exercise above an intensity of 50% of VO$_{2max}$ (for example, Kendall, Hoffman-Goetz, Houston, MacNeil, & Arumugam, 1990; MacKinnon, 1989; Pedersen et al., 1988; Pedersen & Ullum, 1994; Tvede, Kappel, Halkjær-Kristensen, Galbo, & Pedersen, 1993). Following a single episode of intense exercise of long duration, the percentage of NK cells in blood declines relative to preexercise values and occurs within a window of 2–4 h after cessation of exercise.

The functional activity of NK cells (measured either as percentage of cytolysis of tumor target cells, as normalized lytic units, or as killing per NK cell) is either suppressed (Brahmi, Thomas, Park, & Dowdeswell, 1985; Gabriel, Schwartz, Born, & Kindemann, 1992), unchanged (Nieman, 1993; Palmø et al., 1995), or enhanced (Hoffman-Goetz, 1995a; Nieman et al., 1993). These variations in NK cytolytic activity reflect differences in exercise intensity, exercise duration, and timing of sampling. Maximal or supramaximal exercise of a brief duration produces an initial increase in NK cytolytic activity followed by decline 30–60 min postexercise and a recovery to preexercise values within 24 h. Strenuous long-duration exercise or exercise of moderate intensity but long duration results in an immediate increase followed by marked decline in NK cytolytic activity 30 min to 2 h postexercise; these changes are quite transient with recovery to preexercise values at 24 h.

Normally, individuals do not engage in isolated, single sessions of exercise but rather perform exercise or sport on a repeated basis. However, there is only limited data concerning the effect of repeated sessions of exercise on innate immune responses. The first study in this area was by Hoffman-Goetz, Simpson, Cipp, Arumugam, and Houston (1990). Submaximal cycle ergometry exercise (65% of $VO_{2max}$) in healthy male volunteers elicited an increase in the percentage of circulating NK cells that did not differ over five repetitive bouts of cycling if the sessions were separated by 24 h. Nielsen and colleagues (Nielsen, Secher, & Pedersen, 1996), using repeated maximal exercise bouts of 6 min delivered over 2 days, found greater increases in the percentage of CD16+ cells and NK cytolytic activity during the last bout of exercise compared with the first bout of exercise. In contrast, Rohde, MacLean, and Pedersen (1998) showed that in male subjects performing three bouts of submaximal (75% of $VO_{2max}$) cycle exercise lasting 60, 45, and 30 min separated by 2 h of rest had lower LAK activity only after the third exercise session. Taken together, these findings suggest that if the interval between exercise sessions is of sufficient duration to allow recovery to baseline parameters (i.e., 24 h), repeated submaximal work elicits a consistent increase in NK cell numbers immediately postexercise. However, if the intensity and duration of exercise are just at the border in terms of inducing postexercise immune impairment, repeated exercise bouts will induce suppression even at exercise of shorter duration.

## B. Acquired Immune Response

The effect of acute exercise on cellular immune response has been the subject of extensive investigations; the effect on humoural immune responses has received less confirmatory evidence.

Immediately following an episode of acute exercise, a marked lymphocytosis occurs that is primarily due to the recruitment of all major lymphocyte subpopulations (CD4+ T lymphocytes, CD8+ T lymphocytes, and CD19+ B lymphocytes) to the vascular compartment. Lymphocytosis, however, is of relatively greater magnitude for CD8+ T cells than for CD4+ T cells. This greater CD8+ percentage following acute exercise characterizes both healthy subjects and those with lymphoproliferative disease (Mulligan, Wills, & Young, 1990). Moreover, lymphocytes recruited into the vascular compartment following exercise primarily express the CD45RO+ and CD45RO–CD62L– phenotype (Gabriel, Schmidtt, Urhausen, & Kindermann, 1993; H. Bruunsgaard & B. K. Pedersen, unpublished observations). These data suggest that it is the memory (CD45RO+) but not naive (CD45RA+) CD4+ and CD8+ lymphocytes that are rapidly mobilized to blood.

To function in adaptive or acquired immunity, rare antigen-specific lymphocytes need to undergo differentiation and clonal expansion into daughter effector cells of a given antigen specificity. Most exercise studies on lymphocyte proliferative capacity have used polyclonal mitogens such as concanavalin A (Con A) and phytohemagglutinin (PHA) to drive T-cell replication, or pokeweed mitogen (PWM) and lipopolysaccharide (LPS) to drive B cell replication. In general, T lymphocyte responses to mitogens are lower during, and for several hours after, acute exercise (e.g., Kaufman, Harris, Higgins, & Maisel, 1994; MacNeil, Hoffman-Goetz, Kendall, Houston, & Arumugam, 1990; Nielsen & Pedersen, 1997). Waern and Fossum (1993) were unable to demonstrate an effect of repeated short-term treadmill exercise on PHA- or Con A-induced proliferative responses in pig blood lymphocytes. B-lymphocyte proliferative responses to mitogens have been found to be higher after than before exercise (Hoffman-Goetz & Pedersen, 1994).

One index of lymphocyte function is cellular activation as measured by respiratory enzyme activity, expression of soluble receptors, and secondary messengers. Aryl hydrocarbon hydroxylase activity (an isozyme of cyctochrome P-450) was significantly enhanced in human peripheral blood lymphocytes following subjects' performance of acute cardiopulmonary exercise at 85% of predicted maximum heart rate (Moochhala, Fung, Yuen, & Das, 1990). Acute exercise results in increased production of oxygen-based free radicals due to hyperventilation, mitochondrial respiration, and phagocytic respiratory burst activity. We have found a significant increase in lipid peroxides and a depletion of endogenous antioxidant enzymes (superoxide dismutase and catalase) in thymus and spleen following an exhaustive exercise bout; this suggests that oxidative stress occurring within lymphoid tissues during exercise contributes to the reduced functional responses observed through in vitro mitogenesis and cytotoxicity studies (Azenabor & Hoffman-Goetz, 1999a). An increase in intracellular $Ca^{2+}$ ions, generation of oxidative products, and formation of lipid peroxide was observed in thymocytes taken from exhaustively exercised mice (Azenabor & Hoffman-Goetz, 1999b). Using a variety of exercise paradigms, several investigators have reported acute increases in secondary messenger systems, including isoprenaline-induced cAMP synthesis (Graafsma et al., 1990) and $\beta_2$-adrenoreceptor expression (Maisel, Harris, Rearden, & Michel, 1990; Mäki, 1989; Mäki, Naveri, Härkönen, & Kontula, 1988; Mäki, et al., 1990).

In vivo measures of T-lymphocyte function in response to exercise have not been well characterized. Bruunsgaard et al. (1997) reported a reduction in delayed type hypersensitivity responses to skin recall antigens (a measure of T-dependent immunity) in triatheletes following intense exercise of long duration relative to untrained controls who did not participate in exercise. No differences in specific antibody titers to pneumooccal polysaccharide vaccine (a T-independent antigen) were found between triathletes and controls, similar to early findings reported by Eskola, et al. (1978). The effects of either short duration, high intensity or long duration, moderate intensity physical work on in vivo measures of cellular immunity have not been studied.

Of considerable importance in acquired host immunity is that of the humoral response including mucosal immunity. Although immunoglobulin A (IgA) constitutes only 10–15% of total serum immunoglobulins, secretory IgA in secretions (intestinal, bronchial, nasal, genitourinary secretions, saliva, tears, colostrum, and milk) provide local immunity against infectious agents in the gut and respiratory tract, by combining with and neutralizing pathogens before they gain entry into the body. For example, sIgA in nasal secretions helps to protect against infection and reinfection with rhinovirus and influenza virus, whereas gut sIgA provides immunity against enteric microorganisms such as *Escherichia coli*. Generally, salivary IgA is decreased after high intensity swim exercise (Gleeson et al., 1995; Tharp & Barnes, 1990), intense long-duration cycle ergometry exercise (MacKinnon, Chick, van As, & Tomasi, 1987), and running exercise (Muns, Liesen, Riedel & Bergman, 1989; Steerenberg et al., 1997). The decrease in sIgA levels is likely not to change the absolute number or relative percentage of B cells after exercise or actual salivary IgA concentration. Rather, salivary flow rate is reduced after exercise and, hence, total salivary sIgA output is lessened (Steerenberg et al., 1997). The reduction in sIgA in the nasopharynx has been suggested as a contributory mechanism or a cofactor for the higher incidence of self-reported symptoms of upper respiratory tract infections (URTI) following strenuous exercise in athletes (Nieman, Johanssen, & Lee, 1989; Nieman, Johanssen, Lee, & Arabatzis, 1990; Peters & Bateman, 1983). Clinical demonstration of virions in respiratory mucosa or direct linkage of self-reported symptoms to immune status has not been demonstrated.

## III. HORMONAL MECHANISMS IN IMMUNE RESPONSE TO ACUTE EXERCISE

Acute exercise has been well documented to have simultaneous effects on multiple physiological systems including the immune and endocrine systems (e.g., Brooks et al., 1990; Galbo, 1983; Hoffman-Goetz & Pedersen, 1994; Kjaer & Dela, 1996). For example, intense muscular exercise results in elevations in the blood concentration of epinephrine, norepinephrine, growth hormone, $\beta$-endorphins, sex steroids, and cortisol. How do these acute hormonal changes with exercise influence the number, function, and distribution of lymphocytes and other immune competent cells?

The density of $\beta$-adrenergic receptors on individual lymphocyte subpopulations may determine which lymphocytes are mobilized and the magnitude of the lymphocyte trafficking response following exposure to adrenaline and noradrenaline. Different subpopulations of peripheral blood mononuclear cells have different numbers of $\beta$-adrenergic receptors, with NK cells having the highest, CD8+ lymphocytes an intermediate, and CD4+ lymphocytes having the lowest number (Khan, Sansoni, Silverman, Engleman, & Melmon, 1986; Rabin, Moyna, Kusnecov, Zhou, & Shurin, 1996; van Tits & Graafsma, 1991). The expression of $\beta$-adrenergic receptors on these cells roughly correlates with the pattern of lymphocytosis observed after acute, dynamic exercise (i.e., relatively greater increase in blood NK and CD8+ cells; lesser increase in CD4+ cells). Indeed, selective administration of epinephrine at plasma concentrations equivalent to that observed with cycling exercise for 1 h at 75% of $VO_2$ max produced a leukocytosis predominately in NK and CD8+ cells (Tønnesen, Christensen, & Brinkov, 1987; Tvede et al., 1994). Norepinephrine infusion produces a similar but weaker pattern of lymphocyte trafficking responses (Kappel, Poulsen, Galbo, & Pedersen, 1998b). After administration of propranolol exercise resulted in practically no increase in lymphocyte concentration (Ahlborg & Ahlborg, 1970). Furthermore, $\beta_{1+2}$ receptor blockade inhibited head-up-tilt lymphocytosis and increase in NK-cell activity, but did not influence stress-induced neutrocytosis (Klokker et al., 1997b).

Injection of growth hormone to obtain plasma concentrations comparable to those found during exercise induced significant neutrocytosis without influencing lymphocyte numbers or function (Kappel et al., 1993). Blocking growth hormone release by somatostatin also blocked hyperthermia-induced neutrocytosis. (Kappel, Poulsen, Hansen, Galbo, & Pedersen, 1998c).

The secretion of corticosteroids in response to exercise is dependent on the degree of physical work in relation to an individual's maximal work output, rather than the absolute amount of work performed. Short-term exercise of low intensity does not increase plasma cortisol levels whereas high-intensity or long-duration exercise is associated with significant increases in corticosteroids. Glucocorticoid sensitivity changes as a dynamic phenomenon during exercise reflecting regulation of the expression of type I and type II glucocorticoid receptors in peripheral lymphocytes (DeRijk, Petrides, Deuster, Gold & Sternberg, 1996).

Corticosteroids given intravenously induce lymphocytopenia, monocytopenia, eosinopenia, and neutrohilia with a maximum response within 4 h of administration (Rabin, Moyna, Kusnecov, Zhou, & Shurin, 1996). Corticosteroids, especially at high physiological or supraphysiological levels, induce apoptosis in thymocytes but not in mature T lymphocytes (Cohen & Duke, 1984). The percentage of mature splenic lymphocytes expressing early markers of apoptosis (Annexin V) does not increase after intense treadmill exercise despite an increase in blood corticosterone levels (Hoffman-Goetz, Zajchowski, & Aldred, 1998). Recent experiments indicate that in vitro exposure of thymocytes and splenocytes to concentrations of corticosterone observed at near maximal exercise induced significant apoptosis and necrosis within 24 h of culture (Hoffman-Goetz & Zajchowski, 1999). These observations, coupled with the finding that cortisol exerts its effect with a time lag of several hours, suggest that the immediate reductions in lymphocyte proliferation responses postexercise are not mediated by corticosteroids. However, cortisol may play a role in maintaining lymphopenia and contributing to sustained depressions in cellular immunity after prolonged, intense exercise such as that experienced by particpiants in triathlons and iron-man type marathons.

Under resting conditions, circulating concentrations of the endogenous opiod, β-endorphin, are extremely low ($1–100 \times 10^{12}$ M) but increase dramatically in response to exercise above a VO$_2$ max of 50% and in particular to long duration exercise (Goldfarb, Hatfield, Sforzo, & Flynn, 1987; Harber & Sutton, 1984). The role of endogenous opiods in mediating exercise-associated changes in immune function has yet to be clarified. The limited work on β-endorphins and immune function with exercise has involved NK-cell activity. An early study by Fiatarone and colleagues (Fiatarone et al., 1988) showed that when the β-endorphin receptors were blocked by administration of an opioid antagonist, naloxone, the exercise-associated increase in NK activity was no longer significant. However, naloxone did not influence the exercise-induced increase in NK-cell numbers. Employing other stress models, naloxone had no influence on hyperthermia and head-up-tilt-induced increase in NK cells or NK-cell activity (Klokker et al., 1997a). Furthermore, when the exercise-induced increase in β-endorphin was blocked by epidural analgesia, the exercise-induced increases in NK-cell numbers and function were not inhibited (Klokker et al., 1995). Chronic icv infusion of β-endorphin augmented NK-cell activity in vivo, with the action again blocked by naloxone (Jonsdottir et al., 1996). Thus, there is little evidence for a role of endogenous opioids in mediating the acute exercise effects on NK cells, whereas endogenous opioids may influence the NK-cell activity with exercise of long duration.

Based on the above studies, we propose the following model for stress hormones in mediating the exercise-related changes. Catecholamines are largely responsible for mediating initial acute effects on lymphocyte subsets and on NK and LAK activity. Growth hormone and catecholamines mediate the exercise effects on neutrophils. Corticosteroids have a delayed effect on immune responses with exercise and may contribute to the maintenance of lymphopenia, neutrocytosis, and lower proliferative responses after prolonged exercise. β-Endorphin likely does not mediate acute exercise effects on immunity but may play a role in exercise of prolonged duration.

## IV. HEMODYNAMIC MECHANISMS IN IMMUNE RESPONSE TO ACUTE EXERCISE

One of the defining characteristics of physical exercise is the cardiovascular response of increased heart rate and/or stroke volume with a resultant increase in blood flow to skeletal muscle from other organ systems. The movement of leukocytes from intravascular marginal pools and from extravascular storage pools contributes to the leukocytosis of exercise. The neutrocytosis component involves demargination from lung vasculature (Peters et al., 1992). However, this leukocytosis during exercise is not due strictly to an increase in ventilatory movements that occur (Fairbarn, Blackie, Pardy, & Hogg, 1993). This exercise-induced leukocytosis may better reflect the contribution of storage sites in the spleen (Pabst, 1988), although this remains controversial (Iversen, Aavesen, & Benestad, 1994) since splenectomy is still associated with leukocytosis. We suggest that the role of hemodynamic factors in mediating immune changes is limited to differences in the absolute and/or percentage of leukocytes and lymphocytes in circulation. The number of cells that enter or leave the vascular compartment depends on the duration and intensity of the work. Recirculation shifts could potentially contribute to the functional changes in NK-cell activity, in antibody synthesis, and in proliferative responses to mitogens and antigens. In animal models, there is some indication about the organs to which lymphocytes are redistributed after exercise and the proportion of subsets varies with the tissue compartment (Randall Simpson, Hoffman-Goetz, Thorne, & Arumugam, 1989). This redistribution of lymphocytes does not, however, include skeletal muscle (Espersen et al., 1995). The expression of leukocyte adhesion molecules (e.g., LFA-1, L-selectins, VLA-4) is altered by intense exercise (Gabriel, Brechtel, Urhausen, & Kindermann, 1994; Hoffman-Goetz, 1995b; Kurokawa, Shinkai, Torii, Hino, & Shek, 1995; Miles et al., 1998) and this mechanism likely contributes to the hemodynamic shifts from marginated to vascular pools of leukocyte subsets.

## V. CYTOKINE MECHANISMS IN IMMUNE RESPONSE TO ACUTE EXERCISE

Strenuous exercise is associated with increased circulating levels of several cytokines. Initial and insightful studies of Cannon and colleagues (Cannon & Kluger, 1983; Cannon, Evans, Hughes, Meredith & Dinarello, 1986; Evans et al., 1986) described increased levels of IL-1 ("endogenous pyrogen") in plasma obtained after exercise; because early methods of measuring cytokines lacked specificity, the possibility exists that other cytokines were measured. The latter studies were conducted prior to the availability of recombinant IL-1 proteins and there have been a number of studies which failed to detect elevated levels of IL-1 in plasma (Cannon et al., 1991; Northoff & Berg, 1991; Randall Simpson & Hoffman-Goetz,

1991; Sprenger et al., 1992; Ullum et al., 1994). However, IL-6 has been found to be enhanced in several studies (Bruunsgaard et al., 1997; Northoff & Berg, 1991; Ostrowski, Rohde, Zacho, Asp, & Pedersen, 1998b; Sprenger et al., 1992; Ullum et al., 1994) and is followed by an increase in the concentration of the IL-1 receptor antagonist (IL-1ra), a natural occurring inhibitor of IL-1 (Ostrowski, Rohde, Zacho, Asp, & Pedersen, 1998b). Small increases in plasma tumor necrosis factor-$\alpha$ (TNF-$\alpha$) and IL-1$\beta$ are also found after exercise (Ostrowski, Rohde, Asp, Schjerling, & Pedersen, 1999). Recent data suggest that exercise modifies the levels of plasma TNF-$\alpha$ receptors (TNF-$\alpha$R), IL-1, IL-2, and IL-10 (Ostrowski et al., 1998a, 1999). There is also preliminary evidence that the chemokines IL-8, macrophage inflammatory protein (MIP)-1$\alpha$, and MIP-1$\beta$ are increased in response to strenuous exercise (B. K. Pedersen, unpublished observations).

Although exercise induces initiation of the acute phase response, exercise is not followed by a fully developed systemic response including biological effects of the TNF/IL-1/IL-6 system such as myocardial depression, and dysfunction of kidneys, liver, lungs, and brain. This may reflect the fact that exercise induces an increase in pro-inflammatory cytokines and an especially dramatic increase in IL-6 that is balanced by the release of cytokine inhibitors (such as IL-1ra, sTNF-R1+2) and the anti-inflammatory cytokine IL-10, which may restrict the magnitude of the inflammatory cytokine response to exercise.

Bruunsgaard et al. (1997) compared concentric and eccentric exercise and found an association between increased IL-6 level and muscle damage as visualized by the increase in creatine kinase. Postexercise cytokine production may be related to skeletal muscle damage, but demonstration of a causal relationship between muscle damage and cytokine production remains elusive. IL-6-mRNA was present in skeletal muscle biopsies obtained from runners after, but not before, a marathon run (Ostrowski et al.,1998b). The latter data indicate that IL-6 is locally produced in response to strenuous exercise or exercise-induced muscle damage. IL-1ra-mRNA was not present in the skeletal muscle, but was expressed by blood mononuclear cells (BMNC) obtained after, but not before, the marathon. Taken together, these findings indicate that locally produced IL-6 may stimulate a systemic anti-inflammatory response. The mechanisms underlying exercise-induced cytokine production are not known. However, higher IL-6 levels are seen with exercise of long duration and high intensity and particularly if an eccentric component is included.

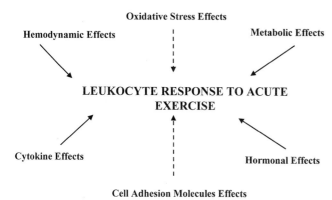

**FIGURE 1**  Schematic representation of the multiple regulatory influences on the immune system during acute exercise. Solid lines indicate mechanisms which have been well characterized empirically. Dashed lines indicate potential mechanisms which require additional experimental evidence.

The cytokine cascade in response to exercise has many similarities to that seen in response to trauma, and, therefore, exercise may be considered a model of trauma (Ostrowski et al., 1998a, 1999).

## VI.  CONCLUSIONS

A single session of acute exercise has an immediate but transient impact on the immune system. The immunological responses to exercise reflect diverse mechanisms including hemodynamic effects and cytokine and classical stress hormone effects. Changes in the expression of cell adhesion molecules or in apoptotic responses to oxidative stress are promising potential mechanisms through which exercise modulates the immune system but additional studies to confirm their exact roles are required. Despite a diverse and complex regulation of lymphocyte numbers and functions to acute exercise (Figure 1), these responses follow patterns similar to those of immune responses observed after other physical, but non-infectious, stressors such as acute trauma. It remains to be determined whether immunological responses to acute exercise are only transient perturbations of homeostasis without clinical relevance or whether the altered immune responses with exercise contribute to subclinical or clinical disease processes.

## Acknowledgments

Preparation of this manuscript was supported in part by research grants from the Natural Sciences and Engineering Research Council of Canada and the Danish National Research Foundation.

## References

Ahlborg, B., & Ahlborg, G. (1970). Exercise leukocytosis with and without beta andrenergic blockade. *Acta Medica Scandinavia,187*, 241–246.

Azenabor, A., & Hoffman-Goetz, L. (1999a). Intrathymic and intrasplenic oxidative stress mediates thymocyte and splenocyte damage in acutely exercised mice. *Journal of Applied Physiology, 86*, 1823–1827.

Azenabor, A., & Hoffman-Goetz, L. (1999b). Effect of exhaustive exercise on membrane estradiol concentration, intracellular calcium, and oxidative damage in mouse thymic lymphocytes. *Free Radical Biology & Medicine* (in press).

Brahmi, Z., Thomas, J. E., Park, M., & Dowdeswell, I. R. (1985). The effect of acute exercise on natural killer-cell acitivity of trained and sedentary human subjects. *Journal of Clinical Immunology, 5*, 321–328.

Brooks, S., Nevill, M. E., Meleagros, L., Lakomy, H. K. A., Hall, G. M., Bloom, S. R., & Williams, C. (1990). The hormonal response to brief maximal exercise in humans. *European Journal of Applied Physiology and Occupational Physiology, 60*, 144–148.

Bruunsgaard, H., Galbo, H., Halkjaer-Kristensen, J., Johansen, T. L., MacLean, D. A., & Pedersen, B. K. (1997). Exercise-induced increase in interleukin-6 is related to muscle damage. *Journal of Physiology (London), 499*, 833–841.

Cannon, J. G., Evans, W. J., Hughes, V. A., Meredith, C. N., & Dinarello, C. A. (1986). Physiological mechanisms contributing to increased interleukin-1 secretion. *Journal of Applied Physiology, 61*, 1869–1874.

Cannon, J. G., & Kluger, M. J. (1983). Endogenous pyrogen activity in human plasma after exercise. *Science, , 617–619*.

Cannon, J. G., Meydani, S. N., Fielding, R. A., Fiatarone, M. A., Meydani, M., Farhangmehr, M., Orencole, S. F., Blumberg, J. B., & Evans, W. J. (1991). Acute phase response in exercise. II. Associations between vitamin E, cytokines, and muscle proteolysis. *American Journal of Physiology, 260*, R1235–R1240.

Cohen, J. J., & Duke, R. C. (1984). Glucocorticoid activation of a calcium-dependent endonuclease in thymocyte nuclei leads to cell death. *Journal of Immunology, 132*, 38–42.

De La Fuente, M., Martin, M. I., & Ortega, E. (1990). Changes in the phagocytic function of peritoneal macrophages from old mice after strenuous exercise. *Comparative Immunology, Microbiology, and Infectious Diseases, 13*, 189–198.

DeRijk, H., Petrides, J., Deuster, P., Gold, P. W., & Sternberg, E. M. (1996). Changes in corticoseroid sensitivity of peripheral blood lymphocytes after strenuous exercise in humans. *Journal of Clinical Endocrinology and Metabolism, 81*, 228–235.

Dziedziak, W. (1990). The effect of incremental cycling on physiological functions of peripheral blood granulocytes. *Biology of Sport, 7*, 239–248.

Eskola, J., Ruuskanen, O., Soppi, E., Viljanen, M. K., Jarvinen, M., Toivonen, H., & Kouvalainen, K. (1978). Effect of sport stress on lymphocyte transformation and antibody formation. *Clinical and Experimental Immunology, 32*, 339–345.

Espersen, E. T., Stamp, I., Jensen, M. L., Elbæk, A., Ernst, E., Kahr, O., & Grunnet, N. (1995). Lymphocyte redistribution in connection with physical activity in the rat. *Acta Physiologica Scandinavica, 155*, 313–321.

Evans, W. J., Meredith, C. N., Cannon, J. G., Dinarello, C. A., Frontera, W. R., Hughes, V. A., Jones, B. H., & Knuttgen, H. G. (1986). Metabolic changes following eccentric exercise in trained and untrained men. *The Journal of Applied Physiology, 61*, 1864–1868.

Fairbarn, M. S., Blackie, S. P., Pardy, R. L., & Hogg, J. C. (1993). Comparison of effects of exercise and hyperventilation on leukocyte kinetics in humans. *Journal of Applied Physiology, 75,* 2425–2428.

Fehr, H. G., Lötzerich, H., & Michna, H. (1989). Human macrophage function and physical exercise: Phagocytic and histochemical studies. *European Journal of Applied Physiology, 58,* 613–617.

Fiatarone, M. A., Morley, J. E., Bloom, E. T., Donna, M., Makinodan, T., & Solomon, G. F. (1988). Endogenous opioids and the exercise-induced augmentation of natural killer cell activity. *Journal of Laboratory and Clinical Medicine, 112,* 544–548.

Gabriel, H., Brechtel, L., Urhausen, A., & Kindermann, W. (1994). Recruitment and recirculation of leukocytes after an ultramarathon run: Preferential homing of cells expressing high levels of the adhesion molecule LFA-1. *International Journal of Sports Medicine, 15,* S148–S153.

Gabriel, H., Schmitt, B., Urhausen, A., & Kindermann, W. (1993). Increased CD45RA+ lymphocytes after exercise. *Medicine and Science in Sports and Exercise 25,* 1352–1357.

Gabriel, H., Schwartz, L., Born, P., & Kindermann, W. (1992). Differential mobilization of leucocyte and lymphocyte subpopulations into the circulation during endurance exercise. *European Journal of Applied Physiology, 65,* 529–535.

Gabriel, H., Urhausen, A., & Kindermann, W. (1992). Mobilization of circulatiang leucocyte and lymphocytes subpopulations during and after short, anaerobic exercise. *European Journal of Applied Physiology, 65,* 164–167.

Galbo, H. (1983). *Hormonal and metabolic adaptation to exercise.* New York. Thieme Verlag.

Gleeson, M., McDonald., W. A., Cripps, A. W., Pyne, D. B., Clancy, R. L., & Fricker, P. A. (1995). The effect on immunity of long-term intensive training in elite swimmers. *Clinical and Experimental Immunology, 102,* 210–216.

Goldfarb, A. H., Hatfield, B. D., Sforzo, G. A., & Flynn, M. G. (1987). Serum β-endorphin levels during a graded exercise test to exhaustion. *Medicine and Science in Sports and Exercise, 19,* 78–82.

Graafsma, S. J., van Tits, L. J. H., Willems, P. H. G. M., Hectors, M. P. C., Rodrigues de Miranda, J. F., de Pont, J. J. H. H. M., & Thien, Th. (1990). β₂-Adrenoceptor up-regulation in relation to cAMP production in human lymphocytes after physical exercise. *British Journal of Clinical Pharmacology, 30,* 142S–144S.

Harber, V. J., & Sutton, J. R. (1984). Endorphins and exercise. *Sports Medicine, 1,* 154–171.

Hoffman-Goetz. L. (1995a). Serine esterase (BLT-esterase) activity in murine splenocytes is increased with exercise but not training. *International Journal of Sports Medicine, 16,* 94–98.

Hoffman-Goetz, L. (1995b). Effect of acute treadmill exercise on LFA-1 antigen expression in murine splenocytes. *Anticancer Research, 15,* 1981–1984.

Hoffman-Goetz, L., & Pedersen, B. K. (1994). Exercise and the immune system: A model of the stress response? *Immunology Today, 15,* 382–387.

Hoffman-Goetz, L., Simpson, J. R., Cipp, N., Arumugam, Y., & Houston, M. E. (1990). Lymphocyte subset responses to repeated submaximal exercise in men. *Journal of Applied Physiology, 68,* 1069–1074.

Hoffman-Goetz, L. & Zajchowski, S. (1999). In vitro apoptosis of lymphocytes after exposure to levels of corticosterone observed following submaximal exercise. *Journal of Sports Medicine and Physical Fitness* (in press).

Hoffman-Goetz, L., Zajchowski, S., & Aldred, A. (1998). Impact of treadmill exercise on early apoptotic cells in mouse spleen and thymus. *Life Sciences, 64,* 191–200.

Iversen, P. O., Arvesen, B. L., & Benestad, H. B. (1994). No mandatory role for the spleen in the exercise-induced leukocytosis in man. *Clinical Sciences (Colch), 86,* 505–510.

Jonsdottir, I. H., Johansson, C., Asea, A., Hellstrand, K., Thorén, P., & Hoffmann, P. (1996). Central β-endorphin administration augments in vivo cytotoxicity in rats. *Regulatory Peptides, 62,* 113–118.

Kappel, M., Hansen, M. B., Diamant, M., Jørgensen, J. O., Gyhrs, A., & Pedersen, B. K. (1993). Effects of an acute bolus growth hormone infusion on the human immune system. *Hormone and Metabolic Research, 11,* 593–602.

Kappel, M., Poulsen, T. D., Galbo, H., & Pedersen, B. K. (1998a). Effects of elevated plasma noradrenaline concentration on the immune system in humans. *European Journal of Applied Physiology, 79,* 93–98.

Kappel, M., Poulsen, T., Galbo, H., & Pedersen, B. K. (1998b). Effect of norepinephrine infusion on immune parameters. *European Journal of Applied Physiology,* in press.

Kappel, M., Poulsen, T., Hansen, M., Galbo, H., & Pedersen, B. K. (1998c). Somatostatin attenuates the hyperthermia induced increase in neutrophil function. *European Journal of Applied Physiology, 77,* 149–156.

Kaufman, J. C., Harris, T. J., Higgins, J., & Maisel, A. S. (1994). Exercise-induced enhancement of immune function in the rat. *Circulation, 90,* 525–532.

Kendall, A., Hoffman-Goetz, L., Houston, M., MacNeil, B., & Arumugam, Y. (1990). Exercise and blood lymphocyte subset responses: Intensity, duration, and subject fitness effects. *Journal of Applied Physiology, 69,* 251–260.

Khan, M. M., Sansoni, P., Silverman, E. D., Engleman, E. G., & Melmon, K. L. (1986). Beta-adrenergic receptors on human suppressor, helper, and cytolytic lymphocytes. *Biochemistry and Pharmacology, 35,* 1137–1142.

Kjær, M., & Dela, F. (1996). Endocrine responses to exercise. In L. Hoffman-Goetz, (Ed.), *Exercise and immune function* (pp. 1–19.) Boca Raton, FL: CRC Press.

Klokker, M., Kjær, M., Secher, N. H., Hanel, B., Worm, L., Kappel, M., Pedersen, B. K. (1995). Natural killer cell response to exercise in humans: Effect of hypoxia and epidural anesthesia. *Journal of Applied Physiology, 78,* 709–16.

Klokker, M., Secher, N. H., Madsen, P., Olesen, H. L., Warberg, J., & Pedersen B. K. (1997a). Influence of naloxone on the cellular immune response to head-up tilt in humans. *European Journal of Applied Physiology, 76,* 415–420.

Klokker, M., Secher, N. H., Olesen, H. L., Madsen, P., Warberg, J., & Pedersen, B. K. (1997b). Adrenergic beta-1-and beta-1+2 receptor blockade suppresses the natural killer cell response during head up tilt. *Journal of Applied Physiology, 83,* 1492–1498.

Kohut, M. L., Davis, J. M., Jackson, D. A., Colberte, L. H., Strasner, A., Essig, D. A., Pate, R. R., Ghaffar, A., & Mayer, E. P. (1998). The role of stress hormones in exercise-induced suppression of alveolar macrophage antiviral function. *Journal of Neuroimmunology, 81,* 193–200.

Kurokawa, Y., Shinkai, S., Torii, J., Hino, S., & Shek, P. N. (1995). Exercise-induced changes in the expression of surface adhesion molecules on circulating granulocytes and lymphocytes subpopulations. *European Journal of Applied Physiology, 71,* 245–252.

Lewicki, R., Tchorzewski, H., Denys, A., Kowalska, M., & Golinska, A. (1987). Effect of physical exercise on some paramters of immunity in conditioned sportsmen. *International Journal of Sports Medicine, 8,* 309–314.

Macha, M., Shlafer, M., & Kluger, M. J. (1990). Human neutrophil hydrogen peroxide generation following physical exercise. *The Journal of Sports Medicine and Physical Fitness, 30,* 412–419.

MacKinnon, L. T., Chick, T. W., van As, A., & Tomasi, T. B. (1987). The effect of exercise on secretory and natural immunity. *Advances in Experirmental Biology and Medicine, 216A*, 869–876.

MacKinnon, L. T. (1989). Exercise and natural killer cells. What is the relationship? *Sports Medicine, 7*, 141–149.

MacNeil, B., Hoffman-Goetz, L., Kendall, A., Houston, M., & Arumugam, Y. (1990). Lymphocyte proliferation responses after exercise in men: Fitness, intensity, and duration effects. *Journal of Applied Physiology, 70*, 179–185.

Maisel, A. S., Harris, T., Rearden, C. A., & Michel, M. C. (1990). β-Adrenergic receptors in lymphocyte subsets after exercise. Alterations in normal individuals and patients with congestive heart failure. *Circulation, 82*, 2003–2010.

Mäki, T. (1989). Density and functioning of human lymphocytic β-adrenergic receptors during prolonged physical exercise. *Acta Physiologica Scandinavica, 136*, 569–574.

Mäki, T., Näveri, H., Leinonen, H., Sovijärvi, A., Lewko, B., Härkönen, M., & Kontula, K. (1990). Effect of propranolol and pindolol on the up-regulation of lymphocytic β adrenoceptors during acute submaximal physical exercise. A placebo-controlled, double-blind study. *Journal of Cardiovascular Pharmacology, 15*, 544–551.

Mäki, T., Näveri, H., Härkönen, M., & Kontula, K. (1988). Propranolol attenuates exercise-induced increment in human lymphocytic β-adrenergic receptors. *Scandinavian Journal of Laboratory and Clinical Investigation, 48*, 357–363.

McCarthy, D. A., & Dale, M. M. (1988). The leucocytosis of exercise: A review and model. *Sports Medicine, 6*, 333–363.

Miles, M. P., Leach, S. K., Kraemer, W. J., Dohi, K., Bush, J. A., & Mastro, A. M. (1998). Leukocyte adhesion molecule expression during intense resistance exercise. *Journal of Applied Physiology, 84*, 1604–1609.

Moochhala, S. M., Fung, K. P., Yuen, R., & Das, N. P. (1990). Effects of acute physical exercise on aryl hydrocarbon hydroxylase activity in human peripheral lymphocytes. *Life Sciences, 47*, 427–432.

Mulligan, S. P., Wills, E. J., & Young, G. A. R. (1990). Exercise-induced CD8 lymphocytosis: A phenomenon associated with large granular lymphocyte leukaemia. *British Journal of Immunology, 75*, 175–180.

Muns, G., Liesen, H., Riedel, H., & Bergman, K. C. (1989). Influence of long-distance running on IgA in nasal secretion and saliva. *Deutsche Zeitung für Sportmedizin, 40*, 94–99.

Nielsen, H. B., & Pedersen, B. K. (1997). Lymphocyte proliferation in response to exercise. *European Journal of Applied Physiology, 75*, 375–379.

Nielsen, H. B., Secher, N., & Pedersen, B. K. (1996). Lymphocytes and NK cell activity during repeated bouts of maximal exercise. *American Journal of Physiology, 271*, R222–R227.

Nieman, D. C., Johanssen, L. M., & Lee, J. W. (1989). Infectious episodes in runners before and after a roadrace. *Journal of Sports Medicine and Physical Fitness, 29*, 289–296.

Nieman, D. C., Johanssen, L. M., Lee, J. W., & Arabatzis, K. (1990). Infectious episodes in runners before and after the Los Angeles Marathon. *Journal of Sports Medicine and Physical Fitness, 30*, 316–328.

Nieman, D. C., Miller, A. R., Henson, D. A., Warren, B. J., Gusewitch, G., Johnson, R. L., Davis, J. M., Butterworth, D. E., & Nehlsen-Cannarella, S. L. (1993). Effects of high- vs. moderate-intensity exercise on natural killer cell activity. *Medicine and Science in Sports and Exercise, 25*, 1126–1134.

Northoff, H., & Berg, A. (1991). Immunologic mediators as parameters of the reaction to strenuous exercise. *International Journal of Sports Medicine, 12*, S9–S15.

Ortaldo, J. R., Mantovani, A., Hobbs, D., Rubinstein, M., Pestka, S., & Herberman, R. B. (1983). Effects of several species of human leukocyte interferon on cytotoxic activity of NK cells and monocytes. *International Journal of Cancer, 31*, 285–289.

Ortega, E., Collazos, M. E., Barriga, C., & De La Fuente, M. (1992). Effect of physical activity stress on the phagocytic process of peritoneal macrophages from old guinea pigs. *Mechanisms of Ageing and Development, 65*, 157–165.

O'Shea, J., & Ortaldo, J. R. (1992). The biology of natural killer cells: insights into the molecular basis of function. In J. R. Lewis, and J. O. McGee, (Eds.), *The natural killer cell* (pp. 1–40). Oxford: Oxford University Press.

Ostrowski, K., Hermann, C., Bangash, A., Schjerling, P., Nielsen, J. N., & Pedersen, B. K. (1998a). A trauma-like elevation in plasma cytokines in humans in response to treadmill running. *Journal of Physiology (London), 508*, 949–953.

Ostrowski, K., Rohde, T., Asp, S., Schjerling, P., & Pedersen, B. K. (1999). Pro- and anti-inflammatory cytokine balance in strenuous exercise in humans. *Journal of Physiology (London), 515*, 287–292.

Ostrowski, K., Rohde, T., Zacho, M., Asp, S., & Pedersen, B. K. (1998b). Evidence that IL-6 is produced in skeletal muscle during intense long-term muscle activity. *Journal of Physiology, 508*, 949–953.

Pabst, R. (1988). The spleen in lymphyocyte migration. *Immunology Today, 9*, 43–45.

Palmø, J., Asp, S., Daugaard, J. R., Richter, E. A., Klokker, M., & Pedersen, B. K. (1995). Effect of eccentric exercise on natural killer cell activity. *Journal of Applied Physiology, 78*, 1442–1146.

Pedersen, B. K., Tvede, N., Hansen, F. R., Andersen, V., Bendix, T., Bendixen, G., Bendtzen, K., Galbo, H., Haahr, P. M., & Klarlund, K. (1988). Modulation of natural killer cell activity in peripheral blood by physical exercise. *Scandinavian Journal of Immunology, 27*, 673–678.

Pedersen, B. K., & Ullum, H. (1994). NK cell response to physical activity: possible mechanisms of action. *Medicine and Science in Sports and Exercise, 26*, 140–146.

Peters, A. M., Allsop, P., Stuttle, A. W., Arnot, R. N., Gwilliam, M., & Hall, G. M. (1992). Granulocyte margination in the human lung and its response to strenuous exercise. *Clinical Sciences, 82*, 237–244.

Peters, E. M. & Bateman, E. D. (1983). Ultramarathon running and upper respiratory tract infections. An epidemiological survey. *South African Medical Journal, 64*, 582–584.

Pincemail, J., Camus, G., Roesgen, A., Dreezen, E., Bertrand, Y., Lismonde, M., Deby-Dupont, G., & Deby, C. (1990). Exercise induces pentane production and neutrophil activation in humans. Effect of propranolol. *European Journal of Applied Physiology, 61*, 319–322.

Rabin, B. S., Moyna, N. M., Kusnecov, A., Zhou, D., & Shurin, M. R. (1996). Neuroendocrine effects on immunity. In L. Hoffman-Goetz, (Ed.), *Exercise and immune function* (pp. 21–37). Boca Raton, FL: CRC Press.

Randall Simpson, J., & Hoffman-Goetz, L. (1991). Exercise, serum zinc, and interleukin-1 concentrations in man: Some methodological considerations. *Nutrition Research, 11*, 309–323.

Randall Simpson, J. A., Hoffman-Goetz, L., Thorne, R., & Arumugam, Y. (1989). Exercise stress alters the percentage of splenic lymphocyte subsets in response to mitogen but not in response to interleukin-1. *Brain, Behavior, and Immunity, 3*, 119–128.

Rodriguez, A. B., Barriga, C., & De la Feunte, M. (1991). Phagocytic function of blood neutrophils in sedentary young people after physical exercise. *International Journal of Spots Medicine, 12*, 276–280.

Rohde, T., MacLean, D., & Pedersen, B. K. (1998). Effect of glutamine on changes in te immune system induced by repeated exercise. *Medicine and Science in Sports and Exercise, 30,* 856–862.

Rohde, T., MacLean, D. A., Richter, E. A., Kiens, B., & Pedersen, B. K. (1997). Prolonged submaximal eccentric exercise is associated with increased levels of plasma IL-6. *American Journal of Physiology, 273,* E85–E91.

Smith, J. A., Gray, A. B., Pyne, D. B., Baker, M. S., Telford, R. D., & Weideman, M. J. (1996). Submaximal exercise causes both priming and activation of neutrophils. *American Journal of Physiology, 39,* R838–R842.

Smith, J. A., McKenzie, S. J., Telford, R. D., & Weidemann, M. J. (1992). Why does moderate exercise enhance, but intense exercise depress, immunity? In Husband, A. J. (Ed.), *Behavior and Immunity* (pp. 155–168). Boca Raton: CRC Press.

Smith, J. A., Telford, R. D., Mason, I. B., & Weidemann, M. J. (1990). Exercise, training, and neutrophil microbicidal activity. *International Journal of Sports Medicine, 11,* 179–187.

Sprenger, H., Jacobs, C., Nain, M., Gressner, A. M., Prinz, H., Wesemann, W., & Gemsa, D. (1992). Enhanced release of cytokines, interleukin-2 receptors, and neopterin after long-distance running. *Clinical Immunology and Immunopathology, 63,* 188–95.

Steerenberg, P. A., van-Aspersen, I. A., van-Nieuw-Amerongen, A., Biewenga, A., Mol, S., & Medema, G. J. (1997). Salivary levels of immunoglobulin A in triathletes. *European Journal of Oral Sciences, 105,* 305–309.

Tharp, G. D., & Barnes, M. W. (1990). Reduction of saliva immunoglobulin levels by swim training. *European Journal of Applied Physiology, 60,* 61–64.

Tønnesen, E., Christensen, N. J., & Brinklov, M. M. (1987). Natural killer cell activity during cortisola nd adrenaline infusion in healthy volunteers. *European Journal of Clinical Investigation, 17,* 497–503.

Tvede, N., Galbo, H., Haahr, P. M., Kjær, M., Linstouw, M., Klarlund, K., & Pedersen, B. K. (1991). Epinephrine can account for the effect of physical exercise on natural killer cell activity. *Journal of Applied Physiology, 70,* 2530–2534.

Tvede, N., Kappel, M., Halkjaer-Kristensen, J., Galbo, H., & Pedersen, B. K. (1993). The effect of light, moderate and severe bicycle exercise on lymphocyte subsets, natural and lymphokine activated killer cells, lymphocyte proliferative response and interleukin-2 production. *International Journal of Sports Medicine, 14,* 275–282.

Tvede, N., Kappel, M., Klarlund, K., Duhn, S., Halkjær Kristensen, J., Kjær, M., Galbo, H., & Pedersen, B. K. (1994). Evidence that the effect of bicycle exercise on blood mononuclear cell proliferative responses and subsets is mediated by epinephrine. *International Journal of Sports Medicine, 15,* 100–104.

Ullum, H., Haahr, P. M., Diamant, M., Palmo, J., Halkjaer Kristensen, J., & Pedersen, B. K. (1994). Bicycle exercise enhances plasma IL-6 but does not change IL-1, IL-1, IL-6, or TNF- pre-mRNA in BMNC. *Journal of Applied Physiology, 77,* 93–7.

van Tits, L. J., & Graafsma, S. J. (1991). Stress influences CD4+ lymphocyte counts. *Immunology Letters, 30,* 141–142.

Voronina, N. P., & Mayanskii, D. N. (1987). Effect of intensive physical exercise on macrophagal functions. *Bulletin of Experimental Biology and Medicine, 104,* 1120–1123.

Waern, M. J., & Fossum, C. (1993). Effects of acute physical stress on immune competence in pigs. *American Journal of Veterinary Research, 54,* 596–601.

Wong, C. W., Thompson, H. L., Thong, Y. H., & Thornton, J. R. (1990). Effect of strenuous exercise stress on chemiluminescence response of equine alveolar macrophages. *Equine Veterinary Journal, 22,* 33–35.

# 36

# Hypnosis and Immunity

ROBERT ZACHARIAE

## I. INTRODUCTION

The growing evidence of possible influences of psychosocial factors on the immune system provided by psychoneuroimmunological research over the past two decades has led some health practitioners to claim that it may be possible to influence the immune system and perhaps even a number of immune-related diseases with the "power of the mind" (Pearsall, 1988). The scientific evidence in support of such claims is, however, limited, and only relatively few well-controlled studies have been conducted so far (Zachariae, 1996). Hypnosis has long been thought to be a particularly "powerful" psychological intervention technique and has been claimed to be effective in the treatment of various physiological and "psychosomatic" disorders (Rossi & Cheek, 1988). In the following, the current data concerning the effects of hypnotic suggestion on immune and inflammatory reactions and possible psychophysiological mediating mechanisms will be reviewed.

## II. WHAT IS HYPNOSIS?

The history of modern hypnosis dates back to the "animal magnetism" practiced by Anton Mesmer in the second half of the 18th century. In line with the Newtonian scientific Zeitgeist at the time, Mesmer is responsible for separating what we today recognize as hypnotic phenomena from those of religion, spirituality, and "exorcism," though he was incorrect in attributing his clinical results to the action of a "magnetic fluid" (Dixon & Laurence, 1992; Hilgard, 1990). The French Royal Commission of Inquiry of 1784 led by Benjamin Franklin concluded that Mesmers' apparent ability to influence his patients was not the result of a physical magnetic force but more likely to be due to "psychological" factors, e.g., the vivid imagination of the patients (Gauld, 1992). While mesmerism lived on, it did so without the acceptance by the establishment, and it was not until late in the 19th century that "hypnotism," a term coined by Braid, was rediscovered by the French. While the renowned Charcot of the Salpetriére in Paris claimed that hypnosis involved neuropathology, Bernheim of the Nancy School emphasized the importance of suggestion and proved him wrong by demonstrating that normal subjects could be hypnotized. While hypnosis was embraced enthusiastically by both the scientific establishment and the public for a 15-year period, the popularity of hypnosis suddenly declined in the late 1890s for reasons that have puzzled writers on the history of hypnosis. One of the reasons may lie in the exaggerated claims of hypnosis as a universally effective method, another in the rise of nonhypnotic psychotherapy, e.g., Freudian psychoanalysis (Hilgard, 1990). Professional interest was revived after the successful use of hypnosis in both World Wars and in the Korean War and, with the advent of standardized tests of hypnotic susceptibility in the 1950s, experimental investigation of hypnotic phenomena became possible by allowing different laboratories to use common measurements in the testing of hypotheses (Dixon & Laurence, 1992).

But, what is hypnosis? How can we know whether a subject is in a hypnotic trance or not, and how can we measure it? It may surprise scientists who are unfamiliar with areas such as hypnosis that, in spite of numerous experimental studies, researchers in hypnosis are currently unable to give a definite answer to such questions. Though hypnosis has been used in the treatment of psychological, psychosomatic, and physiological problems for more than 200 years, what lies behind the commonly observed hypnotic phenomena, is still not agreed upon (Farthing, 1992). Some investigators have subscribed to the view that hypnotic behavior reflects underlying cognitive processes that are unique to the hypnotic context and thus represents a special psychological state or process that is different from waking behavior (Hilgard, 1990). Another position has held that hypnosis does not differ fundamentally from the "normal" psychological state and that any behavior that can be elicited in hypnosis can be elicited outside of hypnosis (Spanos & Chaves, 1989). Proponents of this view have claimed that both overt hypnotic behavior and subjective hypnotic experiences should be regarded as results of social–psychological processes, such as "role-taking," and that the behaviors of "hypnotized" subjects are merely results of their reactions to the demand characteristics inherent in the hypnotic context (Spanos & Coe, 1992). In spite of these theoretical disagreements over the "nature" of hypnosis, researchers generally agree upon a "domain of hypnosis" (Hilgard, 1992), which represents a limited number of phenomena which may occur following some form of direct or indirect hypnotic induction.

First, a hypnotic induction is often accompanied by certain changes in perceptual and cognitive processes, including changes in attention, increased suggestibility, altered sensory perception, vivid imagery or fantasies, and a subjective "dissociated" experience of suggested behaviors as "taking place by themselves" in a nonvolitional manner. It is thus generally accepted that high hypnotic susceptible subjects are able to alter their subjective experience of painful stimuli (Orne, 1983). Several experimental studies have confirmed that suggestions of hypnotic analgesia are accompanied by higher thresholds and increased tolerance to experimentally induced pain (Hilgard & Hilgard, 1983; Hilgard, 1986). It has also been shown that hypnotic analgesia differs markedly from a placebo response in high hypnotic

susceptible subjects (Van Dyck & Hoogduin, 1990; Evans, 1990).

Second, a widely accepted observation about hypnosis is that some subjects seem to be far more capable hypnotic subjects than others, even though it is still only partially known how these high hypnotic susceptible subjects differ from their less responsive counterparts (Woody, Bowers, & Oakman, 1992). Hypnotic susceptibility is usually measured using one of several different hypnotic susceptibility scales, e.g., the Stanford Hypnotic Susceptibility Scale, Form C (SHSS:C) (Weitzenhoffer & Hilgard, 1962) or the Harvard group Scale of Hypnotic Susceptibility, Form A (HGSHS:A) (Shor & Orne, 1962). Hypnotic susceptibility appears to be a rather stable measure (Perry, Nadon, & Button, 1992), and a longitudinal study has even shown a test–retest correlation of .71 over a 25-year period (Piccione, Hilgard, & Zimbardo, 1989). While scores on different hypnotic susceptibility scales generally show moderate to high intercorrelations, hypnotic susceptibility appears to be only weakly correlated to other known personality traits. In one study, a number of psychological trait measures, including absorption and social desirability, thus only accounted for 9% of the variance in hypnotic susceptibility (Kumar, Pekala, & Cummings, 1996).

Third, the hypnotic context, i.e., labeling the situation as "hypnosis" and including some form of formal or informal hypnotic induction, seems necessary for eliciting hypnotic responses (Woody et al., 1992). Why these contextual factors are of such importance has yet to be explained. That contextual and expectational factors are not sufficient to explain hypnotic phenomena has been demonstrated by the so-called "real-simulator" design (Orne, 1959). In this experimental design, high hypnotic susceptible subjects are given hypnotic suggestions in the traditional fashion, while low or nonsusceptible subjects are instructed to behave just as they believe an excellent hypnotic subject would behave and asked not to reveal that they are unaffected by hypnosis. Researchers using this design have been able to show several behavioral differences between high and low hypnotic susceptible subjects (Barabasz & Barabasz, 1992). High hypnotic susceptible subjects show lower pain scores during hypnotic analgesia than lows, and highs also exhibit lower pain scores following specific suggestions of hypnotic analgesia when compared to hypnosis only; a finding that does not apply to low susceptible simulators (Miller, Barabasz, & Barabasz, 1991).

Over the years, researchers have studied possible neurophysiological markers of hypnosis and hypnotic susceptibility. Several studies have compared hypnosis with waking conditions and high with low hypnotic susceptible subjects. A number of possible differences in neurophysiological functioning have emerged (Crawford & Gruzelier, 1992). It has been hypothesized that high hypnotic susceptible subjects show greater cognitive flexibility and are more able to shift their attention and cognitive strategies in compliance with the instructions of the hypnotist. EEG studies showing that high hypnotic susceptible subjects exhibit greater hemispheric specificity (depending on task demands), higher theta power, and greater increases in regional cerebral blood flow during hypnotic analgesia than low hypnotic susceptible subjects, support the hypothesis that hypnotic susceptibility reflects special attentional abilities (Crawford, 1989; Crawford & Gruzelier, 1992; De Pascalis & Perone, 1996). This view is also supported by findings that high hypnotic susceptible subjects are able to reduce event-related brain potentials induced by painful stimuli (Arendt-Nielsen, Zachariae, & Bjerring, 1990; Zachariae & Bjerring, 1994). Taken together, the results from these and other studies indicate that high hypnotic susceptible subjects are especially capable of focusing their attention and disattending other stimuli and that behavioral differences related to hypnotic susceptibility are correlated with neurophysiological mechanisms (Crawford & Gruzelier, 1992). This provides some support for the view of hypnotic susceptibility as a trait—a trait that might even involve a heritability component (Morgan, 1973).

Although recent results indicate a number of possible neurophysiological indicators of hypnotic processes and hypnotic ability, objective analogues for hypnosis do not exist. We must bear in mind, however, that many experiments have been done to evaluate factors, e.g., stressors and stress, that are not easily measured (Olness, 1990). Other psychological intervention techniques, e.g., relaxation, guided imagery, or meditation, may share some characteristics with hypnosis and hypnotic suggestion. However, there seem to be sufficient grounds for claiming that hypnosis is a distinct phenomenon to be differentiated from other psychological techniques. Hypnotic procedures may involve suggestions to relax or to engage in imagery, but relaxation or guided imagery procedures do not necessarily involve hypnosis. In the following, we shall focus only on studies which either explicitly claim to have included some type of formal or informal hypnotic induction procedure or have included some measure of hypnotic susceptibility.

## III. HYPNOTHERAPY AND IMMUNE-RELATED DISORDERS

Hypnosis and hypnotherapy have been found to be useful in the treatment of several psychological, physiological, and "psychosomatic" disorders, including anxiety, sleep disorders, obesity, addictive behaviors, and pain-related and gastrointestinal disorders (Cheek & Le Cron, 1968; Brown & Fromm, 1987). In the following, the efficacy of hypnosis in the treatment of some immune-related and inflammatory diseases will be reviewed.

A number of disorders, though not characterized as "autoimmune" in the strictest sense of the term, are characterized by lesions, e.g., of the skin, caused by a dysfunctional "upregulation" of the immune function and inflammatory reaction. These disorders include skin diseases such as urticaria, psoriasis, and atopic dermatitis, and have, along with other skin disorders, long been considered to involve etiological factors of "psychosomatic" origin (Wittkower, 1946; Whitlock, 1976). Although research has been unable to pinpoint personality traits or variables of etiological importance; psychosocial factors, e.g., stressful life events and emotional distress, are generally thought to play a role in both onset and exacerbation of diseases such as urticaria (Graham, 1950; Shelley & Shelley, 1985) and psoriasis (Farber, Bright, & Nall, 1968; Baughman & Sobel, 1971; Invernizzi et al., 1988). Although it is generally believed that hypnosis is effective in the treatment of such disorders (Kroger & Fezzler, 1976; Brown & Fromm, 1987), and although there are numerous clinical case reports, only relatively few controlled clinical trials have been conducted.

Shertzer and Lookingbill (1987) investigated the effects of hypnotherapy on 15 patients with chronic urticaria. In a cross-over design, half of the patients received hypnotherapy first and then psychological testing, while the other half received psychological testing first and then hypnotherapy. Following hypnotic suggestions of deep relaxation, the patients received direct suggestions for decreased itching and the disappearance of their hives. Although there were no differences found in the number of wheals immediately following hypnosis, 6 of the patients were clear of all their hives after 14 months, and 7 showed some improvement. Immediate improvement was not found to be associated with hypnotic susceptibility, and data on the relationship between long-term improvement and hypnotic susceptibility are not available. High hypnotic susceptible patients did, however, report greater itching and were more likely to attribute their disease to stress.

There have over the years been several case-study reports of reductions of psoriasis severity following hypnosis and hypnotherapy (Kline, 1954; Kohli, 1967; Frankel & Misch, 1973; Waxman, 1973), but controlled studies have been lacking. In a more recent study (Zachariae, Øster, Bjerring, & Kragballe, 1996), 50 patients with stable psoriasis were randomized to either a control group or a treatment group receiving psychological intervention in the form of stress management, relaxation, and hypnosis-like imagery suggestions for localized analgesia and reduction of erythema, scaling, and itching. The patients in the treatment group participated in 8 individual therapy sessions over 12 weeks and psoriasis severity was monitored with 3-week intervals in both groups using Psoriasis Area Severity Index and laser Doppler skin blood flow measurements. Significant, but moderate, improvement was found for psoriasis severity in the treatment group, with no changes seen in the control group. After termination of the treatment, hypnotic susceptibility was assessed using the HGSHS:A (Shor & Orne, 1962; Zachariae, Molay, & Sommerlund, 1996), but no association between hypnotic susceptibility scores and improvement in psoriasis activity was found.

Several clinical studies on the effect of hypnosis on immune-related skin disorders have focused on the treatment of common warts. In an early study by Sinclair-Gieben and Chalmers (1959), 6 patients with bilateral warts were given hypnotic suggestions that their warts would gradually disappear, but only on one side of the body, which they did. A replication of this study with 17 patients was conducted by Surman, Sheldon, Gottlieb, Hackett, and Silverberg (1973). A little more than half the patients in the treatment group improved, while no improvement was seen in the control group. The improvement following hypnosis was, however, not restricted to one side of the body. No data are available on the role of hypnotic susceptibility in the improvement. In a study investigating the role of formal hypnotic induction, Johnson and Barber (1978) compared the effects of direct hypnotic suggestions that the warts would disappear with the same suggestions given without a formal hypnotic induction. The results were interpreted by the authors to indicate that "believed-in-efficacy" and motivation were more important factors in wart relief than hypnosis in itself. In a later study, Spanos, Stenstrom, and Johnson (1988) found similar results. In an attempt to differentiate more clearly between the effects of hypnosis and expectation, Spanos, Williams, and Gwynn (1990) assigned 40 patients to four experimental conditions: hypnotic suggestions, an over-the-counter wart treatment med-

ication, a placebo medication, and a no-treatment control. Although there were no differences between the three treatment groups in treatment effectiveness expectations, only the hypnosis group showed a significant posttreatment improvement. The results suggest that hypnosis does in fact contribute to the treatment effect—in addition to expectation and suggestions for wart disappearance.

Diseases characterized by hyperreactivity, e.g., asthma, share a number of clinical and pathophysiological characteristics. Asthma may be triggered and exacerbated by several factors, including infection and exposure to irritants and allergens, but allergen-IgE-mediated asthma is thought to occur in only 10–20% of the adult asthmatic population (Calabrese & Wilde, 1991). Although asthma has long been thought to include a "psychosomatic" component (Clarkson, 1937; Alexander, 1950), recent studies have generally failed to identify personality traits specific to asthma (Wistuba, 1986; Sokhey, Vasudeva, & Kumar, 1989; Reiter, Goldstein, & Vezza, 1989). Asthmatic or hay fever reactions may, however, be triggered in particularly sensitive individuals by psychosocial stimuli such as emotional distress or suggestions. The classical case of "rose cold" induced by an artificial rose (MacKenzie, 1886) and an experiment in which hay fever attacks were induced in sensitive patients by the presentation of a picture of a hay field (Hill, 1930) are often cited. In a review of 20 experimental studies of the effects of suggestion on asthmatic symptoms, Isenberg, Lehrer, and Hochron (1992) conclude that brochoconstriction to a placebo can be induced by suggestion. The authors found that the proportion of asthmatic reactors varied from approximately 20 to 40% across studies and that the ability of subjects to respond appeared to be independent of whether the subject responded to specific allergens or not. The role of hypnotic susceptibility remains uncertain since this factor had not been adequately assessed in any of the studies reviewed. The findings seem to confirm the hypothesis that allergic reactions may be learned and elicited by nonallergenic stimuli (Ader & Cohen, 1991).

Since asthma attacks can be induced by suggestion, it seems likely that hypnosis generally will be effective in the treatment of asthma (Wadden & Anderton, 1982; Frankel, 1987), and several case studies seem to support this hypothesis. Collison (1975) conducted a retrospective analysis of 121 cases treated with hypnotherapy. Of the total number, 21% became completely free of their asthma and a further 33% showed a decrease in frequency or severity of asthma attacks. Hypnotic susceptibility, as evaluated by the ability to go into a "deep trance," was found to

**TABLE II** Hypnotic Suggestion, Hypnotic Susceptibility, and Delayed Type Hypersensitivity

| Study | N | Control | Subject characteristics | Hypnotic susceptibility (measure) | Stimulus/ method | Suggestions | Time | Induration | p | Effect size(r) | Additional results |
|---|---|---|---|---|---|---|---|---|---|---|---|
| Black et al., 1963 | 4 | (+) | Psychosomatic history, trained | High (2) Medium (3) | Tuberculin (PPD) (challenge) | ↓ | 48 h | ↓ | (.04) | .57 | Lymphocyte infiltration ↔ |
| Beahrs et al., 1970 | 3 | (+) | Healthy volunteers | High | Mumps antigen (challenge) | ↓↑ | 24 h | ↔ | (.50) | — | — |
| Oker-Blom et al., 1981 | 6 | (+) | Patients referred to hypnotic treatment | ? | Tuberculin (PPD) (challenge) | ↓↑ | 48, 72 h | — | — | — | In vitro PPD reaction (cell count and fluid volume)↓↑ (7 of 12Ss) |
| Locke et al., 1987 | 42 | + | Healthy volunteers | High (HGSHS:A; SHSS:C) | Multitest (a panel of antigens) (challenge) | ↓-↑-↔ | 24, 48 h | ↔ | (.50) | .00 | Lymphocyte infiltration ↔ |
| Zachariae et al., 1989 | 18 | + | Healthy volunteers | High (HGSHS:A) | Tuberculin (PPD) (challenge) | ↓↑ | 72 h | ↓↑ | .01 | .64 | — |
| Zachariae & Bjerring, 1993 | 20 | (+) | Healthy volunteers | High (HGSHS:A) | Dinittrochlorobenzene (DNCB) and diphenylcyclopropenone (DCP) (sensitization, challenge) | ↓↑ During sensitization | 6 weeks 48 h | ↓↑ | .01 | .66 | — |
| Locke et al., 1994 | 24 | (+) | Healthy volunteers | High (HGSHS:A) Ss who responded to suggestions to change skin temperature | Varicella–zoster antigen (challenge) | ↓-↑-↔ | 24, 48 h | ↔ | (.99) | .00 | — |
| Zachariae et al., 1997 | 73 | + | Healthy volunteers | High (42) low (42) (HGSHS:A) | Diphenylcyclopropenone (DCP) (sensitization, challenge) | Relaxation during sensitization and/or challenge | 5 weeks 48 h | ↓, ↑ | .05 (Intervention compared to control) .05 (high compared to low) | .47 .36 | Degree of relaxation associated with induration ($r = .40, p < .05$) |

Note. +, control group; (+), Ss served as their own controls; ?, unknown or not reported; ↓, suggestions to suppress the reaction/decreased reaction; ↑, suggestions to enhance the reaction/enhanced reaction; ↓↑, comparing suggestions to enhance in one arm and suppress in another; ↓-↑, suggestions to enhance and suppress at different times; ↔, no change; HGSHS:A, Harvard Group Scale of Hypnotic Susceptibility; SHSS:C, Stanford Hypnotic Susceptibility Scale; (p), calculations based on data reported; (r), Estimated effect size.

audiotaped version of the hypnotic suggestions and instructed to listen to the tapes once a day for 5 days, after which the chambers were to be removed. Six weeks later, the subjects returned for allergen challenge and had two rows of four dilutions of both allergens placed side by side on one arm, again in a double-blind manner. The challenge did not involve hypnosis or hypnotic suggestions. Forty-eight hours later, the responses to the challenge were quantitated by visual scores and by ultrasound measurements of the induration. These measurements were also performed double-blind. Differences between the reactions to DNCB and DCP were calculated and the results showed that the differences in visual scores were significantly greater for subjects who had received suggestions to enhance the reaction to DNCB and inhibit the reaction to DCP than for subjects who had received suggestions in the opposite direction. Similar results, approaching the significance level ($p = .055$), were seen for the ultrasound measurements. These data suggest that hypnotic suggestions given during sensitization can affect the reactions during the subsequent challenge.

Hypnotic induction procedures usually, but not necessarily, include suggestions of relaxation and pleasant feelings of comfort. It is therefore possible that the element of relaxation in hypnosis is partly responsible for the physiological effects of hypnotic suggestions. In a study attempting to determine the effect of relaxation on DTH reactions (Zachariae, Jørgensen, Christensen, & Bjerring, 1997), 42 high and 42 low hypnotic susceptible subjects were randomly assigned to four groups. The subjects in Group 1 were sensitized with DCP and instructed to listen to audiotaped relaxation instructions during the 6-day sensitization period. When they returned 5 weeks later for allergen challenge, they listened to the relaxation tape twice daily for the next 48 h, after which they had their DTH reactions measured. Subjects in Group 2 followed the same procedure during sensitization, but did not listen to the relaxation tape during challenge. Group 3 did not listen to the tape during sensitization, but listened to the tape during challenge. Group 4 did not listen to relaxation tapes at any time during the experimental procedure. There were no differences between groups in hypnotic susceptibility, age, or perceived stress during the 5–6 weeks that the experiment lasted. Diaries kept by the participants showed that high hypnotic susceptible subjects generally experienced a greater degree of relaxation while listening to the tape. There were no differences in the degree of perceived relaxation between groups. When analyzing the results, a significant difference was found between Groups 1

and 3 for ultrasound measurements of the induration. The results indicated that relaxation during sensitization *and* challenge resulted in greater DTH reactions than relaxation during challenge alone. It is possible that the training during sensitization resulted in a more effective relaxation during challenge in Group 1. There were, however, no differences between the two groups in the number of times subjects listened to the tapes during challenge or in the degree of perceived relaxation. Another explanation could therefore be that a form of *conditioning* or perhaps *state-dependent learning* had taken place. State dependency refers to well-known phenomenon that behavior learned in one physiological state is better remembered when retention is tested in the same physiological state (Stewart, Krebs, & Kaczender, 1967; Ho, Richards, & Chute, 1978). While state-dependency generally refers to human memory and behavior, it could perhaps apply to immune "memory and behavior" as well. The results also showed a significant effect of hypnotic susceptibility with high hypnotic susceptible subjects exhibiting greater DTH responses than low hypnotic susceptible, regardless of the experimental condition. The correlation found between induration and both scores on the HGSHS:A and the degree of perceived relaxation suggests that the effect of hypnotic susceptibility may work through the influence of this trait on the ability of the subject to experience relaxation. However, a trend toward greater reactivity in highs was also seen in the control group, and the possibility that high hypnotic susceptible subjects are generally more reactive to allergens needs to be investigated. Taken together, the results of the two studies suggest that the reaction to the challenge may be influenced by psychological intervention during the sensitization.

In three of the eight published studies, no effects of hypnotic suggestion on delayed-type hypersensitivity were found. In the study by Beahrs and colleagues (1970), three experienced, high hypnotic susceptible volunteers were tested with mumps antigen to ensure that they would react to the antigen. After a second injection in each arm, they were hypnotized and given suggestions that one arm would be "cool" and "insensitive" and not react to the antigen, while the other would be "warm" and "sensitive" and would react to the antigen. There were no differences between the mean reactions of the two arms. We are unable to tell whether there were any differences between-subjects since the authors do not report the variance or the results for the individual subjects. The authors suggest that the normal skin responses of the healthy subjects investigated could explain the contrasting results to those reported by Black and his collaborators (1963) who had recruited patients with a history of psychosomatic symptoms.

Locke and colleagues (1987) studied 12 high hypnotic susceptible, but untrained, volunteers randomized to four hypnotic conditions, during which they were given suggestions to suppress or enhance the reaction in either the left or the right arm, while no reaction was suggested for the other. Thirty control subjects, who received no hypnotic suggestions, also had their DTH reactions measured in both arms. Skin testing was done, using the Multitest CMI system, which administered seven antigens (e.g., tetanus, tuberculin, and *Candida*) and a negative control (glycerin). The results were assessed using caliper measurements at 24 and 48 h after hypnosis, and the suggestions were reinforced twice during the first 24 h with audiotapes. In addition, skin biopsies of one test site were taken from each arm at both 24 and 48 h. When the indurations of the target and the control arm were compared, only one subject exhibited changes in the expected directions. The results from the skin biopsies also failed to show any changes in the expected directions. The authors list several factors, which might explain the negative result: (1) the subjects were healthy and lacked the psychosomatic history, (2) the use of untrained subjects, and (3) the DTH-testing device did not deliver the antigens in a reliable and uniform way. They also suggest that the hypothesis that it is possible to alter DTH unilaterally may be false and that the previous positive findings are a result of a general suppressive effect of hypnosis and not of specific suggestions to suppress the response in one arm. When the authors designed a second experiment (Locke et al., 1994), several of these factors were taken into consideration. Since the previous negative study was based on the assumption that the ability to influence DTH is randomly distributed in the population, the authors carefully screened the volunteers for hypnotic susceptibility and selected 24 high hypnotic susceptible subjects who, as a part of the screening procedure, showed the ability to respond to hypnotic suggestions to enhance and suppress peripheral skin temperature in the suggested direction. The previous studies, which had showed positive results, had used tuberculin (PPD) as antigen. Since the subjects, who were relatively young students, were unlikely to have antibodies against tuberculin, varicella–zoster (VZ) antigen was chosen as the stimulus. This choice was based on the previous findings by Smith, McKenzie, Marmer, and Steele (1985), who had used VZ in a case study showing the DTH response to VZ to be modulated by meditation. The subjects were tested on one arm 24 and 48 h under four experimental conditions: (1) no hypnosis, (2) hypnosis without any specific suggestions, (3) hypnotic suggestions to enhance the DTH response, and (4) hypnotic suggestions to suppress the DTH response. The subjects listened to audiotaped instructions four times during the 48 h after the hypnotic procedure. The results were assessed blindly using the caliper method and DTH responses were measured as the diameter of the indurations. The results were negative, showing only one of the 24 subjects to be able to alter the DTH response in the expected direction.

## 2. Comparing and Combining Results

As a whole, the results for hypnosis and DTH reactions are contradictory. Five studies show results indicative of some effect on DTH reactions, while three studies, including two particularly well-designed studies, are unable to show any effect at all on DTH reactions. There are, however, several methodological differences, including both the type and the dosage of antigen used, which could explain the contradictory findings. The first study by Locke and colleagues (1987) used a multitest device, which may, as suggested by the authors, have been unreliable. The second study by Locke and collaborators (1994) used VZ antigen, which may be a measure that is considerably more difficult to influence by healthy subjects than tuberculin. VZ is a virus which may remain latent after the acute infection is over and responsivity may therefore depend on the continuous inner balance between the virus and the immune system. This is not the case for tuberculin, and the challenge may therefore more easily be influenced by psychosocial factors. This hypothesis seems supported by the finding that all studies on the effect of various psychological interventions which have used PPD have found an effect, while the results from studies using VZ have been negative or inconclusive (Locke et al., 1994; Zachariae, 1996).

If sensory feedback is important, as was suggested for the ITH reactions, then the size of the response may be of importance. In the study by Zachariae and colleagues (1989), large doses of PPD were used to ensure a response, and the resulting erythemas were approximately four times larger than those obtained in the study by Beahrs and colleagues (1970), in which mumps antigen was used, and almost 10 times larger than those found in the study by Locke and collaborators (1994), in which VZ was used as antigen. Similarly, large doses of DCP and DNCB were used in the studies of Zachariae and Bjerring (1993) and Zachariae and colleagues (1997), which yielded positive results. If the hypothesis of the mediating role of sensory feedback response in inflammatory skin responses is true, then the wording of the suggestions given may also be of importance. While suggestions to enhance and suppress the DTH skin responses were given simultaneously for both arms in the study of Zachariae and colleagues (1989) and Zachariae and Bjerring (1993), they were given as separate conditions one week or more apart in the negative studies by Locke and colleagues. It could be easier for a subject to discriminate between the suggestions to suppress and enhance when they are given simultaneously than when given weeks apart. Other more subtle differences in the wording of the suggestions may also play a role. Since large doses of antigen were injected or applied in the Zachariae and colleagues (1989) and Zachariae and Bjerring (1993) studies, it was, prior to the experiment, assumed to be unlikely that the subjects would be able to produce a 100% reduction of the DTH response. Care was therefore taken to give suggestions that would allow the subjects to experience a skin reaction without interpreting it as a failure to respond to the suggestions. The subjects were therefore instructed that they would react, but that the reaction would be smaller than expected under normal conditions. Beahrs and collaborators (1970), on the other hand, gave suggestions that the subjects would not respond at all, and sensory information that skin reactions were actually occurring could have convinced the subjects that the suggestions were ineffective and the suggestions not to react at all could therefore have been counterproductive.

As suggested by both Beahrs and colleagues (1970) and Locke and colleagues (1987, 1994), the characteristics of the subjects may also be of importance. While Black and his collaborators (1963) and Oker-Blom and colleagues (1981) used subjects with a history of psychosomatic problems or subjects referred to hypnotic treatment for other problems, the remaining studies used healthy volunteers. In the two studies by Locke and colleagues (1987 and 1994), the subjects were even carefully screened to exclude any subjects with possible immune-related problems. Such careful screening procedures may be biased in favor of selecting subjects with a well-regulated immune system and may thus unintentionally exclude subjects who are psychologically and psychophysiologically more likely to respond to the suggestions.

If we chose to disregard the methodological differences between the studies and calculate the combined $p$ value for the studies as described above, an unweighted $p$ value of .0001 (two-tailed) was found. The calculation is based on the reported $p$ values and $p$ values based on the available data (see Table II). If such data were unavailable, a $p$ value of .50 was chosen for the negative studies. The positive findings of Oker-Blom and colleagues (1981) were not included in the analysis since the authors did not report sufficient data to estimate a $p$ value. When using the square root of the sample sizes as weights, a weighted $p$ value of .0007 was found. The many methodological differences should, however, caution us not to draw any firm conclusions; further investigations are clearly needed.

### 3. Mediating Mechanisms

As mentioned above, the DTH reaction is a local inflammatory reaction produced by the release of inflammatory cytokines by T cells. The effects of hypnotic suggestion, which may be found for at least some antigens, may, however, not necessarily be a result of a specific effect on T cells or the antigen-presenting cells. While the DTH reaction in itself is a reaction which is seen only in individuals who have acquired immunity to the injected antigen, this does not necessarily mean that the differences in the inflammatory response found after hypnosis are related to effects on cell-mediated immunity. The changes found in blood vessel permeability after hypnosis may be results of mechanisms similar to those which were found likely to mediate ITH and similar early inflammatory responses. This hypothesis is supported by the findings of localized changes, e.g., differences between responses in the two arms, and by the findings of Black and associates (1963) and Locke and his collaborators (1987), who were unable to demonstrate any changes in lymphocyte infiltration, regardless of the positive or negative results found in the two studies. While Oker-Blom and colleagues (1981) did report changes in lymphocyte infiltration and in the in vitro responsiveness of the cells found in the infiltrate, the lack of detailed information in their report does not allow any conclusions to be drawn. The finding by Zachariae and Bjerring (1993) that hypnotic suggestions given during sensitization differentially affected the response to the subsequent challenge, where no hypnotic suggestions were given, does lend some support to the hypothesis that hypnotic suggestion may affect the specific responsiveness of the cells. The initial mechanism may, however, still be nonspecific and it is possible that the subsequent differences found in responsiveness are a result of increased or decreased blood flow or vascular permeability following suggestions to react more or less during sensitization, thereby causing more or fewer cells to be exposed to the allergen. Changes following nonspecific suggestions, e.g., suppressed DTH reactions following suggestions to relax (Zachariae et al., 1997), could involve several mechanisms, and changes in peripheral skin blood flow, as discussed above, are only one possibility. Dhabhar and McEwen (1997) have suggested that the enhanced and suppressed DTH reactions seen after acute and chronic stressors, respectively (Kelley, Greenfield, Evermann, Parish, & Perryman, 1982; Gmünder et al., 1994), could be mediated by changes in leukocyte trafficking. Alterations in lymphocyte redeployment may play an important role in the effects of nonspecific hypnotic suggestions on cell-mediated immunity measured in vivo.

## C. Other Immune Measures

### 1. Investigations

In contrast to the 21 separate experiments reviewed above, in which effects of hypnotic suggestion or hypnotic susceptibility on in vivo skin measures of immune or inflammatory activity were studied, the remaining eight studies focused on various in vitro immune measures, e.g., white blood cell counts, immunoglobulins, monocyte chemotaxis, and functional measures such as mitogen-induced proliferative responses and natural killer cell activity. The subjects studied in these experiments were all normal, healthy adults (seven experiments) or healthy children (one experiment). The designs and results of these studies are summarized in Table III.

Four studies measured changes in counts or percentages of white blood cells and different subpopulations. Bongartz, Lyncker, and Kossman (1987) studied 12 high hypnotic susceptible healthy subjects, each participating in three experimental conditions: (1) a music-assisted hypnosis condition including suggestions to imagine relaxing scenes, (2) a film session, during which the subjects viewed a historical film about Anton Mesmer, and (3) a mental arithmetic stressor, during which the subjects were instructed to add two four-digit numbers for 20 min. All three conditions lasted 25 min. White blood cell counts including leukocytes, monocytes, and lymphocytes, catecholamines, blood pressure, and heart rate were measured prior to and immediately after the experimental conditions. Total and differential cell counts were generally reduced after the hypnosis–relaxation session when compared to the two other sessions, as were heart rate and blood pressure. Only one of the catecholamine measures (urine concentrations of vanillyl mandelic acid) showed an effect of condition, and no associations were found between immune changes and changes in catecholamines or

autonomic responses. Ruzyla-Smith, Barabasz, Barabasz, and Warner (1995) also studied short-term changes in enumerative measures. In this study, 55 high and low hypnotic susceptible healthy subjects were randomized to: (1) a condition, in which they, prior to a 25-min pre/post experiment, had practiced hypnosis for one week with suggestions to imagine a strong immune response; (2) a relaxation condition requiring subjects to participate in two 25-min "restricted environmental stimulation therapy" (REST) sessions one week apart in which the subjects float in an enclosed tank with water at 34°C; and (3) a control group which received suggestions to enhance the immune response without hypnosis. The results showed no pre/post effects of condition for any of the immune cell counts, but further statistical analyses yielded effects of experimental condition and interactions between condition and hypnotic susceptibility for some of the measures. The subjects showed higher B-cell and CD4+ T-helper-cell counts after hypnosis than those examined after the two other conditions, and high hypnotic susceptible subjects showed higher or lower T-cell counts depending on the experimental condition to which they were exposed. The results do not allow us to conclude whether the observed differences are due to an enhancing effect of hypnosis or suppressing effect of relaxation, and while the interactions found for high hypnotic susceptibility and condition could suggest an effect of hypnotic susceptibility, the results are unclear as to what these effects may be. In a similar study (Hall, Minnes, Tosi, & Olness, 1992) of the effect of specific hypnotic suggestions to increase neutrophil adherence (see later), no long- or short-term differences in total white blood cell, neutrophil, or monocyte counts were found between hypnosis and a control condition.

While the previous investigations studied *short-term* changes in white blood cell counts, Whitehouse and collaborators (1996) investigated the effect of self-hypnosis and relaxation on white blood cell counts, lymphocyte proliferative responses to mitogens (LPR), and natural killer cell activity (NKCA) over the course of 19 weeks. Twenty-one subjects were randomly selected from a group of 35 first-year medical students and taught the use of self-hypnosis and relaxation. Blood samples were drawn at four time points: (1) baseline, (2) late semester, (3) examination period, and (4) postsemester recovery. Significant increases in stress and fatigue were observed over the course of the semester and these changes in stress levels were associated with increased counts of B lymphocytes, activated T lymphocytes, LPR, and NKCA. The subjects in the self-hypnosis/relaxation group reported significantly

**TABLE III**  Effects of Hypnotic Suggestion and Hypnotic Susceptibility on Other Immune Parameters

| Study | N | Control | Subject characteristics | Hypnotic susceptibility (measure) | Hypnotic suggestions | Other techniques | Time/ sampling | Dependent measures | Results | p< | Effect size (r) | Additional results |
|---|---|---|---|---|---|---|---|---|---|---|---|---|
| Bongartz et al., 1987 | 12 | (+) | Healthy volunteers | High to medium (HGSHS:A) | Relaxation | Mental arithmetic, Film | Prepost (25 min) | Leukocytes; lymphocytes; polym. leukocytes; monocytes; | ↓ ↓ ↓ ↓ | .05 .05 .05 .05 | .47 .48 .36 .42 | ↓ Catecholamines (vanillyl mandelic acid); ↓ blood pressure; ↓ heart rate |
| Olness et al., 1989 | 57 | + | Healthy children 6–12 years | (SCHSS) | A ($n = 19$): relaxation B ($n = 19$): sugg. to enhance SIgA C ($n = 19$): control | — | 0; 25; 35 min | SIgA | ↔ A ↑ B ↔ C | .94 .007 .53 | .01 .43 .11 | No association between SCHSS scores and SIgA |
| Zachariae et al., 1991 | 11 | (+) | Healthy volunteers | High (HGSHS:A) | Experiencing anger, depression, and happiness | — | Pre; after every emotion (10 min duration); post | Monocyte chemotactic activity; IL-2 receptors | ↓ Depression ↑ Anger ↑Happiness ↔ | .02 to .001 ns. | .69 to .85 — | No changes in cortisol, epinephrine, norepinephrine, DOPA, and DOPAC |
| Hall et al., 1992 | 45 | + A ($n = 15$): trained Ss B ($n = 15$): untrained Ss C ($n = 15$): control | Healthy volunteers | (PSSH) | Increase in neutrophil adherence or SIgA | — | Prepost (30 min) | Neutrophil adherence; SIgA; cell counts | ↑ A ↔ ↔ | .05 ns ns | .46[c] — — | Immune changes associated with PSSH scores in 1 of 6 sessions |
| Zachariae et al., 1994 (study 1) | 30 | + Imagery ($n = 10$) relaxation ($n = 10$) control ($n = 10$) | Healthy volunteers High (15) low (15) (HGSHS:A) | — | Imagery or relaxation | Prepost (60 min); week 1,2,3 | Lymphocyte proliferation (PHA, Con A, PWM); Monocyte chemotaxis | ↓-↑[a] PHA | .05 | .64[a] | Significant within-subject difference, but not between imagery and relaxation |

| Study | | Population | Susceptibility | Imagery or relaxation | Prepost | Natural killer cell activity | $\downarrow$–$\uparrow^{b}$ NKCA | | | Significant within-subject difference, but not between imagery and relaxation |
|---|---|---|---|---|---|---|---|---|---|---|
| Zachariae et al., 1994 (study 2) | 30 + Imagery (n = 10) relaxation (n = 10) control (n = 10) | Healthy volunteers | High (15) low (15) (HGSHS:A) | — | Prepost (60 min); week 1, 2, 3 | | NKCA | .05 | .36[a] | Significant within-subject difference, but not between imagery and relaxation |
| Ruzyla-Smith et al., 1995 | 55 + REST (n = 19) hypnosis (n = 20) control (n = 16) | Healthy volunteers | High (29) low (26) (SHSS:C) | Imagine enhanced immune response REST Relaxation | Prepost (25 min); post interv. after 1 week | B cells T cells CD4+ cells CD8+ cells | $\uparrow$ (hypn) $\uparrow\downarrow$ (high) $\uparrow$ (hypn) $\leftrightarrow$ | .02[d] .02[d] .05[d] ns | .70[e] — .54[e] — | — |
| Whitehouse et al., 1996 | 35 + Self-hypnosis (n = 21) control (n = 14) | Healthy volunteers (medical students) | High: 7 medium: 14 (ISH) (HGSHS:A) | — | Four samples over a 19-week period | B-cell counts; T-cell counts; PHA; PWM; Con A; natural killer cell activity | $\leftrightarrow$ $\leftrightarrow$ $\leftrightarrow$ $\leftrightarrow$ $\leftrightarrow$ | ns ns ns ns ns | .07 .00 .15 .03 .16 .23 | $\downarrow$ Distress; relaxation associated with natural killer cell activity and NK-cells ($p < .05$); no association between immune changes and HGSHS:A or ISH |

Note. +, control group included; (+), s's serving as their own controls; ?, not reported; Results: $\downarrow$, decrease; $\uparrow$, increase; $\downarrow$–$\uparrow$, increase, decrease, or significant difference; $\leftrightarrow$, no observed change or difference; HGSHS:A, Harvard Group Scale of Hypnotic Susceptibility; SHSS:C, Stanford Hypnotic Susceptibility Scale; CIS, Creative Imagination Scale; PSSH, Pennsylvania State Scale of Hypnotizability; SCHSS, Stanford Children's Hypnotic Susceptibility Scale; ISH, Inventory of self-hypnosis; REST, Restricted Environmental Stimulation Therapy;

[a] Results shown for hypnotic susceptibility only.
[b] Effect in pooled imagery and relaxation group.
[c] Effect in group C only.
[d] Effects of condition, but no prepost difference.
[e] Comparing hypnosis with REST + Control.

less distress and anxiety than the control group, but no differences in immune measures were observed between the two groups. However, increases in perceived relaxation were significantly associated with increased NKCA and NK cell numbers. No short-term changes, e.g., immediately after a self-hypnosis training session, were assessed, and we are therefore unable to tell whether the negative results are due to characteristics of the specific student sample investigated, e.g., medium hypnotic susceptibility or whether hypnosis is less likely to affect long-term than short-term immune function in healthy subjects. Since the suggestions given primarily involved self-instructions to relax, it is also possible that the negative results reflect the lack of long-term changes following relaxation rather than effects of hypnotic suggestions. Finally, self-hypnosis may of course be less efficient than hypnosis involving direct interaction between subject and hypnotist. Although assessments of hypnotic susceptibility were done using two separate hypnotic susceptibility measures, the HGSHS:A and the Inventory of Self-Hypnosis (ISH), hypnotic susceptibility was not a significant predictor of any of the immune measures included in the investigation.

The differential effects of nonspecific self-hypnosis and self-hypnosis with specific hypnotic suggestions to alter immune function were investigated by Olness, Culbert, and Uden (1989). A group of 59 children, ages 6 to 12 years, were randomly assigned to three conditions of: (1) self-hypnosis-induced relaxation; (2) self-hypnosis-induced relaxation with specific suggestions to enhance their immune function, and (3) a no-hypnosis control group that engaged in conversation for 25 min. The results showed significant increases in salivary immunoglobulin A (SIgA) in the immune-specific hypnotic suggestion group 35 min after termination of the hypnosis. No differences were observed in the two other groups, suggesting that the effect of specific suggestions to enhance immune function differs from hypnosis with general suggestions to relax. The reliability of SIgA as a measure of immunocompetence has previously been questioned, mainly due to difficulties in controlling salivary flow rates (Stone, Cox, Valdimarsdottir, Jandorf, & Neale, 1987). It is unclear whether salivary flow rates were controlled for in the study by Olness and colleagues. A review of the nine published studies of the effects of psychological intervention on SIgA (Zachariae, 1996) revealed that eight of the studies showed increased SIgA levels following intervention, regardless of whether the interventions used were a humorous video, relaxation, guided imagery, or self-hypnosis. The effects of stress, on the other hand, vary, with

some studies showing decreased SIgA levels following examination stress (Deinzer & Schüller, 1998) or undesirable life events (Stone et al., 1994) and others showing increases following a stressor, e.g., competition stress or a mental arithmetic stressor (Zeier, Brauchli, & Joller-Jemelka, 1996; Kugler, Reintjes, Tewes, & Schedlowski, 1996; Willemsen et al., 1998). The unclear dynamics of SIgA over time and its interaction with changes in salivary flow rates make it difficult to interpret results of studies using SIgA as the dependent measure.

The study by Hall and his collaborators (1992) also investigated effects of specific suggestions to enhance immune function. Thirty subjects received specific hypnotic suggestions to increase neutrophil adherence. The migration of leukocytes, such as monocytes and neutrophils, out of the blood vessels, is known to depend on adhesive interactions activated by the release of inflammatory mediators. The suggestions given included instructions to imagine the neutrophils becoming sticky, e.g., as "ping pong balls with honey oozing out of the surface." After the first hypnosis session, half the subjects practiced hypnosis for two weeks prior to a second session, and another 15 subjects served as controls. While no differences were found between groups after the first session, a significant increase in neutrophil adherence was seen in the trained hypnosis group after the second session. When examining the pre- and postexperimental data for each session provided by the authors, a moderate positive effect size of $r = .46$ was found for Session 2, while a small negative effect size, i.e., a decrease, of $-.26$ was seen for the first session in the training group. There is no specific information about how the neutrophil assay was performed, e.g., whether it was performed for all conditions and sessions together or for each session or group separately. If the latter is the case, day-to-day assay variability could be a serious confounder.

The results seem to indicate that specific suggestions to increase neutrophil adherence resulted in a specific change in the expected direction. This hypothesis is supported by the results of an earlier study (Rider & Achterberg, 1989), which used nonhypnotic guided imagery techniques, instructing subjects in one training group to imagine that their lymphocytes became more active and subjects in another that the adhesiveness of their neutrophils increased. The results showed decreased lymphocyte but not neutrophil count in the lymphocyte imagery group, and decreased neutrophil but not lymphocyte count in the neutrophil imagery group. The methodology used in this study remains, however, unclear and details about the imagery instructions given are not reported. When analyzing the pre-experimental neutrophil adherence for Sessions 1 and 2 in the study by Hall and colleagues (1992), the results show a significant ($p < .05$) decrease prior to the second session, suggesting that the 2-week hypnosis training to enhance neutrophil adherence may have had a suppressive effect on this measure. This finding of opposite effects of hypnotic suggestions, depending on the time frame studied, seems to suggest that the changes in neutrophil adherence attributed to hypnosis are more likely to be nonspecific and a result of general effects of hypnosis, e.g., an effect of relaxation on homeostasis, rather than specific effects on the immune function studied. If a relaxation control condition with no specific suggestions to alter immune function had been included, it would have been possible to discriminate between the effects of specific and nonspecific suggestions on immune function.

This question of differential effects of specific instructions to enhance the immune function and general instructions to relax was the main focus of two separate experiments comparing a number of measures of immune function in high and low hypnotic susceptible volunteers (Zachariae et al., 1994). Fifteen high and 15 low hypnotic susceptible subjects participated in each experiment. In both experiments the subjects were selected for three groups with 5 high and 5 low hypnotic susceptible subjects in each group: (1) an imagery group, which was instructed to concentrate and imagine their white blood cells becoming increasingly active; (2) a relaxation group, which received relaxation instructions without any reference to their immune system, and (3) a resting control group, which sat quietly for the 30 min allotted for each experimental condition. The experimental sessions took place on the same weekday and the same time of day for 3 weeks in the first experiment and for 3 weeks with a 4 follow-up session 1 month later in the second experiment. The subjects in Groups 1 and 2 listened to audiotaped instructions between sessions. In the first experiment, the dependent immune measures were formyl-methyl-leucine-peptide-induced monocyte chemotaxis and phytohemagglutinin (PHA), concanavalin A (Con A), and pokeweed mitogen (PWM) induced lymphocyte proliferative responses (LPR). In the second, the dependent measure was whole blood NKCA. A significant increase in monocyte chemotaxis was found after both the first imagery and the first relaxation session but not after the resting control condition. No differences were seen over the following weeks. Although not all differences reached statistical significance, a general response pattern

emerged for mitogen-induced LPR with decreased responses immediately after each imagery or relaxation session. There were no changes observed in the resting control group. In the second experiment, 15 high and 15 low hypnotic susceptible subjects who had not participated in the previous experiment were studied. The same response pattern was seen for NKCA as for LPR in the previous experiment, with decreased NKCA after each experimental session throughout the study. There were no significant effects of condition, as NKCA was also seen to decrease after the resting control condition. A statistically significant effect of hypnotic susceptibility was seen for PHA LPR in the first experiment, and in the second experiment, a consistent pattern of greater percentage decreases in NKCA was observed in the high hypnotic susceptible group. The results indicate that there were no differences between the effects of specific instructions to enhance immunity and effects of general relaxation on the immune measures studied, but they also support the hypothesis that high hypnotic susceptible subjects may be more reactive to psychosocial stimuli than low hypnotic susceptible subjects.

Most experimental studies of the effects of emotional states on immunity have used films (McClelland & Kirshnitt, 1988) or role-playing methods (Futterman, Kemeny, Shapiro, & Fahey, 1994) to induce emotional states. Films may be a standardized method of inducing emotions, but one cannot be certain that subjects will respond in a uniform matter to a standardized stimulus. Another possibility involves the use of hypnotic suggestions. It is generally believed that hypnosis is associated with greater use of imagery, more vivid imagery, and increased availability of emotional involvement (Crawford & Allen, 1983; Kahn, Fromm, Lombard, & Sossi, 1989), and hypnotic suggestions seem to be a safe and valid way of inducing relatively specific emotional states of considerable intensity (Weiss, Blum, & Gleberman, 1987; Zachariae, Bjerring, Arendt-Nielsen, Nielsen, & Gotliebsen, 1991a). In a study of the effects of hypnotically induced emotions on immunity, Zachariae and colleagues (1991b) measured monocyte chemotactic activity in sera prior to hypnosis and after hypnotically induced emotions of depression, happiness, and outward expression of anger in 12 high hypnotic susceptible subjects. Chemotaxis is an important factor in the motility of leukocytes, e.g., the attraction of phagocytes to the vicinity of invading pathogens. Chemotaxis is stimulated by a number of chemoattractants, including cytokines secreted by white blood cells. In this study, the general chemotactic activity in the sera of the subjects was measured by stimulating monocytes from control subjects with sera obtained from blood samples after each experimental condition. Emotional states were induced by giving suggestions to the subjects to recall a specific situation associated with each of the three emotional states. The emotional states were induced in randomized order and lasted 10 min with blood samples drawn after each emotional state. The results showed significant increases in monocyte chemotactic activity after the conditions of anger and happiness when compared to the condition of hypnotically induced depression. Based on the results of both previous and later studies, one would expect negative emotions such as depression to be associated with immunosuppression, e.g., lowered NK cell numbers and NKCA (Herbert & Cohen, 1993; Valdimarsdottir & Bovbjerg, 1997), while positive emotions such as happiness would be associated with enhanced immune function, e.g., increased SIgA (Dillon & Baker, 1985; Rein, Atkinson, & McCraty, 1995). The relative enhancement of chemotactic activity in anger is also in agreement with previous results, e.g., increased NKCA found in subjects scoring high on hostility (Christensen et al., 1996). The results also seem supportive of the hypothesis of an association between immunosuppression and suppressed anger (Pettinggale, Greer, & Tee, 1977) and with more general findings of enhanced immune function following disclosure of negative emotions (Pennebaker, Kiecolt-Glaser, & Glaser, 1988; Petrie, Booth, Pennebaker, Davidson, & Thomas, 1996). Although the results thus seem to support the hypothesis that positive emotions and outward expression of anger are associated with immune enhancement, effects of positive and negative emotions on immune and inflammatory parameters are, however, not unidirectional. Thus inflammation as measured by histamine flare reactions seems to be enhanced by negative emotions and suppressed by positive emotions (Laidlaw, Booth, & Large, 1994, 1996) and cytokines such as IL-2 and IL-6 have been likewise shown upregulated in major depression (Maes et al., 1995). The interpretation of such results is further complicated by possible differences between short-term, intermediate, and long-term effects.

## 2. Comparing Studies

When reviewing the eight studies of immune measures other than ITH and DTH, we are struck by the many differences in methodology. Some studies include specific suggestions to enhance the immune response, while others merely study the effects of hypnotically induced relaxation or emo-

tional states. The immune measures studied vary, ranging from white blood cell counts to functional immune measures such as NKCA or mitogen induced LPR. Comparisons are also complicated by the differences in the timing of the blood samples. In some experiments short-term immune responses, e.g., after 20–30 min, are measured, while other investigators monitored changes over several weeks or months. Though all subjects studied were healthy volunteers, they may differ with respect to other sample characteristics. Some subjects had been trained in hypnosis, while others were untrained. Although all studies included some measure of hypnotic susceptibility, the measures used differ and hypnotic susceptibility scores are not reported for all experiments.

Short-term changes in immune measures differed depending on the suggestions given and the immune measures assessed. The studies that included suggestions of or a condition of relaxation generally showed decreases in white blood cell counts and functional measures such as NKCA and LPR, findings that are consistent with results from studies investigating the effects of other relaxation techniques and also consistent with studies showing increases after short-term stressors (Van Rood, Bogaards, Goulmy, & Houweilingen, 1993; Zachariae, 1996). Two studies indicated short-term enhancements for SIgA (Olness et al., 1989) and for neutrophil adherence (Hall et al., 1992). The results for SIgA are consistent with the results of nine other studies which, with the exception of the study by Hall and colleagues (1992), found increased SIgA levels after psychological intervention, regardless of the intervention technique used (Zachariae, 1996). There were no indications of any long-term effects of hypnosis.

With respect to the influence of hypnotic susceptibility, the results are contradictory. Zachariae and collaborators (1994) and Ruzyla-Smith and her colleagues (1995) found greater changes in immune response in high hypnotic susceptible subjects. Whitehouse and colleagues (1996) and Olness and her collaborators (1989) found no effects of hypnotic susceptibility and Hall and colleagues (1992) found an association in only one of six experimental sessions. The studies which did find an effect of hypnotic susceptibility all specifically compared high and low hypnotic susceptible subjects selected on the basis of extreme hypnotic susceptibility scores. The remaining studies did not specifically select for this characteristic. It is possible that assessment and selection on the basis of hypnotic susceptibility prior to inclusion in a study could influence the results through effects on expectation. In the two experiments by Zachariae and colleagues (1994), hypnotic susceptibility assessments had been done up to two years prior to recruitment, and special care had been taken in avoiding any mentioning of hypnotic susceptibility or hypnosis, thus reducing the possible effects of expectation.

In 5 of the studies, specific suggestions to enhance the immune function were given either as the only experimental condition or in comparison with non-specific instructions to relax. In the remaining three studies, only nonspecific suggestions or instructions were given. Though two studies (Olness et al., 1989; Hall et al., 1992) indicated a specific effect of hypnotic suggestions, the lacking control for possible confounders, e.g., salivary flow rates and nonspecific effects of relaxation, does not allow us to draw any clear conclusions. Taken together with the lack of differences between specific imagery instructions and general relaxation found in two other experiments (Zachariae et al., 1994), it seems less likely that the effects found are results of specific instructions to "enhance immunity."

### 3. Mediating Mechanisms

With regard to possible mediating mechanisms, only two studies included other relevant measures. Bongartz and colleagues (1987) measured both cate-cholamines and autonomic responses in the form of heart rate and blood pressure and found decreased responses after hypnosis, suggesting a decrease in sympathetic activity. The observed changes in white blood cell counts were, however, not correlated with changes in autonomic activity. In the study of the effects of hypnotically induced emotional states on monocyte chemotactic activity, Zachariae and colleagues (1991b) also measured catecholamine levels. The results showed that changes in monocyte chemotactic activity were correlated with changes in plasma DOPA levels. A subsequent in vitro analysis, however, showed that DOPA did not in itself exhibit monocyte chemotactic properties. The results suggest that the changes in DOPA were probably not directly responsible for the observed changes in chemotactic activity. We are thus generally left in the dark with respect to the possible mediating psychophysiological mechanisms involved in the changes in enumerative and functional immune measures found after hypnosis.

## V. CONCLUSIONS AND PERSPECTIVES

Taken together, the results from the available studies suggest that ITH wheal reactions and perhaps also flare reactions can be suppressed by hypnosis.

The available data also suggest that DTH reactions to certain antigens, e.g., tuberculin, but not others, e.g., varicella–zoster, may be altered following hypnosis. Though hypnosis seemed to affect both enumerative and functional immune measures, the many different immune parameters investigated in a relatively small number of studies do not allow us to draw any conclusions. The results from the available studies raise several important issues.

One question is whether the results found are related to effects of specific hypnotic suggestions to enhance or suppress the immune or inflammatory parameter in question, or whether they are merely related to nonspecific psychophysiological effects, e.g., of the general relaxed state often associated with hypnosis. In the majority of the studies, it is not possible to distinguish between effects of the hypnotic state itself and effects of the specific suggestions given in the hypnotic state. A few studies found effects of simultaneous suggestions to react and not react (Ikemi & Nakagawa, 1962) or enhance and suppress (Zachariae et al., 1989) in the expected directions, suggesting that hypnotic suggestions may produce specific, localized changes in skin inflammatory reactions.

Another question is whether the results found are related to effects of hypnotic suggestions on specific immune mechanisms or whether they reflect changes in nonspecific immune or even nonimmune physiological processes. With respect to ITH and early inflammatory responses, it seems more than likely that the effects found are due to influences on the neurogenic component of the inflammatory reaction, and it is also likely that localized changes in cutaneous blood flow represent the main mediating mechanism behind the observed changes. With respect to DTH reactions, it is possible that the effects observed are related to similar changes in cutaneous blood flow or perhaps even vascular permeability. Such mechanisms may still, if they occur during sensitization, influence the specific responsivity of the immune cells at subsequent challenges. The results from the few studies which included hormonal measures such as cortisol and catecholamines do not indicate that these hormones provide a major mediating mechanism. With respect to enumerative and functional measures, we are still left in the dark, but it seems likely that the observed changes are due to nonspecific effects, e.g., of relaxation on general homeostasis.

The question whether hypnosis is more effective than other types of psychological intervention, e.g., relaxation or guided imagery techniques, has yet to be answered. Studies of effects of psychological intervention on ITH and DTH reactions have almost exclusively used hypnosis (Zachariae, 1996) and the results from the few studies which included techniques other than hypnosis are inconclusive. Another way of addressing this question is by comparing results in high and low hypnotic susceptible subjects. While results of several of the studies indicated an effect of hypnotic susceptibility, others were unable to demonstrate such an effect. Studies distinctly selecting subjects on the basis of extreme hypnotic susceptibility scores were more likely to show an effect than studies where no preselection was conducted. In several of the negative studies, hypnotic susceptibility scores have not been reported and the different hypnotic susceptibility measurements used also limit the comparability of the results.

Effects of hypnotic suggestions were reported in all but one (Fry et al., 1964, Study 2) of the 10 experiments which included subjects with allergies, urticaria, asthma, or a history of psychosomatic complaints. Though effects were also found in the majority of experiments using healthy subjects, the results are more mixed, suggesting that subject characteristics may be of importance. It may be more difficult to influence a healthy well-regulated immune system than a dysregulated immune system, and it is possible that careful screening for both mental and physical illness could introduce a bias in favor of negative results. Only one study in which both healthy subjects and patients were included reported no differences (Levine et al., 1966).

Differences in hypnotic procedures may also play a role. From a methodological viewpoint, standardized procedures, e.g., the use of manuscripts or taped instructions, would be preferred. Such standardization could, however, also introduce a bias in favor of negative or reduced effects. It has been suggested that the specific techniques used in different psychotherapeutic approaches are of less importance for the efficacy of therapy than a number of *nonspecific* factors that characterize the psychotherapeutic relationship in general (Frank, 1973). Such factors include the empathetic abilities of the therapist and the degree of rapport obtained in the relationship between therapist and patient. Rapport depends, among other factors, on the ability of the therapist to respond to the particular needs, thoughts, and feelings of the patient as they are expressed, sometimes in the form of minimal cues. When special care is taken to eliminate intersubject variation, e.g., when hypnotic suggestions are given using a prepared manuscript or taped instructions, rapport may be diminished, thereby reducing the ability of the hypnotist to influence the subject.

In conclusion, there are no data to support the hypothesis that it is possible to specifically "strengthen" the immune system "at will." When specific changes in the suggested direction do occur, it seems possible that specific localized changes in cutaneous inflammatory reactions are responsible. While it may be possible for certain patients to influence local psychophysiological and inflammatory reactions, it has not been confirmed that it should be possible to stimulate or suppress selected immune responses directly by hypnotic suggestion. Several unresolved questions need to be addressed in future research: (1) To what degree are the effects of hypnotic suggestions to suppress inflammatory or immune reactions a result of specific suggestions or nonspecific effects of the hypnotic state itself? (2) Are the effects of hypnosis different from the results of other psychological techniques? (3) Are the reactions of patients, e.g., allergy patients, more easily influenced than those of healthy subjects? (4) Are the responses to certain antigens, e.g., tuberculin, more readily affected than the reactions to others, e.g., varicella–zoster? To answer these questions, future studies should address the problem of differences in methodology, e.g., measurements of immune and inflammatory reactions and assessments of hypnotic susceptibility, and attempt to increase the comparability of results across studies.

# References

Ader, R., & Cohen, N. (1991). The influence of conditioning on immune responses. In R. Ader, D. L. Felten, & N. Cohen. (Eds.), *Psychoneuroimmunology*, (2nd ed.). (pp. 611–642) New York: Academic Press.

Alexander, F. (1950). *Psychosomatic medicine*. New York: Norton.

Arendt-Nielsen, L., Zachariae, R., & Bjerring, P. (1990). The effect of painful argon laser stimulation on human evoked potentials during hypnotically induced hyperalgesia and analgesia. *Pain, 42*, 243–251.

Aronoff, G. M., Aronoff, S., & Peck, L. W. (1975). Hypnotherapy in the treatment of bronchial asthma. *Annals of Allergy, 34*, 356–362.

Auerbach, J. E., Oleson, T. D., & Solomon, G. F. (1992). A behavioral medicine intervention as an adjunctive treatment for HIV-related illness. *Psychology and Health, 6*, 325–334.

Barabasz, A. F., & Barabasz, M. (1992). Research designs and considerations. In E. Fromm, & M. R. Nash (Eds.), *Contemporary hypnosis research* (pp.173–201). New York: Guilford.

Barber, T. X. (1984). Changing "unchangeable" bodily processes by (hypnotic) suggestions: A new look at hypnosis, cognitions, imagining, and the mind–body problem. In A.E. Sheikh (Ed.), *Imagination and healing* (pp. 69–127). New York: Baywood.

Baughman, R., & Sobel, R. (1971) Psoriasis, stress, and strain. *Archives of Dermatology, 103*, 599–605.

Beahrs, J. O., Harris, D. R., & Hilgard, E. R. (1970). Failure to alter skin inflammation by hypnotic suggestion in five subjects with normal skin reactivity. *Psychosomatic Medicine, 32*, 627–631.

Ben-Zvi, Z., Spohn, W. A., Young, S. H., & Kattan, M. (1982). Hypnosis for exercise-induced asthma. *American Review of Respiratory Diseases, 125,* 392–395.

Black, S. (1963a). Inhibition of immediate-type hypersensitivity response by direct suggestion under hypnosis. *British Medical Journal, 1,* 1649–1652.

Black S. (1963b). Shift in dose-response curve of Prausnitz–Kustner reaction by direct suggestion under hypnosis. *British Medical Journal, 1,* 990–992.

Black, S., & Friedman, M. (1965). Adrenal function and the inhibition of allergic responses under hypnosis. *British Medical Journal, 1,* 562–567.

Black, S., Humphrey, J. H., & Niven, J. S. (1963). Inhibition of mantoux reaction by direct suggestion under hypnosis. *British Medical Journal, 6,* 1649–1652.

Blatt, S. P., Hendrix, C. W., Butzin, C. A., Freeman, T. M., Ward, W. W., Hensley, R. E., Melcher, G. P., Donovan, D. J., & Boswell R. N. (1993). Delayed-type hypersensitivity skin testing predicts progression to AIDS in HIV-infected patients. *Annals of Internal Medicine, 119,* 177–184.

Bongartz, W., Lyncker, I., & Kossman, K. T. (1987). The influence of hypnosis on white blood cell count and urinary levels of catecholamines and vanillyl mandelic acid. *Hypnos, 14,* 52–61.

Brown, D. P., & Fromm, E. (1987). *Hypnosis and behavioral medicine.* Hilsdale, NJ: Erlbaum Associates.

Calabrese, J. R., & Wilde, C. (1991). Alterations in immunocompetence during stress: A Medical perspective. In N. Plotnikoff, A. Murgo, R. Faith, & J. Wybran (Eds.), *Stress and immunity* (pp. 81–97). Boca Ranton, FL: CRC Press.

Chapman, L. F., & Godell, H. (1964). The participation of the nervous system in the inflammatory reaction. *Annals of the New York Academy of Science, 116,* 990–1017.

Chapman, L. F., Goodell, H., & Wolff, H. G. (1959). Changes in tissue vulnerability during hypnotic suggestion. *Journal of Psychosomatic Research, 4,* 99–105.

Christensen, A. J., Edwards, D. L., Wiebe, J. S., Benotsch, E. G., McKelvey, L., Andrews, M., & Lubaroff, D. M. (1996). Effect of verbal self-disclosure on natural killer cell activity: Moderating influence of cynical hostility. *Psychosomatic Medicine, 58,* 150–155.

Clarkson, A. K. (1937). The nervous factor in juvenile asthma. *British Medical Journal, 2,* 845–850.

Collison, D. R. (1975). Which asthmatic patients should be treated by hypnotherapy? *Medical Journal of Australia, 1,* 776–781.

Crawford, H. J. (1989). Cognitive and physiological flexibility: Multiple pathways to hypnotic responsiveness. In V. Ghorghui, P. Netter, H. Eysenck, & R. Rosenthal (Eds.), *Suggestion and suggestibility: Theory and research* (pp. 155–168) Berlin: Springer Verlag.

Crawford, H. J., & Allen, S. H. (1983). Enhanced visual memory during hypnosis as mediated by hypnotic responsiveness and cognitive strategies. *Journal of Experimental Psychology, 112,* 662–685.

Crawford, H. J., & Gruzelier, J. H. (1992). A midstream view of the neuropsychophysiology of hypnosis: Recent research and future directions. In E. Fromm & M. R. Nash (Eds.), *Contemporary hypnosis research* (pp. 227–268). New York: Guilford.

De Pascalis, V., & Perrone, M. (1996). EEG asymmetry and heart rate during experience of hypnotic analgesia in high and low hypnotizables. *International Journal of Psychophysiology, 21,* 163–175.

Deinzer, R., & Schüller, N. (1998). Dynamics of stress-related decrease of salivary immunoglobulin A (sIgA): Relationship to symptoms of the common cold and studying behavior. *Behavioral Medicine, 23,* 161–169.

Dennis, M., & Philippus, M. J. (1965). Hypnotic and non-hypnotic suggestion and skin response in atopic patients. *American Journal of Clinical Hypnosis, 7,* 342–345.

Dhabhar, F. S., & McEwen, B. S. (1997). Acute stress enhances while chronic stress suppresses cell-mediated immunity in vivo: A potential role for leukocyte trafficking. *Brain, Behavior, and Immunity, 11,* 286–306.

Dillon, K. M., & Baker, K. H. (1985–1986). Positive emotional states and the enhancement of the immune system. *International Journal of Psychiatry in Medicine, 15,* 13–18.

Dixon, M., & Laurence, J.-R. (1992). Two hundred years of hypnosis research: Questions resolved? Questions unanswered! In E. Fromm & M. R. Nash (Eds.), *Contemporary hypnosis research* (pp. 34–67). New York: Guilford.

Evans, F. J. (1990). Hypnosis and pain control. Australian Journal of Clinical Experimental Hypnosis, 18, 21–33.

Ewer, T. C., & Stewart, D. E. (1986). Improvement in bronchial hyper-responsiveness in patients with moderate asthma after treatment with a hypnotic technique: A randomised controlled trial. *British Medical Journal,* (Clinical Research Edition), *293,* 1129–1132.

Farber, E. M., Bright, R. D., & Nall M. L. (1968). Psoriasis. A questionnaire survey of 2,144 patients. *Archives of Dermatology, 98,* 248–259.

Farthing, G. W. (1992). *The psychology of consciousness.* Englewood Cliffs, NJ: Prentice-Hall.

Förster, C., Greiner, T., Nischik, M., Schmelz, M., & Handwerker H. O. (1995). Neurogenic flare responses are heterogeneous in superficial and deep layers of human skin. *Neuroscience Letters, 185,* 33–36.

Frank, J. (1973). *Persuasion and healing: A comparative study of psychotherapy.* Baltimore: Johns Hopkins University Press.

Frankel, F. H. (1987). Significant developments in medical hypnosis during the past 25 years. *International Journal of Clinical and Experimental Hypnosis, 35,* 231–247.

Frankel, F. H., & Misch, R. C. (1973). Hypnosis in a case of long-standing psoriasis in a person with character problems. *International Journal of Clinical and Experimental Hypnosis, 21,* 121–130.

Fry, L., Mason, A. A., & Pearson, R. S. B. (1964). Effect of hypnosis on allergic skin responses in asthma and hay-fever. *British Medical Journal, 1,* 1145–1148.

Futterman, A. D., Kemeny, M. E., Shapiro, D., & Fahey, J. L. (1994). Immunological and physiological changes associated with induced positive and negative mood. *Psychosomatic Medicine, 56,* 499–451.

Gauld, A. (1992). *A history of hypnotism.* Cambridge: Cambridge University Press.

Good, R. A. (1981). Foreword: Interaction of the body's major networks. In R. Ader (Ed.), *Psychoneuroimmunology* (pp. xvii–xix). New York: Academic Press.

Graham, D. T. (1950). The pathogenesis of hives: Experimental study of life situations, emotions, and cutaneous vascular reactions. *Annals of Research of Nervous and Mental Disease (Proceedings), 29,* 987–1009.

Gmünder, F. K., Konstantinova, I., Cogoli, A., Lesnyak, A., Bogomolov, W., & Grachov, A. W. (1994). Cellular immunity in cosmonauts during long duration spaceflight on board the orbital MIR station. *Aviation and Space Environment Medicine, 65,* 419–423.

Hajek, P., Jakoubek, B., Kyhos, K., & Radil T. (1992). Increase in cutaneous temperature induced by hypnotic suggestions of pain. *Perceptual and Motor Skills, 74,* 737–738.

Hall, H. R., Minnes, L., Tosi, M., & Olness, K. (1992). Voluntary modulation of neutrophil adhesiveness using a cyberphysiologic strategy. *International Journal of Neuroscience, 63,* 287–297.

Hammarlund, A., Olsson, P., & Pipkorn, U. (1991). Dermal blood flow after local challenges with allergen, histamine, bradykinin and compound 48/80 . *Clinical and Experimental Allergy, 21*, 333–342.

Herbert, T. B., & Cohen, S. (1993). Stress and immunity in humans: A meta-analytic review. *Psychosomatic Medicine, 55*, 364–379.

Hilgard, E. R. (1986). Hypnosis and pain. In R. A. Sternbach (Ed.), *The psychology of pain*. New York: Raven Press.

Hilgard, E. R. (1990). Hypnosis in perspective. In Van Dyck et al. (Eds.), *Hypnosis, current theory, research, and practice* (pp. 1–16), Amsterdam: VU University Press.

Hilgard, E. R. (1992). Dissociation and theories of hypnosis. In E. Fromm and M. R. Nash. (Eds.), *Contemporary hypnosis research* (pp. 69–101). New York: Guilford.

Hilgard, E. R., & Hilgard, J. R. (1983). *Hypnosis in the relief of pain*. Los Altos CA: Kaufmann.

Hill, L. E. (1930). *Philosophy of a biologist*. London: Arnold.

Ho, B., Richards, D., & Chute, D. (1978). *Drug discrimination and state-dependent learning*. New York: Academic Press.

Hokfelt, T., Skirboll, L., Lundberg, J. M., Dalsgaard, C.-J., Johansson, O., Pernow, B., & Jancso, G. (1983). Neuropeptides and pain pathways. In J. J. Bonica (Ed.), *Advances in pain research and therapy* (pp. 227–246). New York: Raven Press.

Ikemi, Y., & Nakagawa, S. (1962). A psychosomatic study of contagious dermatitis. *Kyushu Journal of Medical Science, 13*, 335–350.

Invernizzi, G., Gala, C., Bovio, L., Conte, G., Manca, G., Polenghi, M., & Russo R. (1988). Onset of psoriasis: The role of life events. *Medical Science Research, 16*, 143–144.

Isenberg, S. A., Lehrer, P. M., & Hochron S. (1992). The effects of suggestion and emotional arousal on pulmonary function in asthma: A review and a hypothesis regarding vagal mediation. *Psychosomatic Medicine, 54*, 192–216.

Jancsó, N., Jancsó-Gábor, A., & Szolcsányi, J. (1967). Direct evidence for neurogenic inflammation and its prevention by denervation and by pretreatment with capsaicin. *British Journal of Pharmacology, 31*, 138–151.

Janeway, C. A., & Travers, P. (1997). *Immunobiology: The immune system in health and disease*. New York: Garland Publishing.

Johnson, R. F. Q., & Barber, T. X. (1978). Hypnosis, suggestions, and warts: An experimental investigation implicating the importance of "believed-in efficacy." *American Journal of Clinical Hypnosis, 20*, 165–174.

Kahn, S. P., Fromm, E., Lombard, L. S., & Sossi M. (1989). The relation of self-reports of hypnotic depth in self-hypnosis to hypnotizability and imagery production. *International Journal of Clinical, & Experimental Hypnosis, 37*, 290–304.

Kelley, K. W., Greenfield, R. E., Evermann, J. F., Parish, S. M., & Perryman, L.E. (1982). Delayed-type hypersensitivity, contact sensitivity, and phytohemagglutinin skin-test responses of heat- and cold-stressed calves. *American Journal of Vetenary Research, 43*, 775–779.

Kemppainen, P., Leppänen, H., Jyväsjärvi, E., & Pertovaara, A. (1994). Blood flow increase in the orofacial area of humans induced by painful stimulation. *Brain Research Bulletin, 33*, 655–662.

Kline, M. V. (1954). Psoriasis and hypnotherapy: A case report. *Journal of Clinical and Experimental Hypnosis, 2*, 318–322.

Kohli, D. R. (1967). Psoriasis, a physiopathologic adaptive reaction: Six year cure by retraining. *Northwestern Medicine, 66*, 33–39.

Kroger, W. S., & Fezler, W. D. (1976). *Hypnosis and behavior modification: Imagery conditioning*. Philadelphia, PA: Lippincott.

Kugler, J., Reintjes, F., Tewes, V., & Schedlowski, M. (1996). Competition stress in soccer coaches increases salivary. Immunoglobin A and salivary cortisol concentrations. *Journal of Sports Medicine and Physical Fitness, 36*, 117–120.

Kumar, V. K., Pekala, R. J., & Cummings, J. (1996). Trait factors, state effects, and hypnotizability. *International Journal of Clinical & Experimental Hypnosis, 44*, 232–249.

Laidlaw, T. M., Booth, R. J., & Large, R. G. (1994). The variability of hypersensitivity reactions: The importance of mood. *Journal of Psychosomatic Research, 38*, 51–61.

Laidlaw, T. M., Booth, R. J., & Large, R. G. (1996). Reduction in skin reactions to histamine after a hypnotic procedure. *Psychosomatic Medicine, 58*, 242–248.

Laidlaw, T. M., Richardson, D. H., Booth, R. J., & Large R. G. (1994) Immediate-type hypersensitivity reactions and hypnosis: Problems in methodology. *Journal of Psychosomatic Research, 38*, 569–580.

Levine, M. I., Geer, J. H., & Kost, P. F. (1966). Hypnotic suggestion and the histamine wheal. *Journal of Allergy, 37*, 246–250.

Locke, S. E., Ransil, B. J., Covino, N. A., Toczydlowski, J., Lohse, C. M., Dvorak, H. F., Arndt K. A., & Frankel F. H. (1987). Failure of hypnotic suggestion to alter immune response to delayed-type hypersensitivity antigens. *Annals of the New York Academy of Science, 496*, 745–749.

Locke, S., Ransil, B., Zachariae, R., Molay, F., Tollins, K., Covino, N.A., & Danforth D. (1994). Effect of hypnotic suggestion on the delayed-type hypersensitivity response. *Journal of the American Medical Association, 272*, 47–52.

Lynn, B. (1988). Neurogenic inflammation. *Skin Pharmacology, 1*, 217–224.

Lynn, B., Pini, A., & Baranowski R. (1987). Injury of somatosensory afferents by capsaicin: Selectivity and failure to regenerate. In L. M. Pubols, & B. J. Sessle (Eds.), *Effects of injury on trigeminal and spinal somatosensory systems*. New York: Liss.

MacKenzie, J. N. (1886). The production of the so-called "rose-cold" by means of an artificial rose. *American Journal of Medical Science, 91*, 45–57.

Maes, M., Meltzer, H. Y., Bosmans, E., Bergmans, R., Vandoolaeghe, E., Ranjan, R., & Desnyder, R. (1995). Increased plasma concentrations of interleukin-6, soluble interleukin-6, soluble interleukin-2 and transferrin receptor in major depression. *Journal of Affective Disorders, 34*, 301–309.

Maslach, C., Marshall, G., & Zimbardo, P. G. (1972). Hypnotic control of peripheral skin temperature: A case report. *Psychophysiology, 9*, 600–605.

McClelland, D. C., & Kirshnitt, C. (1988). The effect of emotional arousal through films on salivary immunoglobulin A. *Psychology and Health, 2*, 31–52.

Miller, M. F., Barabasz, A. F., & Barabasz, M. (1991). Effects of active alert and relaxation hypnotic inductions on cold pressor pain. *Journal of Abnormal Psychology, 100*, 223–226.

Morgan, A. H. (1973). The heritability of hypnotic susceptibility in twins. *Journal of Abnormal Psychology, 82*, 55–61.

Morgan, A. H., & Hilgard, J. R. (1978–1979). The Stanford Hypnotic Clinical Scale for adults. *American Journal of Clinical Hypnosis, 21*, 134–147.

Morrison, J. B. (1988). Chronic asthma and improvement with relaxation induced by hypnotherapy. *Journal of Research in Social Medicine, 81*, 701–704.

Murphy, A. I., Lehrer, P. M., Karlin, R., Swartzman, L., Hochron, S., & McCann, B. (1989). Hypnotic susceptibility and its relationship to outcome in the behavioral treatment of asthma: Some preliminary data. *Psychological Reports, 65*, 691–698

Oker-Blom, N., Cedercreutz, C., Willebrandt E. V., Häyry, P., Kiistala, U., & Mustakallio, K. (1981). Psychical factors in infectious disease and immunological response. *Psychiatrica Fennica, Supplement*, 195–196.

Olness, K. (1990). Pediatric psychoneuroimmunology: Hypnosis as a possible mediator. In Dyck Rv (Eds.), *Hypnosis, current theory and practice* (pp.71–81). Amsterdam: VU University Press.

Olness, K., Culbert, T., & Uden D. (1989). Self-regulation of salivary immunoglobulin A in children. *Pediatrics, 83*, 66–71.

Orne, M. T. (1959). The nature of hypnosis: artifact and essence. *Journal of Abnormal and Social Psychology, 58*, 277–299.

Orne, M. T. (1983). Hypnotic methods for managing pain. In J. J. Bonica (Ed.), *Advances in pain research and therapy*, (vol. 5). New York: Raven Press.

Pearsall, P. (1988). *Superimmunity—Master your emotions and improve your health*. New York: Fawsett Book Group.

Pennebaker, J. W., Kiecolt-Glaser, J. K., & Glaser R. (1988). Disclosure of traumas and immune function—Health implications for psychotherapy. *Journal of Consulting and Clinical Psychology, 56*, 239–245.

Perry, C., Nadon, R., & Button, J. (1992). The measurement of hypnotic ability. In E. Fromm and M. R. Nash (Eds.), *Contemporary hypnosis research* (pp. 459–489). New York: Guilford.

Petersen, L. J., Church, M. K., & Skov, P. S (1997). Platelet-activating factor induces histamine release from human skin mast cells in vivo, which is reduced by local nerve blockade. *Journal of Allergy and Clinical Immunology, 99*, 640–647.

Petrie, K. J., Booth, R. J., Pennebaker, J. W., Davison, K. P., & Thomas M G. (1995). Disclosure of trauma and immune response to a hepatitis B vaccination program. *Journal of Consulting and Clinical Psychology, 63*, 787–792.

Pettingale, K. W., Greer, S., & Tee, D. E. H. (1977). Serum IgA and emotional expression in breast cancer patients. *Journal of Psychosomatic Research, 21*, 395–399.

Piccione, C., Hilgard, E. R., & Zimbardo P. G. (1989). On the degree of stability of measured hypnotizability over a 25-year period. *Journal of Personality and Social Psychology, 56*, 289–295.

Raynaud, J., Michaux, D., Bleirad, G., Capderou, A., Bordachar, J., & Durand, J. (1983). Changes in rectal and mean skin temperature in response to suggested heat during hypnosis in man. *Physiology and Behavior, 33*, 221–226.

Rein, G., Atkinson, M., & McCraty, R. (1995). The physiological and psychological effects of compassion and anger. *Journal of Advancement in Medicine, 8*, 87–105.

Reiter, H. H., Goldstein, F., & Vezza, M. E. (1989). Personality patterns of allergic and nonallergic college students *Psychological Studies, 34*, 59–60.

Rider, M. S., & Achterberg, J. (1989). Effect of music-assisted imagery on neutrophils and lymphocytes. *Biofeedback and Self-Regulation, 14*, 247–57.

Roberts, A. H., Schuler, J., Bacon, J. G., Zimmermann, R. L., & Patterson, R. (1975). Individual differences and autonomic control: Absorbtion, hypnotic susceptibility, and the unilateral control of skin temperature. *Journal of Abnormal Psychology, 84*, 272–279.

Rosenthal, R. (1991). Meta-analysis: A review. *Psychosomatic Medicine, 53*, 247–271.

Rosenthal, R., & Rubin, D. B. (1982). A simple, general purpose display of magnitude of experimental effect. *Journal of Educational Psycholology, 74*, 166–169.

Rossi, E. L., & Cheek, D. B. (1988). *Mind–body therapy: Methods of ideodynamic healing in hypnosis*. New York: Norton.

Ruzyla-Smith, P., Barabasz, A., Barabasz, M., & Warner D. (1995). Effects of hypnosis on the immune response: B-cells, T-cells, helper- and suppressor cells. *American Journal of Clinical Hypnosis, 38*, 71–79.

Shelley, W. B., & Shelley, E. D. (1985). Adrenergic urticaria: A new form of stress-induced hives. *Lancet, 2*, 1031–1033.

Shertzer, C. L., & Lookingbill, D. P. (1987). Effects of relaxation therapy and hypnotizability in chronic urticaria. *Archives of Dermatology, 123*, 913–916.

Shor, R. E., & Orne, E. C. (1962). *Harvard group scale of hypnotic susceptibility, Form A*. Palo Alto, CA: Consultant Psychologists Press.

Sinclair-Gieben, A. H. C., & Chalmers, D. (1959). Evaluation of treatment of warts by hypnosis. *Lancet, 2*, 480–482.

Smith, G. R., McKenzie, J. M., Marmer, D. J., & Steele, R. W. (1985). Psychologic modulation of the human immune response to varicella zoster. *Archives of Internal Medicine, 145*, 2110–2112.

Sokhey, G., Vasudeva, P., & Kumar L. (1989). Certain personality correlates of the allergic population with different levels of skin reactivity. *Journal of Personality and Clinical Studies, 5*, 227–231.

Spanos, N. P., & Chaves, J. F. (1989). The cognitive-behavioral alternative in hypnosis research. In N. P. Spanos, & J. F. Chaves (Eds.), *Hypnosis: The cognitive–behavioral perspective* (pp. 9–16). Buffalo, NY: Prometheus Books.

Spanos, N. P., & Coe, W. C. (1992). A social-psychological approach to hypnosis. In E. Fromm and M. R. Nash. (Eds.), *Contemporary hypnosis research* (pp. 102–130). New York: Guilford.

Spanos, N. P., Stenstrom, R. J., & Johnston J. C. (1988). Hypnosis, placebo, and suggestion in the treatment of warts. *Psychosomatic Medicine, 5*, 245–260.

Spanos, N. P., Williams, R. J., & Gwynn, J. C. (1990). Effects of hypnotic, placebo, and salicylic acid treatments on wart regression. *Psychosomatic Medicine, 52*, 109–114.

Stewart, J., Krebs, W. H., & Kaczender, E. (1967). State-dependent learning produced with steroids. *Nature, 216*, 1233–1234.

Stone, A. A., Cox, D. S., Valdimarsdottir, H., Jandorf, L., & Neale JM. (1987). Evidence that secretory IgA antibody is associated with daily mood. *Journal of Personality and Social Psychology, 52*, 988–993.

Stone, A. A., Neale, J. M., Cox, D. S., Napoli, A., Valdimarsdottir, H., & Kennedy-Moore, E. (1994). Daily events are associated with a secretory immune response to an oral antigen in men. *Health Psychology, 13*, 440–446.

Surman, O. S., Sheldon, K., Gottlieb, K., Hackett, T. P., & Silverberg, E. L. (1973). Hypnosis in the treatment of warts. *Archives of General Psychiatry, 28*, 439–441.

Taylor, D. N. (1995). Effects of a behavioral stress-management program on anxiety, mood, self-esteem, and t-cell count in HIV-positive men. *Psychological Reports, 76*, 451–457.

Thestrup-Pedersen, K. (1975). Suppression of tuberculin skin reactivity by prior tuberculin skin testing. *Immunology, 28*, 342–348.

Ullman, M. (1947). Herpes simplex and second degree burn induced under hypnosis. *American Journal of Psychiatry, 103*, 828–830.

Valdimarsdottir, H. B., & Bovbjerg, D. H. (1997). Positive and negative mood: association with natural killer cell activity. *Psychology and Health, 12*, 319–327.

Van Dyck, R., & Hoogduin, K. (1990). Hypnosis: Placebo or nonplacebo? *American Journal of Psychotherapy, 44*, 396–404.

Van Rood, Y. R., Bogaards, M., Goulmy, E., & Houweilingen, H. C. V. (1993). The effects of stress and relaxation on the in vitro immune response in man: A meta-analytic study. *Journal of Behavioral Medicine, 16*, 163–181.

Wadden, T. A., & Anderton, C. H. (1982). The clinical use of hypnosis. *Psychological Bulletin, 91*, 215–243.

Waxman, D. (1973). Behavior therapy of psoriasis—a hypnoanalytical and counter-conditioning technique. *Postgraduate Medical Journal, 49*, 591–595.

Weiss, F., Blum, G. S., & Gleberman, L. (1987). Anatomically based measurement of facial expressions in simulated versus hypnotically induced affect. *Motivation and Emotion, 11,* 67–81.

Weitzenhoffer, A. M., & Hilgard, E. R. (1962). *Stanford hypnotic susceptibility scale, form C.* Palo Alto, CA: Consulting Psychologists Press.

Whitehouse, W. G., Dinges, D. F., Orne, E. C., Keller, S. E., Bates, B. L., Bauer, N. K., Morahan, P., Haupt, B. A., Carlin, M. M., Bloom, P. B., Zaugg, L., & Orne, M. T. (1996). Psychosocial and immune effects of self-hypnosis training for stress management throughout the first semester of medical school. *Psychosomatic Medicine, 58,* 249–263.

Whitlock, F. A. (1976). *Psychophysiological aspects of skin disease.* London: Saunders.

Willemsen, G., Ring, C., Carroll, D., Evans, P., Clow, A., & Hucklebridge, F. (1998). Secretory immunoglobulin A and cardiovascular reactions to mental arithmetic and cold pressor. *Psychophysiology, 35,* 252–259.

Wistuba, F. (1986). Significance of allergy in asthma from a behavioral medicine viewpoint. *Psychotherapy and Psychosomatics, 45,*186–194.

Wittkower, E. (1946). Psychological aspects of psoriasis. *Lancet,* 566–569.

Woody, E. Z., Bowers, K. S., & Oakman, J. M. (1992). A conceptual analysis of hypnotic responsiveness: Experience, individual differences, and context. In E. Fromm & M. R. Nash (Eds.), *Contemporary hypnosis research* (pp. 3–34). New York: Guilford.

Zachariae, R. (1996). *Mind and immunity: Psychological modulation of immunological and inflammatory parameters.* Copenhagen: Munksgaard-Rosinante.

Zachariae, R., & Bjerring, P. (1990). The effect of hypnotically induced analgesia on flare reaction of cutaneous histamine prick test. *Archives of Dermatological Research, 282,* 539–543.

Zachariae, R., & Bjerring, P. (1993). Increase and decrease of cutaneous reactions obtained by hypnotic suggestions during sensitization—studies on dinitrochlorobenzene (DNCB) and diphenylcyclopropenone (DCP). *Allergy, 48,* 6–11.

Zachariae, R., & Bjerring, P. (1994). Laser-induced pain-related brain potentials and sensory pain ratings in high and low hypnotizable subjects during hypnotic suggestions of relaxation, dissociated imagery, focused analgesia, and placebo. *International Journal of Clinical & Experimental Hypnosis, 42,* 56–80.

Zachariae, R., Bjerring, P., & Arendt-Nielsen, L. (1989). Modulation of Type I immediate and Type IV delayed immuno reactivity using direct suggestion and guided imagery during hypnosis. *Allergy, 44,* 537–542.

Zachariae, R., Bjerring, P., Arendt-Nielsen, L., Nielsen, T., & Gotliebsen K. (1991a). The effect of hypnoticaly induced emotional states on brain protentials evoked by painful argon laser stimulation. *Clinical Journal of Pain, 7,* 130–138.

Zachariae, R., Bjerring, P., Zachariae, C., Arendt-Nielsen, L., Nielsen, T., Eldrup, E., Larsen, C.S., & Gotliebsen K. (1991b). Monocyte chemotactic activity in sera after hypnotically induced emotional states. *Scandinavian Journal of Immunology, 34,* 71–79.

Zachariae, R., Hansen, J. B., Andersen, M., Jinquan, T., Petersen, K.S., Simonsen, C., Zachariae, C., & Thestrup-Pedersen, K. (1994). Changes in cellular immune function after immune specific guided imagery and relaxation in high and low hypnotizable subjects. *Psychotherapy and Psychosomatics, 61,* 74–92.

Zachariae, R., Jørgensen, M. M., Christensen, S., & Bjerring, P. (1997). Effects of relaxation on the delayed-type hypersensitivity reaction to diphenylcyclopropenone (DCP). *Allergy, 52,* 760–764

Zachariae, R., Molay, F., & Sommerlund, B. (1996). Danish norms for the Harvard Group Scale of Hypnotic Susceptibility, Form A (HGSHS:A). *International Journal of Clinical and Experimental Hypnosis, 44,* 140–152.

Zachariae, R., Øster, H., & Bjerring, P. (1994). Effects of hypnotic suggestions on UV-B-radiation induced erythema and skin blood flow. *Photodermatology, Photoimmunology and Photomedicine, 10,* 154–160.

Zachariae, R., Øster, H., Bjerring, P., & Kragballe K. (1996). Effects of psychological intervention on psoriasis: A preliminary investigation. *Journal of the American Academy of Dermatology, 34,* 1008–1015.

Zeier, H., Brauchli, P., & Joller-Jemelka, H. I. (1996). Effects of work demands on immunoglobulin A and cortisol in air traffic controllers. *Biological Psychology, 42,* 413–423.

# 37

# Alternative Medicine and the Immune System

NICHOLAS R. S. HALL

## I. INTRODUCTION

In the United States and elsewhere, a growing segment of the population is turning to alternative therapies despite uncertainty as to how they work, convinced that such approaches will counter a plethora of medical ailments. A state of uncertainty is further encountered when attempting to define the concept in a manner acceptable to all who refer to it, in part because the word "alternative" is relative. Acupuncture is an alternative approach in the United States, but certainly not in Asia. The same is true of herbal remedies prescribed in Germany, but not endorsed by the dominant medical authority in the United States. Even the designation "alternative" is shunned by many who consider it judgmental, preferring instead "complementary." When considering that many protocols are used as adjuncts to conventional practices, complementary certainly reflects more accurately the manner in which such medical strategies are employed. Another term used is "traditional." Preserving the remedy in its natural form and administering it in a manner consistent with

tradition may be a valued part of the protocol. Advocates of such practices will often cite a thousand-year or longer history as evidence of a treatment's value. It is important to recognize that while such interventions may have a time-honored tradition, seldom are adjustments made based upon experience—the defining characteristic of conventional medical practices that are subject to scientific inquiry. The latter may be embraced one moment, but rejected the next when the cost–benefit ratio is found to be harmful. For the purpose of this review, the term alternative will be employed not because it is necessarily the most descriptive or best adjective, but because of common usage. It will be defined in the following way: poorly understood, difficult to assess medical intervention that is embraced by some as having efficacy, but which is not formally accepted by the regional, legally designated medical authority. However, this definition will not encompass the "off-label" use of prescription drugs in the United States even though their use for such purposes—while legal—may lack both scientific validity and formal acceptance by the Food and Drug Administration.

Alternative medical interventions are commonly embraced with a passion not always warranted by scientific data. Some do have the capacity to improve the overall health of the person using it. However, while it is clear that engaging in the behaviors associated with a particular treatment may have a desirable health outcome, it is not always clear that the mechanism of action is as postulated. In this chapter, representative protocols have been chosen to illustrate the varied mechanisms whereby the immune system might be impacted by alternative remedies. It will begin with examples of interventions that modulate health and immunity in part through psychotherapeutic processes. This will be followed by a description of plants containing hormone-receptor modifiers which in turn can influence host defense. Finally, Echinacea will serve as an example of an intervention capable of directly modifying cytokine production and lymphocyte function. Instead of focusing upon a large number of specific interventions, a few have been selected to illustrate the varied ways by which an alternative approach to treatment may modify the immune system. All medical treatments are multifactorial. This is especially true of the complex remedies associated with herbs or the sequences of rituals incorporated into some behavioral interventions. Just as the progression of disease is multifactorial—dependent upon genetic, physiological, and psychological factors—so is the successful treatment of disease dependent upon a variety of factors.

## II. INDIRECT AND PSYCHOTHERAPEUTIC ACTIONS

Alternative therapies are able to impact the course of immune system mediated disease through a variety of potential mechanisms. Some botanical remedies may work directly upon lymphocytes or through the production of cytokines. Other interventions, such as massage, may alter the activity of immunomodulatory pathways such as neuroendocrine circuits or the autonomic nervous system. For example, massage may induce a state of relaxation which would serve to counter the adverse effects of generalized stress. Massage has been found to reduce anxiety and depression in those suffering from chronic fatigue syndrome (Field et al., 1997), in adolescent mothers (Field, Grizzle, Scafidi, & Schanberg, 1996a) and in those who are HIV-positive (Field et al., 1996b; Ironson et al., 1996). This may explain the correlation between massage and elevated natural killer cell activity and CD8 cell levels in those diagnosed with HIV (Ironson et al., 1996). Others have reported a correlation between massage and elevated levels of $\beta$-endorphin (Kaard & Tostinbo, 1989), while an effect upon the lymphatics and lymphocye trafficking has also been suggested (Elkins, Herrick, & Grindlay, 1953). Regardless of whether the effects are direct or indirect, massage certainly has been found to have positive effects in treating a variety of immunologic

illness such as asthma, chronic fatigue syndrome, pediatric dermatitis, and HIV (Field, 1998).

There may be psychotherapeutic effects associated with some alternative interventions which may indirectly speed recovery from disease. For example, being involved in the negotiation of a treatment helps to counter a feeling of helplessness and speed recovery from illness (Greenfield, 1985). When a person becomes involved in deciding their care, their prognosis improves. Rodin and Langer demonstrated that when patients were able to chose a remedy, they did better with that intervention then with individuals doing the same thing but in response to a physician's orders (Rodin, 1986; Rodin & Langer, 1977). People who use alternative therapies are involved in their treatment. They have perceived control over a part of the environment that they can influence, thereby reducing their sense of helplessness. They are no longer at the mercy of a health care system which may have little to offer among the limited arsenal of accepted conventional drugs. Furthermore, a remedy would be chosen based upon the belief that it will be effective. Independent of any other mechanism, the belief in the efficacy of any medical intervention will enhance its biological activity (White, Turskey, & Schwartz, 1985). The placebo effect, as it is referred to, is more than just artifact. In the context of clinical trials undertaken by the pharmaceutical industry, it is necessary to separate placebo-driven effects from those due to a particular chemical configuration. However, placebos result in measurable biological changes. Therefore, the placebo effect is a viable mechanism whereby virtually any medical intervention may be partially explained. It also offers a compelling argument that there is a clinically relevant link between the mind and body.

Participating in healing rituals, especially with others, may constitute an additional explanation as to why alternative remedies are sometimes effective. Involvement in psychosocial support groups significantly increases the life expectancy of cancer patients (Spiegel, Bloom, Kraemer, & Gottheil, 1989). Hope also can tilt the balance between good health and disease. This has been shown in HIV positive women who continued to find meaning in life by transcending self-image (Coward, 1995). Negative expectations, reflecting a loss of hope and pessimism, are correlated with a worse prognosis for HIV-positive individuals—especially when accompanied by bereavement (Kemeny, 1996). Conversely, a fighting spirit along with increased internal locus of control has been correlated with increases in immune system measures and improved prognosis in cancer patients practicing guided imagery (Gruber et al.,1993; Hall & O'Grady, 1991). At the very least, alternative interventions provide hope. When no options remain within the arsenals of conventional medicine, through alternative channels there will often be an explanatory model accompanying a claimed treatment. Regardless of the remedy, hope remains an undeniable component of the treatment.

Some beneficial effects of alternative medicine may be psychotherapeutic. Green tea contains over 300 constituents, including catechin, which has been shown to induce apoptosis in cancerous cells (Mukhtar, 1997). The presence of antioxidants may also help to reduce the burden of free-radicals which in turn have been linked with a wide variety of chronic illnesses (Halliwell & Gutteridge, 1993). However, preparing an infusion can constitute a healing ritual. Water has to be boiled. Then it is added to the leaves or flower. A prescribed amount of time is required as the heat extracts the chemicals which will function as drugs. Additional time is required as the tea begins to cool and it is slowly sipped. The preparation and consumption of tea requires enough attention to constitute a respite from a stressful environment, but not so much attention that the task becomes an additional burden. Since many herbal drugs are prepared as either infusions or decoctions, the psychotherapeutic benefits have to be weighed when considering the mechanism of action. Only when engaging in all the behaviors associated with the acquisition and preparation of a therapy may the full healing potential be realized.

Classical conditioning may be another important variable, especially when alternative interventions are simultaneously paired with conventional therapies. Concern about adverse side-effects prompts many consumers to reject some powerful drugs. That is because, while present, the adverse effects of alternative therapies are often milder than those associated with conventional remedies. For this reason, patients may be motivated to wean themselves from the conventional drug while simultaneously administering the alternative therapy. The conventional drug could serve as the unconditioned stimulus while the alternative therapy becomes the conditioned stimulus. Through association, the alternative therapy could then acquire biological activity similar to that triggered by the unconditioned stimulus. In the manner that Pavlov was able to induce dogs to salivate and experience gastric secretions in response to the ringing of a bell, so may a person experience a desired clinical outcome after pairing a purported remedy (conditioned stimulus) with one having known

efficacy (unconditioned stimulus). While it is not recommended that a person combine herbal drugs with conventional interventions because of potential adverse effects, it could be argued that such pairing may enhance the efficacy of a weak remedy. There is ample documentation that classical conditioning can serve as a powerful modulator of the immune system (Ader & Cohen, 1975; see Ader this volume).

If conditioning is a viable mechanism, it follows that certain reinforcement regimens may be better than others. First, periodic reinforcement with continued pairing of the conditioned and unconditioned stimuli would be required to retain the effect, especially on a partial reinforcement schedule. This is quite likely to occur. A person who might find a diminished effect associated with the alternative therapy might well resort to the conventional drug during times of severe symptoms. This would serve to reinforce the conditioned effect. Thus, a biologically ineffective treatment could acquire efficacy while a treatment with a lesser potency could be strengthened.

## III. INTERVENTION-SPECIFIC EFFECTS

Botanical remedies lend themselves more readily to scientific assessment since the chemical constituents can be isolated and quantified. For that reason, representatives of this rapidly growing branch of alternative medicine have been chosen to illustrate how such interventions may impact the immune system directly or through well documented endocrine pathways. Rather than present an exhaustive review of an inconclusive literature, this section instead will focus upon potential mechanisms whereby such therapies may work. Inclusion of an intervention should not be construed as an endorsement of that strategy any more than omission of an approach reflects rejection.

### A. Reproductive Steroids

A number of plants are used in various cultures as womens' tonics. This is mostly due to the presence of phytoestrogens and phytoprogestins. Of the large number of herbs used to treat health problems, those containing the highest amounts of estrogen-binding chemicals are soy, licorice, red clover, thyme, tumeric, hops, and verbena (Zava, Dollbaum, & Blem,1998). Many of the plant-derived estrogens function as agonists when tested for bioactivity. Therefore, they may impact the immune system in a manner similar to natural ovarian estrogen. Soy, for example, contains ginsenosides that are sufficiently powerful to reduce the health risks associated with menopause as well as lengthen the reproductive cycle of women. While the evidence is limited, there is no reason that the same biologically active chemical would not modulate immunologic activities known to be altered by ovarian estrogen.

Many women consume sources of phytoestrogens for their ability to protect against the health risks associated with menopause. Included among these are osteoporosis, heart disease, and Alzheimer's disease. Coupled with genetic and biological variables, the cessation of ovarian estrogen and progesterone production sets a physiological stage enabling the symptoms of these conditions to manifest themselves. Some of the protective effects of estrogen may well be via proinflammatory cytokines. Specifically, interleukin (IL)-1, IL-11, and interferon (IFN)-$\gamma$ are known to influence osteoclasts and osteoblasts. Recently, the cytokine IL-6, which increases with age and menopause, has been identified as a bone-reactive agent which may play a central role in bone resorption (see Ershler, Harman, & Keller 1997).

Various studies have revealed that estrogen can modulate cytokine production, including inflammatory cytokines from murine splenic macrophages. 17 $\beta$-Estradiol decreases lipopolysaccharide-induced IL-1$\alpha$, IL-6, and tumor necrosis factor (TNF)-$\alpha$ production, but not IL-10, IL-12, or macrophage inflammatory protein. (Deshpande, Khalili, Pergolizzi, Michael, & Chang,1997). It is also able to inhibit inducible major histocompatibility complex class II antigen expression in allografts. (Saito, Foegh, Motomura, Lou, Kent, & Ramwell, 1998). One of the few studies that has examined the biological activity of a plant estrogen upon the immune system examined the ability of genistein, the primary phytoestrogen present in soy, to modulate the interleukin-1$\beta$ gene in a monocytic cell line. 17$\beta$-estradiol (E2) enhanced lipopolysaccharide-induced IL-1$\beta$ promoter-driven CAT activity and in a dose-dependent manner. While lacking the potency of 17 $\beta$-estradiol, genistein was, nonetheless, able to function as an agonist using this model (Ruh, Bi, Cox, Berk, Howlett, & Bellone, 1998). It also synergized with LPS to enhance IL-1$\beta$ promoter activity. Thus, while not as powerful as other environmental estrogens such as those associated with pollutants, the soy derived estrogen was able to alter IL-1 gene expression.

Some effects may be age and gender-specific. When estrogen receptors were studied in young and old, male and female C57BL/6J mice, differences were observed (Kohen et al., 1998). Thymocytes from all the animals studied exhibited evidence of estrogen receptors, however, in vivo treatment with estradiol increased the specific activity of thymic creatine kinase in only the female mice. Male thymocytes responded only to dihydrotestosterone. Thus, while present, the estrogen receptor does not appear to be functional in the males. Estrogen treatment was also found to increase the cellularity of cultured thymocytes from young, but not old animals. Consequently, if phytoestrogens are shown to be immunomodulatory, similar differences would be expected. They might have an even greater impact upon the immune system if exposure were to occur during early development.

A survey of 170 DES daughters revealed a significantly greater incidence of infectious disease as adults compared with 123 non-DES-exposed women. Highly significant were the incidences of measles and bladder infection (Vingerhoets, Assies, Goodkin, Van Heck, & Bekker,1998). Many of the developmental milestones that occur in utero in humans take place during the first few days postpartum in rodents. Therefore, it may be relevant that female mice injected with estrogen during the first 3 days after birth never ovulated and had CD8-positive thymocytes and splenocytes that were always fewer than in noninjected females (Deshpande, Chapman, & Michael, 1997). Similar changes were observed in mice exposed to estrogen from days 3 to 6; however, by 32 weeks they were comparable to control values. Thus, exposure to estrogen during a critical window of development may have an even greater impact than when exposure occurs as an adult. This has to be a consideration when exposing young children to excessive amounts of phytoestrogen-containing plants.

There also is the potential for phytoestrogens to modulate the course of autoimmune disease directly via antibody production. Long-term exposure of mice to estrogen results in the production of not only immunoglobulin-producing cells, but autoantibody-producing cells (Verthelyi & Ahmed, 1998). This observation is consistent with the fact that autoimmune disease is more prevalent in women. Systemic lupus erythematosis affects women at a ratio of 9:1 compared with men. Women also have an increased risk of developing rheumatoid arthritis and multiple sclerosis (Jansson & Holmdahl, 1998). A role for sex hormones is suggested by the decline in the intensity of symptoms after menopause. Another role for estrogen is revealed by the observation that this steroid increases calcineurin mRNA expression in cultured T cells from lupus patients, but not from age matched, healthy women (Rider, Foster, Evans, Suenaga, & Abdou, 1998). In addition, estrogen has been shown to potentiate the generation of self-reactive T cells and granulocytes in the liver and other organs (Narita, et al., 1998). In short, it would appear that estrogens should be avoided by those with susceptibility to autoimmune disease. Nonetheless, clinical experience clearly reveals that estrogen replacement therapy is often well tolerated (Buyon, 1998) despite the potential for exacerbation of symptoms following the administration of estrogen including possibly those derived from plants.

In other instances, estrogen may render the organism more susceptible to toxins. This is suggested by the observation that rats treated with estrogen 24 h prior to a sublethal dose of LPS died within 24 h, while none of the control rats succumbed (Ikejima et al., 1998). Correlated with the estrogen administration were increased levels of plasma nitrite levels and inducible nitric oxide synthase in the liver. In addition, Kupffer cells produced about twice as much TNF-$\alpha$ and nitrite in response to the estrogen treatment. Whether in high enough concentration phytoestrogens would also be able to override B-cell tolerance and induce autoreactive cells can only be the subject of speculation. It is also possible that some effects of estrogen upon the immune system may be countered by other interventions. Many individuals who embrace alternative therapies also take dietary supplements of vitamins. $\beta$-Carotene, which has been found to enhance NK cell cytolysis of YAC-1 malignant cells by 65% has been found to counter the inhibition observed following estrone exposure in athymic mice (Fernandes-Carlos, Riondel, Glise, Guiraud, & Favier, 1997).

A considerable amount of interest has focused on the role of environmental estrogens upon health (see Golden et al., 1998). As briefly reviewed, estrogen exposure during critical periods of development may leave a permanent biological footprint upon both the reproductive and the immune systems of the organism. Alone or in combination, compounds acting as weak estrogens have been linked with increased susceptibility to gonadal steroid-dependent cancers, altered patterns of sexual behavior, fertility problems, cognitive difficulties, and adverse effects upon immune and thyroid function. While there is no question that certain estrogenic compounds, such as DES, can have profound effects upon the adult organism after prenatal exposure, there is insufficient evidence to suggest that the small amounts of weak estrogenic compounds in plants would exert the same effect, especially since some act as estrogen receptor agonists while others function as antagonists. Yet, while biologically unlikely, it is not an unreasonable question to pose.

Androgens represent another category of reproductive steroids which play a role in regulating the immune system, including the balance of Th1/Th2 cytokines. Testosterone receptors have been identified on the surface of CD4 and CD8 lymphocytes (Benton et al., 1999), while androgen exposure induces T-cell lines to secrete less IFN-gamma and more IL-10 than untreated cells (Bebo, Schuster, Vandenbark, & Offner, 1999). Consequently, Saw palmetto, which is able to block the conversion of testosterone into dihydrotestosterone might be expected to indirectly impact the immune system via disruption of normal androgen pathways. High testosterone levels and/or low estrogen levels appear to be responsible for the opposite reactions that males and females have to trauma-induced hemorrhage. Males exhibit depressed immune function while females exhibit enhanced function with the effects correlating with the relative amounts of testosterone and estradiol (Angele, Ayala, Cioffi, Bland, & Chaudry, 1998). Whether Saw palmetto will prove to be capable of modulating the immune system cannot be determined without more data.

Defense against infection is critically dependent upon the expression of Fc-$\gamma$ receptors on macrophages which can be decreased with both glucocorticoids and a variety of synthetic and natural progestins (Gomez, Ruiz, Briceno, Lopez, & Michan, 1998). While phytoprogestins are usually ingested in the context of hormone replacement therapy, a potential immuno-modulatory role has to be considered. Since progestins associated with oregano, verbena, tumeric, thyme, red clover, and damiana have been found to either function as progesterone receptor antagonists or remain neutral, the clinical outcome would be highly variable depending upon the biological characteristics of the phytoprogesterone being considered (Zava, Dollbaum, & Blem, 1998). Progesterone also inhibits the conversion of cholesterol into cholesteryl ester in monocyte-derived human macrophages as well as cortisol-induced increases in cholesteryl ester (Cheng, Lau, & Abumrad, 1999).

## B. Glucocorticoids

Ginseng is used as an alternative therapy to ameliorate a variety of stress-related ailments. A limited body of evidence suggests that it may act in part upon glucocorticoid production. This might explain why it has been used in both Asian and Native American traditions as an adaptogen, enabling the consumer to better cope with stressors. However, a direct mechanism upon glucocorticoid production would provide an explanation as to how ginseng may modulate the immune system. Glucocorticoids play an important immunomodulatory role and thus have utility in treating autoimmune and inflammatory disorders along with serving as anti-inflammatory agents in preventing transplant rejection. Some effects of ginseng are direct via modulation of membrane-associated signal transduction, the expression of certain adhesion molecules, and the synthesis and release of cytokines. For example, glucocorticoids have been shown to downregulate circulating and macrophage derived IL-6 thereby having an immunoprotective effect in burn injury (Faunce, Gregory, & Kovacs, 1998). Hydrocortisone, at low concentrations, has further been shown to inhibit granulocyte-macrophage colony-stimulating factor (GM-CSF) production from normal human blood mononuclear cells and T-cells by inhibiting the expression of GM-CSF mRNA, while higher concentrations inhibit the expression of GM-CSF mRNA and also decrease T-lymphocyte count (Chikkappa, Lansing, Chu, & Pasquale, 1998). By selectively blocking the production of Th1 cytokines, glucocorticoids may enhance Th2 activity. They also influence transcriptional and post transcriptional events by binding to cytosol receptors which in turn can attach to the promotor region of cytokine genes as well as interact with nuclear factors and thereby influence gene expression (see Almawi, Hess & Rieder, 1998, and elsewhere in this volume)

Considerable evidence supports the hypothesis that ginseng is able to act at the level of the brain to modulate glucocorticoid production. Intracerebroventricular injection of a number of ginsenosides has been found to block stress-induced increases in corticosterone in mice. This inhibition was blocked by $N(G)$-nitro-L-arginine methyl ester, suggesting that the inhibition is mediated by nitric oxide (Kim et al., 1998).

Some effects of ginseng may be indirectly mediated by the gut. Aqueous solutions of ginseng root, when applied to an in vitro brain stem–gastric preparation resulted in a dose-dependent inhibition of neuronal discharge frequency, suggesting that this root may play a role in modulating digestive processes and brain-stem activity (Yuan, Wu, Lowell, & Gu, 1998). Furthermore, the ginsenoside Rb1 has been found to protect hippocampal CA1 neurons against lethal ischemic damage possibly by scavenging free radicals (Lim et al., 1997). Additional data reveal that an extract of Indian ginseng (*Withania somnifera*) can increase cortical muscarinic acetylcholine receptor capacity (Schliebs, Liebmann, Bhattacharya, Kumar, Ghosal, & Bigl, 1997), while others have demonstrated that the ginsenoside, Rb1, is able to facilitate

acetylcholine metabolism in the hippocampus (Benishin, Lee, Wang, & Liu, 1991). These findings might partly explain ginseng's use in some cultures to treat memory loss. In addition, ginseng may exert biphasic effects depending upon the age of the individual. Oral ingestion of ginseng significantly reduces dopamine levels in the striatum of old rats which also exhibited increased spontaneous motor activity during the dark phase of the day. Opposite changes in dopaminergic activity were observed in young rats (Watanabe, Ohta, Imamura, Asakura, Matoba, & Matsumoto, 1991).

While not necessarily through dampening of the glucocorticoid response, it is noteworthy that ginseng has a protective effect upon stress-induced memory loss. Ginseng has been found to prevent learning impairment and neuronal loss in guinea pigs subjected to forebrain ischemia (Wen, Yoshimura, Matsuda, Lim, & Sakanaka, 1996) and to protect hippocampal neurons from anoxic injury (Wang, Ding, & Liu, 1995). Ginseng extract also has been found to ameliorate the memory acquisition impairment stemming from bilateral lesions of the amygdala (Nishiyama, Zhou, & Saito, 1994). However, while choline acetyltransferase was significantly decreased in lesioned mice, administration of ginseng did not alter this measure. Memory loss can also occur secondary to thymectomy. Using this paradigm, a Chinese medical prescription containing ginseng has been found to improve performance in both a passive avoidance and a spatial memory task (Zhang, Saito, & Nishiyama, 1994).

## IV.  DIRECT IMMUNE INTERVENTIONS

While significant changes in a biological system can be identified using an extract of a botanical species, clinical relevance may be difficult to establish when a particular preparation is arbitrarily selected for a clinical trial. For example, Echinacea has been found in many investigations to stimulate cytokine release from human macrophages. Concentrations as low as 0.012 µg/mL stimulate a significant increase in the production of IL-1, TNF-$\alpha$, IL-6, and IL-10 (Burger, Torres, Warren, Caldwell, & Hughes, 1997). Others have reported similar effects, noting differences depending upon the manner in which the plant was prepared. Melchart et al. (1995) compared intravenous homeopathic preparations of *Echinacea purpurea* with oral alcohol and non-alcohol extracts. Two of the five protocols resulted in significant increases in phagocytic activity compared with placebo treatment, while the other regimens resulted in no change. Natural killer cell activity also can be enhanced with 0.1 µg/kg of *E. purpurea* administered to both healthy volunteers as well as those with depressed cellular immunity (see, Broumand, Sahl, & Tilles, 1997). The clinical relevance of such in vitro studies is difficult to assess; however, since some of the cytokines stimulated by Echinacea can suppress others. A high-molecular-weight extract of polysaccharides from *Echinacea angustifolia* has been found to exert anti-inflammatory effects when applied topically to mice (Tragni et al., 1988; Tragni, Tubaro, Melis, & Galli, 1985). This latter effect may be mediated by induction of IL-10 which has been found to inhibit inflammatory cytokine production by activated macrophages (Fiorentino, Zlotnik, Mosmann, Howard, & O'Garra, 1991). It is also possible that the induction of IL-10 may negate the effects of the other cytokines which might explain the failure to demonstrate an ability of Echinacea to prevent the common cold. This does not mean Echinacea is not effective in treating any immunologically mediated disorder. It simply means that more information is required before drawing conclusions, especially when assessing in vitro studies.

While a number of studies have demonstrated that Echinacea can modulate measures of the immune system, it is not clear which of the eight species is most effective, nor which part of the plant would be optimal. Neither is anything known about the appropriate dose to administer. Compounding the problem even further is the fact that commercial preparations often contain other herbs as well as zinc. Similar problems plague studies of other botanical remedies. For example, hyperacin is thought to be the anti-depressive chemical in St. John's wort which is present at highest concentration in the flower (Bisset, 1997). Some studies, though, suggest that a flavonoid may suppress cytokine production which can potentiate the symptoms of depression. Thus, St. John's wort may help to alleviate those forms of depression due to chronic immune system activation.

## V. INTERPRETATION ISSUES

There are numerous difficulties in interpreting the results of studies designed to evaluate the drugs found in herbs. Foremost is the formidable task of determining cause and effect. Many herbal preparations contain complex mixtures of chemicals which vary from one supplier to another depending upon growth conditions, maturity of the plant when harvested, or part of the plant being administered.

Potency also varies depending upon soil and other growing conditions, duration of storage, handling, and preparation. In addition to the natural ingredients, contaminants may be present, especially heavy metals and pesticides, which have an affinity for herbs (Bisset, 1997). Furthermore, virtually all herbal products have a tendency to accumulate pollutants such as pesticides and heavy metals. A Chinese patent medicine, Jin bu huan, has been linked with several cases of liver damage in the United States, while Hai ge fen has been linked with lead and other heavy metal poisonings. Ephedrine alkaloids—found in Ma huang—and the presence of animal-derived endocrine glands in other mixtures further confounds the interpretation of data. Either the natural ingredients or contaminants may be responsible for both desirable and undesirable effects, such as anaphylaxis and hyperthyroidism (Mullins, 1998; Eliason, Donenier, & Nuhlicek, 1994 ). Therefore, changes observed during empirical testing may not necessarily be due to the constituent of interest.

Different preparations are often used in clinical protocols and sometimes prepared in a manner that departs from the tradition from which it arose. When used as a remedy for nervous conditions, the flower of St. John's wort was traditionally prepared as an infusion or tea, although when applied as an antiseptic, it was prepared as a poultice. However, it is commonly available in the United States as a dried preparation administered in a capsule. A 1998 survey by the Los Angeles times revealed considerable variability between preparations of St. Johns wort being sold through retail outlets. In addition to the flower, stems and leaves were often present which have varying amounts of hyperacin and other ingredients.

Herbal remedies may appear to modulate immunity, but instead directly impact the growth of microbial pathogens. Garlic, tea tree oil, propolis, and grapefruit seed extract are each being marketed as antibiotics, while Echinacea is promoted as both an antibiotic and inducer of cytokine production. Antiviral, parasitic, and fungal properties have been associated with a large number of botanical species, especially those of the African tradition (Oliver-Bever, 1986). Other botanicals may help to alleviate symptoms of infection without necessarily altering bacterial cell division or the immune system. For example, ginger and licorice are used to loosen mucus. Other botanicals are used to alleviate the symptoms of allergies. Ma huang and Albizzia are each promoted as treatments for asthma while Baical skullcap and Quercetin are touted as anti-histamine and anti-inflammatory agents, respectively. The average person would be concerned about only an alleviation of symptoms and therefore might erroneously attribute a remedy to impacting immunity when in fact it is exerting a direct effect upon either the expression of symptoms or the proliferation of a pathogen. This may explain the popularity of Echinacea. By increasing IL-10, it may alleviate "sickness behaviors" by blocking other cytokines, while having minimal impact upon those immune system pathways that might be required to eliminate a pathogen.

The method of preparation also can result in biphasic effects. *Valerianae radix* when prepared as a tea has been administered as a sedative in some cultures. Valerenic acid is a muscle relaxant while related sequiterpenes are thought to inhibit the degradation of gamma amino butyric acid. (Bisset, 1997). However, isolated valepotriates in prepared medications may have the opposite effect, serving as psychostimulants. Similarly, the relative concentrations of arbutin and tannins varies considerably depending upon whether bearberry leaves are first boiled or extracted cold. In the kidney, arbutin is claimed to be activated as an antiseptic which then is thought to promote recovery from urinary tract infection. When prepared as an infusion, equal amounts of tannin and arbutin will be obtained. However, if prepared as a maceration, the ratio of tannin to arbutin increases. This is not necessarily undesirable. It has been found that tannins in cranberry juice may prevent bacteria from adhering to the cell wall of the urinary tract. These observations clearly underscore the fact that method of preparation may have a profound impact upon efficacy.

Unfortunately, many questions concerning the safety and pharmacokinetics of herbal drugs will continue to remain unknown. That is because of a lobbying effort that resulted in the passage of the Food Supplement Act of 1994. The Food and Drug Administration sought authority to start testing herbal and other remedies for safety and efficacy. This attempt prompted the largest letter writing campaign since the Vietnam conflict regarding a policy issue. Manufacturers protested that being required to bear the financial burden of testing herbal drugs was unfair since their product could not be protected with a patent. The clear message sent to the United States Congress was to leave herbal remedies readily available with minimal restrictions regarding their marketing. Some remedies may be more effective when taken with food. Time of day when the remedy is taken may influence others. Efficacy as well as side-effects may vary depending upon the dose or whether other types of medications are being consumed. This and related information simply are not known, so statements regarding clinical effectiveness are based largely upon marketing claims and traditional beliefs rather than a solid foundation of scientific literature. It does not mean that the claims are incorrect. It means only that there are few objective criteria by which to assess their validity.

## VI. POLITICAL ISSUES

The fervor with which some individuals embrace alternative remedies is not dissimilar to that expressed by those who embrace a fundamentalist religious philosophy. This is not surprising. Many people turn to alternative therapies out of desperation. They are told by their physician that there are no options available through conventional medicine, or they may not be able to afford the drugs that have been prescribed for their ailment. The choice may be limited to an unproven treatment or no treatment— the option of doing something or assuming a posture of helplessness. A judgement concerning an alternative treatment becomes a commentary about the intervention, the person's belief system, as well as their sense of hope. It is no wonder that such a large amount of passion envelops the practice of alternative medicine. There also is an enormous amount of conflict between the practitioners of conventional and alternative medicine with fault on both sides.

Many claims are embellished with sweeping statements having little validity. This is reflected in the message on an envelope sent out by a marketer proclaiming, "the all natural healing secrets doctors don't tell you." It does not specify whether these are psychiatrists or naturopaths, or whether they are family doctors or neurologists. It just says "doctors." The purported implication is that all doctors are part of a well organized global conspiracy that includes the pharmaceutical industry and the National Institutes of Health, supposedly conspiring to keep the American people from having natural remedies readily available. This is simply not true. There are many doctors researching this topic and making recommendations for herbal interventions to their patients. Over half the medical schools in the United States now include information about alternative medicine as part of their curriculum. This is because medical educators recognize the clinical value of some of the interventions and the need to understand what patients are using for self-medication, whether scientifically sound or not.

The fault is not among only the practitioners of alternative medicine. It is to be found among the more conservative element of the medical profession. *"The fact that para-herbalists fail to develop or accept accurate*

# Behavioral Genetics
# and Immunity

JOHN M. PETITTO

## I. INTRODUCTION

Whether certain behavioral traits may render individuals more vulnerable to some immune-related disease states is an intriguing question at the heart of psychoneuroimmunology. Despite considerable theorizing about the relationship of heritable personality variables to disease susceptibility (e.g., Fox, 1978; Hagnell, 1966; Solomon, 1981; Wellisch & Yager, 1983), there are only limited data from controlled experiments relating immune status parameters to complex behavioral traits. The potential effects of various developmental and experiential states on immune status and the biological mechanisms involved are well documented in the literature and reviewed elsewhere in this text. In psychoneuroimmunology research, the influence of individual differences in behavior on immunity has focused on determining if such behavioral differences may govern the physiological response of the individual (e.g., hypothalamic–pituitary–adrenal reactivity, sympathetic autonomic nervous system reactivity) to particular developmental, experiential or stressful psychosocial conditions (states). Elsewhere in this edition, Drs. Kemeny and

Laudenslager discuss relevant research pertaining to such neurobehavioral influences on individual differences in immunological reactivity in animals and humans. The pages that follow, by contrast, will focus on examining the basis for the hypothesis that particular genetically determined differences in parameters of behavior and immunity (traits) may be co-heritable variables.

The aim of this chapter is to examine some of the salient data that address a genetic hypothesis, that is, that subsets of genes involved in the expression of complex behavioral and immunological traits may be physically linked, interactive at the level of the genome, or shared by the brain and the immune system. Since the data available to test this hypothesis are quite limited, a good portion of this chapter is theoretical, examining ideas and strategies applicable to ongoing and future genetic studies in the field. It is a formidable challenge to address such questions in humans, and as is often the case, animal models can provide valuable research paradigms to disentangle multifactorial behavioral-immune relationships. Although most of the data described herein are from studies using rodent models, translation of such findings to humans is possible. Enormous strides are being made in molecular genetics and there is striking homology between the organization of human and mouse (and more recently rat) genomes. Thus, genes of interest, specific chromosomal loci, and linkages identified in the rodent may be found in homologous regions of the human genome.

## II. SELECTIVE BREEDING

### A. Background and Theory

The behavioral traits associated with parameters of immunity examined throughout this chapter fall within the behavioral domains of emotionality and of learning and memory. Although beyond the scope of this chapter, there is a large literature that has used selective breeding and other approaches (e.g., recombinant inbred strains) to study the genetics of behavioral responses and differential sensitivity of animals to psychotropic drugs and various drugs of abuse, in particular, alcohol (Crabbe, Belknap, & Buck, 1994). The potential genetic relationship between traits such as susceptibility to alcohol and other drugs of abuse and immunity may be a significant area of inquiry in psychoneuroimmunology (Bonneau, Mormede, Vogler, McClearn, & Jones, 1998). Selected behavioral traits related to drug responsiveness have also been found to be associated with differences in parameters of immune status in mice and rats (Fride, McIntyre, Skolnick, & Arora, 1993; Friedman, Irwin, & Overstreet, 1996; Petitto, McIntyre, McRae, Skolnick, & Arora, 1990).

The strategy of selective breeding has provided valuable models to study the neurobiological basis of trait differences including alcohol sensitivity (Crabbe et al., 1994; Fuller & Thompson, 1978), active avoidance learning (Brush, Froehlich, & Sakellaris, 1979), emotionality (Broadhurst, 1958), open-field activity (DeFries, Gervais, & Thomas, 1978), and aggression (Cairns, MacCombie, & Hood, 1983; Lagerspetz, Tirri, & Lagerspetz, 1968; Sandnabba, 1995; Van Oortmerssen & Baker, 1981). Selective breeding has also been used to study the genetic regulation of immune responsiveness (e.g., Biozzi et al., 1979). Selectively bred animal lines are also valuable in that they provide models to study how different genotypes may interact with environmental factors (e.g., developmental and experiential conditions) to produce phenotypes or traits.

In selective breeding experiments, outbred animals are selected for high and low levels of expression of a phenotype of interest (e.g., an observable behavioral or physiological characteristic). The animals selected from the high and low ends of the distribution are then mated among themselves (high phenotype animals with high phenotype animals, and low phenotype animals with low phenotype animals). Following multiple successive generations of systematic selection and breeding, a wide divergence results in the selected phenotypic response. At the "selection limit," the high and low lines are con-sidered to be homozygous at the various polymorphic gene alleles involved in encoding high versus low levels of the selected trait. Inbreeding is proscribed in selective breeding (no sibling and cousin mating) and if rigorous methodological procedures are followed (e.g., using large numbers of breeding pairs, maintaining careful control of environmental conditions across generations), genes that are not involved in encoding the selected trait should assort randomly. Said another way, all of the remaining gene alleles that are not associated with the selected trait of interest, are expected to occur at the same frequency in the high and low lines (Fuller & Thompson, 1978). If it is found that the two lines also differ significantly in an unselected second trait, a genetic correlation may exist between the selected trait (e.g., behavioral) and the second, associated trait (e.g., immunological). Such an outcome suggests that either a common group of genes may be involved in encoding both the selected and the associated traits (referred to as pleiotropy) or that each trait may be encoded by different but neighboring genes that are physically linked and cosegregating on the same chromosome. As discussed in subsequent sections, other factors may also be involved and potentially confounding factors must be carefully ruled out before it is concluded that a true genetic correlation exists between the two traits (Crabbe, Phillips, Kosobud, & Belnap, 1990; Henderson, 1989).

### B. Selective Breeding for Behavioral Traits: Association with Line Differences in Immune Status

As seen in Table I, several studies have sought to determine if mice and rats that have been selectively bred for differences in certain emotional and cognitive traits also differ in parameters of immune status and/or disease susceptibility. Sandi and colleagues examined immune status measures in two lines of Wistar rats selected for high and low levels of active avoidance learning (Sandi, Castanon, Vitiello, Neveu, & Mormede, 1991). These rat lines are referred to as the Roman high and low avoidance lines. These lines had previously been found to differ in stress-induced brain monoamine turnover in prefrontal cortex and in stimulated HPA axis activity, which led these investigators to examine if immune functioning might also differ between the Roman high and low avoidance lines. They found that the high avoidance line has lower splenic NK cell activity against YAC-1 tumor cells in vitro. Across effector to tumor target cell ratios, NK cells from the high avoidance line showed activity levels of approxi-

TABLE I   Selective Breeding Experiments for Differences in Emotional and Cognitive Domains of Behavior: Association with Line Differences in Immune Status

| Species | Selectively bred trait | Immune/disease status variables | References |
|---|---|---|---|
| Rat | High and low active avoidance | High line has lower NK cell activity and mitogen-induced T lymphocyte proliferation<br>No line differences in mitogen- induced B cell proliferation or antibody responses to SRBC | Sandi et al., 1991<br>Castanon et al., 1992 |
| Mouse | High and low isolation-induced aggression | Low line is more susceptible to chemical carcinogen-induced tumor development and has lower NK cell activity, mitogen-induced T lymphocyte proliferation, IL-2 and IFN-$\gamma$ production<br>No line differences in mitogen-induced B cell proliferation | Petitto et al., 1993, 1994, 1999 |
| Rat | High and low open field reactivity | No line differences in chemical carcinogen-induced tumor development | Eysenck, 1983 |

Note. NK, natural killer; SRBC, sheep red blood cell; IFN, interferon.

mately one-half those of the low avoidance line. These line differences in NK activity were increased somewhat in splenocytes from animals immediately following the behavioral challenge of a shuttle box avoidance paradigm. The magnitude of this difference, however, was similar to the differences observed between unchallenged animals of the high and low lines. In addition, the high avoidance line was found to have significantly reduced splenic T cell proliferative responses to the mitogens concanavalin A (Con A) and phytohemagglutinin (PHA), with [$^3$H]thymidine incorporation ranging from levels of approximately two-thirds to one-half the levels of the low avoidance line. These differences were found for both males and females of the high vs. low avoidance lines. No line differences were seen in B lymphocyte proliferative responses to lipopolysaccharide (LPS) stimulation, nor for the primary or secondary antibody responses to sheep red blood cell (SRBC) antigens.

In a follow-up study, Castanon and colleagues were unable to link the immune differences between the Roman high and low avoidance lines to differences in HPA axis function (Castanon, Dulluc, LeMoal, & Mormede, 1992). The endocrine measures tested included basal HPA axis activity as well as activity following corticotropin-releasing factor (CRF) and novel environments used as acute stressors. Basal and challenge-related activity in ACTH, corticosterone, and aldosterone did not differentiate the lines, indicating that the HPA axis was not responsible for mediating the robust difference in cellular immune status between the Roman high and low avoidance rats. Although they did find that exposure to a novel open field resulted in significant differences in prolactin secretion between the lines, basal prolactin levels were not different. Since the marked differences in NK cell activity (Castanon et al., 1992; Sandi et al., 1991)

and mitogen stimulated T lymphocyte proliferation (Sandi et al., 1991) in the lines were seen under basal conditions, it unlikely that prolactin was responsible for the line differences in cellular immune activity.

Sandi et al. (1991) also examined the NK cell activity of the first filial generation (F1) of a cross between the high and the low avoidance lines. As predicted for a phenotypic outcome in a cross of high and low lines, in the nonsegrating F1 generation, NK cell activity levels were intermediate between the high and the low avoidance parental lines. Maternal developmental influences (i.e., whether the mother of a high-low mating pair was from the high or low avoidance line) also influenced the NK activity of the F1 offspring. Specifically, they found that maternal developmental influences (unidentified pre- and postnatal maternal influences) transmitted from high avoidance mothers resulted in lower NK activity. Thus, the NK activity phenotype of the F1 mice was shown to be the result of an interaction between environmental factors (maternal developmental influences) and genetics.

As summarized in Table I, selective breeding for differences in aggression has also been found to be associated with differences in immunity (Petitto et al., 1993, 1999; Petitto, Lysle, Gariepy, & Lewis, 1994). Our group has used two lines of Institute for Cancer Research (ICR) mice that were selectively bred for high and low levels of aggression. Aggression was assessed in a neutral test chamber following post-weaning social isolation of the selectively bred animal. Partner animals were group housed, non-selected ICR mice. The original breeding program by Cairns and colleagues was aimed at developing lines with both high and low aggressive characteristics. Relatively little change in isolation-induced attack, however, has been observed across generations in the high aggressive (NC900) line relative to the foundational stock and to nonselected, randomly bred mice derived from the same ICR stock. By contrast, considerable decreases in attack were observed across generations of the low aggressive (NC100) line (Cairns, MacCombie, & Hood, 1983). Therefore, the selective breeding program has led to a line of mice (NC100) that fails to exhibit the isolation-induced aggression expected of this mouse strain (Gariepy, Hood, & Cairns, 1988). Moreover, the line differences in behavior appear to be selective to social contexts since several domains of nonsocial behavior including fear-motivated behaviors in response to novelty, reactivity to tactile stimulation, and overall motor activity do not reliably differentiate the lines (Gariepy, Hood, & Cairns, 1988; Petitto et al., 1993). In a study which compared levels of splenic NK cell activity and susceptibility to 3-methylcholanthrene (3-MC)-induced tumor development, the low aggressive line had significantly lower NK cell activity and increased occurrence of tumor development relative to the high aggressive line (Petitto et al., 1993). In the low aggressive line (NC100), NK cell activity against YAC-1 tumor target cells was less than one-half of that of the high aggressive line (NC900). Interestingly, there were no differences in NK activity between high aggressive (NC900) mice and randomly bred mice (nonselected ICR mice, referred to as NC600). By 17 weeks following 3-MC tumor induction, all of the low aggressive line had developed tumors, compared to 44% of the high aggressive line. In addition, the low aggressive mice exhibited evidence of greater tumor burden, with 30% of the mice having tumors weighing 3 g or more, whereas none of the high aggressive mice had tumors that large. Additional studies have revealed that, in addition to NK activity, the low aggressive line also had lower levels of splenic T-cell responsiveness (Petitto et al., 1994). The low aggressive line had significantly reduced splenic T-cell proliferative responses to Con A, with stimulation indices ranging from approximately two-thirds to one-half the levels of the high aggressive mice. The low aggressive line also produced lower levels of the Th1 cytokines, interleukin-2 and interferon-$\gamma$, than the high aggressive line; the effect sizes for these immune measures, however, were modest compared to those seen for NK activity and mitogen-induced T-cell proliferation. No line differences were found in B lymphocyte proliferation following LPS stimulation. Basal serum corticosterone concentrations and splenic norepinepherine concentrations do not differ between the lines (Petitto et al., 1993, 1999). Although systematic investigation of other potential neurobiological pathways that may be involved has not been

performed, these data suggest that the robust differences in immune status are not attributable to differences in tonic control by adrenal corticosterone or splenic norepinepherine.

In our studies of the high aggressive (NC900) and low aggressive (NC100) mice, we have attempted to dissect further this novel association by performing experiments designed to test two competing hypotheses. The first hypothesis was that the phenotypic expression of the line differences in NK cell activity are dependent on and regulated by the expression of high and low levels of aggressive behavior in the lines. The alternative hypothesis was that the differences in immune status are independent of the expression of aggression by the lines, suggesting linkage between a subset of genes involved in determining these complex behavioral and imunological traits or pleiotropy. In these experiments the immunological assessment focused on NK cell activity because we have found robust differences between the lines across several generations, suggesting that this would be a reliable dependent measure. Behaviorally, isolation is the "state" under which the most robust line differences in social behavior are observed in a dyadic social interaction test of aggression in males (Cairns, Hood, & Midlam, 1985). By contrast, group housing attenuates the magnitude of the line differences in male aggressive behavior in a dyadic social interaction test (Cairns et al., 1983, 1985; Gariepy et al., 1988). Thus, three conditions of postweaning social experience (mice singly housed, group housed within line, or group housed between lines) were tested in males to determine whether experiential conditions which modify the expression of aggression would, in turn, modify the line differences in NK cell activity (Petitto et al., 1999). The results showed that the difference in NK cell activity between high aggressive and low aggressive male mice was attributable to line only. The different postweaning social conditions examined had no effect on modifying the differences in NK activity. Moreover, the social dominance hierarchy among group housed males did not correlate with levels of NK cell activity.

These two competing hypotheses were examined further in studies that compared NK cell function in males versus females of the high and low aggressive lines. Because males of the two lines exhibit differences in aggressive behavior across social contexts, females were tested. Testing females of the lines provided an opportunity to examine the hypothesis that the line differences in NK cell activity would be observed independent of aggressive experience or the conditions associated with the expression of aggression (Hood & Cairns, 1988). Once again, the data showed that only line accounted for the marked differences in NK cell activity seen between NC900 and NC100 mice. Females of the low aggressive line had low levels of NK activity compared to high aggressive females and the magnitude of the line difference was comparable to that between males of the high and those of the low lines. Taken together, these experiments lend support to the hypothesis that this association may be due to genetics. In contrast to the Roman high and low avoidance rat lines described earlier, the line differences in NK cell function in the high aggressive (NC900) and low aggressive (NC100) mouse lines appears to be largely independent of post-weaning environmental factors which modify the behavior of the lines. Although postnatal experience did not modify the line differences in NK cell activity, it is possible that pre- and perinatal factors could be important. Pre- and perinatal experience can have long-term effects on behavior (e.g., Denenberg & Rosenberg, 1967), neuroendocrinology (e.g., Levine, 1967), and immunity (e.g., Denenberg et al., 1991; Miyawki, Moriya, Nagoki, & Taniguchi, 1981; Solomon, Levine, & Kraft, 1968). Therefore, the impact of these forms of experience cannot be ruled out in the high and low aggressive lines and may warrant further investigation.

Eysenck (1983) studied the vulnerability of rats selectively bred for emotional reactivity to develop tumors following 3,4-benzpyrene. These lines, referred to the Maudsley reactive and nonreactive rats, were originally selectively bred by Broadhurst (1976) for differences in defecation in a novel open field. In that experiment, Eysenck and co-workers were testing the hypothesis that exposure of the Maudsley reactive and nonreactive lines to an identical stressor (footshock prior to tumor implantation) would result in differences in tumor development. As seen in table 1, no differences were found in tumor development between the lines, either between unstressed rats of the reactive versus nonreactive lines or between stressed rats of the reactive and those of the nonreactive lines. Several potentially interesting interactions between the variables were observed, however, suggesting that further study of the Maudsley reactive and nonreactive rats may be informative.

### C. Genetic Correlations between Behavioral and Immunological Variables?

The selective breeding studies just described illustrate some of the caveats and shortcomings encountered in selectively breeding experiments where two traits (the selected trait and a second, nonselected trait) appear to be correlated. First, it is interesting that in both the studies of Sandi and co-workers in rats selectively bred for high and low active avoidance learning and Petitto and colleagues in mice selected for high and low aggression, similar immunological differences were seen between these two sets of high and low lines. In both cases, the high and low lines exhibited differences in NK cell activity and T-lymphocyte responsiveness to Con A stimulation, whereas neither set of lines differed in B-lymphocyte responsiveness to LPS stimulation. Although extensive immunological assessments have not been conducted in either of these sets of selectively bred lines, the outcome that similar immunological differences between the two sets of lines has occurred is intriguing. Interestingly, in both cases the robust line differences in basal NK and T-cell activity in un-challenged animals were not readily attributable to differences in HPA axis activity (although it is possible that dynamic changes in prolactin secretion could be involved in the high and low avoidance rats; Castanon et al., 1992). Although similar immunological correlates were seen between the Roman high and low avoidance lines and the NC high and low aggressive lines, the contribution of genetic versus developmental/experiental influences appears to differ between these two sets of selected lines. In the Roman high and low avoidance lines, Sandi et al. (1991) found that maternal developmental influences make a significant contribution. As noted by Henderson (1989), in an extreme scenario it is possible in selective breeding studies that a second trait (e.g., an immune status parameter) that is found to be correlated with the selected trait (e.g., a behavioral trait) could be determined largely by maternal environmental factors and not accounted for to any significant degree by genetics.

By contrast, in the NC high and low aggressive mice, we have found that developmental rearing conditions postweaning that modify the magnitude of the behavioral differences had no effect on the magnitude of the immunological differences (Petitto et al., 1994, 1999). Thus, the association between these complex behavioral and immunological traits could represent a true genetic correlation, although several notable caveats must first be considered. It is also possible that this association is a fortuitous one. Nonrandom association of gene alleles can occur in randomly bred and selectively bred laboratory colonies due to genetic drift toward homogeneity at some gene loci. Rather than being polymorphic, such gene alleles may become inbred or fixed in selected lines. The genes involved in determining an immune outcome such as NK activity may have been fixed during selective breeding and the association between these traits may not represent a true genetic correlation (Crabbe et al., 1994; Henderson, 1989). Henderson (1989) suggests that in order to estimate whether a second trait associated with a selected trait is a true genetic correlate or due to other factors such as genetic drift, selective breeding strategies should employ the use of a second set of replicate lines. Unfortunately, this is not commonly performed in selective breeding experiments, in part, due to the considerable expense involved.

Using the converse strategy, Vidal and Rama (1994) examined the behavioral characteristics of mice selectively bred for differences in immune status. They test several measures of emotional behavior in the Biozzi high and low antibody responder lines that were bred for serum agglutinin response to SRBC (Biozzi et al., 1979). The high and low antibody responder lines were found to differ in two of the emotional behavioral paradigms tested. The low antibody responder line had higher responses in rearing behavior in an open field (under conditions of dim but not bright lighting) and in a behavioral response-to-capture paradigm. To determine whether a genetic correlation was present between level of the antibody response and the emotional behavioral measures, Vidal et al. (1994) examined the immune–behavior relationship in the genetically segregating (segregation for the formation of recombinant chromosomes) second filial generation (F2) mice of a cross mating between the high and low antibody responder lines. They found that antibody response levels and the behavior were not correlated in F2 mice. This finding may indicate a fortuitous association between the immune and the behavioral traits seen in the parental lines. On the other hand, since multiple genes are involved in determining complex traits, as described in the sections that follow, not all of the loci involved in producing many complex traits cosegregate (e.g., multiple genes, located on a handful of different chromosomes control each of the various pathogenetic steps in a disease like autoimmune diabetes). Thus, in lines selectively bred for differences in a specific behavior, if the lines are also found to differ in a second trait such as susceptibility to a disease, all of the genetic loci involved in producing the associated disease susceptibility trait may not cosegregate in the F2 generation of a cross between the high and low lines. Therefore, if only the presence or absence of disease is examined in the F2 generation and no association between the behavioral and the disease traits are found, one would conclude that the two traits are not genetically correlated. It is possible,

however, that some of the component loci that each encode different processes that together result in the expression of the disease trait may actually cosegregate with the behavioral measure.

## III. MECHANISMS BY WHICH BEHAVIORAL AND IMMUNOLOGICAL TRAITS CO-VARY?

### A. Conceptualization

As alluded to in the preceding sections, there are several ways by which behavioral and immunological traits may be associated and co-vary. These are depicted in the simple schematic diagrams in Figure 1 and summarized briefly. First, genetically determined differences in behavior (traits) may differentially modify the physiological response (e.g., HPA axis reactivity, sympathetic autonomic nervous system reactivity) of individuals to particular developmental or experiential conditions (states), which, in turn, can differentially modify immune physiology. This is depicted in Figure 1A. In this scenario, the genes involved in controlling the behavioral and immune responses of interest are not physically linked to one another (behavioral gene 1 and immune response gene 1 are depicted here on separate chromosomes). The second way in which behavioral and immunological traits may be associated and co-vary is that they are linked (gene loci physically close or adjacent to each other on the same chromosome). This is illustrated in Figure 1B, where a gene involved in determining a behavioral trait (behavioral gene 2) and one determining an immunological trait (immune gene 2) neighbor one another on the same chromosome. The closer in proximity to one another, the less the likelihood for recombination events and the greater the probability that these two genes will cosegregate. Such examples are the topic of the following section. In the third scenario, a gene (or set of genes) may be involved in encoding a process common to both the expression of a behavioral and that of an immunological trait (pleiotropic gene effects that influence both traits). This is depicted in Figure 1C as a common pathway gene. As noted in other chapters in this textbook, perhaps the simplest examples of this would occur in the case where a particular gene is knocked out, and the loss of this gene product is found to result in alterations in both the central nervous and the immune systems. In studies performed in my laboratory, for example, we have demonstrated that in addition to producing marked effects on the immune system, IL-2 gene

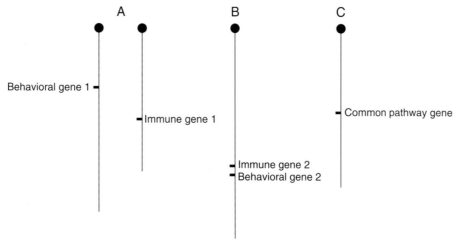

**FIGURE 1**  Simple schematic diagram illustrating three ways by which behavioral and immunological traits may be associated and co-vary.

deletion produces robust impairments in spatial learning and alterations in hippocampal cytoarchitecture (Petitto, McNamara, Gendreau, Huang, & Jackson, 1999). Another interesting example is seen in mice with the nude mutation. In addition to the immunological abnormalities (e.g., athymic, NK deficient), this mutation has also been reported to modify ambulatory activity in an open field and the response to a conspecific in a social interaction paradigm (Vidal, 1996). The nude mutation has also been associated with deficits in thyroxine, estradiol, and progesterone secretion (Kopf-Maier & Mboneko, 1990).

## B. Behavioral Quantitative Trait Loci (QTL) and Linked Immune-related Genes or Intervals

Most complex behavioral traits do not follow simple Mendelian inheritance patterns, but are commonly multigenically controlled. Some multigenically controlled complex traits can be either discontinuous traits (e.g., such as the presence or absence of disease) or continuous traits (exhibiting a continuous phenotypic distribution). In most cases, it appears that complex behavioral traits are continuous. For a continuous trait, none of the individual genes involved is sufficient for the expression of the complex trait, and the trait is determined by the segregation of multiple loci (often on different chromosomes). Each locus makes a quantitative contribution to the total variance in expression of the trait. The individual loci involved in controlling continuous traits, therefore, are referred to as quantitative trait loci (QTL) or polygenes (Crabbe et al., 1994; Tanksley, 1993). The genome

project and other factors have led to recent advances in molecular genetics research. These include combining polymerase chain reaction (PCR)-based genomewide scanning methods using phenotypically neutral genetic markers (e.g., over 7000 such markers have been identified in the mouse) referred to as simple sequence length polymorphisms (SSLPs) and computer-based statistical modeling software (Dietrich et al., 1996). This permits researchers to identify the chromosomal addresses of loci involved as well as estimate their relative contribution to the expression of a complex trait (Lander & Kruglyak, 1995; Tanksley, 1993).

To determine if specific candidate immunological genes and/or immune-related disease susceptibility loci might be physically linked to QTL for emotional or learning and memory behavioral traits, these behavioral QTL were obtained by searching the available behavioral genetics literature using Medline. The Mouse Genome Database was then searched for immune genes or loci that might be candidates for linkage to each significant behavioral QTL (performed in the Fall, 1998). The results are summarized in Tables II and III. Linkage is expressed as the frequency of recombination between two loci. As mentioned earlier, the closer in proximity to one another, the less the likelihood for recombination events and the greater the probability that two loci will cosegregate. By definition, the distance of 1 centimorgan (cM) on genome maps is associated with a recombination frequency of 1%, which corresponds to approximately 1 Mb (Lander & Schork, 1994; Lander & Kruglyak, 1995). In generating these tables, a map distance of ≤10 cM was adopted as the operational definition for potential linkage candidates (e.g., a marker interval size of 10 cM is common in genome-wide scans and is sufficient to assess linkages in most experiments where sample size and other methodological conditions are met; Zeng, 1994). In general, where it was possible to ascertain, a QTL that did not meet conservative estimates of linkage (e.g., Lander & Kruglak, 1995) was not included. The two tables are organized by behavioral trait (emotional behaviors in Table II, and learning and memory in Table III), and the data presented in them is generally self-explanatory.

It is noteworthy that a QTL for learning in a contextual fear conditioning paradigm (Owen, Christensen, Paylor, & Wehner, 1997) and emotional behavior in a Y-maze (Flint et al., 1995) were localized to the same location on chromosome 12 in two independent studies. In the fear conditioning study by Owen and colleagues (1997), the specific behavioral measure that was localized to this area of chromosome 12 was freezing behavior in an altered context. It may be that the genes in this interval are involved in controlling the freezing response to novelty rather than controlling learning per se in this paradigm. Like Y-maze activity that was also localized to this same area of chromosome 12, freezing behavior commonly falls within the domain of

TABLE II    Emotional Behavioral Quantitative Trait Loci (QTL) and Linked Immune Genes
or Susceptibility Loci within 10 cM Distance on a Chromosome

| Location (chromosome, cM) | Behavioral QTL | Reference | Linked immune genes/Loci | Position (cM) |
|---|---|---|---|---|
| 1, 73.2 | Open field behavior | Gershenfeld & Paul, 1997 | Intracisternal A particle, lymphocyte specific 3-1 | 66.6 |
| | | | Chemokine receptor 4 | 67.4 |
| | | | Interleukin-10 | 69.9 |
| | | | B-cell translocation gene 2, anti-proliferation | 71.0 |
| | | | Sjogren syndrome antigen A2 | 78.7 |
| | | | Trypanosome infection response 3 | 81.6 |
| 1, 100.0 | Covarying tests: Open field activity and defecation, Y-maze activity, elevated plus (open arm entries) | Flint et al., 1995 | Lupus NZB × NZW 7 | 90.0 |
| | | | Fc receptor IgG, low affinity IIb | 92.3 |
| | | | Intracisternal A particle, lymphocyte specific 2-38 | 92.5 |
| | | | Cytotoxic T lymphocyte response 1 | 92.7 |
| | | | Non-MHC restricted killing associated | 93.0 |
| | | | Lymphocyte stimulating determinant | 93.1 |
| | | | CD48 antigen, Fc receptor IgE high affinity gamma polypeptide, and lymphocyte antigen 9 | 93.3 |
| | | | Fc receptor high affinity I alpha polypeptide | 94.2 |
| | | | New Zealand Black autoimmunity 2 | 95.0 |
| | | | Interferon activated genes 201, 203, and 204 | 95.2 |
| | | | Histocompatibility 25 | 100.0 |
| | | | Colon tumor susceptibility 3, and transforming growth factor beta 2 | 101.5 |
| | | | Tumor necrosis factor receptor-associated factor 5 | 105.0 |
| | | | CD34 antigen, complement receptor 2 and complement related protein | 106.6 |
| | | | Autoimmune orchitis resistance 4 | 110.0 |
| 10, 72.1, and 74.1 | Light-to-dark transition | Gershenfeld & Paul, 1997 | Interferon gamma | 67.0 |
| | | | CD63 antigen | 72.0 |
| | | | Neuro-oncological ventral antigen related sequence 3 | 72.5 |
| 12, 4.0 | Y-maze activity | Flint et al., 1995 | Cytokine induced activation 2 | 1.0 |
| | | | Tumor necrosis factor alpha converting enzyme | 3.0 |
| 15, 14.0 | Open field activity | Flint et al., 1995 | Leukemia inhibitory factor receptor | 4.6 |
| | | | Intracisternal A particle, lymphocyte specific probe 3-45 | 22.7 |

TABLE III  Learning and Memory Behavioral Quantitative Trait Loci (QTL) and Linked Immune Genes or Susceptibility Loci within 10 cM Distance on a Chromosome

| Location (chromosome, cM) | Behavioral QTL | Reference | Linked immune genes/loci | Position (cM) |
|---|---|---|---|---|
| 1, 29.0 | Contextual fear conditioning (freezing during contextual task) | Caldarone et al., 1997 | Interleukin-1 receptor types I and II | 19.5 |
| | | | Autoimmune orchitis resistance 5 | 20.0 |
| | | | Lymphocyte antigen 84 | 20.6 |
| 1, 60.8 | Contextual fear conditioning (freezing during contextual task) | Owen et al., 1997 | Chemokine orphan receptor 1 | 55.6 |
| | | | Intracisternal A particle, lymphocyte specific 1-31 | 60.2 |
| | | | Intracisternal A particle, lymphocyte specific 3-1 | 60.6 |
| | | | Chemokine receptor 4 | 67.4 |
| | | | Interleukin-10 | 69.9 |
| 1, 65.0 | Contextual fear conditioning (freezing during contextual task) | Caldarone et al., 1997 | B-cell translocation gene 2, antiproliferation (plus the 5 preceding immune genes/loci) | 71.0 |
| | | | Complement component factor h | 74.1 |
| 10, 16.0 | Contextual fear conditioning (freezing during contextual task) | Wehner et al., 1997 | Intracisternal particle A, lymphocyte specific 3-21 | 9.0 |
| | | | Interferon gamma receptor | 15.0 |
| | | | CD24a antigen | 26.0 |
| 12, 6.0 | Contextual fear conditioning (freezing during altered context task) | Owen et al., 1997 | Cytokine induced activation 2 | 1.0 |
| | | | Tumor necrosis factor alpha converting enzyme | 3.0 |
| 16, 58.0 | Contextual fear conditioning (freezing during contextual task) | Wehner et al., 1997 | Interleukin-10 receptor beta | 61.0 |
| | | | Invasion inducing TIAM1 | 61.8 |
| | | | Interferon alpha/beta receptor | 64.0 |
| | | | Interferon gamma receptor 2 | 65.0 |
| 17, 35.0 | Contextual fear conditioning (freezing during contextual task) | Owen et al., 1997 | Intracisternal A particle, lymphocyte specific 1-3 | 25.0 |
| | | | Thymus cell antigen 2 | 27.8 |
| | | | Transplantation specific integration cluster 1 | 29.0 |
| | | | Macrophage migration inhibitory factor, pseudogene 8 | 30.5 |
| | | | Complement component 3 | 34.3 |
| | | | Immune response 5 | 37.1 |
| | | | Leukemia associated gene, related sequence 2 | 38.9 |
| | | | Intracisternal A particle, lymphocyte specific 3-24 | 44.2 |
| | | | T-cell integration locus | 45.0 |

emotional behaviors. It is also possible that genes in this area may control processes common to the expression of emotional behavior and learning and memory. Similarly, although QTL related to drug or stress responsiveness were not included as part of this chapter, it is also interesting that stress-induced changes in rearing behavior in an open field, an emotional response, was localized to the same interval on chromosome 1 as two QTLs (60–65 cM) detected for contextual fear conditioning (Tarricone, Hingtgen, Belknap, Mitchell, & Nurnberger, 1995; Caldarone, Saavedra, Tartaglia, Wehner, Dudek, & Flaherty, 1997; Owen et al., 1997). Of the various

studies assessing these emotional behavioral and learning and memory QTLs, a significant strength of the study of Flint et al. (1995) was that they employed a group of covarying behavioral tests which load on the emotional behavioral domain. Of five behavioral measures examined, four were associated with QTLs on the distal portion of chromosome 1 ($100 \pm$ several cM). It can be seen from Table II that a significant number of immune genes or disease susceptibility loci are found in this area of the distal portion of chromosome 1. Likewise, it is interesting that a QTL for contextual fear conditioning (at 35 cM) on chromosome 17, which contains the major histocompatibility complex (MHC), is located close to a number of loci involved in immune function (Table III).

## C. Evolutionary Significance: Opposites Attract and Families Stick Together

Functional genetic relationships between behavior and immunity are not unprecedented. Several lines of investigation address the potential evolutionary significance of genetic mechanisms linking adaptive behavioral and immunological processes in vertebrate species. There is extraordinary diversity of MHC alleles in vertebrates, in some instances more than 100 alleles per coding locus. It has traditionally been theorized that this diversity may be due to pathogen-driven selection processes whereby MHC heterozygotes and/or rare MHC genotypes have enhanced resistance against infectious diseases. Since pathogens readily evolve mechanisms to evade common forms of MHC-dependent immunity, by expressing a wider array and less common MHC genes, heterozygotes are thought to be better able to combat infectious diseases, although few relationships between susceptibility to specific infectious diseases and MHC genotypes have been documented (Potts & Wakeland, 1993).

Studies of laboratory mice and other vertebrates have also shown that these diverse MHC gene alleles control certain individual odors. These odor profiles can influence mating preferences by smell (Andrews & Boyse, 1978; Beauchamp et al., 1985; Boyse, Beauchamp, Bard, & Yamazaki, 1991; Singh, Brown, & Roser, 1987). It is theorized that MHC based disassortative mating, which preferentially produces heterozygotes, has evolved to reduce homozygosity in the MHC and throughout the genome. From an evolutionary perspective, this leads to increased "fitness" in that the offspring of MHC-based disassortative matings are more resistant to infectious diseases and less prone to inbreeding depression due to the heterozygosity of their MHC alleles (Potts and Wakeland, 1993; Potts, Manning, & Wakeland, 1991; Tanksley, 1993). Studying components of selection in populations of wild-derived mice, Potts and colleagues demonstrated that mating patterns are influenced by MHC genotype (Potts, Manning, & Wakeland, 1991). They observed that mating preferences among mice resulted in 27% fewer MHC homozygous offspring than expected from random mating. Moreover, that study indicated that these mating preferences were strong enough to account for most of the genetic diversity of the MHC.

Olfactory cues in mice such as urine and glandular secretions have effects on reproductive biology (e.g., reproductive maturity, the estrous cycle) and pregnancy block, the termination of pregnancy prior to implantation of the embryo after exposure to an unfamiliar male (e.g., a male mouse differing from the stud male with whom she has mated). The incidence of pregnancy block has been shown to be significantly higher when the stud male and the unfamiliar male differ in their MHC haplotypes. This indicates that MHC-based chemosensory recognition may also affect the reproductive hormonal status of a pregnant female mouse and her likelihood of carrying the fetus to term (Yamazaki et al., 1983). It has also been hypothesized that chronic spontaneous abortions in humans result from MHC homozygosity, and some data suggest that aborting couples share a greater proportion of MHC alleles than expected from random matings (Thomas, Harger, Wagener, Rabin, & Gill, 1985).

MHC genes have also been implicated in kinship recognition (Manning, Wakeland, & Potts, 1992). Related female mice in the wild and in seminaturalistic settings form communal nests in which they care for their progeny. According to kinship theory, related females preferentially form communal nests among themselves to reduce the likelihood of exploitation and increase fitness of the offspring (Wilkinson & Baker, 1988). It has been postulated, for example, that this serves to protect infant pups from predators (e.g., infanticide by a conspecific) as well as provide the family offspring with other homeostatic and physiologic advantages (e.g., improved nutrition, cross-immunization, thermoregulation). The hypothesis that MHC gene alleles play a role in communal nesting patterns in house mice was examined in seminatural populations of wild derived mice by Manning and colleagues (1992). Their study demonstrated that MHC similarity among chosen communal nesting partners was significantly greater than expected by random chance, consistent with the hypothesis that MHC similarity is a genetic mechanism used to detect kin for cooperative behaviors such as care and survival of related offspring. These data indicate that MHC gene polymorphisms which control individual odor profiles are sensory markers that serve to modify both mating and communal behaviors. In mating choices, they follow MHC disassortative preferences whereby nonrelated individuals mate to promote diversity of the gene pool, and in kin recognition they follow MHC assortative preferences to ensure that related individuals share in the survival of their offspring and thus their common genes. In addition to these studies in vertebrates, related systems have also been described in invertebrates (Scofield, Schlumpberger, West, & Weissman, 1982; Grosberg & Quinn, 1986).

## D. Models of Complex Autoimmune Traits: Relevance to Behavioral Genetics and Immune Correlates of Certain Neuropsychiatric Disorders

Remarkable progress is being made in dissecting the fundamental genetics of complex autoimmune diseases, in particular insulin-dependent diabetes (IDDM) and systemic lupus erythematosus (SLE). Murine models are being used to identify the relative contribution of multiple genes involved in the expression of complex, polygenic autoimmune diseases. In the NOD mouse model of IDDM, for example, 16 genomic intervals on 13 different chromosomes associated with diabetes susceptibility have been identified (Leiter, 1998). A unique MHC haplotype, H2$^{g7}$, is the primary locus contributing to the development of autoimmune diabetes. For murine SLE, as many as 22 genomic susceptibility intervals have been identified (Wakeland, Morel, Mohan, & Yui, 1997). Depending on the size of the particular susceptibility interval characterized (e.g., 10–50 cM), one to several hundred genes may be contained within the susceptibility interval. Many susceptibility intervals for these autoimmune diseases are non-MHC loci. A number of congenic strains have been produced (often using newer, efficient PCR-based marker-assisted speed congenic methods) where an interval of interest is introgressed onto a particular genomic background. To determine the unique contribution of a susceptibility interval in the pathogenesis of diabetes, susceptibility intervals have been introgressed onto an autoimmune disease-resistant genomic background (C57BL/6 background) (Yui et al., 1996). Conversely, intervals from a disease-resistant background have been introgressed onto the NOD background, thus replacing the NOD interval (Leiter, 1998; Serreze, 1998). Using these strategies, congenic strains containing multiple combinations of susceptibility intervals (e.g., bi-, tri-, tetra-cogenic strains, etc.) can be used to piece together or take apart the pathogenetic steps involved in autoimmune diabetes. In a model of SLE, different genomic intervals have found to each contribute component phenotypes (e.g., antinuclear autoantibodies in the absences of significant nephritis, amplification of T helper cells) or act as negative modifiers which can suppress autoimmunity (Morel et al., 1997; Morel & Wakeland, 1998; Wakeland et al., 1997). In autoimmune disease models of experimental allergic encephalomyelitis, disease susceptibility between strains may be determined, in part, by differences in the genetics associated with the HPA axis (MacPhee, Antoni, & Mason, 1989; Mason 1991; Mason, McPhee, & Antoni, 1990). Hence, it is possible that genes that control endocrine responsiveness may actually serve as susceptibility genes or disease modifiers for some complex autoimmune diseases.

There has been recurrent interest in the theory that autoimmune-like processes may be operative in neuropsychiatric diseases, in particular schizophrenia. Support for the theory comes largely from non-specific correlative data. In many instances, although the mean values of patient groups for various laboratory measures of immune status (e.g., proinflammatory cytokines, elevated CD5$^+$ lymphocytes) have differed significantly from the group means of comparison control subjects in many studies, for the most part the actual values themselves fall within the range of normal limits. On the other hand, some of the same issues that researchers are struggling with in this field are similar to those being grappled with by researchers studying systemic autoimmune disorders. Chronic schizophrenic individuals (including never medicated subjects) have been found to have a significantly higher frequency of antinuclear antibodies than control subjects (e.g., Spivak et al., 1995). Antinuclear antibodies are also found in certain systemic autoimmune disorders, and it is often unclear what role they play in the pathogenesis of autoimmunity against the tissue targeted in the disease (e.g., inflammation and destruction of the pancreas in autoimmune diabetes). Many autoantibodies are found to be nonspecific (Atkinson, 1997). Thus, is has been unclear whether the various autoimmune-like findings in neuropsychiatric disorders such as schizophrenia represent evidence of pathophysiological steps involved in autoimmunity or are epiphenomena.

The meaning of such immune correlates of schizophrenia may be derived from these autoimmune models. Congenic mice bearing certain diabetes-susceptibility intervals, for example, can express nonspecific autoantibodies but show no evidence of damage to the target organ of autoimmune destruction, the pancreas. Multiple susceptibility genes appear to be required to produce sufficient target organ damage to result in insulin deficiency (Leiter, 1998; Serreze, 1998). Thus, by analogy, populations of schizophrenic individuals could possess several of the autoimmune susceptibility intervals found in autoimmune diabetes or SLE; they exhibit a laboratory correlate (e.g., a nonspecific autoantibodies) but lack the other autoimmune disease genes necessary to express systemic autoimmune disease. It is plausible that susceptibility genes unique to schizophrenia in concert with one or more autoimmune susceptibility intervals, may result in immune-associated abnormalities of brain development (e.g., alterations in brain cytokines). Therefore, some common genetic processes may be operative in schizophrenia as well as autoimmune diseases such as SLE and diabetes.

## IV. CONCLUDING REMARKS

Genetic research in psychneuroimmunology has been limited to date. The currently available literature suggests that subsets of genes involved in the expression of complex behavioral and immunological traits may be physically linked, interactive at the level of the genome, or shared by the brain and immune system. There is intriguing evidence that a handful of behavioral QTLs involved in emotionality and learning and memory are linked to a subset of immune genes or susceptibility loci. The functional significance of these linkages remains to be determined. It is noteworthy that for many genomic intervals identified as susceptibility intervals for complex autoimmune traits (e.g., diabetes, SLE), the specific suceptibility genes within the interval are yet unidentified. From the perspective of a psychoneuroimmunologist, it is reasonable to speculate that some of these intervals may contain behavioral, neural, or endocrine genes serving as susceptibility genes and thus contributing to the expression of complex immunological traits (e.g., either a discontinuous trait like diabetes, or a continuous trait such as a parameter of immune responsiveness). Intriguing data in both nonverterbrates and vertebrates suggest potential evolutionary value for co-varying inheritance of some genes participating in the expression of certain behavioral and immunological traits. Although this chapter attempted to focus on genetics, it is clear from some of the data reviewed here and elsewhere in this text, that it is often a challenge to disentangle genetic from environmental contributions and the effects of their interactions. The lines separating genetic and environmental effects are sometimes blurred. In "genetic" animal models, for example in NOD mice, penetrance rates of diabetes often differ widely between animal colonies apparently due to varying degrees of largely unknown environmental triggers that influence the expression of this complex trait. Nonetheless, it is clear that there is enormous potential for molecular genetic strategies to bring critical understanding of behavioral–immune interactions to the field of psychoneuroimmunolgy. Given

the striking homology between the organization of the human and mouse genomes, for example, findings elucidating actions and linkages of key genes involved in the expression of correlated behavioral and immunological traits in experimental models may be translated to humans. This knowledge could provide vital new clues into the pathogenesis and treatment of psychosomatic illnesses and major neuropsychiatric disorders such as schizophrenia.

## References

Andrews, P. W., & Boyse, E. A. (1978). Mapping of an H-2-linked gene that influences mating preferences in mice. *Immunogenetics*, 6, 265–268.

Atkinson, M. A. (1997). Molecular mimicry and the pathogenesis of insulin-dependent diabetes mellitus: still just an attractive hypothesis. *Annals of Medicine*, 29, 393–399.

Beauchamp, G. K., Yamazaki, K., Wysocki, C. J., Slotnick, B. M., Thoms, L., & Boyse, E. A. (1985). Chemosensory recognition of mouse major histocompatibility types by another species. *Proceedings of the National Academy of Science USA*, 82, 4186–4188.

Biozzi, G., Mouton, D., Heumann, A. M., Bouthillier, Y., Stiffel, C., & Mevel, J. C. (1979). Genetic analysis of antibody responsiveness to sheep erythrocytes in crosses between lines of mice selected for high or low antibody synthesis. *Immunology*, 36, 427–438.

Bonneau, R. H., Mormede, P., Vogler, G. P., McClearn, G. E., & Jones, B. C. (1998). A genetic basis for neuroendocrine—immune interactions. *Brain, Behavior, and Immunity*, 12, 83–89.

Boyse, E. A., Beauchamp, G. K., Bard, J., & Yamazaki, K. (1991). Behavior and the major histocompatibility complex of the mouse. In R. Ader, D. L. Felten, & N. Cohen (Eds.), *Psychoneuroimmunology* (pp. 831–846). New York: Academic Press.

Broadhurst, P. L. (1958). Determinants of emotionality in the rat III. strain differences. *Journal of Comparative and Physiological Psychology*, 51, 55–59.

Broadhurst, P. L. (1976). The maudsley reactive and nonreactive strains of rats: A clarification. *Behavioral Genetics*, 6, 363–365.

Brush, F. R., Froehlich, J. C., & Sakellaris, P. (1979). Genetic selection for avoidance learning in the rat. *Behavioral Genetics*, 9, 309–316.

Cairns, R. B., Hood, K., & Midlam, J. (1985). On fighting in mice: is there as sensitive period for isolation effects? *Animal Behavior*, 33, 166–180.

Cairns, R. B., MacCombie, D. J., & Hood, K. E. (1983). A developmental-genetic analysis of aggressive behavior. *Journal of Comparative Psychology*, 97, 69–89.

Caldarone, B., Saavedra, C., Tartaglia, K., Wehner, J. M., Dudek, B. C., & Flaherty, L. (1997). Quantitative trait loci analysis affecting contextual conditioning in mice. *Nature Genetics*, 17, 335–337.

Castanon, N., Dulluc, J., Le Moal, M., & Mormede, P. (1992). Prolactin as a link between behavioral and immune differences between the roman rat lines. *Physiology and Behavior*, 51, 1235–1241.

Crabbe, J. C., Belknap, J. K., & Buck, K. J. (1994). Genetic animal models of alcohol and drug abuse. *Science*, 264, 1715–1723.

Crabbe, J. C., Phillips, T. J., Kosobud, A., & Belknap, J. K. (1990). Estimation of genetic correlation: Interpretation of experiments using selectively bred and inbred animals. *Alcoholism: Clinical and Experimental Research*, 14, 141–151.

DeFries, J. C., Gervais, M. C., & Thomas, E. A. (1978). Response to 30 generations of selection for open-field activity in laboratory mice. *Behavioral Genetics*, 8, 3–13.

Denenberg, V. H., Morbraaten, L. E., Sherman, G. F., Morrison, L., Schrott, L. M., Waters, N. S., Rosen, G. D., Behan, P. O., & Galaburda, A. M. (1991). Effects of the autoimmune uterine/maternal environment upon cortical ectopias, behavior and autoimmunity. *Brain Research, 563*, 114–122.

Denenberg, V. H., & Rosenberg, K. M. (1967). Nongenetic transmission of information. *Nature (London), 216*, 549–550.

Dietrich, W. F., Miller, J., Steen, R., Merchant, M. A., Damron-Boles, D., Husain, Z., Dredge, R., Daly, M. J., Ingalls, K. A., & O'Connor, T. J. (1996). A comprehensive genetic map of the mouse genome. *Nature, 380*, 149–152.

Eysenck, H. J. (1983). Stress, disease, and personality: The "inoculation effect." In C. L. Cooper (Ed.), *Stress research* (pp. 121–146). New York: Wiley.

Flint, J., Corley, R., DeFries, J. C., Fulker, D. W., Gray, J. A., Miller, S., & Collins, A. C. (1995). *Science, 269*, 1432–1435.

Fox, B. H. (1978). Premorbid psychological factors as related to cancer incidence. *Behavioral Medicine, 1*, 45–63.

Fride, E., McIntyre, T. Skolnick, P., & Arora, P. K. (1993). Immunocompetence in the long sleep and short sleep mouse lines: Baseline versus primed responses. *Brain, Behavior and Immunity, 7*, 231–242.

Friedman, E. M., Irwin, M. R., & Overstreet, D. H. (1996). Natural and cellular immune responses in flinders sensitive and resistant line rats. *Neuropsychopharmacology, 15*, 314–322.

Fuller, J. L., & Thompson, W. R. (1978). *Foundations of behavior genetics.* Saint-Louis, 140: Mosby.

Gariepy, J. L., Hood, K. E., & Cairns, R. B. (1988). A developmental-genetic analysis of aggressive behavior in mice: III. Behavioral mediation by heightened reactivity or increased immobility? *Journal of Comparative Psychology, 102*, 392–399.

Gershenfeld, H. K., & Paul, S. M. (1997). Mapping quantitative trait loci for fear-like behaviors in mice. *Genomics, 46*, 1–8.

Grosberg, R. K., & Quinn, J. F. (1986). The genetic control and consequences of kin recognition by the larvae of a colonial marine invertebrate. *Nature, 322*, 456–459.

Hagnell, O. (1966). The premorbid personality of persons who develop cancer in a total population investigated in 1947 and 1957. *Annals of the New York Academy of Science, 125*, 846–855.

Henderson, N. D. (1989). Interpreting studies that compare high- and low-selected lines on new characters. *Behavioral Genetics, 19*, 473–501.

Hood, K. E., & Cairns, R. B. (1988). A developmental-genetic analysis of aggressive behavior in mice II. Cross-sex inheritance. *Behavioral Genetics, 18*, 605–619.

Kopf-Maier, P., & Mboneko, V. F. (1990). Anomalies in the hormonal status of athymic nude mice. *Journal of Cancer Research and Clinical Oncology, 116*, 229–231.

Lagerspetz, K. Y. H., Tirri, R., & Lagerspetz, K. M. J. (1968). Neurochemical and endocrinological studies of mice selectively bred for aggressiveness. *Scandinavian Journal of Psychology, 9*, 157–160.

Lander, E., & Kruglyak, L. (1995). Genetic dissection of complex traits: Guidelines for interpreting and reporting linkage results. *Nature Genetics, 11*, 241–247.

Lander, E. S., & Schork, N. J. (1994). Genetic dissection of complex traits. *Science, 265*, 2037–2048.

Leiter, E. H. (1998). Genetics and Immunogenetics of NOD mice and related strains. In Leiter & Atkinson (Eds.), *NOD mice and related strains: Research applications in diabetes, AIDS, cancer, and other diseases* (pp. 37–70). Austin, TX: R. G. Landes.

Levine, S. (1967). Maternal and environmental influences on the adrenocortical response to stress in weanling rats. *Science, 156*, 258–260.

MacPhee, I. A., Antoni, F. A., & Mason, D. W. (1989). Spontaneous recovery of rats from experimental allergic encephalomyelitis is dependent on regulation of the immune system by endogenous adrenal corticosteroids. *Journal of Experimental Medicine, 169*, 431–445.

Manning, C. J., Wakeland, E. K., & Potts, W. K. (1992). Communal nesting patterns in mice implicate mhc genes in kin recognition. *Nature, 360*, 581–583.

Mason, D. (1991). Genetic variation in the stress response: Susceptibility to experimental allergic encephalomyelitis and implications for human inflammatory disease. *Immunology Today, 12*, 57–60.

Mason, D, MacPhee, I., & Antoni, F. (1990). The role of the neuro-endocrine system in determining genetic susceptibility to experimental allergic encephalomyelitis in the rat. *Immunology, 70*, 1–5.

Miyawki, T., Moriya, N., Nagoki, T., & Taniguchi, N. (1981). Maturation of B-cell differentiation ability and T-cell regulatory function in infancy and childhood. *Immunological Reviews, 57*, 61–87.

Morel, L., Mohan, C., Yu, Y., Croker, B. P., Tian, N., Deng, A., & Wakeland, E. K. (1997). Functional dissection of systemic lupus erythematosus using congenic mouse strains. *Journal of Immunology, 158*, 6019–6028.

Morel, L., & Wakeland, E. K. (1998) Susceptibility to lupus nephritis in the NZB/W model system. *Current Opinions in Immunology, 10*, 718–725.

Owen, E. H., Christensen, S. C., Paylor, R., & Wehner, J. M. (1997). Identification of quantitative trait loci involved in contextual and auditory-cued fear conditioning in bxd recombinant inbred strains. *Behavioral Neuroscience, 111*, 292–300.

Petitto, J. M., Gariepy, J. L., Gendreau, P. L., Rodriguiz, R. M., Lewis, M. H., & Lysle, D. T. (1999) Differences in NK cell function in mice bred for high and low aggression: genetic linkage between complex behavioral and immunological traits? *Brain, Behavior, and Immunity, 13*, 175–186.

Petitto, J. M., Lysle, D. T., Gariepy, J. L., Clubb, P. H., Cairns, R. B., & Lewis, M. H. (1993). Genetic differences in social behavior: Relation to natural killer cell function and susceptibility to tumor development. *Neuropsychopharmacology, 8*, 35–43.

Petitto, J. M., Lysle, D. T., Gariepy, J. L., & Lewis, M. H. (1994). Association of genetic differences in social behavior and cellular immune responsiveness: Effects of social experience. *Brain, Behavior, and Immunity, 8*, 111–122.

Petitto, J. M., McIntyre, T. D., McRae, B. L., Skolnick, P., & Arora, P. K. (1990). Differential immune responsiveness in mouse lines selectively bred for high and low sensitivity to ethanol. *Brain, Behavior, and Immunity, 4*, 39–49.

Petitto, J. M., McNamara, R., Gendreau, P. L., Huang, Z., & Jackson A. (1999). Impaired learning and memory and altered hippocampal neurodevelopment resulting from IL-2 gene deletion. *Journal of Neuroscience Research, 56*, 441–446.

Potts, W. K., Manning, C. J., & Wakeland, E. K. (1991). Mating patterns in seminatural populations of mice influenced by MHC genotype. *Nature, 352*, 619–621.

Potts, W. K., & Wakeland, E. K. (1993). Evolution of mhc genetic diversity: A tale of incest, pestilence and sexual preference. *Trends in Genetics, 9*, 408–412.

Sandi, C., Castanon, N., Vitello, S., Neveu, P. J., & Mormede, P. (1991). Different responsiveness of spleen lymphocytes from two lines of psychogenetically selected rats (Roman high and low avoidance). *Journal of Neuroimmunology, 31*, 27–33.

Sandnabba, N. K. (1995). Predatory aggression in male mice selectively bred for isolation-induced intermale aggression. *Behavioral Genetics, 25*, 361–366.

Scofield, V. L., Schlumpberger, J. M., West, L. A., & Weissman, I. L. (1982). Protochordate allorecognition is controlled by a MHC-like gene system. *Nature, 295,* 499–502.

Serreze, D. V. (1998). The identity and ontogenic origins of autoreactive T lymphocytes in NOD mice. In Leiter & Atkinson (Eds.), *NOD mice and related strains: Research applications in diabetes, AIDS, cancer, and other diseases* (pp. 71–100). Austin, TX: R. G. Landes.

Singh, P. B., Brown, R. E., & Roser, B. (1987). MHC antigens in urine as olfactory recognition cues. *Nature (London) 327,* 161–164.

Solomon, G. F. (1981). Emotional and personality factors in the onset and course of autoimmune disease, particularly rheumatoid arthritis. In R. Ader (Ed.), *Psychoneuroimmunology* (pp. 159–184). New York: Academic Press.

Solomon, G. F., Levine, S., & Kraft J. K. (1968). Early experience and immunity. *Nature, 220,* 821–822.

Spivak, B., Radwan, M., Bartur, P., Mester, R., & Weizman, A. (1995). Antinuclear autoantibodies in chronic schizophrenia. *Acta Psychiatry Scandanavia, 92,* 266–269.

Tanksley, S. D. (1993). Mapping polygenes. *Annual Review of Genetics, 27,* 205–233.

Tarricone, B. J., Hingtgen, J. N., Belknap, J. K., Mitchell, S. R., & Nurnberger, J. L. (1995). Quantitative trait loci associated with the behavioral response of BXD recombinant inbred mice to restraint stress: A preliminary communication. *Behavioral Genetics, 25,* 489–495.

Thomas, M. L., Harger, J. H., Wagener, D. K., Rabin, B. S., & Gill, T. J., III (1985). HLA sharing and spontaneous abortion in humans. *American Journal of Obstetrics and Gynecology, 151,* 1053–1058.

Van Oortmerssen, G. A., & Baker, T. C. M. (1981). Artificial selection for short and long attack latencies in wild Mus musculus domesticus. *Behavioral Genetics, 11,* 115–126.

Vidal, J. (1996). Differences of nu/+ and nu/nu mice in some behaviors reflecting temperament traits. *Physiology and Behavior, 59,* 341–348.

Vidal, J., & Rama, R. (1994). Association of the antibody response to hemocyanin with behavior in mice bred for high or low antibody responsiveness. *Behavioral Neuroscience, 108,* 1172–1178.

Wakeland, E. K., Morel, L., Mohan, C., & Yui, M. (1997). Genetic dissection of lupus nephritis in murine models of sle. *Journal of Clinical Immunology, 17,* 272–281.

Wehner, J. M., Radcliffe, R. A., Rosmann, S. T., Christensen, S. C., Rasmussen, D. L., Fulker, D. W., & Wiles, M. (1997). Quantitative trait locus analysis of contextual fear conditioning in mice. *Nature Genetics, 17,* 331–334.

Wellisch, D. K., & Yager, J. (1983). Is there a cancer-prone personality? *CA, 33,* 145–153.

Wilkinson, G. S., & Baker, A. M. (1988). Communal nesting among genetically similar house mice. *Ethology, 77,* 103–114.

Yamazaki, K., Beauchamp, G. K., Wysocki, C. J., Bard, J., Thomas, L., & Boyse, E. A. (1983). Recognition of H-2 types in relation to the blocking of pregnancy in mice. *Science, 221,* 186–188.

Yui, M. A., Muralidharan, K., Moreno-Altamirano, B., Perrin, G., Chestnut, K., & Wakeland, E. K. (1996). Production of congenic mouse strains carrying NOD-derived diabetogenic genetic intervals: An approach for the genetic dissection of complex traits. *Mammalian Genome, 7,* 331–334.

Zeng, Z.-B. (1994). Precision mapping of quantitative trait loci. *Genetics, 136,* 1457–1468.

# STRESS AND IMMUNITY

# Effects of Stress on Immune Functions:
# An Overview

MASSIMO BIONDI

## I. INTRODUCTION

In 1936, Selye reported that laboratory animals presented a common response to noxious stimuli such as heat, cold, epinephrine, strenuous muscular exercise, and X-rays and used the term "stress" to indicate it (Selye, 1936). Stress was defined as "the nonspecific response of the body to any demand." He termed "stressors" all stimuli able to induce it. If stress exposure lasted several days or weeks, a characteristic triad consisting of three subsequent phases, i.e., activation, resistance, and exhaustion, could be observed, which Selye called "general adaptation syndrome" (GAS) (Selye, 1946). Selye first reported alterations to immune organs and cells after stress, such as atrophy of the thymus and other lymphatic structures, lymphocytopenia, with increased morbidity, mortality, and susceptibility to infection. Hundreds of further investigations provided detailed knowledge of the mechanisms of the stress response and of possible consequences that result in adaptation of the whole organism to stressors or different disease conditions (1950).

The original concept of stress, however, has been the object of confusion and controversy (Selye, 1976); Lazarus (1971) and Mason (1971) argued against the concept of its aspecificity. The utility of the stress concept has been questioned also in psychosomatic medicine as an excessively inclusive label, descriptive rather than explanatory of mediating mechanisms (Ader, 1980). Nonetheless the stress concept has been pivotal to psychosomatic medicine (Gunderson & Rahe, 1974; Levi, 1971; Pancheri, 1984; Wolff, Wolf, & Hare, 1950). As concerns immune-related disorders, Wolff applied the life stress concept to bodily disease, introducing the method of Meyer's "Life Chart" to measure life events, and testing the hypothesis that disease, including allergy, hay fever, and infectious disease, might be a consequence of the failure of adaptation to life stress. Holmes and Rahe (1967) developed the Social Readjustment Rating Scale, aimed at the objective measurement and weighting of life stress events. Retrospective and prospective studies reported that an increase of life stress preceded several diseases, including miscellaneous infectious (such as common cold, bronchitis, mononucleosis, gonorrhea, pneumonia, and hepatitis) and allergic disorders (Petrich & Holmes, 1977; Wyler, Masuda, & Holmes, 1971). Ader and Friedman (1964) first demonstrated that early experiences could affect susceptibility to transplanted tumor in animals, opening a window on the relationship between the psychobiology of development and the response of the immune system in the adult. Finally, although the possible contribution of psychological factors to cancer was suspected by physicians of the 18th and 19th centuries (Le Shan & Worthington, 1956), the study of the psychobiological aspects of cancer is increasingly carried out by investigating the stress–immunity link (Bahnson, 1969; Bahnson & Kissen, 1966). As concerns autoimmune disorders, Solomon and Moos advanced the idea that emotional stress might play a role in the pathogenesis and course of rheumatoid arthritis (1964).

Further developments in the past 20 years have confirmed clinical intuitions and shown immune function to be stress-sensitive, raising the question of whether acute or chronic stressful life events could contribute to the pathogenesis of immune-related diseases. After seminal work in the late 1970s, psychoneuroimmunology (Ader, 1981) was established as a new, actively growing field in both the United States and Europe and in many university programs, despite some difficulties (Ader, 1996). Hundreds of animal studies contributed to the knowledge of neural-immune interactions (Madden & Felten, 1995) and as a framework for human research animals served as models of the pathogenesis of stress-induced diseases (Monjan, 1981; Moynihan & Ader, 1996).

With advancing research, stress models evolved. Individual cognitive appraisal of stimuli (Lazarus & Folkman; 1984), emotional arousal (Mason, 1975), and psychosocial stimuli as stress determinants rather than stressors (Levi, 1971) were recognized as mediators of the stress response in man and as contributing factors to its possible health consequences. Psychological stimuli and stressors can induce modifications in the central nervous (CNS) (Biondi, 1997; Stone, 1988), autonomic nervous (ANS) (Grings & Dawson, 1981), and neuroendocrine systems (Biondi & Picardi, 1999). The neurobiology of psychological stress at all these levels is a key step to the understanding of stress-induced changes of immune functions (Felten, Cohen, Ader, Felten, Carlson, & Roszman, 1991; Felten & Felten, 1994).

The present chapter will review the main findings in the psychoneuroimmunology of human stress, the effect of different types of acute and chronic stress on immune function, and their possible role in susceptibility to disease and deal with questions that are still open to debate.

## II. PSYCHOLOGICAL STRESS AND IMMUNE FUNCTION

The number of studies on psychological stress-related immune changes in humans has been steadily growing since the early 1970s. A previous review published in 1995 covered 46 human research studies between 1972 and 1992 (Biondi & Pancheri, 1995). Between 1972 and 1976 we find only three studies (Canter, Cluff, & Imboden 1972; Fischer, Daniels, Levin, Kimzey, Cobb, & Ritzman 1972; Palmblåd et al., 1976). The methodological quality of the published papers has been improving steadily. One might also wonder if, at this phase in the evolution of psychoneuroimmunology, redundant methodological rigor could in some instances restrain further developments and downplay serendipitous findings, inhibiting innovative and divergent views, while permitting only refinement of already established paradigms.

This chapter reviews nearly 120 experimental studies in humans. Papers on psychiatric disorders are not included. Table I reviews the methodology and findings of 50 studies on the effects of chronic or longitudinal stressors on immune functions, while Table II summarizes the methodology and findings of 61 studies focusing on immune function during or after short-term or acute stress.

### A. Sampling, Age, and Sex

Due to the costs of immune assessments, psychoneuroimmunological research sample sizes are generally small.

The majority of studies observed physically and psychologically healthy subjects, if we exclude studies on psychiatric or AIDS patients which are not explicitly focused on stress. About one-third of the investigations concerned individuals under 30 years of age. The standard deviation of age is often small; this might limit the generalizability of findings. Another third of the studies concerned the age range between 30 and 40 years. Although an interest in aging is increasing in other fields of medicine and the subject of aging and immunity has been dealt with in depth since the early 1960s, psychoneuroimmunologic studies on elderly subjects are rare. Animal studies suggest that older rats are less susceptible than younger rats to immune response impairment induced by a 6-month stress (Odio, Brodish, & Ricardo, 1987). Few studies exist on endocrine stress reactivity differences between young and elderly subjects, but they show, for instance, stronger reactivity of growth hormone (GH) and a weakened hypothalamo-pituitary-adrenal (HPA) axis response in the elderly subject as compared to the young (Delle Chiaie, De Cesare, Biondi, Stagi, & Pancheri, 1990). A study of elderly Alzheimer's disease caregivers confirms that such a chronic life stress does not alter plasma cortisol, but rather increases norepinephrine, which

**TABLE I** Summary of Studies on Chronic or Longitudinal Stress and Immune Functions in Humans (1972–1999)

| Authors | Sample | Stressor | Immune assessment | Results |
|---|---|---|---|---|
| Arnetz et al., 1987 | Three groups of women (9 unemployed—no support (A), 8 unemployed with psychosocial support (B), 8 with safe job (C) | Unemployment | Lymphocyte stimulation tests phytohemoagglutinin (PHA), protein purified derivate (PPD)) | Decreased reactivity of lymphocytes to PHA and PPD in groups A and B; no changes in group C |
| Bartrop et al., 1977 | 26 Bereaved subjects, 26 normal subjects | Bereavement | E-, EAC-rosettes, response to mitogens, IGs, T- and B-cells | Bereaved subjects show reduced response to mitogens |
| Benschop et al., 1994 | 27 Subjects and 20 controls | Subjects reporting extremely low- or high everyday problems are exposed to acute stress (learning process) | Endocrine, cardiovascular and immune variables | Acute psychological stress is associated with increase in the plasma levels of epinephrine and of natural killer (NK) and T cells in the low hassles group; NK cells remain unchanged in high hassle group after stress, while T cells decrease |
| Biondi et al., 1993 | 50 Healthy air crew | Life stress events, job stress, mood anxiety | Lymphocytes subsets, NK-cell activity | Minor daily chronic stressors are not related to immune changes; NK-cell activity positively correlated with social introversion; hypomania inversely correlated with lymphocyte T CD11$^+$ and NK cell count |
| Biondi et al., 1994 | 24 Healthy adults | Life stress, psychological changes over an 8-month period | Prolactin, cortisol, growth hormone plasma levels. T helper, T cytotoxic and T CD11$^+$ percentage; NK-cell counts and activity | Decrease in CD11$^+$ cell percentage is related to a reduction in the scores of the Minnesota Multiphasic Personality Inventory (MPPI) scales of Subtle Defensiveness and Social Introversion; positive correlation between prolactin and T helper lymphocyte percentage |
| Boyce et al., 1993 | 20 Children | Earthquake | Th CD4$^+$, T-suppressors CD8$^+$ | Substantial changes in CD4+/CD8+ ratio predict changes in respiratory illness after the earthquake period; children showing upregulation of immune parameters at school entrance have significant increase in respiratory illness incidence after earthquake |
| Brosschot et al., 1994 | 86 Male teachers; 24–55 years | Life stress and daily hassles | Monocytes, T lymphocytes, HLA-DR$^+$ cells and NK cell number | High numbers of daily hassles are associated with decreases of T- and NK-cell numbers in peripheral blood; HLA-DR$^+$ cells decrease only slightly during stressor but increase during the control condition |
| Canter et al., 1972 | 313 Normal subject "vulnerable" vs "non vulnerable" | Perceived stress | Immunization test | Hypersensitivity reaction to immunization more frequent in the vulnerable group |
| Castle et al., 1995 | Elderly caregiver wives of demented patients | Stress of caregiving | Immune cell phenotype and cell proliferative capacity | Strongest association between stress parameters and impaired T-cell proliferative capacity; depression is also most strongly associated with a shift in T cell populations with an increase in CD8+ T cells, and reduction in NK cells as well as the percentage of CD56+ of the CD8+; findings could help to explain the higher risk of disease and mortality of caregivers |

*(Continues)*

**TABLE I** (*Continued*)

| Authors | Sample | Stressor | Immune assessment | Results |
|---|---|---|---|---|
| DeGucht et al., 1999 | 60 Nurses | Professional stress | Lymphocyte subpopulations, expression of IL-2 receptor, neopterin | Chronic professional stress seems associated with signs of immune activation (increased number of cells expressing the IL-2 receptor) and possibly immune suppression (decrease in percentage of NK cells); high stress and high psychopathology are associated with decrease in CD8+ CD11+ B cells |
| Di Gennaro et al., 1997 | Mothers of low birth weight infants | Caregiving to very low birthweight infants | Lymphocyte transformation tests, NK | Decreased lymphocyte response to mitogens is related to anxiety; no influence on NK cells |
| Dimsdale et al., 1994 | 16 Healthy normotensive and 9 untreated hypertensive subjects | Life stress (homelessness) | Lymphocyte $\beta$-adrenergic receptors | High life stress subjects have less lymphocytic $\beta$-adrenoceptors |
| Esterling et al., 1996 | 28 Caregivers of Alzheimer's disease patients and 29 control subjects | Psychological stress | Natural killer cell cytotoxicity | Reduced as compared to controls |
| Fawzy et al., 1990 | 61 Cancer and 35 psychiatric patients, 26 controls | Cancer diagnosis | T-helper, T-suppressor, NK cell and large granular lymphocyte number; NK-cell activity | At 6 weeks the intervention group shows higher anger than the control group; low anxiety and depression are related to higher LGLs and NK-cell percentage and NK-cell activity. At 6 months, the difference between groups persists |
| Fischer et al., 1972 | 21 Normal healthy air crew | Space flight | Peripheral lymphocyte count, immune response mitogen (PHA) | Mean lymphocyte numbers and immune reactivity to PHA during spaceflight are in the normal range |
| Glaser et al., 1992 | 48 Students | Academic examinations and Hepatitis-B vaccine injection | Antibody titers to HBsAg and blastogenic response to HBsAg peptide (Sag) | Early seroconverters (seroconverted after the first vaccine) have lower anxiety and perceived stress levels than later seroconverters; at the third vaccine inoculation, high social support scores are related to higher antibody titers and blastogenic response to Sag |
| Greene et al., 1978 | 33 Normal subjects | Life events | Interferon, antibody titer cytotoxicity | Negative correlation between cellular immunity and LCU-Vigor score |
| Heisel et al., 1986 | 111 Students (78 men and 33 women) | Not considered | NK-cell activity | High MMPI scores ($T>70$) are related with NK values below the sample median; higher MMPI scales (Hy, D, Pd, Mf, Pa, Pt, Sc, Ma, Ego strength, maladjustment) scores are related to lower NK-cell activity |
| Ironson et al., 1990 | | Status notification HIV-1 antibody | T-helper, T-inducer subset and NK cell numbers; immune response to mitogens (PHA, PWM); NK-cell activity; HIV-1 antibody titer | Seropositive subjects show increased anxiety, high avoidance and intrusion scores (IES), and decreased NK-cell activity at the time of seropositive status notification and, 1 week later, unchanged immune response to PHA and PWM; seronegative subjects show depressed immune response to PHA and PWM at baseline; at 5 weeks, all measures returned to their initial, non-clinical baseline levels in both the seropositive and seronegative groups |

| Reference | Sample | Stressor | Immune measure | Findings |
|---|---|---|---|---|
| Ironson et al., 1997 | Community sample damaged by hurricane | Hurricane Andrew (1–4 months later) | Lymphocyte subsets, Natural killer cell cytotoxicity, | Overall the community sample is significantly lower in natural killer cell cytotoxicity, CD4 and CD8 number and higher in NK cell number compared to laboratory controls; natural killer cell cytotoxicity is negatively related to both damage and psychological variables (loss, intrusive thoughts, posttraumatic stress symptoms); white blood cell counts significantly positively related with the degree of loss |
| Irwin et al., 1986 | 12 Widows, 16 with ill husbands, 11 controls | Disease of spouse, stressful life events | NK-cell activity | High depression scores and many life changes are correlated with impaired NK-cell activity |
| Irwin et al., 1988 | 9 Recently bereaved women; 11 anticipating death of husband; 8 controls | Bereavement | NK-cell activity | Reduced NK-cell activity in bereaved and bereavement-anticipating women |
| Jamner et al., 1988 | 312 Outpatients classified as repressive (REP, $n = 79$) defensive high-anxious (DEF, $n = 69$), true high anxious (Ha, $n = 124$), and true low- anxious (LA, $n = 40$) | | Monocyte and eosinophil count | REP patients show lower monocyte counts than LA patients; higher eosinophil counts than LA and HA patients; more medication reactions than all other groups; DEF patients show lower monocyte levels than HA patients |
| Jemmott et al., 1983 | 64 Students | Academic stress | Secretory IgA (s-IgA) | The s-IgA secretion rate is significantly lower in high stress than in low stress period for the whole group |
| Kang et al., 1996 | 64 Healthy and asthmatic adolescents | Academic examinations | Leucocytes, lymphocyte proliferation, cytolytic responses | Several changes in lymphocyte subsets and marked alterations in the three functional measures in students, without aggravation in asthmatic students |
| Kasl et al., 1979 | 1400 Cadets | Academic stress | Appearance of Epstein–Barr virus antibodies and/or mononucleosis | High academic motivation and poor performance predict clinical mononucleosis |
| Kang et al., 1997 | 21 Asthmatic adolescents and 13 healthy controls | Academic stress | IFN-γ, IL-2, IL-4, IL-5 | Cells from asthmatic subjects release significantly more IL-5 during examination, whereas cells from healthy controls release more IL-2 during the same period. IL-4 and IL-5 show marked decrease during and after examination in healthy controls |
| Kiecolt-Glaser et al., 1984 | 75 Students | Academic exam | NK-cell activity, IgA, IgM, IgG | NK-cell activity declines under examination stress |
| Kiecolt-Glaser et al., 1984 | 33 Psychiatric inpatients | Loneliness | NK-cell activity, immune reactivity to PHA | High loneliness group shows lower NK-cell activity and PHA response |
| Kiecolt-Glaser et al., 1988 | 64 Men; 32 separated/divorced, 32 married | Separation/ divorce | Antibody titers to Epstein–Barr virus and herpes simplex virus type-1 (HSV-1) | Separated/divorced group vs married group: more illness are reported in the former, higher antibody titers to EBV and HSV-1 (poor cellular immune system control over virus latency) |

(Continues)

**TABLE I** (*Continued*)

| Authors | Sample | Stressor | Immune assessment | Results |
|---|---|---|---|---|
| Kubitz et al., 1986 | 30 Subjects | Perceived stress | Secretory IgA (s-IgA) | The s-IgA levels inversely correlate with high internal locus of control levels; no difference between high- and low-stress groups |
| Levy et al., 1985 | 75 Breast cancer patients | Perceived stress | NK-cell activity | High distress is related to higher NK-cell activity |
| Levy et al., 1990 | 120 Breast cancer patients | Life-threatening illness | NK-cell activity | High social support is related with high NK-cell activity and a fair tumor status |
| Locke et al., 1977 | 124 Students | Perceived stress | Antibody titers to flu vaccine | No relationship |
| Maes et al., 1999 | Posttraumatic stress disorder patients (PTSD) and normal controls | Accidental man-made traumatic events | Serum interleukin 6 (IL-6), soluble IL-6 Receptor (R), IL-6 signal transducing protein, sCD8, CC16 (an endogenous anticotokine) | PTSD patients have serum IL-6 and soluble IL-6 R concentrations significantly higher than controls; findings suggest that PTSD is associated with increased IL-6 signaling |
| McClelland et al., 1980 | 27 College males | Inhibition in the need for power | Salivary IgA (S-IgA), epinephrine (E) excretion rates, illness reports | More of the high in power stress subjects than other subjects show above average E excretion rates in urine and below average concentrations of IgA in saliva; higher rates of E excretion are significantly associated with lower S-IgA concentrations; lower S-IgA concentrations are significantly associated with reports of more frequent illness reports |
| Mills et al., 1997 | 37 Elderly wives, caregivers to Alzheimer patients | Life stress | $\beta$-2 adrenergic sensitivity and density in lymphocytes | Caregivers with high life chronic stress have higher plasma norepinephrine levels but no change in plasma cortisol; chronic high stress may be associated with changes in adrenoceptors and provide a mechanism through which chronic stress alters cellular immunity |
| Nakano et al., 1998 | Randomly selected male taxi drivers | Job stress after severe economic crisis | Lymphocyte proliferative responses to phytohemoagglutinin (PHA), concanavalin A, Pokeweed, PHA-induced IL-2, IL-4 | Stress of severe economic crisis is associated with reduction of mitogen responses and IL-2 production, while production of IL-4 is increased as compared to assessments 1 year before crisis. |
| Pariante et al., 1997 | 18 Female caregivers of disabled individuals and 18 age- and sex-matched controls | Psychological stress of caregiving | T-cells, T-helper, T-suppressor/cytotoxic number and function, antibody titers and inflammation markers | In the caregiver population, severity of stress correlates positively with T suppressor/cytotoxic cells and inversely with T suppressor ratio |
| Pettingale et al., 1981 | 57 Breast cancer patients | Life-threatening illness | IgM, IgG, IgA | Increase of IgA is associated with emotional repression; increase of IgM is associated with denial |
| Schleifer et al., 1983 | 20 Normals | Bereavement | B- and T-cell counts, Phytohemoagglutinin (PHA), concanavalin A (Con A), Pokeweed mitogen (PWM) reactivity | Suppressed reactivity to PHA, Con A, and PKW |

| Study | Subjects | Stressor | Immune measures | Findings |
| --- | --- | --- | --- | --- |
| Segerstrom et al., 1998 | 47 Hospital employees | Earthquake | Autonomic measures, lymphocytes population, natural killer (NK) cells | At three follow-up points, subjects with scores above the median on a trait worry measure have fewer NK cells than those with worry scores below the median. Worry may have a detrimental effect on NK cells under stress |
| Solomon et al., 1997 | 68 Employees | Earthquake | Lymphocyte subsets-total T, Th, cytotoxic T cells, NK cells, lymphoid cell mitogenesis (PHA) | Low distress subjects have higher numbers of total T and T-cytotoxic cells and higher proliferative response to PHA; high distress subjects have highest levels of total T and T-cytotoxic cells |
| Szckeklik et al., 1996 | 149 Patients (81 undergoing coronary artery bypass, 33 chest surgery, 17 cholecystectomy, 18 inguinal hernia repair), 30 healthy control | Surgery | Serum IgE levels | IgE serum levels rise shortly after surgery in all groups except controls, reach a peak by the 5th postoperative day, and then gradually decline |
| Taylor et al., 1986 | 41 Astronauts | Space flight | Monocyte, B-lymphocyte, and T-lymphocyte counts; T-helper and T-suppressor number; T-helper/T-suppressor ratio; mitogenic responses | Decreased monocytes, decreased B-lymphocytes, decreased T-lymphocytes, increased T-helper cells, T-suppressor cells slightly decreased, increased T-helper/T suppressor ratio, and decreased T-cell blastogenic response |
| Thomas et al., 1985 | 256 Healthy elderly adults (54% men and 46% women) | Stressful life events and social bonds | Total lymphocyte | Strong social support (defined in this study as satisfying, confident relationships) is related to higher lymphocyte counts and mitogenic responses |
| Totman et al., 1980 | 52 Normal subjects | Life stress events | Antibody titer to experimental common cold | Introverts develop more severe symptoms and infections than extroverts |
| Udelmann, 1982 | 10 Normal subjects | Threat of loss | B- and T-cell counts | Immune measures are correlated with hope and antidepressants |
| Vedhara et al., 1999 | 50 Spouses of dementia patients | Caregiving of a family member with a chronic and severe disease | IgG antibody titers, flu vaccine, cortisol | Elderly caregivers of spouses with dementia have increased cortisol and a poor antibody response to influenza vaccine; caregivers may be more vulnerable to infectious disease than the population of similar age |
| Weiss et al., 1996 | 22 Male subjects | Missile attack during Persian Gulf war | Lymphocyte subset, NK-cell number and activity, lymphocyte transformation tests | NK-cell activity and cell-mediated lympholysis are significantly increased during war; mitogen responses are reduced |

**TABLE II   Summary of Studies on Acute or Short-Term Stress and Immune Functions in Humans, 1972–1999**

| Authors | Sample | Stressor | Immune assessment | Results and conclusions |
|---|---|---|---|---|
| Aragona et al., 1996 | 106 Breast cancer patients and 37 patients with benign breast cancer (controls) | Stressful life events (hospital admission, uncertain diagnosis, awaiting surgery) | Catecholamine excretion and blood cortisol levels. CD3$^+$, CD4$^+$, CD8$^+$, CD16$^+$ lymphocyte percentage | Breast cancer patients show increased 24-h catecholamine excretion and a positive correlation between blood cortisol and lymphocyte percentage |
| Bachen et al., 1995 | Normal subjects | Laboratory mental stress | Lymphocyte subsets, natural killer (NK) cells number and activity, T cell response to mitogens; sympathetic activation and blockade by labetolol | Treatment with adrenoceptor antagonist labetolol reduces immune changes, increases peripheral NK cell number and cytotoxicity, lowers mitogenic response to PHA and Con A, reduces ratio CD4/CD8 after acute psychological stress, suggesting a mediatory role of the sympathetic system |
| Baker et al., 1984 | 35 Students in their first days of medical course, 28 second-year medical students as controls | First week in a new college | Leucocyte and lymphocyte counts | Students in their first week in a new college have significantly greater anxiety, serum cortisol concentration, and increased percentage of OKT4 (helper/inducer) cells than second-year students |
| Biondi & Pancheri, 1984 and 1991 | 25 Female inpatients | Awaiting breast surgery | E-rosettes, phytohemagglutinin (PHA), skin test | Subjects with significantly reduced PHA lymphoproliferative responses, reduced skin test reactivity, and reduced E rosette formation have significantly higher scores of depression, social introversion, and coping styles with stress based on repression-denial, than subjects with normal immune values under the stress of waiting for surgery |
| Bosch et al., 1996 | 28 Dental students | Academic examination | Salivary IgA (s-IgA), effect of whole saliva on the aggregation of Streptococcus Gondii | Increase of s-IgA, significant reduction of aggregation of Streptococcus gondii under stress is related to state anxiety; reduced bacterial aggregation under stress may impair oral health |
| Boyce et al., 1995 | 39 Five-year-old children | Starting school | Immunization with pneumococcal vaccine, CD4+, CD8+, CD19+, lymphoproliferative responses to pokeweed (PWM), pneumococcal antibody response (ABR), salivary cortisol | CD4+ cells increase, response to PWM decreases, salivary cortisol rises after kindergarten entry; change in cortisol is positively associated with change in CD19+ |
| Breznitz et al., 1998 | 50 Normal male volunteers | Anticipation of mild shock | CD4, CD8, NK cells | Anticipatory threat lead to significant elevations of NK cell numbers and cytotoxic activity, with a reduction of CD4/CD8 ratio. The changes are very rapid |
| Brohee et al., 1990 | Nine normal subjects; five men and four women | Pharmacological stress (epinephrine and hydrocortisone intravenously) | T-helper, T-suppressor, T-11, T-3, NK and monocyte numbers; immune reactivity to PHA, PWM, LPS | At 10 min, all leukocytes increase, particularly T-suppressor and NK cells; at 1 h, moderate lymphopenia and monocytopenia; at 6 h, neutrophilia and eosinopenia; unchanged mitogenic reactivity throughout the study |

| Reference | Subjects | Stressor/Condition | Measures | Results |
| --- | --- | --- | --- | --- |
| Brosschot et al., 1992 | 86 Normal subjects: 50 experimental group; 30 control group | Three dimensional unsolvable puzzle (experimental group) vs. reading popular magazine (control group) | Mononuclear cell counts, lymphocyte subsets, immune response to mitogens (PHA, PWM, and antigen cocktail) | Experimental subjects show increased NK cells, T suppressors, and cytotoxic cells after the stress period. No change in the immune response to mitogens |
| Brosschot et al., 1998 | Subjects perceiving high or low control over stressors | Three acute interpersonal stressors | Lymphocyte subsets | Subjects perceiving low control over stress exhibit decreased T helper cells, while subjects perceiving high control show an increase in B cells number |
| Burleson et al., 1998 | 55 Postmenopausal women (16 on estrogen alone, 14 on estrogen and progesteron, 25 controls) | Speech and arithmetic tasks | Quantitative and functional immune tests, cardiovascular and neuroendocrine assessments | Long-term estrogen replacement therapy is associated with higher overall levels and smaller stress-induced reductions of mitogen-stimulated blastogenesis, suggesting upregulated T cell function; estrogen replacement therapy enhances parasympathetic response to acute stress |
| Buske-Kirschbaum et al., 1992 | 24 Students divided in three groups: epinephrine controls, saline controls and conditioned | Conditioning procedure neutral sherbet sweet paired with a subcutaneous injection of epinephrine | NK-cell activity | Increased NK-cell activity in epinephrine and conditioned groups; no change in the saline group |
| Cacioppo et al., 1995 | 22 Aged women | Laboratory stressor | Immune function, plasma catecholamine levels, cortisol plasma levels | Brief psychological stressors raises catecholamine and cortisol concentrations and affect the cellular immune response |
| Cacioppo et al., 1998 | 27 Women caring for Alzheimer spouse and 37 controls | Laboratory stressor | Cellular immune functions | Diminished proliferative responses and heightened NK cell cytotoxicity, suggesting that although the stress of caregiving diminishes immune cellular functions, the effects of acute stress on cellular immune responses is modest |
| Cohen et al., 1999 | 39 Healthy women | Life events, acute and chronic stressors | NK cell cytotoxicity, CD4 and CD8 T-cell subsets | Immune outcomes are differentially assessed by acute and chronic stressors; an optimistic perspective seems to buffer acute stress and changes of immune parameters; however, when stress persists at high levels, optimists show more subsequent immune decrements than pessimists |
| Cole et al., 1999 | 36 Adults with functional bowel disease or fibromialgia | Conditions of high and low social engagement | Delayed type hypersensitivity to intradermal tetanus toxoid (ITT) | Under high engagement conditions, socially inhibited individuals show significantly increased induration in response to ITT |
| Davidson et al., 1999 | Healthy subjects | Positive and negative film clips, in a not stressful period and during the subject's most important final examination | NK cell number and activity, prefrontal EEG symmetry | Subjects with greater relative EEG right-sided activation at baseline show greater decrease in NK function during the final exam period compared to the baseline period, while subjects with EEG left-sided activation show a larger increase in NK function from before to after the positive film clip |

(Continues)

**TABLE II** (*Continued*)

| Authors | Sample | Stressor | Immune assessment | Results and conclusions |
|---|---|---|---|---|
| Decker et al., 1996 | 45 Patients with symptomatic cholelithiasis | Laparoscopic (LPC) surgery vs. traditional cholecistectomy (CCE) | Type 1/type 2 T-helper cell balance | Shift in the Th1/Th2 balance toward Th2 cells that evoke production of IL-4 more after CCE than LCE |
| Fittschen et al., 1990 | 61 Students | Academic stress | Large immunocyte number (LI); antibody titer against Herpes simplex virus (HSV) | No stress-induced change in HSV-Ab; increased LI percentage; high perceived stress is related to higher antibody titer |
| Fricchione et al., 1996 | 10 Patients and 35 nonsurgical controls | Psychological anticipatory stress under cardiac surgery | Immunocyte desensitization | Surgical anticipatory stress response may precipitate granulocyte monocyte desensitization |
| Fry et al., 1994 | 5 Men | Intensive sport training sessions | Quantitative parameters, lymphocyte subpopulations | Overtrained state is accompanied by fatigue, immune system deficits, mood disturbance, physical complaints across two weeks of training |
| Futterman et al., 1996 | 24 Partners of patients undergoing bone marrow transplantation (BMT) | Impact of waiting bone marrow transplantation in partner or spouse | Lymphocyte subsets, NK cells, NK-cell cytotoxicity | Greatest abnormalities of immune parameters was detected before BMT; less psychological escape-avoidance coping predicted better immune functioning |
| Geenen et al., 1998 | 22 Patients with rheumatoid arthritis (RA) of recent onset (under medication) and 23 healthy controls | Task with mental and physical effort | Lymphocyte subsets, plasma cortisol, cardiovascular parameters | Experimentally induced changes in peripheral blood lymphocytes as well as cortisol are normal in patients with early RA who are receiving long-term medication |
| Grazzi et al., 1993 | Three groups of subjects: swimmers, controls, splenectomized | Physical exercise | White blood cells (WBC), lymphocyte subsets, plasma catecholamine (NE), cortisol levels | Increase of WBC, lymphocyte, and NK after exercise in all the three groups; reduction of cortisol in swimmers and controls; increased NE levels in all subjects |
| Halvorsen et al., 1987 | 23 Students | Academic stress | Lymphocyte stimulation tests (PHA, IL-2, *D. farinae*), T-helper, T-suppressor, large T-helper, and large T-suppressor numbers; monocyte count | During acute examination stress: increased monocytes, decreased large lymphocytes, T-helpers and T-suppressors, no change in T-helper and T-suppressor total numbers; reduced response to IL-2; after examination: reduced response to antigen (*D. farinae*) and mitogen (PHA) |
| Hisano et al., 1997 | 26 Patients | Chest or abdominal surgery | IL-6 and soluble IL-6 receptor (sIL-6R) level in blood and drainage fluid | High quantity of sIL-6R is constantly produced in other areas than the operative fields, so surgical stress may involve sIL-6R and its ligand IL-6 |
| Kang et al., 1997 and 1998 | Three type of students (*n* = 88), healthy, mild asthma, severe asthma | Final exam | Lymphocyte subpopulations, NK-cell activity, lymphocyte transformation test, neutrophil superoxide release | NK-cell activity declines during final exam; social support appears to attenuate the magnitude of the exam-induced reduction; lymphocyte transformation and neutrophil superoxide release are increased after exam, suggesting continuous stress-induced activation of inflammatory cell function |
| Irwin et al., | 23 Healthy subjects | Partial sleep deprivation between 3 and 7 AM | Quantitative measures, NK-cell activity, EEG | NK-cell activity is reduced in 18 of the 23 subjects, returning to baseline levels after a night of resumed sleep |

| Reference | Subjects | Stressor | Measures | Findings |
|---|---|---|---|---|
| Kiecolt-Glaser et al., 1986 | 34 Students (22 men and 12 women) | Academic stress | T-helper, T-suppressor, and NK-cell activity | Decreased T-helper numbers and T4/T8 ratio; low NK-cell activity on the day of examination |
| Kiecolt-Glaser et al., 1993 | 90 Couples | Marital conflict, problem-solving behavior | Lymphocyte subsets, NK-cell activity, blastogenic response to mitogens, antibody titer to Epstein Barr virus, intergeron-2γ | Subjects who exhibited more negative or hostile behavior during a 30-min discussion of marital problems show greater decrements on natural killer cell lysis, blastogenic response to mitogens, larger increases in total T lymphocytes and T helper lymphocytes, higher antibody titers to latent Epstein–Barr virus; women are more likely to show negative immunological changes than men |
| Linn et al., 1987 | 24 Healthy men undergoing hernia repair | Life stress events, pre- and post-operative and surgical stress, cold pressure test | Immune response to mitogens (PHA, Con A, PWM) | High responders to life stress have significantly less response to PHA than low responders; high responders to cold pressure test have lower PWN responses. High responders to cold pressure test have significantly lower PWN response after the stress of surgery, indicating some T-B cell interaction defect |
| Locke et al., 1984 | 114 Students (79 men and 35 women) | Life stress events; Perceived stress | NK-cell activity | Low perceived stress scores and high life stress events scores are related with high NK-cell activity |
| Maes et al., 1999 | 38 University students | Difficult academic examination | Lymphocytic subsets, Peripheral blood mononuclear cells | Student high reactors to stress at the PSS have a significant increase in the number of neutrophils, monocytes, CD8+, CD2+, CD26+, CD2+HLADr+ cells, CD19+ B cells and significant reductions in the CD4/CD8+ T cell ratio, findings indicate immune activation under acute stress, probably orchestrated by a stress-induced production of cytokines |
| Marchesi et al., 1989 | 14 Students, 9 men and 5 women | Academic examination | T-helpers, T-suppressors, T-11, T-3, and IL-2 | Six students with high anxiety scores show decreased lymphocyte subsets |
| Marshall et al., 1999 | 16 Healthy medical students | Exam stress | Type-1 (IFN-γ) and type-2 (IL-10) cytokines from 72-h PHA/PMA-stimulated peripheral cells | Decreased IFN-γ accompanied by increased IL-10 during exam stress, resulting in a decreased IFN-γ: IL-10 ratio, stressful situations seem to shift type-1/type-2 cytokine balance, this might explain the increased incidence of type-2 mediated reactions such as increased viral infections, latent viral expression, allergic reactions and autoimmunity during high stress |
| Marsland et al., 1995a | 30 Young men | Acute mental stress (speech task) | Lymphocyte proliferative responses, lymphocyte subsets | Speech stressor elicits diminished proliferative responses to mitogens (PHA and con A), a decrease in CD8 and CD19, and an increase in CD8 and CD56 lymphocytes; these changes are stable across two sessions (2 weeks apart) |
| Marsland et al., 1995b | 22 Male volunteers and 11 unstressed control subjects | Mental stress: frustrating laboratory task | T suppressor/cytotoxic and NK cell number | Increase of T-suppressor/cytotoxic cells and NK percentage in subjects subjected to stressor |

(Continues)

**TABLE II** (Continued)

| Authors | Sample | Stressor | Immune assessment | Results and conclusions |
|---|---|---|---|---|
| Matthews et al., 1995 | 19 Women | 3 min of public speaking | T helper and NK cells | The stress-induced decrease in CD4+ percentage and the increase in NK cell number and cytolitic activity are only apparent among the high reactors |
| McClelland et al., 1985 | 46 Students (29 men and 17 women) | Academic stress | Secretory IgA | Increase in serum IgA |
| Mills et al., 1995 | 24 Healthy males | Speaking stressor | Lymphocyte subsets | Stressor causes significant increases in total WBC, NK cells, T-suppressor/cytotoxic cells and decreases T-helper/suppressor ratio; findings are only moderately stable in two sessions 6 weeks apart |
| Mills et al., 1995 | 110 Subjects | Naturalistic speaking stressor | Total WBC, NK cells, CD4, CD8, B and T cells, $\beta$-2 receptor lymphocyte sensitivity | Speaking task causes marked increase in total WBC, NK cells, T-suppressor/cytotoxic cells, and a decrease of T-helper and B cells; immune activation seems mediated by sympathetic mechanisms |
| Mizutani et al., 1996 | 20 Patients with cancer of bladder, renal pelvis, urethra or kidney | Surgical stress | Serum immunoglobulin levels and immunosuppressive acid protein (IAP) | Surgical stress may result in both suppression and stimulation of host immunity |
| Naliboff et al., 1991 | 23 Women divided in two groups: young group ($n = 12$) and aged group ($n = 11$) | Laboratory stress: mental arithmetic task and videotaped lecture on a health topic | NK-cell activity and mitogen response (PHA), T-helpers, T-suppressors and other lymphocyte subsets | Increased T-suppressor and NK cells number in both age groups; increased NK-cell activity only in the younger group; no changes in T-helper number |
| Naliboff et al., 1995 | 20 Healthy young men | Video-watching control task | NK cells number and reactivity, CD4, CD8 | Increase in NK cytotoxicity, and of CD8; naloxone does not block immune changes under stress, suggesting that opioids do not mediate them |
| Natelson et al., 1996 | Seven men | Exhausting physical exercise | Cytokine levels | Relative decrease of TNF-$\alpha$; no change in IL-1, IL-2, IL-4, IL-6, IL-10 and IFN-$\gamma$ levels |
| Osuka et al., 1996 | 70 Patients | Neurosurgery | IL-1$\beta$, IL-6, IL-8, TNF-$\alpha$, and INF-$\gamma$ concentration | No significant change in IL-1$\beta$, IL-8, TNF-$\alpha$ and IFN-$\gamma$ concentration; maximum concentration level of IL-6 peaking at postoperative day 1 and then gradually decreasing |
| Palmblad et al., 1976 | Five normal subjects | Laboratory stress | Granulocyte phagocytosis and turnover | Reduced phagocytosis and higher turnover during stress followed by increase |
| Palmblad et al., 1979 | 12 Normal subjects | Sleep deprivation | Immune response to mitogen (PHA) and polymorphonuclear leukocyte number | Decreased immune response to PHA |
| Pettingale et al., 1977 | 160 Women admitted for breast tumor biopsy | Waiting operation | Serum immunoglobulins | Both in cancer patients and those with benign breast disease serum IgA levels are higher in patients who suppress anger than in patients who express it |
| Pike et al., 1997 | 12 Male volunteers with and 11 without chronic stress | 12-Min laboratory stressor | Epinephrine, norepinephrine, ACTH, cortisol, NK-cell distribution | Peak sympathomedullary reactivity during acute psychological stress in subjects with chronic life stress are associated with decrements in individual NK-cell function |

| Reference | Subjects | Stressor | Measures | Findings |
|---|---|---|---|---|
| Redmond et al., 1994 | 44 Patients with cholelithiasis | Laparoscopic surgery versus traditional cholecistectomy | Monocyte release of $O_2$ and tumor necrosis factor (TNF), neutrophil release of $O_2$ and chemotaxis, WBC counts, cortisol and C-reactive protein levels | Increase in monocyte $O_2$ and TNF release, in $O_2$ neutrophil release and chemotaxis; in open lapascopic cholecystectomy |
| Sauer et al., 1995 | 18 Students | Academic stress | Lymphocyte cortisol sensitivity | Positive correlation between lymphocyte DNA synthesis and control inhibition; decreased lymphocyte sensitivity to cortisol |
| Schmid et al., 1998 | 13 Psoriatic patients, 7 healthy controls | Mental arithmetic | Catecholamine, cortisol, DHEA, T cells, NK cells | Mental stress increases NK cell numbers (CD+16 and CD+56) but not T lymphocytes in healthy and psoriatic patients |
| Sgoutas Emch et al., 1994 | Normal subjects, high and low heart rate reactors | Speech stressor, noise, mental arithmetic | Lymphocyte subpopulations, mitogenic responses, NK cells | Speech stress reduces con A response, increases NK cell number and cytotoxicity, absolute numbers of CD8+ T lymphocytes, noradrenaline and adrenaline levels, heart rate and blood pressure; cortisol and NK cytotoxicity differentiate high and low heart rate reactors; findings suggest interactions between the sympathetic nervous and the immune systems under stress |
| Song et al., 1999 | 38 University students | Academic examination | Serum concentrations of interleukin (IL)-1 receptor (R) antagonist, soluble(s) IL-2R, s IL-6R, soluble glycoprotein 130 (sgp 130) Clara cell protein, sCD8, sCD14, cortisol | Academic examination was associated with increases in cortisol, PSS, STAI scores, sgp 130, sCD8 values, decreases sCD14 in students with high, but not low, stress perception; psychological acute stress is associated with immune-inflammatory changes, decreased anti-inflammatory capacity of the serum, and monocytic activation |
| Tanabe, 1993 | Patients with gastric cancer | Surgery | Suppressor inducer T, T-suppressors, T-lymphokine activated killer cells (LAK) | Significant increase of suppressor inducers and T suppressors; significant decrease of LAK cells |
| Tonnesen et al., 1987 | Surgery patients | Coronary artery bypass grafting | Lymphocyte subsets, NK-cell activity, immune response to mitogens | Increase of NK-cell activity while awaiting surgery; decreased immune response to PHA |
| Vadhara & Nott, 1996 | 16 Students and 12 controls | School examination | Delayed skin test | High stress subjects have poorer reaction than low stress subjects |
| Van der Pompe et al., 1998 | 23 Breast cancer patients and 15 controls | Speech task | Lymphocyte subsets | Stressor induces marked increase of NK and CD8 cells and of NK-cell activity; no significant differences between healthy subjects and patients |

accounts for downregulation of lymphocyte $\beta_2$-adrenergic receptor, suggesting possible effects on cellular immunity (Mills et al., 1997). Little is known of whether and to what extent immune changes also differ in young versus elderly populations under stress (Naliboff et al., 1991). A recent metaanalysis, however, concluded that young versus old women do not differ in stress-induced immune changes after acute psychological stress (Benschop et al., 1998). Given the evidence of alterations in sympathetic noradrenergic innervation of lymphoid organs with age (Madden, Thyagarajan, & Felten, 1998), this should be a topic of interest for the future.

Given the complexity and cost of psychoneuroimmunological studies, the large majority of published papers comes from wealthy regions of the world, thus increasing the possibility of underestimating possible cultural or racial differences on stress-induced immune changes.

Sexual dimorphism within the immune system is an established finding, together with evidence that women have greater antibody response to antigens, higher levels of immunoglobulins, and higher incidence of autoimmune diseases (such as systemic lupus erythematosus, Hashimoto's thyroiditis, Grave's disease) than males (Gaillard & Spinedi, 1998). Male/female differences in immunity and sex– and stress–steroid interactions are parallel to hypothalamic (hence, neuroendocrine) sexual dimorphism (Gaillard & Spinedi, 1998; McCruden & Stimson, 1991). However, few studies have specifically investigated the possible influence of gender on responsiveness to acute psychological stress (Caudell & Gallucci, 1995; Matthews et al., 1995; Mills, Berry, Dimsdale, Ziegler, Nelesen, & Kennedy, 1995). Another study reported a limited influence of gender (Mills, Ziegler, Dimsdale, & Parry, 1995); although the menstrual cycle seems not to have affected immune changes after acute stress in this study, the change of endocrine profile across the cycle appears to limit the enrollment of study subjects. It appears that interindividual, rather than gender-related, factors might play a role in acute psychological stress-induced norepinephrine surge and consequent lymphocytosis (Mills et al., 1995). Some studies reported gender differences; sex hormones may modify stress-induced immune-inflammatory responses (Song et al., 1999), while female students on oral contraceptives showed significantly higher stress-induced changes in leukocyte, neutrophil and CD19+ B cell numbers than male and oral contraceptive-free female students (Maes et al., 1999).

From an experimental standpoint, more recent studies adopt strict inclusion criteria in order to keep confounding variables to a minimum. The typical experimental subject in psychoimmunology is a young, male, Caucasian, healthy, medical or psychology student, probably a light or nonsmoker, consuming little or no alcohol or coffee, with no history of allergy or recent infectious disease, not taking anti-inflammatory or other drugs, including minor tranquilizers. The other typical subject is of variable age, in good physical, but not psychological, health, with serious emotional problems (but not specific DSM-IV diagnosis) related to loss, marital or occupational problems, or impending medical or surgical procedures. In these cases, inclusion criteria are larger.

As a whole, sampling characteristics of psychoneuroimmunology studies are satisfactory, with limits common to all experimental research in psychoneuroendocrinology of stress or experimental psychiatry. The relatively small sample sizes and the high homogeneity of the subject populations yield reliable findings in terms of the control of confounding variables, but one could argue that it might limit the generalizability of the findings. In other words, the question remains as to whether stressors can induce larger changes in general population subjects under real-life stress, where many other common confounding variables might come into play. Further studies are needed to show whether experimental studies to date underreport or overestimate the magnitude of stress-induced changes.

## B. Nature of Stressors

Real-life and laboratory stressors are two competing strategies in the study of human stress physiology. They investigate profoundly different conditions, which depend in part on the objective characteristics of the stimulus itself and in part on the emotional arousal that field or laboratory stimuli can elicit. Real-life and field stressors entail poorer control of experimental setting and variables but are associated with greater stimulus impact than laboratory stressors; on the other hand, the latter imply better control of variables but less physiological challenge (Dimsdale, 1984). Real-life stressors are often enduring ones and, although not exclusively, they may be associated with chronic stress conditions (Table III). Some real-life stressors are associated with acute, short-term stress (Table IV). Both stressors can induce changes in immune function. Finally, stressors delivered in laboratory settings may induce acute stress reactions with possible changes of immune functions.

**TABLE III   Examples of Real-Life Stressors in Human Psychoneuroimmunology**

| | |
|---|---|
| Loss and bereavement | Bartrop et al., 1977; Schleifer et al., 1983; Udelmann, 1982 |
| Separation and divorce | Kiecolt-Glaser et al., 1988, 1993 |
| Marital stress | Kiecolt-Glaser et al., 1997 and 1998 |
| Disease of a spouse | Irwin et al., 1986; Mills et al., 1998 |
| Caregiving of demented | Castle et al., 1995; Glaser et al., 1998; Esterling et al., 1996; Kiecolt-Glaser et al., 1996; Mills et al., 1997; Vedhara et al., 1999 |
| Caregiving of severe disabled | Pariante et al., 1997 |
| Loneliness | Kiecolt-Glaser et al., 1984; Thomas et al., 1985 |
| Homelessness | Dimsdale et al., 1994; Esterling et al., 1996 |
| Academic stress | Alvorsen et al., 1987; Kasl et al., 1979; McClelland et al., 1980 |
| Children starting school | Boyce et al., 1995 |
| Earthquake | Boyce et al., 1993; Solomon et al., 1997; Segerstrom et al., 1998 |
| Unemployment | Arnetz et al., 1987 |
| Job-related stress | Nakano et al., 1998, De Gucht et al., 1999 |
| Life stress events | Biondi et al., 1993; Biondi et al., 1994; Brosschot et al., 1994; Byrnes et al., 1998; Canter et al., 1972; Castle et al., 1995; Cole et al., 1999; Evans & Edgerton, 1991; Greene et al., 1978; Gonzalez-Quijano et al., 1998; Kubitz et al., 1986; Leserman et al., 1999; Levy et al.; 1985, Linne et al., 1987; Locke et al., 1977; Locke et al., 1984; Logans et al., 1998; Mills et al., 1997; Potter & Zautra, 1997; Snyder et al., 1993; Stone et al., 1992; Thomas et al., 1985; Totman et al., 1980 |
| Daily hassles | Benschop et al., 1994; Brosschot et al., 1994; Kubitz et al., 1986 |
| Caregiving to low birth weight infants | DiGennaro et al., 1997 |
| Post-traumatic stress disorder | Boyce et al., 1993; Ironson et al., 1997; Maes et al., 1999; Solomon et al., 1997; Wilson et al., 1999 |
| Waiting for bone marrow transplantation of spouse | Futterman et al., 1996 |

**TABLE IV   Examples of Acute Psychic Stressors of Human Research in Psychoneuroimmunology**

| | |
|---|---|
| Space flight | Fischer et al., 1972; Levine & Greenleaf, 1998; Taylor et al., 1986 |
| School examination | Baker et al., 1984; Davidson et al., 1999; Fittschen et al., 1990; Glaser et al., 1992; Kang et al., 1996; Kang et al., 1997; Kiecolt-Glaser et al., 1984; Kiecolt-Glaser et al., 1986; Maes et al., 1999; Marchesi et al., 1989; Marshall et al., 1998; Marucha et al., 1998; McClelland et al., 1985; Sauer et al., 1995; Vedhara & Nott, 1996 |
| Hospital admission | Aragona et al., 1996 |
| Awaiting surgery | Biondi et al., 1981; Cacioppo et al., 1995; Tonnesen et al., 1987 |
| Surgical stress | Decker et al., 1996; Hisano et al., 1997; Mizutani et al., 1996; Osuka et al., 1996; Redmond et al., 1994; Szckelik & Jawien, 1996; Tanabe, 1993; Taylor et al., 1986; Tonnesen et al., 1987 |
| Severe disease notification | Aragona et al., 1996; Fawzy et al., 1990; Ironson et al., 1990; Lewy et al., 1990; Pettingale et al., 1981 |
| Public speaking or speech task | Burleson et al., 1998; Matthews et al., 1995; Mills et al., 1995a; Mills et al., 1995b; van der Pompe et al., 1998 |
| Threat of missile attack | Weiss et al., 1996 |
| Exposure to phobic stimulus | Segerstrom et al., 1999 |
| Social engagement | Cole et al., 1999 |

### 1. Real-Life Stressors

Real-life stressor studies (Table III) often employ longitudinal experimental designs with immune function assessments across two or more observation points. In some cases, they assess immune functions at only one time point in a sample of subjects exposed to long-standing stressors. Serial assessments in longitudinal studies are usually set apart by weeks or months, as, for example, in the seminal studies on immune correlates of bereavement by Bartrop, Lazarus, Luckhurst, and Kiloh (1977), Schleifer, Keller, Camerino, Thornton, and Stein (1983), and Irwin, Daniels, Bloom, and Weiner (1988); in studies of recurrent oral herpes outbreaks (Logan, Lutgendorf, Hartwig, Lilly, & Barberich, 1998); or in assessing possible immune changes associated with intervening psychological changes over several months (Biondi et al., 1994). Some studies suggest a moderate temporal stability of at least certain individual differences in cellular immunity only under acute stress (Mills, Haeri, & Dimsdale, 1995; Marsland, Manuck, Fazzari, Stewart, & Rabin, 1995).

☞ Immune functions seem sensitive to long-standing emotional stress related to waiting for an important school examination, life crises such as divorce or separation, bereavement, caregiving to a family member with severe illness, waiting for surgery or medical procedures, unemployment, life-threatening illness, and cumulative life events (see Table III). All these studies are of interest because they represent common, naturally occurring situations. Real-life stressors differ in at least two dimensions, i.e., duration and severity. Some stressors, such as waiting for surgery or taking school examinations, are of relatively short duration, and they represent a source of acute arousal. They are rated as low- or medium-impact in life events scales or in the psychosocial stress scale of the DSM. Examination stress is largely the most adopted model, with about 15 studies (Table IV). Other stressors, such as bereavement and, to a lesser extent, divorce or separation are long-standing. They are rated as severe stressors on life events scales. Although it may be an oversimplification, acute stress is frequently associated with transient immune activation, while chronic stress is associated with immune downregulation or depression (Olff, 1999). Studies of the psychobiological aspects of loss-induced depression suggest that long-lasting feelings of despair and conflicted mourning can alter neurotransmitter and receptor status in the brain and can contribute to peripheral neuroendocrine and immune changes (Biondi & Picardi, 1996). Epidemiological studies suggested increased morbidity and mortality associated with bereavement (Jacobs & Ostfeld, 1972), such as the increased mortality due to the so called "broken heart" (Parkes, Benjamin, & Fitzgerald, 1969). It is under study whether immune changes might contribute to other causes of increased morbidity. A decreased lymphocyte response to mitogens persisting several months during bereavement was reported in man (Bartrop et al., 1977; Schleifer et al., 1983). The cross-sectional and prospective studies of Irwin and Weiner (1987), Irwin, Daniels, Risch, and Weiner (1988), showing endocrine and NK cell changes in bereaved subjects, are of particular interest and may have prominent health implications. Studies in Alzheimer's caregivers found impairment of T-cell proliferative capacity (Castle, Wilkins, Heck, Tanzy, & Fahey, 1995) and impaired response to immunization (Vedhara et al., 1999) with possible increased risk of morbidity.

A few studies investigated extreme events including space flights, earthquake, civilians under missile attack, or events leading to posttraumatic stress disorder (PTSD). The impact of events on PTSD may result in exceptionally long-standing stress. Endocrine and neural long-lasting changes have been reported, such as enhanced suppression of cortisol to low doses of dexamethasone (Yehuda, Giller, Levengood, Southwick, & Siever, 1995) and long-standing total and free triiodothyronine increases (Mason et al., 1995). Little is known of the immune correlates of PTSD and the possible health consequences with respect to immunological disorders. A community sample exposed to and damaged by hurricane Andrew, 1–4 months later had significantly lower NK cell cytotoxicity (NKCC), and CD4 and CD8 numbers, as well as higher NK cell numbers as compared to controls. NKCC was correlated inversely with damage, psychological loss, and PTSD symptoms such as intrusive thoughts (Ironson et al., 1997). A study found serum interleukin-6 (IL-6) and soluble IL-6 receptor significantly higher in civilian PTSD patients than controls, suggesting that consequences of severe psychological trauma may be associated with increased interleukin-6 signaling and stress-induced secretion of proinflammatory cytokines (Maes et al., 1999a). Another study confirms evidence of chronic immune activation (Wilson, van der Kolk, Burbridge, Fisler, & Kradin, 1999). Immune correlates of PTSD seem thus to confirm that trauma may have also subtle, chronic consequences at brain and neuroendocrine levels. This is a promising field of investigation.

**TABLE V  Laboratory Stressors in Human Psychoneuroimmunology**

| | |
|---|---|
| Sleep deprivation | Palmblad et al., 1979; Irwin et al., 1994 |
| Mental stress | Ackerman et al., 1998; Bachen et al., 1995; Cacioppo et al., 1998; Marsland et al., 1995a; Marsland et al., 1995b; Naliboff et al., 1991 |
| Laboratory stress | Breznitz et al., 1998; Brosschot et al., 1992; Brosschot et al., 1998; Buske-Kirschbaum et al., 1992; Cacioppo et al., 1995; Cacioppo et al., 1998; Naliboff et al., 1995; Palmblad et al., 1976; Pike et al., 1997; Sgoutas et al., 1994 |
| Acute physical overtraining | Fry et al., 1994; Grazzi et al., 1993 |

## 2. Laboratory Stressors

Laboratory stressors provide the experimenter with near total control of setting and experimental variables. In particular, they have been adopted in cardiovascular psychophysiology and neuroendocrine assessment of acute stressful stimuli, as they allow for standardized control and differing conditions of emotional arousal of experimental subjects (Steptoe, 1983). Stimuli delivered in laboratory settings are, however, of limited potency, short duration (minutes or hours), with transient effects and rapid recovery. Typical stimuli include cognitive performance tests, problem solving, mental stress, anticipation of mild cutaneous shocks, and partial sleep deprivation (Table V). Measures of autonomic and psychophysiologic reactivity (skin conductance, brain bioelectrical activity, heart rate, peripheral vasoconstriction, etc.) show high and moment-to-moment sensitivity to these stressors. Minor laboratory stressors, such as mental arithmetic or anticipation of mild painful electric shock, also seem able to induce some immune changes. As the elegant study by Breznitz et al. (1998) showed, threat of a mild electrical shock is also able to induce a small, but significant, transient elevation of NK cells and increase in the CD4/CD8 ratio.

Laboratory stressors are of interest in the investigation of the timing and mechanism of acute stress-induced immune changes. Their potential impact on health, however, is an open question.

## 3. Cumulative Life Changes

Studies assessing the cumulative stress of life by means of life events questionnaires and schedules, such as the Schedule of Recent Experiences by Holmes and Rahe (1967), the Life Experiences Survey by Sarason, Johnson, and Siegel (1978), and Paykel's Life Events Scale (1978), or other methods of assessment are largely represented, with about 20 investigations (Table III). A previous review of the literature (Biondi & Pancheri, 1985) reported that about one-fourth of human stress studies included a life events scale as a method of assessment and "scoring" previous life stress, mainly occurring during the prior 6 or 12 months. They seem to be decreasing slightly in recent years. Many reasons could account for this apparent reduction of interest. Low reliability of life events scales filled out by the subject might be a first reason. Difficulties in the control of the life setting of the individual and confounding variables (variability of sleep habits and biorhythms, changes in health-related behavior, level of activity, and use of psychotropic medications) might be another reason. Weak or inconclusive findings as concern immune changes and the difficulty to precisely correlate life stress scoring to laboratory immune parameters might be a third reason. However, careful collection of life events with structured interviews, better definition of the time period under investigation, and recognition of the subjective impact of negative and positive events (instead of a standard, predetermined scoring of events) might prove useful in some research areas, such as specific population screening, or as an additional method for assessing global stress level. Life stress, in particular a high number of daily hassles, could affect immunological reactivity after acute psychological stress, reducing peripheral T and NK cells (Brosschot et al., 1994). High daily hassle levels were reported to influence the sensitivity of immunologic responsiveness to an acute psychological stress (Benschop et al., 1994). Psychological distress related to life events was associated with reduced primary cellular immune response 3 weeks after immunization (Snyder, Roghmann, & Sigal, 1993).

In summary, real-life stressors have been largely investigated in human studies. Together with investigations on cumulative life change and specific life stress events, such as bereavement, divorce, natural disaster, etc., they represent both acute and chronic conditions with significant impact potential on immune function. They are probably more relevant than laboratory stress studies to the understanding of immune mediation between stress and disease. Laboratory stress studies have been increasing recently; they provide new and valid information on the mediating mechanisms of stressor exposure-induced acute immune changes.

## C.  Individual Variability and Stress-Related Immune Changes

Most of the studies of stress and immune changes in humans focus on mean and group values, underestimating interindividual psychological variability. Since the first years of psychoimmunology, it has been stressed that "one simple, universal observation underlies psychosomatic research...the observation that when a population of individuals is exposed to the same environmental pathogens only some individuals manifest disease...for the psychosomatist, such variability is the starting point of his research" (Ader, 1980). Only recently the issue of individual variability appears to have received due attention in psychoneuroimmunology (Cohen, 1999; Kemeny & Laudenslager, 1999), as related to cognitive factors (Biondi, 1991), or to a subject's ways of dealing with stress and affective state (Olff, 1999), or to social support (Uchino, Cacioppo, & Kiecolt-Glaser, 1996).

The possible sources of interindividual variability are several. Physical variables, such as gender, ethnicity, age, weight, biorhythms, health and nutritional status are a first major source of variability. Experimental studies almost always control for this kind of variability. A second source of variability depends on stimulus or situation characteristics, such as acute *versus* chronic, predictable *versus* unescapable. A third source of variance is interindividual variability due to psychological factors, such as personality, mood states, defense mechanisms, control over or coping with the situation, and availability of social support. Investigators in psychophysiology and psychosomatics tried in the past to recognize if and to what extent this third source of variability could affect biological reactivity under stress. Parameters such as anxiety levels, introversion *vs.* extroversion, levels of hostility, field-dependence or -independence, and the possibility and degree of coping, all contributed to the profiles of psychophysiological responses and to differences among individuals (Greenfield & Sternbach, 1972).

Cognitive appraisal of stimuli is basic to psychological stress adaptation and may explain interindividual variability of response (Lazarus, 1971). The process of cognitive appraisal gives subjective meaning to stimuli and life events. It determines the type,

direction, and intensity of the stress-related emotions, such as anxiety, anger, guilt, sadness, shame, envy, and disgust (Lazarus, 1993). Type and efficacy of psychological defense and coping can reduce acute emotional arousal and endocrine stress responses to real-life stressors such as parachute jumping (Ursin, Schytte Blix, & Rosseland, 1987), breast biopsy (Gorzynski et al., 1980), and fatal pediatric illness (Wolff, Friedman, Hofer, & Mason, 1964). Under the acute stress of poor performance-related frustration in a difficult computerized task paradigm, social support provided by the experimenters to the subject prevents blood pressure rise and blocks stress-related cortisol increases (Biondi et al., 1986). Psychological differences among individuals, coping and support thus contribute to the variability in both endocrine and associated immune reactivity during stress.

### 1. Anxiety

As concerns anxiety level, subclinically anxious normal male college freshmen show significantly lower lymphocyte proliferative responses to the mitogen concanavalin A (Con A) and lower levels of circulating interleukin-1. Subjects with a more negative attribution style for aversive events also have reduced blastogenic T-cell responses and levels of circulating interleukin-2 (Zorrilla, Redei, & DeRubeis, 1994). Students with high anxiety scores under examination stress may show altered lymphocyte subset (Marchesi, Cotani, Santone, DiGiuseppe, Bartocci, & Montroni, 1989), while students in their first week in a new college have high serum cortisol and increased percentage of OKT4 (helper/inducer) (Baker et al., 1984). High scores of anxiety have been related to decreased lymphocyte response to mitogens in undergraduate students (Gonzales-Quijano, Martin, Millan, & Lopez-Calderon 1998), in children starting school (Boyce, Adams, Tschann, Cohen, Wara, & Gunnar, 1995), and in mothers of low-birthweight infants, with no effect on Natural Killer (NK) cells (Di Gennaro, Fehder, Nuamah, Campbell, & Douglas, 1997).

Given that anxiety is often associated with sympathetic activation, individual differences in ANS reactivity might contribute to individual immune variability under acute stress. Acute psychological stress can induce short-term catecholamine increases which may result in lymphocytosis and leukocytosis (Benschop, Rodriguez-Feuerhahn, & Schedlowski, 1996). Changes in NK-cell and T-lymphocyte function during acute stress appear to be mainly mediated by sympathetic activation (for a review see Madden, Sanders, & Felten 1995). High- but not low-sympathetic reactors to the stress of public speaking, showed increased NK-cell number and reactivity (Matthews et al., 1995). High- *versus* low autonomic cardiac activation has been reported to be correlated with heterogeneity of endocrine and immune responses under acute stress (Cacioppo et al., 1995). Other studies confirm that interindividual differences in sympathetic nervous system reactivity have a significant role in acute immune system activation under naturalistic public speaking stress (Mills et al., 1995a, b).

Higher scores on a trait measure of worry has been associated with fewer natural killer cells after the stress of earthquake. The authors suppose that the cognitive style of persistent worry may be associated with persistent dysregulation of the autonomic nervous system, which may extend to the immune system (Segerstrom, Solomon, Kemeny, & Fahey, 1998). High worry subjects exposed to feared phobic stimuli showed increased heart rate and skin conductance, but not the increase of peripheral blood NK cells shown by control subjects (Segerstrom, Glover, Craske, & Fahey, 1999a). Under the threat of missile attack, civilians were more anxious than in pre- and postwar assessment. NK-cell activity and cell-mediated lympholysis were significantly elevated (Weiss et al., 1996).

### 2. Perceived Stress

High perceived stress has been repeatedly associated with altered immune function. High reactors to acute stressors seem to show significantly larger immune changes (Brosschot, Godaert, Benschop, Olff, Ballieux, & Hejinen, 1998; Linn & Linn, 1987; Maes et al., 1999a; Marchesi et al., 1989; Matthews et al., 1995). Some studies also suggest a tendency to immune activation under acute conditions in high stress reactors, such as higher antibody titer under academic stress (Fittschen, Schulz, Schulz, Raedler, & Kerekjarto, 1990), neutrophile, monocyte, CD8+, CD2+, and CD26+ increase, and reduction of CD4/ CD8 ratio (Maes et al., 1999b). Low perceived stress has been associated with high NK-cell activity (Locke, Kraus, Leserman, Hurst, Heisel, & Williams, 1984). Perceived controllability may have immunomodulating effects, with subjects perceiving low control over stress exhibiting decreased T helper cells and subjects perceiving high control an increase in B cell number (Brosschot et al., 1998).

### 3. Personality and Coping

Several studies explored the relationships between personality, affective state, coping, and immune changes under stress. They were, however, methodo-

logically different as concerns psychometric assessment or personality dimensions tested.

A naturalistic study in women the day before breast surgery found that subjects with subclinical depression (high scores on the Depression scale of the Minnesota Multiphasic Personality Inventory [MMPI]) and social introversion (high scores on the Social Introversion scale of the MMPI) had statistically significant decreases in blastogenic T-lymphocyte response, rosette-E formation, and skin test reactivity to common antigens compared to control subjects in the same situation (Biondi & Pancheri, 1985). Severity of depressive symptoms has been also associated with impairment of NK-cell activity, loss of suppressor/ cytotoxic cells and an increase in the ratio of the T helper to T suppressor cytotoxic cells in women who experienced major life changes (Irwin & Weiner, 1987). A strong association was also reported in caregivers of demented patients between severity of depression and impairment of T-cell proliferative capacity, with an increase in CD8+ cells and reduced percentages of CD38+ and NK cells. According to the authors, the reduction of CD38+, a signal transduction factor, is interestingly correlated with impaired T-cell function and proliferation, and these findings could contribute to the higher risk of disease in the caregivers (Castle et al., 1995). Depressive symptoms and life stress were related to reduced phagocytosis and reduced killing of *Staphylococcus aureus* in children (Bartlett, Demetrikopoulos, Schleifer, & Keller, 1997).

Subjects high in social inhibition displayed heightened delayed type hypersensitivity under conditions of high social engagement, suggesting a relationship between social inhibition and physiologic hyperresponsiveness (Cole, Kemeny, Weitzman, Schoen, & Anton, 1999). Higher scores on the Minnesota Multiphasic Personality Inventory (*T* scores on the Depression, Psychopathic deviation, Paranoia, Schizophrenia, and Hypomania scales higher than 70), which suggest soft psychopathology or distress, were related to lower NK-cell activity in a sample of normal college students (Heisel, Locke, Kraus, & Williams 1986). Low extroversion, but not neuroticism, has been associated with higher NK-cell cytotoxicity, a finding accounted for by epinephrine levels (Miller, Cohen, Rabin, Skoner, & Doyle, 1999). Lower lymphocyte response to PHA has been reported in introverted with respect to extroverted undergraduate students (Gonzales-Quijano et al., 1998). In the same study, lymphocyte response to PHA was lower in students with high life events compared to those with low events. In the group with high scores of independence of personality, however, a high accumulation of life events was not associated with low lymphoproliferation. This finding suggests that an independent personality could buffer the association between high life stress and reduced lymphocyte proliferation.

Optimistic attitude seems to buffer changes of immune parameters under acute stress, although if stress persists at high levels, pessimists show less immune changes than optimists (Cohen et al., 1999). A prospective study in law students reported that optimism is associated with better mood, higher number of T cells, and higher NK-cell cytotoxicity. Better mood accounted for the optimism–T cell relationship, and perceived stress accounted for the optimism–cytotoxicity relationship (Segerstrom, Taylor, Kemeny, & Fahey, 1999b). Pessimism might also be a risk factor for cervical cancer, according to a study which found that greater pessimism was related to lower natural killer cell cytotoxicity and cytotoxic/suppressor cells in a sample of black women infected with human immunodeficiency virus type 1 and human papilloma virus; according to the authors, such an immune impairment could lead to an increased risk of progression of cervical dysplasia to cervical cancer (Byrnes et al., 1998).

Coping style and defense mechanisms affect emotional arousal and the response to stressful stimuli. They can affect ANS and endocrine changes under stress (Biondi & Picardi, 1999; Mason, 1975) and might also contribute to immune changes (Olff, 1999). In waiting for breast surgery, subjects with higher score at the repression-denial scale of the Reaction Scheme Test (measuring defense mechanisms and prevalent behavioral coping styles in stressful situations) had a significantly reduced lymphocyte proliferation response to PHA than subjects with lower scores (Biondi & Pancheri, 1991). A repressive defensive high-anxious coping style has been related to decreased monocyte count, while repressive coping has been associated with elevated eosinophil counts (Jamner, Schwartz, & Leigh, 1988). Escape-avoiding coping style was predictive of worse immune functioning during the stress of waiting for blood marrow transplantation of one's partner or spouse (Futterman, Wellisch, Zighelboim, Luna-Raines, & Weiner, 1996).

Locus of control is a personality dimension which can affect coping responses. A study of the effects of daily hassles on humoral immunity reported that individuals high in internal locus of control had less salivary IgA than subjects low in internal locus of control, suggesting that high internal individuals might be especially vulnerable to high levels of stress (Kubitz, Peavey, & Moore, 1986). Locus of control, however, did not affected immune response to a mild interpersonal stressor (Brosschot et al., 1994).

Perceived uncontrollability under acute stress might have immunomodulating properties that are, at least in part, independent of the type of stressor (Brosschot et al., 1998).

Finally, electrophysiological study of brain activity, which might be related to mood and coping, suggests a lateralized brain modulation of the ANS, endocrine, and immune response under stress, probably by mediation of lateralized brain neurotransmitter activity (Neveu, Delrue, Deleplanque, D'Amato, Puglisi-Allegra, & Cabib, 1994). Changes in NK-cell activity and lymphocyte proliferation to mitogens after acute laboratory stress in adolescents were found to be associated only among subjects with previous negative life events and greater left frontal cortical activation in resting EEG (Liang, Jemerin, Tschann, Wara, & Boyce, 1997). Right-sided prefrontal activation asymmetry at the EEG predicted lower levels of basal NK function and a greater decrease during the final exam period as compared to the baseline period (Davidson, Coe, Dolski, & Donzella, 1999). These findings seem to invite further investigation of the correlations between personality, brain, and immune system under stress.

### 4. Social Support, Loss, and Loneliness

Nonhuman primate studies show that social separation can significantly affect some immune functions, such as decreased lymphocyte proliferation responses, but that immune changes occur in those who exhibit the most severe response to separation, with despair, distress vocalizations, and agitation (Coe, 1993). The presence of a preferred companion attenuates the profound stress that female rhesus monkeys show after removal from their social group, with smaller changes of CD4+, CD8+ cell numbers and CD4/CD8 ratio (Gust, Gordon, Brodie, & McClure, 1994). Both individual psychological variability and social support seem, therefore, to characterize immune correlates of disrupted attachment in nonhuman primates.

Several studies found immunodepression after the death of a loved one (Bartrop et al., 1977; Irwin & Weiner, 1987; Schleifer et al., 1983); immune downregulation was also found in separating and divorcing male subjects, as compared to stably married individuals (Kiecolt-Glaser et al., 1988). Although studies reported mean group values, clinical experience suggests that significant differences among individuals could exist. Irwin and Weiner (1987) found that T helper/T suppressor ratio, but not NK-cell activity, strongly correlated with severity of depression on the Hamilton Depression Scale in bereaved subjects. A further study by the Kiecolt-Glaser group found that subjects who exhibited more negative or hostile behaviors (which suggest a more negative, intense but conflicting emotional involvement toward separation) during an interview had downregulated immune function (Kiecolt-Glaser et al., 1993). Individual psychological differences after loss of a loved one could affect both psychiatric and somatic complications of emotional loss and bereavement (Biondi & Picardi, 1996; Jacobs & Ostfeld, 1977).

Again, loss of property and damage after a hurricane seem able to affect immune function. NK cytotoxicity has been found to correlate negatively with the degree of perceived loss and damage after a hurricane in a community sample (Ironson et al., 1997).

Social support attenuates the magnitude of examination-induced reduction in NK activity, suggesting a possible buffering of immunological impairment during stress (Kang, Coe, Karaswenski, & McCarthy, 1998). In an elderly sample, high support positively correlated with total lymphocyte counts and mitogen responses in women, but not in men. Findings were thought to confirm the hypothesis that social support mitigates the effects of stressful stimuli in day-to-day life (Thomas, Goodwin, & Goodwin, 1985). High social support has been related to high NK-cell activity in breast cancer patients (Levy et al., 1990). On the other hand, high perceived stress, demoralization, and low perceived support have been related to increased episodes of reported upper respiratory infections in previous months (Biondi, Manganaro, & Procaccio, 1991). Loneliness, which may be considered a condition of chronic low support, has been related to lower NK-cell activity and PHA response in psychiatric patients (Kiecolt-Glaser et al., 1984).

### 5. Is There an Individual Immune Response Specificity?

Several studies in the past proposed specificity of psychophysiological response to stimuli (stimulus-response specificity) *versus* specificity of the response of each individual to the same stimulus (individual-response specificity) (Engel, 1960). Clinical experience notes that some individuals seem to react during periods of life crisis and stress with blood pressure increases, others with gastrointestinal symptoms, and others with muscular tension and headache, low back pain, and other autonomic symptoms. Although not supported as a primary mechanism in the pathogenesis of psychosomatic disease (Weiner, 1977), the theory of "response specificity," however, could be

further explored in psychoneuroimmunology. Could the increased susceptibility to some immune-related disease, such as the common cold, upper respiratory infections, dermatitis, or allergy or recurrence of chronic infections such as herpes virus be mediated by physiological specificity of immune response under stress? Or could it be only a matter of the immune function as *locus minoris resistentiae* of the organism? Mechanisms of visceral learning (Miller, 1969), which have been demonstrated for the immune system since 1975 (Ader & Cohen, 1975) could account for the former; and nonspecific stress-associated immune function impairment could account for the latter, as the Selye stress model predicts. An original perspective suggests a stance for specificity within the individual in psychoneuroimmunological research (Stein, 1986). These are at present interesting questions to be answered.

In summary, findings seem to suggest that personality, coping, and affective state could account for considerable variability of immune changes among individuals under the same stress condition. It is difficult, however, to draw overall conclusions, because in research carried out to date there is little overlap concerning stress models and experimental design used, stressor type, timing, and immune functions assessed. Considering these limitations, persistent distress or worry, depressive symptoms after major life events, low social support and loneliness, reduced coping ability, and repression of emotional reactions were found associated with a decrease in some immunological parameters, such as lymphocyte transformation tests and NK-cell activity. On the contrary, preliminary findings suggest that optimistic attitude and independent personality might buffer negative effects of acute stress on immune function. Taken together, these psychoneuroimmunologic studies seem to agree with those suggesting augmented ANS psychophysiological reactivity in behavioral inhibition (Reznick, 1994) and increased disease risk under stress-induced behavioral inhibition (Pancheri & Benaissa, 1976; Laborit, 1989, 1991). Current data on immune correlates of personality traits, such as extroversion and locus of control, are scanty; these aspects of psychoneuroimmunology deserve further investigation.

### D. Immune Parameters

As Tables I and II show, human studies investigated parameters of cellular more than humoral immunity. Tables VI and VII summarize common immune correlates of, respectively, acute and chronic psychological stress in humans.

**TABLE VI   Common Immune Correlates of Acute Psychological Stress in Humans**

| | |
|---|---|
| Transient increase in leukocyte count | Brohee et al., 1990; Grazzi et al., 1993; Maes et al., 1999; Mills et al., 1995 |
| Moderate lymphopenia | Brohee et al., 1990; Halvorsen et al., 1987 |
| Increase of monocytes | Halvorsen et al., 1987; Maes et al., 1999 |
| Transient increase of natural killer cells number and activity | Bachen et al., 1995; Breznitz et al., 1998; Brosschot et al., 1992 Buske-Kirschbaum et al., 1992; Grazzi et al., 1993; Marsland et al., 1995b; Matthews et al., 1995; Mills et al., 1995a and 1995; Naliboff et al., 1991 and 1995; Schmid et al., 1998; Sgoutas et al., 1994; Tonnesen et al., 1987; van der Pompe et al., 1998 |
| Reduced CD4/CD8 ratio | Bachen et al., 1995; Breznitz et al., 1998; Kiecolt-Glaser et al., 1986; Matthews et al., 1995; Mills et al., 1995a and 1995b |
| Increase of T suppressor/cytotoxic cells | Marsland et al., 1995b; Mills et al., 1995b; Naliboff et al., 1991; Sgoutas et al., 1994; Tanabe et al., 1993; van der Pompe et al., 1998 |
| Decrease of T helper cells | Brosschot et al., 1998; Kiecolt-Glaser et al., 1986; Mills et al., 1995b |
| Decrease of lymphocyte response to in vitro mitogens | Bachen et al., 1995; Biondi et al., 1991; Brosschot et al., 1992; Linn et al., 1987; Marsland et al., 1995; Palmblad et al., 1979; Sgoutas et al., 1994; Tonnesen et al., 1987 |
| Decrease of skin tests reactivity | Biondi & Pancheri, 1984; Vedhara & Nott, 1996 |

Overall, lymphocyte subsets, natural killer cell number and activity, and lymphoproliferative responses to mitogens were the most investigated parameters. Humoral immunity was assessed more frequently in studies on chronic than acute stress. Several investigations on chronic stress assessed basal immunoglobulins titers (Bartrop et al., 1977; Greene, Betts, Ochitill, Iker, & Douglas, 1978; Pariante et al., 1997; Pettingale et al., 1981), serum IgE levels (Koh & Hong, 1993; Szckeklik & Jawien, 1996), and salivary IgA (Jemmott et al., 1983; Kubitz et al., 1986; McClelland, Floor, Davidson, & Saron, 1980). Stress exposure was associated with reduced antibody titers to specific infectious challenges, such as flu vaccine (Locke & Heisel, 1977; Vedhara et al., 1999), the common cold (Totman, Kliff, Reed, & Craig, 1980), HbsAg (Glaser et al., 1992), and a novel antigen (Snyder et al., 1983). Acute stress studies assessed antibody titer against herpes simplex virus (Fittschen et al., 1990), secretory IgA (McClelland, Ross, & Patel,

1985), and serum immunoglobulin levels (Mizutani, Terachi, Okada, & Yoshida, 1996).

Cytokines were investigated only in few chronic (Kang, Coe, McCarthy, & Ershler, 1997; Kang et al., 1998; Maes et al., 1999; Nakano et al., 1998) and acute stress studies (Hisano, Sakamoto, Ishiko, Kamohara, & Okawa, 1997; Marshall, Agarwal, Lloyd, Cohen, Henninger, & Morris, 1998; Natelson et al., 1996; Osuka, Suzuki, Saito, Takayasu, & Shibuya, 1996; Song et al., 1999).

Only three studies assessed skin test response (Biondi & Pancheri, 1994; Vedhara & Nott, 1996; Cole et al., 1999).

In summary, common changes reported in response to an acute psychological stressor are diminished proliferative responses to mitogens, temporary increases of NK cells number and activity, an increase in CD8+ cells, and a decrease or, in some cases, an increase of T helpers and B cells (see Table VI). There is, however, evidence that acute psychological stress

**TABLE VII   Common Immune Correlates of Chronic Psychological Stress in Humans**

| | |
|---|---|
| Decrease of T lymphocytes | Brosschot et al., 1994; Castle et al., 1995; Taylor et al., 1986 |
| Decrease of natural killer cells number and activity | Brosschot et al., 1994; DeGucht et al., 1999; Esterling et al., 1996; Ironson et al., 1990; Irwin et al., 1986 and 1988; Kiecolt-Glaser et al., 1984a and 1984b; Segerstrom et al., 1998 |
| Increased natural killer cells number and activity | Weiss et al., 1996 |
| Decreased response to in vitro mitogens | Arnet al., 1987; Bartrop et al., 1977; Castle et al., 1995; DiGennaro et al., 1997; Kiecolt-Glaser et al., 1984b; Schleifer et al., 1983; Weiss et al., 1996 |
| Lower soluble IgA secretion | Jemmott et al., 1983 |
| Higher interleukin-6 | Maes et al., 1999 |
| Higher interleukin-4 | Nakano et al., 1998 |

may be associated with transient immune activation, while chronic stress and life events-induced depression are more often associated with immunodepression (Olff, 1999). Prolonged or subacute stress is consistently associated with a decrease of mitogen responses and reduced NK cell number and activity (see Table VII). Depression levels in caregivers of demented patients is associated with a strong reduction of NK cells, increase of CD8+ cells (Castle et al., 1995), increased serum cortisol and decreased antibody titer to influenza vaccine (Vedhara et al., 1999).

## III. PERSPECTIVES FOR THE STRESS-DISEASE CONNECTION

The possible link between neural, endocrine and immune systems deserves particular interest in view of its potential relevance to health maintenance and to its etiopathogenetic implication in several diseases (Moynihan, Kruszewska, Brenner, & Cohen 1998). Animal models in psychoneuroimmunology demonstrated that stress can modulate susceptibility to disease (Moynihan & Ader, 1996). Evidence on stress-induced immune changes could significantly contribute to further advancement of psychosomatic medicine (Ader, 1994). At the present state of knowledge, apart from psychiatry, main areas of potential clinical interest in psychoneuroimmunology are cancer, infectious, autoimmune diseases, inflammatory bowel disease, multiple sclerosis, and wound healing.

### A. Cancer

Recent studies provide evidence of the multistep nature of cancer, for example, studies on p53 (Hollstein, Sidransky, Vogelstein, & Harris, 1991). The p53 is a tumor-suppressor gene involved in transcription, DNA repair, genomic stability and control of the cell cycle and apoptosis, and it is functionally inactivated by viral, mutational, and cellular mechanisms in many human neoplasms (Wang & Harris, 1997). If cancer develops due to suprathreshold damage to specific genes regulating cell growth, with alteration or loss of chromosomal fragments leading to damaged DNA and expression of the cancer phenotype, what, if any, is the role of psychological factors and stress?

Although controversial, the contribution of psychoimmunological factors in the pathophysiology, course, and treatment of cancer is receiving increasing attention (Lewis, O'Sullivan, & Barraclough, 1994). Although some studies reported conflicting findings, several investigations since 1960 have suggested that

psychological stress might favor, mainly but not exclusively, through neuroimmunomodulation, cancer growth in animals (Bammer & Newberry, 1981; Riley, 1981). A recent review noted that "chemically induced cancers are more likely to be inhibited and transplanted tumors and metastases are more likely to be promoted by stress" (Newberry, Gordon, & Meehan, 1991) and concluded that "our belief that stress-induced immunosuppression can mediate tumor enhancement is growing, albeit slowly" (ibid., p. 39). In mice bearing Lewis lung carcinoma, psychological stress facilitates metastasis and decreases the survival of experimental animals with respect to controls (Giraldi, Perissin, Zorzet, Piccini, & Rapozzi, 1989). It has also been shown that psychological stress reduces the effectiveness of antitumor drugs in mice (Giraldi, Perissin, Zorzet, & Rapozzi, 1994). Data on psychological factors and cancer in humans are controversial, although several authors cautiously agree that, to some extent, they may contribute to disease manifestation and progression (Biondi, Costantini, & Grassi, 1995; Cooper & Watson, 1991; Levenson, Bemis, & Presberg, 1994; Stoll 1979). Human studies seem to suggest that stress and psychological factors, such as coping (Watson & Ramirez, 1991) and social support (Bloom, Kang, & Romano, 1991), may contribute to the course and progress of cancer and that they cannot be ignored.

We could take two examples, colon and breast cancer, to discuss the connection between stress, genes, and cancer. Two epidemiological studies found that life stress could be a risk factor for the development of colorectal cancer. The Swedish study by Courtney, Longnecker, Theorell, and Gerhardsson-de-Verdier (1993) is a case–control study conducted in Stockholm between 1986 and 1988 on 569 incident cases and 510 controls. Serious work-related problems in the prior 10 years were strongly associated with colorectal cancer, with an odds ratio of 5.5. Increased odds of colorectal cancer were associated with death of a spouse. The Melbourne Colorectal Cancer Study by Kune, Kune, Watson, and Rahe (1991) included 715 histologically confirmed colorectal cancers over a 12-month period in Melbourne, Australia, and 727 age- and sex-matched controls. Major illness and death of a close family member, and major work or family problems were significantly more frequent over the 5 years prior to diagnosis in cancer patients with respect to controls. In both studies, after multivariate analysis, the risk associated with life events was independent of dietary risk factors and physical activity. Recent investigations suggest that genetic instability and chromosomal aberrations are two molecular mechanisms found in the genesis of colorectal cancer. Genomic instability permits the accumulation of a sufficient amount of genetic damage and the emergence of the neoplastic phenotype (Boland et al., 1998). It could be that a long-term stress condition induced by loss or major life changes reduces anti-tumor immunity and defense against such damaged cells (Biondi et al., 1995).

The hypothesis of a possible relationship between psychological stress and some cases of breast cancer was put forward several decades ago. Sir James Paget and 18th- and 19th-century physicians working with cancer patients reported that great emotional loss and hopelessness occurred before the first symptoms of cancer appeared (Le Shan & Worthington, 1956). Although some modern studies reported negative findings (Roberts, Newcomb, Trenthan-Dietz, & Storer, 1996), several other investigations found a high risk associated with major life stress in the years preceding disease diagnosis. In a study on 99 breast cancer cases and 99 matched controls, women in the highest quartile of life change and distress over the past 10 years had 4.67 times the risk of developing breast cancer as compared with those in the lowest quartile (Ginsberg, Price, Ingram, & Nottage, 1996). Confirming the findings of a previous investigation (Geyer, 1993), a British case–control study using a standardized life event interview found that severe life events in the 5-year period preceding the diagnosis increased the risk of breast cancer with an odds ratio of 3.2, which rose after adjustment for age and menopausal status to 11.6 (Chen et al., 1995). It should be further assessed if negative findings of other studies are related to methodological issues, such as telephone interviews for the assessment of events, selection of only a limited number of events, and exploration of only the 2 past years preceding the diagnosis (Roberts et al., 1996), which might not fit the needs of the questions to be answered. However, the possible role of loss events as a risk factor seems questioned by a retrospective study in Norway, including 4491 breast cancer cases and 44,910 controls between 1935 and 1954, which found no increased risk of breast cancer in divorced women after the divorce or death of the husband (Kvikstad, Vatten, Tretli, & Kvinnsland, 1994), suggesting that a loss event per se, independently of considerations of its meaning for the subject, might not be a risk factor.

As psychosomatics suggests (Weiner, 1977; Ader, 1980), it is the meaning of the lost object and its relation to the single individual that influence the impact of the loss event and of its possible consequences on CNS neurotransmitters, neuroendocrine modifications, and risk of loss-induced depression (Biondi & Picardi, 1996). Therefore we should not expect that all breast cancer cases have an event as antecedent. As in the field of loss-induced depressions (Biondi & Picardi, 1996), so too in psychoneuroimmunology of cancer it might be that not loss events per se but only loss perceived as irreparable (such as in the death of an only child) and persistence of unresolved grief could profoundly alter CNS neurotransmitters, psychoneuroendocrine axes, and, ultimately, immune functions. It has been hypothesized that lasting intense grief, despair, or hopelessness due to a severe emotional loss might contribute to the activation of latent breast neoplasia in some women (Biondi, Costantini, & Parisi, 1996). A study carried out in Denmark found at medicolegal autopsy that 20% of healthy women ages 20–54 had foci of latent carcinoma of the breast (Nielsen, Thomson, Primdahl, Direborg, & Andersen, 1987). Bereavement has been associated with persistent immunodepression (Bartrop et al., 1977; Irwin et al., 1988; Schleifer et al., 1983). The incidence of mammary tumors in mice was shown to be a function of emotional stress level (Riley, 1975). Some recent studies appear to confirm that stress-induced suppression of NK activity is sufficient to cause enhanced development of different syngeneic tumors (Ben-Eliyahu, Page, Yirmiya, & Shakhar, 1999). Repeated restraint stress in mice with syngeneic B16 melanoma suppresses tumor-specific CD+4 cell-dependent interferon-gamma production of immunized spleen cells, decreases the potential of spleen cells to turn into antitumor cytotoxic T lymphocytes, and reduces responsiveness of NK cells to an NK activity augmenting stimulus (Li, Harada, Tamada, Abe, & Nomoto 1997). Restraint stress is particularly interesting from a psychological viewpoint, because it maximizes emotional arousal and despair while inhibiting any actions or possible coping response of animals. It might well resemble, better than other laboratory stress models, some kind of unhappy human existence. The hypothesis of a possible interaction between severe emotional stress and activation of latent neoplasia may help to explain why only a subgroup of bereaved subjects might be at risk for cancer and how discrepancies between impressive clinical observations on a single case and negative findings from group studies can be found. The hypothesis that psychological stress in human cancer interferes at an early stage with antitumor immune mechanisms, such as NK-cell function, lymphokine-activated killer cell activity, macrophage function, cytokine production, humoral immunity, and T-cell-mediated cellular immune response (Souberbielle & Dalgleish, 1994), remains open to further investigation.

## B. Infectious Diseases

Subsequent to earlier studies (Friedman, Glasgow, & Ader, 1969), several findings suggest that psychological stress can act as a cofactor in their pathogenesis, course, and outcome of infectious disease in animals and humans (Biondi & Zannino, 1997). Many investigations have reported higher morbidity and mortality through infectious agents in animals exposed to psychophysical and emotional stress with respect to control groups, ranging from poliovirus (Johnson & Rassmussen, 1965; Levinson, Milzer, & Lewin, 1945), Coxsackievirus B3 (Gatmaitan, Chason, & Lerner, 1970), influenza A (Chetverikova, Frolov, Kramskaya, & Polyak, 1987), herpes simplex virus (Bonneau, Sheridan, Feng, & Glaser, 1991; Rasmussen, Marsh, & Brill, 1957), herpes simplex encephalitis (DeLano & Mallery, 1998), encephalomyocarditis virus (Friedman, Glasgow, & Ader, 1970), *Salmonella typhimurium* (Edwards & Dean, 1977), and parasitic infections such as *Hymenolepis nana* (Hamilton, 1973) and *Plasmodium berghei* (Friedman & Glasgow, 1973). Some studies, however, reported no effect of stress or even reduced morbidity or mortality (for review, see Biondi & Zannino, 1997). Findings may be influenced by strain or sex of animals, time of infection with respect to stressor exposure, and the pathogenicity and virulence of the infecting agent. In the case of viral infection in animals, pathophysiologic mechanisms of increased stress-associated morbidity or mortality include increased virus titer in the target tissue, reduced activity of the HSV-specific cytotoxic T lymphocytes and NK cells, reduced migration and activation of memory cytotoxic T lymphocytes (Bonneau et al., 1991; Dobbs, Vasquez, Glaser, & Sheridan, 1993), and interferon production suppression (Chang & Rasmussen, 1965; Chetverikova et al., 1987). Stress can also reactivate in animals latent herpes simplex in lumbar dorsal root ganglia (Bonneau, Aoki, & Glavin, 1993).

Although some studies reported negative findings, human studies suggested a possible role of stress in increasing the risk of tuberculosis (Holmes, Hawkins, Bowerman, Clarke, & Joffe, 1957), the common cold (Cohen, Tyrrel, & Smith, 1991; Evans & Edgerton, 1991; Stone et al., 1992), episodes of upper respiratory infections in adults (Biondi et al., 1991; Jackson et al., 1960) and children (Turner Cobb & Steptoe, 1998), influenza (Clover, Abell, Becker, Crawford, & Ramsey, 1989), genital herpes virus recurrences (Goldmeier & Johnson, 1982; Kemeny, Cohen, Zegans, & Conant, 1989; Vander Plate, Aral, & Magder, 1988), herpes labialis virus recurrences (Katcher, Brightman, Luborsky, & Ship, 1973), and infectious mononucleosis (Kasl, Evans, & Neiderman, 1979). However, prospective studies in humans are very few and some negative findings exist (for detailed review, see Biondi & Zannino, 1997). The possible relationship between stress and immunity should also be integrated in a more complex pattern than the simple stress–disease connection. For instance, a prospective study on herpes simplex and mood with daily self-reports over a 3-month period from 38 subjects with genital herpes and 28 subjects with oral herpes found multiple variables to play a role; recurring genital HSV infection was preceded by reduced overall emotional well-being over a period of 2 weeks. Females showed a marked trend which was related to the menstrual cycle. Conversely, males showed a more marked relationship with reduction of the amount of sleep. The common cold was a significant precipitating factor in oral herpes (Dalkvist, Wahlin, Bartsch, & Forsbeck, 1995).

Amount of life stress, depressive symptoms, and low social support were found to be associated with acceleration in the progress of the HIV infection in a 5-year prospective study (Leserman, Jackson, Petitto, Golden, Silva, Perkins, Cai, Folds, & Evans, 1999).

Pathophysiological links between stress and increased morbidity have been less studied in humans than in animals. Recently, Drummond and Hewson Bower (1997) suggested that increased psychosocial stress could increase susceptibility to respiratory tract infections through reduced salivary IgA. According to the authors, lower sIgA/albumin ratios in these children indicate a deficiency in local mucosal immunity and suggest that stressful experiences could deplete local immune protection against viral invasion of the upper respiratory tract. Similar findings come from a study showing reduced bactericidal, but not phagocytic, activity of polymorphonuclear leukocytes in children with major depression (Bartlett et al., 1997). Chronic depression is associated with a marked decline of cellular immunity to varicella–zoster virus, a finding that helps to explain the increased incidence of herpes zoster with increasing age and psychologic stress (Irwin et al., 1998). Changes in the CD4/CD8 ratio after the severe emotional stress of earthquake predicted increases in episodes of respiratory illness incidence in children (Boyce, Chesterman, Martin, Folkman, Cohen, & Wara, 1993). Chronic stress in elderly caregivers of dementia patients was associated with reduced antibody response to influenza (Vedhara et al., 1999) and hepatitis-B vaccination (Glaser, Kiecolt-Klaser, Malarkey, & Sheridan, 1998), suggesting increased risk of disease in these subjects.

Taken together, these studies impressively suggest that psychological stress and depression could alter susceptibility to several infectious diseases in man, ranging from the common cold and upper respiratory infections to HIV progression. Effects may also be modulated by individual variability as related to personality, affective state, and available support.

## C. Autoimmune Disorders

A possible contribution of psychosocial factors in the pathogenesis and course of specific autoimmune diseases, such as rheumatoid arthritis, ulcerative colitis, and Crohn's disease, has been discussed in classical treatises of psychosomatics (Weiner, 1977, pp. 435–574). The link between psychosocial factors and autoimmune processes is, however, still unknown (Weiner, 1991). The stress-induced changes of the hypothalamo-pituitary-adrenal axis may contribute to modulate processes of immune-mediated inflammation (Chrousos, 1995), which may be relevant in the course of many autoimmune diseases. It has been also suggested that the release of $\beta$-endorphin from lymphocytes directly into inflamed tissue could exert anti-inflammatory and analgesic effects (Stein, 1995, p. 1688). Thus the stress-induced peripheral opioid increase could contribute to modulate mechanisms of pain and inflammation (Jessop, 1998).

Increases in mood disturbances in rheumathoid arthritis (RA) patients were prospectively correlated with decreases in sIL-2R levels and increases in joint pain, suggesting a possible link between immunity, mood, and short-term changes in symptoms of disease (Affleck et al., 1993). This finding seems to be confirmed by a further study, carried out in 41 women with RA, where measures of everyday stressful events, perceived stress, and disease activity were prospectively assessed for 12 weeks. Findings showed that interpersonal stress was associated with increases in disease activity; and in a subgroup of 20 patients significant elevations in DR+CD3 cells, sIL-2R, clinician's rating of disease, and self-reports of joint tenderness were also found during the period of increased stress (Zautra, Hoffman, Potter, Matt, Yocum, & Castro, 1997). In another study the authors found that increased daily stressors were associated with increased joint pain but indirectly with decreased joint inflammation through reduction of soluble IL-2 receptors. They proposed a dual-pathway model of the interaction between stress and RA which suggests that stress might have opposite effects on pain versus inflammation in patients with RA

(Affleck, Urrows, Tenne, Higgins, Pav, & Aloisi, 1997). However, a mental effort-inducing task did not change cortisol plasma levels, nor did it modify peripheral blood lymphocyte mobilization (B-, T-, and NK-cells) in 22 patients with rheumatoid arthritis of recent onset. Negative findings might have several explanations, e.g., patients might not be sufficiently stressed by such a mild laboratory stimuli, or they might be receiving long-term medication for arthritis (Geenen et al., 1998). Physical disability, mood changes, reactive psychological distress, and intervening external life events may be interrelated in a complex way in autoimmune diseases. In a 2-year prospective study in Norway, high levels of disability in 216 patients predicted an increase in depression during the next year, but changes in psychological distress were not predicted by disease-related variables (Smedstadt, Vaglum, Moum, & Kvien, 1997). Male gender, personal coping resources, an extended social network and support, and improved clinical status after treatment emerged as protective factors against depression and psychological distress in the first year after the diagnosis of RA (Evers, Kraaimaat, Geenen, & Bijisma, 1997).

It is at present not known if and to what extent psychosocial variables might affect immune and inflammatory activity in different patients. The expectancy to find a simple, linear relationship between psychological variables, immune parameters and disease activity is probably going to be frustrated by clinical complexity. The stress reaction induced by a severe life event induces several endocrine changes and might not always be detrimental; for example, beta-endorphin release from immune cells during inflammation may be a potent local analgesic (Schafer, Carter, & Stein, 1994). Anecdotal report describes the case of a 53-year-old woman with RA who suffered two unexpected family deaths during a 12-week study. Her disease went on remission the same weeks as the deaths, suggesting that major events might be associated with symptom decreases (Potter & Zautra, 1997).

Less studied are stress-related immune changes in systemic lupus erythematosus (SLE), although high levels of daily hassle and low social support are associated with impaired psychological status (Dobkin et al., 1998); and stress, anxiety, and depression could predict average symptom severity and daily symptom fluctuation, with some individuals appearing as stress-responders, while other did not (Adams, Dammers, Saia, Brantley, & Gaydos, 1994). SLE patients did not respond to mechanical and psychological laboratory stress differently from controls (Hinrichsen, Folsch, & Kirch, 1992).

While life stress and coping responses contribute to the psychological adjustment to multiple sclerosis (MS) (Aikens, Fischer, Namey, & Rudick, 1997), it is controversial whether psychological stress could contribute to clinical exacerbations. The macrophage-derived cytokines IL-1$\beta$ and TNF-$\alpha$ increased during videotaped speech stress in MS subjects (Ackerman, Martino, Heyman, Moyna, & Rabin, 1998). Findings from retrospective and prospective clinical studies, however, are discordant, and "there is not sufficient evidence to accept that psychological stress is able to induce or trigger the onset of the relapses of MS, or to influence its evolution" (Nisipenau & Korczyn, 1995, p. 179).

In summary, at least from the clinican viewpoint, the contribution of stress-related changes to auto-immune disorders is an open question. Further studies are needed to assess thoroughly the interaction between psychological stress and immunemodulation of pain and inflammatory responses in rheumatoid arthritis. The issue of interindividual variability of stress-related immune and inflammatory changes has not been addressed to date. Con- clusions cannot be drawn for systemic lupus erythematosus, since its psychoimmunology has been insufficiently studied, while conflicting evidence exists for multiple sclerosis.

## D. Other Disorders

The role of psychological stress in the pathogenesis or exacerbation of asthma has been often discussed since the pioneering clinical studies of Alexander and the first controlled studies in the 1970s (Weiner, 1977, pp. 223–299). The prevalence of anxiety disorders, intrafamilial stress, and emotional disturbances is higher in children with asthma than seen in a healthy group (Bussing, Burket, & Kelleher, 1996). Mechanisms of bronchoconstriction involve the immunologic extrinsic pathway and CNS–ANS cooperation, and it is to the latter that the possible effects of psychological stress on asthma have been more frequently attributed (Mrazek & Klinnert, 1991). Serum IgE, considered a stable indicator of allergy, was not influenced by stress in a sample of 54 outpatients with bronchial asthma (Koh & Hong, 1993). Students with mild or moderate asthma as well as healthy students show transient declines in NK cell activity during the stress of the final examination (Kang et al., 1998). Asthmatic subjects, however, show significantly higher than normal lymphocyte proliferation and neutrophile superoxide release, suggesting a continuous activation of inflammatory cell function after stressor challenge (Kang et al., 1997).

If confirmed by further studies, this finding could suggest a role of immune-inflammatory mechanisms in stress-mediated asthmatic exacerbations.

Although psoriasis could be exacerbated by psychological stress, laboratory stress induced enhanced autonomic response in psoriatic patients as compared to normal controls but no significant immunological differences, such as modifications of NK-cell number and activity and T-lymphocyte subsets (Schmid et al., 1998).

There is a new perspective in the possible contribution of stress-associated immune changes in irritable bowel disease and peptic ulcer recurrence. Emotional stress has been implicated for many years in the pathogenesis and course of bowel disease, ulcerative colitis, and Crohn's disease (Weiner, 1977, pp. 495–574). Although mucosal immune function in the gut is operationally distinct from the systemic immune system, a brain-gut-immune axis and a "mucosal gut psychoneuroimmunology" have been recently proposed (Shanahan, 1999). The possible contribution of stress-related immune mechanims in this group of diseases is in an early phase of investigation (Anton & Shanahan, 1998; Collins, Barbara, & Vallance, 1999). Although the discovery of *Helicobacter pylorii* as a "cause" of peptic ulcer seemed to rule out psychosomatic explanations, it has been suggested that psychological stress and infection with *Helicobacter pylorii* may interact in the etiopathogenesis and course of many peptic ulcers (Levenstein, 1999). Stress could facilitate ulcer recurrence or impair ulcer healing, for example, by stimulating inflammatory cytokine production, such as interleukin-1$\beta$ and tumor necrosis factor, followed by an increased infiltration of neutrophiles and mononuclear cells (Arakawa et al., 1998).

A new line of research recently focused on another stress-related defect, retarded wound healing, which may be relevant to the defense of the organism against infection in patients after major or minor surgery, diabetes, accidents and other traumatic conditions. The chronic stress of caregivers of Alzheimer's patients is associated with impairment in wound healing (Kiecolt-Glaser, Marucha, Malarkey, Mercado, & Glaser, 1995). A mean 3-day delay of wound healing has been reported in students under acute examination stress, as compared to controls, suggesting that also minor and brief psychological stress can alter repair processes (Marucha, Kiecolt-Glaser & Favagchi, 1998). Stress-related changes seem able to delay wound healing mainly through proinflammatory cytokines (Glaser et al., 1999).

In summary, the effects of psychological stress in bronchial asthma may be mainly mediated by the extrinsic CNS–ANS pathway, although immune-inflammatory mechanisms might contribute to stress-associated exacerbations. Preliminary, but of high interest, is the role of the brain-gut-immune axis in inflammatory bowel disease and ulcer recurrences. Stress-related defects in wound repair may also have a prominent impact on health. Finally, stress-related impairment of wound healing may have a significant effect on repair processes under several clinical conditions.

## E. Are There Treatments for Stress-Related Immune Changes?

Stress treatment could be divided into psychopharmacological and psychological–behavioral. There are endless reports and research papers focusing on the treatment and prevention of stress. The brief review that follows examines only recent, specific data on putative immune system changes (or absence of change) after anti-stress treatments.

Psychopharmacological treatment with benzodiazepines (BDZ) prevents or attenuates the acute stress response. A first pathway is through BDZ central type receptor potentiation of inhibitory GABAergic transmission, which reduces the arousal of the limbic-hypothalamo-pituitary-adrenal cortical axis. A second pathway is at the peripheral BDZ receptors, located on phagocytes and glial cells (Zavala, 1997). Although some animal studies report that potentiation of GABAergic system at the CNS level by means of diazepam has a stimulatory influence on immune reactivity (Devoino, Idova, Alperina, & Cheido, 1994), a systematic review of the literature suggests that benzodiazepines have immunomodulatory properties in animals and humans, but potentiating or inhibiting effects, however, depend on molecule, dose, and immune function considered (Talamonti & Biondi, 1997, p. 317–321). Potentiation of central serotonergic or noradrenergic neurotransmission with different classes of antidepressants (AD) normalizes alterations of HPA axis and immune functions typical of severe depression (Delle Chiaie & Regine, 1997), but it is open to question if they can exert a therapeutic effect on normal subjects undergoing stress challenge. Effects of antidepressants on immune responses differ according to the class of AD and immune parameter (Talamonti & Biondi, 1997, pp. 330–334). For instance, fluoxetine inhibits cellular proliferation at mitogenic ConA doses but stimulates it at submitogenic doses in mice (Kubera, Holan, Basta-Kaim, Roman, Borycz, & Shani, 1998). It inhibits NK cytotoxicity after acute administration, while after chronic administration such effect undergoes tolerance (Pellegrino & Bayer,

1998). Fluoxetine treatment did not change CD4+ values of HIV patients (Rabkin, Wagner & Rabkin, 1999). As data suggest, at the present state of knowledge, the possible use of antidepressants for reducing stress-related immune changes should be further investigated.

Possible immune changes produced by behavioral interventions are still at a preliminary phase of investigation, although they show promise (Kiecolt-Glaser & Glaser, 1992). Relaxation treatment enhances salivary IgA in children, a finding the authors suggest might help against recurrent upper respiratory infections (Hewson-Bower & Drummond, 1996). Biofeedback-assisted relaxation for 4 weeks increased blastogenesis and decreased white blood cells in trained healthy subjects (McGrady, Conran, Dickey, Garman, Farris, & Schumann-Brzezinski, 1992). Other studies yielded inconsistent findings (Zachariae et al., 1994). Moderate physical exercise may have a role in stimulating the immune system, and it could be useful in conditions such as aging, spaceflight, chronic fatigue syndrome, and HIV-infection (Mac-Kinnon, 1998), although further research is needed. On the contrary, the stress of heavy physical training transiently suppresses NK activity, neutrophil oxidative burst activity, and T cell function, increasing the susceptibility of athletes to upper respiratory infections (Nieman, 1998). Citrus fragrance seems able to restore stress-induced immunosuppression in animals (Shibata, Fujiwara, Iwamoto, Matsuoka, & Yokohama, 1991) and, as preliminary data suggest, ameliorates depressive states and immune function in humans (Komori, Fujiwara, Tanida, Nomura, & Yokohama, 1995). Preliminary studies suggest that cancer patients may benefit from behavioral treatment, with associated positive immune changes (Siegel, Septhton, Terr, & Stites, 1998). In stages I and II malignant melanoma patients, for example, a 6-week short-term group psychotherapy reduced distress, favored active coping, and, at 6-months, was associated with increases in NK cells number and cytotoxic activity and of large granular lymphocytes (Fawzy et al., 1990). This group also had significantly better survival rates at 5-year followup than the control group (Fawzy, Fawzy, & Hyun, 1994). Behavioral group treatment in breast cancer patients also increased, in the short- and long-term, the absolute number of white blood cells and reduced cortisol levels (Schedlowski, Tewes, & Schmoll, 1994). Relaxation training in ovarian cancer patients during chemotherapy resulted in higher lymphocyte and white blood cell counts than seen in the control group, with no effect on lymphoproliferative responses and NK cell activity. Among negative findings, imagery techniques or group supports ameliorate stress perception-increased vigor but had no effect on immune measurements such as NK activity, interferon production, IL-$1\alpha$ and -$\beta$ (Richardson, Post-White, Grimm, Moye, Singletany, & Justice, 1997). No modifications of psychological and immune parameters after behavioral interventions, however, have been reported in patients with advanced cancer (de Vries, Schilder, Mulder, Vrancken, Remie, & Garssen, 1997).

## IV. CONCLUSIONS

As the reviewed studies suggest, several naturally occurring situations of psychological stress can alter immune functions. While chronic stress induced by real-life stressors can often be associated with down-regulation of the immune system, with some exceptions (see Tables I and III), acute psychological stressors in laboratory settings can transiently induce an activation of some immune functions (see Tables II and IV). Some specific stress models studied by the Glaser group, such as academic examination, marital stress, and Alzheimer patient caregiving have been the object of continuing progress and improvement and seem particularly fruitful. Bereavement is another important model of stress research in psychoneuroimmunology (Irwin & Weiner, 1987). Several questions, however, remain to be addressed in future research.

First is the issue of interindividual variability of stress-induced endocrine and immune modifications. This still represents a classic problem in psychosomatics (Ader, 1980). Recent research data suggest, with few exceptions, that an individual psychological variability of stress-related immune changes does exist (Cohen, 1999). As a whole, studies show that higher levels of perceived stress, ineffective coping, depression (Olff, 1999), and low social support (Uchino et al., 1996) are associated with greater risk of immune impairment. The design of new research in this field should ideally include (a) psychological instruments to assess the subjective impact of stressors; (b) assessment of emotional responses such as anxiety, depression, and anger; (c) measurement of coping, particularly focusing on inhibition-suppression *versus* efficacy/action dimensions; and (d) measurement of social support.

Second, the findings reviewed introduce the issue of the potential impact on health of stress-related immune changes. Immune correlates of PTSD were, until a few years ago, unknown. Recent studies suggest that changes in immune functions do exist, in particular introducing evidence of immune activation (Ironson et al., 1997; Maes et al., 1999; Wilson et al., 1999). At present, little is known about the risk of immune-related disease in PTSD, and this is an issue to explore.

The potential role of psychological stress in the pathogenesis and progression of cancer has been often debated. Findings in animals were controversial (Bammer & Newberry, 1981) or suggested a possible relationship (Riley, 1981). Recent reviews, both animal (Newberry et al., 1991) and human (Biondi et al., 1995), seriously consider the possibility that stress-induced immunological impairment contributes to neoplasia. Experimental findings in animal cancer (Ben-Eliyahu et al., 1999; Giraldi et al., 1989, 1994) and epidemiological findings in colorectal (Courtney et al., 1993; Kune et al., 1991) and breast cancer (Chen et al., 1995; Geyer, 1993; Ginsberg et al., 1996) seem to give further support to the above possibility, although negative findings exist (Kvikstad et al., 1994).

Although variability of findings may exist in animal studies on the basis of methodological variables such as design, type, and timing of stress, stress-induced changes in immune functions in humans seem able to increase susceptibility to several infectious diseases, ranging from the common cold, influenza, and upper respiratory infections, while psychic factors and stress can modulate herpes virus infection (Biondi & Zannino, 1997). Stress, low social support, and depression can contribute to accelerated progression of HIV infection (Leserman et al., 1999).

The possible contribution of psychological stress-related immune changes to the pathogenesis and course of bronchial asthma and autoimmune diseases, such as rheumatoid arthritis, systemic lupus erythematosus, or multiple sclerosis is still debated. New interesting areas are stress-related immune changes in inflammatory bowel disease (Shanahan, 1999) and wound healing (Glaser et al., 1999).

A third issue concerns the mechanisms involved in the relationship between psychological stress and immune function changes. The central neurobiology of the stress response is essential to an understanding of stress-associated immune changes. Psychological stressors are transduced into modifications of neurotransmitters and neuro- and immunopeptides. The limbic-hypothalamo-pituitary axes and the hypothalamo-sympathetic axes are the two main efferent pathways affecting neuroendocrine, autonomic, and immune functions under stress (Felten et al., 1991; Felten & Felten, 1994). The role of adrenergic mediation in acute stress-related immune changes has been clearly established in the past decade. Human studies which assess in parallel autonomic and immune responses have been a prominent advance in the area (Madden et al., 1995). The role of cytokines as a mediator was also shown in several studies, such as in immune activation in PTSD (Maes et al., 1999) and impaired wound healing (Glaser et al., 1999).

A fourth issue regards possible intervention for stress-related impairment of immune functions. Available data are very limited and preliminary. Anxiolytics protect from acute biological ANS and endocrine effects of stress, including stress-related immune changes (Zavala, 1997). Data on antidepressants are, at least at present, inconsistent. Psychosocial intervention improved psychological status and, in some studies, immune function in cancer patients (Siegel et al., 1998); psychoneuroimmunology of cancer will probably be an area of major research expansion in the next decade.

## References

Ackerman, K. D., Martino, M., Heyman, R., Moyna, N. M., & Rabine, B. S. (1998). Stressor-induced alteration of cytokine production in multiple sclerosis patients and controls. *Psychosomatic Medicine, 60,* 484–491.

Adams, S. G. Jr., Dammers, P. M., Saia, T. L., Brantley, P. J., & Gaydos, G. R. (1994). Stress, depression, and anxiety predict average symptom severity and daily symptom fluctuation in systemic lupus erythematosus. *Journal of Behavioral Medicine, 17,* 459–477.

Ader, R. (1980). Psychosomatic and psychoimmunolgic research. *Psychosomatic Medicine, 42,* 307–321.

Ader, R. (1996). On the teaching of psychoneuroimmunology. *Brain, Behavior, and Immunity, 10,* 315–323.

Ader, R. (Ed.) (1981). *Psychoneuroimmunology.* New York: Academic Press.

Ader, R., & Cohen, N. (1975). Behaviorally conditioned immunosuppression. *Psychosomatic Medicine, 37,* 333–340.

Ader, R., & Friedman, S. B. (1964). Differential early experiences and susceptibility to transplanted tumor in the rat. *Journal of Comparative Physiological Psychology, 59,* 361–364.

Affleck, G., Urrows, S., Tennen, H., Higgins, P., Pav, D., & Aloisi, R. (1997). A dual pathway model of daily stressors effects on rheumatoid arthritis. *Annals of Bevahioral Medicine, 19,* 161–170.

Affleck, G., Urrows, S., Tenne, H., Higgins, P., Zautra, A., & Hoffman, S. (1993). Temporal covariation of soluble interleukin-2 receptor leels, daily stress and disease activity in rheumathoid arthritis. *Arthritis and Rheumatism, 36,* 199–203.

Aikens, J. E., Fischer, J. S., Namey, M., & Rudick, R. A. (1997). A replicated prospective investigation of life stress, coping, and depressive symptoms in multiple sclerosis. *Journal of Behavioral Medicine, 20,* 433–445.

Anton, P. A., & Shanahan, F. (1998). Neuroimmunomodulation in inflammatory bowel disease. How far from "bench" to "bedside"? *Annals of the New York Academy of Sciences, 840,* 723–734.

Aragona, M., Muscatello, M. R., Losi, E., Panetta, S., La Torre, F., Pastura, G., Bertolani, S., & Mesiti, M. (1996). Lymphocyte number and stress parameter modifications in untreated breast cancer patients with depressive mood and previous life stress. *Journal of Experimental Therapy in Oncology, 1,* 354–360.

Arakawa, T., Watanabe, T., Fukuda, T., Higuchi, K., Fujiwara, Y., Kobayashi, K., & Tarnawsi, A. (1998). Ulcer recurrence: Cytokines and inflammatory response-dependent process. *Digestive Disease Science, 43*(Suppl. 9), 61S–66S.

Arnetz, B. B., Wasserman, J., Petrini, B., Brennmer, S. O., Levi, L., Eneroth, P., Salovaara, H., Hjelm, R., Salovaara, L., Theorell, T., & Petterson, L. (1987). Immune function in unemployed women. *Psychosomatic Medicine, 49,* 3–11.

Bachen, E. A., Manuck, S. B., Cohen, S., Muldoom, M. F., Raible, R., Herbert, T. B., & Rabin, B. S. (1995). Adrenergic blockade ameliorates cellular immune responses to mental stress in humans. *Psychosomatic Medicine, 57,* 366–372.

Baker, G. H. B., Byrom, N. A., Irani, M. S., Brewerton, D. A., Hobes, J. R., Wood, R. J., & Nagvekar, N. M. (1984). Stress, cortisol, and lymphocyte subpopulations. *The Lancet, 10,* 574.

Bahnson, C. B. (1969). Second Conference on Psychophysiological Aspects of Cancer. *Annals of the New York Academy of Sciences, 164,* 307–634.

Bahnson, C. B., & Kissen, D. M. (1966). Psychophysiological aspects of cancer. *Annals of the New York Academy of Sciences, 125,* 773–1055.

Bammer, K., & Newberry, B. H. (Eds.). (1981). *Stress and cancer.* Toronto: Hogrefe.

Bartlett, J. A., Demetrikopoulos, M. K., Schleifer, S. J., & Keller S. E. (1997). Phagocytosis and killing of *Staphylococcus aureus*: Effects of stress and depression in children. *Clinical and Diagnostic Laboratory Immunology, 4,* 362–366.

Bartrop, R. W., Lazarus, L., Luckhurst, E., & Kiloh, L. G. (1977). Depressed lymphocyte function after bereavement. *The Lancet, 2,* 834–837.

Ben-Eliyahu, S., Page, G. G., Yirmiya, R., & Shakhar, G. (1999). Evidence that stress and surgical interventions promote tumor development by suppressing natural killer cell activity. *International Journal of Cancer, 80,* 880–888.

Benschop, R. J., Brosschot, J. F., Godaert, G. L., DeSmet, M. B., Geenen, R., Olff, M., Heijnene, C. J., & Ballieux, R. E. (1994). Chronic stress affects immunologic but not cardiovascular responsiveness to acute psychological stress. *American Journal of Physiology, 266,* R75–R80.

Benschop, R. J., Geenen, R., Mills, P. J., Naliboff, B. D., Kiecolt Glaser, J. K., Herbert, T. B., van der Pompe, G., Miller, G. E., Matthews, K. A., Godaert, G. L., Gilmore, S. L., Glaser, R, Hejinen, C. J., Dopp, J. M., Bijlsma, J. W., Solomon, G. F., & Cacioppo, J. T. (1998). Cardiovascular and immune response to acute psychological stress in young and old women, a meta-analysis. *Psychosomatic Medicine, 60,* 290–296.

Benschop, R. J., Rodriguez-Feuerhahn, M., & Schedlowsi, M. (1996). Catecholamine-induced leukocytosis: Early observations, current research, and future directions. *Brain, Behavior, and Immunity, 10,* 77–91.

Biondi, M. (1991). The application of the human stress model to psychoneuroimmunology. *Acta Neurologica, 13,* 328–334.

Biondi, M. (1995). Beyond the mind-brain dichotomy and toward a common organizing principle of psychotherapy and pharmacotherapy. *Psychotherapy and Psychosomatics, 63,* 3–8.

Biondi, M (1997). *Mente, cervello e sistema immunitario.* Milano: McGraw Hill-Italia.

Biondi, M., Costantini, A., & Grassi, L. (1995). *La mente e il cancro. Insidie e risorse della psiche nelle patologie tumorali.* Roma: Il Pensiero Scientifico.

Biondi, M., Costantini, A., & Parisi, A. M. (1996). Can loss and grief activate latent neoplasia? *Psychotherapy and Psychosomatics, 65,* 102–105.

Biondi, M., Manganaro, M., & Procaccio, V. (1991). Stress emozionale soggettivo e malattie infettive. Studio preliminare. *Medicina Psicosomatica, 36,* 217–224.

Biondi, M., & Pancheri, P. (1985). Stress, personality, immunity and cancer, a challenge for psychosomatic medicine. In R. Kaplan & M. Criqui (Eds.), *Behavioral epidemiology and disease prevention* (pp. 271–300). New York: Plenum.

Biondi, M., & Pancheri, P. (1991). Depression and coping style as modulators of immune response under stress. In N. P. Plotnikoff, R. E. Faith, A. J. Murgo, & J. Wybran (Eds.), *Stress and immunity.* Boca Raton, FL: CRC Press.

Biondi, M., & Pancheri, P. (1994). Clinical research strategies in psychoimmunology, a review of 46 human research studies (1972–1992). In B. Leonard & K. Miller (Eds.), *Stress, the immune system and psychiatry* (pp. 85–111). New York: Wiley.

Biondi, M., Pancheri, P., Falaschi, P., Teodori, A., Paga, G., Delle Chiaie, R., Di Cesare, G., & Proietti, A. (1986). Social support as a moderator of the psychobiological stress response. *New Trends in Experimental and Clinical Psychiatry, 2,* 173–183.

Biondi, M., Peronti, M., Pacitti, F., Pancheri, P., Pacifici, R., Altieri, I., Paris, L., & Zuccaro, P. (1994). Personality, endocrine and immune changes after eight months in healthy individuals under normal daily stress. *Psychotherapy and Psychosomatics, 62,* 176–184.

Biondi, M., & Picardi, A. (1996). Clinical and biological aspects of bereavement and loss-induced depression, a reappraisal. *Psychotherapy and Psychosomatics, 65,* 229–245.

Biondi, M., & Picardi A. (1999). Psychological stress and neuroendocrine functions in humans, the last two decades of research. *Psychotherapy and Psychosomatics, 68,* 114–150.

Biondi, M., & Zannino L. G. (1997). Psychological stress, neuroimmunomodulation and susceptibility to infectious diseaseas in animal and man, a review. *Psychotherapy and Psychosomatics, 66,* 3–26.

Biondi, M., Zuccaro, P., Paolucci, G. P., Palma, A., Pacifici, R., & Pancheri, P. (1993). Psychoneuroimmunological status and subjective stress in air crew healthy persons. *Zacchia, 66,* 105–128.

Blondeau, J. M., Aoki, F. Y., & Glavin, B. (1993). Stress-induced reactivation of latent herpes simplex virus infection in rat lumbar dorsal root ganglia. *Journal of Psychosomatic Research, 37,* 843–849.

Bloom, J. R., Kang, S. H., & Romano, P. (1991). Cancer and stress, the effect of social support as a resource. In C. L. Cooper & N. Watson (Eds.), *Cancer and stress. Psychological, biological and coping studies* (pp. 95–124). New York: Wiley.

Boland, C. R., Sato, J., Saito, K., Carethers, J. M., Marra, G., Laghi, L., & Chauhan, D. P. (1998). Genetic instability and chromosomal aberrations in colorectal cancer, a review of the current models. *Cancer, Detection and Prevention, 22,* 377–382.

Bosch, J. A., Brand, H. S., Ligtenberg, T. J., Bermond, B., Hoogstraten, J., & Amerongen, A. V. (1996). Psychological stress as a determinant of protein levels and salivary-induced aggregation of Streptococcus gordonii in human whole saliva. *Psychosomatic Medicine, 58,* 374–382.

Bounneau, R. H., Sheridan, J. F., Feng, N., & Glaser, R. (1991). Stress-induced suppression of herpes simplex virus-specific cytotoxic T lymphocyte and natural killer cell activity and enhancement of acute pathogenesis following local HSV infection. *Brain, Behavior, and Immunity, 5,* 170–192.

Boyce, W. T., Adams, S., Tschann, J. M., Cohen, F., Wara, D., & Gunnar, M. R. (1995). Adrenocortical and behavioral predictors of immune responses to starting school. *Pediatric Research, 38,* 1009–1017.

Boyce, W. T., Chesterman, E. A., Martin, N., Folkman, S., Cohen, F., & Wara, D. (1993). Immunologic change occurring at kindergarten entry predict respiratory illness after the Loma Prieta earthquake. *Journal of Developmental and Behavioral Pediatrics, 14,* 296–303.

Breznitz, S., Ben Hur, H., Berzon, Y., Weiss D. W., Levitan, G., Tarcic, N., & Lischinsky, S. (1998). Experimental induction and termination of acute psychological stress in human volunteers, effects on immunological, neuroendocrine, cardiovascular, and psychological parameters. *Brain, Behavior, and Immunity, 12,* 34–52.

Brohee, D., Vanhaeverberbeek, M., Kennes, B., & Neve, P. (1990). Leukocyte and lymphocyte subsets after a short pharmacological stress by intravenous epinephrine and hydrocortisone in healthy humans. *International Journal of Neuroscience, 53,* 53–62.

Brosschot, J. F., Benschop, R. J., Godaert, G. L., Olff, M., De Smet, M., Heijnen, C. J., & Ballieux R. E. (1994). Influence of life stress on immunological reactivity to mild psychological stress. *Psychosomatic Medicine, 56,* 216–224.

Brosschot, J. F., Godaert, G. L., Benschop, R. J., Olff, M., Ballieux, R. E., & Heijnen, C. J. (1998). Experimental stress and immunological reactivity, a closer look at perceived uncontrollability. *Psychosomatic Medicine, 60,* 359–361.

Burleson, M. H., Malarkey, W. B., Cacioppo, J. T., Poehlmann, K. M., Kiecolt Glaser, J. K., Bernston, G. G., & Glaser, R. (1998). Postmenopausal hormone replacement, effects on autonomic, neuroendocrine and immune reactivity to brief psychological stressor. *Psychosomatic Medicine, 60,* 17–25.

Buske–Kirschbaum, A., Kirschbaum, C., Stierle, H., Lehnert, H., & Hellhammer, D. (1992). Conditioned increase of natural killer cell activity (NKCA) in humans. *Psychosomatic Medicine, 54,* 123–132.

Bussin, R., Burket, R. C., & Kelleher, E. T. (1996). *Psychosomatics, 37,* 108–115.

Byrnes, D. M., Antoni, M. H., Goddkin, K., Efanis-Potter, J., Asthana, D., Simon, T., Munajj, J., Ironson, G., & Fletcher, M. A., (1998). Stressful events, pessimism, natural killer cell cytotoxicity, and cytotoxic/suppressor T cells in HIV+ black woman at risk for cervical cancer. *Psychosomatic Medicine, 60,* 714–722.

Cacioppo, J. T., Malarkey, W. B., Kiecolt-Glaser, J. K., Uchino, B. N., Sgoutas-Emch, S. A., Sheridan, J. F., Bernston, G. G., & Glaser R. (1995). Heterogeneity in neuroendocrine and immune response to brief psychological stressors as a function of autonomic cardiac activation. *Psychosomatic Medicine, 57,* 154–164.

Canter, A., Cluff, L. E., & Imboden, J. B. (1972). Hypersensitive reaction to immunization inoculation and antecedent psychological vulnerability. *Journal of Psychosomatic Research, 16,* 99–101.

Castle, S., Wilkins, S., Heck, E., Tanzy, K., & Fahey, J. (1995). Depression in caregivers of demented patients is associated with altered immunity, impaired proliferative capacity, increased CD8+ and a decline in lymphocytes with surface signal transduction molecules (CD38+) and a cytotoxity marker (CD56+ CD8+). *Clinical and Experimental Immunology, 101,* 487–493.

Chang, S. S., & Rasmussen, A. F. (1965). Stress-induced suppression of interferon production in virus-infected mice. *Nature, 205,* 623–624.

Chen, C. C., David, A. S., Nunnerley, H., Michell, M., Dawson, J. L., Berry, H., Dobbs, J., & Fahy, T. (1995). Adverse life events and breast cancer: Case-control study. *British Medical Journal, 311,* 1527–1530.

Chetverikova, L. K., Frolov, B. A., Kramskaya, T. A., & Polyak, R. Y. (1987). Experimental influenza infection, influence of stress. *Acta Virologica, 31,* 424–433.

Chrousos, G. P. (1995). The hypothalamic-pituitary-adrenal axis and immune-mediated inflammation. *New England Journal of Medicine, 332,* 1351–1362.

Clover, R. D., Abell, T., Becker, L. A., Crawford, S., & Ramsey, J. N. C. (1989). Family functioning and stress as predictors of influenza B infection. *Journal of Family Practice, 28 ,* 535–539.

Coe, C. L. (1993). Psychosocial factors and immunity in nonhuman primates: A review. *Psychosomatic Medicine, 55,* 298–308.

Cohen, J. J. (1999). Individual variability and immunity. *Brain, Behavior, and Immunity, 13,* 76–79.

Cohen, F., Kearney, K. A., Zegans, L. S., Kemeny, M. E., Neuhaus, J. M., & Stites, D. P. (1999). Differential immune system changes with acute and persistent stress for optimist and pessimists. *Brain, Behavior, and Immunity, 13,* 155–174.

Cohen, S., Tyrrel, D. A. J., & Smith, A. P. (1991). Psychological stress and susceptibility to common colds. *New England Journal of Medicine, 325,* 606–612.

Cole, S. W., Kemeny, M. E., Weitzman, O. B., Schoen, M., & Anton, P. A. (1999). Socially inhibited individuals show heightened DHT response during intense social engagement. *Brain, Behavior, and Immunity, 13,* 187–200.

Collins, S. M., Barbara, G., & Vallance, B. (1999). Stress, inflammation and the irritable bowel syndrome. *Canadian Journal of Gastroenterology, 13*(Suppl. A), 47A–49A.

Cooper, C. C., & Watson, M. (Eds.) (1991). *Cancer and stress.* New York: John Wiley.

Courtney, J. G., Longnecker, M. P., Theorell, T., & Gerhardsson-de-Verdier, M. (1993). Stressful life events and the risk of colorectal cancer. *Epidemiology, 4,* 407–414.

Dalkvist, J., Wahlin, T. B., Bartsch, E., & Forsbeck, M. (1995). Herpes simplex and mood: A prospective study. *Psychosomatic Medicine, 57,* 137.

Davidson, R. J., Coe, C. C., Dolski, I., & Donzella, B. (1999). Individual differences in prefrontal activation asymmetry predict natural killer cell activity at rest and in response to challenge. *Brain, Behavior and Immunity, 13,* 93–108.

De Gucht, V., Fischler, B., & Demanet, C. (1999). Immune dysfunction associated with chronic professional stress in nurses. *Psychiatry Research, 85,* 105–111.

Deker, D., Schondorf, M., Bidlingmaier, F., Hirner, A., & von Ruecker, A. A. (1996). Surgical stress induces a shift in the type 1/type 2 T-helper cell balance, suggesting down regulation of cell-mediated and up regulation of antibody mediated immunity commensurate to the trauma. *Surgery, 119,* 316–325.

DeLano, R. M., & Mallery, S. R. (1998). Stress-related modulation of central nervous system immunity in a murine model of herpes simplex encephalitis. *Journal of Neuroimmunology, 89,* 51–58.

Delle Chiaie, R., De Cesare, G., Biondi, M., Stagi, L., & Pancheri, P. (1990). Psychoneuroendocrine reactivity in the aged, a controlled study. In G. Nappi (Ed.), *Stress and the aging brain* (pp. 121–129). New York: Raven Press.

Delle Chiaie, R., & Regine, F. (1997). Modificazioni immunitarie nelle malattie mentali: elementi per un'interpretazione transnosografica. In M. Biondi (Ed.), *Mente, cervello e sistema immunitario* (pp. 225–248). Milano: McGraw-Hill Italia.

Devoino, L., Idova, G., Alperina, & Cheido, M. (1994). Brain neuromediator systems in the immune response control: Pharmacological analysis of pre- and postsynaptic mechanisms. *Brain Research, 633,* 267–274.

De Vries, M. J., Schilder, J. N., Mulder, C. L., Vrancken, A. M., Remie, M., & Garssen, B. (1997). Phase II study of psychotherapeutic intervention in advanced cancer. *Psychooncology, 6,* 29–37.

Di Gennaro, S., Fehder, W., Nuamah, I. F., Campbell, D. E., & Douglas, S. D. (1997). Caregiving to very low birthweight infants, a model of stress and immune response. *Brain, Behavior, and Immunity, 11,* 201–215.

Dimsdale, J. E. (1984). Generalizing from laboratory studies to field studies of human stress physiology. *Psychosomatic Medicine, 46,* 463–468.

Dimsdale, J. E., Mills, P., Patterson, T., Ziegler, M., & Dillon, E. (1994). Effects of chronic stress on beta adrenergic receptors in the homeless. *Psychosomatic Medicine, 56,* 290–295.

Dobbs, C. M., Vasquez, M., Glaser, R., & Sheridan, J. F. (1993). Mechanisms of stress-induced modulation of viral pathogenesis and immunity. *Journal of Neuroimmunomodulation, 48,* 151–160.

Dobkin, P. L., Fortin, P. R., Joseph, L., Esdaile, J. M., Danoff, D. S., & Clarke, A. E. (1998). Psychosocial contributors to mental and physical health in patients with systemic lupus erythematosus. *Arthritis Care and Research, 11,* 23–31.

Drummond, P. D., & Hewson Bower, B. (1997). Increased psychosocial stress and decreased mucosal immunity in children with recurrent upper respiratory tract infections. *Journal of Psychosomatic Research, 43,* 271–278.

Edwards, E. A., & Dean, L. M. (1977). Effects of crowding of mice on humoral antibody formation and protection to lethal antigenic challenge. *Psychosomatic Medicine, 39,* 19–24.

Engel, B. T. (1960). Stimulus-response and individual-response specificity. *Archives of General Psychiatry, 2,* 305–313.

Esterling, B. A., Kiecolt-Glaser, J. K., & Glaser, R. (1996). Psychosocial modulation of cytokine induced natural killer cell activity in older adults. *Psychosomatic Medicine, 58,* 264–272.

Evans, P. D., & Edgerton, N. (1991). Life-events and mood as predictors of the common cold. *British Journal of Medical Psychology, 64,* 35–44.

Evers, A. W., Kraaimat, F. W., Geene, R., & Bijsma, J. W. (1997). Determinants of psychological distress and its course in the first year after diagnosis in rheumatoid arthritis patients. *Journal of Behavioral Medicine, 20,* 489–504.

Fawzy, F. I., Fawzy, N. W., & Hyun, C. S. (1994). Short-term psychiatric intervention for patients with malignant melanoma: Effects on psychological state, coping and the immune system. In Lewis, C. E., O'Sullivan, C., & J. Barraclough (Eds), *The psychoimmunology of human cancer* (pp. 291–319). Oxford; UK: Oxford University Press.

Fawzy, I., Kemeny, M. E., Fawzy, N. W., Elashoff, R., Morton, D., Cousins, N., & Fahey, J. L. (1990). A structured psychiatric intervention for cancer patients. *Archives of General Psychiatry, 47,* 729–735.

Felten, D. L., Cohen, N., Ader, R., Felten S. Y., Carlson, S. L., & Roszman, T. L. (1991). Central neural circuits involved in neural-immune interactions. In R. Ader, D. L. Felten, & N. Cohen (Eds.), *Psychoneuroimmunology* (pp. 1–20). New York: Academic Press.

Felten, S. Y., & Felten D. L. (1994). Neural-immune interactions. *Progress in Brain Research, 100,* 157–162.

Fischer, C. L., Daniels, J. C., Levin, W. C., Kimzey, S. L., Cobb, E. K., & Ritzmann, S. E. (1972). Effects of the space flight environment on man 5 immune system. II. Lymphocyte counts and reactivity. *Aerospace Medicine, 43,* 1122–1125.

Fittschen, B., Schulz, K. H., Schulz, H., Raedler, A., & Kerekjarto, M. (1990). Chances of immunological parameters in healthy subjects under examination stress. *International Journal of Neuroscience, 51,* 241–242.

Fricchione, G., Bilfinger, T. V., Jandorf, L., Smith, E. M., & Stefano, G. B. (1996). Surgical anticipatory stress manifests itself in immunocyte desensitization, evidence for autoimmunoregulatory involvement. *International Journal of Cardiology*, 26(Suppl. 53), 65–73.

Friedman, S. B., & Glasgow, L. A. (1973). Interaction of mouse strain and differential housing upon resistance to Plasmodium Berghei. *Journal of Parasitology*, 59, 851–854.

Friedman, S. B., Glasgow, L. A., & Ader, R. (1969). Psychosocial factors modifying host resistance to experimental infections. *Annals of the New York Academy of Sciences*, 164, 381–393.

Friedman, S. B, Glasgow, L. A., & Ader, R. (1970). Differential susceptibility to a viral agent in mice housed alone or in groups. *Psychosomatic Medicine*, 32, 285–299.

Fry, R. W, Grove, J. R., Morton, A. R., Zeroni, P. M., Gaudieri, S., & Keast, D. (1994). Psychological and immunological correlates of acute overtraining. *British Journal of Sports Medicine*, 28, 241–246.

Futterman, A. D., Wellisch, Zighelboim, J., Luna–Raines, M., & Weiner, H. (1996). Psychological and immunological reactions of family members to patients undergoing bone marrow transplantation. *Psychosomatic Medicine*, 58, 472–480.

Gaillard, R. C., & Spinedi, E. (1998). Sex- and stress-steroids interactions and the immune system, evidence for a neuroendocrine-immunological sexual dimorphism. *Domestic Animal Endocrinology*, 15, 345–352.

Gatmaitan, B. G., Chason, J. L., & Lerner, A. M. (1970). Augmentation of the virulence of murine Coxsackievirus B3 myocarditis by exercise. *Journal of Experimental Medicine*, 131, 1121–1136.

Geenen, R., Godaert, G. L., Heijnen, C. J., Vianen, M. E., Wenting, M. J., Nederhoff, Mg. G., & Bijisma, J. W. (1998). Experimentally induced stress in rheumatoid arthritis of recent onset: Effects on peripheral blood lymphocytes. *Clinical and Experimental Rheumatology*, 16, 553–559.

Geyer, S. (1993). Life events, chronic difficulties and vulnerability factors preceding breast cancer. *Social Science and Medicine*, 37, 1545–1555.

Ginsberg, A., Price, S., Ingram, D., & Nottage, E. (1996). Life events and the risk of breast cancer: A case–control study. *European Journal of Cancer*, 32A, 2049–2052.

Giraldi, T., Perissin, L., Zorzet, S., Piccini, P., & Rapozzi, V. (1989). Effect of stress on tumor growth and metastasis in mice bearing Lewis lung carcinoma. *European Journal of Cancer and Clinical Oncology*, 25, 1583–1588.

Giraldi, T., Perissin, L., Zorzet, S., & Rapozzi, V. (1994). Rotational stress reduces the effectiveness of antitumor drugs in mice. *Annals of the New York Academy of Sciences*, 741, 234–243.

Glaser, R., Kiecolt-Glaser, J. K., Bonneau, R. H., Malarkey, W., Kennedy, S., & Hughes, B. (1992). Stress-induced modulation of the immune response to recombinant hepatitis B vaccine. *Psychosomatic Medicine*, 54, 22–29.

Glaser, R., Kiecolt-Glaser, J. K., Malarkey, W. B., & Sheridan, J. F. (1998). The influence of psychological stress on the immune response to vaccines. *Annals of the New York Academy of Sciences*, 840, 649–655.

Glaser, R., Kiecolt-Glaser, J. K., Marucha, P. T., MacCallum, R. C., Laskowski, B. F., & Malarkey, W. B. (1999). Stress-related changes in proinflammatory cytokine production in wounds. *Archives of General Psychiatry*, 56, 450–456.

Goldmeier, D., & Johnson, A. (1982). Does psychiatric illness affect the recurrence rate of genital herpes? *British Journal of Venereal Disease*, 58, 40–43.

Gonzales-Quijano, M. I., Martin, M., Millan, S., & Lopez-Calderon, A. (1998). Lymphocyte response to mitogens, influence of life events and personality. *Neuropsychobiology*, 38, 90–96.

Gorzynski, J. G., Holland, J., Katz, J. K., Weiner, H., Zumoff, B., Fukushima, D., & Levin J. (1980). Stability of ego defenses and endocrine responses in women prior to breast biopsy and ten yeras later. *Psychosomatic Medicine*, 42, 323–328.

Grazzi, L., Salmaggi, A., Dufour, A., Ariano, C., Colangelo, A. M., Parati, E., Lazzaroni, M., Nespolo, A., Bordin, G., & Castellazzi, C. (1993). Physical effort induced changes in immune parameters. *International Journal of Neuroscience*, 68, 133–140.

Greene, W. A., Betts, R. F., Ochitill, H. N., Iker, H. P., & Douglas, R. G. (1978). Psychosocial factors and immunity, a preliminary report. *Psychosomatic Medicine*, 40, 87.

Greenfield, N. S., & Sternbach, R. A. (Eds.) (1972). *Handbook of psychophysiology*. New York: Holt, Rinehart & Winston.

Grings, W. W., & Dawson, M. E. (1978). *Emotions and bodily responses*. New York: Academic Press.

Gunderson, E. K., & Rahe, R. H. (Eds.) (1974). *Life stress and illness*. Springfield, II: Charles C. Thomas.

Gust, D. A., Gordon, T. P., Brodie, A. R., & McClure, H. M. (1994). Effect of a preferred companion in modulating stress in adult female monkeys. *Physiology and Behavior*, 55, 681–684.

Halvorsen, R., & Vassend, O. (1987). Effects of examination stress on some cellular immunity functions. *Journal of Psychosomatic Research*, 31, 693–697.

Hamilton, D. R. (1973). Immunosuppressive effects of predator induced stress in mice with acquired immunity to Hymenolepis nana. *Journal of Psychosomatic Research*, 18, 143–150.

Heisel, B. S., Locke, S. F., Kraus, L. B., & Williams, R. M. (1986). Natural killer cell activity and MMPI scores of a cohort of college students. *American Journal of Psychiatry*, 163, 1382–1386.

Hewson-Bower, B., & Drummond, P. D. (1996). Secretory immunoglobulin A increases during relaxation in children with and without recurrent upper respiratory infections. *Journal of Development and Behavioral Pediatrics*, 17, 311–316.

Hinrichsen, H., Folsch, U., & Kirch, W. (1992). Modulation of the immune response to stress in patients with systemic lupus erythematosus: Review of recent studies. *European Journal of Clinical Investigation*, 22(Suppl. 1), 21–25.

Hisano, S., Sakamoto, K., Ishiko, T., Kamohara, H., and Ogawa, M. (1997). IL-6 and soluble IL-6 receptor levels change differently after surgery both in the blood and in the operative field. *Cytokines*, 9, 447–452.

Hollstein, M., Sidransky, D., Vogelstein, B., & Harris, C. C. (1991). The multistep nature of cancer. *Science*, 253, 49–53.

Holmes, T. H., Hawkins, N. G., Bowerman, C. E., Clarke, E. R., & Joffe, J. R. (1957). Psychosocial and physiological studies of tuberculosis. *Psychosomatic Medicine*, 19, 134–143.

Holmes, T. H., & Rahe, R. H. (1967). The Social Readjustment Rating Scale. *Journal of Psychosomatic Research*, 11, 213–218.

Ironson, G., La Perriere, A., Antoni, M., O'Rearn, P., Schneiderman, N., Klimas, N., & Fletcher, M. A. (1990). Changes in immune and psychological measures as a function of anticipation and reaction to news of HIV-1 antibody status. *Psychosomatic Medicine*, 52, 247–270.

Ironson, G., Wynings, C., Schneidermann, N., Baum, A., Rodriguez, M., Greedwood, D., Benight, C. Antoni, M., LaPerriere, A., Huang, H. S., Klimas, N., & Fletcher, M. A. (1997). Posttraumatic stress symptoms, intrusive thought, loss, and immune function after hurricane Andrew. *Psychosomatic Medicine*, 59, 128–141.

Irwin, M., Costlow, C., Williams, H., Artin, K, H., Chan, C. Y., Stinson, D. L., Levin, M. J., Hayward, A. R., & Oxman, M. N. (1998). *Journal of Infectious Diseases*, 178 (Suppl. 1), S104–S108.

Irwin, M., Daniels, M., Bloom, E. T., & Weiner, H. (1986). Life events, depression and natural killer cell activity. *Psychopharmacology Bulletin*, 22, 1093–1096.

Irwin, M., Daniels, M., Risch, S. C., & Weiner, H. (1988). Plasma cortisol and natural killer cell activity during bereavement, *Biological Psychiatry, 24*, 173–178.

Irwin, M., Mascovich, A., Gillin, J. C., Willoghby, R., & Smith, T.-L., (1994). Partial sleep deprivation reduces natural killer cell activity in humans. *Psychosomatic Medicine, 56*, 493–498.

Irwin, M., & Weiner, H. (1987). Depressive symptoms and immune function during bereavement. In S. Zisook (Ed.), *Biopsychosocial aspects of bereavement*. Washington; DC: American Psychiatric Press.

Jackson, G. C., Dowling, H. F., Anderson, T., Riff, L., Saporta, M. S., & Turck, M. (1960). Susceptibility and immunity to common upper respiratory viral infections. *Annals of Internal Medicine, 53*, 719–738.

Jacobs, S. C., & Ostfeld, A. (1977). An epidemiological review of the mortality of bereavement. *Psychosomatic Medicine, 39*, 344–357.

Jamner, L. D., Schwartz, G. F., & Leigh, H. (1988). The relationship between repressive and defensive coping styles and monocyte, eosinophil, and serum glucose levels, support for the opioid peptide hypothesis of repression. *Psychosomatic Medicine, 50*, 567–575.

Jemmott, J. B., Borysenko, J. Z., Borysenko, M., McClelland, D. C., Champman, R., Meyer, D., & Benson, H. (1983). Academic stress, power motivation, and decrease in secretion rate of salivary secretory immunoglobulin A. *Lancet, 2*, 1400–1402.

Johnson, T., & Rassmussen, A. F., Jr. (1965). Emotional stress and susceptibility to polyomyelitis virus infection in mice. *Archivs Gesamte Virusforsch, 17*, 392–397.

Jessop, J. (1998). Beta-endorphin in the immune system, mediator of pain and stress? *The Lancet, 351*, 1828–9.

Kang, D. H., Coe, C. L., Mc Carthy, D. O., Jarjour, N. N., Kelly, E. A., Rodriguez, R. R., & Busse, W. W. (1997). Cytokine profiles of stimulated blood lymphocytes in asthmatic and healthy adolescents across the school year. *Journal of Interferon and Cytokine Research, 17*, 481–487.

Kang, D. H., Coe, C. L., Karaszweski, J., & McCarthy, D. O. (1998). Relationship of social support to stress responses and immune function in healthy and asthmatic adolescents. *Research Nursing Health, 21*, 117–128.

Kang, D. H., Coe, C. L., & McCarthy, D. O. (1996). Academic examinations significantly impact immune responses, but not lung function in healthy and well-managed asthmatic adolescents. *Brain, Behavior, and Immunity, 10*, 164–181.

Kang, D. H., Coe, C. L., McCarthy, D. O., & Ershler, W. B. (1997). Immune responses to final exams in healthy and asthmatic adolescents. *Nursing Research, 46*, 12–19.

Kasl, S. V., Evans, A. S., & Neiderman, J. C. (1979). Psychosocial risk factors in the development of infectious mononucleosis. *Psychosomatic Medicine, 41*, 445–466.

Katcher, A. H., Brightman, V. J., Luborky, L., & Ship, I. (1973). Prediction of the incidence of recurrent herpes labialis and systemic illness from psychological measurement. *Journal of Dental Research, 52*, 49–58.

Kemeny, M. E., Cohen, F., Zegans, L. A., & Conant, M. A. (1989). Psychological and immulogical predictors of genital herpes recurrence. *Psychosomatic Medicine, 51*, 195–208.

Kemeny, M. E., & Laudenslager, M. L. (1999). Introduction beyond stress, the role of individual difference factors in psychoneuroimmunology. *Brain, Behavior, and Immunity, 13*, 73–75.

Kiecolt-Glaser, J. K., Garner, W., Speicher, C., Penn, G. M., Holliday, J., & Glaser, R. (1984). Psychosocial modifiers of immunocompetence in medical students. *Psychosomatic Medicine, 46*, 7–14.

Kiecolt-Glaser, J. K., & Glaser, R. (1992). Psychoneuroimmunology: Can psychological interventions modulate immunity? *Journal of Consulting and Clinical Psychology, 60*, 569–575.

Kiecolt-Glaser, J. K., Glaser, R., Cacioppo, J. T., & Malarkey, W. B. (1998). Marital stress: Immunologic, neuroendocrine, and autonomic correlates. *Annals of the New York Academy of Sciences, 840*, 656–663.

Kiecolt-Glaser, J. K., Glaser, R., Cacioppo, J. T., McCallum, R. C., Snydersmith, M., Kim, C., & Malarkey, W. B. (1997). Marital conflict in older adults: Endocrinological and immunological correlates. *Psychosomatic Medicine, 59*, 339–349.

Kiecolt-Glaser, J. K., Glaser, R., Gravenstein, S., Malarkey, W. B., & Sheridan, J. (1996). Chronic stress alters the immune response to influenza virus vaccine in older adults. *Proceedings of the National Academy of Sciences USA, 93*, 3043–3047.

Kiecolt-Glaser, J. K., Glaser, R., Strain, E. C., Stout, J. C., Tarr, K. L., Holliday, J. E., & Speicher, C. E. (1986). Modulation of cellular immunity in medical students. *Journal of Behavioral Medicine, 9*, 5–21.

Kiecolt-Glaser, J. K., Kennedy, S., Malkoff, S., Fisher, L., Speicher, C. F., & Glaser, R. (1988). Marital discord and immunity in males. *Psychosomatic Medicine, 50*, 3–29.

Kiecolt-Glaser, J. K., Malarkey, W. B., Chee, M., Newton, T., Cacioppo, J. T., Mao, H. Y., & Glaser, R. (1993). Negative behavior during marital conflict is associated with immunological down-regulation. *Psychosomatic Medicine, 55*, 395–409.

Kiecolt-Glaser, J. K., Marucha, P. T., Malarkey, W. B., Mercado, A. M., & Glaser, R. (1995). Slowing of wound healing by psychological stress. *Lancet, 346*, 1194–1196.

Kiecolt-Glaser, J. K., Ricker, D., George, J., Messik, G., Speicher, C. E., Garner, W., & Glaser, R. (1984). Urinary cortisol levels, cellular immunocompetency and loneliness in psychiatric inpatients. *Psychosomatic Medicine, 46*, 15–23.

Koh, K. B., & Hong, C. S. (1993). The relationship of stress with serum IgE level in patients with bronchial asthma. *Yonsei Medical Journal, 34*, 166–174.

Komori, T., Fujiwara, R., Tanida, M., Nomura, J., & Yokohama, M. M. (1995). Effects of citrus fragrance on immune function and depressive states. *Neuroimmunomodulation, 2*, 174–180.

Kubitz, K. A., Peavey, B. S., & Moore, B. S. (1986). The effect of daily hassles of humoral immunity, an interaction moderated by locus of control. *Biofeedback and Self-Regulation, 11*, 115–123.

Kune, S., Kune, G. A., Watson, L. F., & Rahe, R. H. (1991). Recent life changes and large bowel cancer. Data from the Melbourne Colorectal Cancer Study. *Journal of Clinical Epidemiology, 44*, 57–68.

Kvikstad, A., Vatten, L. J., Tretli, S., & Kvinnsland, S. (1994). Death of a husband or marital divorce related to risk of breast cancer in middle-aged women. *European Journal of Cancer, 30A*, 473–477.

Laborit, H. (1989). *L'inhibition de l'action*. Paris, Masson.

Laborit, H. (1991). The major mechanism of stress. In G. Jasmin & L. Proschek (Eds.), *Stress revisited. 2. Systemic effects* (pp. 1–26). Basel: Karger-Verlag.

Lazarus, R. (1971). The concept of stress and disease. In L. Levi, (Ed.), *Society, stress and disease* (pp. 53–58). London: Oxford Univ. Press.

Lazarus, R. (1993). Coping theory and research, past, present and future. *Psychosomatic Medicine, 55*, 234–247.

Lazarus, R. S., & Folkman, S. (1984). Stress, appraisal and coping. New York: Springer Verlag.

Lekander, M., Furst, C. J., Rotstein, S., Hursti, T. J., & Frederikson, M. (1997). Immune effects of relaxation during chemotherapy for ovarian cancer. *Psychotherapy and Psychosomatics, 66*, 185–191.

Levenson, J. L., Bemis, C., & Presberg, B. A. (1994). The role of psychological factors in cancer onset and progression, a critical appraisal. In C. E. Lewis, C. O'Sullivan, & J. Barraclough (Eds.), *The psychoimmunology of cancer* (pp. 246–265). Oxford: Oxford Univ. Press.

Levenstein, S. (1999). Stress and peptic ulcer: Life beyond helicobacter. *British Medical Journal, 316*, 538–541.

Levi, L. (Ed.) (1971). *Society, stress and disease*. London: Oxford Univ. Press.

Levine, D. S., & Greenleaf, J. E. (1998). Immunosuppression during spaceflight deconditioning. *Aviation Space and Environmental Medicine, 69*, 172–177.

Levinson, S. O., Milzer, A., & Lewin, P. (1945). Effect of fatigue, chilling and mechanical trauma on resistance to experimental polyomyelitis. *American Journal of Hygiene, 42*, 204–213.

Levy, S. M., Herberman, R. B., Maluish, A. M., Schlien, B., & Lippman, M. (1985). Prognostic risk assessment in primary breast cancer by behavioural and immunological parameters. *Health Psychology, 4*, 99–113.

Levy, S. M., Herberman, R. B., Whiteside, T., Sanzo, K., Lee, J., & Kirkwood, J. (1990). Perceived social support and tumor estrogen/progesterone receptor status as predictors of natural killer cell activity in breast cancer patients. *Psychosomatic Medicine, 52*, 73–85.

Lewis, J. W., Morgan, M. M., & Marek, P. (1989). Stress-induced analgesia. In H. Weiner, I. Florin, R. Murison, & D. Hellhammer (Eds.), *Frontiers of stress research* (pp. 21–36). Toronto: Huber.

Lewis, C. E., O'Sullivan, C., & J. Barraclough (Eds.) (1994). *The psychoimmunology of human cancer*. Oxford, UK: Oxford Univ. Press.

Li, T., Harada, M., Tamada, K., Abe, K., & Nomoto, K. (1997). Repeated restraint stress impairs the antitumor T cell response through suppressive effect on Th1-type CD4+ T cells. *Anticancer Research, 17*, 4259–4268.

Liang, S. W., Jemerin, J. M., Tschann, J. M., Wara, D. W., & Boyce, W. T. (1997). Life events, frontal electroencephalogram laterality and functional immune status after acute psychological stressors in adolescents. *Psychosomatic Medicine, 59*, 178–186.

Linn, B. S., & Linn, M. W. (1987). The effects of psychophysical stress on surgical outcome. *Psychosomatic Medicine, 49*, 210. [abstract]

Locke, S. F., & Heisel, B. S. (1977). The influence of stress and emotions on the human immune response. *Biofeedback and Self Regulation, 2*, 320.

Locke, S. F., Kraus, L., Leserman, B., Hurst, M. W., Heisel, B. S., & Williams, R. M. (1984). Life change stress, psychiatric symptoms and natural killer cell activity. *Psychosomatic Medicine, 46*, 441–453.

Logan, H. L., Lutgendof, S., Hartwig, A., Lilly, J., & Berberich, S. L. (1998). Immune, stress, and mood markers related to recurrent oral herpes outbreaks. *Oral Surgery, Oral Pathology, Oral Radiology and Endodontology, 86*, 48–54.

MacKinnon, L. T. (1998). Future directions in exercise and immunology: Regulation and integration. *International Journal of Sport Medicine, 19*(Suppl. 3), s205–s209.

Madden, K. S., & Felten, D. L. (1995). Experimental basis for neural-immune interactions. *Physiological Review, 75*, 77–106.

Madden, K. S., Sanders, V. M., & Felten, D. L. (1995). Catecholamine influences and sympathetic neural modulation of immune responsiveness. *Annual Review of Pharmacology and Toxicology, 35*, 417–448.

Madden, K. S., Thyagarajan, S., & Felten, D. L. (1998). Alterations in sympathetic noradrenergic innervation in lymphoid organs with age. *Annals of the New York Academy of Sciences, 840*, 262–268.

Maes, M., Lin, A. H., Delmeire, L., Van Gastel, A., Kenis, G., De Jongh, R., & Bosmans, E. (1999a). Elevated serum interleukin-6 (IL-6) and IL-6 receptor concentrations in posttraumatic stress disorder following accidental man-made traumatic events. *Biological Psychiatry, 45*, 833–839.

Maes, M., Van Bockstaele, D. R., Gastel, A., Song, C., Schotte, C., Neels, H., DeMeester, I., Scharpé, S., & Janca, A. (1999b). The effects of psychological stress on leucocyte subset distribution in humans, evidence of immune activation. *Neuropsychobiology, 39*, 1–9.

Marchesi, G. F., Cotani, P., Santone, G., Di Giuseppe, S., Bartocci, C., & Montroni, M. (1989). Psychological and immunological relationships during acute academic stress. *New Trends in Experimental and Clinical Psychiatry, 5*, 5–22.

Marshall, G. D., Jr., Agarwal, S. K., Lloyd, C., Cohen, L., Henninger, E. M., & Morris, G. J. (1998). Cytokine dysregulation associated with exam stress in healthy medical students. *Brain, Behavior, and Immunity, 12*, 297–12,307.

Marsland, A. L., Manuck, S. B., Fazzari, T. V., Stewart, C. J., & Rabin, B. S. (1995). Stability of individual differences in cellular immune responses to acute psychological stress. *Psychosomatic Medicine, 57*, 295–298.

Marsland, A. L., Manuck, S. B., Wood, P., Rabin, B. S., Muldoon, M. F., & Cohen, S. (1995). Beta 2 adrenergic receptor density and cardiovascular response to mental stress. *Physiology and Behavior, 57*, 1163–1167.

Marucha, P. T., Kiecolt-Glaser, J. K., & Favagchi, M. (1998). Mucosal wound healing is impaired by examination stress. *Psychosomatic Medicine, 60*, 362–365.

Marx, C., Ehrhart-Bornstein, M., Scherbaum, W. A., & Bornstein, S. R. (1998). Regulation of adrenocortical function by cytokines—Relevance for immuno-endocrine interaction. *Hormone and Metabolism Research, 30*, 416–420.

Mason, J. W. (1971). A re-evalutaion of the concept of "nonspecificity" in stress theory. *Journal of Psychiatry Research, 8*, 323–333.

Mason, J. W. (1975). Emotions as reflected in patterns of endocrine integration. In L. Levi (Ed.) *Emotions—Their parameters and measurement*. New York: Raven Press.

Mason, J. W., Wang, S., Yehuda, R., Bremner, J. D., Riney, S. J., Lubin, H., Johnson, D. R., Southwick, S. M., & Charney, D. S. (1995). Some approaches to the study of the clinical implications of thyroid alterations in post-traumatic stress disorder. In M. J. Friedman, D. S. Charney, & A. Y. Deutch (Eds.), *Neurobiological and clinical consequences of stress* (pp. 367–380). Philadelphia: Lippincott.

Matthews, K. A., Caggiula, A. R., McAllister, C. G., Berga, S. L., Owens, J. F., Flory, J. D., & Miller, A. L. (1995). Sympathetic reactivity to acute stress and immune response in women. *Psychosomatic Medicine, 57*, 564–571.

McClelland, D. C., Floor, F., Davidson, R. B., & Saron, C. (1980). Stressed power motivation, sympathetic activation, immune function, and illness. *Journal of Human Stress, 6*, 11–19.

McClelland, D. C., Ross, G., & Patel, V. (1985). The effect of an academic examination on salivary norepinephrine and immunoglobulin levels. *Journal of Human Stress, 11*, 52–59.

McCruden, A. B., & Stimson, W. H. (1991). Sex hormones and immune function. In R. Ader, D. L. Felten, & N. Cohen (Eds.), *Psychoneuroimmunology* (pp. 475–488). New York: Academic Press.

McEwen, B. S. (1998). Protective and damaging effects of stress mediators. *New England Journal of Medicine, 338*, 171–179.

McGrady, A., Conran, P., Dickey, D., Garman, D., Farris, E., & Schumann-Brzezinski, C. (1992). The effects of biofeedback-assisted relaxation on cell-mediated immunity, cortisol, and white blood cell count in healthy adult subjects. *Journal of Behavioral Medicine, 15*, 343–353.

Miller, N. E. (1969). Learning of visceral and glandular responses. *Science, 163*, 434–445.

Miller, G. E, , Cohen, S., Rabin, B. S., Skoner, D. P., & Doyel, W. J. (1999). Personality and tonic cardiovascular, neuroendocrine and immune parameters. *Brain, Behavior, and Immunity, 13*, 109–123.

Mills, P. J., Berry, C. C., Dimsdale, J. E., Ziegler, M. G., Nelesen, R. A., & Kennedy, B. P. (1995a). Lymphocyte subset redistribution in response to acute experimental stress, effects of gender, ethnicity, hypertension, and the sympathetic nervous system. *Brain, Behavior, and Immunity, 9*, 61–69.

Mills, P. J., Haeri, S. L., & Dimsdale, J. E. (1995b). Temporal stability of acute stressor-induced changes in cellular immunity. *International Journal of Psychophysiology, 19*, 287–290.

Mills, P. J., Ziegler, M. G., Dimsdale, J. E., & Parry, B. L. (1995c). Enumerative immune changes following acute stress: Effect of the menstrual cycle. *Brain, Behavior, and Immunity, 9*, 190–195.

Mills, P. J., Ziegler, M. G., Patterson, T., Dimsdale, J. E., Hauger, R., Irwin, M., & Grant, I. (1997). Plasma catecholamine and lymphocyte beta 2 receptor alterations in elderly Alzheimer caregivers under stress. *Psychosomatic Medicine, 59*, 251–256.

Mizutani, Y., Terachi, T., Okada, Y., & Yoshida, O. (1996). Effect of surgical stress on immune function in patients with urologic cancer. *International Journal of Urology, 3*, 426–434.

Monjan, A. A. (1981). Stress and immunologic competence: Studies in animals. In R. Ader (Ed.), *Psychoneuroimmunology* (pp. 185–228). New York: Academic Press.

Monroe, S. M., & Kelley, J. M. (1995). Measurement of stress apparaisal. In S. Cohen, R. C. Kessler, & L. U. Gordon (Eds.), *Measuring stress* (pp. 122–147). New York: Oxford Univ. Press.

Moynihan, J. A., & Ader, R. (1996). Psychoneuroimmunology, Animal models of disease. *Psychosomatic Medicine, 58*, 546–558.

Moynihan, J. A., Kruszeska, B., Brenner, G. J., & Cohen, N. (1998). Neural, endocrine, and immune system interactions. Relevance for health and disease. *Advances in Experimental Medicine and Biology, 438*, 541–549.

Mrazek, D. A., & Klinnert, M. (1991). Asthma, psychoneuroimmunologic considerations. In R. Ader, D. L. Felten, & N. Cohen (Eds.), *Psychoneuroimmunology* (pp. 1013–1035). New York: Academic Press.

Nakano, Y., Nakamura, S., Hirata, M., Harada, K., Ando, K., Tabuchi, T., Matunaga, I., & Oda, H. (1998). Immune function and lifestyle of taxi drivers in Japan. *Industrial Health, 36*, 32–39.

Naliboff, B. D., Bendon, D., Solomon, G. F., Morley, J. E., Fahey, J. L., Bloom, E. T., Makinodan, T., & Gilmore, S. L. (1991). Immunological changes in young and old adults during brief laboratory stress. *Psychosomatic Medicine, 53*, 121–132.

Naliboff, B. D., Solomon, G. F., Gilmore, S. L., Benton, D., Morley, J. E., & Fahey, J. L. (1995). The effects of the opiate antagonist naloxone on measures of cellular immunity during rest and brief psychological stressor. *Journal of Psychosomatic Research, 39*, 345–359.

Natelson, B. H., Zhou, X., Ottenweller, J. E., Bergen, M. T., Sisti, S. A., Drastal, S., Tapp, W. N., & Gause, W. L. (1996). Effects of acute exausting exercise on cytokine gene expression in men. *International Journal of Sports Medicine, 17*, 299–302.

Neveu, P. J., Delrue, C., Deleplanque, B., D'Amato, F. R., Puglisi-Allegra, S., & Cabib, S. (1994). Influence of brain and behavioral lateralization in brain. Monoaminergic, neuroendocrine and immune stress responses. *Annals of the New York Academy of Sciences, 741*, 271–283.

Newberry, B. H., Gordon, T. L., & Meehan, S. M. (1991). Recent animal studies of stress and cancer. In C. L. Cooper & N. Watson (Eds.), *Cancer and stress. Psychological, biological and coping studies* (pp. 27–46). New York: Wiley.

Nielsen, M., Thomson, J. L., Primdahl, S., Direborg, U., & Andersen J. A. (1987). Breast cancer and atypia among young and middle-aged women. A study of 110 medicolegal autopsies. *British Journal of Cancer, 56*, 814–819.

Nieman, D. C. (1998). Exercise and resistance to infection. *Canadian Journal of Physiology and Pharmacology, 76*, 573–580.

Nisipeanu, P., & Korczyn, A. D. (1995). Psychological stress and multiple sclerosis. In B. Leonard & K. Miller (Eds), *Stress, the immune system and psychiatry* (pp. 165–181). Chichester: Wiley.

Odio, M., Brosish, A., & Ricardo, M. J. (1987). Effects on immune responses by chronic stress are modulated by aging. *Brain, Behavior, and Immunity, 1*, 204–215.

Olff, M. (1999). Stress, depression and immunity, the role of dedenses and copyng styles. *Psychiatry Research, 18*, 7–15.

Osuka, K., Suzuki, Y., Saito, K., Takayasu, M., & Shibuya, M. (1996). Changes in serum cytokine concentrations after neurosurgical procedures. *Acta Neurochirurgica (Wien), 138*, 970–976.

Paget, J. (1870). *Surgical pathology*. London: Longman.

Palmblåd, J., Cantell, K., Strander, H., Froberg, J., Carlsson, C., Levi, L., Granström, M., & Unger, P. (1976). Stressors exposure and immunological response in man. Interferon producing capacity and phagocytosis. *Journal of Psychosomatic Research, 20*, 193–199.

Palmblåd, J., Petrini, B., Wassermann, B., & Åkerstedt, T. (1979). Lymphocyte and granulocyte reactions during sleep deprivation. *Psychosomatic Medicine, 41*, 273–278.

Pancheri, P. (Ed.) (1984). *Trattato di medicina psicosomatica*. Firenze: USES.

Pancheri, P., & Benaissa, C. (1976). Stress and psychosomatic illness. In C. D. Spielberger & I. G. Sarason (Eds.), *Stress and anxiety*, Washington: Hemisphere.

Pancheri, P., & Biondi, M. (1990). Biological and psychological correlates of anxiety, the role of psychoendocrine reactivity as a marker of the anxiety response. In N. Sartorius (Ed.), *Anxiety, Psychobiological and clinical perspectives* (pp. 101–113). Washington: Hemisphere.

Papez, J. W. (1937). A proposed mechanism of emotion. *Archives of Neurology and Psychiatry, 38*, 725–744.

Pellegrino, T. C., & Bayer, B. M. (1998). Modulation of immune cell function following fluoxetine administration in rats. *Pharmacology, Biochemistry, and Behavior, 59*, 151–157.

Pettingale, K. W., Philalithis, A., Tee, D. E. H., & Gree, H. 5. (1981). The biological correlates of psychological responses to breast cancer. *Psychosomatic Research, 25*, 453-458.

Parkes, C. M., Benjamin, B., & Fitzgerald, R. G. (1969). Broken heart: A statistical study of the mortality among widowers. *British Medical Journal, 1*, 740-743.

Pariante, C. M., Carpinello, B., Orrù, M. G., Sitzia, R., Piras, A., Farci, A. M., Del Giacco, G. S., Piludu, G., & Miller, A. H. (1997). Chronic caregiving stress alters peripheral blood immune parameters: The role of age and severity of stress. *Psychotherapy and Psychosomatics, 66*, 199–207.

Paykel, E. S. (1974). Life stress and psychiatric disorders, Applications of the clinical approach. In B. S. Dohrenwend, & B. P. Dohrenwend (Eds.), *Stressful life events—Their nature and effects*. (pp. 135–159). New York: Wiley.

Petrich, J., & Holmes, T. H. (1977). Life change and onset of illness. *Medical Clinics of North America, 61*, 825–838.

Pettingale, K. W., Greer, S., & Tee, D. E. H. (1977). Serum IgA and emotional expression in breast cancer patients. *Journal of Psychosomatic Research, 21*, 395–399.

Pike, J. L., Smith, T. L., Hauger, R. L., Nicassio, P. M., Patterson, T. L., McClintick, L., Costlow, C., & Irwin, M. R. (1997). Chronic life stress alters sympathetic, neuroendocrine and immune responsivity to an acute psychological stressor in human. *Psychosomatic Medicine, 59,* 447–457.

Potter, P. T., & Zautra, A. J. (1997). Stressful life event's effects on rheumatoid arthritis disease activity. *Journal of Consulting and Clinical Psychology, 65,* 319–323.

Rabkin, J. G., Wagner, G. J., & Rabkin, R. (1999). Fluoxetine treatment for depression in patients with HIV and AIDS: A randomized, placebo-controlled trial. *American Journal of Psychiatry, 156,* 101–107.

Rasmussen, A. F. Jr., Marsh, J. T., & Brill, N. Q. (1957). Increased susceptibility to herpes simplex in mice subjected to avoidance-learning stress or restraint. *Proceedings of the Society for Experimental Biology and Medicine, 96,* 183–189.

Redmond, H. P., Watson, R. W., Houghton, T., Condron, C., Watson, R. G., & Bouchier-Hayes, D. (1994). Immune function in patients undergoing open *vs* laparoscopic cholecystectomy. *Archives of Surgery, 129,* 1240–1246.

Reznick, J. S. (Ed.) (1994). *Perspectives on behavioral inhibition.* London: Univ. of Chicago Press.

Richardson, M. A., Post-White, J., Grimm, E. A., Moye, L. A., Singletary, S. E., & Justice, B. (1997). Coping, life attitudes, and immune responses to imagery and group support after breast cancer treatment. *Alternative Therapy and Health Medicine, 3,* 62–70.

Riley, V. (1975). Mouse mammary tumors: Alteration of incidence as apparent function of stress. *Science, 189,* 465–467.

Riley, V. (1981). Psychoneuroendocrine influences on immunocompetence and neoplasia. *Science, 212,* 1100–1109.

Roberts, F. D., Newcomb, P. A., Trentham-Dietz, A., & Storer, B. E. (1996). Self-reported stress and risk of breast cancer. *Cancer, 77,* 1089–1093.

Sarason, I. G., Johnson, J. H., & Siegel, J. M. (1978). Assessing the impact of life changes, Development of the Life Experience Survey. *Journal of Consulting and Clinical Psychology, 46,* 932–946.

Sauer, J., Polack, E., Wikinski, S., Holsboer, F., Stalla, G. K., & Arzt, E. (1995). The glucocorticoid sensitivity of lymphocyte changes according to the activity of the hypothalamic pituitary adrenocortical system. *Psychoneuroendocrinology, 20,* 269–280.

Schafer, M., Carter, L., & Stein, C. (1994). Interleukin 1beta and CRF inhibit pain by releasing opioids from immune cells in inflammation. *Proceedings of the National Academy of Sciences USA, 91,* 4219–4223.

Schedlowski, M., Tewrs, U., & Schmoll, H. J. (1994). The effects of psychological intervention on cortisol levels and leukocyte numbers in the peripheral blood of breast cancer patients. In C. E. Lewis, C. O'Sullivan, & J. Barraclough (Eds.), *The psychoimmunology of human cancer* (pp. 336–348). Oxford, UK: Oxford Univ. Press.

Schleifer, S. J., Keller, S. E., Camerino, M., Thornton, J. C., & Stein, M. (1983). Suppression of lymphocyte stimulation following bereavement. *Journal of the American Medical Association, 250,* 31–37.

Schmale, A., & Iker, H. (1996). The psychological setting of uterine cervical cancer. *Annals of the New York Academy of Sciences, 125,* 807–814.

Schmid, O. G., Jacobs, R., Jager, B., Wolf, J., Werfel, T., Kapp, A., Schurmeyer, T., Lamprecht, F., Schmidt, R. E., & Schedlowski, M. (1998). Stress-induced endocrine and immunological changes in psoriasis patients and healthy controls. A preliminary study. *Psychotherapy and Psychosomatics, 67,* 37–42.

Segerstrom, S. C., Glover, D. A., Craske, M. G., & Fahey, J. L. (1999a). Worry affects the immune response to phobic fear. *Brain, Behavior, and Immunity, 13,* 80–92.

Segerstrom, S. C., Solomon, G. F., Kemeny, M. E., & Fahey, J. L. (1998). Relationship of worry to immune sequelae of the Northridge earthquake. *Journal of Behavioral Medicine, 21,* 433–450.

Segerstrom, S. C., Taylor, S. E., Kemeny, M. E., & Fahey, J. L. (1999b). Optimism is associated with mood, coping and immune change in response to stress. *Journal of Personality and Social Psychology, 74,* 1646–1655.

Selye, H. (1936). A syndrome produced by diverse nocuous agents. *Nature, 138,* 32.

Selye, H. (1946). The general adaptation syndrome and the diseases of adaptation. *Journal of Clinical Endocrinology, 6,* 117–230.

Selye, H. (1950). *Stress.* Montreal: Acta.

Selye, H. (1976). *The stress of life,* 2nd ed. New York: McGraw-Hill.

Sgoutas-Emch, S. A., Cacioppo, J. T., Uchino, B. N., Malarkey W., Pearl, D., Kiecolt-Glaser J. K., & Glaser, R. (1994). The effects of an acute psychological stressor on cardiovascular, endocrine and cellular immune response, a prospective study of individuals high and low in heart rate reactivity. *Psychophysiology, 31,* 264, 271.

Shanahan, F. (1999). Brain-gut axis and mucosal immunity: A perspective on mucosal psychoneuroimmunology. *Seminars in Gastrointestinal Disease, 10,* 8–13.

Shibata, H., Fujiwara, R., Iwamoto, M., Matsuoka, H., & Yokohama, M. M. (1991). Immunological and behavioral effects of fragrance in mice. *International Journal of Neuroscience, 57,* 151–159.

Siegel, D., Sephton, S., Terr, A. I., & Stites, D. P. (1998). Effects of psychosocial treatment in prolonging cancer survival may be mediated by neuroimmune mechanisms. *Annals of the New York Academy of Sciences, 840,* 674–683.

Smedstad, L. M., Vaglum, P., Moum, T., & Kvien, T. K. (1997). The relationship between psychological distress and traditional clinical variables, a 2-year prospective study of 216 patients with early rheumatoid arthritis. *British Journal of Rheumatology, 36,* 1304–1311.

Snyder, B. K., Roghmann, K. J., & Sigal, L. H. (1983). Stress and psychosocial factors, effects on primary cellular immune response. *Journal of Behavioral Medicine, 16,* 143–161.

Solomon, G. F., Segerstrom, S. C., Grohr, P., Kemeny, M., & Fahey, J. (1997). Shaking up immunity, psychological and immunologic changes after a natural disaster. *Psychosomatic Medicine, 59,* 114–127.

Song, C., Kenis, G., van Gastel, A., Bosmans, E., Lin, A., de Jong, R., Neels, H., Scharpe, S., Janca, A., Yakusawa, K., & Maes, M. (1999). Influence of psychological stress on immune-inflammatory variables in normal humans. II. Altered serum concentrations of natural anti-inflammatory agents and soluble membrane antigens of monocytes and T lymphocytes. *Psychiatry Research, 85,* 293–303.

Souberbielle, B., & Dalgleish, A. (1994). Anti-tumour immune mechanisms. In C. E. Lewis, C. O'Sullivan, & J. Barraclough (Eds.), *The psychoimmunology of human cancer* (pp. 267–289). Oxford: Oxford Univ. Press.

Stein, M. (1986). A reconsideration of specificity in psychosomatic medicine: From olfaction to the lymphocyte. *Psychosomatic Medicine, 48,* 3–22.

Stein, M. (1995). The control of pain in peripheral tissue by opioids. *New England Journal of Medicine, 332,* 1685–1690.

Steptoe, A. (1983). Stress, helplessness and control, the implications of laboratory studies. *Journal of Psychosomatic Research, 27,* 361–367.

Stoll, B. A. (Ed.) (1979). *Mind and cancer prognosis.* New York: Wiley.

Stone, E. (1988). Stress and brain neurotransmitter receptors. In A. K. Sen, & T. Lee (Eds.), *Receptors and ligands in psychiatry.* Cambridge, U.K.: Cambridge Univ. Press.

Stone, A. A., Bovbjerg, D. H., Neale, J. M., Napoli, A., Valdimarsdottir, H., Cox, D., Hayden, F. G., & Gwaltney, J. M., Jr. (1992). Development of common cold symptoms following experimental rhinovirus infection is related to prior stressful life events. *Behavioral Medicine, 18,* 115–120.

Szczeklik, A., & Jawien, J. (1996). Immunoglobulin E in acute phase response to surgical stress. *Clinical and Experimental Allergy, 26,* 303–307.

Taché, Y., Monniknes, H., Bonaz, B., & Rivier, J. (1993). Role of CRF in stress-related alterations of gastric and colonic motor function. *Annals of the New York Academy of Sciences, 697,* 233–243.

Taché, J., & Selye, H. (1978). On stress and coping mechanisms. In C. D. Spielberger, & I. G. Sarason (Eds.), *Stress and anxiety* (pp. 3–23). Washington: Hemisphere.

Talamonti, F., & Biondi, M. (1997). Psicofarmaci e sistema immunitario. In M. Biondi (Ed.), *Mente, cervello e sistema immunitario* (pp. 291–364). Milano: McGraw-Hill Italia.

Tanabe, H. (1993). Study of effects of surgical stress on immunity in patients with gastrointestinal cancer. *Nippon Geka Hokan, 62,* 145–152.

Taylor, G. R., Neale, L. S., & Dardano, B. (1986). Immunological analyses of U.S. Space Shuttle crewmembers. *Aviation, Space and Environmental Medicine, 57,* 213–217.

Talamonti, F., & Biondi, M. (1997). Psicofarmaci e sistema immunitario. In M. Biondi (Ed.), *Mente, cervello e sistema immunitario* (pp. 291–362). Milano: McGraw-Hill Italia.

Thomas, P. D., Goodwin, J. M., & Goodwin, J. G. (1985). Effect of social support on stress-related changes in cholesterol level, uric acid level, and immune function in an elderly sample. *American Journal of Psychiatry, 162,* 735–737.

Tonnesen, E., Brinklov, M. M., Christensen, N. J., Olesen, A. S., & Madsen, T. (1987). Natural killer cell activity and lymphocyte function during and after coronary artery bypass grafting in relation to the endocrine stress response. *Anesthesiology, 68,* 526–533.

Totman, R., Kliff, J., Reed, S. E., & Craig, J. W. (1980). Predicting experimental colds in volunteers from different measures of recent life stress. *Journal of Psychosomatic Research, 24,* 155–163.

Turner Cobb, J. M., & Steptoe, A. (1998). Psychosocial influences on upper respiratory infectious illness in children. *Journal of Psychosomatic Research, 45,* 319–330.

Uchino, B. N., Cacioppo, J. T., & Kiecolt-Glaser, J. K. (1996). The relationship between social support and physiological processes: A review with emphasis on underlying mechanisms and implications for health. *Psychological Bulletin, 119,* 488–531.

Udelman, D. L. (1982). Stress and immunity. *Psychotherapy and Psychosomatics, 37,* 176–184.

Ursin, H., Baade, E., & Levine, S. (Eds.) (1987). *Psychobiology of stress. A study of the coping men.* New York: Academic Press.

Ursin, H., Schytte Blix, A., & Rosseland, S. (1987). Subjects and the methods used in the field phase of the experiment. In H. Ursin, E. Baade, & S. Levine (Eds.), *Psychobiology of stress. A study of coping men* (pp. 23–33). New York: Academic Press.

Vander Plate, C., Aral, S. O., & Magder, L. (1988). The relationship among genital herpes virus, stress, and social support. *Health Psychology, 7,* 159–168.

Van der Pompe, G., Antoni, M. H., Visser, A., & Hejinen, C. J. (1998). Effect of mild acute stress on immune cell distribution and natural killer cell activity in breast cancer patients. *Biological Psychology, 48,* 21–35.

Vedhara, K., Cox, N. K. M., Wilcock, G. K., Perks, P., Hunt, M., Anderson, S., Lightman, S., & Shanks, N. M. (1999). Chronic stress in elderly carers of dementia patients and antibody response to influenza vaccination. *The Lancet, 353,* 627–631.

Vedhara, K., & Nott, K. (1996). The assessment of the emotional and immunological consequences of examination stress. *Journal of Behavioral Medicine, 19,* 467–478.

Yehuda, R., Giller, E. L., Levengood, R. A., Southwick, S. M., & Siever, L. Y. (1995). Hypothalamic–pituitary–adrenal functioning in post-traumatic stress disorder. In M. J. Friedman, D. S. Charney, & A. Y. Deutch (Eds.), *Neurobiological and clinical consequences of stress* (pp. 351–365). Philadelphia: Lippincott-Raven.

Wang, X. W., & Harris, C. C. (1997). p53 tumor-suppressor gene, clues to molecular carcinogenesis. *Journal of Cell Physiology, 173,* 247–255.

Watson, M., & Ramirez, A. (1991). Psychological factors in cancer prognosis. In C. L. Cooper & N. Watson (Eds.), *Cancer and stress. Psychological, biological and coping studies* (pp. 47–72). New York: Wiley.

Weiner, H. (1977). *Psychobiology and human disease.* New York: Elsevier.

Weiner, H. (1991). Social and psychobiological factors in autoimmune disease. In R. Ader, D. L. Felten, & N. Cohen (Eds.), *Psychoneuroimmunology* (2nd ed., pp. 955–1005). New York: Academic Press.

Weiss, D. W., Hirt, R., Tarcic, N., Ben-Zur, H., Bresznitz, S., Glaser, B., Grover, N. B., Baras, M., & O'Dorisio, T. M. (1996). Studies in psychoneuroimmunology, psychological, immunological and neuroendocrinological parameters in Israeli civilians during and after a period of Scud missile attacks. *Behavioral Medicine, 22,* 5–14.

Wilson, S. N., van der Kolk, B., Burbridge, J. Fister, & Kradin, R. (1999). Phenotype of blood lymphocytes in PTSD suggests chronic immune activation. *Psychosomatics, 40,* 222–225.

Wolff, H. G., Wolf, S., & Hare, C. E. (1950). *Life stress and bodily disease.* Baltimore: Williams & Wilkins.

Wolff, C. T., Friedman, S. B., Hofer, M. A., & Mason, J. W. (1964). Relationship between psychological defenses and mean urinary 17-OHCS excretion rates. I. A predictive study of parents of fatally ill children. *Psychosomatic Medicine, 25,* 576–591.

Wyler, A. R., Masuda, M., & Holmes, T. H. (1971). Magnitude of life events and seriousness of illness. *Psychosomatic Medicine, 33,* 115–121.

Zachariae, R., Hansen, J. B., Andersen, M., Jinquan, T., Petersen, K. S., Simonsen, C., Zachariae, C., & Thestrup-Pedersen, K. (1994). Changes in cellular immune function after immune specific guided imagery and relaxation in high and low hypnotiable healthy subjects. *Psychotherapy and Psychosomatics, 61,* 74–92.

Zautra, A. J., Hoffman, J., Potter, P., Matt, K. S., Yocum, D., & Castro, L. (1997). Examination of changes in interpersonal stress as a factor in disease exacerbations among women with rheumatoid arthritis. *Annals of Behavioral Medicine, 19,* 279–286.

Zavala, F. (1997). Benzodiazepines, anxiety and immunity. *Pharmacology and Therapeutics, 75,* 199–216.

Zorrilla, E. P., Redei, E., & DeRubeis, R. J. (1994). Reduced cytokine levels and T-cell function in healthy males, relation to individual differences in subclinical anxiety. *Brain, Behavior, and Immunity, 8,* 293–312.

CHAPTER

# 40

# Mechanisms of Stress-Induced Modulation of Immunity in Animals

JAN A. MOYNIHAN, SUZANNE Y. STEVENS

## I. INTRODUCTION

The purpose of this chapter is to highlight advances that have been made in understanding the mechanisms underlying stress-induced modulation of immune function. To accomplish this task—if this is really at all possible—will require examination of the topic from both the neuroendocrine and immunological perspectives. That is, we will consider what is noteworthy with respect to stress-induced changes in neurocircuitries and neuroendocrinology that have known or inferred consequences for a variety of immune effector functions. Documentation that stressors can alter pathophysiological processes dates back well over 100 years (reviewed by Biondi & Zannino, 1997; Chrousos, 1998) and since that time, it has been clearly established that stress-induced changes in disease progression may (and in other cases may not) be mediated via altered immune function. There are certainly scores of original articles and reviews that discuss this ever-growing body of literature; however, it is the intention of this chapter to highlight relevant examples from the literature that attempt to determine mechanisms of stress-induced changes in immunity.

Paramount to the discussion of mechanisms of stress-induced changes in immune function is the definition of what is stressful. For the present purposes, a stressor is defined as a stimulus that causes an organism to deviate from baseline functioning or homeostasis. The stress response is an adaptive response that redirects energy to appropriate sites to maintain survival in the face of a challenge, as in the fight-or-flight response of Cannon (Cannon, 1932). A stressor will evoke behavioral and physiological responses from an organism in the organism's attempt to survive, and then to regain equilibrium (Selye, 1950). Decades of research provide evidence that stressors evoke central nervous system (CNS) responses that are principally mediated via the hypothalamo-pituitary-adrenal (HPA) axis and the highly interconnected autonomic, i.e., sympathetic and parasympathetic, nervous system.

The CNS constantly receives and integrates neurosensory signals and signals from the blood. As elegantly reviewed by Chrousos (Chrousos & Gold, 1992; Webster, Elenkov, & Chrousos, 1997; Chrousos, 1995, 1998), Dunn (Dunn, 1995), and others (Berczi, 1998; Biondi & Zannino, 1997; Sternberg, 1998; McEwen, 1998), these signals are ultimately received in the paraventricular nucleus (PVN) of the hypothalamus, as well as the locus ceruleus-noradrenergic center. In response to stressors, the hypothalamus secretes corticotropin-releasing hormone (CRH) and arginine vasopressin (AVP). From the PVN, CRH-containing neurons have efferent pathways to the median eminence and also projections to noradrenergic centers in the brain stem and spinal cord. CRH release further activates the HPA axis, leading to release of peptides from the pituitary produced by the differential cleavage of pro-opiomelanocortin (POMC), most notably adrenocorticotropic hormone (ACTH) and $\beta$-endorphin (Chrousos, 1992; Chrousos & Gold, 1992). ACTH induces downstream release of glucocorticoids from the adrenal cortex. CRH and noradrenergic neurons in the CNS innervate and stimulate each other. Activation of the noradrenergic pathways by CRH results in secretion of norepinephrine (NE) by the peripheral sympathetic nervous system and release of NE and epinephrine (EPI) from the adrenal medulla.

A wide variety of immunomodulatory hormones/transmitters can be enhanced or suppressed by stressful stimuli and these have all been shown to be immunomodulatory. Currently, this list includes glucocorticoids, opioids, catecholamines, acetylcholine, CRH, benzodiazepines, sex hormones, ACTH, growth horm, prolactin, vasoactive intestinal peptide, somatostatin, substance P, thyroid hormones, melatonin, vasopressin, oxytocin, and thymic hormones (reviewed by Khansari, Murgo, & Faith, 1990). The majority of the research to date describing stress-induced changes in immune function is focused, however, on four major stress hormones/transmitter systems: catecholamines, CRH, opioids, and glucocorticoids (cortisol in humans and corticosterone in rodents). To a large extent, this chapter will focus on the immunological consequences of changes in these four mediators.

It should be noted that for a number of years, it was thought that glucocorticoids were the most important of the stress hormones, mediating the majority of the reported changes in immune function. Although increased corticosteroid levels have been associated with altered immune function in many reports (e.g., Blecha, Kelley, & Satterlee, 1982; Coe, Rosenberg, Fisher, & Levine, 1987; Dobbs, Feng, Beck, & Sheridan, 1996; Okimura, Ogawa, Yamauchi, & Sasaki, 1986), it is also very clearly the case that stress-induced changes in immune function can occur in adrenalectomized or hypophysectomized animals (Blecha et al., 1982; Esterling & Rabin, 1987; Keller, Weiss, Schleifer, Miller, & Stein, 1983; Rabin, Cunnick, & Lysle, 1990; Scott, 1993a) and that altered immunity can be documented in cases where there is no detectable stress-induced increase in glucocorticoids (Jessop, Gale, & Bayer, 1987; Moynihan, Koota, Brenner, Cohen, & Ader, 1989). Further, stress-induced elevations in glucocorticoids can occur in the absence of detectable changes in immune function (Flores, Hernandez, Hargreaves, & Bayer, 1990; Mormede, Dantzer, Michaud, Kelley, & LeMoal, 1988). Thus, investigators have been forced to look elsewhere for, and have been unable to define, the "magic" stress hormone that is so detrimental to immunity. At this point, it seems very likely that the effects of stress on immune function are due to *interactions* among numerous hormones/transmitters, perhaps each with immunomodulatory potential.

Indeed, it is clear from reviewing hundreds of papers on stress and immune function that the response of an organism to a stressor will depend on a variety of factors, including the chronicity of the stressor; the nature and intensity of the stressor; the species, strain, and sex of the animal; the life history of the animal; the timing of the stressor in relation to the immune response; and the immune parameter or effector function(s) examined. In particular, it is very often the case that following stressor administration, lymphocyte responses may differ depending upon the site being examined—peripheral blood versus spleen, for example (Lysle, Lyte, Fowler, & Rabin, 1987). In addition, studies documenting stress-induced changes in immunity have examined both cell-mediated immunity (mediated by T lymphocytes) and humoral immunity (mediated by B lymphocyte secretion of soluble antibody), both antigen-specific responses. As many studies have investigated innate, nonspecific effector functions mediated by natural killer (NK) cells and monocyte/macrophages. Also, much of the literature has focused on the role of leukocyte-derived cytokines, soluble proteins that are pivotal for inducing the growth, differentiation, and function of both antigen-specific and nonspecific effector cells.

## II. THE MECHANISMS OF ACTION OF STRESSORS ON T HELPER CELL RESPONSES

The elucidation of two types of mature T helper (Th) cells has provided some new insight into how it is that immune effector functions are not necessarily all affected by stressors in either the same direction or the same magnitude. T lymphocytes express either the cell surface antigen CD8 (a marker for cytotoxic T cells) or CD4 (which delineates Th cells). Th1 and Th2, found in rodents and humans, are defined by the cytokines they produce following antigenic stimulation (Adorini, Guery, & Trembleau, 1996; Cacopardo et al., 1996; Chehimi et al., 1996; Crucian, Dunne, Friedman, Ragsdale, Pross, & Widen, 1996; D'Elios et al., 1997; Gorham et al., 1996; Hussell, Spender, Georgiou, O'Garra, & Openshaw, 1996; Lamont & Adorini, 1996; Lord & Lamb, 1996; Nuemann, Gitgesell, Fliegert, Bonifer, & Herrmann, 1996; Nichoolson & Kuchroo, 1996; Paul & Seder, 1994; Pawelec, Rehbein, Schlotz, Friccius, & Pohla, 1996; Powrie & Coffman, 1993; Romagnani, 1996; Romagnani, 1997; Scott, 1993a,b). Differentia-tion into distinct Th1 or Th2 cells appears to be a property of mature effector T cells. Th1 cells typically produce interleukin (IL)-2, tumor necrosis factor (TNF)-$\beta$, and interferon (IFN)-$\gamma$, which are important cytokines for the generation of cell-mediated immunity. Th2 cells produce IL-4, IL-5, IL-6, IL-9, IL-10, and IL-13, and these cytokines promote humoral immune responses. Both types of cell produce TNF-$\alpha$, IL-3, and granulocyte/monocyte-colony stimulating factor (GM-CSF). Production of these cytokines is, however, not limited to Th1 and Th2 cells—although investigators often refer to a Th1-dominant state (without actually measuring cytokines produced by purified CD4+ T cells). In addition to Th1 and Th2 cells, there are uncommitted or non-polarized Th0 cells that secrete cytokines of both types which may be either undifferentiated precursor cells or a separate population of differentiated T cells

(reviewed by O'Garra & Murphy, 1996; Romagnani, 1997). Thus, the Th1 and Th2 cytokines are perhaps more correctly referred to as type 1 and type 2 cytokines, respectively.

Preferential skewing toward a Th1- or a Th2-dominant response is important for the generation of an adaptive immune response. Th1 responses are often critical for viral clearance, whereas Th2 cells are important for immune responses to parasites in mice and in humans (Cacopardo et al., 1996; Chehimi et al., 1996; Hussell et al., 1996; Moran, Isobe, Fernandez-Sesma, & Schulman, 1996; O'Garra & Murphy, 1996; Pawelec et al., 1996; Romagnani, 1996; Romagnani, 1997; Sharma, Ramsay, Maguire, Rolph, & Ramshaw, 1996). In addition, dominant Th1 versus Th2 responses play a role in autoimmune disease in humans (Adorini et al., 1996; Chen et al., 1996; Crucian et al., 1996; de Vries & Yssel, 1996; Kallman et al., 1997; Lord & Lamb, 1996; Romagnani, 1997). The balance or ratio of production of Th1-derived versus Th2-derived cytokines is important for the generation of an adaptive immune response to antigens (including parasites and a number of viruses). Antigen concentration and route of inoculation (Bretscher, Wei, Menjon, & Bielefeldt-Ohmann, 1994; Golding, Zaitseva, & Golding, 1994; Guery, Galbiati, Smiroldo, & Adorini, 1996; Hosken, Shibuya, Heath, Murphy, & O'Garra, 1995; Paul & Seder, 1994; Scott, 1993a), as well as host factors such as the strain of the experimental subject (Belosevic, Finbloom, van der Meade, Slayter, & Nacy, 1989; Bretscher et al., 1994; Heinzel, Sadick, Holaday, Coffman, & Locksley, 1989; Sadick, Heinzel, Holaday, Pu, Dawkins, & Locksley, 1990), influence production of Th1 versus Th2 cytokines.

Th1 and Th2 cells can be cross-inhibitory. IFN-$\gamma$ can directly suppress the synthesis of Th2-derived cytokines (Paul & Seder, 1994; O'Garra & Murphy, 1996; Scott, 1993a, b). Suppression by Th2 cells of Th1-derived IFN-$\gamma$ production appears to be more complicated, occurring via IL-10-induced suppression of IL-12 synthesis by monocyte/macrophages and B cells (Hsieh et al., 1993; Scott, 1993b; Trinchieri, 1993). IL-12 is a key cytokine for cellular immune regulation (Lamont & Adorini, 1996), is required for optimal production of IFN-$\gamma$ (Hsieh et al., 1993; Paul & Seder, 1994; Scott, 1993b; Trinchieri, 1993), and may be the basis for the observed dominance of Th1- derived versus Th2-derived cytokines by different mouse strains (Guler et al., 1996; Noben-Trauth & Muller, 1996). Thus, there is an established cytokine network that biases the overall immune effector functions activated following antigen stimulation.

## III. STRESSOR-INDUCED CHANGES IN TH1/TH2 CYTOKINE PRODUCTION

Another factor that can alter the balance between Th1 and Th2 cell function or cytokine production is stressor administration. Olfactory cues have been shown by our laboratory (Cocke, Moynihan, Cohen, Grota, & Ader, 1993; Moynihan, Karp, Cohen, & Cocke, 1994) and others (Matthes, 1963; Rogers et al., 1980; Shibata, Fujiwara, Iwamoto, Matsuoka, & Yokoyama, 1990; Zalcman, Kerr, & Anisman, 1991) to alter immune function. We have determined that exposure to the odors produced by stressed BALB/c mice results in a highly significant elevation of keyhole limpet hemocyanin (KLH)-specific production of the Th2 cytokine IL-4 in vitro following immunization with KLH in vivo, with no change in production of IL-2 or IFN-$\gamma$ (Moynihan et al., 1994). Interestingly, this increase in IL-4 production is associated with an increase in serum IgM and IgG anti-KLH antibody titers. This pheromone-induced change in Th2 cell activity may have a genetic component to it, since these changes were not observed in C57Bl/6 mice.

Fleshner and colleagues have also observed effects of stressors on one type of Th cell but not necessarily on the other. Using an inescapable tail shock paradigm, they observed that shocked rats failed to expand Th1-like cells following immunization with KLH. These rats also produced less serum IgM and IgG anti-KLH antibody. The suppression of IgG appeared to be due to decreased production of Th1 cell-driven IgG2a; no decrease in Th2 cell-driven IgG1 was observed (Fleshner, Brennan, Nguyen, Watkins, & Maier, 1996). In addition, lymphocytes from rats subjected to inescapable tail shock produced less IFN-$\gamma$ following stimulation with the T cell mitogen concanavalin A (Con A). Support for stress-induced depression of Th1 cell responses, with no change in Th2 cell responses, comes from the laboratory of Iwakabe and his colleagues (Iwakabe et al., 1998). These investigators observed that BALB/c or C57Bl/6 splenic natural killer (NK) cell cytotoxicity and mitogen-induced production of IFN-$\gamma$, but not IL-4, were suppressed in mice restrained for 10–24 h. In contrast, however, Dobbs and colleagues (Dobbs et al., 1996) observed that 16 h of restraint administered for a total of 7 days (1 day preinfection and 6 days postinfection) significantly diminished both the Th1 (IL-2 and IFN-$\gamma$)- and the Th2-derived (IL-10) cytokine responses following infection of C57Bl/6 mice with influenza virus. It is easy to reconcile the differences reported in cytokines observed following restraint in these two studies since Iwakabe and

colleagues (Iwakabe et al., 1998) did not immunize their experimental mice, but examined responses in resting spleen cell populations, whereas Dobbs (Dobbs et al., 1996) examined the effects of restraint in virus-infected mice. Probably more important, however, the Iwakabe study examined the effects of a single restraint session, whereas Dobbs and his associates used multiple restraint sessions.

Taken altogether, these data suggest that some of the observed differential effects of stressors on immune parameters might be due to differential neuroendocrine responses that trigger changes in only one, but not necessarily both, types of Th cells. This differential triggering, which may interact with the activational state of lymphocytes, might have downstream consequences on some, but not all, effector functions. In our pheromone model, Th2 responses appear to be preferentially upregulated, with either concomitant downregulation (Cocke et al., 1993) or no change (Moynihan et al., 1994) in Th1 responses, whereas others have observed decreases in only Th1-derived cytokines (Fleshner et al., 1995b, 1996; Maier, 1995b; Fleshner, Nguyen, Cotter, Watkins, & Maier, 1998; Iwakabe et al., 1998) or decreases in both Th1 and Th2 cytokine production (Dobbs et al., 1996).

The production of Th1- and Th2-derived cytokines can be dramatically altered by the classic stress hormones glucocorticoids administered either in vivo or in vitro. Glucocorticoids can alter cytokine production in a number of ways: inducing apoptosis in lymphocytes (Gonzalo, Gonzalez-Garcia, Martinez, & Kroemer, 1993; Penninger & Mak, 1994; Schwartzman & Cidlowski, 1994), indirectly inactivating NF-$\kappa$B response elements that are cytokine promoters (Scheinman, Cogswell, Lofquist, & Baldwin, 1995), suppressing transcription of the IL-2 gene (Northrup, Crabtree, & Mattial, 1992; Vacca et al., 1992), and downregulating major histocompatibility complex (MHC) class II expression (Celada, McKercher, & Maki, 1993). The work of Daynes and Araneo and their colleagues (Daynes & Araneo, 1989, 1992; Daynes, Dudley, & Araneo, 1990) suggests that glucocorticoids suppress IL-2 and IFN-$\gamma$ production, whereas IL-4 production is enhanced due to relief from the cross-inhibitory effects of IFN-$\gamma$. These findings are somewhat controversial; Ramirez (Ramirez, Fowell, Puklavec, Simmonds, & Mason, 1996) has published data in support of Daynes and his colleagues, and other investigators have shown that the synthetic glucocorticoid dexamethasone (DEX) or corticosterone suppresses both Th1 and Th2 cytokine production in vitro in a dose-dependent fashion (Dobbs et al., 1996; Moynihan, Callahan, Kelley, &

Campbell, 1998; Wu, Fargeas, Nakajima, & Delepesse, 1991). Further, Elenkov (Elenkov, Papanicolaou, Wilder, & Chrousos, 1996) observed that incubation of human whole blood with DEX suppressed lipopolysaccharide (LPS)-induced production of IL-12, but did not affect production of the Th2-like cytokine IL-10.

Elevated levels of glucocorticoids were observed in rats subjected to inescapable tail shock (Fleshner et al., 1995a), and acute administration of the type II glucocorticoid receptor antagonist RU486 blocked the shock-induced suppression of IgM, IgG, and IgG2a (Fleshner et al., 1996). Of interest is the observation that injection of corticosterone at a dose that mimicked shock-induced levels did not suppress antibody responses. These data suggest that there is an interaction between glucocorticoids and some other hormone(s) increased during stress. In support of the hypothesis that glucocorticoids are permissive for, but not sufficient by themselves to induce the changes in immune responses, we (Moynihan et al., 1994) determined that, although RU486 administration abrogated the stress odor-induced increase in IL-4 production (but not the increase in antibody titer), glucocorticoids were not significantly increased by pheromone exposure (unpublished data). Thus, we hypothesize that endogenous levels of these steroids are interacting with other hormones or transmitters produced in response to stress pheromones. In contrast to our findings, elevated corticosterone levels were observed in influenza virus-infected and re-strained mice (Dobbs et al., 1996; Iwakabe et al., 1998), and RU486 administration ameliorated the suppression of Th1 and Th2 cytokines in the study by Dobbs and colleagues (Dobbs et al., 1996). In addition, incubation of lymphocytes in vitro with corticosterone and influenza virus mimicked the in vivo response to stress; i.e., Th1 and Th2-derived cytokine production was suppressed in a dose-dependent fashion.

Taken together, it is clear that glucocorticoids alter production of cytokines by Th cells, and that steroids may exert their effects on or both types of Th cells. It would also appear to be the case that other neuro-modulators may also be involved in regulation of cytokines following stressor administration; the nature and mechanisms of these additional mediators remains elusive.

## IV. EFFECTS OF CATECHOLAMINES AND OTHER NEUROPEPTIDES ON TH1/TH2 CYTOKINE PRODUCTION

The role of catecholamines in the phenomenon of stress-induced changes in Th1 and Th2 cell activity is still relatively unexplored, but there is good reason for speculating that there is an important contribution of these neurotransmitters. An extensive literature documents the expression of adrenergic receptors on surfaces of lymphoid cells (reviewed by Sanders, 1995); more importantly, Sanders and her associates (Ramer-Quinn, Baker, & Sanders, 1997; Sanders, Baker, Ramer-Quinn, Kasprowicz, Fuchs, & Street, 1997) have documented that murine Th1 clones, but not Th2 clones, express $\beta_2$-adrenergic receptors. Incubation of clones with $\beta_2$-adrenergic receptor agonists induces an increase in cAMP in Th1, but not Th2 cells. These investigators (Ramer-Quinn et al., 1997) also determined that incubation of resting Th1 cell clones with the $\beta$-adrenergic receptor agonist terbutaline resulted in suppression of IFN-$\gamma$ production, and IgG2a antibody production by cocultured B cells. In contrast, when T-cell clones were activated by anti-CD3 antibody prior to incubation with terbutaline, production of IL-2, but not IFN-$\gamma$, was suppressed (Sanders et al., 1997). These effects were prevented by the addition of $\beta$-adrenergic receptor antagonists.

In the in vitro study of Elenkov and colleagues (Elenkov et al., 1996) physiological concentrations of NE or EPI suppressed LPS-induced production of IL-12 (an inducer of Th1-derived cytokines), and enhanced production of the Th2-derived cytokine IL-10 by human whole blood cells, illustrating the cross-inhibitory nature of these cell types. These authors speculated that catecholamines released during a stress response would alter the balance of production of the Th1 and Th2 cytokines, increasing an individual's risk for viral infection or tumor growth.

In addition to catecholamines, various neuropeptides that are often induced by a variety of stressors have been shown to modify the secretion of Th1 and Th2 cell-derived cytokines. For example, somatostatin, calcitonin gene-related peptide, substance P, and neuropeptide Y all exert effects on murine Th1 and Th2 cytokine production and may even, in fact, drive T cell clones to produce cytokines of the "forbidden" phenotype, i.e., secretion of Th2 cytokines from a Th1 clone (Levite, 1998).

The production of IL-2, IFN-$\gamma$, IL-12, IL-10, and IL-4 can be regulated by neurohormones/transmitters, including glucocorticoids and catecholamines, during a stress response. Not only does this occur in vivo in stressed rodents, but also in humans, as illustrated by a recent paper by Decker and colleagues (Decker, Schondorf, Bidlingmaier, Hirner, & vonRuecker, 1996). In this paper, the authors document a decrease in IFN-$\gamma$ production and an increase in IL-4 production by peripheral blood mononuclear cells (PBMC) from patients undergoing an invasive surgical procedure. In contrast, however, Maes and associates (Maes et al., 1998) observed that PBMC from medical students with high anxiety levels while undergoing examination stress produced more IFN-$\gamma$ and less IL-10 following stimulation with phytohemagglutinin (PHA) and LPS. This suggests that in some situations, stress induces a Th1-like response, which may be considered to be an adaptive stress response.

## V. CONSEQUENCES OF STRESSOR-INDUCED TH1/TH2 CYTOKINE CHANGES FOR IMMUNE EFFECTOR FUNCTION AND DISEASE: ROLE OF THE HPA AXIS

In a recent review by Webster et al. (Webster et al., 1997), it is noted that cases in which the HPA axis is hyperactive, such as Cushing's disease or the third trimester of pregnancy, are associated with suppressed resistance to infectious disease, suggesting a diminished Th1 response. A shift from the Th1 to the Th2 state has been documented in pregnant female rodents and humans (Lin et al., 1993; Robertson, Seamark, Guilbert, & Wegmann, 1994; Wegmann, Lin, Guilbert, & Mosmann, 1993). In contrast, hypoactivity of the HPA axis is associated with an increased resistance to infection, suggesting a shift in favor of Th1 responses. In addition to infection and tumorigenesis, HPA axis activity is correlated with risk for development of autoimmune diseases that are cell-mediated (Webster et al., 1997).

### A. Infectious Disease

The effects of restraint stress on infectious disease in mice have been evaluated using a number of different agents, including influenza virus, herpes simplex virus-type 1 (HSV), and *Mycobacterium avium*. These studies, along with others, have been important for establishing that the effects of stress on pathogenesis can often be mediated by suppression of immune responses, and for determining some of the HPA axis pathways that are involved.

### 1. Influenza

As discussed above, restraint stress can inhibit production of both Th1 and Th2 cytokines in influenza-infected C57Bl/6 mice (Dobbs et al., 1996), and this response appears to be mediated by glucocorticoids. Restraint for 16 h/day beginning 1 day before and 7 days after intranasal infection

with the PR8 strain of influenza resulted in decreased pulmonary inflammation compared to controls (Hermann, Beck, & Sheridan, 1995; Sheridan, Dobbs, Brown, & Zwilling, 1994; Sheridan, Feng, Bonneau, Allen, Huneycutt, & Glaser, 1991). No effect of restraint stress on the magnitude of the anti-influenza antibody response was observed; however, the kinetics of the antibody response lagged in restrained animals (Feng et al., 1991; Hermann et al., 1995).

In another study, these investigators examined the strain dependence of the response to restraint in C57Bl/6, DBA/2, and C3H/HeN male mice infected intranasally with the LD$_{50}$ of the PR8 strain of influenza (Dobbs et al., 1996). Experimental mice were restrained for 12 h/day for 1 day before and 10 days after infection. Increased corticosterone levels were observed in all three strains of mice on day 10 postinfection. DBA/2 mice had higher corticosteronelevels than the other two strains. Restraint resulted in decreased survival only in the DBA/2 strain and was not associated with changes in virus titer in lung tissue or with pulmonary inflammation on day 10 in any of the strains of mice. However, restraint did suppress virus-specific IL-2 production in all three strains on day 10 postinfection; again, the magnitude of the anti-influenza antibody response was unaffected by restraint. These studies highlight the role of genetic factors in determining the effects of stressful life experiences on pathophysiologic processes and the value of examining strain differences in behavioral and neurochemical responses to stressful experiences when attempting to understand the possible immunological mediation of such effects.

### 2. Herpes Simplex Virus

Sheridan and his colleagues have also used restraint to study neural influences on the immune response to herpes simplex virus (HSV)-type 1 infection (Bonneau, Sheridan, Feng, & Glaser, 1991b; Bonneau, Sheridan, Feng, & Glaser, 1993; Kusnecov et al., 1992). Restraint was observed to result in reduced anti-HSV cytotoxic T lymphocyte (CTL) responses in C57Bl/6 male mice, suppressed NK cell activity, reduced popliteal lymph node cellularity, suppressed activation of CTL memory cells, and increased infectious virus at the site of infection (Bonneau et al., 1991b).

These same investigators have determined that both catecholamines and corticosterone play a role in the suppressed anti-HSV responses (Bonneau et al., 1993). The nonselective $\beta$-adrenergic receptor antagonist nadolol did not restore the suppression in lymph node cell number in restrained mice, but partially restored CTL activation in lymph nodes from restrained mice, suggesting a role for catecholamines in the restraint-induced suppression. The glucocorticoid receptor antagonist RU486 abrogated the restraint stress-induced suppression of lymph node cellularity, but not the suppression of the CTL response. Combined β-adrenergic receptor and glucocorticoid receptor blockade fully restored both the lymph node cell numbers and the CTL activity of popliteal lymph node cells. These data clearly indicate that both catecholamines and corticosterone play a role in regulating the cell-mediated immune response to HSV.

Studies of stress and HSV infection are of interest in that they provide a potential model for examining the role of stress, HPA axis activation, and sympathetic outflow on virus reactivation. Although stress has long been thought to be a factor in reactivation of latent HSV in humans, until recently there has been no good experimental basis for this belief. Recently, however, Padgett, and colleagues (Padgett et al., 1998b) and Noisakran, Halford, Veress, and Carr (1998) have demonstrated stressor-induced reactivation of HSV in murine models. Interestingly, Padgett and colleagues demonstrated reactivation of latent virus in 40% of mice using disruption of social hierarchy as the stressor, which was associated with increased corticosterone levels. Restraint stress, which also results in HPA axis activation as described above, was not associated with reactivation.

Noisakran and colleagues (Noisakran et al., 1998) utilized a hyperthermia model to examine HSV reactivation in latently infected (greater than 30 days after primary infection) CD-1 mice. This model requires mice to be restrained during a 10-min period of immersion to neck level in a 43°C water bath. Trigeminal ganglia (TG) were removed 0–24 h following stressor. Approximately 29% of mice subjected to hyperthermic stress had evidence of reactivation as measured by infectious virus in the TG. This was accompanied by a time-dependent increase in IL-6 mRNA, but not IL-1 mRNA, and a decrease in CD8 transcript. A significant decrease in CD8+ T cells, MAC-3+ macrophages, and DX5+ NK cells in the TG was also observed. It was not clear what the source of the IL-6 mRNA was from dendritic cells, macrophages, Schwann cells, or neurons. Finally, the reactivation of HSV appeared to be abrogated in a dose-dependent fashion by prestress treatment of mice with the corticosterone synthesis inhibitor cyanoketone. Activation of the HPA axis, therefore, plays a permissive role in reactivation of latent HSV; however, dexamethasone by itself did not appear to be sufficient to induce reactivation.

### 3. Mycobacterium

Resistant and susceptible congenic strains of BALB/c mice were restrained for 18 h/day for 1, 5, or 10 days and a significant increase in mycobacterial growth was detected in both the spleen and the lungs of BALB/c.Bcg[s] (disease sensitive) male mice, but not in the organs of congenic BALB/c.Bcg[r] (disease resistant) mice (Brown, Sheridan, Pearl, & Zwilling, 1993). Even a single session of restraint resulted in suppressed class II MHC expression by macrophages from sensitive, but not resistant, mice (Zwilling et al., 1990). Splenic macrophages (which ingest mycobacterium during infection) obtained from restrained sensitive mice were less protective against the in vitro growth of *M. avium*. The effects of restraint on mycobacterium growth were abrogated by adrenalectomy; replacement of basal concentrations of *d*-aldosterone and epinephrine, plus high levels of corticosterone, partially restored the increase in mycobacterial growth. Daily administration of the glucocorticoid receptor antagonist RU486, beginning 2 days prior to restraint, fully abrogated the effects of restraint on mycobacterium growth (Brown et al., 1993). Thus, it is clear that stressful life experiences, mediated at least in part by corticosterone, can contribute to the growth of mycobacterium in sensitive hosts.

## B. Experimental Allergic Encephalomyelitis

Experimental autoimmune encephalomyelitis (EAE) is a demyelinating, paralytic disease induced in mice and rats that is a useful model for a relapse of multiple sclerosis (MS) (Bukilica, Djordjevic, Maric, Dimitrijevic, Markovic, & Jankovic, 1991; Griffin, Lo, Wolny, & Whitacre, 1993; Jankovic & Maric, 1987; Khoury, Hancock, & Weiner, 1992; Kuroda, Mori, & Hori, 1994; Levine & Saltzman, 1987; Levine, Strebel, Wenk, & Harman, 1962; Liblau, Singer, & McDevitt, 1995; MacPhee, Day, & Mason, 1992; Mason, 1992; Mason, MacPhee, & Antoni, 1992; McCombe, deJersey, & Pender, 1992; Munck & Guyre, 1991; Powrie & Coffman, 1993). Approximately 10–12 days following injection of adjuvants and myelin basic protein (MBP), emulsified guinea pig spinal cord, or the relevant MBP peptide, susceptible rats develop a progressive ascending, but transient, paralysis (McCombe et al., 1992). EAE is an autoimmune, CNS inflammatory response, and can be conferred by adoptive transfer of MBP-specific CD4+ T cells alone (Levine & Saltzman, 1987).

It was established over 30 years ago by Levine and associates (Levine et al., 1962) and then others

(Griffin et al., 1993; Kuroda et al., 1994) that multiple, prolonged sessions of physical restraint administered prior to, and following, the induction of EAE decreased the incidence and clinical severity of disease in male and female rats. Further, restraint could prevent relapses of disease that had been observed in female Lewis rats (Levine & Saltzman, 1987). Daily sessions of electric shock also decreased the incidence and severity of histological lesions in EAE-susceptible DA rats when shock was administered after, but not before, injection of guinea pig spinal cord (Bukilica et al., 1991). These studies did not include immunological outcomes. Supporting data (Bukilica et al., 1991; Griffin et al., 1993; Kuroda et al., 1994; McCombe et al., 1992) suggested that stressful experiences affect the outcome of EAE in susceptible strains of rats via direct effects on the immune system.

The HPA axis plays a major role in EAE, and the effects of stress on disease severity appear to be partly mediated by glucocorticoids. Much of the work on EAE has been done in Lewis rats, which have a decreased HPA axis and sympathetic nervous system response to stress, resulting in decreased output of corticosterone and catecholamines (Sternberg et al., 1989). Lewis rats with symptoms of EAE had elevated serum corticosterone levels, recovery from disease began when corticosterone levels were at their peak (Sternberg et al., 1989; Sternberg et al., 1992), and adrenalectomy inhibited spontaneous recovery from EAE. In addition, exogenous glucocorticoid administration was associated with decreases in clinical severity of the disease. EAE-resistant PVG rats developed EAE following adrenalectomy (Mason et al., 1992). The opioid methionine-enkephalin given in a high concentration also inhibited clinical symptoms of EAE and reduced histological lesions; however, a low dose of the same compound yielded the opposite effect (Jankovic & Maric, 1987, 1994). It is not clear from these studies, however, whether glucocorticoids and opioids were influencing the development of disease via direct or indirect effects on the immune system. Despite the potential role of decreased HPA axis activity in development of EAE in Lewis rats, however, it does not appear to be the case that MS patients differ from controls in terms of baseline or acute stress-induced elevations in autonomic and cortisol response, or peripheral blood immunological parameters (Ackerman, Martino, Heyman, Moyna, & Rabin, 1996).

EAE is a cell-mediated disease. MBP-specific Th1 cells induce EAE, but Th2 cells specific for the same peptide–MHC complexes do not (Liblau et al., 1995). During the peak of the disease, the Th1 cytokines IL-2, IFN-$\gamma$, and tumor necrosis factor (TNF)-$\alpha$ are upre-

gulated in CNS tissues; IL-4 and IL-10 are absent (Khoury et al., 1992). Conversely, recovery is associated with dominant expression of IL-10 messenger RNA (mRNA) and IFN-$\gamma$ mRNA is absent (Kennedy, Torrance, Picha, & Mohler, 1992). Rats can be made tolerant to MBP and, in the CNS, these tolerant rats show high expression of IL-4, but not IL-2 or IFN-$\gamma$ (Levine & Saltzman, 1987). In addition, spontaneous recovery from the disease is associated with production of MBP-specific antibody, a Th2-driven effector function (MacPhee et al., 1992). Development of antibody is inversely correlated with severity of EAE; indeed, serum from rats recovering from EAE can confer protection when passively administered to rats at the time of immunization with MBP (MacPhee et al., 1992; Mason, 1992). Thus, there is good evidence that the onset of, and recovery from, EAE is orchestrated by Th1 and Th2 cytokine production and can be regulated by glucocorticoids and opioids.

## C. Atopic Dermatitis

Atopic dermatitis (AD) is a chronic, remitting inflammatory skin disease that affects humans beginning in early childhood; it is considered to be due to dysregulation of immunity; characterized by high levels of IgE secretion and increased Th2-like cytokine responses. There is a great deal of accumulating evidence that AD is causally related to dysregulated HPA axis activation in those afflicted (Buske-Kirschbaum, Jobst, & Helhammer, 1998). Recently, Buske-Kirschbaum and her associates (Buske-Kirschbaum et al., 1997) examined the effects of stress (public speech and mental arithmetic tasks) in two populations of children, normal controls and children with AD who were, at that time, not taking medication and who were in remission. Although heart rate responses to the stressor were similar in the two groups, the children with AD had a significantly lower cortisol responses. Although this study does not demonstrate cause and effect, it strongly suggests that children with AD have blunted HPA axis responses to stressors, which may be linked to their dysregulated immune responses.

## D. Adjuvant-Induced Arthritis

Studies in humans strongly suggest that stressful life events are associated with the onset and/or increased severity of rheumatoid arthritis (RA) (Robinson, 1957; Shochet et al., 1969). Stressor administration has been documented to affect animal models of arthritis as well. Glucocorticoids are the most conspicuous of the neuroendocrine responses that influence these inflammatory responses, although elevated glucocorticoids levels have not been observed in all studies of stress-induced changes in arthritis (Amkraut, Solomon, & Kraemer, 1971; Rogers et al., 1980). Sternberg and colleagues (Sternberg et al., 1989, 1992; Sternberg, Wilder, Gold, & Chrousos, 1990; Zelazowski, Patchev, Zelazowska, Chrousos & Gold, 1993; Zelazowski, Smith, Gold Chrousos, Wilder, & Sternberg, 1992) have focused on abnormal behavioral and neuroendocrine responses in the susceptibility of female Lewis rats to streptococcus cell wall (SCW)-induced arthritis. In addition to an attenuation of corticosterone responses following the injection of SCW and/or a variety of physical/psychosocial stressors, Lewis female rats have attenuated levels of plasma ACTH, as well as decreased CRH mRNA in the hypothalamic PVN compared to MHC syngeneic Fischer rats, which have only a mild, transient SCW-induced arthritis (Sternberg et al., 1992). These data suggest that the blunted HPA axis reactivity of the Lewis rat results in their susceptibility to the inflammatory SCW preparation, whereas the intact HPA response of the Fischer rats is protective against the same challenge. Fischer rats treated with a corticosterone receptor antagonist develop the disease, and treating Lewis rats with glucocorticoids makes them resistant to challenge.

Other neuropeptides have also been implicated in exacerbation of inflammatory disease. Injections of the opioid Met-enkephalin significantly reduced the inflammatory response to adjuvant injection (Jankovic & Maric, 1994). Greater inflammatory involvement of distal joints has been correlated with a higher density of substance P-containing afferent nerve fibers to these areas. In support of substance P-induced inflammatory responses, using a cold water stress paradigm, elevations of substance P were correlated with increased production of the proinflammatory cytokine IL-6 (Zhu et al., 1996) and this cold water stress also increased prostaglandin E2 (PGE2) and IL-1 production by peritoneal macrophages (Cheng, Morrow-Tesch, Beller, Levy, & Black, 1990). Finally, focal neural lesions alter the bilateral symmetry of arthritis, and arthritic inflammation does not occur in the limb paralyzed by a prior CNS lesion (Levine, Clark & Devor, 1984), again supporting neural influences on inflammatory processes.

## VI. CORTICOTROPIN-RELEASING HORMONE AND SYMPATHETIC ACTIVATION: ROLE IN STRESS-INDUCED IMMUNOMODULATION

There is a large literature implicating CRH as an immunoregulatory factor, with both central and peripheral effects (reviewed by (Tsagarakis & Grossman, 1994; Webster et al., 1997; Chrousos, 1995)). CRH has important regulatory roles in the CNS, serving to activate the HPA axis and activating the SNS as well. Much of this chapter highlights stressors which induce changes in immune responses that appear to be mediated either by glucocorticoids, NE, or both. Therefore, in addition to the direct role that peripheral CRH plays in inflammatory responses in particular, central CRH plays an indirect role in immunomodulation. Generally, the central effects of CRH are immunosuppressive. A series of studies by Irwin demonstrates that central infusion of CRH affects peripheral immunity (Irwin, Hauger, Brown, & Britton, 1988; Irwin, Hauger, & Brown, 1990; Strasbaugh & Irwin, 1992; Irwin, Vale, & Britton, 1987; Irwin, 1994). CRH administered intracerebroventricularly (icv) decreased spleen and peripheral blood NK-cell activity, antibody production to KLH, and in vitro lymphocyte proliferation to Con A. In addition, Irwin demonstrated that central CRH-induced decrease of NK-cell activity was mediated via the SNS by blocking SNS signaling with intracerebroventricular injection of chlorisondamine (Irwin et al., 1988) or by denervation with the neurotoxin 6-hydroxydopamine (6-OHDA)(Irwin, 1994). Irwin also observed that CRH administered subcutaneously did not alter NK-cell activity or antibody production to KLH (Friedman & Irwin, 1999; Irwin et al., 1987). Further, in a number of studies employing stressors, Irwin and his colleagues have observed that immunosuppressive effects of stress can be driven by central CRH induction (Friedman & Irwin, 1995, 1999; Irwin, 1993, 1994). These data suggest that at least some of the immunosuppressive effects of stress are mediated by central CRH acting via the sympathetics, not via the HPA axis.

Aside from its presence in the CNS, CRH has been located in the periphery in association with lymphoid tissue (Aird, Clevenger, Prystowsky, & Redei, 1993; Brouxhon, Prasad, Joseph, Felten, & Bellinger, 1998; Muglia, Jenkins, Gilbert, Copeland, & Majzoub, 1994; Webster, Tracey, Jutila, Wolfe, & DeSouza, 1990), and CRH receptors have been identified on macrophages and T cells (Webster et al., 1990; Webster & DeSouza, 1988; Audhya, Jain, & Hollander, 1991). It is becoming well established that there are peripheral sources of CRH. Both CRH peptide and CRH mRNA have been found in rat and mouse thymus and spleen and in human peripheral blood (Aird et al., 1993; Muglia et al., 1994; Stephanou, Jessop, Knight, & Lightman, 1990; Tsagarakis & Grossman, 1994; Webster et al., 1997). In addition, high levels of CRH have been measured in inflamed synovia in rats. Peripheral CRH injection induces release of the proinflammatory cytokine cascade (in particular, IL-1 and IL-6) and oxygen reactive species and induces chemotaxis by mononuclear leukocytes (reviewed by Webster et al., 1997; Salas, Brown, Perone, Castro, & Goya, 1997; Paez Pereda et al., 1995). IL-1 production by activated macrophages was inhibited by CRH, however (Paez Pereda et al., 1995). Administration of anti-CRH antibody systemically suppresses arthritis symptoms when used therapeutically in a number of experimental arthritis models (reviewed by (Webster et al., 1997)). In addition to the inflammatory effects of CRH, CRH has been observed to increase human PBL T-cell proliferation and increase IL-2 receptor expression with or without mitogen stimulation (Singh, 1989). In rats, however, blocking endogenous CRF with antisense oligonucleotides decreased Con A-induced spleen cell proliferation (Jessop, Harbuz, Snelson, Dayan, & Lightman, 1997).

## VII. SYMPATHETIC NERVOUS SYSTEM REGULATION OF LYMPHOCYTE TRAFFICKING AND FUNCTION

Of the most marked consequences of acute stress or elevated catecholamines, such as occurs during a stress response, is a rapid, transient leukocytosis in peripheral blood (Carlson, Beiting, Kiani, Abell, & McGillis, 1996; Carlson, Fox, & Abell, 1997). Catecholamines reduce binding of lymphocytes to vascular endothelium, leading to detachment of cells in tissues and increasing the trafficking into the circulation (Benschop et al., 1997). Mills and colleagues (Mills et al., 1997; Mills, Ziegler, Rehman, & Maisel, 1998) and Carlson and colleagues (1996) showed that this process occurred without decreases in expression of cellular adhesion molecules by leukocytes.

In humans, redistribution of leukocytes during exercise-to-exhaustion resulted in lymphocytosis, particularly increased T cells and NK cells, and a marked increase in soluble intracellular cellular adhesion molecule (ICAM). The increase in soluble ICAM was hypothesized to be due to shedding from the cell surface, which could then act as a competitor for binding to endothelial surfaces (Mills et al., 1997). These effects were largely abrogated by pretreatment with the $\beta$-adrenergic receptor antagonist propranolol or metopropol. Data obtained from these studies suggest that the critical factor for determining overall level of lymphocyte redistribution during stress are baseline levels of plasma catecholamines and $\beta$-adrenergic receptor expression. The transient nature of this response to catecholamines or stress is worth reiterating. Indeed, the significance of this redistribution is unknown, and NK cell numbers and soluble ICAM levels return to baseline within 1 h of exercise (Mills et al., 1997). In contrast to the findings of Benschop, Carlson, Mills, et al. (Benschop et al., 1997; Carlson et al., 1996, 1997; Mills et al., 1997), it has also been reported that acute stress can result in a rapid and transient decrease in numbers of rat PBMC (Dhabhar & McEwen, 1997; Horan, Taylor, Yamamura, & Porreca, 1992) and an hypothesized redistribution of these cells to other organs, including the bone marrow, lymph nodes, and the skin.

Despite the evidence for transient leukocytosis, reports of effects of stress or injection of catecholamines on cell-mediated immune responses by PBL have been mixed. For example, NK-cell activity in PBMC following stress/elevated catecholamines has been shown to be suppressed (Shakhar & Ben-Eliyahu, 1998; Stefanski & Ben-Eliyahu, 1996), elevated (Schedlowski et al., 1993a, b), or unchanged (Bachen et al., 1995). Ben-Eliyahu and colleagues (Shakhar & Ben-Eliyahu, 1998) determined that independent of, or perhaps in spite of, the observed transient increase in NK-cell number in rat peripheral blood following injection of catecholamines, there was a dose-dependent decrease in NK-cell activity. However, in this paper, NK-cell function was measured 1 h after catecholamine injection, when NK-cell numbers had returned to baseline levels. Using a social confrontation model to suppress NK-cell function, however, it was observed that propranolol only partially restored NK-cell activity in rat peripheral blood (Stefanski & Ben-Eliyahu, 1996).

Studies utilizing stressors, injection of catecholamines, and chemical sympathectomy all suggest that NE and peptides that are colocalized in the sympathetic nerves throughout the periphery, especially in lymphoid organs, have robust immunoregulatory capabilities. As is true for all of the hormones/transmitters discussed in this chapter thus far, however, the outcome of elevated catecholamine levels on an immune response will be dependent upon the total neuroendocrine milieu, the immune cell types involved in the response, the site of the response, the lymphoid organ investigated, and myriad other factors, including baseline levels of receptor expression. Indeed, a perfect example of this is the effects of $\beta$-adrenergic receptor stimulation on B lymphocyte activation (reviewed by Sanders, 1995). B cell stimulation by $\beta$-adrenergic receptor agonists in the presence of LPS or anti-immunoglobulin to cross-link receptors results in inhibition of B cell proliferation, whereas the nonspecific activational response to phorbol myristate acetate (PMA) and ionomycin is enhanced. Further, in antigen-driven T cell–B cell interactions, $\beta$-adrenergic receptor triggering of B cells can boost the effectiveness of B cells in activating T cells, thereby increasing T cell help to B cells, resulting in increased production of antibody.

## VIII. OPIOIDS AS IMMUNOMODULATORS

The opioid peptides (proopiomelanocortin (POMC) peptides, the enkephalins, and the dynorphins) are derived from the hypothalamus, pituitary, and adrenal medulla, as well as from lymphocytes (reviewed by Carr, Rogers, & Weber, 1996; Stefano et al., 1996; Weigent & Blalock, 1994). The best characterized opiate receptors in the nervous system are the $\mu$, $\kappa$, and $\delta$ receptors; there is evidence of expression of these receptors on cells of the immune system (reviewed by Madden, Whaley, & Ketelson, 1998; Mellon & Bayer, 1998b; Sharp, Roy, & Bidlack, 1998; Stefano et al., 1996). Opioids, which many investigators currently view as cytokines acting within the CNS and immune system (Peterson, Molitor, & Chao, 1998), are clearly immunomodulatory; their effects on immune function are dependent upon concentration as well as the immune parameter being investigated. With respect to opioid-induced immunomodulation, most of what is known has been determined by administration of exogenous morphine.

The in vivo effects of exogenous opioids are generally immunosuppressive. Phagocytic and other monocyte/macrophage function (reviewed by Eisenstein & Hilburger, 1998; Stefano et al., 1996), NK cell activity (Carr & France, 1993; Hsueh, Chen, Huang, Ghanta, & Hiramoto, 1996; Lysle, Coussons, Watts, Bennett, & Dykstra, 1993; Shavit, 1991; Shavit et al., 1987; Shavit, Lewis, Terman, Gale, & Liebeskind, 1984; Yeager et al., 1995) mitogen-induced proliferation (Fecho, Dykstra, & Lysle, 1993; Fecho, Maslonek, Dykstra, & Lysle, 1996a; Hernandez, Flores, & Bayer, 1993; Lysle et al., 1993; Mellon & Bayer, 1998a, b), CTL activity (Carpenter & Carr, 1995), and IL-2 and IFN production (Lysle et al., 1993) were all observed to be decreased following injection of morphine. In contrast, $\beta$-endorphin has been shown to increase T-cell proliferation (Bocchini, Bonnano, & Canevari, 1983; Gilmore & Weiner, 1988; Stefano, Leung, Bilfinger, & Scharrer, 1995) and IL-2 production (Gilmore & Weiner, 1988) in vitro. Further, polyclonal Ig secretion (reviewed by Eisenstein & Hilburger, 1998; Mellon & Bayer, 1998a) was enhanced following chronic morphine injection (Carr & France, 1993), whereas splenic

antibody forming cell responses (Pruett, Han, & Fuchs, 1992), polyclonal Ig secretion following stimulation with *Staphylococcus aureus* Cowen I (SAC) in vitro (Morgan, 1956), and in vivo antibody responses to KLH (Lockwood et al., 1994; Lockwood et al., 1996) were suppressed by morphine or selective opioid receptor agonists.

A review of the literature on opioid effects on immunity highlights the complexity of the mechanisms of action. The effects of exogenous morphine on immune function have frequently been demonstrated to be centrally mediated (Fecho et al., 1996a; Hernandez et al., 1993; Mellon & Bayer, 1998a, b) and to be mediated predominantly through $\mu$ opioid receptors expressed in the periaqueductal gray of the mesencephalon. Evidence exists for either $\beta$-adrenergic (Fecho et al., 1993; Fecho, Maslonek, Dykstra, & Lysle, 1996b) and/or glucocorticoid involvement in morphine-induced changes in immune function (Fecho et al., 1996b; Freier & Fuchs, 1994; Pruett et al., 1992). Morphine injection can be associated with an increase in glucocorticoids (Bayer, Daussin, Hernandez, & Irvin, 1990; Lockwood et al., 1994; Mellon & Bayer, 1998b); however, the glucocorticoid increase does not always appear to correlate with decreased immune responses (Lockwood et al., 1994). In addition, effects of morphine administered into the lateral ventricle of rats can produce decreases in peripheral blood lymphocyte proliferation at 20 times less than the concentration required for increasing glucocorticoid levels (Mellon & Bayer, 1998b). However, there is also evidence of direct receptor-mediated actions of opioids on leukocytes (reviewed by Carr et al., 1996; Eisenstein & Hilburger, 1998; Sharp et al., 1998; Stefano et al., 1996) and ample evidence for the expression of opioid receptors on lymphocytes (Carr et al., 1996; Sharp et al., 1998; Stefano et al., 1996; Wybran, Applebloom, Famaey, & Govaerts, 1979).

The effects of stress-induced endogenous opioids on immune function have been largely focused on NK-cell activity and tumor growth (Shavit, 1991; Shavit et al., 1984, 1987). Recent data, however, suggest that endogenous $\beta$-endorphin plays a physiological role in immune regulation. $\beta$-Endorphins suppress NK-cell activity and mitogen-induced proliferation and increase allograft survival time (Panerai, Sacerdote, Bianchi, & Manfredi, 1997; Panerai, Manfredi, Granucci, & Sacerdote, 1995). In addition, $\beta$-endorphin may be involved in downregulation of EAE in rats (Panerai et al., 1994) and Chron's disease in humans (Wiedermann et al., 1994). Panerai and his colleagues have hypothesized that opioids, in particular $\beta$-endorphin that can be elevated during a stress response, induce increased production of Th2 cytokines, thus exerting a tonic inhibitory effect on the cell-mediated immune system (Panerai & Sacerdote, 1997). However, high levels of $\beta$-endorphin do not always result in suppression of immune function (Flores et al., 1990), and stress-induced changes in NK-cell activity can be induced in the absence of opioid involvement (Ben-Eliyahu, Yirmiya, Shavit, & Liebeskind, 1990).

## IX.  ACUTE STRESSOR-INDUCED IMMUNOMODULATION—ADAPTIVE OR MALADAPTIVE?

The stress response is fundamentally adaptive for an organism. The response is a complex series of behavioral and physiological reactions that are crucial for maintaining survival; this is underscored by the finding that the stress response and the neuroendocrine components are highly conserved throughout evolution (reviewed by Ottaviani & Franceschi, 1996). In a recent review by Ottaviani and colleagues (Ottaviani, Franchini, & Francheschi, 1997), the authors postulate that the most critical signal molecules that mediate the adaptive stress response (catecholamines, neuropeptides, hormones and neurohormones, cytokines, and nitric oxide) have been most remarkably conserved throughout evolution and exist even in lower invertebrate species.

In response to a stressor, oxygen and nutrients are shunted to the CNS and appropriate peripheral sites; cardiovascular activity, gluconeogenesis, and lipolysis are all increased to provide substrates for rapid responses to acute challenge. In response to stressors, there is increased arousal, attention, cognition, and aggression, whereas appetite and reproductive behavior are suppressed.

Is this stress response good or bad for an organism's ability to mount an immune response? The answer to this question is that it may be either. That is, there are instances in which the same immune effector functions (e.g., NK-cell activity) can be enhanced and suppressed by stressors, and we are only beginning to understand the basis for such differential regulation of immunity. Clearly, the nature of the immune response and the chronicity and intensity of the stressor are important in determining the overall immune response to stressors.

Sapolsky (Sapolsky, 1994) and others (Dhabhar, 1998; Dhabhar & McEwen, 1996; Dhabhar, Miller, McEwen & Spencer, 1995; McEwen, 1998) would predict that acute stress might enhance, whereas chronic stress might suppress, immunity. Of course, this leads to some discussion as to the definition of

chronic versus acute stressors—for the sake of this chapter, we will consider acute to involve a single exposure to stressor, albeit for differing lengths of time. Chronic stress will refer to multiple sessions of stressor over longer periods of time (days to weeks).

From a teleological perspective, the hypothesis that acute stress will enhance immune function may be true for innate responses and false for acquired immunity. It is important to highlight that innate responses are the critical first line of defense against invading microorganisms, as encountered through a bite or other wound received during fight–flight. Wound healing has three stages (Martin, 1997), the first being an inflammatory stage, involving platelet aggregation, blood coagulation, and recruitment of polymorphonuclear (PMN) leukocytes and monocytes to the wound. Indeed, the neutrophil is the first cell to arrive at a site of damage, and plays a critical role in the inflammatory process. The second stage is proliferative, involving recruitment and proliferation of keratinocytes, endothelial cells, and fibroblasts. The final stage is one of remodeling. This is an orchestrated series of events that requires changes in adhesion molecule expression and secretion of chemokines, cytokines, and growth factors. Key components of the response are the early influx of PMN and monocytes to the wound, and the production of proinflammatory cytokines, including IL-6 and IL-1. During a fight–flight or acute stress response, it would "make sense" to provide energy for potential wound healing. However, there should be little adaptive value to providing energy for the generation of *primary* specific immune responses, either cell-mediated or humoral. Such primary responses would require days to be of any significant benefit to the organism.

Is there support in the literature for the hypothesis that acute stress enhances innate immunity and suppresses cell-mediated and humoral immunity? There are numerous examples in the literature of increased monocyte/macrophage function following acute stressors. Following acute hyperthermic stress, increased IL-6 mRNA was detected in the TG ganglia of stressed mice, although the cellular source of this proinflammatory cytokine (macrophage versus T cell) is unknown (Noisakran et al., 1998). Increased nitric oxide (NO) production by Con A-stimulated spleen cells, which was correlated with the presence of plastic adherent cells (most of which are macrophage/monocytes), was observed following presentation of a conditioned stimulus previously paired with electric shock (Coussons-Read, Maslonek, Fecho, Perez, & Lysle, 1994). Increased NO was detected in supernatants from Con A-stimulated spleen and mesenteric lymph node cells from rats that were subjected to acute inescapable tailshock (Fleshner et al., 1998). Finally, Lyte and colleagues (Lyte, Nelson & Thompson, 1990) observed that following acute social conflict, there was a significant increase in innate immunity, as measured by phagocytosis by splenic leukocytes from DBA/2J mice (269% increase in phagocytosis) or C57Bl/6J mice (412% increase in phagocytosis). Therefore, it would appear to be the case that short duration stress results in enhanced innate responses.

NK cells spontaneously lyse virally infected cells and tumor cells. NK cell activity, however, can be augmented by IFN-$\gamma$ produced largely by T cells, although NK cells themselves can make IFN-$\gamma$. Thus, while they are innate, they are also under some control by T helper cells. The effects of acute stress on NK cell function are largely suppressive (Ben-Eliyahu et al., 1990, 1991; Cunnick, Lysle, Armfield, & Rabin, 1988; Shavit, 1991; Shavit et al., 1984; Stefanski & Ben-Eliyahu, 1996).

The effects of acute stressors on T and B cell function have been examined in a variety of studies. Acute exposure to electric shock suppressed rat spleen cell responses to the mitogen Con A, and this suppressed response appeared to be attenuated with additional or chronic shock sessions (Lysle et al., 1987). Suppression of mitogen responses by peripheral blood lymphocytes (PBL) was also observed by these investigators following a single shock session, and no recovery of this suppression was observed with increasing shock sessions. Mitogen responses by rat lymphocytes were suppressed following a single session of footshock only when the shock was intermittent, but not when shock was continuous (Panerai, Sacerdote, Bianchi, & Manfredi, 1997; Shavit 1991; Shavit et al., 1984, 1987) this suppression of the mitogen response was dependent upon production of $\beta$-endorphin, but was independent of elevated levels of corticosterone, which were observed with both intermittent and continuous shock (Panerai et al., 1997). Keller and his colleagues (Keller et al., 1983) similarly observed that unpredictable tailshock induced a suppression of phytohemagglutinin (PHA) responses by rat PBL and that adrenalectomy did not abrogate the effects of shock. Fleshner and her colleagues also observed suppressed antibody responses and Th1-like cytokine production following a single session of acute tailshock, but that the effects were partially abrogated by glucocorticoid receptor antagonist administration (Fleshner et al., 1995a, 1998). Finally, Zalcman and his associates (Zalcman, Minkiewicz-Janda, Richter, & Anisman, 1989) observed that plaque forming cell responses and serum

antibody titer to sheep red blood cells were suppressed in mice following a single footshock session, but only in mice that were subjected to footshock 72 h after immunization. Other acute stressors can suppress immunity, such as the single restraint protocol of Iwakabe and others (Iwakabe et al., 1998) described earlier. These investigators observed that splenic NK cell cytotoxicity (which we might have considered to reflect innate processes) and mitogen-induced production of IFN-$\gamma$ were suppressed in mice restrained for 10–24 h.

Few studies have carefully examined the response to a stressor over time, although Lysle and his colleagues did observe habituation to footshock over a short range of time points (Lysle et al., 1987). There is, however, a classic study that examined the dynamic of the response to stressors over approximately 6 weeks. The 1977 study of Monjan and Collector (1977) highlights a biphasic interaction of stress and time on cell-mediated immune response. In this study, splenic T- and B-cell mitogen responses, as well as the cytotoxic response of primed spleen cells to the P815 tumor line were examined in mice exposed nightly to 100 dB noise. Although initially (1–10 days) responses were observed to be suppressed compared to baseline following acute noise stress, they were enhanced with increasing time, after approximately 20 days of noise stress. Parenthetically, the data of Monjan and Collector (1977) mimic the general adaptation syndrome of Selye (Selye, 1950). This syndrome is characterized by an initial suppressed response (resistance phase) to stressor, followed by recovery and an enhanced response (the alarm reaction) for some period of time. Finally, the exhaustion phase of the response occurs in which resistance declines; death would be the final outcome.

As we have come to expect from our review of studies of stress and neural-immune interactions, there are also some paradigms in which acute stressors appear to enhance cell-mediated or humoral acquired immunity. Lysle and others (Lysle, Cunnick, & Rabin, 1990) determined that the Con A response of spleen cells was enhanced following a single session of electric footshock in some, but not all, strains of inbred mice, as opposed to the suppressed responses observed in rats (Lysle et al., 1987). The enhancement in mitogen response was dependent upon the intensity of the footshock (0.3–1.2 mA), and became attenuated as a function of days of shock. Moynihan and her colleagues (Moynihan et al., 1994) observed serum antibody responses to KLH to be enhanced following an acute (24 h) exposure to stress odors. Again, using KLH as the immunogen, Wood and associates (Wood, Karol, Kusnecov, & Rabin, 1993) observed that a single session of footshock enhanced IgM and IgG anti-KLH antibody titers depending upon when the shock was administered (day 0 or 1) in relation to immunization. It would be tempting to argue that these last two experiments suggest an increased Th2 response at the expense of Th1 response in stressed rats. However, Wood and associates (1993) subcutaneously challenged immunized stressed and control rats with KLH and, although there were no differences between the groups in the size of the induration at the site of challenge, a greater cellular infiltrate and edema was observed in tissue sections from stressed rats. The authors believe the infiltrate to be mononuclear, suggesting to them an enhanced T-cell-mediated delayed type hypersensitivity (DTH) response. Whether the cells were really mononuclear, and certainly that they were T cells, may be debatable. Perhaps what was considered to be a cell-mediated response is actually an exaggerated Arthus ·reaction, which precedes the development of a DTH response. An Arthus reaction is a type III hypersensitivity reaction mediated by antigen-specific IgG and the formation of immune complexes; monocytes and neutrophils subsequently being recruited to the site. This might be likely, since the stressed rats had increased antibody production to KLH.

Dhabhar and colleagues have documented that a single acute stressor presentation of either restraint, shaking, or both together for 2–5 h resulted in significantly increased ear swelling when rats were challenged 2 h later by painting ear pinnae with the contact sensitizer dinitro-fluorobenzene (DNFB) (Dhabhar & McEwen, 1996, 1997). Although the authors argue that this increase in pinnae swelling indicates that there is an increase in cutaneous cell-mediated immunity, they do not have good verification that this response is, in fact, T-cell-mediated. Although this protocol has been used by others to study T-cell function, the changes in responsiveness that these investigators observed might be due to early increases in recruitment of neutrophils and monocytes to the skin. Indeed, the peak of the hypersensitivity reaction they measured occurred at or before 24 h (Dhabhar & McEwen, 1997), when the immune complex-mediated Arthus reaction could be at its peak. The investigators did examine cellularity in tissue samples and, while there does appear to be increased cellularity, from the published photomicrographs it is not possible to determine if the cells are mononuclear or PMNs (Dhabhar & McEwen, 1996). Thus, an alternative interpretation of the interesting data obtained by Dhabar and McEwen (1996, 1997) as well

as Wood and colleagues (1993), is that the enhanced ear swelling in acutely stressed rats is due to enhanced Arthus reaction (due to an increased Th2 humoral response and innate responses), rather than DTH, a Th1-cell-mediated response. In these models, it would be most interesting to carefully examine shifts in Th1/Th2 cell function.

Dhabhar and associates have observed that their acute 2 h restraint stress paradigm is associated with a rapid decrease in absolute numbers of monocytes, NK cells, T cells, and B cells from the peripheral blood (Dhabhar, Miller, McEwen, & Spencer, 1995), which appears to be correlated with increased corticosterone levels; indeed, adrenalectomy abrogated much of the redistribution of cells. Further, the effects appear to be mediated through the type II adrenal receptor (Dhabhar, Miller, McEwen, & Spencer, 1996). This is quite interesting in light of other studies documented above that have observed rapid, stress- or catecholamine-induced increases in peripheral blood lymphocytes (Carlson et al., 1996, 1997). Dhabhar hypothesizes that this decrease in cell numbers represents a redistribution or redeployment of lymphocytes to other organs of the body, in particular the skin, lymph nodes, and bone marrow—where they might be needed. What is of almost greater interest, however, is that following cessation of the stressor, both the increased corticosterone levels and the decreased leukocyte numbers rapidly returned to normal levels (measured 1 and 3 h following cessation). The real question that remains to be addressed is this: if PB leukocyte levels have returned to baseline levels at about the time of challenge with DNFB in the experiments described above, what then is the relationship between redeployment of lymphocytes and increased cutaneous hypersensitivity?

It is of added interest that Kawaguchi and colleagues (Kawaguchi, Okada, Fujino, Asai, & Ito, 1997) observed a time-dependent reduction in DTH in BALB/c mice restrained for 1–8 h immediately before sensitization, but not before challenge, with fluorescein isothiocyanate (FITC). Ear thickness was measured 24 h following challenge. In this study, skin from the dorsal trunk of restrained and control mice was biopsied; class II-positive cells (predominantly Langerhans cells (LC)) and T cells were enumerated. Numbers of Thy 1-positive T cells did not differ between the groups. Although numbers of class II (Ia)-positive LC were the same in the two groups, the morphology of the LC was significantly different, cells from restrained mice were smaller, with few and shorter of the characteristic dendrites. Finally, the investigators observed a dramatic increase in expression of calcitonin gene-related peptide (CGRP)-containing nerve fibers, which is known to inhibit LC antigen presentation.

Finally, Rinner and associates (Rinner, Schauenstein, Mangge, Porta, & Kvetnansky, 1992) observed that 150 min of acute immobilization led to decreased leukocyte numbers in rat peripheral blood and decreased Con A, PHA, and pokeweed mitogen (PWM, a B cell mitogen) responses; there was no evidence of habituation of these responses over a period of 6 days of immobilization, and responses were observed to recover within 24 h of immobilization. Spleen cell responses to Con A and PWM were examined and, although splenic responses following immobilization stress appear to be enhanced, these data are difficult to interpret within the context of acute stressor administration because all of the rats were also subjected to either adrenalectomy or sham surgery prior to immobilization. In any case, adrenalectomy appeared to abrogate the effects of immobilization on PBL and spleen cells.

In summary, innate and acquired immune responses to acute stressors have been observed to be either suppressed or enhanced. From PBL trafficking data obtained following either injection of catecholamines, acute exercise, or acute restraint and/or shaking (Benschop et al., 1997; Carlson et al., 1996, 1997; Schedlowski et al., 1993a, b), however, it is clear that the change in PBL number in response to acute stressors is dynamic; the number drops initially, recovers quickly to baseline, and perhaps could even be observed to overshoot baseline depending upon the stressor, etc. Thus, differences observed throughout the literature might be due to the time at which responses are measured (immediately following versus two hr after stressor, for instance), as well as the response examined. Although they are costly and often tedious, some solid parametric experiments might well address these questions.

## X. THE EFFECTS OF CHRONIC STRESS ON IMMUNITY

The literature reviewed earlier on the effects of restraint stress on the immune response to HSV, influenza, and *M. avis* would all indicate that multiple restraint sessions negatively affect immune response and disease progression (Bonneau et al., 1991b, 1993; Bonneau, Sheridan, Feng, & Glaser, 1991a; Brown et al., 1993; Dobbs et al., 1996; Feng, Pagniano, Tovar, Bonneau, Glaser, & Sheridan, 1991; Sheridan et al., 1991; Zwilling et al., 1990). In addition, this chronic restraint paradigm slows cutaneous wound healing in mice. In a recent paper by Padgett and colleagues

(Padgett, Marucha, & Sheridan, 1998a), restraint for 3 days before and 5 days after a 3.5-mm punch biopsy resulted in delayed wound healing and delayed cellularity of the wounds compared to control SKH (hairless) mice. The delayed wound healing was correlated with increased levels of glucocorticoids, and the delay was abrogated by treatment of the restrained mice with the glucocorticoid receptor antagonist RU40555. These data provide support for studies documenting delayed wound healing in either students undergoing examination stress (Marucha, Kiecolt-Glaser, & Favagehi, 1998) or Alzheimer's patient caregivers (Kiecolt-Glaser, Marucha, Malarkey, Mercado, & Glaser, 1995; Kiecolt-Glaser, Page, Marucha, MacCallum, & Glaser, 1998).

With respect to innate immunity, there are reports that 3 days of footshock stress (but not a single session) appeared to significantly enhance the ability of rat PMNs to phagocytose viable *Staphylococcus aureus*. However, it also appeared that PMN from stressed rats were less able to kill the ingested bacteria; therefore, it would seem difficult to actually discriminate between increased ingestion versus decreased killing. Others have observed that mice exposed to cold water stress for 4 days showed an increased production of PGE2 and IL-1 by proteose peptone-elicited macrophages (Cheng et al., 1990), yet decreased IFN-$\gamma$-induced class II expression.

In the study of Cheng (Cheng et al., 1990), 4 days of cold water stress administered twice daily for 1 min resulted in significantly decreased splenic NK cell cytotoxicity and Con A-induced proliferative responses. In contrast to these findings, however, Jain and Stevenson (Jain & Stevenson, 1991) observed that 11, 22, and 33 days of restraint (14 h/day during the light portion of the light cycle) generally resulted in enhanced immune responses in rats. Specifically, 11 days of restraint stress was associated with a significant enhancement of splenic NK cell cytotoxicity, and 11, 22, and 33 days of restraint associated with enhanced spleen cell responses to Con A, but not LPS. Most interesting was the finding that restraint for 11–33 days was associated with no weight gain in the young rats over the period of the experiment, whereas control rats gained approximately 100 g. Jain and Stevenson speculate that the long (greater than 11 days) period of restraint administration might have been associated with hyperadaptation in the form of enhanced cellular immunity, as was observed by Monjan and Collector (1977). It is interesting to reflect on how this experimental protocol compares to the studies of Sheridan, Zwilling, Padgett, and others (Dobbs et al., 1996; Padgett et al., 1998a; Bonneau et al., 1993; Sheridan et al., 1991; Brown et al., 1993). Three obvious differences are the species used as the experimental subject in these studies (rats versus mice), the use of in vitro measures versus in vivo measures and infection (by the investigators from Ohio State), and the administration of stressor during the light portion of the light:dark cycle versus the dark portion by the Ohio State investigators, the active time for a rodent.

## XI. CNS-DERIVED CYTOKINES AS THE MESSENGERS OF THE STRESS RESPONSE

Although we have focused in this chapter on the role of "traditional" hormones and transmitters as the purveyors of the stress response from the CNS to the immune system, in closing we would like to highlight some evidence that one of the important centrally derived mediators of the stress response is IL-6, a cytokine that is not only produced by leukocytes, but also by the hypothalamus, anterior pituitary, and adrenal cortex (reviewed by Turnbull & Rivier, 1995). A study by Zhou and colleagues (Zhou, Kusnecov, Shurin, DePaoli, & Rabin, 1993) documented that following restraint or footshock stress, or exposure to an aversive conditioned stimulus, male Lewis rats had significantly increased levels of plasma IL-6 as well as increased ACTH and corticosterone. These investigators hypothesize that the source of the IL-6 was the adrenals, because PBMC from these stressed rats produced decreased IL-6 compared to controls when stimulated in vitro. Adrenalectomy abolished the increased plasma levels of IL-6. These data suggested that IL-6 production by the adrenals, along with corticosterone production, may be an important part of the classic stress response. Further, Noisakran and colleagues (1998) speculated that hyperthermic stress, via HPA axis activation, induced expression of IL-6 and IL-6 receptors in the trigeminal ganglion by resident, perhaps nonlymphoid cells.

Manfredi and colleagues (Manfredi, Sacerdote, Gaspari, Poli, & Panerai, 1998) have recently used IL-6 knockout mice to evaluate the role of IL-6 in the known stress-induced changes in immune function. In this study, mice were restrained for 16 h prior to sacrifice. Splenic NK cell cytotoxicity, and Con A-induced IL-2 production and proliferation were examined. Unstressed knockout mice were shown to have decreased levels of NK cell function and Con A-induced IL-2 production, which was expected because of the role of IL-6 as a T- and B-cell-growth/differentiation factor. The presence or absence of IL-6 was not a factor in the restraint-stress induced suppression of immune parameters. The authors conclude that IL-6 is important for development of normal immune responses, but that in the absence of IL-6, other neurohormones or transmitters compensate for the putative HPA axis-derived IL-6. Of course, this does not elucidate what the role of HPA axis-derived IL-6 is in an intact or normal animal.

## XII. CONCLUDING REMARKS

In this time when we have reached a state of acceptance of the integration of the mind and body in maintaining the immune system and health, we also acknowledge that we have a long road ahead in terms of understanding the mechanisms involved in this integration. What we know is that stress affects immunity, and that the signals originating from the CNS to the immune system are mediated via HPA axis activation and/or SNS activation. In this chapter, we have attempted to highlight that the ultimate immune outcome is dependent upon a plethora of factors, including the chronicity, intensity, and other characteristics of the stressor; the species, sex, and strain of the experimental subject; the type of immune response measured, i.e., innate versus acquired, cell-mediated versus humoral; and the timing of the measurement in relation to stressor administration.

## References

Ackerman, K. D., Martino, M., Heyman, R., Moyna, N. M., & Rabin, B. S. (1996). Immunologic response to acute psychological stress in MS patients and controls. *Journal of Neuroimmunology, 68,* 85–94.

Adorini, L., Guery, J. C., & Trembleau, S. (1996). Manipulation of the Th1/Th2 cell balance: An approach to treat human autoimmune diseases? *Autoimmunity, 23,* 53–68.

Aird, F., Clevenger, C. V., Prystowsky, M. B., & Redei, E. (1993). Corticotropin-releasing factor mRNA in rat thymus and spleen. *Proceedings of the National Academy of Science USA, 90,* 7104–7108.

Audhya, T., Jain, R., & Hollander, C. S. (1991). Receptor mediated immunomodulation by corticotropin releasing factor. *Cellular Immunology, 134,* 77–84.

Amkraut, A. A., Solomon, G. F., & Kraemer, H. C. (1971). Stress, early experience and adjuvant-induced arthritis in the rat. *Psychosomatic Medicine, 33,* 203–214.

Bachen, E. A., Manuck, S. B., Cohen, S., Muldoon, M. F., Raible, R., Herbert, T. B., & Rabin, B. S. (1995). Adrenergic blockade ameliorates cellular immune responses to mental stress in humans. *Psychosomatic Medicine, 57,* 366–372.

Bayer, B. M., Daussin, S., Hernandez, M., & Irvin, L. (1990). Morphine inhibition of lymphocyte activity is mediated by an opioid-dependent mechanism. *Neuropharmacology, 29,* 369–374.

Belosevic, M., Finbloom, D. S., van der Meade, P., Slayter, M. V., & Nacy, C. A. (1989). Administration of monoclonal anti-IFN-γ antibodies in vivo abrogates natural resistance of C3H/HeN mice to infection with Leishmania major. *Journal of Immunology, 143,* 266–274.

Ben-Eliyahu, S., Yirmiya, R., Liebeskind, J. C., Taylor, A. N., & Gale, R. P. (1991). Stress increases metastatic spread of a mammary tumor in rats: Evidence for mediation by the immune system. *Brain, Behavior, and Immunity, 5,* 193–205.

Ben-Eliyahu, S., Yirmiya, R., Shavit, Y., & Liebeskind, J. C. (1990). Stress-induced suppression of natural killer cell cytotoxicity in the rat: A naltrexone-insensitive paradigm. *Behavioral Neuroscience, 104,* 235–238.

Benschop, R. J., Schedlowski, M., Wienecke, H., Jacobs, R., & Schmidt, R. E. (1997). Adrenergic control of natural killer cell circulation and adhesion. *Brain, Behavior, and Immunity, 11,* 321–332.

Berczi, I. (1998). The stress concept and neuroimmunoregulation in modern biology. *Annals of the New York Academy of Science, 851,* 3–12.

Biondi, M., & Zannino, L. (1997). Psychological stress, neuroimmunomodulation, and susceptibility to infectious diseases in animals and man: A review. *Psychotherapy and Psychosomatics, 66,* 3–26.

Blecha, F., Kelley, K. W., & Satterlee, D. G. (1982). Adrenal involvement in the expression of delayed-type hypersensitivity to DNFB in mice. *Proceedings of the Society of Experimental Biology and Medicine, 169,* 247–252.

Bocchini, G., Bonnano, G., & Canevari, A. (1983). Influence of morphine and naloxone on human peripheral blood T lymphocytes. *Drug and Alcohol Dependency, 11,* 233–237.

Bonneau, R. H., Sheridan, J. F., Feng, N. G., & Glaser, R. (1991a). Stress-induced effects on cell-mediated innate and adaptive memory components of the murine immune response to herpes simplex virus infection. *Brain Behavior and Immunity, 5,* 274–295.

Bonneau, R. H., Sheridan, J. F., Feng, N. G., & Glaser, R. (1991b). Stress-induced suppression of herpes simplex virus (HSV)-specific cytotoxic T lymphocyte and natural killer cell activity and enhancement of acute pathogenesis following local HSV infection. *Brain Behavior, and Immunity, 5,* 170–192.

Bonneau, R. H., Sheridan, J. F., Feng, N., & Glaser, R. (1993). Stress-induced modulation of the primary cellular immune response to herpes simplex virus infection is mediated by both adrenal-dependent and independent mechanisms. *Journal of Neuroimmunology, 42,* 167–176.

Brenner, I., Shek, P. N., Zamecnik, J., & Shephard, R. J. (1998). Stress hormones and the immunological responses to heat and exercise. *International Journal of Sports Medicine, 19,* 130–143.

Bretscher, P. A., Wei, G., Menjon, J. N., & Bielefeldt-Ohmann, H. (1994). Establishment of stable, cell-mediated immunity that makes "susceptible" mice resistant to Leishmania major. *Science, 257,* 539–542.

Brouxhon, S. M., Prasad, A. V., Joseph, S. A., Felten, D. L., & Bellinger, D. L. (1998). Localization of corticotropin-releasing factor in primary and secondary lymphoid organs of the rat. *Brain, Behavior, and Immunity, 12,* 107–122.

Brown, D. H., Sheridan, J., Pearl, D., & Zwilling, B. S. (1993). Regulation of mycobacterial growth by the hypothalamus-pituitary-adrenal axis: Differential responses of Mycobacterium bovis BCG-resistant and -susceptible mice. *Infection and Immunity, 61,* 4793–4800.

Bukilica, M., Djordjevic, S., Maric, I., Dimitrijevic, M., Markovic, B. M., & Jankovic, B. D. (1991). Stress-induced suppression of experimental allergic encephalomyelitis in the rat. *International Journal of Neuroscience, 59,* 167–175.

Buske-Kirschbaum, A., Jobst, S., & Hellhammer, D. H. (1998). Altered reactivity of the hypothalamus-pituitary-adrenal axis in patients with atopic dermatitis: Pathologic factor or symptom? *Annals of the New York Academy of Science, 840,* 747–754.

Buske-Kirschbaum, A., Jobst, S., Psych, D., Wustmans, A., Kirschbaum, C., Rauh, W., & Hellhammer, D. (1997). Attenuated free cortisol response to psychosocial stress in children with atopic dermatitis. *Psychosomatic Medicine, 59,* 419–426.

Cacopardo, B., Nigro, L., Preiser, W., Fama, A., Satariano, M. I., Braner, J., Celesia, B. M., Weber, B., Russo, R., & Doerr, H. W. (1996). Prolonged Th2 cell activation and increased viral replication in HIV-Leishmania co-infected patients despite treatment. *Transactions of the Royal Society for Tropical Medicine and Hygeine, 90,* 434–435.

Cannon, W. B. (1932). *The wisdom of the body.* Norton, New York,

Carlson, S. L., Beiting, D. J., Kiani, C. A., Abell, K. M., & McGillis, J. P. (1996). Catecholamines decrease lymphocyte adhesion to cytokine-activated endothelial cells. *Brain, Behavior, and Immunity, 10,* 55–67.

Carlson, S. L., Fox, S., & Abell, K. M. (1997). Catecholamine modulation of lymphocyte homing to lymphoid tissues. *Brain, Behavior, and Immunity, 11,* 307–320.

Carpenter, G. W., & Carr, D. J. J. (1995). Pretreatment with β-funaltrexamine blocks morphine-mediated suppression of CTL activity in alloimmunized mice. *Immunopharmacology, 29,* 129–140.

Carr, D. J. J., & France, C. P. (1993). Immune alterations in morphine-treated Rhesus monkeys. *Journal of Pharmacology and Experimental Therapeutics, 267,* 9–15.

Carr, D. J. J., Rogers, T. J., & Weber, R. J. (1996). The relevance of opioids and opioid receptors on immunocompetence and immune homeostasis. *Proceedings of the Society for Experimental Biology and Medicine, 213,* 248–257.

Celada, A., McKercher, S., & Maki, R. A. (1993). Repression of major histocompatibility complex IA expression by glucocorticoids: The glucocorticoid receptor inhibits the DNA binding of the X box DNA binding proteins. *Journal of Experimental Medicine, 177,* 691–698.

Chehimi, J., Ma, X., Chouaib, S., Zyad, A., Nagashunmugam, T., Wojcik, L., Chehimi, S., Nissim, L., & Frank, I. (1996). Differential production of interleukin 10 during human immunodeficiency virus infection. *AIDS Research and Human Retroviruses, 12,* 1141–1149.

Chen, Y., Inobe, J., Kuchroo, V. K., Baron, J. L., Janeway, C. A., & Weiner, H. L. (1996). Oral tolerance in myelin basic protein T-cell receptor transgenic mice: Suppression of autoimmune encephalomyelitis and dose-dependent induction of regulatory cells. *Proceedings of the National Academy of Science, 93,* 388–391.

Cheng, G. J., Morrow-Tesch, J. L., Beller, D. I., Levy, E. M., & Black, P. H. (1990). Immunosuppression in mice induced by cold water stress. *Brain, Behavior, and Immunity, 4,* 278–291.

Chrousos, G. P. (1992). Regulation and dysregulation of the hypothalamic-pituitary-adrenal axis: The corticotropin-releasing hormone perspective. *Neuroendocrinology, 21,* 833–858.

Chrousos, G. P. (1995). The hypothalamic-pituitary-adrenal axis and immune-mediated inflammation. *New England Journal of Medicine, 332,* 1351–1362.

Chrousos, G. P. (1998). Stressors, stress, and neuroendocrine integration of the adaptive response. The 1997 Hans Selye Memorial Lecture. *Annals of the New York Academy of Science, 851,* 311–335.

Chrousos, G. P., & Gold, P. W. (1992). The concepts of stress and stress system disorders. *Journal of American Medical Society, 267,* 1244–1252.

Cocke, R., Moynihan, J. A., Cohen, N., Grota, L. J., & Ader, R. (1993). Exposure to conspecific alarm chemosignals alters immune responses in BALB/c mice. *Brain, Behavior, and Immunity, 7,* 36–46.

Coe, C. L., Rosenberg, L. T., Fisher, M., & Levine, S. (1987). Psychological factors capable of preventing the inhibition of antibody responses in separated infant monkeys. *Child Development, 58,* 1420–1430.

Coussons-Read, M. E., Maslonek, K. A., Fecho, K., Perez, L., & Lysle, D. T. (1994). Evidence for the involvement of macrophage-derived nitric oxide in the modulation of immune status by a conditioned aversive stimulus. *Journal of Neuroimmunology, 50,* 51–58.

Crucian, B., Dunne, P., Friedman, H., Ragsdale, R., Pross, S., & Widen, R. (1996). Detection of altered T helper 1 and T helper 2 cytokine production by peripheral blood mononuclear cells in patients with multiple sclerosis utilizing intracellular cytokine detection by flow cytometry and surface marker analysis. *Clinical Diagnosis and Laboratory Medicine, 3,* 411–416.

Cunnick, J. E., Lysle, D. T., Armfield, A., & Rabin, B. S. (1988). Shock-induced modulation of lymphocyte responsiveness and natural killer cell activity: Differential mechanisms of induction. *Brain, Behavior, and Immunity 2,* 102–113.

D'Elios, M. M., Manfhetti, M., DeCarli, M., Costa, F., Baldari, C. T., Burroni, D., Telford, J. L., Romagnani, S., & DelPrete, G. (1997). T helper 1 effector cells specific for Helicobacter pylori in the gastric antrum of patients with peptic ulcer disease. *Journal of Immunology,* 962–967.

Daynes, R. A., & Araneo, B. A. (1989). Contrasting effects of glucocorticoids on the capacity of T cells to produce the growth factors interleukin 2 and interleukin 4. *European Journal of Immunology, 19,* 2319–2325.

Daynes, R. A., & Araneo, B. A. (1992). Natural regulators of T cell lymphokine production in vivo. *Journal of Immunotherapy, 12,* 174–179.

Daynes, R. A., Dudley, D. J., & Araneo, B. A. (1990). Regulation of murine lymphokine production in vivo. II. Dehydroepiandrosterone is a natural enhancer of interleukin 2 synthesis by helper T cells. *European Journal of Immunology, 20,* 793–802.

Decker, D., Schondorf, M., Bidlingmaier, F., Hirner, A., & vonRuecker, A. A. (1996). Surgical stress induces a shift in the type-1/type-2 T-helper cell balance, suggesting down-regulation of cell-mediated and up-regulation of antibody-mediated immunity commensurate to the trauma. *Surgery, 119,* 316–325.

de Vries, J. E., & Yssel, H. (1996). Modulation of the human IgE response. *European Respiratory Journal, 22,* 58s–62s.

Dhabhar, F. S. (1998). Stress-induced enhancement of cell-mediated immunity. *Annals of the New York Academy of Science, 840,* 359–372.

Dhabhar, F. S., & McEwen, B. S. (1996). Stress-induced enhancement of antigen-specific cell-mediated immunity. *Journal of Immunology, 156,* 2608–2615.

Dhabhar, F. S., & McEwen, B. S. (1997). Acute stress enhances while chronic stress suppresses cell-mediated immunity in vivo: A potential role for leukocyte trafficking. *Brain, Behavior, and immunity, 11,* 286–306.

Dhabhar, F. S., Miller, A. H., McEwen, B. S., & Spencer, R. L. (1995). Effects of stress on immune cell distribution. Dynamics and hormonal mechanisms. *Journal of Immunology, 154,* 5511–5527.

Dhabhar, F. S., Miller, A. H., McEwen, B. S., & Spencer, R. L. (1996). Stress-induced changes in blood leukocyte distribution. *Journal of Immunology, 157,* 1638–1644.

Dobbs, C. M., Feng, N., Beck, M., & Sheridan, J. F. (1996). Neuroendocrine regulation of cytokine production during experimental influenza viral infection: Effects of restraint stress-induced elevation in endogenous corticosterone. *Journal of Immunology, 157,* 1870–1877.

Dunn, A. J. (1995). Psychoneuroimmunology, stress and infection. In Friedman and Klein (Eds.), *Psychoneuroimunology, stress, and infection,* pp. (25–45). Boca Raton, FL: CRC.

Eisenstein, T. K., & Hilburger, M. E. (1998). Opioid modulation of immune responses: Effects on phagocyte and lymphocyte populations. *Journal of Neuroimmunology, 83,* 36–44.

Elenkov, I. J., Papanicolaou, D. A., Wilder, R. L., & Chrousos, C. P. (1996). Modulatory effects of glucocorticoids and catecholamines on human interleukin-12 and interleukin-10 production: Clinical implications. *Proceedings of the Association of American Physicians, 108,* 374–381.

Esterling, B., & Rabin, B. S. (1987). Stress-induced alteration of T-lymphocyte subsets and humoral immunity in mice. *Behavioral Neuroscience, 101,* 115–119.

Fecho, K., Dykstra, L. A., & Lysle, D. T. (1993). Evidence for beta adrenergic receptor involvement in the immunomodulatory effects of morphine. *Journal of Pharmacology and Experimental Therapeutics, 265,* 1079–1087.

Fecho, K., Maslonek, K. M., Dykstra, L. A., & Lysle, D. T. (1996a). Assessment of the involvement of central nervous system and peripheral nervous system opioid receptors in the immunomodulatory effects of acute morphine treatment in rats. *Journal of Pharmacology and Experimental Therapeutics, 276,* 626–636.

Fecho, K., Maslonek, K. A., Dykstra, L. A., & Lysle, D. T. (1996b). Evidence for sympathetic and adrenal involvement in the immunomodulatory effects of acute morphine treatment in rats. *Journal of Pharmacology and Experimental Therapeutics, 277,* 633–645.

Feng, N., Pagniano, R., Tovar, C. A., Bonneau, R. H., Glaser, R., & Sheridan, J. F. (1991). The effect of restraint stress on the kinetics, magnitude, and isotype of the humoral immune response to influenza virus infection. *Brain, Behavior, and Immunity, 5,* 370–382.

Fleshner, M., Brennan, F. X., Nguyen, K., Watkins, L. R., & Maier, S. F. (1996). RU-486 blocks differentially suppressive effect of stress on in vivo anti-KLH immunoglobulin response. *American Journal of Physiology, 271,* R1344–R1352.

Fleshner, M., Deak, T., Spencer, R. L., Laudenslager, M. L., Watkins, L. R., & Maier, S. F. (1995a). A long term increase in basal levels of corticosterone and a decrease in corticosteroin-binding globulin after acute stressor exposure. *Endocrinology, 136,* 5336–5342.

Fleshner, M., Hermann, J., Lockwood, L. L., Laudenslager, M. L., & Watkins, L. R. (1995b). Stressed rats fail to expand the CD45RC+CD4+ (Th1-like) T cell subset in response to KLH: Possible involvement of IFN-gamma. *Brain, Behavior, and Immunity, 9,* 101–112.

Fleshner, M., Nguyen, K. T., Cotter, C. S., Watkins, L. R., & and Maier, S. F. (1998). Acute stressor exposure both suppresses acquired immunity and potentiates innate immunity. *American Journal of Physiology, 275,* R870–R878.

Flores, C. M., Hernandez, M. D., Hargreaves, K. M., & Bayer, B. M. (1990). Restraint stress-induced elevations in plasma corticosterone and beta-endorphin are not accompanied by alterations in immune function. *Journal of Neuroimmunology,. 28,* 219–225.

Freier, D. O., & Fuchs, B. A. (1994). A mechanism of action for morphine-induced immunosuppression: Corticosterone mediates morphine-induced suppression of natural killer cell activity. *Journal of Pharmacology and Experimental Therapeutics, 271,* 1127–1133.

Friedman, E. M., & Irwin, M. R. (1995). A role for CRH and the sympathetic nervous system in stress-induced immunosuppression. *Annals of the New York Academy of Science, 771,* 396–418.

Gilmore, W., & Weiner, L. P. (1988). β-endorphin enhanced interleukin-2 (IL-2) production in murine lymphocytes. *Journal of Neuroimmunology, 18,* 125–138.

Golding, B., Zaitseva, M., & Golding, H. (1994). The potential for recruiting immune responses toward type 1 or type 2 T cell help.

*American Journal of Tropical Medicine and Hygeine, 50*(Suppl.), 33–40.

Gonzalo, J. A., Gonzalez-Garcia, A., Martinez, C., & Kroemer, G. (1993). Glucocorticoid-mediated control of the activation and clonal deletion of peripheral T cells in vivo. *Journal of Experimental Medicine, 177*, 1239–1246.

Gorham, J. D., Guler, M. L., Steen, R. G., Mackey, A. J., Daly, M. J., Frederick, K., Dietrich, W. F., & Murphy, K. M. (1996). Genetic mapping of a murine locus controlling development of T helper 1/T helper 2 type responses. *Proceedings of the National Academy of Science USA, 93*, 12467–12472.

Griffin, A. C., Lo, W. D., Wolny, A. C., & Whitacre, C. C. (1993). Suppression of experimental allergic encephalomyelitis by restraint stress: Sex differences. *Journal of Neuroimmunology, 44*, 103–116.

Guery, J.-C., Galbiati, F., Smiroldo, S., & Adorini, L. (1996). Selective development of T helper (Th)2 cells induced by continuous administration of low dose soluble proteins to normal and $\beta$2-microglobulin-deficient BALB/c mice. *Journal of Experimental Medicine, 183*, 485–497.

Guler, M. L., Gorham, J. D., Hsieh, C., Mackey, A. J., Steen, R. G., Dietrich, W. F., & Murphy, K. M. (1996). Genetic susceptibility to Leishmania: IL-12 responsiveness in TH1 cell development. *Science, 271*, 984–987.

Heinzel, F. P., Sadick, M. D., Holaday, B. J., Coffman, R. L., & Locksley, R. M. (1989). Reciprocal expression of interferon-$\gamma$ or interleukin-4 during the resolution of murine Leishmaniasis. *Journal of Experimental Medicine, 169*, 59–72.

Hermann, G., Beck, F. M., & Sheridan, J. F. (1995). Stress-induced glucocorticoid response modulates mononuclear cell trafficking during an experimental influenza viral infection. *Journal of Neuroimmunology, 56*, 179–186.

Hernandez, M., Flores, L. R., & Bayer, B. M. (1993). Immunosuppression by morphine is mediated by central pathways. *Journal of Pharmacology and Experimental Therapeutics, 267*, 1336–1341.

receptor-$\alpha\beta$-transgenic model. *Journal of Experimental Medicine, 182*, 1579–1584.

Hsieh, C. S., Macatonia, S. E., Tripp, C. S., Wolf, S. F., O'Garra, A., & Murphy, K. M. (1993). Development of TH1 CD4+ T cells through IL-12 produced by Listeria-induced macrophages. *Science, 260*, 547–549.

Hsueh, C., Chen, S., Huang, H., Ghanta, V. K., & Hiramoto, R. N. (1996). Activation of $\mu$-opioid receptors are required for the conditioned enhancement of NK cell activity. *Brain Research, 737*, 263–268.

Hussell, T., Spender, L. C., Georgiou, A., O'Garra, A., & Openshaw, P. J. (1996). Th1 and Th2 cytokine induction in pulmonary T cells during infection with respiratory syncytial virus. *Journal of General Virology, 77*, 2447–1455.

Irwin, M. (1993). Stress-induced immune suppression. Role of the autonomic nervous system. *Annals of the New York Academy of Science, 697*, 203–218.

Irwin, M. (1994). Stress-induced immune suppression: Role of brain corticotropin-releasing hormone and autonomic nervous system mechanisms. *Advances in Neuroimmunology, 4*, 29–47.

Irwin, M., Hauger, R., & Brown, M. (1990). Sympathetic nervous system mediates central corticotropin-releasing factor induced suppression of natural killer cell cytotoxicity. *Journal of Phrmacology and Experimental Therapeutics, 255*, 101–107.

Irwin, M., Hauger, R. L., Brown, M., & Britton, K. T. (1988). CRF activates autonomic nervous system and reduces natural killer cell cytotoxicity. *American Journal of Physiology, 255*, R744–R747

Irwin, M. R., Vale, W., & Britton, K. T. (1987). Central corticotropin-releasing factor suppresses natural killer cell cytotoxicity. *Brain, Behavior and Immunity, 1*, 81–87.

Iwakabe, K., Shimada, M., Ohta, A., Yahata, T., Ohmi, Y., Habu, S., & Nishimura, T. (1998). The restraint stress drives a shift in Th1/Th2 balance toward Th2-dominant immunity in mice. *Immunology Letters, 62*, 39–43.

Jain, S., & Stevenson, J. R. (1991). Enhancement by restraint stress of natural killer cell activity and splenocyte responsiveness to concanavalin A in Fischer 344 rats. *Immunological Investigations, 20*, 365–376.

Jankovic, B. D., & Maric, D. (1987). Enkephalins and autoimmunity: Differential effect of methionine-enkephalin on experimental allergic encephalomyelitis in Wistar and Lewis rats. *Journal of Neuroscience Research, 18*, 88–94.

Jankovic, B. D., & Maric, D. (1994). Enkephalins as regulators of inflammatory immune responses. In B. Scharrer, E. M. Smith, & G. B. Stefano (Eds.), *Neuropeptides and immunoregulation* (pp. 76–100). New York: Springer-Verlag.

Jessop, D. S., Harbuz, M. S., Snelson, C. L., Dayan, C. M., & Lightman, S. L. (1997). An antisense oligoneucleotide complementary to corticotropin-releasing hormone mRNA inhibits rat splenocyte proliferation in vitro. *Journal of Neuroimmunology, 75(1–2)*, 135–140.

Jessop, J. J., Gale, K., & Bayer, B. M. (1987). Enhancement of rat lymphocyte proliferation after prolonged exposure to stress. *Journal of Neuroimmunology, 16*, 261–271.

Kallman, B. A., Huther, M., Tubes, M., Feldkamp, J., Bertrams, J., Gries, F. A., Lampeter, E. F., & Kolb, H. (1997). Systemic bias of cytokine production toward cell-mediated immune regulation in IDDM and toward immunity in Graves' disease. *Diabetes, 46*, 237–243.

Kawaguchi, Y., Okada, T., Fujino, M., Asai, J., & Ito, A. (1997). Reduction of the DTH response is related to morphological changes of Langerhans cells exposed to acute immobilization stress. *Clinical and Experimental Immunology, 109*, 397–401.

Keller, S. E., Weiss, J. M., Schleifer, S. J., Miller, N. E., & Stein, M. (1983). Stress-induced immunosuppression of immunity in adrenalectomized rats. *Science, 221*, 1301–1304.

Kennedy, M. K., Torrance, D. S., Picha, K. S., & Mohler, K. M. (1992). Analysis of cytokine mRNA in the central nervous system of mice with experimental autoimmune encephalomyelitis reveals that IL-10 mRNA expression correlates with recovery. *Journal of Immunology, 149*, 2496–2505.

Khansari, D. N., Murgo, A. J., & Faith, R. E. (1990). Effects of stress on the immune system. *Immunology Today, 11*, 170–175.

Khoury, S. J., Hancock, W. W., & Weiner, H. L. (1992). Oral tolerance to myelin basic protein and natural recovery from experimental autoimmune encephalomyelitis are associated with downregulation of inflammatory cytokines and differential upregulation of transforming growth factor $\beta$, interleukin 4, and prostaglandin E expression in the brain. *Journal of Experimental Medicine, 176*, 1355–1364.

Kiecolt-Glaser, J. K., Marucha, P. T., Malarkey, W. B., Mercado, A. M., & Glaser, R. (1995). Slowing of wound healing by psychological stress. *The Lancet, 346*, 1194–1196.

Kiecolt-Glaser, J. K., Page, G. G., Marucha, P. T., MacCallum, R. C., & Glaser, R. (1998). Psychological influences on surgical recovery. *American Psychologist, 53*, 1209–1218.

Kuroda, Y., Mori, T., & Hori, T. (1994). Restraint stress suppresses experimental allergic encepthalomyelitis. *Brain Research Bulletin, 34*, 15–17.

Kusnecov, A. V., Grota, L. J., Schmidt, S. G., Bonneau, R. H., Sheridan, J. F., Glaser, R. M., & Moynihan, J. A. (1992). Decreased herpes simplex viral immunity and enhanced pathogenesis following stressor administration in mice. *Journal of Neuroimmunology, 38,* 129–137.

Lamont, A. G., & Adorini, L. (1996). IL-12: A key cytokine in immune regulation. *Immunology Today, 17,* 214–217.

Leung, D. Y. (1997). Atopic dermatitis: immunobiology and treatment with immune modulators. *Clinical and Experimental Immunology, 107,* 25–30.

Levine, J. D., Clark, R., & Devor, M. (1984). Intraneuronal substance P contributes to the severity of experimental arthritis. *Science, 226,* 547–549.

Levine, S., & Saltzman, A. (1987). Nonspecific stress prevents relapse in experimental allergic encephalomyelitis. *Brain, Behavior, and Immunity, 1,* 336–341.

Levine, S., Strebel, R., Wenk, E. J., & Harman, P. J. (1962). Suppression of experimental allergic encephalomyelitis by stress. *Proceedings of the Society for Experimental Biology and Medicine, 109,* 294–298.

Levite, M. (1998). Neuropeptides, by direct interaction with T cells, induce cytokine secretion and break the commitment to a distinct helper phenotype. *Proceedings of the National Academy of Science USA, 95,* 12544–12549.

Liblau, R. S., Singer, S. M., & McDevitt, H. O. (1995). Th1 and Th2 CD4+ T cells in the pathogenesis of organ-specific autoimmune diseases. *Immunology Today, 16,* 34–38.

Lin, H., Mosmann, T. R., Guilbert, L., Tuntipopipat, S., & Wegmann, T. G. (1993). Synthesis of T helper 2-type cytokines at the maternal–fetal interface. *Journal of Immunology, 151,* 4562–4573.

Lockwood, L. L., Silbert, L. H., Fleshner, M., Laudenslager, M. L., Watkins, L. R., & Maier, S. F. (1994). Morphine-induced decreases in in vivo antibody responses. *Brain, Behavior, and Immunity, 8,* 24–36.

Lockwood, L. L., Silbert, L. H., Fleshner, M., McNeal, C., Watkins, L. R., Laudenslager, M. L., Rice, K. C., Weber, R. J., & Maier, S. F. (1996). Morphine-induced alterations in antibody levels: receptor and immune mechanisms. *Journal of Pharmacology and Experimental Therapeutics, 278,* 689–696.

Lord, C. J., & Lamb, J. R. (1996). TH2 cells in allergic inflammation: A target of immunotherapy. *Clinical and Experimental Allergy, 26,* 756–765.

Lysle, D. T., Coussons, M. E., Watts, V. J., Bennett, E. H., & Dykstra, L. A. (1993). Morphine-induced alterations of immune status: Dose dependency, compartment specificity, and antagonism by naltrexone. *Journal of Pharmacology and Experimental Therapeutics, 265,* 1071–1078.

Lysle, D. T., Cunnick, J. E., & Rabin, B. S. (1990). Stressor-induced alteration of lymphocyte proliferation in mice: Evidence for enhancement of mitogenic responsiveness. *Brain, Behavior, and Immunity, 4,* 269–277.

Lysle, D. T., Lyte, M., Fowler, H., & Rabin, B. S. (1987). Shock-induced modulation of lymphocyte reactivity: Suppression, habituation, and recovery. *Life Sciences, 41,* 1805–1814.

Lyte, M., Nelson, S. G., & Thompson, M. L. (1990). Innate and adaptive immune responses in a social conflict paradigm. *Clinical Immunology and Immunopathology, 57,* 137–147.

MacPhee, I. A. M., Day, M. J., & Mason, D. W. (1992). The role of serum factors in the suppression of experimental autoimmune encephalomyelitis: Evidence for immunoregulation by antibody to the encephalitogenic peptide. *Immunology, 70,* 527–534.

Madden, J. J., Whaley, W. L., & Ketelsen, D. (1998). Opiate binding sites in the cellular immune system: Expression and regulation. *Journal of Neuroimmunology, 83,* 57–62.

Maes, M., Song, C., Lin, A., De Jongh, R., Van Gastel, A., Kenis, G., Bosmans, E. D., Benoy, I., Neels, H., Demedts, P., Janca, A.,

Scharpe, S., & Smith, R. S. (1998). The effects of psychological stress on humans: Increased production of pro-inflammatory cytokines and a Th1-like response in stress-induced anxiety. *Cytokine, 10,* 313–318.

Manfredi, B., Sacerdote, P., Gaspari, L., Poli, V., & Panerai, A. E. (1998). IL-6 knock-out mice show modified basal immune functions, but normal immune responses to stress. *Brain, Behavior, and Immunity, 12,* 201–211.

Martin, P. (1997). Wound healing—Aiming for perfect skin regeneration. *Science, 276,* 75–81.

Marucha, P. T., Kiecolt-Glaser, J. K., & Favagehi, M. (1998). Mucosal wound healing is impaired by examination stress. *Psychosomatic Medicine, 60,* 362–365.

Mason, D. (1992). Genetic variation in the stress response: Susceptibility to experimental allergic encephalomyelitis and implications for human inflammatory disease. *Immunology Today, 12,* 57–60.

Mason, D. M., MacPhee, I. A. M., & Antoni, F. (1992). The role of the neuroendocrine system in determining genetic susceptibility to experimental allergic encephalomyelitis in the rat. *Immunology, 70,* 1–5.

Matthes, T. (1963). Experimental contribution to the question of emotional stress reactions to tumor growth. *Proceedings of the Eighth Anti-Cancer Congress, 3,* 1608–1610.

McCombe, P. A., deJersey, J., & Pender, M. P. (1992). Inflammatory cells, microglia, and MHC class II antigen-positive cells in the spinal cord of Lewis rats with acute and chronic relapsing experimental allergic encephalomyelitis. *Journal of Neuroimmunology, 149,* 2496–2505.

McEwen, B. S. (1998). Stress, adaptation, and disease. Allostasis and allostatic load. *Annals of the New York Academy of Science, 840,* 33–44.

Mellon, R. D., & Bayer, B. M. (1998a). Evidence for central opioid receptors in the immunomodulatory effects of morphine: Review of potential mechanism(s) of action. *Journal of Neuroimmunology, 83,* 19–28.

Mellon, R. D., & Bayer, B. M. (1998b). Role of central opioid receptor subtypes in morphine-induced alterations in peripheral lymphocyte activity. *Brain Research, 789,* 56–67.

Mills, P. J., Ziegler, M. G., Patterson, T., Dimsdale, J. E., Hauger, R., Irwin, M., & Grant, I. (1997). Plasma catecholamine and lymphocyte beta 2-adrenergic receptor alterations in elderly Alzheimer caregivers under stress. *Psychosomatic Medicine, 59,* 251–256.

Mills, P. J., Ziegler, M. G., Rehman, J., & Maisel, A. S. (1998). Catecholamines, catecholamine receptors, cell adhesion molecules, and acute stressor-related changes in cellular immunity. *Advances in Pharmacology, 42,* 587–590.

Monjan, A. A., & Collector, M. I. (1977). Stress-induced modulation of the immune response. *Science, 196,* 307–309.

Moran, T. M., Isobe, H., Fernandez-Sesma, A., & Schulman, J. L. (1996). Interleukin-4 causes delayed virus clearance in influenza virus-infected mice. *Journal of Virology, 70,* 5230–5235.

Morgan, E. L. (1956). Regulation of human B lymphocyte activation by opioid peptide hormones: Inhibition of IgG production by opioid receptor class ($\mu$-, $\kappa$-, and $\delta$-) selective agonists. *Journal of Neuroimmunology, 65,* 21–30.

Mormede, P., Dantzer, R., Michaud, B., Kelley, K., & LeMoal, M. (1988). Influence of stressor predictability and behavioral control on lymphocyte reactivity, antibody responses, and neuroendocrine activation in rats. *Physiology and Behavior, 43,* 577–583.

Moynihan, J. A., Callahan, T. A., Kelley, S. P., & Campbell, L. M. (1998). Adrenal hormone modulation of type 1 and type 2 cytokine production by spleen cells: Dexamethasone and dehydroepiandrosterone suppress interleukin-2, interleukin 4, and interferon-$\gamma$ production in vitro. *Cellular Immunology, 184,* 58–64.

Moynihan, J. A., Karp, J. D., Cohen, N., & Cocke, R. (1994). Alterations in interleukin-4 and antibody production following pheromone exposure: Role of glucocorticoids. *Journal of Neuroimmunology, 54,* 51–58.

Moynihan, J. A., Koota, D., Brenner, G. J., Cohen, N., & Ader, R. (1989). Repeated intraperitoneal injections of saline attenuate the antibody response to a subsequent intraperitoneal injection of antigen. *Brain, Behavior, and Immunity, 3,* 90–96.

Muglia, L. J., Jenkins, N. A., Gilbert, D. J., Copeland, N. G., & Majzoub, J. A. (1994). Expression of the mouse corticotropin-releasing hormone gene in vivo and targeted inactivation in embryonic stem cells. *Journal of Clinical Investigation, 93,* 2066–2072.

Munck, A., & Guyre, P. M. (1991). Glucocorticoids and immune function. In R. Ader, D. L. Felten, and N. Cohen (Eds.), *Psychoneuroimmunology* (pp. 447–474). New York: Academic Press.

Nichoolson, L. B., & Kuchroo, V. K. (1996). Manipulation of the Th1/Th2 balance in autoimmune disease. *Current Opinion in Immunology, 8,* 837–842.

Noben-Truth, N. K. P., & Muller, I. (1996). Susceptibility to Leishmania major infection in interleukin-4-deficient mice. *Science, 271,* 987–990.

Noisakran, S., Halford, W. P., Veress, L., & Carr, D. J. (1998). Role of the hypothalamic pituitary adrenal axis and IL-6 in stress-induced reactivation of latent herpes simplex virus type 1. *Journal of Immunology, 160,* 5441–5447.

Northrup, J. P., Crabtree, G. R., & Mattial, P. S. (1992). Negative regulation of interleukin 2 transcription by the glucocorticoid receptor. *Journal of Experimental Medicine, 175,* 1235–1245.

Nuemann, C., Gutgesell, C., Fliegert, F., Bonifer, R., & Herrmann, F. (1996). Comparative analysis of the frequency of house dust mite specific and non-specific Th1 and Th2 cells in skin lesions and peripheral blood of patients with atopic dermatitis. *Journal of Molecular Medicine, 74,* 401–406.

O'Garra, A., & Murphy, K. (1996). Role of cytokines in development of Th1 and Th2 cells. *Chemical Immunology, 63,* 1–13.

Okimura, T., Ogawa, M., Yamauchi, T., & Sasaki, Y. (1986). Stress and immune responses IV. Adrenal involvement of antibody responses in adrenalectomized rats. *Japanese Journal of Pharmacology, 41,* 237–245.

Ottaviani, E., & Franceschi, C. (1996). The neuroimmunology of stress from invertebrates to man. *Progress in Neurobiology, 48,* 421–440.

Ottaviani, E., Franchini, A., & Franceschi, C. (1997). Pro-opiomelanocortin-derived peptides, cytokines, and nitric oxide in immune responses and stress: An evolutionary approach. *International Review of Cytology, 170,* 79–141.

Padgett, D. A., Marucha, P. T., & Sheridan, J. F. (1998a). Restraint stress slows cutaneous wound healing in mice. *Brain, Behavior, and Immunity, 12,* 64–73.

Padgett, D. A., Sheridan, J. F., Dorne, J., Berntson, G. G., Candelora, J., & Glaser, R. (1998b). Social stress and the reactivation of latent herpes simplex virus type 1. *Proceedings of the National Academy of Science, 95,* 7231–7235.

Paez Pereda, M., Sauer, J., Perez Castro, C., Finkelman, S., Stalla, G. K., Holsboer, F., & Arzt, E. (1995). Corticotropin-releasing hormone differentially modulates the interleukin-1 system according to the level of monocyte activation by endotoxin. *Endocrinology 136(12),* 5504–5510.

Panerai, A. E., Manfredi, B., Granucci, F., & Sacerdote, P. (1995). The beta-endorphin inhibition of mitogen-induced splenocytes proliferation is mediated by central and peripheral paracrine/

autocrine effects of the opioid. *Journal of Neuroimmunology, 58,* 71–76.

Panerai, A. E., Radulovic, J., Monastra, G., Manfredi, B., Locatelli, L., Sacerdote, P. (1994). Beta-endorphin concentrations in brain areas and peritoneal macrophages in rats susceptible and resistant to experimental allergic encephalomyelitis: A possible relationship between tumor necrosis factor alpha and opioids in the disease. *Journal of Neuroimmunology, 51,* 169–176.

Panerai, A. E., & Sacerdote, P. (1997). $\beta$-endorphin in the immune system: A role at last? *Immunology Today, 18,* 317–319.

Panerai, A. E., Sacerdote, P., Bianchi, M., & Manfredi, B. (1997). Intermittent but not continuous inescapable footshock stress and intracerebroventricular interleukin-1 similarly affect immune responses and immunocyte beta-endorphin concentrations in the rat. *International Journal of Clinical Pharmacological Research, 17,* 115–116.

Paul, W. E., & Seder, R. A. (1994). Lymphocyte responses and cytokines. *Cell, 76,* 241–251.

Pawelec, G., Rehbein, A., Schlotz, E., Friccius, H., & Pohla, H. (1996). Cytokine modulation of TH1/TH2 phenotype differentiation in directly alloresponsive CD4+ human T cells. *Transplantation, 62,* 1095–1101.

Penninger, J. M., & Mak, T. W. (1994). Signal transduction, mitotic catastrophes, and death in T-cell development. *Immunological Reviews, 142,* 248–275.

Peterson, P. K., Molitor, T. W., & Chao, C. C. (1998). The opioid-cytokine connection. *Journal of Neuroimmunology, 83,* 63–69.

Powrie, F., & Coffman, R. L. (1993). Cytokine regulation of T cell function: potential for therapeutic intervention. *Immunology Today, 14,* 270–274.

Pruett, S. B., Han, Y., & Fuchs, B. A. (1992). Morphine suppresses primary humoral immune responses by a predominantly indirect mechanism. *Journal of Pharmacology and Experimental Therapeutics, 262,* 923–928.

Rabin, B. S., Cunnick, J. E., & Lysle, D. T. (1990). Stress-induced alteration of immune function. *NeuroendocrinImmunology, 3,* 116–124.

Ramer-Quinn, D. S., Baker, R. A., & Sanders, V. M. (1997). Activated T helper 1 and T helper 2 cells differentially express the $\beta$2-adrenergic receptor. *Journal of Immunology, 159,* 4857–4867.

Ramirez, F., Fowell, D. J., Puklavec, M., Simmonds, S., & Mason, D. (1996). Glucocorticoids promote a Th2 cytokine response by CD4+ T cells in vitro. *Journal of Immunology, 156,* 2406–2412.

Rinner, I., Schauenstein, K., Mangge, H., Porta, S., & Kvetnansky, R. (1992). Opposite effects of mild and severe stress on in vitro activation of rat peripheral blood lymphocytes. *Brain, Behavior, and Immunity, 6,* 130–140.

Robertson, S. A., Seamark, R. F., Guilbert, L. J., & Wegmann, T. G. (1994). The role of cytokines in gestation. *Critical Review of Immunology, 14,* 239–292.

Robinson, C. E. (1957). Emotional factors and rheumatoid arthritis. *Canadian Medical Association Journal, 77,* 344–345.

Rogers, M. P., Trentham, E., McCune, J., Ginsburg, B., Rennke, H., Reich, P., & David, J. (1980). Effects of psychosocial stress on the induction of arthritis in the rat. *Arthritis and Rheumatism, 23,* 1337–1342.

Romagnani, S. (1996). Th1 and Th2 in human diseases. *Clinical Immunology and Immunopathology, 80,* 225–235.

Romagnani, S. (1997). The Th1/Th2 paradigm. *Immunology Today, 18,* 263–266.

Sadick, M. D., Heinzel, F. P., Holaday, B. J., Pu, R. T., Dawkins, R. S., & Locksley, R. M. (1990). Cure of murine leishmaniasis with anti-interleukin-4 monoclonal antibody. *Journal of Experimental Medicine, 171,* 115–127.

Salas, M. A., Brown, O. A., Perone, M. J., Castro, M. G., & Goya, R. G. (1997). Effect of the corticotrophin releasing hormone precursor on interleukin-6 release by human mononuclear cells. *Clinical Immunology and Immunopathology, 85*, 35–39.

Sanders, V. M. (1995). The role of adrenoceptor-mediated signals in the modulation of lymphocyte function. *Advances in Neuroimmunology, 5*, 283–298.

Sanders, V. M., Baker, R. A., Ramer-Quinn, D. S., Kasprowicz, D. J., Fuchs, B. A., & Street, N. E. (1997). Differential expression of the β 2-adrenergic receptor by Th1 and Th2 clones. *Journal of Immunology, 158*, 4200–4210.

Sapolsky, R. M. (1994). *Why zebras don't get ulcers: A guide to stress, stress-related diseases, and coping.* New York: Freeman.

Schedlowski, M., Falk, A., Rohne, A., Wagner, T. O., Jacobs, R., Tewes, U., & Schmidt, R. E. (1993a). Catecholamines induce alterations of distribution and activity of human natural killer (NK) cells. *Journal of Clinical Immunology, 13*, 344–351.

Schedlowski, M., Jacobs, R., Alker, J., Prohl, F., Stratmann, G., Richter, S., Hadicke, A., Wagner, T. O., Schmidt, R. E., & Tewes, U. (1993b). Psychophysiological, neuroendocrine and cellular immune reactions under psychological stress. *Neuropsychobiology, 28*, 87–90.

Scheinman, R. I., Cogswell, P. C., Lofquist, A. K., & Baldwin, A. S. (1995). Role of transcriptional activation of IκBα in mediation of immunosuppression by glucocorticoids. *Science, 270*, 283–290.

Schwartzman, R. A., & Cidlowski, J. A. (1994). Glucocorticoid-induced apoptosis of lymphoid cells. *International Archives of Allergy and Immunology, 105*, 347–354.

Scott, P. (1993b). IL-12: Initiation cytokine for cell-mediated immunity. *Science, 260*, 496–497.

Scott, P. (1993a). Selective differentiation of CD4+ T helper cell subsets. *Current Opinion in Immunology, 5*, 391–397.

Selye, H. (1950). *Stress.* Montreal: ACTA.

Shakhar, G., & Ben-Eliyahu, S. (1998). In vivo b-adrenergic stimulation suppresses natural killer activity and compromises resistance to tumor metastasis in rats. *Journal of Immunology, 160*, 3251–3258.

Sharma, D. P., Ramsay, A. J., Maguire, D. J., Rolph, M. S., & Ramshaw, I. A. (1996). Interleukin-4 mediates down regulation of antiviral cytokine expression and cytotoxic T-lymphocyte responses and exacerbates vaccinia virus infection in vivo. *Journal of Virology, 70*, 7103–7107.

Sharp, B. M., Roy, S., & Bidlack, J. M. (1998). Evidence for opioid receptors on cells involved in host defense and the immune system. *Journal of Neuroimmunology, 83*, 45–56.

Shavit, Y. (1991). Stress-induced immunomodulation in animals: Opiates and endogenous opioid peptides. In R. Ader, D. L. Felten, and N. Cohen (Eds.), *Psychoneuroimmunology* (pp. 789–806). New york: Academic Press.

Shavit, Y., Lewis, J. W., Terman, G. W., Gale, R. P., & Liebeskind, J. C. (1984). Opioid peptides mediate the suppressive effects of stress on natural killer cell activity. *Science, 223*, 188–190.

Shavit, Y., Martin, F. C., Yirmiya, R., Ben-Eliyahu, S., Terman, G. W., Gale, R. P., & Liebeskind, J. C. (1987). Effects of a single administration of morphine or footshock stress on natural killer cell cytotoxicity. *Brain, Behavior, and Immunity, 1*, 318–328.

Sheridan, J. F., Dobbs, C., Brown, D., & Zwilling, B. (1994). Psychoneuroimmunology: Stress effects on pathogenesis and immunity during infection. *Clinical Microbiological Reviews, 7*, 200–212.

Sheridan, J. F., Feng, N. G., Bonneau, R. H., Allen, C. M., Huneycutt, B. S., & Glaser, R. (1991). Restraint stress differentially affects anti-viral cellular and humoral immune responses in mice. *Journal of Neuroimmunology, 31*, 245–255.

Shibata, H., Fijiwara, R., Iwamoto, M., Matsuoka, H., & Yokoyama, M. M. (1990). Recovery of PFC in mice exposed to high pressure stress by olfactory stimulation with fragrance. *International Journal of Neuroscience, 51*, 245–247.

Shochet, B. R., Lisansky, E. T., Schubart, A. F., Fiocco, V., Kurland, S., & Pope, M. (1969). A medical-psychiatric study of patients with rheumatoid arthritis. *Psychosomatics, 10*, 271–279.

Singh, V. K. (1989). Stimulatory effect of corticotropin-releasing neurohormone on human lymphocyte proliferation and interleukin-2 receptor expression. *Journal of Neuroimmunology, 23* (3), 257–262.

Stefano, G. B., Leung, M. K., Bilfinger, T. V., & Scharrer, B. (1995). Effect of prolonged exposure to morphine on responsiveness of human and invertebrate immunocytes to stimulatory molecules. *Journal of Neuroimmunology, 63*, 175–181.

Stefano, G. B., Scharrer, B., Smith, E. M., Hughes, T. K., Magazine, H. I., Bilfinger, T. V., Hartman, A. R., Fricchione, G. L., Liu, Y., & Makman, M. H. (1996). Opioid and opiate regulatory processes. *Critical Reviews of Immunology, 16*, 109–144.

Stefanski, V., & Ben-Eliyahu, S. (1996). Social confrontation and tumor metastasis in rats: Defeat and beta-adrenergic mechanisms. *Physiology and Behavior, 60*, 277–282.

Stephanou, A., Jessop, D. S., Knight, R. A., & Lightman, S. L. (1990). Corticotrophin-releasing factor-like immunoreactivity and mRNA in human leukocytes. *Brain, Behavior, and Immunity, 4*, 67–73.

Sternberg, E. M. (1998). Introduction: Overview of the conference and field. *Annals of the New York Academy of Science, 851*, 1–8.

Sternberg, E. M., Glowa, J. R., Smith, M. A., Calogero, A. E., Listwak, S. J., Chrousos, G. P., Wilder, R. L., & Gold, P. W. (1992). Corticotropin releasing hormone related behavioral and neuroendocrine responses to stress in Lewis and Fischer rats. *Brain, Research, 570*, 54–60.

Sternberg, E. M., Wilder, R. L., Gold, P. W., & Chrousos, G. P. (1990). A defect in the central component of the immune system—Hypothalamic-pituitary-adrenal axis feedback loop is associated with susceptibility to experimental arthritis and other inflammatory diseases. *Annals of the New York Academy of Science, 594*, 289–292.

Sternberg, E. M., Young, W. S., Bernardini, R., Calogero, A. E., Chrousos, G. P., & Wilder, R. L. (1989). A central nervous system defect in biosynthesis of corticotropin-releasing hormone is associated with susceptibility to streptococcal cell wall-induced arthritis in Lewis rats. *Proceedings of the National Academy of Science, 86*, 4771–4775.

Strasbaugh, H., & Irwin, M. (1992). Central corticotropin-releasing hormone reduces cellular immunity. *Brain, Behavior, and Immunity, 6*, 11–17.

Trinchieri, G. (1993). Interleukin 12 and its role in the generation of TH1 cells. *Immunology Today, 14*, 335–338.

Tsagarakis, S., & Grossman, A. (1994). Corticotropin-releasing hormone: Interactions with the immune system. *Neuroimmunomodulation, 1*, 329–334.

Turnbull, A. V., & Rivier, C. (1995). Regulation of the HPA axis by cytokines. *Brain Behavior, and Immunity, 9*, 253–275.

Vacca, A., Felli, M. P., Farina, A. R., Martinotti, S., Maroder, M., Screpanti, I., Meco, D., Petrangeli, E., Frati, L., & Gulino, A. (1992). Glucocorticoid receptor-mediated suppression of the interleukin 2 gene expression through impairment of the cooperativity between nuclear facto of activated T cells and AP-1 enhancer elements. *Journal of Experimental Medicine, 175*, 637–646.

Webster, E. L., Elenkov, I. J., & Chrousos, G. P. (1997). The role of corticotropin-releasing hormone in neuroendocrine-immune interactions. *Molecular Psychiatry, 2*, 368–372.

Webster, E. L., Tracey, D. E., Jutila, M. A., Wolfe, S. A., Jr., & De Souza, E. B. (1990). Corticotropin-releasing factor receptors in mouse spleen: Identification of receptor-bearing cells as resident macrophages. *Endocrinology, 127*, 440–452.

Wegmann, T. G., Lin, H., Guilbert, L., & Mosmann, T. R. (1993). Bidirectional cytokine interactions in the maternal-fetal relationship: Is successful pregnancy a TH2 phenomenon? *Immunology Today, 14*, 353–356.

Weigent, D. A., & Blalock, J. E. (1994). Role of neuropeptides in the bidirectional communication between the immune and neuroendocrine systems In B. Scharrer, E. M. Smith, and G. B. Stefano (Eds.), *Neuropeptides and immunoregulation* (pp. 14–27). New York: Springer-Verlag.

Wiedermann, C. J., Sacerdote, P., Propst, T., Judmaier, G., Kathrein, H., Vogel, W., & Panerai, A. E. (1994). Decreased beta-endorphin content in peripheral blood mononuclear leukocytes from patients with Crohn's disease. *Brain, Behavior, and Immunity, 8*, 261–269.

Wood, P. G., Karol, M. H., Kusnecov, A. W., & Rabin, B. S. (1993). Enhancement of antigen-specific and cell-mediated immunity by electric footshock stress in rats. *Brain, Behavior, and Immunity, 7*, 121–134.

Wu, C. Y., Fargeas, C., Nakajima, T., & Delespesse, G. (1991). Glucocorticoids suppress the production of interleukin 4 by human lymphocytes. *European Journal of Immunology, 21*, 2645.

Wybran, J., Applebloom, T., Famaey, J., & Govaerts, A. (1979). Suggestive evidence for receptors for morphine and methionine-enkephalin on normal human blood T lymphocytes. *Journal of Immunology, 123*, 1068–1071.

Yeager, M. P., Colacchio, T. A., Yu, C. T., Hildebrandt, L., Howell, A. L., Weiss, J., & Guyre, P. M. (1995). Morphine inhibits spontaneous and cytokine-enhanced natural killer cell cytotoxicity in volunteers. *Anesthesthesia, 83*, 500–508.

Zalcman, S., Kerr, L., & Anisman, H. (1991). Immunosuppression elicited by stressors and stress-related odors. *Brain, Behavior, and Immunity, 5*, 262–274.

Zalcman, S., Minkiewicz-Janda, A., Richter, M., & Anisman, H. (1989). Alterations of immune functioning following exposure to stressor related cues. *Brain, Behavior, and Immunity, 3*, 99–110.

Zelazowski, P., Patchev, V. K., Zelazowska, E. B., Chrousos, G. P., & Gold, P. W. (1993). Release of hypothalamic corticotropin-releasing hormone and arginine-vasopressin by interleukin 1 beta and alpha MSH: Studies in rats with different susceptibility to inflammatory disease. *Brain Research, 631*, 22–26.

Zelazowski, P., Smith, M. A., Gold, P. W., Chrousos, G. P., Wilder, R. L., & Sternberg, E. M. (1992). In vitro regulation of pituitary ACTH secretion in inflammatory disease susceptible Lewis (LEW/N) and inflammatory disease resistant Fischer (F344/N) rats. *Neuroendocrinology, 56*, 474–482.

Zhou, D., Kusnecov, A. W., Shurin, M. R., DePaoli, M., & Rabin, B. S. (1993). Exposure to physical and psychological stressors elevates plasma interleukin 6: Relationship to the activation of hypothalamic-pituitary-adrenal axis. *Endocrinology, 133*, 2523–2530.

Zhu, G. F., Chancellor-Freeland, C., Berman, A. S., Kage, R., Leeman, S. E., Beller, D. I., & Black, P. H. (1996). Endogenous substance P mediates cold water stress-induced increase in interleukin-6 secretion from peritoneal macrophages. *Journal of Neuroscience, 16*, 3745–3752

Zwilling, B. S., Brown, D., Christner, R., Faris, M., Hilburger, M., McPeek, M., & Hartlaub, B. A. (1990). Differential effect of restraint stress on MHC class II expression by murine peritoneal macrophages. *Brain, Behavior, and Immunity, 4*, 330–338.

# Nitric Oxide and Neural–Immune Interactions

DONALD T. LYSLE

The discovery of nitric oxide as a simple gaseous molecule with ubiquitous biological activity is both profound and interesting. Prior to 1987, nitric oxide was best known as a constituent of car exhaust fumes, contributing to the smog of large cities. This perspective changed dramatically when it was shown that nitric oxide was the long sought "endothelium-derived relaxing factor" (Palmer, Ferrige, & Moncada, 1987). Since that discovery, it quickly became apparent that nitric oxide is produced by many cell types and mediates diverse biological functions, including the cytotoxic activity of macrophages, inhibition of platelet adhesion and aggregation, and neurotransmission.

## I. NITRIC OXIDE: PRODUCTION AND FUNCTION

Nitric oxide is formed from the guanidino nitrogen group of L-arginine by a group of isozymes termed nitric oxide synthases (NOS). Although the nomenclature varies, there are three known genes of NOS, neuronal NOS (nNOS), endothelial NOS (eNOS), and inducible NOS (iNOS). These genes have been identified in at least four species: mouse, rat, rabbit, and human. Among the three NOS isoforms, the neuronal and endothelial genes are constitutively expressed, and the expression of the inducible gene is dependent upon external factors as its name suggests.

### A. Neuronal Nitric Oxide Synthase

The nNOS has been identified in specific neurons of the central nervous system and spinal cord (Dun, Dun, Forstersmann, & Tseng, 1992). It also is found in sympathetic ganglia, the adrenal gland, and peripheral nerves (Dun, Dun, Wu, & Forstermann, 1993; Hassall et al., 1992; Saffrey et al., 1992; Sheng et al., 1993). In addition, nNOS is expressed by the epithelial cells of the lung, uterus, and stomach, pancreatic islet cells, and the macula densa cells of the kidney (Asano et al., 1994; Schmidt et al., 1992a; Schmidt, Warner, Ishii, Sheng, & Murad, 1992b). Although the function of nNOS remains largely unknown, it has been shown to play an important role in numerous neuronal functions. Growing evidence suggests that nNOS plays an important role in learning and memory. For example, rats that received intrahippocampal injections of the nitric oxide synthase inhibitor, $N^G$-nitro-L-arginine (L-NAME) had a significantly higher number of errors in a working memory task (Ohno, Yamamoto, & Watanabe, 1993). Passive avoidance learning induces a significant increase in hippocampal NOS activity, and intrahippocampal administration of the NOS antagonist, nitro-arginine, at the time of training significantly impairs performance of the passive avoidance task 24 h later (Bernabeu, Stein,

Fin, Izquierdo, & Medina, 1995). Similarly, other investigators have shown that inhibition of nitric oxide production results in deficits in acquisition of place-navigation learning and in memory recall of recently explored objects (Cobb, Ryan, Frei, Guel-Gomez, & Mickley, 1995; Estall, Grant, & Cicala, 1993).

nNOS also appears to be involved in complex behaviors like aggression and sexual behavior. Mice with targeted disruption of the gene for nNOS display exaggerated aggressive behavior and excessive inappropriate sexual behavior (Nelson et al., 1995). Likewise, antagonist studies show that mice treated with 7-nitroindazole, an nNOS selective antagonist, display substantially increased aggression, as compared to control animals, when tested in both a test of resident–intruder aggression and a test of grouped aggression in a neutral arena (Demas et al., 1997). Thus, nNOS plays an important role in behavior.

## B. Endothelial Nitric Oxide Synthase

The endothelial form of NOS has been primarily localized to arterial and venous endothelial cells in many tissues (Pollock et al., 1993). The major function of eNOS in the vascular endothelium is the regulation of vascular tone, with nitric oxide inducing vasodilation (Joannides et al., 1995; Vallance, Collier, & Moncada, 1989). The release of nitric oxide from the endothelium regulates the circulatory adaptation to a variety of physiological stimuli, such as isometric exercise (Gilligan et al., 1994). Mental stress tasks induce a vasodilatory response in the forearm that is mediated by the local release of nitric oxide (Cardillo, Kilcoyne, Quyyumi, Cannon, & Panza, 1997; Dietz et al., 1994). The endothelial form of NOS also has been detected in syncytiotrophoblasts of human placenta (Myatt, Brockman, Eis, & Pollock, 1993), LLC-PK$_1$ kidney tubular epithelial cells (Tracey, Pollock, Murad, Nakane, & Forstermann, 1994), and interstitial cells of the canine colon (Xue, Pollock, Schmidt, Ward, & Sanders, 1994). Interestingly, eNOS also has been found in neurons of the rat hippocampus and other brain regions (Dinnerman, Dawson, Schell, Snowman, & Snyder, 1994). The widespread distribution of eNOS suggests that the nitric oxide production by this enzyme may be involved in an extensive number of physiological activities, perhaps serving functions in addition to vasodilation.

## C. Inducible Nitric Oxide Synthase

The inducible form of NOS requires calmodulin for its activity in a manner similar to eNOS and nNOS,

but in contrast to the other isoforms, iNOS tightly binds calmodulin and therefore does not require any further addition of calmodulin to exert its full biological activity (Cho et al., 1992). Thus, iNOS is not regulated by intracellular calcium levels and the consequence is that iNOS produces large amounts of nitric oxide for a long period of time relative to eNOS and nNOS (Nathan, 1992). Under normal physiological conditions, iNOS is not expressed in mammalian cells, but it is induced by proinflammatory stimuli, such as bacterial lipopolysaccharide or the cytokines tumor necrosis factor, interleukin-1, and interferon-$\gamma$. Immunohistochemical localization of iNOS in rats treated with LPS demonstrated the enzyme in many tissues: macrophages, occasional lymphocytes, neutrophils, and eosinophils of the spleen; Kupffer's cells, endothelial cells and hepatocytes in the liver; alveolar macrophages in the lung; macrophages and endothelial cells in the adrenal gland; and histiocytes, eosinophils, mast cells, and endothelial cells in the colon (Bandaletova et al., 1993). The generation of large amounts of nitric oxide by cells of the immune system, particularly the macrophage, provides a substantial degree of microbial resistance (Green, Meltzer, Hibbs, & Nacy, 1990; Green & Nacy, 1993; James & Glaven, 1989; Vincendeau et al., 1992). Indeed, mice lacking the gene for iNOS have markedly reduced resistance to parasitic and bacterial infections (MacMicking et al., 1995; Wei et al., 1995). The large quantities of nitric oxide produced by macrophages also provide resistance to viral infection and exert tumoricidol effect (Green & Nacy, 1993; Hibbs, Tiantor, & Vavrin, 1987; Karapiah et al., 1993). As each of these examples demonstrates, the production of nitric oxide by iNOS is an important component of innate immunity, being independent of specific antigen recognition mechanisms.

Although the formation of nitric oxide through iNOS participates in immunological defense against infection, inappropriate induction of iNOS plays a role in a number of pathophysiological conditions. The circulatory failure associated with endotoxic shock has been attributed in part to enhanced production of nitric oxide (Kilbourn et al., 1991; Nussler & Billiar, 1993). The development of autoimmune disease also is linked to alterations in the expression of iNOS. Spontaneous autoimmune disease in MRL-*lpr*/*lpr* mice is dependent upon enhanced expression of iNOS (Weinberg et al., 1994). Patients with rheumatoid arthritis show increased levels of nitrite in synovial fluid and serum, possibly related to the induction of iNOS (Farrell, Blake, Palmer, & Moncada, 1992). Inhibition of iNOS attenuates the inflammatory responses and some of the clinical manifestations of arthritis in animal models (McCartney-Francis et al., 1993; Stefanovic-Racic, Stadler, & Evans, 1993). Enhanced formation of nitric oxide derived from iNOS also has been implicated in chronic inflammatory bowel disease (Middleton, Sorthouse, & Hunter, 1993; Miller, Sadowska-Krowicka, Chotinaruemol, Kakkis, & Clark, 1993), in immune complex-mediated alveolitis and dermal vasculitis (Mulligan, Hevel, Marletta, & Ward, 1991), and in streptozotocin-induced diabetes (Corbett et al., 1992; Kolb, Kiesel, Kroncke, & Bachofen, 1991; Lukic, Stosic-Grujicic, Ostojic, Chan, & Liew, 1991).

In addition to nitric oxide's beneficial role in conferring resistance to infectious organisms and its pathophysiological role in autoimmunity and septic shock, nitric oxide also has important regulatory functions in the immune system. Evidence strongly supports a role for nitric oxide in the suppression of antibody formation to tetanus toxoid and sheep red blood cells after immunization with *Salmonella typhimurium* (Al-Ramadi, Meissler, Huang, & Eisenstein, 1992; Eisenstein, Huang, Meissler, & Al-Ramadi, 1994). Furthermore, numerous studies have shown that nitric oxide limits the proliferative activity of lymphocytes (Albina & Henry, 1991; Fu & Blankenhorn, 1992; Pascual, Pascual, Bost, McGhee, & Oparil, 1992) and so appears to play a fundamental role in controlling the onset and duration of cellular immune responses.

Thus, nitric oxide is produced by the enzyme NOS in virtually all areas of the body and participates in a diverse array of biological functions. Given the ubiquitous nature of nitric oxide, the study of the regulation of this simple molecule may provide important new insights into the understanding of neural–immune interactions. Our work in this area has focused on the impact that stressful events and drugs of abuse have on the production of nitric oxide by cells of the immune system.

## II. NITRIC OXIDE IN NEURAL–IMMUNE INTERACTIONS

The study of neural–immune interactions involves many different approaches as witnessed by the diversity of research in the present volumes. These approaches range from the molecular identification of common communication molecules between the nervous and the immune systems, to the influence of complex human behaviors on immune status. One common approach to the study of these interactions is to investigate the impact of stressful events, and the accompanying neuroendocrine activity, on the status of the immune system. Animal research in the area has shown that behavioral responses to various aversive physical stimuli can have pronounced effects on immune status. For example, presentations of electric footshock to rats decrease the proliferative responsiveness of splenic and blood lymphocytes to mitogens, the cytotoxicity of natural killer cells, and the production of keyhole limpet hemocyanin (KLH)-specific antibodies (Laudenslager et al., 1988; Lysle, Lyte, Fowler, & Rabin, 1987; Shavit, Lewis, Terman, Gale, & Liebeskind, 1984). Such findings have led investigators to suggest that immune alterations induced by behavioral responses to aversive stimuli can influence the pathogenesis of disease. This hypothesis is supported by the demonstration that electric shock increases susceptibility to tumor challenge and alters the development of experiment allergic encephalomyelitis, an animal model of multiple sclerosis (Lewis, Shavit, Terman, Gale, & Liebeskind, 1983/84; Lewis et al., 1983; Bukilica 1991).

Research in our laboratory has focused on the immunomodulatory effects of Pavlovian aversive conditioned stimuli. Classic work by Ader and Cohen (1975) showed that an innocuous, saccharin-flavored, drinking solution can acquire immunomodulatory properties through pairings with the immunosuppressive drug cyclophosphamide. Ader and Cohen extended their findings to show that exposure to a conditioned stimulus that had been established through pairings with cyclophosphamide can alter the development of an autoimmune condition similar to systemic lupus-erythematosus in mice (Ader & Cohen, 1982). Our work showed that the presentation of an inherently nonaversive environmental stimulus, such as an auditory, visual, or contextual cue, which previously has been paired with electric shock, can suppress the responsiveness of T and B lymphocytes to mitogens, decrease natural killer cell activity, decrease the number of antibody forming cells, diminish production of interferon-$\gamma$ and interleukin-2, and decrease the development of adjuvant-induced arthritis (Luecken & Lysle, 1992; Lysle, Luecken, & Maslonek, 1992a, b). These studies also demonstrate that the immune alterations are the result of a learned state induced by the conditioned stimulus and are not due to prior electric shock experience itself, handling, or exposure to the type of stimulus used as the conditioned stimulus. Moreover, conditioned suppression of lymphocyte responsiveness can be attenuated by two manipulations known to reduce the expression of a Pavlovian conditioned response, extinction and preexposure, thereby confirming that these immune alterations result from associative learning (Lysle, Cunnick, Fowler, & Rabin, 1988; Lysle, Cunnick, Kucinski, Fowler, & Rabin, 1990).

## A. Stress-Induced Modulation of Nitric Oxide Production

Given the well-established immunosuppressive effect of aversive conditioned stimuli on immune responses like lymphocyte proliferation and cytokine production, we were interested in determining the impact of Pavlovian conditioning processes on the production of inducible nitric oxide by cells of the immune system. In an initial study, rats received two conditioning sessions, each of which consisted of 10 presentations of a footshock, delivered on a variable time schedule, in a conditioning apparatus (Coussons-Read, Maslonek, Fecho, Perez, & Lysle, 1994). Our prior work used extensive control manipulations to demonstrate that this procedure establishes the conditioning chamber as an aversive, immunomodulatory, conditioned stimulus (Lysle et al., 1990). Following a 12-day rest period, during which animals remained undisturbed in their home cages, half of the animals were reexposed to the conditioning chamber for 40 min. No electric shock was administered during this test session. Immediately after the test session, the spleen of each rat was removed and the splenocytes were stimulated with concanavalin A (Con A). Supernatants from the Con A-stimulated splenocyte cultures then were tested for the presence of nitrite, a degradation product of nitric oxide. Direct measurement of nitric oxide production in supernatant is difficult because this molecule is rapidly metabolized. Nitrite is a more stable molecule that results from the metabolism of nitric oxide and can be measured readily in culture supernatants. Importantly, nitrite concentrations have been shown to correlate with concentrations of nitric oxide (Goretski & Hollocher, 1988; Green et al., 1982; Iyengar, Stuehr, & Marletta, 1987; Pellat, Henry, & Drapier, 1990).

Figure 1 shows the production nitric oxide, as measured by nitrite concentration, by unstimulated or Con A-stimulated splenocytes from rats exposed to the aversive conditioned stimulus or control procedures. The results show a significant elevation in the production of nitric oxide by Con-A stimulated splenocytes from rats exposed to the aversive conditioned stimulus. This finding indicates that a psychological stressor can induce an enhancement in nitric oxide production by splenocytes.

Stress-induced enhancement of nitric oxide production has been demonstrated using other types of

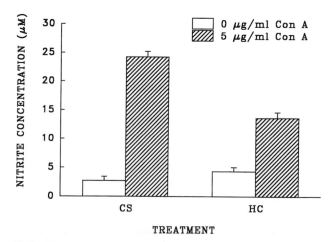

**FIGURE 1** Nitrite concentration in supernatants generated by culturing splenocytes with culture medium alone (open bars) or with the optimal concentration of 5. 0 μg/mL Con A (hatched bars). Animals were either reexposed to the conditioned stimulus (CS) or remained undisturbed in their home cages (HC) on the test day. Data are expressed as mean (±SE) of the averaged duplicate nitrite determinations. (From Coussons-Read, Maslonek, Fecho, Perez, & Lysle, *Journal of Neuroimmunology, 50,* 54, 1994 with permission from Elsevier Science).

stressors. For example, peritoneal exudate cells from mice exposed to acute cold stress show enhanced production of nitric oxide (Kizaki, Oh-Ishi, & Ohno, 1996). Moreover, mice given laparoscopic surgery, an operative stress, show markedly elevated nitrite production by peritoneal macrophages 24 h to at least 5 days after the procedure (Iwanaka, Iwanaka, Arkovitz, Arya, & Ziegler, 1997). Although these results indicate the generality of stress-induced enhancement of nitric oxide by cells of the immune system, there is some evidence to the contrary. The production of nitric oxide by alveolar macrophages was found to be reduced following exposure of rats to a series of mild electric footshocks (Persoons, Schornagel, Breve, & Berkenbosch, 1995). Whether these discrepant findings reflect differences in the neural regulation of the immune compartments, or differences between splenic, peritoneal, and alveolar macrophages remains to be determined. Another possibility is that different stressor paradigms have different effects on the production of nitric oxide.

## B. Consequence of Stressor-Induced Enhanced Nitric Oxide Production

The finding that stress enhances nitric oxide production by macrophages has important implications for the interpretation of how stress influences immune status. We hypothesized that elevations in the production of nitric oxide by macrophages may be

the key factor responsible for stress-induced alterations of lymphocyte function. To test this hypothesis,
we conducted several manipulations designed to both
remove the cells responsible for nitric oxide production from mixed cell cultures and to directly block the
production of nitric oxide in vitro (Coussons-Read
et al., 1994).

Our first investigation showed that removal of
adherent cells from splenocyte cultures completely
eliminates stress-induced suppression of lymphocyte
proliferation, suggesting that the adherent cell population is responsible for the suppression of lymphocyte proliferation. Figure 2 shows that there is no
significant effect of the conditioned stimulus in the
cultures of nonadherent cells, using two cell dilutions
to control for the level of proliferation. These results
provide evidence that the presence of adherent cells,
presumably macrophages, is essential for the expression of conditioned alterations of Con A-stimulated
lymphocyte proliferation.

To support the claim that nitric oxide is essential
for stress-induced alterations of lymphocyte function,
we evaluated the effect of the addition of a competitive inhibitor of iNOS, $N^G$-mono-methyl-L-arginine
(L-NMMA), to cultures of unfractionated splenocyte
suspensions from rats exposed to an aversive conditioned stimulus. Figure 3 shows that the addition of
the L-NMMA dose-dependently attenuates the suppression of mitogen stimulated lymphocyte proliferation induced by the aversive conditioned stimulus.

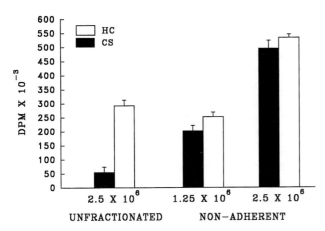

**FIGURE 2**  Proliferative response of cultured unfractionated
splenocytes and of nonadherent splenic lymphocytes to Con A
(5.0 µg/mL). The cell dilution/mL is displayed under the respective
bars. [³H]Thymidine incorporation is expressed as the mean (±SE)
of the averaged triplicate disintegrations per minute (dpm). CS
represents animals reexposed to the conditioned stimulus on the
test day, and HC (home cage) represents cultures from animals that
remained in their home cages on the test day. (From Coussons-
Read, Maslonek, Fecho, Perez, & Lysle, *Journal of Neuroimmunology*,
*50*, 55, 1994 with permission from Elsevier Science).

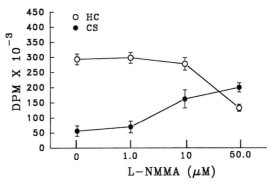

**FIGURE 3**  Proliferative response of cultured splenocytes to the
optimal concentration of Con A (5.0 µg/mL) and increasing concentrations of L-NMMA. [³H]Thymidine incorporation is expressed as the
mean (±SE) of the averaged triplicate disintegrations per minute
(dpm). CS represents animals reexposed to the conditioned stimulus
on the test day, and HC (home cage) represents cultures from animals
that remained in their home cages on the test day. (From Coussons-
Read, Maslonek, Fecho, Perez, & Lysle, *Journal of Neuroimmunology, 50,*
55, 1994 with permission from Elsevier Science).

The results indicate that alterations in the L-arginine-
dependent nitric oxide production underlie the stress-
induced suppression of lymphocyte proliferation.
Furthermore, excess L-arginine, the preferred substrate for NOS, counters the L-NMMA-induced attenuation of suppression in the proliferative response of
lymphocytes. This finding is confirmation of the
involvement of the L-arginine-dependent, nitric-oxide
synthesizing pathway. In contrast to the effect of L-
arginine, increasing the concentration of the inactive
enantiomer of L-arginine, D-arginine, did not significantly influence the effect of L-NMMA. Together, these
experiments provide the first evidence that nitric
oxide production is related to stress-induced changes
in T-lymphocyte proliferation (Coussons-Read et al.,
1994).

Given the strong evidence that nitric oxide plays an
important role in primary host defense responses
associated with a number of microbial infections, an
interesting question is whether stress-induced immunomodulatory effects increase or decrease host resistance to infection. The present data suggest that
decreases in measures of immune status, such as
mitogenic responsiveness of lymphocytes, may be
secondary to increases in nitric oxide production.
Stress-induced elevation of nitric oxide production
might enhance resistance to infection; however,
uncontrolled elevation of nitric oxide might produce
detrimental effects to host tissue. To complicate
understanding of the impact of enhanced nitric oxide
production, recent evidence suggests a role for nitric
oxide in the apoptosis or programmed cell death of
immune cells. Apoptosis serves an important role in
promoting the resolution of immune responses. For

example, the apoptosis of inflammatory neutrophils serves as a signal for macrophage phagocytosis of these cells, which then limits tissue damage and promotes healing (Haslett, 1992; Savill, 1997). Stress-induced elevation of nitric oxide production might promote the apoptosis of inflammatory neutrophils and thereby promote the resolution of an inflammatory response, or it might promote the apoptosis of macrophages and thereby block the resolution of the inflammatory response (Messmer, Reimer, Reed, & Brune, 1996; Singhal et al., 1998). Either possibility could be beneficial to the host if the response is initiated at a critical time in the overall inflammatory response. The disruption of the inflammatory response by untimely apoptosis could just as well be detrimental to the host defense system. Collectively, these investigations tell us that the health consequences of stress-induced immune alterations, including alterations in nitric oxide production, must be derived from the totality of the sequelae of cellular events involved in the cascade of the immune response.

## C. Mechanisms of Stressor-Induced Alteration of Nitric Oxide Production

Although there is evidence for the neural modulation of iNOS production by cells of the immune system, there is little understanding of the mechanisms mediating this relationship. There is absolutely no shortage of potential mechanisms governing this relationship. The central nervous system can signal the immune system in many ways. First, neural–immune interactions can occur indirectly, through the endocrine products resulting from activation of the hypothalamo-pituitary-adrenal axis and/or the adrenal medulla. The central nervous system also can directly influence the immune system via sympathetic nerve fiber connections with cells in primary and secondary lymphoid compartments (Felten et al., 1985). Both adrenocortical hormones and catecholamines have been shown to modulate lymphocyte function, providing evidence for the influence of both systems on immunoregulation (Onsrud & Thorsby, 1981; Crabtree, Munck, & Smith, 1980).

Over the past few years substantial attention has been given to the role of endogenous opioids in the modulation of immune status. Opioid receptors have been detected on lymphocytes and may provide a basis for the effects of opioids on immune status (Carr, 1991; Carr et al., 1989; Madden, Donahoe, Zwemer-Collins, Shafer, & Falek, 1987; Wybran, Applebloom, Famaey, & Gavaerts, 1979). Indeed, the responses of immune cells in culture are altered by the addition of endogenous opioids (Froelich & Bankhurst, 1984; Gilmore & Weiner, 1988; Mandler, Biddison, Mandler, & Serate, 1986; Mathews, Froelich, Sibbitt, & Bankhurst, 1983; McCain, Lamster, Bozzone, & Grbic, 1982; Van Epps & Saland, 1984). In vivo studies link the immunomodulatory effects of aversive stimulation to endogenous opioid activity. For example, the presentation of inescapable electric shock to rats not only produces opioid-mediated analgesia, but also reduces the proliferative responsiveness of splenic lymphocytes to mitogen (Laudenslager, Ryan, Drugan, Hyson, & Maier, 1983). Visintainer, Volpicelli, and Seligman (1982) utilized a similar electric shock paradigm to show that electric shocks that induce elevations in opioid activity also enhance tumor development. The correlational design of these studies makes it difficult to conclude that opioid activity is directly responsible for the immune alterations observed following shock because the responses of many physiological systems also are altered during the presentation of this aversive stimulus. More direct support for the involvement of opioids in immunomodulatory effects of electric shock is provided by research showing that the opioid receptor antagonist, naltrexone, blocks the suppression of natural killer cell activity induced by inescapable electric shock (Shavit et al., 1984).

Our laboratory examined the effectiveness of the opioid antagonist naltrexone in blocking the immunomodulatory effect of an aversive conditioned stimulus (Lysle et al., 1992a). The experiment involved development of an aversive conditioned stimulus by pairing a conditioning chamber with presentations of electric footshock. On a subsequent test day, subjects received a subcutaneous injection of either saline or different doses of naltrexone prior to exposure to the aversive conditioned stimulus or home cage control treatment. Immunologic assessments were performed immediately following exposure to the conditioned stimulus or home cage treatment. The mitogenic responsiveness of lymphocytes from the spleen was measured using T- and B-cell mitogens. The cytotoxic activity of natural killer cells derived from the spleen also was assessed. Naltrexone administration prior to presentation of the conditioned stimulus dose-dependently attenuated the conditioned suppression of the proliferative response of splenic lymphocytes and the conditioned reduction in natural killer cell activity. This study indicates that activity at opioid receptors is involved in the immunomodulatory effects of an aversive conditioned stimulus, but does not provide enough information to discern the location of the receptors at which naltrexone is acting. As previously mentioned, there is evidence suggesting that opioid receptors located directly on the surface of cells of the immune system may be involved in the effect. Alternatively, opioid receptors located in the central nervous system can regulate the neural system and endocrine factors can influence the immune system. To investigate these alternatives, we assessed the ability of N-methylnaltrexone, a naltrexone derivative that does not cross the blood-brain barrier (Brown & Goldberg, 1985), to block the immunosuppressive effects of the aversive conditioned stimulus. Peripheral administration of N-methylnaltrexone did not significantly alter the conditioned immunomodulatory effects, even at doses 1 log unit higher than an effective dose of naltrexone. Given the ability of naltrexone to cross the blood-brain barrier and the ineffectiveness of N-methylnaltrexone, these findings provide evidence that central endogenous opioid activity is involved in the immunomodulatory effects of an aversive conditioned stimulus (Lysle et al., 1992a)

The involvement of endogenous opioids in stress-induced immunomodulation suggested that exogenous opioids also would produce immunomodulatory effects. In fact, there is now substantial evidence that opioid agonists are highly efficacious in producing immunomodulatory effects (Lysle, Coussons, Watts, Bennett, & Dykstra, 1993; Shavit et al., 1986). Together, these studies raise the possibility that opioid activity may be important in the regulation of iNOS production by cells of the immune system. To begin to investigate this possibility, our laboratory assessed the effect of morphine, a prototypical opioid agonist, on nitric oxide production (Fecho, Maslonek, Coussons-Read, Dykstra, & Lysle, 1994; Fecho, Maslonek, Dykstra, & Lysle, 1995). In those investigations, rats received a single injection morphine or saline followed by the assessment of nitric oxide production by cultured splenocytes. Figure 4 shows concentrations of nitrite in supernatants generated by culturing splenocytes with culture medium alone or with Con A. Nitrite concentrations in Con A cultures from morphine-treated animals are higher than those in cultures from saline-injected control animals. These results indicate that the administration of morphine induces a pronounced elevation in the production of nitric oxide by splenocytes, similar to that observed following stress.

Subsequent investigations showed that removal of adherent cells from splenocyte cultures eliminates morphine-induced suppression of lymphocyte proliferation, suggesting that nitric oxide production by splenic macrophages present in the adherent cell population is responsible for the suppression of lymphocyte proliferation (Fecho et al., 1994). In

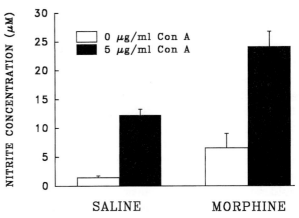

**FIGURE 4** Nitrite concentration in supernatants generated by culturing splenocytes with culture medium alone (open bars) or with the optimal concentration of 5.0 µg/mL Con A (Shaded bars). Animals were inject with either saline or morphine (15 mg/kg). Data are expressed as mean (±SE) of the averaged duplicate nitrite determinations. (From Fecho, Maslonek, Coussons-Read, Dykstra, & Lysle, *Journal of Immunology*, *152*, 5848, 1994 with permission Copyright © 1994 The American Association of Immunologists).

support of this suggestion, additional experiments showed that the addition of L-NMMA, to cultures of unfractionated spleen cell suspensions dose-dependently attenuates the suppression of lymphocyte proliferation to mitogen induced by morphine, indicating the involvement of nitric oxide. The attenuation of morphine-induced suppression afforded by addition of L-NMMA to culture was countered by addition of excess L-arginine. These observations indicate that morphine-administration modulates the production of nitric oxide by macrophages, and that this alteration in nitric oxide production is related to morphine-induced changes in lymphocyte proliferation (Fecho et al., 1994, 1995).

To further our understanding of how opioids modulate nitric oxide production, we assessed the effect on splenic nitric oxide production of administration of opioid agonists, which are highly selective for the different types of opioid receptors (Schneider & Lysle, 1998). At least three main types of opioid receptors exist: $\mu$, $\delta$, and $\kappa$. We tested the effects of in vivo and in vitro administration of [D-Ala[2],N-Me-Phe[4],Gly-ol[5]] enkephalin (DAMGO), a $\mu$- selective opioid agonist, [D-Pen [2,5]] enkephalin (DPDPE), a $\delta$-selective agonist, and U69,593, a $\kappa$- selective agonist. These compounds were chosen because they show greater than 100 times the affinity for their target receptor than for other opioid receptor types (Emmerson, Liu, Woods, & Medzihradsky, 1994; Goldstein, 1987). We measured the production of nitric oxide by splenic macrophages and the lymphocyte proliferation in response to the superantigen, toxic shock syndrome toxin (TSST-1) in vitro. The use of TSST-1 in the present study provides an examination of a more refined immune response than that measured by mitogen-induced stimulation, for it involves both macrophages and T cells, as well as T-cell receptor recognition (Drake & Kotzin, 1992; Marrack & Kappler, 1990; Schwab, Brown, Aderle, & Schlievert, 1993; White et al., 1989).

For the initial study, rats with cannulae directed at the lateral ventricle received microinjection of the $\mu$-selective agonist, DAMGO. In these experiments, intracerebroventrical (icv) injection was used to test the additional hypothesis that the opioid receptors involved in the regulation of splenic iNOS regulation are located within the central nervous system. One hour following the injection of DAMGO splenocyte cultures were prepared for immunologic assessment. Total nitrite was measured in splenocyte cultures after incubation. The proliferative response of splenic lymphocytes to TSST-1 was also measured.

Figure 5A shows that the icv injection of the $\mu$-selective opioid receptor agonist, DAMGO, induces a dose-dependent increase in the production of nitric oxide by splenocytes, as determined by nitrite levels produced in response stimulation by increasing concentrations of TSST-1. Figure 5B shows that the injection of DAMGO induces a dose-dependent decrease in the proliferative response of splenocytes to TSST-1. The effect of DAMGO is apparent across all concentrations of TSST-1. The proliferative response was virtually eliminated at the 1.0-$\mu$g dose of DAMGO.

To determine whether the DAMGO-induced increase in nitric oxide production is related to the suppression of proliferation to TSST-1, the nitric oxide synthase inhibitor, N-monomethyl-L-arginine (L-NMMA), was added to the splenocyte cultures stimulated with TSST-1. As predicted, the addition of L-NMMA antagonizes the suppressive effect of DAMGO on proliferation induced by TSST-1, as shown in Figure 6. Figure 6 also shows that the effect of L-NMMA is stereoselective, for the addition of the inactive enantiomer, D-NMMA, does not attenuate the suppressive effect of DAMGO.

To verify that DAMGO was modulating immune status through the classic $\mu$-opioid receptor, an antagonism study was conducted administering N-methylnaltrexone and DAMGO icv and measuring nitric oxide production and lymphocyte proliferation in splenocyte cultures. Those studies showed that N-methylnatrexone blocks the effects of DAMGO, indicating that the agonist is acting at $\mu$ opioid receptor in the CNS to modulate splenic nitric oxide production and lymphocyte proliferation.

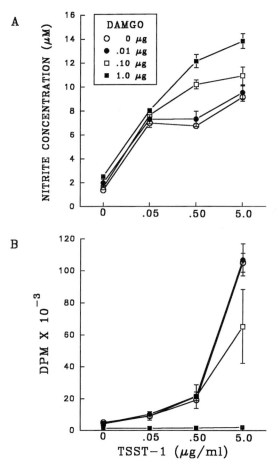

**FIGURE 5** Results from Icv microinjection of DAMGO. (A) Nitrite present in supernatant from TSST-1 stimulated splenocyte cultures from rats that received Icv administration of DAMGO. The data are expressed for each group of rats as the mean (±SE) of the averaged duplicate nitrite determinations. (B) Proliferative responses of splenocytes to increasing concentrations of TSST-1 following ICV administration of DAMGO. [³H]Thymidine incorporation is expressed as the mean (±SE) of the averaged triplicate disintegrations per minute (dpm). (From Schneider & Lysle, *Journal of Neuroimmunology*, *89*, 153, 1998 with permission from Elsevier Science).

To determine the involvement of $\kappa$- and $\delta$- opioid receptors in the regulation of nitric oxide, we assessed the effects of microinjection of the $\kappa$-selective agonist, U69,593 and $\delta$-selective opioid agonist, DPDPE, on nitric oxide production. The results show that microinjection of either U69,593 or DPDPE has no significant effect on the production of nitric oxide by splenocytes, as determined by nitrite levels produced in response stimulation by TSST-1. Moreover, U69,593 and DPDPE do not alter the proliferative response of splenocytes to TSST-1. These results suggest that $\kappa$- and $\delta$-opioid receptors within the central nervous system are not involved in the regulation of nitric oxide production or proliferative responses of splenocytes. Additional studies found that addition of

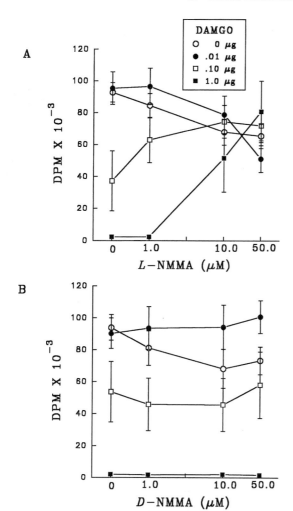

**FIGURE 6** Results from the addition of L-NMMA and D-NMMA to splenocyte cultures. Following Icv administration of DAMGO splenocytes were activated with the optimal concentration of TSST-1 (5.0 μg/mL) and increasing concentrations of L-NMMA were added to culture. [$^3$H]Thymidine incorporation is expressed as the mean (±SEM) of the averaged triplicate disintegrations per minute (dpm). (B) Displays the results of the addition of D-NMMA in place of L-NMMA. (From Schneider & Lysle, *Journal of Neuroimmunology*, **89**, 157, 1998 with permission from Elsevier Science).

DAMGO, U69,593, or DPDPE to cultures, in concentrations as high $10^{-4}$ M, has no effect on splenocyte nitric oxide production or lymphocyte proliferation (Schneider & Lysle, 1998). Together, these results indicate that central, but not the peripheral, μ-opioid receptors are involved in the modulation of nitric oxide production and lymphocyte proliferation.

Studies designed to determine the role of activity at μ- κ- and δ-opioid receptors in conditioned immuno-modulation have found effects parallel to what has been reported using selective opioid agonists (Perez Lysle, 1997). These studies evaluated the effects of selective opioid receptor antagonists on conditioned stimulus-induced alterations in immune status. The results show that icv administration of naltrexone or the μ$_1$- selective opioid antagonist naloxonazine blocks conditioned alterations of immune status, indicating that activity at μ-opioid receptors is involved in conditioned immunomodulation. Further support for the involvement of μ-opioid receptors within the central nervous system is provided by data showing that peripheral administration of naloxonazine, at doses shown to be effective when administered icv, had no effect on conditioned alterations of immune status. Ventricular administration of the κ-selective receptor antagonist nor-binaltorphimine does not antagonize the immunomodulatory effects of the conditioned stimulus. Moreover, administration of the δ receptor antagonist naltrindole also does not antagonize the conditioned alterations of immune status. The results of this study indicate that the alterations of immune status produced by an aversive conditioned stimulus require activity at μ-opioid receptors, possibly at the μ$_1$ receptor subtype, within the central nervous system.

Although the prior data indicate that endogenous opioid activity within the central nervous system can modulate nitric oxide production, these studies are based strictly on in vitro assessments of nitric oxide production. To test whether the in vivo induction of iNOS expression involves endogenous opioid activity within the central nervous system, we evaluated the effect of ICV administration of the opioid receptor antagonist, *N*-methylnaltrexone, on LPS-induced expression of iNOS by splenocytes (Lysle & How, 1999). LPS is a potent stimulator of iNOS in vivo (Liu, Ian, Old, Barnes, & Evans, 1993; Liu, Barnes, & Evans, 1997). Our hypothesis, which was based largely on our prior work, was that blockage of opioid receptors in the central nervous system would inhibit the expression of iNOS by splenocytes following injection with LPS. To measure nitric oxide production in vivo, RT-PCR and Western blotting techniques were used to measure iNOS mRNA and protein expression in spleen tissue, and Griess reagent was used to measure nitrite/nitrate in plasma. Naltrexone induces a pronounced dose-dependent reduction in iNOS mRNA and protein expression by splenocytes, and reduces the level of nitrate/nitrite in the plasma. The modulation of iNOS expression occurs *via* central opioid receptors, since icv but not peripheral administration of *N*-methylnaltrexone reduces the expression of iNOS. These findings, displayed in Figure 7, indicate that central opioid receptors are involved in the in vivo regulation of splenic nitric oxide production.

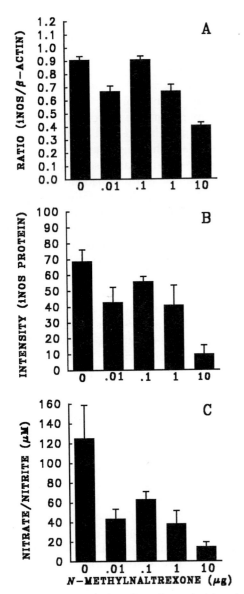

**FIGURE 7**   Results show the effect of icv administration of *N*-methylnaltrexone (0, .01, .1, 1.0,10) on LPS-induced expression of nitric oxide. *N*-methylnaltrexone was injected at the same time as LPS, and the same dose of *N*-methylnaltrexone was administered again 4 h later. Rats were sacrificed 8 h following the injection of LPS. Figure 6A shows the effect of *N*-methylnaltrexone on the ratio of iNOS/β-actin mRNA expression as determine by RT-PCR. Figure 6B shows the results of the densitometric analysis of the bands from the Western blot for iNOS protein. Figure 6C shows the effect of *N*-methylnaltrexone on serum nitrate/nitrite levels in the plasma expressed in μM. (From Lysle & How, *Journal of Pharmacology and Experimental Therapeutics*, 1999 with permission).

## III.  IMPLICATIONS

The research reported in this chapter provides only a brief overview of the continuously expanding field of investigation into the role of nitric oxide in neural-immune interactions. Over the past few years, there has been tremendous growth in the understanding of the factors controlling the activation of NOS and the functional significance of the production of this class of enzymes. The story is more complex than anyone would have previously thought with the list of functional consequences rapidly growing. Recent advances in molecular biology have facilitated the pioneering efforts to elucidate the signals that influence the production and actions of nitric oxide, and further understanding of the numerous physiological and pathophysiological processes of nitric oxide will benefit from the recognition that neural-immune interactions are important to these processes.

The study of nitric oxide also has led the way for the investigation of the role of other gaseous molecules in neural-immune interactions. Carbon monoxide is produced as a by-product of heme catabolism to biliverdin by the enzyme heme oxygenase and has many of the same biological properties as nitric oxide. Like nitric oxide, carbon monoxide stimulates the production of cGMP by interacting with the heme moiety of guanylyl cyclase (Ramos, Lin, & McGrath, 1989) and causes blood vessel relaxation and platelet inhibition through a cGMP-dependent mechanism (Brune & Ullrich, 1987; Graser, Vedernikov, & Li, 1990). Recent reports indicate that vascular smooth muscle cells express two isoforms of heme oxygenase, an inducible form, heme oxygenase-1, and a constitutive form, heme oxygenase-2 (Christodoulides, Durante, Kroll, & Schafer, 1995). Heme oxygenase-1 is found in macrophages, and in vivo heme oxygenase-1 activity increases in a model of acute inflammation in the rat induced by injection of carageenin into the peritoneal cavity (Willis, Moore, Frederick, & Willoughby, 1996). Thus, there is tremendous similarity between nitric oxide and carbon monoxide, and the future of nitric oxide and the larger class of biologically formed gaseous molecules has yet to be realized.

## Acknowledgments

This research was supported by grants from the National Institute on Drug Abuse (DA10167; DA07481). Donald T. Lysle is the recipient of a Research Scientist Development Award (DA00334) from the National Institute on Drug Abuse.

## References

Albina, J. E., & Henry, W. L. (1991). Suppression of lymphocyte proliferation through the nitric oxide synthesizing pathway. *Journal of Surgical Research, 50*, 403–409.

Ader, R., & Cohen, N. (1975). Behaviorally conditioned immunosuppression. *Psychosomatic Medicine, 37*, 333–340.

Ader, R., & Cohen, N. (1982). Behaviorally conditioned immuno-suppression and murine systemic lupus erythematosus. *Science, 215*, 1534–1536. .

Al-Ramadi, B. K., Meissler, J. J., Huang, D., & Eisenstein, T. K. (1992). Immunosuppression induced by nitric oxide and its inhibition by interleukin-4. *European Journal of Immunology, 22*, 2249–2254.

Asano, K., Chee, C., Gaston, B., Lilly, C. M., Gerard, C., Drazen, J. M., & Stamler, J. S. (1994). Constitutive and inducible nitric oxide synthase gene expression, regulation, and acitvity in human lung epithelial cells. *Proceedings of the The National Academy of Sciences USA, 91*, 10089–10093

Bandaletova, T., Brouet, I., Bartsch, H., Sugimura, T., Esumi, H., & Ohshima, H. (1993). Immunohistochemical localization of an inducible form of nitric oxide synthase in various organs of rats treated with Propionibacteriumacnes and lipopolysaccharide. *Apmis, 101*, 330–336.

Bernabeu, R., Stein, M. L., Fin, C., Izquierdo, I., & Medina, J. H. (1995). Role of hippocampal NO in acquisition and consolida-tion of inhibitory avoidance learning. *Neuroreport, 6*, 1498–1500.

Brown, D. R., & Goldberg, L. I. (1985). The use of quaternary narcotic antagonists in opiate research. *Neuropharmacology, 24*, 181–191.

Brune, B., & Ullrich, V. (1987). Inhibition of platelet aggregation by carbon monoxide is mediated by activation of guanylate cyclase. *Molecular Pharmacology, 32*, 497–504.

Bukilica, M., Djordjevic, S., Maric, I., Dimitrijevic, M., Markovic, B. M., & Jankovic, B. D. (1991). Stress-induced suppression of Experimental allergic encephalomyelitis in the rat. *International Journal of Neuroscience, 59*, 167–175.

Cardillo, C., Kilcoyne, C. M., Quyyumi, A. A., Cannon, R. O., & Panza, J. A. (1997). Role of nitric oxide in the vasodilator response to mental stress in normal subjects. *American Journal of Cardiology, 80*, 1070–1074.

Carr, D. J. (1991). The role of endogenous opioids and their receptors in the immune system. *Proceedings of The Society of Experimental Biology and Medicine, 198*, 710–720.

Carr, D. J. J., DeCosta, B. R., Kim, C. H., Jacoben, A. E., Rice, K. C., & Blalock, J. E. (1989). Opioid receptors on cells of the immune system: Evidence for delta and kappa classes. *Journal of Endocrinology, 122*, 161–168.

Cho, H. J., Xie, Q., Calaycay, J., Mumfors, R. A., Swiderek, K. M., Lee, T. D., & Nathan, C. (1992). Calcodulin as a tightly bound subunit of calcium-, calmodulin-independent nitric oxide synthase. *Journal of Experimental Medicine, 176*, 599–604.

Christodoulides, N., Durante, W., Kroll, M. H., & Schafer, A. I. (1995). Vascular smooth muscle cell heme oxygenases generate guanylyl cyclase-stimulatory carbon monoxide. *Circulation, 91*, 2306–2309.

Cobb, B. L., Ryan, K. L., Frei, M. R., Guel-Gomez, V., & Mickley, G. A. (1995). Chronic administration of L-name in drinking water alters working memory in rats. *Brain Research Bulletin, 38*, 203–207.

Corbett, J. A., Tilton, R. G., Chang, K., Hasan, K. S., Ido, Y., Wang, J. L., Sweetland, M. A., Lancaster, J. R., Jr., Williamson, J. R., & McDaniel, M. L. (1992). Aminoguanidine, a novel inhibitor of nitric oxide formation, prevents diabetic vascular dysfunction. *Diabetes, 41*, 552–556.

Coussons-Read, M. E., Maslonek, K. A., Fecho, K., Perez, L., & Lysle, D. T. (1994). Evidence for the involvement of macrophage-derived nitric oxide in the modulation of immune status by a conditioned aversive stimulus. *Journal of Neuroimmunology, 50*, 51–58.

Crabtree, G. R., Munck, A., & Smith, K. A. (1980). Glucocorticoids and lymphocytes. II. Cell-cycle dependent changes in glucocor-ticoid receptor content. *Journal of Immunology, 125*, 13–17.

Demas, G. E., Eliasson, M. J. L., Dawson, T. M., Dawson, V. L., Kriegsfeld, L. J., Nelson, R. J., & Snyder, S. H. (1997). Inhibition of neuronal nitric oxide synthase increases aggressive behavior in mice. *Molecular Medicine, 3*, 610–616.

Dietz, N. M., Rivera, J. M., Eggener, S. E., Fix, R. T., Warner, D. O., & Joyner, M. J. (1994). Nitric oxide contributes to the rise in forearm blood flow during mental stress in humans. *Journal of Physiology, 480*, 361–368.

Dinerman, J. L., Dawson, T. M., Schell, M. J., Snowman, A., & Snyder, S. H. (1994). Endothelial nitric oxide synthase localized to hippocampal pyramidal cells: Implications for synaptic plasticity. *Proceedings of The National Academy of Sciences USA, 91*, 4214–4218.

Drake, C. G., & Kotzin, B. L. (1992). Superantigens: Biology, immunology, and potential role in disease. *Clinical Immunology, 12*, 149–162.

Dun, N. L., Dun, S. L., Forstersmann, U., & Tseng, L. F. (1992). Nitric oxide synthase immunoreactivity in rat spinal cord. *Neuroscience Letters, 147*, 217–220.

Dun, N. J., Dun, S. L. Wu, S. Y., & Forstermann, U. (1993). Nitric oxide synthase immunoreactivity in rat superior cervical ganglia and adrenal glands. *Neuroscience Letters, 158*, 51–54.

Eisenstein, T. K., Huang, D. Meissler, J. J., & Al-Ramadi, B. (1994). Macrophage nitric oxide mediates immunosuppression in infectious inflammation. *Immunobiology, 191*, 493–502.

Emmerson, P. J., Liu, M. R., Woods, J. H., & Medzihradsky, F. (1994). Binding affinity and selectivity of opioids at mu, delta and kappa receptors in monkey brain membranes. *Journal of Pharmacology and Experimental Therapeutics, 271*, 1630–1637.

Estall, L. B., Grant, S. J., & Cicala, G. A. (1993). Inhibition of nitric oxide (NO) production selectively impairs learning and memory in the rat. *Pharmacology, Biochemistry, and Behavior, 46*, 959–962.

Farrell, A. J., Blake, D. R., Palmer, R. M. J., & Moncada, S. (1992). Increased concentrations of nitrite in synovial fluid and serum samples suggest increased nitric oxide synthesis in rheumatic diseases. *Annals of Rheumatic Diseases, 51*, 1219–1222.

Fecho, K., Maslonek, K. A., Coussons-Read, M. E., Dykstra, L. A., & Lysle, D. T. (1994). Macrophage-derived nitric oxide is involved in the depressed Con A-responsiveness of splenic lymphocytes from rats administered morphine in-vivo. *Journal of Immunology, 152*, 5845–5852.

Fecho, K., Maslonek, K. A., Dykstra, L. A., & Lysle, D. T. (1995). Mechanisms whereby macrophage-derived nitric oxide is involved in morphine-induced suppression of splenic lympho-cyte proliferation. *Journal of Pharmacology and Experimental Therapeutics, 272*, 477–483.

Felten, D. L., Felten, S. Y., Carlson, S. L., Olschowka, J. A., & Livnat S. (1985). Noradrenergic and peptidergic innervation of lym-phoid tissue. *Journal of Immunology, 135*, 755s–765s.

Froelich, C. J., & Bankhurst, A. D. (1984). The effect of β-endorphin on natural cytotoxicity and antibody dependent cellular cyto-toxicity. *Life Sciences, 35*, 261–265.

Fu, Y., & Blankenhorn, E. P. (1992). Nitric oxide-induced anti-mitogenic effects in high and low responder strains. *Journal of Immunology, 148*, 2217–2222.

Gilligan, D. M., Panza, J. A., Kilcoyne, C. M., Waclawiw, M. A., Casion, P. R., & Quyyumi, A. A. (1994). Contribution of endo-thelium-derived nitric oxide to exercise-induced vasodilation. *Circulation, 90*, 2853–2858.

Gilmore, W., & Weiner, L. P. (1988). Beta-endorphin enhances interleukin-2 production in murine lymphocytes. *Journal of Neuroimmunology, 18*, 125–130.

Goldstein, A. (1987). Binding selectivity profiles for ligands of multiple receptor types: Focus on opioid receptors. *Trends in Pharmacological Sciences, 8*, 456–466.

Goretski, J., & Hollocher, T. C. (1988). Trapping of nitric oxide produced during denitrification by extracellular hemoglobin. *Journal of Biological Chemistry, 263*, 2316–2323.

Graser, T., Vedernikov, Y. P., & Li, D. S. (1990). Study on the mechanism of carbon monoxide induced endothelium-independent relaxation in porcine coronary artery and vein. *Biomedical and Biochemical Acta, 49*, 293–296.

Green, L. C., Wagner, D. A., Glogowski, J., Skipper, P. L.,Wishnok, J. S., & Tannenbaum, S. R. (1982). Analysis of nitrate, nitrite, and [$^{15}$N]nitrate in biological fluids. *Analytic Biochemistry, 126*, 131–136.

Green, S. J., Meltzer, M. S. Hibbs, J. B., & Nacy, C. A. (1990). Activated macrophages destroy intracellular *Leishmania major* amastigotes by an L-arginine-dependent killing mechanism. *Journal of Immunology, 144*, 278–283.

Green, S. J., & Nacy, C. A. (1993). Antimicrobial and immuno-pathologic effect of cytokine-induced nitric oxide synthesis. *Current Opinions on Infectious Diseases, 6*, 384–396.

Haslett, C. (1992). Resolution of acute inflammation and the role of apoptosis in tissue fate of graulocytes. *Clinical Science, 83*, 639–648.

Hassall, C. J., Saffrey, M. J., Belai, A., Hoyle, C. H., Moules, E. W., Moss, J., Schmidt, H. H., Murad, F., Forstermann, U., & Burnstock, G. (1992). Nitric oxide synthase immunoreactivity and NADPH-diaphorase activity in a subpopulation of intrinsic neurones of the guinea-pig heart. *Neuroscience Letters, 143*, 65–68.

Hibbs, J. B., Tiantor, R. R., & Vavrin, Z. (1987). Macrophage cytotoxicity: Role for L-arginine deaminase and iminonitrogen-oxidation of nitrite. *Science, 235*, 473–476.

Iwanaka, T., Arkovitz, M. S., Arya, G., & Ziegler, M. M. (1997). Evaluation of operative stress and peritoneal macrophage function in minimally invasive operations. *Journal of American College of Surgery, 184*, 357–363.

Iyengar, R., Stuehr, D. J., & Marletta, M. A. (1987). Macrophage synthesis of nitrite, nitrate, and *N*-nitrosamines: Precursors and role of the respiratory burst. *Proceedings of The National Academy of Sciences, USA, 84*, 6369–6373.

James, S. L., & Glaven, J. (1989). Macrophage cytotoxicity against schistosomula of *Schistosoma mansoni* involves arginine-dependent production of reactive nitrogen intermediates. *Journal of Immunology, 143*, 4208–4212.

Joannides, R., Haefeli, W. E., Linder, L., Richard, V., Bakkali, E. H., Thuillez, C., & Luscher, T. F. (1995). Nitric oxide is responsible for flow-dependent dilatation of human peripheral conduit arteries in vivo. *Circulation, 91*, 1314–1319.

Karapiah, G., Xie, Q., Buller, R. M. L., Nathan, C., Duarte, C., & MacMicking, J. D. (1993). Inhibition of viral replication by interferon gamma induced nitric oxide synthase. *Science, 261*, 1445–1448.

Kilbourn, R. G., Jubran, A., Gross, S. S., Griffith, O. W., Levi, R., Adams, J., & Lodato, R. F. (1991). Reversal of endotoxin-mediated shock by $N^g$-methyl-L arginine, an inhibitor of nitric oxide synthesis. *Biochemical and Biophysical Research Communications, 172*, 1132–1138.

Kizaki, T., Oh-Ishi, S., & Ohno, H. (1996). Acute cold stress induces suppressor macrophages in mice. *Journal of Applied Physiology, 81*, 393–399.

Kolb, H., Kiesel, U., Kroncke, K. D., & Bachofen, V. (1991). Suppression of low doses of streptozocin induced diabetes in mice by administration of a nitric oxide synthase inhibitor. *Life Sciences, 49*, 213–217.

Laudenslager, M. L., Fleshner, M., Hofstadter, P., Held, P. E., Simons, L., & Maier, S. F. (1988). Suppression of specific antibody production by inescapable shock: Stability under varying conditions. *Brain, Behavior, and Immunity, 2*, 92–101.

Laudenslager, M. L., Ryan, S. M., Drugan, R. C., Hyson, R. L., & Maier, S. F. (1983). Coping and immunosuppression: inescapable but not escapable shock suppresses lymphocyte proliferation, *Science, 221*, 568–570.

Lewis, J. W., Shavit, Y., Terman, G. W., Gale, R. P., & Liebeskind, J. C. (1983/84). Stress and morphine affect survival of rats challenged with a mammary ascites tumor (MAT 13762B), *Natural Immunity and Cell Growth Regulation, 3*, 43–50.

Lewis, J. W., Shavit, Y., Terman, G. W., Nelson, L. R., Gale, R. P., & Liebeskind, J. C. (1983). Apparent involvement of opioid peptides in stress-induced enhancement of tumor growth. *Peptides, 4*, 635–638.

Liu, S., Barnes, P. J., & Evans, T. W. (1997). Time course and cellular localization of lipopolysaccharide-induced inducible nitric oxide synthase messenger RNA in the rat in vivo. *Critical Care Medicine, 25*, 512–518.

Liu, S., Ian, M., Old, R. W., Barnes, P. J., & Evans, T. W. (1993). Lipopolysaccharide treatment in-vivo induces widespread tissue expression of inducible nitric oxide synthase mRNA. *Biochemical and Biophysical Research Communications, 196*, 1208–1213.

Luecken, L. J., & Lysle, D. T. (1992). Evidence for the involvement of $\beta$-adrenergic receptor in conditioned immunomodulation. *Journal of Neuroimmunology, 38*, 209–220.

Lukic, M. L., Stosic,-Grujicic, S., Ostojic, N., Chan, W. L., & Liew, F. Y. (1991). Inhibition of nitric oxide generation affects the induction of diabetes by streptozocin in mice. *Biochemical and Biophysical Research Communications, 178*, 913–920.

Lysle, D. T., Coussons, M. E., Watts, V. J., Bennett, E. H., & Dykstra, L. A. (1993). Morphine-induced alterations of immune status: Dose-dependency, compartment specificity and antagonism by naltrexone. *Journal of Pharmacology and Experimental Therapeutics, 265*, 1071–1078.

Lysle, D. T., Cunnick, J. E., Fowler, H., & Rabin B. S. (1988). Pavlovian conditioning of shock-induced suppression of lymphocyte reactivity: Acquisition, extinction, and preexposure effects, *Life Sciences, 42*, 2185–2194.

Lysle, D. T., Cunnick, J. E., Kucinski, B. J., Fowler, H., & Rabin, B. S. (1990). Characterization of immune alterations induced by a conditioned aversive stimulus, *Psychobiology, 18*, 220–226.

Lysle, D. T., & How T. (1999). Endogenous opioids regulate the expression of inducible nitric oxide synthease by splenocytes. *Journal of Pharmacology and Experimental Therapeutics, 288*, 502–508.

Lysle, D. T., Luecken, L. J., & Maslonek, K. A. (1992a). Modulation of immune status by a conditioned aversive stimulus: Evidence for the involvement of endogenous opioids. *Brain, Behavior, and Immunity, 6*, 179–188.

Lysle, D. T., Luecken, L. J., & Maslonek, K. A. (1992b). Suppression of the development of adjuvant arthritis by a conditioned aversive stimulus. *Brain, Behavior, and Immunity, 6*, 64–73.

Lysle, D. T., Lyte, M., Fowler, H., & Rabin, B. S. (1987). Shock-induced modulation of lymphocyte reactivity: suppression, habituation, and recovery. *Life Sciences, 41*, 1805–1814. .

MacMicking, J. D., Nathan, C., Hom, G. Chartrain, N., Fletcher, D. S., Trumbauer, M., Stevens, K., Xie, Q. W., Sokol, K., Hutchinson, N. Chen, H., & Mudgett, J. S. (1995). Altered responses to baterial infection and endotoxic shock in mice lacking inducible nitric oxide syntase. *Cell*, *81*, 641–650.

Madden, J. J., Donahoe, R. M., Zwemer-Collins, J., Shafer, D. A., & Falek, A. (1987). Binding of naloxone to human T-lymphocytes. *Biochemical Pharmacology*, *36*, 4103–4109.

Mandler, R. N., Biddison, W. E., Mandler, R., & Serate, S. (1986). β-endorphin augments the cytolytic activity and interferon production of natural killer cells. *Journal of Immunology*, *136*, 934–936.

Marrack, P., & Kappler, J. (1990). The staphylococcal enterotoxins and their relatives. *Science*, *248*, 705–711.

Mathews, P. M., Froelich, C. J., Sibbitt, W. L., & Bankhurst, A. D. (1983). Enhancement of natural cytotoxicity by β-endorphin. *Journal of Immunology*, *130*, 1658–1662.

McCain, H. W., Lamster, I. B., Bozzone, J. M., & Grbic, J. T. (1982). β-endorphin modulates human immune activity via non-opiate receptor mechanisms. *Life Sciences*, *31*, 1619–1624.

McCartney-Francis, N., Allen, J. N., Mizel, D. E., Albina, J., Xie, Q. W., Nathan, C. F., & Wahl, S. M. (1993). Suppression of arthritis by an inhibitor of nitric oxide synthase. *Journal of Experimental Medicine*, *178*, 749–753.

Messmer, U. K., Reimer, D. M., Reed, J. C., & Brune, B. (1996). Nitric oxide induced poly(ADP-ribose) polymerase cleavage in RAW264. 7 macrophage apoptosis is blocked by Bcl-2. *Federation of European Biochemical Societies Letters*, *384*, 162–166.

Middleton, S. J., Sorthouse, M., & Hunter, J. O. (1993). Increased nitric oxide synthesis in ulcerative colitis. *Lancet*, *341*, 465–466.

Miller, M. J. S., Sadowska,-Krowicka, H., Chotinaruemol, S., Kakkis, J. L., & Clark, D. A. (1993). Amelioration of chronic iletis by nitric oxide syntheASE inhibition. *Journal of Pharmacology and Experimental Therpeutics*, *264*, 11–16.

Mulligan, M. S., Hevel, J. M., Marletta, M. A., & Ward, P. A. (1991). Tissue injury caused by deposition of immune complexes is l-arginine dependent. *Proceedings of the National Academy of Sciences USA*, *88*, 6338–6342.

Myatt, L., Brockman, D. E., Eis, A., & Pollock, J. S. (1993). Immunohistochemical localization of nitric oxide synthase in the human placenta. *Placenta*, *14*, 487–495.

Nathan, C. (1992). Nitric oxide as a secretory product of mammalian cells. *Federation of American Societies for Experimental Biology Journal*, *6*, 3051–3064.

Nelson, R. J., Demas, G. E., Huang, P. L., Fishman, M. C., Dawson, V. L., Dawson, T. M., & Synder, S. H. (1995). Behavioural abnormalities in male mice lacking neuronal nitric oxide synthase. *Nature*, *378*, 383–386.

Nussler, A. K., & Billiar, T. R. (1993). Inflammation, immunoregulation and inducible nitric oxide synthase. *Journal of Leukocyte Biology*, *54*, 171–178.

Ohno, M., Yamamoto, T., & Watanabe, S. (1993). Deficits in working memory following inhibition of hippocampal nitric oxide synthesis in the rat. *Brain Research*, *632*, 36–40.

Onsrud, M., & Thorsby, E. (1981). Influence of in vivo hydrocortisone on some human blood lymphocyte populations. I. effect on natural killer cell activity. *Scandanavian Journal of Immunology*, *13*, 573–579.

Palmer, R. M. J., Ferrige, A. G., & Moncada, S. (1987). Nitric oxide accounts for the biological activity of endothelium-derived relaxing factor. *Nature*, *327*, 524–526.

Pascual, D. W., Pascual, V. H., Bost, K. L., McGhee J. R., & Oparil, S. (1992). Nitric oxide mediates immune dysfunction in the spontaneously hypertensive rat. *Hypertension*, *21*, 185–194.

Pellat, C., Henry, Y., & Drapier, J. C. (1990). IFN-γ activated macrophages: detection by electron paramagnetic resonance of complexes between L-arginine- derived nitric oxide and non-heme iron proteins. *Biochemical and Biophysical Research Communications*, *166*, 119–125.

Perez, L., & Lysle, D. T. (1997). Conditioned immunomodulation: investigations of the role of endogenous activity at μ, κ, and δ opioid receptor subtypes. *Journal of Neuroimmunology*, *79*, 101–112.

Persoons, J. H. A., Schornagel, K., Breve, J., & Berkenbosch, F. (1995). Acute stress affects cytokines and nitric oxide production by alveolar macrophages differently. *American Journal of Respiratory and Critical Medicine*, *152*, 619–624.

Pollack, J. S., Nakane, M., Buttery, L. K., Martinez, A., Springall, D., Polak, J. M., Forstermann, U., & Murad, F. (1993). Characterization and localization of endothelial nitric oxide synthase using specific monoclonal antibodies. *American Journal of Physiology*, *265*, C1379–C1387.

Ramos, K. S., Lin, H., & McGrath, J. J. (1989). Modulation of cyclic guanosine monophosphate levels in cultured smooth muscle cells by carbon monoxide. *Biochemical Pharmacology*, *38*, 1368–1370.

Saffrey, M. J., Hassall, C. J., Hoyle, C. H., Belai, A., Moss, J., Schmidt, H. H., Forstermann, U., Murad, F., & Burnstock, G. (1992). Colocalization of nitric oxide synthase and NADPH-diaphorase in cultured myenteric neurons. *Neuroreport*, *3*, 333–336.

Savill, J. (1997). Apoptosis in resolution of inflammation. *Journal of Leukocyte Biology*, *61*, 375–380.

Schmidt, H. H. H. W., Gagne, G. D., Nakane, M., Pollock, J. S., Miller, M. F., & Murad, F. (1992a). Mapping of neural nitric oxide synthase in the rat suggests frequent colocalization with NADPH diaphorase but not with soluble guanylyl cyclase, and novel paraneural functions for nitrinergic signal transduction. *Journal of Histochemistry and Cytochemistry*, *40*, 1439–1456.

Schmidt, H. H. H. W., Warner, T. D., Ishii, K., Sheng, H., & Murad, F. (1992b). Insulin secretion from pancreatic B cells caused by l-arginine-derived nitrogen oxides. *Science*, *255*, 721–723.

Schneider, G. M., & Lysle, D. T. (1998). Role of central mu-opioid receptors in the modulation of nitric oxide production by splenocytes. *Journal of Neuroimmunology*, *89*, 150–159.

Schwab, J. H., Brown, R. B., Aderle, S. K., & Schlievert, P. M. (1993). Superanitgen can reactivate bacterial cell wall-induced arthritis. *Journal of Immunology*, *150*, 4151–4159.

Shavit, Y., DePaulis, A., Martin, F. C., Terman, G. W., Pechnick, R. N., Zane, C. J., Gale, R. P., & Liebeskind, J. C. (1986). Involvement of brain opiate receptors in the immune-suppressive effect of morphine. *Proceedings of the National Academy of Sciences USA*, *83*, 7114–7117.

Shavit, Y., Lewis, J. W., Terman, G. W., Gale, R. P., & Liebeskind, J. C. (1984). Opioid peptides mediate the suppressive effect of stress on natural killer cell cytotoxicity, *Science*, *223*, 188–190.

Sheng, H., Gagne, G. D., Matsumoto, T., Miller, M. F., Forstermann, U., & Murad, F. (1993). Nitric oxide synthase in bovine superior cervical ganglion. *Journal of Neurochemistry*, *61*, 1120–1126.

Singhal, P. C., Sharma, P., Kapasi, A. A., Reddy, K., Franki, N., & Gibbons, N. (1998). Morphine enhances macrophage apoptosis. *Journal of Immunology*, *160*, 1886–1893.

Stefanovic-Racic, M., Stadler, J., & Evans, C. (1993). Nitric oxide and arthritis. *Arthritis and Rheumatism*, *36*, 1037–1044.

Tracey, W. R., Pollock, J. S., Murad, F., Nakane, M., & Forstermann, U. (1994). Identification of a type III (endothelial-like) particulate nitric oxide synthase in LLC-PK1 kidney tubular epithelial cells. *American Journal of Physiology*, *266*, C22–C26.

Vallance, P., Collier, J., & Moncada, S. (1989). Effects of endothelium-derived nitric oxide on peripheral arteriolar tone in man. *Lancet*, *2*, 997–1000.

Van Epps, D. E., & Saland, L. (1984). Beta-endorphin and met-enkephalin stimulate human peripheral-blood mononuclear cell chemotaxis, *Journal of Immunology, 132,* 3046–3053.

Vincendeau, P., Daulouede, S., Veyret, B., Darde, M. L., Bouteille, B., & Lemesre, J. L. (1992). Nitric oxide-mediated cytostatic activity on *Trypanosoma brucei gambiense* and *Trypanosoma brucei brucei. Experimental Parasitology, 75,* 353–360.

Visintainer, M. A., Volpicelli, J. R., & Seligman, M. E. P. (1982). Tumor rejection in rats after inescapable or escapable shock. *Science, 216,* 437–439.

Wei, X. Q., Charles, I. G., Smith, A., Ure, J., Feng, G. J., Huang, F. P., Xu, D., Muller, W., Mocado, S., & Liew, F. Y. (1995). Altered immune responses in mice lacking inducible nitric oxide synthase. *Nature, 375,* 408–411.

Weinberg, J. B., Granger, D. L., Pisetsky, D. S., Seldin, M. F., Misuknois, M. A., Mason, S. N., Pippen, A. M., Ruiz, P. Wood, E. R., & Gilkeson., G. S. (1994). The role of nitric oxide in the pathogenesis of spontaneous murine autoimmune disease: Increased nitric oxide production and nitric oxide synthase expression in MRL-lpr/lpr mice, and reduction of spontaneous glomerulonephritis and arthritis by orally administered $N^G$-monomethyl-Larginine. *Journal of Experimental Medicine, 179,* 651–660.

White, H., Herman, A., Pullen, A. M., Kubo, R., Kappler, J. W., & Marrack, P. (1989). The V$\beta$ specific superantigen staphylococcal enterotoxin B: Stimulation of mature T cells and clonal deletion in neonatal mice. *Cell, 56,* 27–35.

Willis, D., Moore, A. R., Frederick, R., & Willoughby, D. A. (1996). Heme oxygenase: A novel target for the modulation of the inflammatory response. *Nature and Medicine, 2,* 87–90.

Wybran, J., Applebloom, T., Famaey, J. P., & Gavaerts, A. (1979). Suggestive evidence for receptors for morphine and methionine enkephalin on normal human peripheral blood T-lymphocytes. *Journal of Immunology, 123,* 1068–1070.

Xue, C., Pollock, J., Schmidt, H. H. H. W., Ward, S. M., & Sanders, K. M. (1994). Expression of nitric oxide synthase immunoreactivity by interstitial cells of the canine proximal colon. *Journal of The Autonomic Nervous System, 49,* 1–14.

# Immunologic Effects of Acute versus Chronic Stress in Animals

ALEXANDER W. KUSNECOV, ALAN SVED, BRUCE S. RABIN

I. IMPORTANT ISSUES RELATING TO ACUTE AND
 CHRONIC STRESSORS
II. ACUTE AND CHRONIC STRESS AND
 IMMUNE FUNCTION
III. CONCLUSION

It is now a well documented fact in animal and human research that stress impacts on the immune system (Anisman, Zalcman, & Zacharko, 1993; Glaser & Kiecolt-Glaser, 1998; Kusnecov & Rabin, 1994; Miller, 1998). However, the sobering and frustrating reality is that it remains very difficult to predict what manner of immunological outcomes will ensue following exposure to specific stressors. Such a problem should be less apparent with animal research, where investigators have more latitude in controlling a considerable number of experimental variables. Nonetheless, the multitude of different experimental approaches (e.g., variations in animal subjects, types of stressors, variations in stressor application, types of immune measures) and findings is somewhat daunting and, viewed globally, presents a perplexing array of heterogeneous and seemingly incoherent information. Historically, such a situation jeopardizes the viability of a specific research field, unless some semblance of order can be discerned.

In preparing this chapter, and from our own experience (Cunnick, Lysle, Armfield, & Rabin, 1988; Esterling & Rabin, 1987; Kusnecov et al., 1995; Shanks & Kusnecov, 1998), there is little question that in experimental animals "stressful stimuli" alter the activity of a variety of components of the immune system (e.g., antibody production or lymphocyte mitogenic function). However, it was also clear that apparently similar experiential events result in null or opposite immunological effects. The lack of systematic studies designed to address "contradictory" or seemingly incompatible results exemplifies the obstacles still present in achieving a full appreciation and understanding of the impact of stress on immune function. As we and others have already stated, there are many levels of analysis—e.g., gender, age, genotype—that are required to achieve the typical scientific goals of understanding and prediction (Ader & Cohen, 1993; Kusnecov & Rabin, 1994; Moynihan & Ader, 1996). In the present chapter, we have attempted to examine the vast literature dealing with stress-evoked immune alterations from the perspective of acute and chronic stress.

How do we define acute and chronic stress in a physiologically (or pathophysiologically) relevant manner? How do we study the immune altering effect of acute or chronic stress in a rigorous and controlled way? Equally critical is the concern regarding which of the numerous aspects of immune function have biological relevance when altered by stress? Answers to these questions can only be derived empirically, although we will examine some of the issues we believe to be relevant, reviewing in the process some studies that have nominally attempted to compare acute and chronic stressor effects on immune function.

# I. IMPORTANT ISSUES RELATING TO ACUTE AND CHRONIC STRESSORS

## A. The Concepts of Acute and Chronic

The issue of acute and chronic stress is an essential derivative of studies aimed at understanding how stress affects immunobiological function. Perusal of the literature on acute and chronic stress studies reveals that such research is conducted with the understanding that these terms are used in a relative sense, delineating essentially how often the experimental subject is exposed to the designated stressor stimulus. Thus, a session of electric shock, restraint, cold swim, etc., is an acute stressor, while multiple sessions are referred to as chronic stressors. However, could not the initial impact, within milliseconds, of any of these stressors just as easily be referred to as "acute" and as the exposure is prolonged shifted to "chronic?" This determination cannot be made unless there is a biological marker for a change from acute to chronic. Possible markers could include the electrical activity of single neurons in areas of the brain that are activated by the stressor, the concentration of stress hormones in plasma, or the function of cells of the immune system. Simply to designate seconds as acute and minutes, hours, or days as chronic does not suffice. Furthermore, given that chronic stress is typically used as an instance of repeated exposure to the same acute stress, what assurances are there that the qualitative aspects of the stressor stimulus have not changed? Restraint as a novel imposition on an animal's life has all the elements of surprise and threat. However, the lack of surprise, the predictability of being restrained if repeated enough times, and foreknowledge of the outcome of each restraint session (i.e., return to the home cage), are all variables that differ from the initial restraint episode. Hence, while the physical dimensions of a stressor may have the same characteristics, learning and perceptual elements alter the meaning of a chronic stressor to the animal. This may have a profound impact on biological outcomes observed under so-called acute and chronic stress conditions.

Some researchers have tried to overcome such habituation effects by using stress regimens in which animals are exposed to *heterotypic* (i.e., different stressor stimuli on alternating days or within the same stress session—see Dhabhar and McEwen, 1998) as opposed to *homotypic* stressors (i.e., the same stressor stimulus on each day). This would then assess the impact on behavior and the nervous and immune systems of persistent stressful challenges that vary in form and nature, thereby forcing animals to maintain vigilant states that otherwise would be relaxed if animals acquired prior knowledge of the biological outcome of a given stressor exposure.

Here it is worth commenting on a recent study in which mice exposed daily to conflict stress (i.e., fighting with an intruder mouse) showed no signs of habituated brain c-*fos* expression, a measure of neural activation (Matsuda, Peng, Yoshimura, Wen, Fukuda, & Sakanaka, 1996). This contrasts considerably with other findings of repeated immobilization leading to complete absence of c-*fos* mRNA increases (and presumably c-Fos protein) (Melia, Ryabinin, Schroeder, Bloom, & Wilson, 1994; Watanabe, Stone, & McEwen, 1994). Thus, whereas repeated immobilization has certain predictive properties after multiple exposures (e.g., no further stimulation other than physical confinement and eventual removal and return to the home cage), conflict stress is unlikely to have such predictive value. Indeed, this was demonstrated using chronic restraint stress, in which habituation of c-*fos* expression was prevented by imposing unpredictable characteristics on the repeated stressor (e.g., shaking) (Watanabe, Stone, & McEwen, 1994).

The impact on the immune system may reflect these different psychological experiences. Presuming that stressor-induced immune modulation is mediated by increased concentrations of blood hormones and peripheral nervous system neurotransmitters and neuropeptides, the reactivity of these mechanisms to higher-order events invoked by stressor exposure may fluctuate erratically and inconsistently under chronic stress conditions that fail to result in habituation. Consequently, sensitive components of the immune system may also fail to habituate, since there is no predictive level of stress-induced increase in the concentration of relevant neuroendocrine factors with repeated exposure to the stressor. That is, as the animal copes with repeated exposure to a homotypic stressor by learning consistent parameters such as onset and duration, this translates into consistent and declining degrees of neuroendocrine activation. However, if such learning were not possible (as with a heterotypic stress regimen), central habituation mechanisms would not be implemented and the neuroendocrine resources may be evoked at consistently high levels.

As with the concept of stress itself, discussion about its acute and chronic aspects can persist without satisfactory closure. For instance, to study chronic stress, is it truly necessary to use a heterotypic approach? Indeed, there are many examples in life where different challenges (all "stressful") arrive one after the other. Alternatively, the same or similar challenge (e.g., academic examination, child rearing, caregiving) arises consistently. Therefore, homotypic approaches are equally justified. In fact, under these circumstances it is possible to ask questions relating to coping or control, wherein failure to habituate may reflect impaired coping abilities.

## B. Physiological Baseline

Another difficult but important problem is characterizing the physiological parameters that exist in a subject at the time an acute or a chronic stress regimen is experienced. The question relates to whether there is ever a time when an experimental subject is not experiencing physiological processes associated with stress. If there are stress hormones present in plasma and tissue, even though an individual is not consciously experiencing a stressor, do the concentrations of hormones present modify in a causal manner the subsequent response to an acute stressor? Furthermore, with respect to studies addressing the effects of stress on antigen specific immune responses, it is important to be aware that an immune reaction to an antigen can modulate peripheral concentrations of stress sensitive neuroendocrine hormones and central neurotransmitter systems that constitute part of the stress circuitry of the brain (Anisman et al., 1993; Besedovsky & del Rey, 1996). Therefore, different stress regimens may constitute additional stimuli to the brain, which already may be under the influence of cytokines emanating from an ongoing immune response. For example, it was demonstrated that a single stressor exposure during the peak phase of the primary antibody response to sheep erythrocytes attenuated the antibody response, whereas acute stressor exposure at other times during the immune response had no effect (Zalcman, Minkiewicz-Janda, Richter, & Anisman, 1988). Interestingly, the same laboratory showed alterations in central monamine neurotransmitters during the peak phase of the antibody response (Zalcman, Shanks, & Anisman, 1991).

While the latter example involved interactions between experimentally induced phenomena, it raises serious concerns about whether the immunologic baseline of animals affects the brain and consequently their reactivity to stress. It is possible to rear animals under germ-free conditions where exposure to antigen is eliminated, but in such animals there is a paucity of lymphoid tissue development. It is likely that the cytokines whose production is elicited by an antigen are important for maturation of the immune system. Finding an environment similar to a germ-free environment in order to limit stimulation of stress

hormone production by baseline immunological processes would be difficult. The baseline to which an acute stress is applied is not a true baseline, but rather a baseline that has been activated to a greater or lesser degree by the environment in which the experimental study subjects reside. Therefore, it is likely that anytime an acute stress is studied in an experimental system, some degree of chronic stimulation is present. The critical question is how much stimulation is present and how that stimulation modifies the response to the acute stressor.

Obviously, appropriate control groups in an experiment provide an estimate of baseline physiological function. However, baselines vary according to housing conditions, and the impact of a stressor (acute or chronic) may differ in terms of immunological outcome. For example, housing either one or five mice in a cage would appear to be a benign event that would not be expected to have a significant impact on how the immune system functions. However, housing different numbers of animals in a cage can markedly influence several components of immune system function (Rabin, Lyte, Epstein, & Caggiula, 1987; Salvin, Rabin, & Neta, 1990). For example, the immune response to sheep erythrocytes requires the CD4 T helper lymphocyte to interact with the antibody producing B lymphocyte before antibody to the sheep erythrocytes will be produced. Thus, by using sheep erythrocytes as an antigen the functional activity of T helper lymphocytes and B lymphocytes can be evaluated. The number of B lymphocytes in the spleen producing antibody to sheep erythrocytes was significantly lower in C3H/HeJ male mice that were housed five per cage in comparison to that seen in those housed alone. To determine whether the T lymphocyte or the B lymphocyte (or both) is functionally altered by the housing conditions, mice were immunized with a T-independent antigen that does not require the participation of a CD4 T helper lymphocyte for antibody production. The antigen used was a carbohydrate that directly interacts with B lymphocytes and causes them to synthesize and release antibody. When the mice were injected with this carbohydrate antigen, equal numbers of antibody-producing B lymphocytes were produced in the spleen of animals housed either one or five per cage. Thus, B-lymphocyte functional activity was not directly altered by the differential housing conditions. However, when a T helper lymphocyte was required to facilitate antibody production, less antibody production occurred in the group housed animals. Therefore, the decrease in antibody production in the group housed mice was due to an altered function of the CD4 T helper lymphocyte population.

These results show that the environment in which one resides may influence the function of the immune system. Similar results in terms of differential immune reactivity to protein antigen in differentially housed mice have been reported by others (Karp, Moynihan, & Ader, 1993, 1997). Therefore, these findings suggest that it is possible that the baseline immune and hormone parameters that are present when antigen is injected likely differed between the group and individually housed animals. Whether one set of housing conditions represents more of a chronic stress condition than the other is not clear; however, the data indicate that the immune system does not function independently of basic living parameters such as the number of cage mates. Differences in housing conditions do not necessarily constitute stressors but ways of existing that impact on the baseline status of the immune system. The impact of stress under such conditions may reveal important differences.

Another example of the influence of the environment on the immune system is provided by studying the effect of social rank on immune function (Cunnick et al., 1991). Male cynomolgus monkeys were housed in groups of five in large pens, with access to the outdoors. Experimental animals were reorganized at 4-week intervals so that each monkey was rehoused with three or four new animals each month. Social rank was determined by observing whether or not a monkey won or lost when fighting with another monkey. The most dominant monkey won all of their fights and the animal that lost all of their fights was the least dominant (submissive). All monkeys, regardless of rank, had access to adequate amounts of food. The immune response measured was the amount of antibody produced subsequent to immunization with tetanus toxoid. For analysis of the data, the monkeys that were ranked numbers 1 and 2, the dominant monkeys, were grouped together and the animals ranked 3, 4, and 5, the subordinate monkeys, were grouped together. Differences in antibody response were not random but were influenced by the social rank of the monkeys. A significant difference in the amount of IgG antibody produced to tetanus was detected between the two groups with the subordinate monkeys producing significantly more antibody. Possibly, the submissive monkey was under the least amount of stress as it knew its place and therefore did not worry about its lowly role. The dominant monkey had to fight to maintain dominance and was experiencing stress because of this. The stress may have decreased the ability of the dominant monkey to produce antibody. Alternatively, the submissive monkey may have been experiencing more stress than the dominant monkey and the stress response enhanced the antibody response.

The baseline physiology that exists in an individual at the time of experiencing a stressor will influence the physiological alterations that are induced. For example, an acute stressor may not produce the same changes in an individual who is experiencing chronic stress as an individual who is not experiencing chronic stress (Pike et al., 1997). Clearly, it is not just experiencing an acute stressor that influences the central nervous system and hormonal response; the background upon which the acute stressor is applied contributes to the characteristics of the response.

Regardless of the explanation for the above findings based on housing and social rank (Cunnick et al., 1991; Karp et al., 1993; Rabin et al., 1987), it is highly likely that some degree of "chronic" stress may always be present. Obtaining unambiguous interpretations of the effect of acute and chronic stress on the immune system will be highly dependent on the experimental conditions and baseline physiologic parameters.

## C. Response to the Same or Different Stressors: Habituation and Sensitization

As already mentioned above repeated stressor application can lead to habituation of a physiological response. However, this does not mean that the ability to react to a new stimulus has declined. For example, repeated exposure to the same stress may decrease the amount of NE released in the brain and into plasma. Alternatively, repeated exposure to the same stress and then exposure to a novel stressor may result in increased release of NE that is significantly greater than the amount of NE released when a nonstressed animal is exposed to the novel stressor (Gresch, Sved, Zigmond, & Finlay, 1994; Konarska, Stewart, & McCarty, 1989; Nisenbaum, Zigmond, Sved, & Abercrombie, 1991). This is termed sensitization. Chronic stress must therefore be evaluated in regard to the declining uniqueness of being exposed repeatedly to the same stressor and the imposition of additional new stressors. Does the chronic stress in an individuals life consist of a prolonged duration of a single stressor or a random exposure to different, heterotypic stressors? Being stressed by one's spouse for a week, financial concerns the next week a medical problem the next week, and job performance the following week may produce different effects in the brain and on the immune system than months of worrying whether your managed care health plan will cover your latest round of medical bills.

An acute response to a stressor may also have a different influence on altering the function of the immune system in a physically fit subject in comparison to a sedentary subject. Exercise produces many of the same hormonal and immune alterations as does psychological stress (Moyna et al., 1996). It is possible that an acute stressor in a physically fit subject is acting on a background that is already experiencing chronic stress and which has achieved a certain degree of habituation. However, it is also possible, depending on the conditions of exercise and stress intensity, that physical fitness may be associated with an enhanced catecholamine response to an acute stress (Levenson & Moore, 1998).

The above considerations are important because different pathways may be involved in conveying the presence of different stressors to the brain and different stressors may be initially perceived in different areas of the brain (for example, noise vs. pain). If pain and chronic loud noise initially activate different neurons but then have a merging of pathways so that they stimulate the same neurons which innervate and alter the function of the immune system, different chronic stressors may invoke the same pathways in their ability to modify the effect of an acute stressor on immune function.

Determination of habituation of glucocorticoid production with repeated or chronic stress has been evaluated in studies of stressor-induced immune alteration. Although the studies were performed in humans, they provide important information that is applicable to animal studies. For example, parachute jumping was utilized as a stressor in humans to evaluate whether habituation of cortisol production occurred with repeated jumping (Deinzer, Kirschbaum, Gresele, & Hellhammer, 1997). After the third jump some of the subjects had significantly lower cortisol responses than after the first and second jumps. However, there were subjects who maintained a high response after the third jump. Thus, habituation does occur in some individuals at a time when it does not occur in others. This suggests a lack of uniformity of glucocorticoid responses in different individuals when experiencing repeated stress. Thus, it can be anticipated that different responses to repeated stress will be elicited in experimental studies. Different species, strains, and genders of animals may respond differently to the process of habituation.

## D. Acute and Chronic Effects in the Brain

The hormonal response to stress may have a direct effect on the anatomy of the brain. Severe acute stress may change the size of the hippocampus (Gurvits et al., 1996) as may high levels of chronic stress (Bremner et al., 1997). Chronic elevation of glucocorticoids, possibly induced by stress, may produce anatomic and functional alterations of hippocampal neurons (Sapolsky, 1996). However, whether this anatomic change alters the subsequent response to stress needs to be determined.

Differential alterations in CNS function after either acute or chronic stress are well documented. For example, neurons in the locus coeruleus (LC) increase their activity in response to acute presentation of stressful stimuli (Aston-Jones, Rajkowski, Kubiak, Valentino, & Shipley, 1996), but this response can be modified by chronic stress exposure.

Alterations in CNS function after either acute or chronic stress are well documented. Several examples of this follow:

1. Exposure of cats to a loud noise activates the LC but the electrical activity decreases with repeated exposures to the noise (Abercrombie & Jacobs, 1987). This suggests that repeated exposure to the same stressor modifies the ability of the LC to become activated.

2. Activation of the LC either by stress or injection with corticotropin-releasing hormone (CRH) has been shown to alter the reactivity of the LC to subsequent exposure to the activating stimulus or another stimulus. If a rat is given a single session of footshock stress the response of the LC to localized CRH injection is altered as the LC has a reduction of its normal electrical activation to CRH injection. However, if the rat is given five stress sessions, the sensitivity of the LC to low concentrations of CRH is increased but the magnitude of activation is decreased (Curtis, Pavcovich, Grigoriadis, & Valentino, 1995).

3. Injection of CRH into the LC alters its reactivity to subsequent injections of CRH (Conti & Foote, 1995). A single CRH injection attenuated the response of the LC to a second injection of CRH for 72 h. Rats given eight daily injections of CRH into the LC had a decreased LC reactivity to subsequent CRH injection 7 days later. The data indicate that reactivity of the LC to an acute stressor will be altered if the LC experiences prolonged CRH exposure induced by chronic stress. How this alteration of LC activity relates to immune differences in response to acute and chronic stress remains to be determined though a single injection of CRH into the LC has been demonstrated to reduce lymphocyte mitogenic responses (Rassnick, Sved, & Rabin, 1994).

It is clear that within the CNS, there are progressive changes in specific neurochemical or neurophysiological alterations when a stressor is continuously applied. In some cases, there is habituation; in others habituation is lacking (Matsuda et al., 1996; Watanabe et al., 1994). Stressor-induced modulation of immune function is predicated on an initial triggering of peripheral endocrine and autonomic pathways by higher order central systems (e.g., nuclei within the brain stem such as the LC). Therefore, it is likely that stressor-induced changes in immune reactivity might not persist or perhaps change direction as a result of habituation processes within the brain.

## II. ACUTE AND CHRONIC STRESS AND IMMUNE FUNCTION

Having addressed some of the issues to keep in mind regarding acute and chronic stress studies, we turn to an examination of studies that have addressed this topic with reference to immunological effects. The immune system is a complex biological entity, the functional status of which is assessed using a wide variety of in vitro and in vivo procedures that may or may not evaluate similar processes. Within the stress literature, the major immune parameters assessed under noninfectious conditions are mitogenic stimulation of lymphocyte transformation, natural killer cell activity, and antibody responses to antigen [(Kusnecov & Rabin, 1994); for infectious disease studies see the chapter by Sheridan and Bonneau in Volume III]. As stressors, investigators have utilized footshock, restraint/immobilization, conditioned fear, forced swim, social conflict, social reorganization, maternal deprivation, and a host of other stressors chosen as a means to perturb or threaten the equanimity of the organism and, in so doing, affect a specific immune parameter. Insofar as animal studies are concerned, this has been done in mice, rats, monkeys, and in rare cases agricultural animals such as pigs, cattle, and fowl. The general consensus from all of these studies is that stress does affect the immune system. However, predicting the direction of the effect (e.g., suppression or enhancement) has proven difficult. In part this is due to the highly intricate paracrine and autocrine regulation that exists within the immune system and how it self-regulates its response to specific antigens. However, this lack of predictive precision is not necessarily a lamentable state, since the immune system in and of itself is heavily compartmentalized and in some ways resembles a black box that yields a particular result—either up, down, or no change without researchers seeming

to understand why. This should not be taken as cause for confusion, but rather an important indicator of how different sets of experimental conditions (e.g., species, stressor, antigen, etc.) can result in varying types of outcome. The challenge is in designing the right experimental approaches to reveal consistent relationships between stressor *input* and immunobiological *output*.

From this perspective, and in spite of numerous publications, stress research on immune function is actually in its infancy and, as with all emergent fields, is confounded by numerous procedural differences between laboratories. Table I lists some of the studies conducted over the past decade addressing "acute" and "chronic" stress effects on immune function. Of course, there are appreciably more studies on the effects of stress on immune function (see other chapters in this volume), but only these particular studies considered the impact of exposing animals to variable numbers of a given stress manipulation. It can be clearly seen from Table I that there are considerable differences between different laboratories in the choice of species, immune parameters assessed, and stressor type and regimen. The most commonly used immune measures were antibody responses to antigen and lymphocyte transformation in response to mitogens. Our categorization of stressor exposure as acute or chronic was highly arbitrary and, in essence, should be read as discriminating between single (or "less") and repeated (or "more") exposure.

### A. B Cell Antibody Production

An important issue in regard to the effects of stress (chronic or acute) on in vivo immune responsiveness to a specific antigen is timing of stressor application in relation to antigenic challenge. Prior to antigen entry in vivo, naive B cells are for all intents and purposes in a "resting" state. However, once an immunizing antigen encounters the immune system, a dynamic process is initiated that involves cognate interactions between antigen-presenting cells, T cells, and B cells. This evolves over a period of days to weeks into an accumulation of antibody levels produced by differentiated antigen-specific B cells. The B cell immune response therefore involves a series of temporally defined steps that are all potentially susceptible to stressor influences. Clearly, studying the impact of a stressor on an antigen-specific immune response does not necessarily have to focus on the moment of antigen administration. Thus, acute stressor application can be administered hours to days (or even weeks) prior to or after administration of antigen.

**TABLE I** Summary of Findings from Studies that Investigated the Immunological Effects of Varying the Number of Exposures to an Experimental Stressor

| Immune parameter | Species | Stressor | "Acute" parameters | "Chronic" parameters | Outcome | Authors |
|---|---|---|---|---|---|---|
| Primary IgM to KLH | Mice | Social Conflict | One session | Multiple sessions over days | Acute: Ø<br>Chronic: ↓ | Lyte et al., 1990 |
| Primary IgM to PVP (T-independent Ag) | Mice | Social Conflict | One session | Multiple sessions over days | Acute: Ø<br>Chronic: Ø | Lyte et al., 1990 |
| Primary IgM antibody to SRBC | Mice | Grouped to individual housing | 5–10 Days isolation | 15–30 Days isolation | Acute: ↓<br>Chronic: Ø | Shanks et al., 1994 |
| Primary PFC to SRBC | Rats | Cold in neonatally handled and unhandled | Single session | 21 Daily sessions | Acute (H): ↓<br>Chronic (H): ↓<br>Acute (NH): ↓<br>Chronic (NH): ↓ | Bhatnagar et al., 1996 |
| Primary antibody titre to SRBC | Rats | Restraint | 2 Days | 4 Days | Acute: ↑<br>Chronic: Ø | Millan et al., 1996 |
| Primary IgM to SRBC | Mice | Footshock | Single session | 13–15 Daily sessions | Acute: Ø or ↓ Ab*<br>Chronic: Ø | Zalcman & Anisman, 1993 |
| Delayed type hypersensitivity | Rats | Restraint | Single session | 3–5 Weeks daily sessions | Acute: ↑ DTH<br>Chronic: ↓ DTH | Dhabar & McEwen, 1997 |
| IL-2 production to influenza virus | Mice | Restraint | Single session | 2–8 Days | Acute: Ø<br>Chronic: ↓IL-2 | Sheridan et al., 1991 |
| Lymphocyte proliferation to PHA and LPS | Rats | Grouped to individual housing | 1–7 Days isolation | 8–35 Days isolation | Acute: ↓ Blood and Spleen<br>Chronic: ↑ Blood and Spleen | Jessop & Bayer, 1989 |
| Lymphocyte proliferation to Con A | Rats | Footshock | Single session | 3–5 Daily sessions | Acute: ↓ Blood and Spleen<br>Chronic: ↓ Blood; Spleen attenuated suppression or Ø | Lysle et al., 1987 |
| Lymphocyte proliferation to Con A or LPS or IL-2 production | Rats | 4° or 15°C swim | Three sessions over a period of 12 hrs | Three daily sessions for 5 days | Acute: ↓ Bld, Spln<br>Chronic: ↑ Bld, Spln | Shu et al., 1993 |
| Peripheral blood lymphocyte proliferation to PHA, Con A, PWM | Rats | Immobilization | One session | 6–7 Days | Acute: ↓<br>Chronic: ↓ | Rinner et al., 1992 |
| Splenocyte proliferation to con A or LPS | Mice | Loud noise | 1–7 Days | 8–39 Days | Acute: ↓<br>Chronic: Ø (at 3 weeks), ↑ (at 4–5 weeks) | Monjan & Collector, 1977 |

**TABLE I** (*Continued*)

| Immune parameter | Species | Stressor | "Acute" parameters | "Chronic" parameters | Outcome | Authors |
|---|---|---|---|---|---|---|
| Con A activated intracellular calcium changes | Mice | Immobilization | One session | 3–21 Daily sessions | Acute: ↓ CD4 ↑ CD8<br>Chronic: ↓ CD4 (3–7 sessions) Ø CD8 | Sei et al., 1991 |
| Lymphocyte proliferation to Con A | Rats | Restraint | Two daily sessions | Four daily sessions | Acute: ↓ Bld Ø spln<br>Chronic: ↓ Bld Ø spln | Millan et al., 1996 |
| Lymphocyte proliferation and IL-2 production to Con A and PHA | Rats | Restraint + tail shock | One session | 7 and 14 Daily sessions | Acute: ↓ PHA, Ø con A, ↓ IL-2<br>Chronic: ↓ PHA ↓ con A, ↓ IL-2 | Batuman et al., 1990 |
| Spleen cell proliferation to Con A and LPS | Mice | Footshock or predator exposure | One session | 14 Daily sessions | Acute: ↑ LPS, Ø con A<br>Chronic: Ø LPS and con A | Lu et al., 1999 |

Note. ↑ or ↓, Immune parameter was significantly enhanced or reduced, respectively, relative to control group; Ø, no effect on immune parameter; Ig, immunoglobin; SRBC, sheep red blood cell; PFC, plaque-forming cell; PHA, phytohemagglutinin; LPS, lipopolysaccharide; Con A, concanavalin A.
* See text for more detail.

Indeed, this has been done by several laboratories with interesting results.

In terms of the number of antibody-forming cells (e.g., plaque-forming cells, PFC, against sheep erythrocytes, SRBC), it appears that when the antigen is SRBC, brief or acute exposure to isolated housing, cold exposure or electric footshock is suppressive in both rats and mice (Bhatnagar, Shanks, & Meaney, 1996; Shanks, Renton, Zalcman, & Anisman, 1994; Zalcman & Anisman, 1993). Suppressive effects on the number of antibody releasing B cells were noted in the case of cold or footshock administered several days after immunization (Zalcman & Anisman, 1993; Bhatnagar et al., 1996), therefore exerting some neurally mediated action on ongoing antigen-specific immunological processes. Acute application of the stressor at the time of immunization or a day or two before or afterward had no effects on the number of antibody producing cells (Zalcman & Anisman, 1993). These findings of acute stressor application contrast with those of others in which exposure to a single stress session (tail shock, footshock, or restraint) just prior to or after primary immunization enhanced or reduced the concentration of antibody titers or number of antibody forming cells against sheep erythrocytes or the commonly used protein antigen, keyhole limpet hemocyanin (KLH) (Berkenbosch, Wolvers, & Derijk, 1991; Fleshner, Brennan, Nguyen, Watkins, & Maier, 1996; Laudenslager et al., 1988; Millan et al., 1996; Persoons, Berkenbosch, Schornagel, Thepen, & Kraal, 1995; Shanks & Kusnecov, 1998). Given that these studies differed in terms of the mouse and rat strains used, as well as the particular types of stressors (even footshock varied in terms of session length, intensity and number of footshocks), it is virtually impossible to comment meaningfully on the discrepancies. However, if we base comparisons on the particular antigen used, it appears that most studies utilizing KLH as the antigen observe an enhancing effect of a single stress session on the antibody response (Persoons et al., 1995; Shanks & Kusnecov, 1998; Wood et al., 1993). Where inhibitory effects were observed (Fleshner et al., 1996), it is possible that stressor severity and lack of opportunity to elicit motoric responses (e.g., jumping) may play a role. Furthermore, in other studies using SRBC as the antigen, if an acute stressor was administered at the time of immunization, an enhanced response was observed (Berkenbosch et al., 1991).

What these studies suggest is that primary humoral immune responses may be refractory to suppressive acute stressor influences when these coincide with antigen exposure. This is not to say that if the stressor is severe enough (e.g., a compound stressor involving restraint and tail shock—see Fleshner et al., 1996) or administered for more than several hours that it will not have suppressive influences. Nonetheless, the weight of evidence in both rats and mice does point to the conclusion that cognate interactions between antigen presenting cells and B and T cells may be resistent to acute stressor effects, such that the antibody response remains unaltered or is actually augmented. Alternatively, if an acute stressor is applied several days after cognate interactions that establish an antibody response, there is suppression of antibody producing cell numbers. The reduction in numbers is a deviation from normal ongoing responsiveness, and assuming that this is not due to shunting of primed B cells into different lymphoid organs (in the studies referred to, the spleen served as the source of antibody producing cell determinations), it is possible that once B cells are activated and begin generating antibody, they may become sensitive to acute elevations of neurohormonal factors.

Interestingly, Zalcman and Anisman (1993) observed that if animals were subjected to chronic footshock exposure (a 1-h session for 13–15 days) that terminated 1–2 days prior to immunization, there was no effect on the number of cells producing antibody to SRBC. However, if the chronically stressed animals received one more footshock session 72 h after immunization (which ordinarily suppresses the cells producing antibody), the overall outcome was enhanced antibody titers and antibody forming cell numbers (Zalcman & Anisman, 1993). In fact, even a single footshock session prior to or at the same time as immunization will have the same effect. Furthermore, if in place of actual footshock exposure at 72 h, animals were exposed (at this time) only to the environmental cues associated with prior footshock at the time of immunization, the effect was enhanced antibody forming cell numbers. While no further work has been conducted to pursue an explanation for this complex set of findings, they do suggest that preexposure to stress modifies the effects of subsequent stressor exposure on antigen-specific immune responsiveness. In addition, they also raise the issue of how different stressors varying along psychological dimensions (conditioned versus unconditioned) may exert different effects on the antibody response.

Clearly, if an acute stressor is severe and novel and applied after the immune response has been ongoing for several days, the net effect on B-cell function may be suppressive. However, while chronicity of stressor exposure may imply an eventual inhibitory influence on in vivo antigen-specific immune responsiveness, some studies in Table I suggest otherwise. Shanks et al. (1994) showed that isolation stress in mice for 2–4 weeks did not affect the antibody response to SRBC. This is in contrast to the antibody response being deficient at earlier stages of isolation (5–10 days after rehousing). This highlights the ability of the antibody response to deviate from a reactivity level similar to group-housed animals and then ultimately to recover as animals apparently habituate to their novel housing situation. Using restraint stress, Millan et al. (1996) showed that while two daily exposures to restraint reduced anti-SRBC antibody titers, prolonged exposure (4 days) revealed normalization of the response. While suppression after short-term stress followed by normalization after longer term stressor exposure may not be a universal pattern for immune effects, it is evident that the reactivity of the immune system to antigen does fluctuate with the number of stressor exposures. Indeed, in another study using mice (Lyte, Nelson, & Thompson, 1990) it was shown that the antibody response to KLH was resistant to any modulatory effects of acute conflict stress, while more prolonged exposure actually inhibited the antibody response. This supports the concept that the quality of the humoral immune response changes with repeated stressor exposure.

Where this was not the case was in the study by Bhatnagar et al. (1996), who found that acute and chronic exposure to a cold environment did not differentially affect the PFC response to SRBC. That is, in both cases the response was suppressed. However, it should be mentioned that in this study the immunological readout was based on the ability of a stressor applied several days after immunization to suppress the number of PFCs, as Zalcman et al. (1988) had initially demonstrated. Since chronically stressed animals still showed suppression of PFC, this finding stands in contrast to that of Zalcman and Anisman (1993) who showed that chronic stress prevented the ability of additional stressor exposure to modify the PFC response. These studies differed considerably in terms of the duration of each stress session (1 h vs. 4 h), type of stressor used (cold vs footshock), and species (rat vs mouse). Moreover, dose of antigen differed considerably based on the species used. Further work is required to determine the universality of prior chronic or short-term stress exposure from influencing the immunomodulatory capabilities of subsequent stressors.

## B. Cell-Mediated Immune Responses

A recent study by Dhabar & McEwen (1998) examined the effect of acute and chronic stressor exposure on the delayed type hypersensitivity (DTH) response, an in vivo measure of T-cell-mediated immunity that involves initial sensitization with antigen followed days to weeks later by challenge with the sensitizing antigen. One readout measure in the DTH response is the size of swelling or enlargement of the challenged part of the body (typically the footpad or pinnae of the ear). In the Dhabar and McEwen experiment, it was shown that a single exposure to 2–5 h of restraint just prior to challenge with the sensitizing chemical DNFB, elevated the DTH response in the pinnae of rats. Interestingly, by rendering the acute restraint episode turbulent and presumably more "intense" (i.e., the restraint apparatus was shaken), the DTH response was significantly more enhanced than in acutely restrained animals that were not shaken. Insofar as the DTH response to an antigenic challenge represents a response by memory T cells, these findings are consistent with other in vitro evidence showing that the antigen-specific proliferative response of cholera toxin-sensitized spleen cells was enhanced by acute footshock exposure (Kusnecov & Rabin, 1993). They also confirm one mouse study showing that acute stress enhanced DTH reactivity (Blecha, Barry, & Kelley, 1982), while being in disagreement with another showing that the DTH response to SRBC in the lung is suppressed by acute stress (Blecha & Topliff, 1984). Clearly, the anatomical location of the DTH response may influence the effects of an acute stressor.

Dhabar and McEwen (1998) also showed that chronic stress exposure suppressed the DTH response to DNFB challenge. The chronic stress paradigm differed from the acute stress experiments in that a stress session consisted of a 6-h regimen of restraint, shaking in the home cage and restraint combined with shaking. Different groups of animals were subjected to chronic stress for either 3 weeks (at the end of which sensitization with DNFB occurred), 4 weeks (the 3 weeks before sensitization and one more week after sensitization with DNFB), or 5 weeks (the same as the 4-week group, except that stress continued to be applied for one more week once the animals had been challenged). The results revealed that for all chronically stressed animals, the DTH response was significantly reduced. This was consistent with the concept that acute and chronic stress differentially affect the DTH response. However, this study did not conduct experiments examining the influence of acute stress on sensitization. In the chronic stress experiment, all groups gave the same result (suppressed DTH reactivity), thereby suggesting that the critical effect occurred at the time of sensitization. Previously, these authors had demonstrated that several days of restraint exposure prior to sensitization did not affect the DTH response to DNFB, thereby suggesting that longer term exposure (up to 3 weeks) prior to sensitization will affect generation of memory cells capable of responding to recall antigen. However, the acute experiments conducted above involved stressor exposure just prior to challenge, and hence it would have been interesting to know if more numbers of stress sessions prior to or after challenge would have prevented the acute effect (just prior to challenge) of enhanced DTH reactivity.

A number of studies have examined the effects of acute and repeated stress on in vitro lymphocyte reactivity to mitogens, and in rare cases, antigens. From Table I it is evident that whether the stressor is footshock, immobilization/restraint, forced swim, loud noise, or enforced isolation, the net effect of brief exposure to these stressors is reduction of mitogenic function in response to the nonspecific T lymphocyte mitogens concanavalin A (Con A) or phytohemagglutinin (PHA). This occurs in both the spleen and blood. Agreement wanes, however, when we consider the effects of more prolonged numbers of exposure to these stressors. Whereas less than 1 week of isolation inhibited lymphocyte proliferation in blood and spleen, several weeks of isolation caused an increase in proliferative function (Jessop & Bayer, 1989). A similar finding was observed by Shu, Stevenson, and Zhou (1993) using forced swim as a stressor. They found that as rats were exposed to more sessions of swim stress, the proliferative capacity of splenic and blood lymphocytes actually increased. This bimodal effect (acute suppression to chronic enhancement) was also seen in mice exposed daily to loud noise (Monjan & Collector, 1977). Similarly, in a very recent study using mice, it was found that acute exposure to either a session of footshock or a predator (i.e., rat) enhanced the proliferative response of spleen cells to LPS (Lu, Halyley, Merali, & Anisman, 1999). This effect did not persist if either stressor was presented repeatedly for 14 days, suggesting that B-cell proliferative function is capable of adapting to persistent exposure of the animal to either physical or psychological stressors.

In contrast to these findings of adaptation or reversal of initial acute stressor effects on cellular immune parameters with chronic exposure to stress, other studies utilizing immobilization/restraint or electric shock stress consistently observed that repeated exposure to the stressor continued to reveal depressed splenic and blood lymphocyte proliferative function (Batuman, Sajewski, Ottenweller, Pitman, & Natelson, 1990; Lysle, Lyte, Fowler, & Rabin, 1987; Rinner, Schauenstein, Mangge, Porta, & Kvetnansky, 1992). These studies suggest that the intensity of the stressor and/or how often it is reexposed may be an important variable in determing how long it takes for lymphocyte mitogenic function to rebound from an initial suppression.

## C. Human Studies

There are some important studies conducted using human subjects that bear upon differences between acute and chronic stress. While other chapters in this volume will address human stress research, we briefly consider some relevant studies for completeness. A functional assay of natural killer (NK) cell activity in human subjects exposed to an acute laboratory stressor differed between individuals experiencing high or low levels of stress in their lives. Specifically, NK-cell function decreased significantly more in subjects with high levels of life stress than in those without (Pike et al., 1997). Thus, the definition of immune baseline will have to depend on an individual's own particular experience of stressful life events. In another study, functional alteration of several different immune parameters after acute stress has been studied in subjects who were experiencing high or low levels of stress in their lives. Thus, individuals who experience greater numbers of "hassles" in their lives have a greater decrease of peripheral blood T and NK lymphocytes in comparison to individuals who experience fewer "hassles" in their lives (Brosschot et al., 1994). It has also been reported that an acute stressor may alter some parameters of the immune system in subjects experiencing high levels of life stress but the cardiovascular system of the same individuals responds to the same extent as the cardiovascular system of individuals experiencing a low degree of life stressors (Benschop et al., 1994). Thus, if chronic stress elevates hormones and the concentration and function of hormonal receptors are subsequently altered, it is possible that different tissues undergo different alterations.

A naturally occurring biological situation where the effect of chronic catecholamine elevation on immune function can be assessed is in individuals with congestive heart failure. A study of 38 subjects who had plasma norepinephrine levels approximately twice normal found no quantitative differences of blood lymphocyte subset numbers or nonspecific mitogenic responses in comparison to controls (Hwang, Harris, Wilson, & Maisel, 1993). However, significant differences were present when the proliferative response of lymphocytes to an antigen, tetanus toxoid, was measured with the subjects having significantly less reactivity than the controls. Thus, although nonspecific mitogenic function was normal, a norepinephrine-dependent alteration of antigen presentation or antigen-specific memory T-cell responsiveness may be present in these subjects.

A metaanalysis of studies of the influence of stress on immune function in humans provides interesting data regarding an effect of the duration of a stressor on immune parameters (Herbert & Cohen, 1993). When the effect on quantitative numbers of lymphocyte populations was determined, both acute experimental laboratory stress and long-term stres's experienced as part of ones life had similar effects on the number of circulating CD4 and B lymphocytes, with decreased numbers being found. Lymphocyte responsiveness to stimulation with nonspecific mitogens was decreased by either acute laboratory or naturalistic long duration stress. CD8 lymphocytes showed a different pattern of change in association with acute or long-term stress. CD8 lymphocyte numbers increase in the blood following an acute laboratory stressor, but are decreased in subjects who have a high level of naturalistic stress in their lives.

## III. CONCLUSION

From the little evidence presently available, there appear to be differences in the alteration of immune function elicited by acute and chronic stress. As stressor-induced immune alteration occurs subsequent to changes in hormone concentrations and binding of hormones to specific receptors on lymphoid cells, the hormonal response to either acute or chronic stress may determine the characteristics of the immune alteration. Moreover, as the hormonal alterations induced by stress are dependent upon activation of specific nuclei in the brain, modification of the CNS response to an acute stress by exposure to chronic stress should also influence stressor-induced immune alterations. It is also likely that a subject's early experiences with stress and degree of coping skills will influence the effect of either acute or chronic stress on immune function. Given that there is only limited information from experimental studies in animals and humans regarding the influence of chronic stress on immune function and health, more studies are needed to determine whether chronic stress is associated with a predisposition to immunologically mediated disease. Therefore, the emphasis of animal studies should be toward examining immune responses in vivo and increasing our understanding of the precise cellular targets of stressor-activated neural and hormonal factors. Human studies necessarily are mostly restricted to blood samples, whereas such is not the case with animal studies. Researchers should take advantage of this and focus on how immune responses to natural and endogenous immunological stimuli (i.e., foreign and self-peptide antigens from nonreplicating and infectious sources) are modulated by acute and chronic stress. The effects of stress on in vitro lymphocyte function in nonimmunized animals suggest that in vivo interactions with antigen may similarly be affected, and this is clearly the next logical step that many laboratories have already taken, using both nonreplicating protein antigens and infectious disease models (see specific chapters in Volume III). Clearly, conducting in vivo studies provides considerable challenges in terms of the timing of stressor exposure in relation to immunization (whether primary, secondary, or tertiary, etc). However, we believe that a focus in this direction should lead to a greater uniformity of findings. Although consistency between various laboratories conducting experiments with complex designs may at times be difficult to obtain, we anticipate that at some point results must converge in the form of a conceptual framework that will drive studies of stress and immune function in a meaningful direction.

## References

Abercrombie, E. D., & Jacobs, B. L. (1987). Single-unit response of noradrenergic neurons in the locus coeruleus of freely moving cats. II. Adaptation to chronically presented stressful stimuli. *Journal of Neuroscience, 7,* 2844–2848.

Ader, R. & Cohen, N. (1993). Psychoneuroimmunology: conditioning and stress. *Annual Review of Psychology, 44,* 53–85.

Anisman, H., Zalcman, S., & Zacharko, R. M. (1993). The impact of stressors on immune and central neurotransmitter activity: Bidirectional communication. *Reviews in Neuroscience, 4,* 147–180.

Aston-Jones, G., Rajkowski, J., Kubiak, P., Valentino, R. J., & Shipley, M. T. (1996). Role of the locus coeruleus in emotional activation. *Progress Brain Research, 107,* 379–402.

Batuman, O. A., Sajewski, D., Ottenweller, J. E., Pitman, D. L., & Natelson, B. H. (1990). Effects of repeated stress on T cell numbers and function in rats. *Brain Behavior and Immunity, 4,* 105–117.

Benschop, R. J., Brosschot, J. F., Godaert, G. L., De Smet, M. B., Geenen, R., Olff, M., Heijnen, C. J., & Ballieux, R. E. (1994). Chronic stress affects immunologic but not cardiovascular responsiveness to acute psychological stress in humans. *American Journal of Physiology, 266,* R75–R80

Berkenbosch, F., Wolvers, D. A., & Derijk, R. (1991). Neuroendocrine and immunological mechanisms in stress-induced immunomodulation. *Journal of Steroid Biochemistry and Molecular Biology, 40,* 639–647.

Besedovsky, H. O., & del Rey, A. (1996). Immune-neuro-endocrine interactions: facts and hypotheses. *Endocrine Reviews 17,* 64–102.

Bhatnagar, S., Shanks, N., & Meaney, M. J. (1996). Plaque-forming cell responses and antibody titers following injection of sheep red blood cells in nonstressed, acute, and/or chronically stressed handled and nonhandled animals. *Developmental Psychobiology, 29,* 171–181.

Blecha, F., Barry, R. A., & Kelley, K. W. (1982). Stress-induced alterations in delayed-type hypersensitivity to SRBC and contact sensitivity to DNFB in mice. *Proceedings of the Society for Experimental Biology and Medicine, 169*, 239–246.

Blecha, F., & Topliff, D. (1984). Lung delayed-type hypersensitivity in stressed mice. *Canadian Journal of Comparative Medicine, 48*, 211–214.

Bremner, J. D., Randall, P., Vermetten, E., Staib, L., Bronen, R. A., Mazure, C., Capelli, S., McCarthy, G., Innis, R. B., & Charney, D. S. (1997). Magnetic resonance imaging-based measurement of hippocampal volume in posttraumatic stress disorder related to childhood physical and sexual abuse—A preliminary report. *Biological Psychiatry, 41*, 23–32.

Brosschot, J. F., Benschop, R. J., Godaert, G. L., Olff, M., De Smet, M., Heijnen, C. J., & Ballieux, R. E. (1994). Influence of life stress on immunological reactivity to mild psychological stress. *Psychosomatic Medicine, 56*, 216–224.

Conti, L. H., & Foote, S. L. (1995). Effects of pretreatment with corticotropin-releasing factor on the electrophysiological responsivity of the locus coeruleus to subsequent corticotropin-releasing factor challenge. *Neuroscience, 69*, 209–219.

Cunnick, J. E., Cohen, S., Rabin, B. S., Carpenter, A. B., Manuck, S. B., & Kaplan, J. R. (1991). Alterations in specific antibody production due to rank and social instability. *Brain Behavior and Immunity, 5*, 357–369.

Cunnick, J. E., Lysle, D. T., Armfield, A., & Rabin, B. S. (1988). Shock-induced modulation of lymphocyte responsiveness and natural killer activity: Differential mechanisms of induction. *Brain, Behavior, and Immunity, 2*, 102–113.

Curtis, A. L., Pavcovich, L. A., Grigoriadis, D. E., & Valentino, R. J. (1995). Previous stress alters corticotropin-releasing factor neurotransmission in the locus coeruleus. *Neuroscience, 65*, 541–550.

Deinzer, R., Kirschbaum, C., Gresele, C., & Hellhammer, D. H. (1997). Adrenocortical responses to repeated parachute jumping and subsequent h-CRH challenge in inexperienced healthy subjects. *Physiology and Behavior, 61*, 507–511.

Esterling, B., & Rabin, B. S. (1987). Stress-induced alteration of T-lymphocyte subsets and humoral immunity in mice. *Behavioral Neuroscience, 101*, 115–119.

Fleshner, M., Brennan, F. X., Nguyen, K., Watkins, L. R., & Maier, S. F. (1996). RU-486 blocks differentially suppressive effect of stress on in vivo anti-KLH immunoglobulin response. *American Journal of Physiology, 271*, R1344–R1352.

Glaser, R., & Kiecolt-Glaser, J. K. (1998). Stress-associated immune modulation: Relevance to viral infections and chronic fatigue syndrome. *American Journal of Medicine 105*, 35S–42S.

Gresch, P. J., Sved, A. F., Zigmond, M. J., & Finlay, J. M. (1994). Stress-induced sensitization of dopamine and norepinephrine efflux in medial prefrontal cortex of the rat. *Journal of Neurochemistry, 63*, 575–583.

Gurvits, T. V., Shenton, M. E., Hokama, H., Ohta, H., Lasko, N. B., Gilbertson, M. W., Orr, S. P., Kikinis, R., Jolesz, F. A., McCarley, R. W., & Pitman, R. K. (1996). Magnetic resonance imaging study of hippocampal volume in chronic, combat-related posttraumatic stress disorder. *Biological Psychiatry, 40*, 1091–1099.

Herbert, T. B., & Cohen, S. (1993). Stress and immunity in humans: A meta-analytic review. *Psychosomatic Medicine, 55*, 364–379.

Hwang, S., Harris, T. J., Wilson, N. W., & Maisel, A. S. (1993). Immune function in patients with chronic stable congestive heart failure. *American Heart Journal, 125*, 1651–1658.

Jessop, J. J., & Bayer, B. M. (1989). Time-dependent effects of isolation on lymphocyte and adrenocortical activity. *Journal of Neuroimmunology, 23*, 143–147.

Karp, J. D., Moynihan, J. A., & Ader, R. (1993). Effects of differential housing on the primary and secondary antibody responses of male C57BL/6 and BALB/c mice. *Brain, Behavior, and Immunity, 7*, 326–333.

Karp, J. D., Moynihan, J. A., & Ader, R. (1997). Psychosocial influences on immune responses to HSV-1 infection in BALB/c mice. *Brain, Behavior, and Immunity, 11*, 47–62.

Konarska, M., Stewart, R. E., & McCarty, R. (1989). Sensitization of sympathetic-adrenal medullary responses to a novel stressor in chronically stressed laboratory rats. *Physiology and Behavior, 46*, 129–135.

Kusnecov, A. W., & Rabin, B. S. (1993). Inescapable footshock exposure differentially alters antigen- and mitogen-stimulated spleen cell proliferation in rats. *Journal of Neuroimmunology, 44*, 33–42.

Kusnecov, A. W., & Rabin, B. S. (1994). Stressor-induced alterations of immune function: Mechanisms and issues. *International Archives of Allergy and Immunology, 105*, 107–121.

Kusnecov, A. W., Shurin, M. R., Armfield, A., Litz, J., Wood, P., Zhou, D., & Rabin, B. S. (1995). Suppression of lymphocyte mitogenesis in different rat strains exposed to footshock during early diurnal and nocturnal time periods. *Psychoneuroendocrinology, 20*, 821–835.

Laudenslager, M. L., Fleshner, M., Hofstadter, P., Held, P. E., Simons, L., & Maier, S. F. (1988). Suppression of specific antibody production by inescapable shock: Stability under varying conditions. *Brain, Behavior, and Immunity, 2*, 92–101.

Levenson, C. W., & Moore, J. B. (1998). Response of rat adrenal neuropeptide Y and tyrosine hydroxylase mRNA to acute stress is enhanced by long-term voluntary exercise. *Neuroscience Letters, 242*, 177–179.

Lu, Z. W., Halyley, S., Merali, Z., & Anisman, H. (1999). Influence of psychosocial, psychogenic and neurogenic stressors on several aspects of immune functioning in mice. *Stress*, in press.

Lysle, D. T., Lyte, M., Fowler, H., & Rabin, B. S. (1987). Shock-induced modulation of lymphocyte reactivity: Suppression, habituation, and recovery. *Life Sciences, 41*, 1805–1814.

Lyte, M., Nelson, S. G., & Thompson, M. L. (1990). Innate and adaptive immune responses in a social conflict paradigm. *Clinical Immunology and Immunopathology, 57*, 137–147.

Matsuda, S., Peng, H., Yoshimura, H., Wen, T. C., Fukuda, T., & Sakanaka, M. (1996). Persistent c-fos expression in the brains of mice with chronic social stress. *Neuroscience Research, 26*, 157–170.

Melia, K. R., Ryabinin, A. E., Schroeder, R., Bloom, F. E., & Wilson, M. C. (1994). Induction and habituation of immediate early gene expression in rat brain by acute and repeated restraint stress. *Journal of Neuroscience, 14*, 5929–5938.

Millan, S., Gonzalez-Quijano, M. I., Giordano, M., Soto, L., Martin, A. I., & Lopez-Calderon, A. (1996). Short and long restraint differentially affect humoral and cellular immune functions. *Life Sciences, 59*, 1431–1442.

Miller, A. H. (1998). Neuroendocrine and immune system interactions in stress and depression. *Psychiatric Clinics of North America, 21*, 443–463.

Monjan, A. A., & Collector, M. I. (1977). Stress-induced modulation of the immune response. *Science, 196*, 307–308.

Moyna, N. M., Acker, G. R., Weber, K. M., Fulton, J. R., Goss, F. L., Robertson, R. J., & Rabin, B. S. (1996). The effects of incremental submaximal exercise on circulating leukocytes in physically active and sedentary males and females. *European Journal of Applied Physiology, 74*, 211–218.

Moynihan, J. A., & Ader, R. (1996). Psychoneuroimmunology: animal models of disease. *Psychosomatic Medicine, 58*, 546–558.

Nisenbaum, L. K., Zigmond, M. J., Sved, A. F., & Abercrombie, E. D. (1991). Prior exposure to chronic stress results in enhanced synthesis and release of hippocampal norepinephrine in response to a novel stressor. *Journal of Neuroscience, 11,* 1478–1484.

Persoons, J. H., Berkenbosch, F., Schornagel, K., Thepen, T., & Kraal, G. (1995). Increased specific IgE production in lungs after the induction of acute stress in rats. *Journal of Allergy and Clinical Immunology, 95,* 765–770.

Pike, J. L., Smith, T. L., Hauger, R. L., Nicassio, P. M., Patterson, T. L., McClintick, J., Costlow, C., & Irwin, M. R. (1997). Chronic life stress alters sympathetic, neuroendocrine, and immune responsivity to an acute psychological stressor in humans. *Psychosomatic Medicine, 59,* 447–457.

Rabin, B. S., Lyte, M., Epstein, L. H., & Caggiula, A. R. (1987). Alteration of immune competency by number of mice housed per cage. *Annals of the New York Academy of Sciences, 496,* 492–500.

Rassnick, S., Sved, A. F., & Rabin, B. S. (1994). Locus coeruleus stimulation by corticotropin-releasing hormone suppresses in vitro cellular immune responses. *Journal of Neuroscience, 14,* 6033–6040.

Rinner, I., Schauenstein, K., Mangge, H., Porta, S., & Kvetnansky, R. (1992). Opposite effects of mild and severe stress on in vitro activation of rat peripheral blood lymphocytes. *Brain, Behavior, and Immunity, 6,* 130–140.

Salvin, S. B., Rabin, B. S., & Neta, R. (1990). Evaluation of immunologic assays to determine the effects of differential housing on immune reactivity. *Brain, Behavior, and Immunity, 4,* 180–188.

Sapolsky, R. M. (1996). Stress, Glucocorticoids, and Damage to the Nervous System: The Current State of Confusion. *Stress, 1,* 1–19.

Sei, Y., McIntyre, T., Skolnick, P., & Arora, P. K. (1991). Stress modulates calcium mobilization in immune cells. *Life Sciences, 49*(9), 671–676.

Shanks, N., & Kusnecov, A. W. (1998). Differential immune reactivity to stress in BALB/cByJ and C57BL/6J mice: In vivo dependence on macrophages. *Physiology and Behavior, 65,* 95–103.

Shanks, N., Renton, C., Zalcman, S., & Anisman, H. (1994). Influence of change from grouped to individual housing on a T-cell-dependent immune response in mice: Antagonism by diazepam. *Pharmacology, Biochemistry, and Behavior, 47,* 497–502.

Sheridan, J. F., Feng, N. G., Bonneau, R. H., Allen, C. M., Huneycutt, B. S., & Glaser, R. (1991). Restraint stress differentially affects anti-viral cellular and humoral immune responses in mice. *Journal of Neuroimmunology 31*(3), 245–255.

Shu, J., Stevenson, J. R., & Zhou, X. (1993). Modulation of cellular immune responses by cold water swim stress in the rat. *Development and Comparative Immunology, 17*(4), 357–371.

Watanabe, Y., Stone, E., & McEwen, B. S. (1994). Induction and habituation of c-fos and zif/268 by acute and repeated stressors. *Neuroreport, 5,* 1321–1324.

Wood, P. G., Karol, M. H., Kusnecov, A. W., & Rabin, B. S. (1993). Enhancement of antigen-specific humoral and cell-mediated immunity by electric footshock stress in rats. *Brain, Behavior, and Immunity, 7,* 121–134.

Zalcman, S., & Anisman, H. (1993). Acute and chronic stressor effects on the antibody response to sheep red blood cells. *Pharmacology, Biochemistry, and Behavior, 46,* 445–452.

Zalcman, S., Minkiewicz-Janda, A., Richter, M., & Anisman, H. (1988). Critical periods associated with stressor effects on antibody titers and on the plaque-forming cell response to sheep red blood cells. *Brain, Behavior, and Immunity, 2,* 254–266.

Zalcman, S., Shanks, N., & Anisman, H. (1991). Time-dependent variations of central norepinephrine and dopamine following antigen administration. *Brain Research, 557,* 69–76.

# 43

# Acute and Chronic Effects of Space Flight on Immune Functions

GERALD SONNENFELD, GERALD R. TAYLOR, KEVIN S. KINNEY

## I. INTRODUCTION

### A. Background

Since the earliest manned space missions, researchers have been concerned with the effects of space flight on resistance to infectious illness and cancer induction. Even before the recognition of the profound effects of the neuroendocrine sequelae of stress on immune function, space biologists speculated on the effects of microgravity, radiation exposure, altered nutrition, and other aspects of space travel on immunity. With the now well-established awareness of the interplay between the immune system and the nervous and endocrine systems, the possibility of alterations in resistance to disease as a consequence of space flight become even more likely. Several studies on various aspects of cellular and humoral immunity have been carried out on both humans and research animals in flight. However, due to the extraordinarily difficult logistics encountered, most studies of the effects of space flight on immunity to date have used groundbased models, to determine which of the effects seen in actual flight conditions are attributable to nonunique aspects (i.e., effects which can be

encountered in other conditions besides space flight) of the system.

### B. Rationale

#### 1. Stress, Immune Function, and Space Flight

It is now recognized that the immune system is in constant bidirectional communication with the rest of the body. This being the case, any perturbation in homeostasis has the potential to affect the functioning of the immune system. Space flight imposes a number of such disturbances, often to an extreme degree. Many of these perturbations are ones that are similar to stresses which may be encountered by organisms on the ground, but exaggerated by the constraints of space travel. Such potential stressors include circadian rhythm changes, anxiety, fatigue, confinement, exposure to radiation, nutritional alterations, acceleration and deceleration forces, and possible alterations in hormone levels (Churchill, 1997; Nicogossian, Huntoon, & Pool, 1989; Sonnenfeld & Taylor, 1991).

#### 2. Potential Hazards

In addition to the set of stressors common to groundbased systems, there are relatively unique physiological perturbations that occur during space flight. Perhaps primary among these are the effects of microgravity (technically, vehicles orbiting a planet are in free-fall and experience low, but not zero, gravity, this greatly diminished gravitational attraction is termed microgravity). As a result of microgravity conditions, organisms experience muscle and bone unloading, leading to the bone mineral loss and musculoskeletal changes commonly seen in astronauts. These changes, along with the effects of space flight on other systems, lead to dramatic changes in the levels of various neuroendocrine hormones.

Even brief space missions pose logistic difficulties in avoiding exposure to infectious disease. Equipment failure in waste handling and decontamination systems occasionally occur, thus constituting a potential sourse of pathogens to a crew that may appear disease-free at the inception of the mission. In microgravity, aerosolized infectious particles remain suspended far longer than when under the influence of Earth's gravity. As an additional hazard, the habitable compartments are closed, and possibly crowded, which may promote the spread of infection among crew members. Finally, access to medical supplies and facilities is limited, increasing the risk associated with any infection, and peak performance is generally necessary on space flight missions, mandating avoidance of infection wherever possible.

### 3. Known Immunological Difficulties

Many of the early studies reporting infectious disease problems may actually have involved syndromes such as "space motion sickness" and headward fluid shifts that produced symptoms that, at that time, were indistinguishable from those of the common cold and influenza (Taylor, Konstantinova, Sonnenfeld, & Jennings, 1997). However, there are compelling reasons why it has been, and will continue to be, important to determine the effects of space flight on immune responses. In the Apollo 13 mission, one crew member developed a urinary tract infection with *Pseudomonas aeruginosa*. (Taylor, 1974; Taylor et al., 1997). For this Apollo flight, there was confirmed isolation from the urinary tract infection of *Pseudomonas* in an individual who was normal before flight (Taylor, 1974). This was an indication of possible contamination of an otherwise healthy individual where increased susceptibility to infection could have been related to the great stress of a space flight mission (Apollo 13) where actual survival of the mission was threatened.

In one Mir mission, one cosmonaut was removed from the flight because of possible, but not confirmed, upper respiratory tract infections (I. Konstantinova, pers. commun.; Konstantinova, Rykova, Lesnyak & Antropova, 1993). Therefore, limited, but marked, health problems relating to infectious diseases in astronauts and cosmonauts have been observed (Taylor et al., 1997). Many of the problems reported by U.S. crew members prior to Apollo 14 have been reduced by implementation of a policy of limited crew isolation prior to a mission. Starting with Apollo 14, when restrictions on preflight contact with other personnel was first implemented, crew members had decreased problems with upper respiratory tract infections compared to prior missions where they were not isolated (Taylor, 1974; Taylor et al., 1997).

As space flight in the 21st century is contemplated, there is considerable interest in extended length missions, with an eye toward the development of such projects as a long-term space station, a lunar colony, and a mission to Mars. However, the potential danger of infection increases as the duration of space flight increases. Potential problems over long durations include: (1) development of opportunistic infections if the immune response of space travelers is compromised; (2) transfer of infectious agents from visiting crews to a permanent crew that may be immunocompromised in a space station or colony; and (3) development of infections upon return to Earth in a crew that has been isolated from terrestrial organisms in a multiyear space mission. Therefore, it has become even more crucial for the development of an understanding of the effects of space flight on immune responses, an exploration of the mechanisms involved in these changes, and the potential development of countermeasures to prevent or ameliorate the effects of space flight on immune responses. Additionally, the unique aspects of space flight can be used as a "laboratory" and can contribute to an understanding of the normal mechanisms of immunoregulation on Earth.

## II. RESEARCH ANIMAL STUDIES

Space flight has been shown to have profound effects on immunological parameters of humans, monkeys, and rodents. Among the parameters affected are leukocyte blastogenesis, natural killer cell activity, leukocyte subset distribution, cytokine production—including interferons and interleukins—and macrophage maturation and activity. These changes start to occur only after a few days space flight, and some changes continue throughout long-term space flight. The mechanism(s) for space flight-induced changes in immune responses remain(s) to be established. Certainly, there can be direct effects of the spaceflight environment on cells that play a fundamental role in immune responses. However, it is also clear that there are interactions between the immune system and other physiological systems that play a major role. For example, changes occurring in calcium use in the musculoskeletal system induced by microgravity or lack of use could have great impact on the immune system as a consequence of altered endocrine hormone profiles. The biological significance of space flight-induced changes in immune parameters remains to be established.

## A. Groundbased Studies on Immune Function in Laboratory Animals

Since experimental opportunities are rare and expensive during space flight, model systems have been designed to simulate some effects of space flight on immune responses. All of the models have at least one major deficiency; i.e., it is impossible to replicate sustained microgravity conditions on Earth. Therefore, it is important to recognize the limitations of each model system. Nevertheless, such models are useful for *planning* space flight experiments and for comparison with the results of actual flight experiments, to determine which of the potential immunomodulatory factors are unique.

Many of the nonunique space flight stressors such as crowding, radiation, accelleration, noise, and dietary alterations have been the mainstays of psychoneuroimmunologic stress research for years. The results of these experiments are reviewed elsewhere in this volume, and for the sake of brevity, will not be further examined here. Instead, we will review groundbased experiments which attempt to model the microgravity environment, which is one of the truly unique features of space flight.

First among the models that have been used are rotation of cells is a clinostat (Albrect-Buehler, 1992), an apparatus that allows for rotation of cells so that the direction of the vector of gravity is continually changing. While its use has been accepted for plant cells, which have a known receptor system for gravity, use of the clinostat for animal cells, which lack classical receptors for gravity, has been hotly debated. Nevertheless, rotation of cells in a clinostat has resulted in decreased T-lymphocyte activation (Cogoli & Gmünder, 1991), and decreased leukocyte migration through type 1 collagen (Pellis et al., 1997). Although the mechanisms that cause these changes in the clinostat may be different from those that could occur during space flight, the data obtained could be useful in the planning of experiments to be carried out in space (for a more thorough review of this subject, see Cogoli, 1993).

Antiorthostatic, hypokinetic, hypodynamic suspension (AOS) of rodents has been used to simulate some aspects of microgravity effects on immune responses (Ilyan & Novikovo, 1980; Morey, Sabelman, Turner, &

Baylink, 1979; Musacchia, Deavers, Meininger, & Davis, 1980). This model involves suspension of rats or mice with no load-bearing on the hind limbs and head-down tilt (usually 15–20°), creating a situation where there is bone and muscle disuse and a fluid shift to the head (Taylor, 1993a). Although this configuration does not provide a microgravity environment, it is the best model of the "unloading" aspect of space flight available for long-term rodent studies. One additional benefit of the use of this model is the ability to have orthostatically suspended (confined, with no head-down tilt) rodents as a control for the stress of the model (Berry, Murphy, Smith, Taylor, & Sonnenfeld, 1991; Caren, Mandel, & Nunes, 1980; Chapes, Mastro, Sonnenfeld, & Berry, 1993; Rose, Steffen, Musacchia, Mandel, & Sonnenfeld, 1984; Sonnenfeld et al., 1992a; Sonnenfeld, Morey-Holton, Williams, & Mandel, 1982). Two variants of the model have been used, suspension *via* the tail (Ilyan & Novikovo, 1980; Morey, et al., 1979) and harness suspension (Musacchia, et al., 1980). Although both of these variants have benefits and drawbacks, studies with both models regarding immune responses have shown equivalent results (Berry, Murphy, Smith, Taylor, & Sonnenfeld, 1991; Caren, Mandel, & Nunes, 1980; Chapes et al., 1993; Rose et al., 1984; Sonnenfeld et al., 1992a; Sonnenfeld, et al., 1982).

Mitogen responses to AOS show compartment specificity: response to T-cells mitogens is inhibited in lymph nodes (Armstrong, Nelson, Simske, Luttges, Iandolo, & Chapes, 1993) and peropheral blood (Nash, Bour, & Mastro, 1991), but is apparently enhanced in spleen (Armstrong et al., 1993; Kopydlowski, Mcvey, Woods, Iandolo, & Chapes, 1992). Antiorthostatic supension results in diminished interferon $\alpha/\beta$ production in both mice (Rose et al., 1984; Miller & Sonnenfeld, 1994) and rats (Sonnenfeld et al., 1982) and increases interferon $\gamma$ production by rat lymphocytes (Berry et al., 1991). This last result may be more an effect of the restraint than the complete antiorthostasis model (Taylor, 1993a). Exposure of bone marrow cells from suspended rats to exogenous macrophage colony stimulating factor results in fewer macrohage colonies, relative to similarly treated cells from orthostatic suspencion or control mice (Chapes et al., 1993; Armstrong et al., 1993). Macrophage function, as measured by superoxide production, is depressed in AOS (vs. orthostatic or control mice) mice (Fleming, Rosenkrans, & Chapes, 1990). Natural killer cell function, at least in the spleen, does not apper to be affected by AOS (Armstrong et al., 1993; Chapes et al., 1993). The situation with neutrophil function is less clear; in mice, neutrophil function is inhibited after AOS (Fleming, et al., 1990), while in rats, AOS had no effect on neutrophil oxidative burst (Miller et al., 1994). Reasons for these differences could involve the type of suspension used and the response of different species to suspension. Leukocyte subset distribution and class II histocompatibility molecule expression were not affected by AOS (Chapes et al., 1993; Kopydlowski et al., 1992; Nash et al., 1991). The production of several cytokines (IL-1, IL-2, PGE2, TNF-$\alpha$) were not affected by AOS (Kopydlowski et al., 1992; Nash et al., 1991). The reason for differential effects on immune responses is not clear. In at least one study (Kopydlowski et al., 1992), there was no correlation of corticosterone levels with alterations in immune responses.

AOS has also been shown to affect resistance to infection (Gould & Sonnenfeld, 1987). Female mice normally resistant to infection with the D variant of encephalomyocarditis virus became susceptible to infection after AOS (Gould & Sonnenfeld, 1987). The decreased resistance correlated with the drop in interferon production seen after AOS. In contrast to the diminished resistance to the viral infection, suspended mice showed enhanced immunological memory and resistance to infection with *Listeria monocytogenes* (Miller & Sonnenfeld, 1993, 1994). Therefore, differences in responses of resistance to bacteria and viruses were observed after suspension, and may be related to differences in the effects of AOS on lymphocyte (for the virus) and macrophage (for the bacteria) function (Gould & Sonnenfeld, 1987; Miller & Sonnenfeld, 1993, 1994).

Although mechanisms may or may not be identical between AOS and space flight effects (Sonnenfeld et al., 1992a), the results obtained can be useful for maximizing the return from the limited resources available for space flight studies.

## B. Space Flight Studies on Immune Function in Laboratory Animals

Although not ideal for immunological studies, the mammalian animal of choice for spaceflight studies has been the rat, because housing suitable for space flight has been developed for this species. Multiple modifications are currently under development before housing for space flight will be available for use with mice. Additionally, because of its larger size, the rat has been most useful for studies requiring sharing of tissues among the different groups conducting experiments. It is hoped that experiments involving mice for immunological studies will be carried out in the near future. A very limited number of additional

immunological studies have been performed using Rhesus monkeys as subjects.

Flight experiments have been completed utilizing both Russian and U.S. spacecraft. All flight experiments with laboratory animals have been of relatively short duration, usually from 1 to 2 weeks (Allebban et al., 1994; Congdon et al., 1996; Durnova, Kaplansky, & Portugalov, 1976; Gould, Lyte, Williams, Mandel, & Sonnenfeld, 1987; Ichiki et al., 1996; Lesnyak et al., 1996; Miller, Koebel, & Sonnenfeld, 1995; Nash et al., 1992; Nash & Mastro, 1992; Rykova et al., 1992; Sonnenfeld et al., 1990, 1992a; Sonnenfeld & Miller, 1993). Almost all experiments, except where noted, have been performed immediately (usually within 2–4 h, but sometimes as late as 24 h) after landing of the spacecraft on Earth. Although conditions differ with regard to housing, in-flight environmental conditions, duration and apogee of flight, and landing conditions, results have generally been consistent.

Early studies indicated involution of the thymus of rats after space flight (Durnova et al., 1976). Alterations in thymus and other tissue were later confirmed, but shown to possibly be transient in nature (Congdon et al., 1996; Ichiki et al., 1996). These changes were among the first to suggest that there might be profound effects of space flight on immune responses.

Initial studies which examined rat leukocyte blastogenesis in the Russian Cosmos biosatellite showed no effects of space flight (Mandel & Balish, 1977). Later studies explored this issue further and showed that there was compartmentalization of the effects of space flight on blastogenesis. Leukocytes obtained from lymph nodes of flown animals exhibited diminished mitogenic responses to concanavalin (Con A), but not PHA, nor to B-cell mitogens in one study (Nash & Mastro, 1992), but even the Con A effect was not seen in rat lymph node cells in another (Nash et al., 1992). The Con A effect was apparently not due to a lack of interleukin (IL)-1 or IL-2 production, as addition of these cytokines did not reverse the inhibition (Nash & Mastro, 1992). In contrast, there were no changes seen in any mitogenic responses of spleen cells from the same animals (Nash & Mastro, 1992), although other studies, one of which employed in-flight dissection of animals, found diminished splenic mitogen responses (Lesnyak et al., 1996; Lesnyak et al., 1993).

An experiment with rats flown on the U.S. Space Shuttle mission SL-3 was designed to study cytokine production after landing. Spleens were removed from the rats within a few hours after landing and challenged with mitogen to induce cytokine production (Gould et al., 1987). The interferon-$\gamma$ titer was greatly reduced in culture supernatant fluids from cells obtained from flown animals as compared to controls. However, interleukin-3 measurements made of the same culture supernatant fluids showed no decrease in interleukin-3 production (Cruse et al., 1993; Lesnyak et al., 1996). Later studies showed increases in the production of cytokines such as interleukin-3 (in both thymocytes and splenocytes) and interleukin-6 (in thymocytes only) after space flight (Miller et al., 1995), indicating some compartment-specific effect of space flight on postflight cytokine production. Effects on the production and/ or secretion of other cytokines, such as IL-1 and IL-2 have been mixed. When effects are seen, they appear to return to normal soon after landing (Lesnyak, et al., 1993; Nash & Mastro, 1992; Nash, et al., 1992). Compartmentalization and selectivity of the effects of space flight on blastogenesis and cytokine production indicate that there is not an overall blunting of the immune response after space flight, but, rather, there are selective effects of space flight on immunity. To further complicate matters, the timing of the assays appears to have a major influence on the results. Cells from animals euthanized in flight exhimbited diminished production of IL-1, IL-2, TNF-$\alpha$, and TNF-$\beta$ relative to controls (Lesnyak et al., 1996), but the effects on IL-2 disappeared if animals were euthanized at landing, and the effect in TNF-$\alpha$ reversed itself, becoming an increase.

Studies were also carried out on the effects of space flight on natural killer cell activity. Initial studies on cells from rats flown on the Russian Cosmos biosatellite showed a decrease in the ability of spleen cells to kill YAC-1 cells compared to that seen in controls (Rykova et al., 1992). Later studies showed that this effect was selective, as the ability of natural killer cells from flown animals to kill K-562 cells was not affected (Rykova et al., 1992). These measurements were made in cells from animals euthanized immediately after flight (Rykova et al., 1992). In later experiments, rats were euthanized in flight aboard the U.S. Space Shuttle mission SLS-2 (Lesnyak et al., 1996). This was the first in-flight animal study on the U.S. Space Shuttle. Animals were euthanized 1 day prior to landing, spleens were removed, and refrigerated, and the assay was carried out after landing. In this case, the ability of spleen cells from the rats euthanized in space to kill both YAC-1 and K-562 target cells was inhibited compared to spleen cells from controls euthanized on Earth and maintained at 4°C for the same length of time as the in-flight samples. When spleen cells from animals flown aboard SLS-2 but euthanized immediately upon return to Earth were tested, only the ability to kill

YAC-1 targets was inhibited compared to controls, and there was no effect on the ability to kill K-562 targets (Lesnyak et al., 1996). These unique and important data indicate that in-flight sampling is very important, as there can be changes after landing from the situation during space flight.

Additional studies have centered on colony stimulating factor responsiveness and leukocyte subset distribution (Lesnyak et al., 1993). The response to colony stimulating factors of bone marrow cells from rats flown on several Russian Cosmos biosatellite missions has been examined. The response of cells from flown rats to both granulocyte-macrophage colony stimulating factor and macrophage colony stimulating factor has been shown to be greatly reduced after space flight compared to that seen in cells from control animals housed in normal caging and in caging designed to simulate conditions occurring in the space capsule (Sonnenfeld et al., 1990, 1992a). Additionally, there have been some alterations in leukocyte subset distribution noted after space flight of rats on the Cosmos capsule and the U.S. Space Shuttle, most notably increases in the level of CD4+ helper T cells (Allebban et al., 1994; Ichiki et al., 1996; Sonnenfeld et al., 1990, 1992a).

Studies with Rhesus monkeys have been much more limited, due to the expense and volume considerations regarding the use of primates. Results have been generally consistent with those observed using rats, including diminished proliferative responses and interferon production (Lesnyak et al., 1993). Since experiment conditions differ with each species and each flight, some variation in results is to be expected. Sampling was done of Rhesus monkeys flown in a Russian Cosmos biosatellite mission. Results indicate decreases in interleukin-1 levels, decreases in interleukin-2 receptor levels, and decreases in the ability of bone marrow cells to respond to granulocyte-macrophage colony stimulating factor (Sonnenfeld et al., 1996).

## III. HUMAN STUDIES

### A. Groundbased Studies on Immune Function in Humans

The problems which present themselves regarding space flight studies with research animals are also seen in human studies, compounded by the "normal" problems with studying stress and the human immune response. Several situations have been examined as groundbased models of space flight in humans. The models that have been used for immunological studies have included confinement, exercise, academic stress, isolation, high altitude, and chronic bed rest.

Chronic bed rest is the most frequently used model (Hargans et al., 1983; Konstantinova & Fuchs, 1991; LeBlanc, Schneider, Evans, Englebretson, & Krebs, 1992), and is the bipedal equivalent to AOS (or perhaps vice versa). Most bed rest studies involve lack of load-bearing on limbs and head-down tilt to model fluid shifts seen during space flight (Hargans et al., 1983). Again, since it is impossible to truly model microgravity on Earth, the models have their limitations. Additionally, most of these studies involve very small sample sizes. Results of the various model studies have shown increases in interleukin-1 production and decreases in interleukin-2 production (Schmitt et al., 1996), changes in leukocyte subset distribution that were variable, and alterations in neutrophil and macrophage function (generally inhibited, but also variable) (Dick, Mandel, Warshaver, Conklin, & Jerde, 1977; Konstantinova & Fuchs, 1991; Meehan et al., 1988; Schmitt et al., 1995, 1996; Schmitt and Schaffar, 1993; Sonnenfeld et al., 1992b; Taylor, 1997).

## B. Space Flight Studies on Immune Function in Humans

Ultimately, of course, we are concerned with the state of the immune system of humans under actual space flight conditions. There have been a large number of studies over the years to determine the effects of space flight on immune responses, ranging from investigations of cells in culture to studies on personnel during actual flight conditions.

Many early experiments examined the behavior/phenotype of human cells in culture when sent into space. Although mammalian cells are not known to have receptors for gravity, it was thought that changes in gravity might possibly be sensed as a result of alterations in cell randomness or by changes in fluid dynamics (Cogoli, 1993; Cogoli & Gmünder, 1991; Cogoli, Tschopp, & Fuchs-Bislin, 1984; Cogoli, Valuchi-Morf, Müller, & Breigleb, 1980). It must be noted that isolated cells of immunological importance were out of their normal "milieu" and not subjected to interactions with other body systems such as the neuroendocrine, cardiovascular, and musculoskeletal systems. Therefore, the results observed when isolated cell cultures were exposed to space flight conditions may not be representative of events occurring in vivo.

The seminal studies to show that cells important in immune responses could be affected by spaceflight conditions demonstrated that mitogen-mediated blastogenesis of human peripheral blood leukocytes grown in culture during space flights was severely inhibited (Cogoli, 1993; Cogoli & Gmünder, 1991; Cogoli, et al., 1980, 1984). At first, this was attributed to a possible direct effect of microgravity on lymphocytes (Cogoli, 1993; Cogoli & Gmünder, 1991; Cogoli et al., 1980, 1984). However, other possible mechanisms could be involved. For example, blastogenesis of lymphocytes requires assistance of macrophages as accessory cells. Changes in currents due to microgravity could have prevented necessary interactions between lymphocytes and macrophages that could have resulted in inhibited blastogenesis after space flight (Bechter, Cogoli, Cogoli-Greuter, Müller, & Hunziger, 1992; Gmünder, Kiess, Sonnenfeld, Lee, & Cogoli, 1990). Whatever the mechanism might be, it became clear that space flight inhibited in vitro blastogenesis of leukocytes, an essential immunological function. Later studies indicated that T cell and macrophage functional activities were definitively altered after space flight of cell cultures (Armstrong, Gerren, & Chapes, 1995; Chapes, Morrison, Guikema, Lewis, & Spooner, 1992; Limouse, Manie, Konstantinova, Ferrua, & Schaffar, 1991; Schmitt et al., 1996). Killing of target cells by tumor necrosis factor $\alpha$ was also inhibited in space flight by a mechanism involving protein kinase C. However, no effect on production of superoxide was noted. (Fleming, Edelman, & Chapes, 1991; Woods & Chapes, 1994). Additional studies showed that cultures of human peripheral blood cells challenged in space with an interferon inducer produced markedly enhanced levels of interferon-$\alpha/\beta$ (Tálas et al., 1984). As noted below, however, this only occurred in the in vitro culture situation and not in cells removed after landing from individuals flown in space and challenged with interferon inducers (Tálas et al., 1984). Other studies have shown enhanced interferon-$\gamma$, interleukin-1, interleukin-2, and tumor necrosis factor-$\alpha$ production from cultures of lymphoid cells flown in space (Bechter et al., 1992; Armstrong et al., 1995; Chapes et al., 1992; Limouse et al., 1991; Schmitt et al., 1996; Konstantinova, & Fuchs, 1991; Konstantinova, Rykova, Lesnyak, & Antropova, 1993).

Studies with humans have been constrained due to the necessary limited access to crew members. These studies include data obtained from relatively short-term space flight studies of 2 weeks or less duration, and some results obtained from long-term space flight studies of several months to greater than 1 year (Konstantinova, et al., 1993).

Among those changes observed in samples obtained from crew members of U.S. Space Shuttle flights of relatively short duration decreases in lymphocyte number, decreases in leukocyte blastogenesis, increases in leukocyte number, increases in numbers of B and T lymphocytes, decreases in monocytes, increases in helper T lymphocytes, decreases in cytotoxic T lymphocytes, and an increase in the ratio of CD4 + /CD8 + lymphocytes (Meehan et al., 1992; Meehan, Whitson, & Sams, 1993; Taylor, 1993b; Taylor & Dardano, 1983). There may be some association of these changes with certain neuroendocrine system changes, particularly with changes in catecholamines such as adrenaline and noradrenaline (Meehan, et al., 1993). It must be noted that these are overall values, as there are individual flights where there have been no changes or changes in the opposite direction from those reported in the summary above (Meehan et al., 1992, 1993; Taylor, 1993b; Taylor & Dardano, 1983). Again, it must be noted that conditions in every flight vary, duration of every flight is different, and crew members are genetically diverse; therefore, it is difficult to have a standard effect for every immunological parameter for space flight. The most appropriate comment may be that space flight has profound effects on immunological parameters.

Changes observed in cells obtained from cosmonauts immediately after Russian short-term flights include decreases in natural killer cell activity and decreases in production of interferon-$\alpha/\beta$ (Konstantinova & Fuchs, 1991; Konstantinova, et al., 1993; Tálas et al., 1984). Interestingly, the decreased interferon-$\alpha/\beta$ production was from the same mission and same cosmonauts whose peripheral blood leukocytes were placed in culture and challenged with an interferon inducer in the in vitro space experiment described above (Tálas et al., 1984). In the in vitro experiment, interferon-$\alpha/\beta$ production was markedly enhanced (Tálas et al., 1984). These results reiterate the point that in vitro space flight results may not be representative of the in vivo situation because cells in culture are not in their normal milieu and are not subject to normal interactions with other body systems.

In long-term flights, there have been several major effects on immune responses noted when testing was carried out on samples from cosmonauts immediately upon return to Earth (Konstantinova & Fuchs, 1991; Konstantinova et al., 1993). Among the most prominent are decreases in natural killer cell activity, decreases in leukocyte blastogenesis, and alterations of interleukin-2 production (Konstantinova, & Fuchs, 1991; Konstantinova et al., 1993). There have also been reported increases in the level of serum immunoglobulins (Igs), particularly total serum IgA and IgM, although these studies require confirmation

(Konstantinova, & Fuchs, 1991; Konstantinova et al., 1993). Interestingly, there has been no indication of an effect of relatively short-duration space flight on serum immunoglobulin levels (Taylor, & Dardano, 1983; Voss, 1984). This area requires further investigation.

All of the above studies with humans have been performed on samples obtained shortly after the return of astronauts or cosmonauts to Earth. Recently, there have been some studies carried out involving testing during space flight (Gmünder et al., 1994; Taylor & Janney, 1992). These results were originally reported with data obtained from astronauts during relatively short-term U.S. Space Shuttle flights (Taylor & Janney, 1992), but have been extended to longer-term Mir space station experiments (Gmünder et al., 1994). Delayed-type hypersensitivity responses to common recall antigens of astronauts and cosmonauts have been shown to be decreased when tested during space flights (Gmünder et al., 1994; Taylor & Janney, 1992). These have been the first data to prove that the cell-mediated immune response in humans has been inhibited while the subjects have been in space (Gmünder et al., 1994; Taylor & Janney, 1992).

## IV. SUMMARY

Although it has become clear that space flight can have profound effects on various measures of immune response, and that these effects may prove to have significant consequences to the health of flight crews, there are several major questions that remain unanswered. Many of these questions are unanswered to date because of various logistic obstacles. These obstacles include limited opportunities for flight experiments, technical difficulties, lack of manpower on missions, and the lack of a laboratory in space to carry out the required experiments (and more especially, no completely satisfactory laboratory environment, one mimicking all aspects of space flight, available on the ground).

Because of these logistic difficulties, most space flight studies with humans and, in particular, laboratory animals have involved sharing of specimens by multiple research groups working in multiple disciplines. Experiments have had to be planned to not interfere with or compromise other experiments. Studies involving sensitization to an antigen and determination of antibody levels, therefore, have not been carried out. Additionally, manipulation of animals and access to the crews during flight in current spacecraft is also difficult and has been carried out in only a limited fashion. Therefore, most results covered in the current review have derived from studies conducted immediately upon return of the laboratory animals and crew members to Earth. Reentry acceleration and other forces could have affected results obtained after landing. Only very limited in flight studies have been conducted.

In addition, again owing in part to the coordination of diverse experiments on the same group of subjects, space flight experiments have not always been carried out in consistent fashion between experimental runs (which are often far apart). Timing of launch, sampling, return, and retreival of samples are rarely under the control of the investigators, and must be varied according to other needs. It is hoped that development of the International Space Station will provide the flight opportunities and the required laboratory to answer additional questions which must be answered before long-term space flights to Mars and the possible development of lunar colonies can be attempted.

It still is not apparent what factors induce changes in immunological parameters during and after space flight and whether the factors are stressors which can be encountered in groundbased systems (e.g., accelleration forces, crowding, noise, some radiation components). or are unique to space flight (micravity, the total radiation environment, possibly others). The mechanism(s) of the changes in immunological parameters induced by space flight and models of space flight remain(s) to be established. It is also not clear if the same mechanism(s) are responsible for induction of changes in space flight and in the models used for effects of space flight on Earth. We are not sure how reliable the models are for events occurring during space flight.

A summary of the results of many of the space-flight experiments are given in Tables I and II, which are split into results for short-term and long-term flights. As can be seen, the bulk of the experiments, especially those carried out in laboratory animals, have been short-term (day- long) studies (as opposed to the months-long studies that would be considered long-term). The duration of changes in immunological parameters is not known. It appears from the limited long-duration studies carried out to date that there may be some adaptation of the immune response to space flight (Konstantinova & Fuchs, 1991; Konstantinova et al., 1993). However, there have been no definitive studies to date to determine the duration of the space flight-induced changes in immune responses in space and upon return to normal gravity situations.

**TABLE I**  Acute (Short-Term) Effects of Space Flight on Immune Responses

| Species | Immunological parameter | Effect |
| --- | --- | --- |
| Cell culture | Interferon production | Increased |
| Cell culture | Interleukin production | Increased |
| Cell culture | Leukocyte blastogenesis | Decreased |
| Animal | Interferon production | Decreased |
| Animal | Interleukin production | Increased and decreased |
| Animal | Leukocyte blastogenesis | Decreased or unchanged |
| Animal | Natural killer cell activity | Decreased |
| Animal | Colony stimulating factor responsiveness | Decreased |
| Animal | Leukocyte subset distribution | Altered |
| Human | Interferon production | Decreased |
| Human | Leukocyte blastogenesis | Decreased |
| Human | Leukocyte subset distribution | Altered |
| Human | Delayed hypersensitivity | Decreased |

Most importantly, the biological and biomedical significance of the changes in immunological parameters observed during and after space flight is not known. There have been some infections reported during and after space flight (Taylor, 1974; Taylor, Konstantinova, Sonnenfeld, & Jennings, 1997), although the number of infections has been relatively small and the harm to crews has been limited (Taylor, 1974; Taylor, et al., 1997). However, as the duration of space flight increases, the potential for development of opportunistic infections increases, as incumbent crew members that are potentially immunocompromised are exposed to infectious organisms from replacement crews. The crucial experiments to determine the effects of space flight on the development of immune responses after sensitization or immunization of animals, and the effects of space flight on resistance to infection of animals, have not been carried out and must be done.

**TABLE II**  Chronic (Long-Term) Effects of Space Flight on Immune Responses

| Species | Immunological parameter | Effect |
| --- | --- | --- |
| Human | Delayed hypersensitivity | Decreased |
| Human | Interleukin production | Decreased |
| Human | Leukocyte blastogenesis | Decreased |
| Human | Natural killer cell activity | Decreased |
| Human | Total serum immunoglobulin | Increased |

The increase in serum immunoglobulin levels reportedly observed after long-term flight (Konstantinova & Fuchs, 1991; Konstantinova et al., 1993) could indicate a potential problem with the development of autoimmune diseases. This potential difficulty also requires future exploration, particularly with regard to the duration of any increases in total immunoglobulin levels observed, as well as a determination of the antigenic specificity of the immunoglobulin for which levels are increased.

Another potential danger which must be addressed is increased susceptibility to tumors as a result of alterations in immune responses due to space flight. The relatively short length of time that humans have been in space, the relatively small number of astronauts/cosmonauts that have flown in space and the variation in each mission duration and characteristics has made this problem difficult to assess from an epidemiological basis. However, this must be an area of future consideration as we consider interplanetary travel exposing crew members to levels of cosmic radiation that have never before been encountered.

If the effects of space flight on immune responses proves to be of biomedical significance, then a new issue will arise. If space flight can compromise immune responses and, therefore, crew health, can countermeasures be designed and implemented to prevent any detrimental changes in immune responses? One possible route for countermeasure development would be pharmacological intervention. Therapies with drugs, or other agents such as cytokines, may be developed that could prevent or ameliorate any detrimental effects of space flight on immune responses. Another possible approach could be the use of exercise to prevent or dampen negative effects of space flight on immune responses. Since moderate exercise can have positive effects on immune responses (Nieman, 1997), it is possible that exercise by the crew while in space could have beneficial effects in maintaining a competent immune response. Exercise has been developed as a countermeasure for potential cardiovascular difficulties by both the U.S. and the Russian space programs (Greenleaf, Buibulian, Bernauer, Haskell, & Moore, 1989; Nicogossian et al., 1989). However, since these exercises have been developed to attempt to improve cardiovascular fitness, they have been primarily of an aerobic nature (Churchill, 1997; Greenleaf et al., 1989; Nicogossian et al., 1989). It remains to be seen if exposure of astronauts/cosmonauts to load-bearing exercise during space flight could have beneficial effects on immune responses and bone and muscle changes, or, indeed, if this type of countermeasure would be required to maintain crew health.

It is now very apparent that space flight induces profound changes in immune measures. The biomedical and biological significance of those changes remains to be established, as does the mechanism(s) involved in the induction of these changes. The potential significance of space flight-induced alterations in immune responses increases as the duration of space flights increases. Scientific studies in this area are just beginning, and much more work will be required before pressing questions regarding the integrity of the immune response in long-term space flights can be answered.

## Acknowledgments

Studies performed in the authors' laboratories were funded, in part, by agreements and Grants NCC2-859 and NAG2-933 from the US National Aeronautics and Space Administration.

## References

Albrect-Buehler, G. (1992). The simulation of microgravity conditions on the ground. *American Society for Gravitational and Space Biology Bulletin, 5*, 3–10.

Allebban, Z., Ichiki, A. T., Gibson, L. A., Jones, J. B., Congdon, C. C., & Lange, R. D. (1994). Effects of space flight on the number of rat peripheral blood leukocytes and lymphocyte subsets. *Journal of Leukocyte Biology, 55*, 209–213.

Armstrong, J. W., Gerren, R. A., & Chapes, S. K. (1995). The effect of space and parabolic flight on macrophage hematopoieses and function. *Experimental Cell Research, 216*, 160–168.

Armstrong, J. W., Nelson, K. A., Simske, S. J., Luttges, M. W., Iandolo, J. J., & Chapes, S. K. (1993). Skeletal unloading causes organ-specific changes in immune cell responses. *Journal of Applied Physiology, 75*, 2734–2739.

Bechter, H., Cogoli, A., Cogoli-Greuter, M., Müller, O., & Hunziger, E. (1992). Activation of microcarrier attached lymhocytes in microgravity. *Biotechnology and Bioengineering, 40*, 991–996.

Berry, W. D., Murphy, J. D., Smith, B. A., Taylor, G. R., & Sonnenfeld, G. (1991). Effect of microgravity modeling on interferon and interleukin responses in the rat. *Journal of Interferon Research, 11*, 243–249.

Caren, L., Mandel, A. D., & Nunes, J. (1980). Effect of simulated weightlessness on the immune system in rats. *Aviation Space and Environmental Medicine, 51*, 251–255.

Chapes, S. K., Morrison, D. R., Guikema, J. A., Lewis, M. L., & Spooner, B. S. (1992). Cytokine secretion by immune cells in space. *Journal of Leukocyte Biology, 52*, 104–110.

Chapes, S. K., Mastro, A. M., Sonnenfeld, G., & Berry, W. D. (1993). Antiorthostatic suspension as a model for the effects of space flight on the immune system. *Journal of Leukocyte Biology, 54*, 227–235.

Churchill, S. E. (1997). *Fundamentals of space life sciences*. Malabar, FL: Krieger.

Cogoli, A. (1993). The effect of hypogravity and hypergravity on cells of the immune system. *Journal of Leukocyte Biology, 54*, 259–268.

Cogoli, A., & Gmünder, F. K. (1991). Gravity effects on single cells: techniques, findings and theories. In S. E. Bonting (Ed.), *Advances in space biology and medicine (Vol. 1)*. Greenwich, UK: JAI Press.

Cogoli, A., Tschopp, A., & Fuchs-Bislin, P. (1984). Cell sensitivity to gravity. *Science, 255*, 228–230.

Cogoli, A., Valuchi-Morf, M., Müller, M., & Breigleb, W. (1980). The effect of hypogravity on human lymphocyte activation. *Aviation Space and Environmental Medicine, 51*, 29–34.

Congdon, C. C., Allebban, Z., Gibson, L. A., Kaplansky, A., Strickland, K. M., Jago, T. L., Johnson, D. L., Lange, R. D., & Ichiki, A. T. (1996). Lymphatic changes in rats flown on Spacelab Life Sciences-2. *Journal of Applied Physiology, 81*, 172–177.

Cruse, J. M., Lewis, R. E., Bishop, G. R., Kliesch, W. F., Gaitan, E., & Britt, R. (1993). Decreased immune reactivity and neuroendocrine alterations related to chronic stress in spinal cord injury and stroke patients. *Pathobiology, 61*, 183–192.

Dick, E. C., Mandel, A. D., Warshaver, D. M., Conklin, S. C., & Jerde, R. S. (1977). Respiratory virus transmission at McMurdo Station. *Antarctic Journal, 12*, 2–3.

Durnova, G. N., Kaplansky, A. S., & Portugalov, V. V. (1976). Effect of 22-day space flight on lymphoid organs of rats. *Aviation Space and Environmental Medicine, 47*, 588–591.

Fleming, S. D., Edelman, L. S., & Chapes, S. K. (1991). Effects of corticosterone and microgravity on inflammatory cell production of superoxide. *Journal of Leukocyte Biology, 50*, 69–76.

Fleming, S. D., Rosenkrans, C. F., Jr., & Chapes, S. K. (1990). Test of the antiorthostatic suspension model on mice: Effects on the inflammatory cell response. *Aviation Space and Environmental Medicine, 61*, 327–332.

Gmünder, F. K., Kiess, M., Sonnenfeld, G., Lee, J., & Cogoli, A. (1990). A ground-based model to study the effects of weightlessness on lymphocytes. *Biology of the Cell, 70*, 33–38.

Gmünder, F. K., Konstantinova, I., Cogoli, A., Lesnyak, A., Bogomolov, W., & Grachov, A. W. (1994). Cellular immunity in cosmonauts during long duration space flight on board the orbital MIR station. *Aviation Space and Environmental Medicine, 65*, 419–423.

Gould, C. L., Lyte, M., Williams, J., Mandel, A. D., & Sonnenfeld, G. (1987). Inhibited interferon-gamma but normal interleukin-3 production from rats flown on the space shuttle. *Aviation Space and Environmental Medicine, 58*, 983–986.

Gould, C. L., & Sonnenfeld, G. (1987). Enhancement of viral pathogenesis in mice maintained in an antiorthostatic suspension model: Coordination with effects on interferon production. *Journal of Biological Regulators and Homeostatic Agents, 1*, 33–36.

Greenleaf, J. E., Buibulian, R., Bernauer, E. M., Haskell, W. L., & Moore, T. (1989). Exercise-training protocols for astronauts in microgravity. *Journal of Applied Physiology, 67*, 2191–2204.

Hargans, A. R., Tipton, C. M., Gollnick, P. D., Mubarak, S. J., Tucker, B. J., & Akeson, W. H. (1983). Fluid shifts and muscle function in humans during acute simulated weightlessness. *Journal of Applied Physiology, 54*, 1003–1009.

Ichiki, A. T., Gibson, L. A., Jago, T. L., Strickland, K. M., Johnson, D. L., Lange, R. D., & Allebban, Z. (1996). Effects of space flight on rat peripheral blood leukocytes and bone marrow progenitor cells. *Journal of Leukocyte Biology, 60*, 37–43.

Ilyan, E. A., & Novikovo, V. E. (1980). A stand for the simulation of physiological effects of weightlessness in laboratory experimental rats. *Space Biology and Medicine, 14*, 128–129.

Konstantinova, I. V., & Fuchs, B. B. (1991). *The immune system in space and other extreme conditions.* Chur, Switzerland: Harwood Academic.

Konstantinova, I. V., Rykova, M. V., Lesnyak, A. T., & Antropova, A. A. (1993). Immune changes during long-duration missions. *Journal of Leukocyte Biology, 54*, 189–201.

Kopydlowski, K. M., Mcvey, D. S., Woods, K. M., Iandolo, J. J., & Chapes, S. K. (1992). Effects of antiorthostatic suspension and corticosterone on macrophage and spleen cell function. *Journal of Leukocyte Biology, 52*, 202–208.

LeBlanc, A. D., Schneider, V. S., Evans, H. J., Englebretson, D. A., & Krebs, J. M. (1992). Bone mineral loss and recovery after 17 weeks of bed-rest. *Journal of Bone and Mineral Research, 5*, 843–850.

Lesnyak, A., Sonnenfeld, G., Avery, L., Konstantinova, I., Rykova, M., Meshkov, D., & Orlova, T. (1996). Effect of SLS-2 space flight on immunologic parameters of rats. *Journal of Applied Physiology, 81*, 178–182.

Lesnyak, A. T., Sonnenfeld, G., Rykova, M. P., Meshkov, D. O., Mastro, A., & Konstantinova, I. (1993). Immune changes in test animals during space flight. *Journal of Leukocyte Biology, 54*, 214–226.

Limouse, M., Manie, S., Konstantinova, I., Ferrua, B., & Schaffar, L. (1991). Inhibition of phorbol ester-induced activation in microgravity. *Experimental Cell Research, 197*, 82–86.

Mandel, A. D., & Balish, E. (1977). Effect of space flight on cell-mediated immunity. *Aviation Space and Environmental Medicine, 48*, 1051–1057.

Meehan, R., Whitson, P., & Sams, C. (1993). The role of psychoneuroendocrine factors on space flight-induced immunological alterations. *Journal of Leukocyte Biology, 54*, 236–244.

Meehan, R. T., Duncan, U., Neale, L., Taylor, G., Muchmore, H., Scott, N., Ramsey, K., Smith, E., Rock, P., Goldblum, G., & Houston, C. (1988). Operation Everest 11: Alterations in the immune system at high altitudes. *Journal of Clinical Immunology, 8*, 397–403.

Meehan, R. T., Neale, L. S., Kraus, E. T., Stuart, C. A., Smith, M. L., Cintron, N. M., & Sams, C. F. (1992). Alterations in human mononuclear leucocytes following space flight. *Immunology, 76*, 491–497.

Miller, E. S., Koebel, D. A., Davis, S. A., Klein, J. B., Mcleish, K. R., Goldwater, D., & Sonnenfeld, G. (1994). Influence of suspension on the oxidative burst by rat neutrophils. *Journal of Applied Physiology, 76*, 387–390.

Miller, E. S., Koebel, D. A., & Sonnenfeld, G. (1995). Influence of space flight on the production of interleukin-3 and interleukin-6 by rat spleen and thymus cells. *Journal of Applied Physiology, 78*, 810–813.

Miller, E. S., & Sonnenfeld, G. (1993). Influence of suspension on the expression of protective immunological memory to murine *Listeria monocytogenes* infection. *Journal of Leukocyte Biology, 54*, 578–583.

Miller, E. S., & Sonnenfeld, G. (1994). Influence of antiorthostatic suspension on resistance to murine *Listeria monocytogenes* infection. *Journal of Leukocyte Biology, 55*, 371–378.

Morey, E., Sabelman, E., Turner, R., & Baylink, D. (1979). A new rat model simulating some aspects of space flight. *The Physiologist, 22*, S23–S24.

Musacchia, X. J., Deavers, D., Meininger, G., & Davis, T. (1980). A new model for hypokinesia: Effects on muscle atrophy in the rat. *Journal of Applied Physiology, 48*, 470–476.

Nash, P. V., Bour, B. A., & Mastro, A. M. (1991). Effect of hindlimb suspension simulation of microgravity on in vitro immunological responses. *Experimental Cell Research, 195*, 353–360.

Nash, P. V., Konstantinova, I. V., Fuchs, B. B., Rakhmilevich, A. L., Lesnyak, A. T., & Mastro, A. M. (1992). Effect of space flight on lymphocyte proliferation and interleukin-2 production. *Journal of Applied Physiology, 73*, 186S–190S.

Nash, P. V., & Mastro, A. M. (1992). Variable lymphocyte responses in rats after space flight. *Experimental Cell Research, 202*, 125–131.

Nicogossian, A. E., Huntoon, C. L., & Pool, S. (1989). *Space physiology, & medicine* (2nd ed.). Philadelphia: Lea and Febiger.

Nieman, D. C. (1997). Exercise immunology: Practical applications. *International Journal of Sports Medicine, 18*(Suppl. 1), 91–100.

Pellis, N. R., Goodwin, T. J., Risin, D., McIntyre, B. W., Pizzini, R. P., Cooper, D., Baker, T. L., & Spaulding, G. F. (1997). Changes in gravity inhibit locomotion through type I collagen. *In vitro Cell and Developmental Biology-Animal, 33,* 398–405.

Rose, A., Steffen, J. M., Musacchia, X. J., Mandel, A. D., & Sonnenfeld, G. (1984). Effect of antiorthostatic suspension on interferon alpha/beta production by the mouse. *Proceedings of the Society for Experimental Biology and Medicine, 177,* 253–256.

Rykova, M. P., Sonnenfeld, G., Lesnyak, A. T., Taylor, G. R., Meshkov, D. O., Mandel, A. D., Medvedev, A. E., Berry, W. D., Fuchs, B. B., & Konstantinova, I. V. (1992). Effect of space flight on natural killer cell activity. *Journal of Applied Physiology, 73* (Suppl.), 196S–200S.

Schmitt, D. A., Hatton, J. P., Emond, C., Chaput, D., Paris, H., Levade, T., Cazenave, J. P., & Schaffar, L. (1996). The distribution of protein knase C in human leukocytes is altered in microgravity. *FASEB Journal, 10,* 1627–1634.

Schmitt, D. A., & Schaffar, L. (1993). Isolation and confinement as a model for space flight immune changes. *Journal of Leukocyte Biology, 54,* 209–213.

Schmitt, D. A., Peres, C., Sonnenfeld, G., Tkackzuk, J., Arquier, M., Mauco, G., & Ohayon, E. (1995). Immune responses in humans after 60 days of confinement. *Brain, Behavior, and Immunity, 9,* 70–77.

Schmitt, D. A., Schaffar, L., Taylor, G. R., Loftin, K. C., Schneider, V. S., Koebel, A., Abbal, M., Sonnenfeld, G., Lewis, D. E., Reuben, J. R., & Ferebee, R. (1996). Use of bed rest and head-down tilt to simulate spaceflight-induced immune system changes. *Journal of Interferon and Cytokine Research, 16,* 151–157.

Sonnenfeld, G., Davis, S., Taylor, G. R., Mandel, A. D., Konstantinova, I. V., Lesnyak, A., Fuchs, B. B., Peres, C., Tkackzuk, J., & Schmitt, D. A. (1996). Effect of space flight on cytokine production and other immunologic parameters of rhesus monkeys. *Journal of Interferon and Cytokine Research, 16,* 409–415.

Sonnenfeld, G., Mandel, A. D., Konstantinova, I. V., Berry, W. D., Taylor, G. R., Lesnyak, A. T., Fuchs, B. B., & Rakhmilevich, A. L. (1992a). Space flight alters immune cell function and distribution. *Journal of Applied Physiology, 73*(Suppl.), 191S–195S.

Sonnenfeld, G., Mandel, A. D., Konstantinova, I. V., Taylor, G. R., Berry, W. D., Wellhausen, S. R., Lesnyak, A. T., & Fuchs, B. B. (1990). Effects of space flight on levels and activity of immune cells. *Aviation Space and Environmental Medicine, 61,* 648–653.

Sonnenfeld, G., Measel, J., Loken, M. R., Degioanni, J., Follini, S., Galvagno, A., & Montalbani, M. (1992b). Effects of isolation on interferon production and hematological and immunological parameters. *Journal of Interferon Research, 12,* 75–81.

Sonnenfeld, G., & Miller, E. S. (1993). The role of cytokines in immune changes induced by space flight. *Journal of Leukocyte Biology, 54,* 253–258.

Sonnenfeld, G., Morey-Holton, E. R., Williams, J. A., & Mandel, A. D. (1982). Effect of a simulated weightlessness model on the production of rat interferon. *Journal of Interferon Research, 2,* 467–470.

Sonnenfeld, G., & Taylor, G. R. (1991). Effect of microgravity on the immune system. In *Technical Paper Series No. 911515* Warrendale, PA: Society of Automotive Engineers.

Taylor, G. R. (1974). Recovery of medically important microorganisms from Apollo astronauts. *Aerospace Medicine, 45,* 824–828.

Tálas, M., Bátkai, L., Stöger, I., Nagy, K., Hiros, L., Konstantinova, I., Rykova, M., Mozogovava, J., Guseva, O., & Kozharinov, V. (1984). Results of the space experiment program "Interferon". *Acta Astronautica, 11,* 379–386.

Taylor, G. R., & Dardano, J. R. (1983). Human cellular responsiveness following space flight. *Aviation Space and Environmental Medicine, 54,* S55–S59.

Taylor, G. R., & Janney, R. P. (1992). In vivo testing confirms a blunting of human cell-mediated immune mechanism during space flight. *Journal of Leukocyte Biology, 51,* 129–132.

Taylor, G. R. (1993a). Overview of space flight immunology studies. *Journal of Leukocyte Biology, 54,* 179–188.

Taylor, G. R. (1993b). Immune changes in short-duration missions. *Journal of Leukocyte Biology, 54,* 202–208.

Taylor, G. R., Konstantinova, I. V., Sonnenfeld, G., & Jennings, R. (1997). Changes in the immune system during and after space flight. *Advances in Space Biology and Medicine, 6,* 1–32.

Voss, E. W., Jr. (1984). Prolonged weightlessness and humoral immunity. *Science, 225,* 214–215.

Woods, K. M., & Chapes, S. K. (1994). Abrogation of TNF-mediated cytotoxicity by space flight involves protein kinase C. *Experimental Cell Research, 211,* 171–174.

# 44

# Immunologic Sequelae of Surgery and Trauma

RENÉ ZELLWEGER, MARTIN G. SCHWACHA, IRSHAD H. CHAUDRY

## I. INTRODUCTION

The saga of trauma is a reflection of the story of man. Although it is difficult to visualize early humans' struggle for survival in a hostile environment, the earliest writings suggest that trauma was the main problem. The Edwin Smith Papyrus, written between 3000 and 1600 BC, is a description of 48 cases of trauma described from head to foot, *a capite ad calcem*, an approach that is still in use (Breasted, 1930). Injury must have been frequent, and since most non-fatal injuries are superficial or observable (fractures), trauma must have been the origin of medical practice. Trauma is a multisystem disease, and its treatment and management benefits from almost any advance in medical science. As knowledge about physiology, biochemistry, immunology, and molecular biology has advanced, subsequent management of the trauma victims has improved. Nonetheless, traumatic injury is a costly disease, impacting not only the patient, but

also society as a whole. Furthermore, it remains true today, as it was in the past, that prevention remains the best treatment.

A multitude of studies has examined the relationship between traumatic injury and dysfunction of the immune system. This chapter will focus on the immunological effect of surgery and traumatic injury as well as various therapeutic regimens that have been employed to modulate the potentially fatal consequence of injury, intentional (i.e., surgery) or accidental.

## II. INFLAMMATION AND THE IMMUNE RESPONSE TO INJURY

A great deal has been learned in the past 15 years about the role of the inflammatory and immunologic responses to injury. Recently, the interplay between cellular inflammatory mediators, the neuroendocrine system, and nonspecific and specific immunity has further advanced the understanding of this complex area. The clinical correlates of immunosuppression have become increasingly evident in recent years. Although 50% of patients die of irreversible head injury following trauma to the head, sepsis and multiple organ failure cause 78% of late nonneurologic deaths (Baker, Oppenheimer, Stephens, Lewis, & Trunkey, 1980). Disruption of homeostasis following major elective surgery, major injury, or major illness tends to produce a fairly similar response. Factors affecting the patient's premorbid host resistance and preinjury nutritional status are balanced against the extent of shock, tissue injury, and disruption of normal physiology that occurs with trauma. Following injury, various immune factors (i.e., cytokines, prostaglandins, coagulation factors, and toxic factors) affect the critical elements of gas exchange, energy metabolism, wound healing, and host resistance. It is the effect on these elements that determines the ultimate outcome. If the patient develops sepsis and a treatable cause, such as an abscess, can be found survival is generally feasible. Unfortunately, if the source of sepsis is not identified, mortality follows at a frequency directly proportional to the number of organ systems that have failed (Knaus, Draper, Wagner, & Zimmerman, 1985).

Following a shock-producing insult, cellular potassium and sodium balance is disrupted leading to cell swelling (Sayeed Adler, Chaudry, & Baue, 1981; Shires et al., 1972). The inflammatory mediators of injury, such as tumor necrosis factor-$\alpha$ (TNF) (Tracey et al., 1986a), platelet-activating factor (PAF) (Stahl, Bitterman, Terashita, & Lefer, 1988), leukotrienes (Bitterman, Smith, & Lefer, 1988), and thromboxane $A_2$ (Bitterman, Yanagisawa, & Lefer, 1986), have been implicated in the induction of this membrane dysfunction. In patients with adult respiratory distress syndrome (ARDS) it has been observed, among other conditions, $O_2$ consumption increases as $O_2$ delivery is augmented (Tuchschmidt, Oblitas, & Fried, 1991). This increased $O_2$ consumption occurs despite the depression of peripheral $O_2$ extraction. Furthermore, $O_2$ demand and the arterial lactate concentration are both elevated. Moreover, studies have suggested that tissue hypoxia as a result of injury may be the precipitating factor in flow-dependent $O_2$ consumption (Cabin & Buchman, 1990). Appel and Shoemaker (1992) reported that patient outcome improved when $O_2$ delivery was improved. Nonetheless, conclusive evidence concerning the benefit of $O_2$ delivery on survival remains controversial.

As shown in Figure 1, injury causes dramatic and complex changes in the neuroendocrine system. For example, shock induces massive sympathetic output of norepinephrine and epinephrine via the baroreceptor reflex. In turn, adrenocorticotropic hormone (ACTH) secreted from the pituitary promotes the release of glucocorticoids and, as a result, insulin levels fall and hyperglycemia is seen early after injury, in association with a relative "insulin resistance" (Kinney & Gump, 1982). It has been suggested that this abnormality results from changes in hepatic glucose metabolism, such as increased gluconeogenesis and the inability of the liver to take up glucose

mediated partially by glucagon (Kinney & Gump, 1982).

Physiologic stress leads to the altered release of other neuroendocrine factors, including enkephalins and endorphins (Khansari, Margo, & Faith, 1990). A thorough discussion of the interaction between the hypothalamo-pituitary-adrenal axis (HPA) and the immune system is provided by Lilly and Gann (1992). On the one hand, circulating proinflammatory cytokines (interleukin (IL)-1, IL-6, TNF) from the inflammatory site can directly elicit a response from the HPA (Scarborough, 1990). On the other hand, neuroendocrine factors (endorphins, enkephalins) can exert immunoregulatory effects (Abraham, 1991; Weigent, Carr, & Blalock, 1990). Hence, a two-way communication occurs between the site of injury and the central nervous system (CNS).

A number of metabolic effects occur postinjury. These include increased circulating levels of growth hormone, especially in the anabolic phase of recovery. The utility of growth hormone as well as insulin-like growth factor 1 (IGF-1) (Kupfer, Underwood, Baxter, & Clemmons, 1993) in reversing catabolism following injury appears to depend on adequate caloric intake (Wilmore et al., 1980). Modern techniques have allowed researchers to dissect the complex elements of the metabolic response to injury. Clearly, the insult is proportional to the degree of anatomic disruption with the most severe insult being thermal injury. It is critical, therefore, to concentrate on prompt resuscitation and operative intervention as the potential systemic inflammatory response syndrome (SIRS), with secondary protein catabolism, is associated with high morbidity and mortality.

## A. The Nonspecific Immunoinflammatory Response

Nonspecific immunity involves aspects of the host defense system that respond to foreign material of any type (e.g., a foreign body, necrotic debris, altered protein, etc.). A number of host resistance aspects need to be clarified to permit better understanding of the effects of injury on host defenses. These aspects of resistance can generally be divided into the following categories: (1) mechanical barriers, (2) phagocytosis, (3) the complement system, (4) the kinin system, (5) the coagulation system, (6) toxic factors, (7) heat-shock proteins.

The important mechanical barriers against bacterial invasion are the skin and the mucosal membranes. The skin, in addition to being the largest organ in the body, also has a complex set of host-defense mechanisms. One important barrier aspect of the skin relates

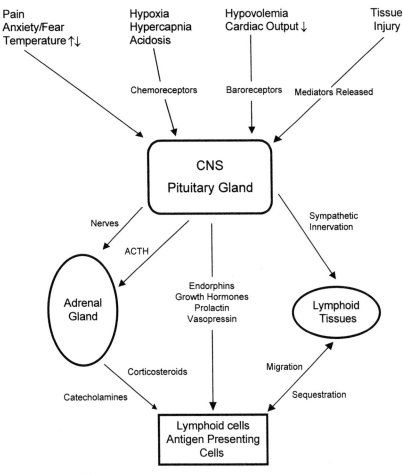

**FIGURE 1**   The neuroendocrine response to injury.

to the low moisture content and low pH of its keratin layer. In addition, a number of natural antimicrobial substances exist in the skin. The most dramatic example of disruption of this mechanical barrier is thermal injury that results in massive suppression of the immune system. In addition, wounds involving the skin and insults that lead to ischemia of the skin can also result in disruption of this important mechanical barrier. The other major mechanical barrier of the body is the mucous membranes, primarily in the respiratory and gastrointestinal tracts. The paradigm for disruption of the mucosal barrier of the respiratory tract is aspiration or inhalation injury. However, a number of factors can disrupt pulmonary homeostasis and precipitate ARDS. It is becoming increasingly clear that metabolites of arachidonic acid and products of endothelial cell damage, acting in concert with white cells, may be involved in the development of ARDS (Demling, 1995; Hechtman, Valeri, & Shepro, 1984). With regards to the gastrointestinal tract, it is now recognized as not merely a

passive organ but rather one that is highly metabolically active. A number of investigators are actively examining the steps that lead to breakdown of the gut mucosal barrier and subsequent bacterial translocation. Three etiologic factors appear important in breakdown of the gut mucosa: direct mucosal injury by toxins or radiation, malnutrition, and decreased mesenteric blood flow. The mechanism for the gut mucosal breakdown, however, may involve multiple mediators other than bacterial endotoxin (Koike et al., 1992). Nonetheless, while supportive evidence for bacterial translocation following injury exists, the role of bacterial translocation as an initiator of organ failure has not been mutually accepted.

The next line of defense to controlling bacterial invasion is the phagocytic system. Although a number of phagocytic cells (neutrophils, eosinophils, monocytes, macrophages) exist, the most important to early host defense is the neutrophil (PMN). Normal phagocytosis occurs in four steps: (1) chemotaxis, the process by which cells migrate to areas of inflammation; (2) opsonization, which involves the recognition and preparation of microbes for ingestion; (3) ingestion, which involves alterations in phagocyte morphology and metabolism; and (4) microbial killing and digestion.

Properdin can activate the alternate pathway of complement leading to the attraction (chemotaxis) of white cells into an area of inflammation. During opsonization, the bacterial wall is made more susceptible to phagocytosis. The two most important opsonins are immunoglobulin G (IgG) and the complement fragment C3b. This latter fragment is a powerful opsonin. These factors cause alterations in bacterial cell wall morphology in preparation of the bacteria for ingestion by phagocytes. After migrating into the area of bacterial invasion and inflammation, the phagocyte forms pseudopodia that surround the bacterium and then join and invaginate to form a phagosome or phagolysosome. A number of metabolic events are associated with phagocytosis. One of these is a tremendous increase in glycolysis and lactate production, resulting in a decrease in pH inside the phagocytic vacuole. Oxygen consumption by the white cell increases, predominantly through activation of the NADPH oxidase and generation of superoxide anion ($O_2^-$). Superoxide can then be reduced to other reactive oxygen species such as $H_2O_2$. Collectively, these events are referred to as the "respiratory burst." All of these substrates are powerful bactericidal agents and, together with lysozymes and other cytoplasmic granule products within the phagolysosome, cause bacterial killing. There are a number of steps in which abnormalities can cause defects in this process, of which several have been demonstrated in burn and trauma patients (Kapur, Jain, & Gidh, 1986; Warden, Mason, & Pruitt, 1974).

The complement system functions in chemotaxis, opsonization, and bacterial killing. These proteins often react in a cascade, much like the coagulation system. Additionally, activation of the complement system induces an inflammatory response and enhances the primary immune reaction.

The complement system also interacts with other inflammatory systems/factors such as fibrin kinin and prostaglandins. The classical complement pathway is initiated by an antigen–antibody complex. Complement receptors are present on a number of different cells, such as erythrocytes, monocytes, eosinophils, PMNs, B cells, and glomerular epithelial cells (Unanue & Benacerraf, 1998). With regard to trauma, serum C3 levels are inversely correlated with the Injury Severity Score (ISS) (Kapur et al., 1986). Moreover, massive activation of complement is associated with increased susceptibility to infection and

development of the sepsis syndrome (Schirmer, Schiermer, Naff, & Fry, 1988; Gardinali et al., 1992) and ARDS (Solomkin, 1990).

The kinin system is another nonspecific aspect of host defense. Kinins are polypeptides of low molecular weight that are released from the inactive substance kininogen by enzymes secreted by granulocytes, or by active kallikrein. The kinin system interacts with both the inflammatory and the coagulation systems. Moreover, kinin can activate phospholipase $A_2$ and C, leading to the generation of prostaglandins (Hartl, Herndon, & Wolfe, 1990), which may have therapeutic implications in modulating traumatic stress. Kinins can also be inactivated by granulocytes, via kininases. The most well known kinin is bradykinin, which is a potent vasoconstrictor and can cause pain, vasodilatation, increased capillary permeability, and the margination of intact granulocytes. In addition to the kinins, histamine (released from basophils and occasionally from leukocytic granules in response to injury) can increase vascular permeability. Moreover, the accumulation of excess bradykinin following trauma is thought to be an important factor in the development of SIRS (Stewart, 1993).

The coagulation and immune systems are interrelated, since activation of the coagulation system may potentiate inflammation (Ryan & Geczy, 1987) and monocytes produce plasminogen activator (PA) leading to plasmin formation. In this regard, Graziano and colleagues have demonstrated alterations in the monocyte production of tissue thromboplastin factor after injury (Graziano, Miller, & Lim, 1980). Furthermore, PA synthesis is depressed in splenectomized patients and burn patients and the depression of synthesis coincided with suppressed T-cell mitogenesis in both groups (Baker, Miller, & Trunkey, 1979) and a direct correlation was found between the ISS and thromboplastin generation in trauma patients (McCullough, Spillert, & Lazaro, 1990). Furthermore, macrophages can express cell-surface procoagulant activity, leading to fibrin deposition by a process mediated through a prostanoid-cyclic AMP-dependent pathway (Williams, Garcia, & Maier, 1993). Animal studies have revealed active interactions between endothelial cells and the coagulation system under inflammatory conditions. Endotoxin, as well as macrophage products, such as TNF and IL-1, induce a phenotypic transformation of endothelial cells from a noninflammatory to a proinflammatory and procoagulant state (Pober and Cotran, 1990; Vane, Anggard, & Botting, 1990). A sequential set of interactions between leukocytes and endothelial cells mediates tissue injury following an inflammatory stimulus

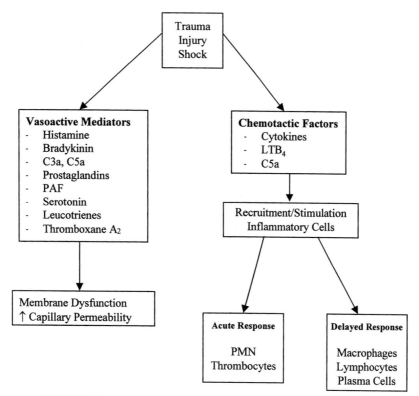

**FIGURE 2**   Trigger points of the inflammatory acute-phase response.

(Butcher, 1991). Leukocytes initially bind by way of adhesion molecules, known as selectins, to receptors on the endothelial cells. Examples of the receptors for selectin include endothelial-leukocyte adhesion molecule-1 (ELAM-1) and intercellular adhesion molecule-1 (ICAM-1) (Ossa, de la Malago, & Gewertz, 1992). This primary binding event is transient and reversible; however, this interaction may activate leukocytes, either via specific chemoattractants or cell contact-mediated signals, leading to the expression of secondary adhesion receptors (e.g., the integrin family CD11/CD18, CD11/CD29; and Mac-1). These secondary receptors facilitate a strong, sustained attachment of leukocytes to the endothelium, thus, completing the recognition process. Simultaneously, the proinflammatory endothelial cells can secrete leukocyte activating factors (IL-1, IL-8, PAF, granulocyte-macrophage colony-stimulating factor [GM-CSF], and granulocyte colony-stimulating factor [G-CSF]). A recent review of PMN-endothelial cell binding was provided by Ossa and colleagues (1992). Following adhesion and binding, leukocytes induce tissue injury by producing reactive oxygen species, proteases, cationic proteins, and collagenases. Interestingly, antibodies to ELAM-1 (Mulligan et al., 1991), Mac-1 (Hill et al., 1992), CD-18 (Mileski et al., 1992), and other adhesion molecules (Harlan, Vedder, Winn, & Rice, 1991) can ameliorate

the extent of organ injury after ischemia and reperfusion. The exact mechanism by which this occurs is not yet clear.

The pathophysiologic changes in the complement, kinin, and coagulation systems after injury are noteworthy for the following points. First, all three of these systems have similar cascade-like structures. Second, these systems share a number of common activators and inactivators. Last, the macrophage plays a key regulatory role in all three systems. It is unclear whether injury induces abnormal activation of these systems, thereby altering macrophage function, or whether macrophage dysfunction is the inciting event in abnormal activation of these systems (Figure 2).

Another aspect of the postinjury milieu is the release of toxic factors that may nonspecifically affect the immune system. Perhaps the most prominent of these is endotoxin. For example, endotoxin in low doses, causes vascular margination and the sequestration of leukocytes, particularly in the capillary bed (Horn & Collins, 1968); however, at higher doses granulocyte destruction is often seen. Furthermore, whereas endotoxin stimulates glycolysis and metabolic effects in the PMN, it also decreases PMN motility and induces cellular aggregation. Many models of "sepsis" have utilized endotoxin, although such models may not be particularly relevant to studies of human sepsis (Wichterman, Baue, & Chaudry, 1980). Recent studies have indicated that a major effect of endotoxin is to liberate TNF, which induces many effects formerly attributed to endotoxin. TNF, produced primarily by macrophages, can have a variety of potent effects (Tracey et al., 1986b).

Heat-shock proteins (HSPs) are polypeptides produced by every type of cell upon exposure to stressful stimuli, such as heat, hypoxia–anoxia, and reactive oxygen metabolites. HSPs are also involved in immune reactions, such as in decreasing TNF-target cell lysis, lymphocyte homing, antigen processing, and autoimmunity. T cells have been shown to be capable of lysing macrophages expressing the processed polypeptides of HSPs (Koga et al., 1989). It has been hypothesized that when present in large concentrations, as in states of severe shock or burns, HSPs can overwhelm T-cell populations and decrease the host's resistance to microbial invasions (Abraham, 1991).

## B. The Specific Immunoinflammatory Response

The four areas to be covered in detail under specific immunity are: (1) lymphokines/monokines, (2) oxygen free radicals, (3) arachidonic acid metabolites, and (4) nitric oxide. The past 10 years have seen an explosion of information about cellular products (cytokines) that modify inflammatory and immune responses. Since there is extensive information on this subject, the key aspects of lymphokines and monokines as they relate to trauma will be described here. The interested reader is directed to an excellent overall review of monocytes and macrophages by Johnston (1988).

Central to the set of processes involving cytokines is the crucial regulatory role of cells of the monocyte-macrophage lineage (Unanue & Allen, 1987). Approximately 100 distinct substances are secreted by macrophages (Nathan, 1987). One of the most important of these is IL-1. IL-1 leads to proteolysis after injury (Baracos, 1983) and stimulates the hepatic synthesis of acute-phase proteins (Dinarello, 1988). Tumor necrosis factor-$\alpha$ (TNF), or cachectin, which is released by monocytes/macrophages in response to various stimuli, has received considerable attention (Beutler, Krochin, & Milsark, 1986). Although TNF mimics many of the effects of IL-1, the two molecules have different receptors and have very little structural homology (Dinarello, 1988). These monokines stimulate procoagulant activity and inhibit PA, which plays a role in the coagulation problems after injury.

IL-2 is produced by T lymphocytes (CD4 +) following stimulation by a number of mitogenic and antigenic factors as well as the monokine IL-1. Dysregulation of IL-2 production following injury has profound implications on cell-mediated immunity and a number of studies using different trauma models have shown suppression in IL-2 production (Chaudry, Ayala, Ertel, & Stephan, 1990).

A great deal of basic and clinical research in the area of trauma has centered on metabolites of arachidonic acid, specifically the prostaglandin, leukotriene, and thromboxane compounds. Probably the most important fact with regard to the arachidonic acid metabolites is that PGE$_2$ is a potent regulatory factor that has, in general, inhibitory effects on monocytes/macropahges, T-helper cells, and B cells. This may not necessarily be a deleterious event, since it may play an important regulatory role in the specific immune response. Faist and co-workers, however, showed that monocytosis occurs postinjury, with resultant excessive PGE$_2$, production, suppression of T-helper cell function, and defects in B-cell maturation (Faist et al., 1987, 1988; Faist, Ertel, Baker, & Heberer, 1989). Another autoregulatory loop involving PGE$_2$, TNF, and cAMP has been described, in which TNF stimulates endogenous PGE$_2$ production, which, in turn, increases intracellular cAMP (Lehmann, Benninghoff, & Dröge, 1988). A recent experimental study showed that in vivo administration of ibuprofen, a cyclooxygenase (the enzyme response for PGE$_2$ production) inhibitor, reversed the TNF-induced shock-like state and reduced mortality (Fletcher et al., 1993).

Platelet-activating factor is an important inflammatory mediator produced by various cells including macrophages, endothelial cells, and PMNs. For example, in an ischemia/reperfusion model, PAF was important in mediating PMN-induced tissue injury (Read, Moore, Moore, Carl, & Banerjee, 1993). Recent studies have shown that administration of the PAF antagonist RO 24-4736 (a thienodiazepine) after hemorrhage and resuscitation prevented the suppression of splenocyte function (Zellweger, Ayala, Schmand, Morrison, & Chaudry, 1995b).

As mentioned, oxygen radical formation by leukocytes is a host-defense mechanism for bactericidal activity. Changes in regulation of this process after injury and/or ischemia and reperfusion may lead to the excessive production of oxygen free radicals, with deleterious effects on organ function (Jaeschke, 1991). A number of investigators have suggested that one of the early effects of injury is complement activation leading to PMN activation and the liberation of oxygen free radicals that induce endothelial-cell damage (Fountain et al., 1980). Injury to the endothelium, in turn, causes platelet and fibrin deposition, microcirculatory ischemia, tissue injury, and further complement activation, causing a vicious cycle of deleterious effects on cell and organ function. This hypothesis is corroborated by several studies of pulmonary function (Fountain, Martin, Musclow, & Cooper, 1980; Ward, Till, Kunkel, & Beauchamp, 1983), hepatic injury (Clemens, McDonagh, Chaudry, & Baue, 1985; Schirmer, Schirmer, Naff, & Fry, 1988), and renal injury (Sumpio, Hull, Baue, & Chaudry, 1986). In experimental models of lung injury, complement depletion protected against bacterial- or endotoxin-induced lung injury (Dehring, Steinberg, & Wismar, 1987; Ward et al., 1983). In addition, pulmonary endothelial damage can be minimized by the prior administration of the oxygen-radical scavengers superoxide dismutase (SOD) and catalase (CAT) (Ward et al., 1983). Numerous studies of pharmacologic manipulation with SOD, CAT, allopurinol, and other antioxidants have strengthened the hypothesis of tissue damage by oxygen free radicals and have further delineated the role of extracellular oxygen free radicals as the principal factors inducing injury (Jaeschke, 1991). In addition, Deitch and coworkers have suggested that bacterial translocation from the gut can be attenuated with xanthine oxidase inhibitors (Deitch, Berg, & Specian, 1987; Deitch, Winterton, & Berg, 1986). Nonetheless, additional studies are required before SOD, CAT, and other means of oxygen-free-radical reduction are routinely utilized clinically.

Nitric oxide (NO) is the simplest known mammalian effector molecule. A paradigm for the development of sepsis syndrome and multiple organ failure involves the potential role of excessive NO production (Moncada, Palmer, & Higgs, 1991; Nava, Palmer, & Moncada, 1991; Teale & Atkinson, 1992). In contrast, a protective role for NO in endotoxemia and hepatic failure has also been suggested (Frederick et al., 1993). This paradox is likely related to the different physiological roles of cNOS and iNOS.

## III. POSTINJURY IMMUNE DYSFUNCTION

Various types of immune dysfunction have been identified following injury (Baker et al., 1979; Chaudry & Ayala, 1992; Deitch et al., 1986; Faist et al., 1987, 1988, 1989; Graziano et al., 1980). The hypothesis derived from these studies is that major trauma produces immunosuppression which can be exacerbated by sepsis. Faist and colleagues (Faist et al., 1987, 1988) demonstrated in trauma patients

that T-cell numbers decreased after injury; however, this reduction in T cells was primarily in the helper (CD4+) rather than in the cytotoxic/suppressor (CD8+) cell population. In addition, IL-2 synthesis and IL-2 receptor expression by T-helper cells was decreased. These findings have recently been confirmed by other clinical studies (McRitchie, Girotti, Rotstein, & Teodorczyk-Injeyan, 1990) and in animal models of shock and sepsis (Zapata-Sirvent et al., 1992; Zellweger, Ayala, DeMaso, & Chaudry, 1995a). Furthermore, IL-2 may be beneficial in limiting the adverse effects of sepsis (Gough, Jordon, Mannick, & Rodrick, 1992). Interestingly, the production of IL-2 in vitro could be augmented (although not completely restored) by blocking $PGE_2$ production with the cyclooxygenase inhibitor, indomethacin. Aberrations in monocytes postinjury have also been suggested. These aberrations include inadequate granulopoiesis (Moore, Peterson, Moore, Rundus, & Poggett, 1990), defective antigen presentation (Ertel, Morrison, Ayala, & Chaudry, 1991), and depressed phagocytic and antimicrobial function (Redmond et al., 1992). In addition, during the early postburn period a population of monocytes with primarily immunosuppressive properties can be detected (Yang & Hsu, 1992).

Patients with severe head injury carry a high risk of mortality and morbidity despite progress in their clinical management. In the United States, approximately 500,000 patients (median age, 25 years) with traumatic brain injury (TBI) require hospitalization annually (Gennarelli, 1993; Jennett, 1996; Kraus, 1993). Patients who survive the initial injury have a mortality rate of greater than 30% during their intensive care period, and survivors are confronted with long-term neurobehavioral and socioeconomic consequences (Jennett, 1996; Ashley, Persel, Clark, & Krych, 1997). The high rate of secondary morbidity and mortality after TBI has been attributed to the posttraumatic inflammatory response within the intracranial compartment (Baethmann, 1997; Holmin, Soberlund, Biderfeld, & Mathiesen, 1998; Kochanek, 1997). This results in cerebral edema, increased intracranial pressure (ICP), and loss of autoregulation of cerebral blood flow (Graham, Adams, & Gennarelli, 1993; Kochanek, 1993; Luer, Rhoney, Hughes, & Hatton, 1996; McIntosh et al., 1996; Regel, 1996). Posttraumatic cerebral ischemia and the intracranial release of neurotoxic mediators also contribute to delayed neuronal cell death (Luer et al., 1996; Regel, 1996; Siesjo, 1993; Wieloch, 1998). Nonetheless, the inflammatory response of the injured brain also has beneficial effects in terms of posttraumatic induction of local neurotrophic factors (Meyer, 1995). In this regard, clinical and experimental studies have shown that the proinflammatory cytokines IL-1$\beta$ (DeKosky et al., 1994, 1996), IL-6 (Kossmann, Hans, Imhof, Trentz, & Morganti-Kossmann, 1996), and      IL-8 (Kossmann et al., 1997) induce the production of the neurotrophin NGF within the injured CNS. Nonetheless, the balance between the detrimental versus beneficial aspects of cerebral inflammation after TBI remains to be elucidated (Kossmann, 1998; Rothwell & Strijbos, 1995).

A traumatic impact to the brain initiates metabolic and inflammatory processes that exacerbate the primary traumatic injury to neurons, leading to secondary brain damage (Baethmann, 1997; Kochanek, 1997; Luer et al., 1996; Regel, 1996). The primary effects of head trauma include diffuse and focal brain injuries, including diffuse axonal injury (DAI), cerebral contusion, and intracranial bleeding (Gennarelli, 1993; Graham et al., 1993; McIntosh et al., 1996). These initial injury patterns lead to the development of secondary cerebral ischemia which is aggravated by the additional presence of systemic hypotension and hypoxia due to shock and pulmonary injury (Doberstein, Hovda, & Becker, 1993). Posttraumatic cerebral ischemia induces a cascade of secondary events leading to decreased cellular energy production followed by pathological membrane depolarization and the release of excitatory amino acids (EAA), such as glutamate and aspartate (Luer et al., 1996; McIntosh et al., 1996; Siesjo, 1993). In addition to ischemia-induced release of neurotransmitters, DAI can directly cause the release of EAA by damaged neurons, thus inducing a cycle of events (Luer et al., 1996; McIntosh et al., 1996; Siesjo, 1993). Membrane depolarization and localized tissue acidosis due to ischemia-related decrease in energy production and elevated extracellular EAA levels contribute to intracellular ion dyshomeostasis by allowing a massive influx of $Ca^{2+}$ and $Na^+$ ions into the injured cells (Luer et al., 1996; Siesjo, 1993; Bullock, 1993). Elevated intracellular $Ca^{2+}$ levels induce the activation of enzymes (i.e., proteases, phospholipases, iNOS, xanthine oxidase), which cause membrane damage via activation of the arachidonic acid cascade and formation of reactive nitrogen and oxygen intermediates (Kochanek, 1997; Luer et al., 1996; Regel, 1996; Siesjo, 1993; Bullock, 1993; Clark et al., 1996). Arachidonic acid metabolites and free radicals induce lipid peroxidation (Homayoun et al., 1997), leading to membrane damage and cell death (Regel, 1996). Additionally, these mediators can damage endothelial cells and astrocytes leading to disruption of the blood-brain barrier (BBB) (Hartl, Medary, Ruge, Arfors, & Ghajar, 1997; Schlosshauer, 1993) and to passive leakage of serum proteins into the intrathecal compartment (Regel, 1996). The posttraumatic intracranial release of proinflammatory cytokines, such as TNF and IL-1 (Kochanek, 1997; Morganti-Kossmann & Kossmann, 1995), further contribute to BBB damage. Furthermore, the release of the chemokine IL-8 into the cerebrospinal fluid (CSF) of patients with severe TBI has been associated with BBB damage (Kossmann et al., 1997). As a result of increased BBB permeability, vasogenic brain edema is induced which increases ICP and decreases cerebral perfusion pressure (CPP), thus aggravating cerebral ischemia (Regel, 1996; Miller, 1993). In the further course of posttraumatic events, blood-derived leukocytes are attracted across the BBB into the subarachnoid space (SAS) (Holmin et al., 1998; Kochanek, 1997). Leukocyte recruitment into the SAS is mediated by upregulation of endothelial and leukocyte adhesion molecules (Kochanek, 1997; Miller, 1993; Clark et al., 1996; Isaksson, Lewen, Hillered, & Olsson, 1997; Pleines, Stover, Kossmann, Trentz, & Morganti-Kossmann, 1998) and by the locally released chemoattractant mediators, $\alpha$- and $\beta$-chemokines (Kossman et al., 1997; Berman, Guida, Warren, Amat, & Brosan, 1996; Ghirnikar, Lee, He, & Eng, 1996; Glabinsky et al., 1996), brain-derived chemotactic factor (Milligan et al., 1995), leukotrienes (Regel, 1996), and activated complement fragments (Kaczorowski, Schiding, Toth, & Kochanek, 1995).

The posttraumatic recruitment of PMNs into the CNS plays an important role in the inflammatory response of the injured brain, since PMNs contribute to tissue damage by release of proteolytic enzymes and reactive oxygen intermediates (Furie & Randolph, 1995). In this regard, a number of experimental studies of meningitis (Tang, Frenette, Hynes, Wagner, & Mayadas, 1996), cerebral ischemia (Chopp et al., 1994; Zhang et al., 1994), and TBI (Miller, 1993; Carlos, 1995) have demonstrated that PMN accumulation in the brain is associated with increased secondary brain damage and adverse outcome. A recent study by Holmin and co-workers (1998) in patients with severe head trauma analyzed the subset of leukocytes invading the perifocal area around brain contusions and demonstrated an early intracranial influx of PMNs within 24 h after injury which persisted for up to 5 days. In this study, other myeloid cells (i.e., monocytes and CD4+ and CD8+ lymphocytes) were barely detected in the CNS during the first 24 h postinjury, but were abundantly present around the brain contusion sites on days 3–5 after TBI (Holmin et al., 1998). PMNs, blood-derived monocytes, and resident CNS immune cells (i.e., astrocytes, microglia) may contribute to inflammation in TBI through the production of proinflammatory cytokines (Kochanek, 1997; Kossmann, 1998) and neurotoxic factors (Giulian, Corpuz, Chapman, Mansouri, & Roberson, 1993; Giulian, Vaca, & Corpuz, 1993). Induction of programmed cell death (PCD; apoptosis) in neurons has been demonstrated in experimental models of TBI (Rink Fung, Trojanowski, Lee, Neugebauer, & McIntosh, 1995; Yakovlev, 1997); however, the mediators inducing neuronal PCD have not been identified.

The complement system contributes to intracranial inflammation in a variety of CNS diseases, including bacterial meningitis (Stahel & Barnum, 1997), multiple sclerosis, and Alzheimer's disease (Morgan, Gasque, Singhrao, & Piddlesden, 1997; Spiegel, Emmerling, & Barnum, 1997). In addition, recent studies have shown that complement contributes to the pathophysiology of TBI (Bellander, van Holst, Fredman, & Svenson, 1996; Kaczorowski et al., 1995; Stahel, Morganti-Kossmann, & Kossmann, 1998; Tornqvist, Liu, Aldskogius, Holst, & Svensson, 1996). The expanding knowledge of the basic cellular and molecular mechanisms responsible for the inflammatory response of the injured brain has evoked new therapeutic approaches in patients with TBI (Bullock, 1993; Luer et al., 1996; Kossmann et al. 1997; Marion et al., 1997; McIntosh, 1993). Nonetheless, to date, efficacious pharmacotherapy has not been developed for TBI patients. Thus, future research should focus on the basic pathological mechanisms of secondary neuronal damage following severe TBI (Doppenberg, Choi, & Bullock, 1997; Faden, 1996; Luer et al., 1996). In this regard, the complement system seems to be involved in the cascade of intracranial pathophysiological events following TBI (Stahel et al., 1998).

## IV. IMMUNOMODULATORY AGENTS THAT MODULATE TRAUMA-INDUCED IMMUNE DYSFUNCTION

Immunomodulators are biologic response-modifying compounds that affect the immune response in either a positive or a negative fashion as shown in Figure 3. An ever-increasing array of potential immunomodulators are being examined for therapeutic benefit in a variety of disorders, including, but not limited to, malignancies, immunodeficiency syndrome (AIDS), and inflammatory diseases. The following section will discuss preclinical and clinical experiences with a number of biologic response modifiers. The net effect of trauma-induced alterations in cell-mediated immunity (CMI) consists of the disruption of the macrophage/T-cell interactions. This phenomenon is caused by an overabundance of "suppressor macrophages" and inadequate T-cell help. Furthermore, the downregulation of CMI mainly results from the immunosuppressive effects of $PGE_2$. $PGE_2$, as well as other mediators associated with specific and nonspecific immunosuppression, exert their effects via a cAMP-dependent pathway. Thus, it has been postulated that cyclooxygenase inhibitors that interfere with this pathway may attenuate the immunosuppression (Baldwin et al., 1986; Ertel, Morrison, Meldrum, Ayala, & Chaudry, 1992; Faist et al., 1987, 1990; Knapp and Baumgartner, 1978; Walker, Kristensen, Bettens, & DeWeck, 1983).

### A. Cyclooxygenase Inhibitors

Inhibitor macrophages can downregulate immune function via the cylcooxygenase product $PGE_2$. Therefore, nonsteroidal anti-inflammatory drugs (e.g., indomethacin) may have a role in limiting the immunosuppressive effects of injury (Ertel et al., 1991; Faist et al., 1986, 1987, 1988; Fletcher et al., 1993, 1986; O'Riordain et al., 1992). Faist and co-workers (Faist et al., 1990) demonstrated increased monocytosis and a reduction in cell surface receptor expression for $CD3^+$, $CD4^+$, $LeuM3^+$, and IL-2 receptor $(R)^+$-positive peripheral blood mononuclear cells in patients undergoing gastrectomy or abdominal aorta reconstruction (Faist et al., 1990). The postoperative administration of indomethacin (a cyclooxygenase inhibitor) resulted in

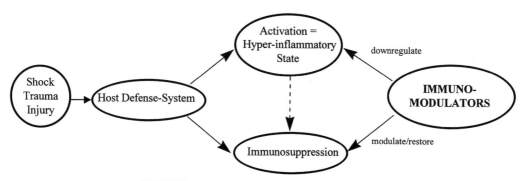

**FIGURE 3**  Possible effects of immunomodulators.

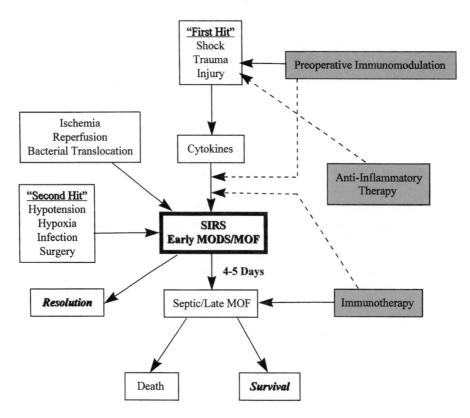

**FIGURE 4**  Therapeutic strategies to prevent postinjury MOF (SIRS, systemetic inflammatory response syndrome; MODS, multiple organ dysfunction syndrom; MOF, multiple organ failure).

significantly reduced postoperative monocytosis and in a protective effect on lymphocyte receptor expression of $CD3^+$, $CD4^+$, and IL-2 receptor-positive cells (Faist et al., 1990).

Several experimental and clinical studies have suggested that after mechanical trauma (Faist et al., 1987) or burn injury (Miller-Graziano, Fink, Wu, Szabo, & Kodys, 1988), $PGE_2$ is responsible for the suppression of CMI (Knapp & Baumgartner, 1978; Walker et al., 1983). Ertel and colleagues (Ertel et al., 1992) demonstrated that administration of the cyclooxygenase inhibitor ibuprofen following hemorrhage and resuscitation significantly improved CMI and increased the overall survival rate of mice following the induction of subsequent sepsis. Experimental studies suggest that macropahges are desensitized to the suppressive effects of $PGE_2$ after thermal injury. However, in vivo administration of indomethacin restored $PGE_2$ sensitivity (Molloy et al., 1993). Thus, blockade of cyclooxygenase activity with ibuprofen decreased the susceptibility to sepsis following hemorrhage and resuscitation. Nonetheless, the overall value of these agents in the treatment of human disease remains to be elucidated.

## B. Thymomimetic Drugs

A number of thymic peptide extracts (i.e., thymosin, thymulin, thymopentin, thymostimulin, and thymic humoral factor) have immunostimulatory properties. With regard to thymulin and thymopentin (TP-5), perioperative subcutaneous injection of TP-5 in patients undergoing open heart surgery have been shown to restore the in vitro lymphocyte proliferative responses as well as the delayed-type hypersensitivity (DTH) skin test responses (Faist et al., 1988).

## C. Cytokines

A number of studies have suggested that lipopolysaccaride (LPS, endotoxin), a cell wall product of Gram-negative bacteria, induces the clinical syndrome of septic shock by stimulating mononuclear phagocytes to release various cellular products (Baumgartner et al., 1985; Ziegler et al., 1982). In this regard, excessive release of TNF, IL-1, and possibly IL-6 appears to play a pivotal role in mediating this aberrant host response to Gram-negative infection. Attempts to modulate this response has led to the development of therapies designed to neutralize endotoxin directly, inhibit cytokine release, or block the actions of cytokines. One of the earliest clinical reports on the use of anti-endotoxin antibodies (Abs) involved a controlled clinical trail of patients with Gram-negative bacteraemia from focal Gram-negative infection (Ziegler et al., 1982). These authors reported a reduced mortality rate (22% versus 39%) with anti-endotoxin treatment. When used prophylactically in high-risk patients this Ab treatment also significantly reduced mortality from Gram-negative sepsis (Baumgartner et al., 1985). Although the results of clinical trials using anti-endotoxin therapy appeared encouraging, these Abs were not found to be useful in the treatment of patients with Gram-positive sepsis.

Recent work has focused on the excessive release of TNF, IL-1, and IL-6 following major thermal or traumatic injury or during infection. Experimental studies with mice, rats, and rabbits suggested that anti-TNF Abs protected these animals against the lethal effects of LPS or Gram-negative bacteria (Beutler, Milsark, & Cerami, 1985; Mullen et al., 1992; Pellicane et al., 1992; Tracey et al., 1987). Further studies using primate models of bacteremic shock have confirmed the ability of anti-TNF Abs to improved survival when given before or following the infusion of a lethal dose of Gram-negative bacteria (Fiedler et al., 1992; Junger et al., 1995; Lowry, 1993; Schlag, Redl, Davies, & Haller, 1994). Anti-TNF Abs also protected against the metabolic consequences of shock and prevented the release of IL-1 and IL-6 in primate models of bacteremia (Fong et al., 1989; Lowry, 1993; Schlag et al., 1994; Junger et al., 1995). Studies of Mullen and co-workers (Mullen et al., 1992) demonstrated that pretreatment with anti-TNF Abs protected pigs from the detrimental hemodynamic and pulmonary consequences of bacteremia. In contrast, other studies (Eskandari et al., 1992) reported that anti-TNF Abs were ineffective in the treatment of polymicrobial sepsis induced by cecal ligation and puncture. Although phase 1 clinical trials in which anti-TNF Abs treatment increased blood pressure in a group with severe septic shock were encouraging (Exley et al., 1990), subsequent clinical trials have failed to demonstrate beneficial effects of anti-TNF Abs treatment on mortality of septic patients (Abraham et al., 1995; Cohen & Carlet, 1996).

A recombinant human IL-1 receptor antagonist (IL-1Ra) blocks the induction of hypotension and leucopenia that follows the intravenous injection of IL-1$\beta$. IL-1Ra also reduced the lethality of LPS or staphylococcal-induced shock in experimental animals, even when given up to 2 h after LPS infusion (Alexander, Doherty, Buresh, Venzon, & Norton, 1991; Ohlsson,

Björk, Bergenfeldt, Hageman, & Thompson, 1990). Preliminary results (Parrillo, 1993) from a small clinical trial using IL-1Ra in sepsis demonstrated improved survival in a dose-dependent fashion. The mortality rate was reduced from 44% in a placebo group to 16% in a group that received a dose of 133 mg/h of IL-1Ra for 72 h. Nonetheless, the results of additional clinical trials with IL-1Ra have not shown similar promise (Fisher et al., 1994).

Among many accessory molecules, CD28 is of critical importance in T-cell activation. CD28, a member of the Ig superfamily, forms a disulfide-linked homodimer of a 44-kDa glycoprotein expressed on the T-cell surface. CD28 and a closely related accessory molecule, CTLA-4, have been shown to modulate the mitogenic response of T-cells (Hara, Fu, & Hansen, 1985; Ledbetter et al., 1985; Linsley & Ledbetter, 1993) by interacting with the costimulatory molecules B7.1 (BB1; CD80) and B7.2 (CD86) on the surface of antigen presenting cells (Linsley, et al., 1994). This function of CD28 has been attributed to its ability to enhance the transcription of cytokine genes, stabilize cytokine mRNA, and inhibit T-cell anergy and apoptosis (Boise et al., 1995; Green & Thompson, 1994; Shi et al., 1995). Wang and co-workers (Wang et al., 1997) found that administration of anti-CD28 Abs prevented septic shock syndrome and death. The protection induced by anti-CD28 Abs was associated with decreased circulating TNF-$\alpha$. In addition, serum from anti-CD28 Ab-treated mice inhibited TNF production by LPS-stimulated bone marrow-derived macrophages, indicating that anti-CD28 Ab induced production of soluble factors that subsequently inhibited the production of TNF. One of these soluble factors was found to be IL-10 (Wang et al., 1997). Furthermore, injection of anti-IL-10 Abs have been shown to abolish the protective effect of anti-CD28 Ab in septic shock and suppress the anti-CD28 Ab-induced inhibition of TNF production, both in vivo as well as in vitro. Thus, this study suggests that ligation of CD28 induces IL-10 production, which in turn suppresses TNF production and prevents the induction of septic shock (Wang et al., 1997).

Malangoni and colleagues (Malangoni, Livingston, Sonnenfeld, & Polk, 1990) showed that interferon-gamma (IFN-$\gamma$), a product of lymphocytes, in combination with cefoxitin reduced the development of polymicrobial soft-tissue infections and Hershman and co-workers (Hershman et al., 1989) found that it enhanced survival after *Klebsiella pneumonia* infection in mice. With regards to traumatic injury, administration of IFN-$\gamma$ following hemorrhagic shock prevented the depression in macrophage MHC class II expression and antigen presentation capacity observed in the absence of treatment (Ertel et al., 1992). The depressed release of IL-1 and TNF and splenocyte proliferation was also increased by IFN-γ treatment following hemorrhagic shock. Furthermore, in these studies, IFN-γ treatment also decreased the lethality from hemorrhage and subsequent sepsis (Ertel et al., 1992). These data, therefore, indicate that IFN-γ is a potent agent for the treatment of hemorrhagic shock-induced immunosuppression and it increases the ability of the host to combat bacterial infections.

## D. Glucan

Glucan is an active component of zymosan, a fungal cell wall product derived from *Saccharomyces cerevisiae* (Williams et al., 1988) and is an immunomodulator that stimulates macrophage activity. In a randomized prospective double-blind study, Browder and co-workers (Browder et al., 1990) investigated the effect of this agent on CMI in patients with multiple injury. They found that glucan treatment resulted in a rapid increase serum IL-1 levels that correlated with conversion of skin tests from anergic to positive. Recently, another glucan product, PGG glucan (Betafectin), was administered pre- and postoperatively in high-risk surgical patients undergoing elective major abdominal surgery. A significant reduction in the number and severity of infections was observed in patients that received PGG glucan (Babineau et al., 1994). Overall glucan products nonspecifically activate macrophages, thereby conferring the resistance against a wide variety of microorganisms.

## E. Growth Hormone and Insulin-Like Growth Factor-1

Growth hormone (GH) is an anabolic hormone belonging to the somatolactogen family of hormones (Arkins, Dantzer, & Kellew, 1993) that improves protein metabolism in critical illness (Chwals & Bristrian, 1991; Voerman, Strack van Schijndel, de Boer, van der Veen, & Thijs, 1992). GH is also the major regulator of IGF-1 synthesis and secretion from various tissues. Moreover, the anabolic effects of GH on protein metabolism are mediated mainly by IGF-1. Studies have recently shown that exogenous GH and IGF-1 increased peritoneal exudate cell numbers, reduced viable bacterial counts in peritoneal lavage fluid and liver, and prolonged survival in a murine sepsis model (Inoue et al., 1995). These authors concluded that administration of GH and IGF-1

effectively improves host defense via immunomodulation, since these hormones affect cytokine production (i.e., TNF, IL-1, IL-6).

## F. Adenosine Triphosphate-Magnesium Chloride (ATP-MgCl₂)

Decreased high-energy phosphates contribute to organ dysfunction following shock and studies (Chaudry, 1983; Grum, Simon, Dantzker, & Fox, 1985) have shown that ATP-MgCl$_2$ treatment after hemorrhagic shock restores tissue ATP levels and organ function. Moreover, ATP-MgCl$_2$ given to anuric multiple organ failure patients had some beneficial effects (Hirasawa, Sugai, & Ohtake, 1990). The effectiveness of this agent is dependent upon its administration following resuscitation, as it reduces afterload (Liebscher et al., 1994). ATP-MgCl$_2$ administration following hemorrhage and resuscitation increased splenocyte ATP levels and restored splenocyte and macrophage function (Meldrum, Ayala, & Chaudry, 1992; Meldrum, Ayala, Wang, Ertel, & Chaudry, 1991b). Furthermore, this laboratory has showed that prolonged sepsis in the mouse caused a significant decrease in lymphocyte ATP levels which correlated with decreased splenocyte proliferative capacity (Meldrum, Ayala, & Chaudry, 1994). However, treatment with ATP-MgCl$_2$ at the onset of sepsis significantly increased lymphocyte ATP levels and the proliferative response. The improvement in splenocyte function correlated with a significant increase in overall survival at day 3 after sepsis. Thus, decreased lymphocyte ATP levels may cause depressed lymphoproliferative responses in late sepsis (Meldrum et al., 1994). A number of studies have demonstrated that ATP-MgCl$_2$ produces beneficial effects following various other circulatory conditions (Harkema, Singh, Wang, & Chaudry, 1992). Wang and Chaudry (1996) demonstrated in a rat sepsis model that administration of ATP-MgCl$_2$ maintained acetylcholine-induced vascular relaxation at 5 and 10 h after CLP (i.e., hyperdynamic stages of polymicrobial sepsis) without altering endothelium-independent vascular relaxation. Whether the salutary effect of ATP-MgCl$_2$ on endothelial cell function extends into the late hypodyamic stage of sepsis or if delayed administration of ATP-MgCl$_2$ after the onset of sepsis produces similar salutary effects on endothelial cell function remains unknown.

## G. Non-anticoagulant Heparin

A novel non-anticoagulant heparin (i.e., GM1892) produces various beneficial effects after hemorrhage and resuscitation, such as improved immune functions as well as improved cardiovascular and hepatocellular function (Wang et al., 1996; Zellweger et al., 1995c). Furthermore, GM 1892 decreased susceptibility to subsequent sepsis (Wang et al., 1996). A recent study indicated that the novel non-anticoagulant heparin prevented vascular endothelial cell dysfunction during hyperdynamic sepsis in rats (Morrison, Wang, & Chaudry, 1996).

## H. Pentoxifylline

Another promising approach to attenuating an excessive systemic inflammatory response consists of the use of xanthine derivatives. Pentoxifylline and related xanthines are widely used clinically and new pharmacologic aspects of these established drugs have been recently demonstrated. Pentoxifylline decreases the susceptibility to sepsis following hemorrhage (Wang, Ba, Zhou, & Chaudry, 1993), possibly through the downregulation of TNF mRNA and TNF production by macrophages as observed in models of endotoxemia (Doherty, Jensen, Alexander, Buresh, & Norton, 1991; Han, Thompson, & Beutler, 1990; Endres et al., 1991). Intracellularly, pentoxifylline appears to exert its pharmacologic effects by inhibiting phoshodiesterase activity, thus increasing the intracellular concentration of cAMP (Strieter, et al., 1988). This is consistent with cAMP-mediated suppression of TNF gene transcription (Strieter et al., 1988). In general, pentoxifylline improved survival in different models of hemorrhagic and endotoxic shock. Furthermore, the effects of pentoxifylline were dose-dependent and effective in a postinjury/insult regime (Hoffmann, Weis, Birg, Schonharting, & Jochum, 1995). The pharmacologic effects of pentoxifylline in humans were studied under controlled conditions of endotoxemia and it was found that pentoxifylline selectively inhibited the formation of TNF without affecting IL-6 and IL-8 (Zabel, Schade, & Schlaak, 1993). Moreover, pentoxifylline counteracted initial leukocytopenia associated with endotoxemia by interfering with the adherence of PMNs in the microvasculature. Pentoxifylline's ability to inhibit TNF production has also been demonstrated under clinical conditions of acute and chronic cytokine-release syndromes (Zabel & Schade, 1994).

## I. Calcium Channel Blockers

A number of investigators (Maitra & Sayeed, 1987; Hess, Warner, Smith, Manson, & Greenfield, 1983; Westfall & Sayeed, 1989) have shown that calcium channel blockers have beneficial effects on cell and

organ function after ischemia or endotoxic shock. These beneficial effects are postulated to be due to inhibition of the massive influx of extracellular calcium into cells after injury or shock. Meldrum and co-workers (Meldrum, Ayala, Perrin, Ertel, & Chaudry, 1991a) examined the effects of diltiazem administration (400–800 μg/kg body wt) on hemorrhage induced immune dysfunction. Their results indicated that the depression in lymphocyte cytokine production following hemorrhage was restored by diltiazem treatment (Meldrum et al., 1991a). Furthermore, diltiazem also improved the survival of animals subjected to hemorrhage and subsequent sepsis to rates comparable to those seen in nonhemorrhaged animals subjected to sepsis. These data suggest that there is an association between low-dose diltiazem treatment, restoration of lymphokine synthesis, Mφ antigen presentation function, and susceptibility to sepsis following hemorrhage. Thus, the adjuvant use of calcium channel blockers, such as diltiazeim, might offer a new therapeutic modality in the treatment of immunosuppression following low-flow conditions.

## J. Chloroquine

Chloroquine, an anti-malarial agent (Rollo, 1980), has also been used for the treatment of rheumatoid arthritis (Freedman, 1956) due to its ability to inhibit the inflammatory events underlying this disease process. Studies by Authi and Tragnor (1979) showed that chloroquine inhibited phospolipase $A_2$ activity leading to decreased production of prostanoids. Chloroquine selectively inhibited macrophage TNF and IL-6 release and decreased the mortality of mice subjected to hemorrhage and subsequent sepsis (Ertel et al., 1991). The inhibition of TNF production by chloroquine appears to be at the level of gene expression (Zhu et al., 1993). Since chloroquine possesses the unique ability to selectively inhibit the release of inflammatory cytokines and prostaglandins, it may be a useful adjunct in the clinical setting for the treatment of shock-induced immunosuppression.

## K. Platelet Activating Factor (PAF)

Bioactive phospholipids, derived from the activation of $PLA_2$, appear to be important in the host systemic inflammatory response to sepsis. Among these, PAF, produced by a variety of cells (endothelial cells, platelets, leucocytes, monocytes, and lymphocytes), is involved in the release of a number of important inflammatory mediators. PAF is expressed rapidly by endothelial cells during shock in response to various stimuli (e.g., thrombin, histamine, leukotrienes) (Schlag & Redl, 1996) and may be partially responsible for the early adherence of PMNs to endothelial cells. Moreover, cytokines such as IL-1, IL-6, and TNF can stimulate PAF synthesis by endothelial cells (Hosford, Koltai, & Barquet, 1993). Increased PAF release has been reported in septic patients (Bussolino, Porcellini, Varese, & Bosia, 1987; Lopez-Diez, Nieto, Fernandez-Gallardo, Gijon, & Sanchez-Crespo, 1989) and high levels of platelet-associated PAF have also been observed in patients with sepsis (Lopez-Diez et al., 1989). Thus, PAF is considered to be an important toxic mediator of septic shock that may be partially responsible for producing the increased membrane permeability under such conditions (Schlag & Redl, 1996).

A number of specific PAF receptor antagonists have been identified. PAF-receptor antagonists inhibit the following: specific binding of PAF to platelets, PAF-induced platelet aggregation, PAF-induced hypotension, and LPS-induced hypotension. PAF inhibitors also appear to attenuate endotoxin-induced pulmonary vascular abnormalities and prevent extravascular fluid accumulation in the lungs. With regard to endotoxin, PAF inhibitors appear to prolong survival in endotoxemic animals (Verhoef, Hustinx, Frasa, & Hoepelman, 1996). Moreover, studies have shown that administration of the PAF antagonist RO 24-4736 after hemorrhage and resuscitation prevented suppression of splenocyte function in mice (Zellweger et al., 1995). In another study, Redl and colleagues (Redl , Vogl, Schiesser, Paul, Thurnher, Bahrami, & Schlag, 1990) evaluated the effect of the PAF antagonist BN 52021 in ovine endotoxin shock and showed that the pulmonary vasculature and lung fluid balance disruption produced by endotoxin was markedly reduced. In a clinical trial involving 120 patients with Gram-negative sepsis, BN-52021 administration was associated with a 42% decrease in mortality, compared to that seen with placebo (Minnard et al., 1994).

## L.  Nitric Oxide (NO)

During sepsis, there appears to be an overproduction of NO that may cause marked reduction in systemic blood pressure which may be responsible for producing the pressor agent-insensitive hypotension (Petros, Bennett, & Vallance, 1991; Thiemermann & Vane, 1990). In addition, studies of patients with the sepsis syndrome have revealed increased levels of NO degradation products (Verhoef et al., 1996). In recent years, the therapeutic implications of inhibition of NO synthesis has been explored. Two laboratories using

murine models demonstrated that NO inhibition could reverse the hyporesponsiveness of the peripheral circulation in sepsis (Evans, Carpenter, Silva, & Cohen, 1994; Minnard et al., 1994). Studies of Wang and colleagues (Wang, Ba, & Chaudry, 1994) in an experimental model of sepsis have raised the question of whether to block or enhance the production of NO during sepsis. Caution should be exercised in blocking NO production since NO is an anticoagulant and its inhibition might lead to disseminated intravascular coagulation (Moncada, Palmer, & Higgs, 1991). Moreover, since NO is an oxygen radical scavenger, blocking NOS activity might lead to increased amount of these oxygen radicals (Minnard et al., 1994).

There is also evidence that the activation of the L-arginine–NO pathway in sepsis may play a role in producing vascular failure (Parratt, 1994). The well-known failure of vascular smooth muscle in response to norepinephrine, termed vasoplegia, may be the cause of peripheral vascular failure, especially during the hypodynamic phase of sepsis. Thus, NO may be a major contributor to the vascular derangement of endotoxemia and sepsis (Parratt, Stoclet, & Furman, 1993). In a baboon model of trauma, high levels of NO degradation products could not detected, though NOS cofactor levels (i.e., neopterin, biopterin) were significantly increased (Schlag et al., 1994). In general, it appears that selective inhibition of iNOS and enhancement of cNOS might be an effective approach for maintaining vascular stability following severe trauma and during sepsis.

## M.  Erythropoietin

Patients with chronic infections and inflammatory diseases often exhibit low serum erythropoietin (Epo) levels in relation to the blood hemoglobin concentration (Means & Krantz, 1992). In vitro studies utilizing Epo-producing human hepatoma cells and isolated perfused rat kidneys have shown that the proinflammatory cytokines IL-1 and TNF inhibit Epo gene expression (Fandrey, Huwiler, Frede, Pfeilschifter, & Jelkmann, 1994; Faquin, Schneider, & Goldberg, 1992; Jelkmann, Pagel, Wolff, & Fandrey, 1992). These proinflammatory cytokines, therefore, are thought to play an important role in the defective production of Epo in distinct acute and chronic inflammatory renal and nonrenal diseases, including nephritis, renal allograft rejection, autoimmune diseases, and malignancies (Jelkman, 1992; Means et al., 1992). There has been one earlier report showing low Epo bioactivity detected in vitro in the plasma of infants with sepsis (Soboleva & Manakova, 1993). In contrast, studies by Abel and colleagues (Abel, Spannbrucker, Fandrey &

Jelkmann, 1996) indicate that Epo production is not generally lowered in septic patients, despite the increased levels of proinflammatory cytokines. However, they proposed that increasingly high Epo levels is a negative prognostic indicator in septic patients since it increases IL-6 levels and APACHE II scores, an indicator of trauma patient morbidity. Septic shock is associated with decreased tissue perfusion and hypoxia (Parrillo, 1993) which may induce Epo gene expression. Alternatively, specific cytokines may stimulate Epo production. For example IL-6, which is produced excessively in septic shock stimulates Epo gene expression in the human hepatic cell line Hep3B (Jelkmann et al., 1992). Since IL-6 can also inhibit Epo production in isolated perfused rat kidneys (Jelkmann et al., 1992; Jelkmann, Fandrey, Frede, & Pagel, 1994), the effects of IL-6 on hepatic Epo synthesis deserve further consideration.

## N. Dietary Manipulation

Recent studies have shown that nutritional therapy can extend well beyond the treatment and prevention of deficiencies of dietary components, as some nutrients can have pharmacologic effects on biological responses. Among these nutrients are the long-chain polyunsaturated fatty acids (PUFAs), arginine, and vitamins A, E, and C, nucleotides, zinc, and selenium. Dietary carbohydrates and proteins appear to be without effect. A number of these nutritional compounds act as immunostimulants, reversing trauma-induced immunosuppression (Alexander, 1993). Current nutritional formulations contain n-6 (PUFAs) as a primary fat source. However, a great deal of attention has been focused recently on the potential use of n-3 PUFAs (i.e., $\omega$-3 fatty acids) which are found in high concentrations in fish oil. Studies have shown that $\omega$-3 fatty acids are rapidly and preferentially incorporated into membrane phospholipids, thereby reducing the production of arachidonic acid metabolites. This effect is thought to be responsible for some of the anti-inflammatory and immunostimulatory effects associated with diets high in $\omega$-3 fatty acids. Experimental studies indicate that the severity of arthritis (Kremer et al., 1985), systemic lupus erythematosus (Robinson, Prickett, Polisson, Steinberg, & Levine, 1985), and amyloidosis (Cathcart, Leslie, Meydani, & Hayes, 1987) are markedly reduced if diets high in $\omega$-3 fatty acids are given. Studies in humans have demonstrated that the synthesis of the inflammatory cytokines TNF and IL-1 are decreased by dietary supplementation with $\omega$-3 fatty acids (Endres et al., 1989). These results are consistent with data from two clinical trials in which dietary fish oil had a restorative effect on the depressed cellular immunity of patients in intensive care units (Cerra et al., 1990) or after major surgery (Leberman, 1990; Cerra et al., 1991). Nonetheless, a significant decrease of infectious complications or mortality in such patients could not be demonstrated. In contrast, a clinical study of burn patients fed a diet containing fish oil demonstrated significantly reduced wound infection, shortened hospital stays, and reduced deaths when compared to that seen with other standard enteral formulations (Alexander Gottschlich, 1990).

## O. Sex Hormone Antagonists

Several clinical and epidemiological studies indicate gender differences in the susceptibility to, and morbidity from, sepsis (Bone, 1992; McGowan, Barnes, & Finland, 1975; Wichmann, Zellweger, DeMaso, Ayala, & Chaudry, 1996; Zellweger, Ayala, Stein, DeMaso, & Chaudry, 1997a). Immune function in normal males and females has been reported to be influenced by sex steroids (Homo-Delarche et al., 1991; Wichmann, Ayala, & Chaudry, 1997). In this regard, it appears that better maintained immune functions in females are not only due to physiologic levels of female sex steroids, but also because of the markedly lower levels of immunosuppressive androgenic hormones (Luster, Pfeifer, & Tucker, 1985). Splenic and peritoneal macrophages from male mice subjected to hemorrhagic shock are markedly decreased in their ability to release IL-1 and IL-6, even though IL-1 and IL-6 mRNA expression was increased, such mice are more susceptible to the lethal effects of subsequent sepsis (Zellweger et al., 1996). Administration of prolactin following hemorrhage, however, attenuated the increased mRNA expression for IL-1$\beta$ and IL-6, restored cytokine release capacity and improved the survival of animals subjected to sepsis after hemorrhage (Zellweger et al., 1996). Furthermore, prolactin as well as metoclopramide (a dopamine antagonist, which to increases prolactin secretion and circulating plasma levels (Ehrenkranz & Ackerman, 1986)) treatment after the onset of sepsis resulted in significant upregulation of constitutive and inducible cytokine (i.e., TNF, IL-1, IL-6) gene expression in macrophages when compared to that seen in septic untreated and sham-operated mice (Zhu, Zellweger, Wichmann, Ayala, & Chaudry, 1997). Thus, prolactin and metoclopramide prevent the depression of macrophage cytokine production and may be useful in improving CMI during sepsis. In line with this is a recent experimental study (Zellweger, Wichmann, Ayala, Stein, DeMaso, &

Chaudry, 1997) in which male and proestrus (a stage at which the female sexual hormones are highest) female mice were subjected to sepsis by cecal ligation and puncture. The results showed that the survival rate of septic female proestrus mice was significantly higher than in comparable male mice. Furthermore, splenocytes isolated 24 h after the onset of sepsis in males were markedly decreased in their proliferative capacity and IL-2 and IL-3 release, whereas splenocytes from comparable females were not suppressed. These results support the concept that the immune response of females differs from males, and that females in the proestrus state are immunologically better positioned to meet the challenge of sepsis (Zellweger et al., 1997). This concept appears to be supported by a recent prospective study of patients with sepsis which demonstrated significantly higher survival in females as compared to males (Schroder, Kahlke, Staubach, Zabel, & Stuber, 1998). Alternatively, to the extent to which androgens contribute to the marked immune depression seen following hemorrhage, recent studies indicate that testosterone receptor blockade in males following hemorrhage and sepsis restored the depressed immune functions and improved survival (Wichmann, Angele, Ayala, Cioffi, & Chaudry, 1997; Angele, Wichmann, Ayala, Cioffi, & Chaudry, 1997).

## V. CLINICAL IMPACT

Inflammation and infection leading to organ dysfunction and failure continue to be the major problems after injury and operations and with intensive care for many diseases and other conditions (Figure 4). When SIRS develops into multiple organ distress syndrome (MODS) and multiple organ failure (MOF), the mortality rate increases, ranging from 30 to 80%. Prospective, randomized, double-blind clinical trials are required to document efficacy of various therapeutic efforts. Unfortunately in this regard, many, if not all, such studies of single "magic bullets" have not been promising (Baue, 1997). Thus, it remains unclear what will make the difference in improving patient care? Would it be, molecular biology, shock research, clinical trials, technologic advances, evidence based medicine or research or all of the above? Recently, several clinical studies showed new aspects for the treatment of severely injured patients. Zimmermann and colleagues (Zimmermann et al., 1996) compared risks and outcomes for intensive care unit (ICU) patients with organ system failure from 1982 to 1990 and found that the most important predictor of mortality was the severity of physiological disturbance on the initial day of organ failure. Christou and co-workers (Christou et al., 1995) provided a 20 year follow-up of 4292 patients in which they studied the delayed-type hypersensitivity skin test and found that overall surgical mortality was 11.4% in the 1970s, 10.2% in the 1980s, and 4% in the 1990s. They concluded that the decrease in mortality was related to improved preoperative, intraoperative, and postoperative care; however, ICU patient mortality did not improve. Regel and associates (Regel et al., 1995) compared morbidity and mortality rates from 1972 to 1981 with those from 1982 to 1991. They discovered that prehospital care had improved immensely, leading to increased survival of severely injured patients early postinjury; however, such patients developed MOF, leading to later death. Thus, this group of injured patients is the one to focus on to increase survival by decreasing the susceptibility to sepsis and MOF. No change in mean age or ISS or crude mortality over a 10-year period was noted at an established trauma center in Seattle, Washington (O'Keefe, Jurkovich, & Maier, 1997). In contrast, the length of hospital stay markedly decreased and cost increased by 16.7%, related likely to the cost of sophisticated monitoring and diagnostic studies. Interestingly, adjustment of the patient population for ISS and abbreviated injury score (AIS) revealed that mortality had decreased by 3% per year in patients with an ISS >16. Therefore, the development of trauma centers and trauma teams has, in fact, improved the outcome of trauma victims.

A number of specific therapeutic modalities have been developed for trauma and surgical patients. In this regard, gastrointestinal (GI) stress bleeding is a potential complication, even though its threat has decreased (Shuman, Schuster, & Zuckermann, 1987). Prophylaxis with sucralfate or omaprazole is commonly used for this complication and it appears to be the best treatment in severely injured or intensive care unit (ICU) patients, particularly ventilated ICU patients (Phillips, Metzler, Palmieri, Huckfeldt, & Dahl, 1996). In contrast, treatment with Ranitidine may increase infectious complications in trauma patients (O'Keefe, Gentilello, & Maier, 1998). Patient with ARDS requiring ventilator support also benefit from rotational kinetic therapy (Stiletto, Bruck, & Bittner, 1998; Badia, Sala, & Rodriguez-Roisin, 1998; Stiletto, 1998). In regard to head trauma, the use of hypertonic solutions appear to be of specific value as such solutions do not increase, and tend to decrease, intracranial pressure (Shackford et al., 1998). Maintenance of body temperature is also important, as normal body temperature intraoperatively appears to decrease wound infections (Kurz, Sessler, &

Lenhardt, 1996). Furthermore, hypothermia does not appear to be of protective value for trauma patients (Gentielello, Jurkovich, Stark, Hassanstash, & O'Keefe 1997).

A number of studies have examined risk factors for the development of MOF in trauma patients. Tran and co-workers (Tran, Cuesta, van Leeuwen Nauta, & Wesdrop, 1993) found that the primary predictors of poor outcome were age, prior chronic disease, malnutrition, coma on admission, the use of an $H_2$-antagonist, the number of blood transfusions, and a potential relationship to shock. Other studies reported that the risk factors were age >55 years, ISS >25, more than 6 units of red blood cells in the first 12 hr, a base deficit >8 mEq/L and lactate levels >2.5 mmol/L (Sauaia et al., 1994). Comparisons between head injury and extracranial injury with regards to morbidity and mortality were made by Gennarelli and co-workers (Gennerelli, Champion, Copes, & Sacco, 1994). They found that while the overall mortality rate following all injuries was 8.3%, the mortality rate in the head injury group was three times higher. These authors concluded, therefore, that head injuries remained the most important single injury contributing to trauma morbidity and mortality. Consideration of these risk factors is important since most of them are beyond the control of surgeons and intensive care physicians. Thus, the best treatment for trauma still remains prevention.

## VI. SUMMARY AND FUTURE DIRECTIONS

The general consensus is that the compensatory mechanisms of the organism for surviving overwhelming trauma are insufficient. In view of this, the principal clinical goal of modern immunotherapy for trauma patients should be to control the development of a SIRS and prevent subsequent sepsis in an immunocompromised host. Several strategic approaches to preventing the development of late MODS/MOF appear to be feasible. As of today, many clinical trials in septic patients with Gram-negative bacterial infections employing therapeutic tools such as antibodies against LPS and TNF, soluble TNF receptors, or IL-1 receptor antagonists have not shown an overall valid, clinically important, reproducible, and statistically significant treatment benefit. Ideally, the intervention employed needs to prevent SIRS from becoming a nonreversible destructive inflammatory response. Furthermore, the intervention/immunomodulation has to be employed in a calculated preventive fashion as early as possible

following trauma and should encompass multiple cellular targets (e.g., lymphocytes, macrophages, granulocytes, and endothelial cells) to protect the host from cell hyperactivation as well as from cell exhaustion. Crucial issues within the complex field of preventive immunotherapy for the control of SIRS and sepsis include patient selection, timing of administration of agents, controlled modulation of the inflammatory responses, and cost. Nonetheless, major advances and reduced mortality following severe injury will become evident by more in-depth investigation of the initiating and perpetuating factors responsible for the transition from manageable to uncontrolled, overzealous inflammatory responses leading to the demise of organs and ultimately the body.

## Acknowledgment

This work was supported by NIH Grant GM 37127.

## References

Abel, J., Spannbrucker, N., Fandrey, J., & Jelkmann, W. (1996). Serum erythropoietin levels in patients with sepsis and septic shock. *European Journal of Haematology, 57*, 359–363.

Abraham, E. (1991). Physiologic stress and cellular ischemia: Relationship to immunosuppression and susceptibility to sepsis. *Critical Care Medicine, 19*, 613–618.

Abraham, E., Wunderink, R., Silverman, H., Perl, T. M., Nasraway, S., Levy, H., Bone, R., Wenzel, R. P., Balk, R., & Allred, R. (1995). Efficacy and safety of monoclonal antibody to human tumor necrosis factor $\alpha$ in patients with sepsis syndrome: A randomized, controlled, double-blind, multicenter clinical trial. *Journal of the American Medical Association, 273*, 934–941.

Alexander, H. R., Doherty, G. M., Buresh, C. M., Venzon, D. J., & Norton, J. A. (1991). A recombinant human receptor antagonist to interleukin 1 improves survival after lethal endotoxemia in mice. *Journal of Experimental Medicine, 173*, 1029–1032.

Alexander, J. W. (1993). Augmentation of host defense reactivity with special nutrients. In E. Faist, J. Meakins, & F. W. Schildberg (Eds.), *Host defense dysfunction in trauma, shock and sepsis* (pp. 995–1001). Berlin: Springer.

Alexander, J. W., & Gottschlich, M. M. (1990). Nutritional immunomodulation in burn patients. *Critical Care Medicine, 18*, S149–S153.

Angele, M. K., Wichmann, M. W., Ayala, A., Cioffi, W. G., & Chaudry, I. H. (1997). Testosterone receptor blockade after hemorrhage in males: Restoration of the depressed immune functions and improved survival following subsequent sepsis. *Archives of Surgery, 132*, 1207–1214.

Appel, P. L., & Shoemaker, W. C. (1992). Relationship of oxygen consumption and oxygen delivery in surgical patients with ARDS. *Chest, 102*, 906–911.

Arkins, S., Dantzer, R., & Kellew, K. W. (1993). Somatolactogens, somatomedins, and immunity. *Journal of Dairy Science, 76*, 2437–2450.

Ashley, M. J., Persel, C. S., Clark, M. C., & Krych, D. K. (1997). Long term follow-up of post acute traumatic brain injury rehabilitation: a statistical analysis to test for stability and predictability of outcome. *Brain Injury, 11*, 677–690.

Authi, K. S., & Tragnor, J. R. (1979). Effects of anti-malarial drugs on phospholipase $A_2$. *British Journal of Pharmacology, 66*, 496–501.

Babineau, T., Marcello, P., Swails, W., Kenler, A., Bistrian B., & Forse, R. A. (1994). Randomized phase I/II trial of a macrophage-specific immunomodulator (PGG–Glucan) in high risk surgical patients. *Annals of Surgery, 22*, 601–609.

Badia, J. R., Sala, E., & Rodriguez-Roisin, R. (1998). Positional changes and drug interventions in acute respiratory failure. *Respirology, 3*, 103–106.

Baethmann, A. (1997). Mechanisms of secondary brain damage in severe head injury: A clinical perspective. In G. Schlag, H. Redl, & D. Traber (Eds.), *Brain damage secondary to hemorrhagic-traumatic shock, sepsis, and traumatic brain injury* (pp. 169–184). Berlin: Springer.

Baker, C. C., Miller, C. L., & Trunkey, D. D. (1979). Identify of mononuclear cells which compromise trauma pateints' resistance. *Journal of Surgical Research, 26*, 478–487.

Baker, C. C., Oppenheimer, L., Stephens B., Lewis, F. R., & Trunkey, D. D. (1980). The epidemiology of trauma death. *American Journal of Surgery, 140*, 144–150.

Baldwin, S. R., Simon, R. H., Grum, C. M., Ketai, L. H., Boxer, L. A., & Devall, L. J. (1986). Oxidant activity in expired breath of patients with adult respiratory distress syndrome. *Lancet, 1*(8471), 11–14.

Baracos, V. (1983). Simulation of muscle protein degradation and prostaglandin-$E_2$ release by leukocytic pyrogen (IL-1). *New England Journal of Medicine, 308*, 553–558.

Baue, A. E. (1997). Multiple organ failure, multiple organ dysfunction syndrome, and the systemic inflammatory response syndrome: Why no magic bullets? *Archives of Surgery, 132*, 703–707.

Baumgartner, J. D., Glanser, M. P., McCutchan, J. A., Ziegler, E. J., van Melle G., Klauber, MR, Vogt, M., Muehlen, E., Luethy, R., Chiolero R., et al. (1985). Prevention of gram-negative shock and death in surgical patients by antibody to endotoxin core glycolipid. *Lancet, 2*(8446), 59–63.

Bellander, B. M., van Holst, H., Fredman, P., & Svenson, M. (1996). Activation of the complement cascade and increase of clusterin in the brain following a cortical contusion in the adult rat. *Journal of Neurosurgery, 85*, 468–475.

Berman, J. W., Guida, M. P., Warren, J., Amat J., & Brosnan, C. F. (1996). Localization of monocyte chemoattractant peptide-1 expression in the central nervous system in experimental autoimmune encephalomyelitis and trauma in the rat. *Journal of Immunology, 156*, 3017–3023.

Beutler, B., Krochin, N., & Milsark, I. M. (1986). Control of cachectin (tumor necrosis factor) synthesis. Mechanisms of endotoxin resistance. *Science, 232*, 977–980.

Beutler, B., Milsark, I. W., & Cerami, A. (1985). Passive immunization against cachectin/tumor necrosis factor protects mice from lethal effect of endotoxin. *Science, 229*, 869–871.

Bitterman, H., Smith, B. A., & Lefer, A. M. (1988). Beneficial actions of antagonism of peptide leukotrienes in hemorrhagic shock. *Circulatory Shock, 24*, 159–168.

Bitterman, H., Yanagisawa, A., & Lefer, A. M. (1986). Beneficial actions of thromboxane receptor antagonism in hemorrhagic shock. *Circulatory Shock, 20*, 1–11.

Boise, L. H., Minn, A. J., Noel, P. J., June, C. H., Accavitti, M. A., Lindsten, T., & Thompson, C. B. (1995). CD28 costimulation can promote T cell survival by enhancing the expression of Bcl-$X_L$. *Immunity, 3*, 87–98.

Bone, R. C. (1992). Toward an epidemiology and natural history of SIRS (systemic inflammatory response syndrome). *Journal of the American Medical Association, 268*, 3452–3455.

Breasted, J. (1930). *The Edwin Smith surgical papyrus*. Chicago, IL: Univ. of Chicago Press.

Browder, W., Williams, D., Pretus, H., Olivero G., Enrichens, F., Mao, P., & Franchello, A. (1990). Beneficial effect of enhanced macrophage function in the trauma patient. *Annals of Surgery, 211*, 605–613.

Bullock, R. (1993). Opportunities for neuroprotective drugs in clinical management of head injury. *Journal of Emergency Medicine, 11*, 23–30.

Bussolino, F., Porcellini, M. G., Varese, L., & Bosia, A. (1987). Intravascular release of platelet-activating factor in children with sepsis. *Thromboxane Research, 48*, 619–620.

Butcher, E. C. (1991). Leukocyte-endothelial cell recognition: three (or more) steps to specificity and diversity. *Cell, 67*, 1033–1036.

Cabin, D. E., & Buchman, T. G. (1990). Molecular biology of circulatory shock. III. Human hepatoblastoma (HEPG2) cells demonstrate two patterns of shock-induced gene expression that are independent, exclusive, and prioritized. *Surgery, 108*, 902–912.

Carlos, T. (1995). Expression of endothelial adhesion molecules after traumatic brain injury in rats. *J Neurotrauma, 12*, 458. [Abstract]

Cathcart, E. S., Leslie, C. A., Meydani, S. N., & Hayes, K. C. (1987). A fish oil diet retards experimental amyloidosis, modulates lymphocyte function, and decreases macrophage arachidonate metabolism in mice. *Journal of Immunology, 139*, 1850–1854.

Cerra, F. B., Lehman, S., Konstantinides, N., Konstantinides, F., Shronts, E. P., & Holman, R. (1990). Effect of enteral nutrient on in vitro tests of immune function in ICU patients: A preliminary report. *Journal of Nutrition, 6*, 84–87.

Cerra, F. B., Lehmann, S., Konstantinides, N., Dzik, J., Fish, J., Konstantinides, F., LiCari, J. J., & Holman, R. T. (1991). Improvement in immune function in ICU patients by enteral nutrition supplemented with arginine, RNA, and Menhaden Oil is independent of nitrogen balance. *Journal of Nutrition, 7*, 193–199.

Chaudry, I. H. (1983). Cellular mechanisms in shock and ischemia and their correction. *American Journal of Physiology, 245*, R117–R134.

Chaudry, I. H., & Ayala, A. (1992). *Immunological aspects of hemorrhage*. Austin, TX: Medical Intelligence Unit, R. G. Landes.

Chaudry, I. H., Ayala, A., Ertel, W., & Stephan, R. N. (1990). Hemorrhage and resuscitation: immunologic aspects. *American Journal of Physiology, 259*, R663–R678.

Chopp, M., Zhang, R. L., Chen, H., Li, Y., Jiang N., & Rusche, J. R. (1994). Postischemic administration of anti-Mac 1 antibody reduces ischemic cell damage after transient middle cerebral artery occlusion. *Stroke, 25*, 869–876.

Christou, N. V., Meakins, J. L., Gordon, J., Yee, J., Hassan-Zahraee, M., Nohr, C. W., Shizgal, H. M., & MacLean, L. D. (1995). The delayed hypersensitivity response and host resistance in surgical patients 20 years later. *Annals of Surgery, 222*(4), 435–548.

Chwals, W. J., & Bistrian, B. R. (1991). Role of exogenous growth hormone and insulin-like growth factor I in malnutrition and acute metabolic stress: A hypothesis. *Critical Care Medicine, 19*, 1317–1322.

Clark, R. S., Carlos, T. M., Schiding, J. K., Bree, M., Fireman, L. A., DeKosky, S. T., & Kochanek, P. M. (1996). Antibodies against Mac-1 attenuate neutrophil accumulation after traumatic brain injury in rats. *Journal of Neurotrauma, 13*, 333–341.

Clark, R. S., Kochanek, P. M., Obrist, W. D., Wong, H. R., Billiar, T. R., Wisniewski, S. R., & Marion, D. W. (1996). Cerebrospinal fluid and plasma nitrite and nitrate concentrations after head injury in humans. *Critical Care Medicine, 24*, 1243–1251.

Clemens, M. G., McDonagh, P. F., Chaudry, I. H., & Baue, A. E. (1985). Hepatic microcirculatory failure after ischemia and reperfusion: Improvement with ATP-MgCl$_2$ treatment. *American Journal of Physiology, 248,* H804–H811.

Cohen, J., & Carlet, J. (1996). Intersept: An international multicenter, placebo-controlled trial of monoclonal antibody to human tumor necrosis factor-$\alpha$ in patients with sepsis. *Critical Care Medicine, 24,* 1431–1440.

Dehring, D. J., Steinberg, S. M., & Wismar, B. L. (1987). Complement depletion in a porcine model of septic acute respiratory disease. *Journal of Trauma, 27,* 615–625.

Deitch, E. A., Berg, R., & Specian, R. (1987). Endotoxin promotes the bacterial translocation from the gut. *Archives of Surgery, 122,* 185–190.

Deitch, E. A., Winterton, J., & Berg, R. (1986). Thermal injury promotes bacterial translocation from the gastrointestinal tract in mice with impaired T cell immunity. *Archives of Surgery, 121,* 97–101.

DeKosky, S. T., Goss, J. R., Miller, J. D., Styren, S. D., Kochanek, P. M., & Marion, D. (1994). Upregulation of nerve growth factor following cortical trauma. *Experimental Neurology, 130,* 173–177.

DeKosky, S. T., Styren, S. D., O'Malley, M. E., Goss, J. R., Kochanek, P. M., Marion, D., Evans, C. H., & Robbins, P. D. (1996). Interleukin-1 receptor antagonist suppresses neurotrophin responses in injured rat brain. *Annals of Neurology, 39,* 123–127.

Demling, R. H. (1995). The modern version of adult respiratory distress syndrome. *Annual Review of Medicine, 46,* 193–202.

Dinarello, C. A. (1988). Interleukin-1. *Digestive Disease Science, 33*(Suppl. 3), 25S.

Doberstein, C. E., Hovda, D. A., & Becker, D. P. (1993). Clinical considerations in the reduction of secondary brain injury. *Annals of Emergency Medicine, 22,* 993–997.

Doherty, G. M., Jensen, J. C., Alexander, H. R., Buresh, C. M., & Norton, J. A. (1991). Pentoxifylline suppression of tumor necrosis factor gene transcription. *Surgery, 110,* 192–198.

Doppenberg, E. M., Choi, S. C., & Bullock, R. (1997). Clinical trials in traumatic brain injury: What can we learn from previous studies? *Annals of the New York Academy of Science, 825,* 305–322.

Ehrenkranz, R. A., & Ackerman, B. A. (1986). Metoclopramide effect on faltering milk production by mothers of premature infants. *Pediatrics, 78,* 614–620.

Endres, S., Fulle, H. J., Sinha, B., Stoll, D., Dinarello, C. A., Gerzer, R., & Weber, P. C. (1991). Cyclic nucleotides differentially regulate the synthesis of tumour necrosis factor-alpha and interleukin-1 beta by human mononuclear cells. *Immunology, 72,* 56–60.

Endres, S., Ghorbani R., Kelley, V. E., Georgilis K., Lonnemann G., van der Meer, J. W., Cannon, J. G., Rogers, T. S., Klempner, M. S., Weber, P. C., et al., (1989). The effect of dietary supplementation with n-3 polyunsaturated fatty acids on the synthesis of interleukin-1 and tumor necrosis factor by mononuclear cells. *New England Journal of Medicine, 320,* 265–271.

Ertel, W., Morrison, M. H., Ayala, A., & Chaudry, I. H. (1991). Insights into the mechanisms of defective antigen presentation following hemorrhage. *Surgery, 110,* 440–447.

Ertel, W., Morrison, M. H., Ayala, A., & Chaudry, I. H. (1991). Chloroquine attenuates hemorrhagic shock induced suppression of Kupffer cell antigen presentation and MHC class II antigen expression through blockade of tumor necrosis factor and prostaglandin release. *Blood, 78,* 1781–1788.

Ertel, W., Morrison, M. H., Ayala, A., Dean, R. E., & Chaudry, I. H. (1992). Interferon-gamma attenuates hemorrhage-induced suppression of macrophage and splenocyte functions and decreases susceptibility to sepsis. *Surgery, 111,* 177–187.

Ertel, W., Morrison, M. H., Meldrum, D. R., Ayala, A., & Chaudry, I. H. (1992). Ibuprofen restores cellular immunity and decreases susceptibility to sepsis following hemorrhage. *Journal of Surgical Research, 53,* 55–61.

Eskandari, M. K., Bolgos, G., Miller, C., Nguyen, D. T., DeForge, L. E., & Remick, D. G. (1992). Anti-tumor necrosis factor antibody therapy fails to prevent lethality after cecal ligation and puncture or endotoxemia. *Journal of Immunology, 148,* 2724–2730.

Evans, T. J., Carpenter, A., Silva, A., & Cohen, J. (1994). Inhibitin of nitric oxide synthase in experimetal gram-negative sepsis. *Journal of Infectious Diseases, 169,* 343–349.

Exley, A. R., Cohen, J., Buurman, W., Owen, R., Hanson, G., Lumley, J., Aulakh, J. M., Bodmer, M., Riddell, A., Stephans, S., & Perry, M. (1990). Monoclonal antibody to TNF in severe septic shock. *Lancet, 335,* 1275–1277.

Faden, A. I. (1996). Pharmacologic treatment of acute traumatic brain injury. *Journal of the American Medical Association, 276,* 569–570.

Faist, E., Ertel, W., Baker, C. C., & Heberer, G. (1989). Terminal B-cell maturation and immunoglobulin synthesis in vitro in patients with major injury. *Journal of Trauma, 29,* 2–9.

Faist, E., Ertel, W., Cohnert, T., Huber, P., Inthorn, D., & Heberer, G. (1990). Immunoprotective effects of cyclooxygenase inhibition in patients with major surgical trauma. *Journal of Trauma, 30,* 8–18.

Faist, E., Ertel, W., Salmen, B., Weiler, A., Ressel, C., Bolla, K., & Heberer, G. (1988). The immune-enhancing effect of perioperative thymopentin administration in elderly patients undergoing major surgery. *Archives of Surgery, 123,* 1449–1453.

Faist, E., Kupper, T. S., Baker, C. C., Chaudry, I. H., Dwyer, J., & Baue, A. E. (1986). Depression of cellular immunity after major injury: Its association with post traumatic complications and its restoration with immunomodulatory agents. *Archives of Surgery, 121,* 1000–1005.

Faist, E., Mewes, A., Baker, C. C., Strasser, T., Alkan, S. S., Rieber, P., & Heberer, G. (1987). Prostaglandin E$_2$ dependent suppression of interleukin-2 production in patients with major trauma. *Journal of Trauma, 27,* 837–848.

Faist, E., Mewes, A., Strasser, T., Walz, A., Alkan, S. S., Baker, C. C., Ertel, W., & Heberer, G. (1988). Alteration of monocyte function following major injury. *Archives of Surgery, 123,* 287–292.

Fandrey, J., Huwiler, A., Frede, S., Pfeilschifter, J., & Jelkmann, W. (1994). Distinct signaling pathways mediate phorbol-ester-induced inhibition of erythropoietin gene expression. *European Journal of Biochemistry, 226,* 335–340.

Faquin, W. C., Schneider, T. J., & Goldberg, M. A. (1992). Effect of inflammatory cytokines on hypoxia-induced erythropoietin production. *Blood, 70,* 1987–1994.

Fiedler, V. B., Loof, I., Sander, E., Voehringer, V., Galanos, C., & Fournel, M. A. (1992). Monoclonal antibody to tumor necrosis factor-alpha prevents lethal endotoxin sepsis in adult rhesus monkeys. *Journal of Laboratory and Clinical Medicine, 120,* 574–588.

Fisher, C. J., Dhainaut, J. F., Opal, S. M., Pribble, J. P., Balk, R. A., Slotman, G. J., Iberti, T. J., Rackow, E. C., Shapiro, M. J., & Greenman, R. L. (1994). Recombinant human interleukin 1 receptor antagonist in the treatment of patients with sepsis syndrome. *Journal of the American Medical Association, 271,* 1836–1843.

Fletcher, J. R., Collins, J. N., Graves, E. D., III, Luterman, A., Williams, M. D., Izenberg, S. D., & Rodning, C. B. (1993). Tumor necrosis factor-induced mortality is reversed with cyclooxygenase inhibition. *Annals of Surgery, 217,* 668–675.

Fong, Y., Tracey, K. J., Moldawer, L. L., Hesse, D. G., Manogue, K. B., Kenney, J. S., Lee, A. T., Kuo, G. C., Allison, A. C., Lowry,

S. F., & Cerami, A. (1989). Antibodies to cachectin/tumor necrosis factor reduce interleukin 1 beta and interleukin 6 appearance during lethal bacteremia. *Journal of Experimental Medicine, 170,* 1627–1633.

Fountain, S. F., Martin, B. A., Musclow, C. E., & Cooper, J. D. (1980). Pulmonary leukostasis and its relationship to pulmonary dysfunction in sheep and rabbits. *Circulation Research, 46,* 175–180.

Frederick, J. A., Hasselgren, P. O., Davis, S., Higashiguchi T., Jacob, T. D., & Fischer, J. E. (1993). Nitric oxide may upregulate in vivo hepatic protein synthesis during endotoxemia. *Archives of Surgery, 128,* 152–157.

Freedman, A. (1956). Chloroquine and rheumatoid arthritis: Short term controlled trial. *Annals of the Rheumatoid Diseases, 15,* 251–257.

Furie, M. B., & Randolph, G. J. (1995). Chemokines and tissue injury. *American Journal of Pathology, 146,* 1287–1301.

Gardinali, M., Padalino, P., Vesconi S, Calcagno, A., Ciappellano, S., Conciato, L., Chiara, O., Agostoni, A., & Nespoli, A. (1992). Complement activation and PMN leukocyte elastase in sepsis. *Archives of Surgery, 127,* 1219–1224.

Gennarelli, T. A. (1993). Mechanisms of brain injury. *Journal of Emergency Medicine, 11,* S5–S11.

Gennerelli, T. A., Champion, H. R., Copes, W. S., & Sacco, W. J. (1994). Comparison of mortality, morbidity, and severity of 59,713 head injured patients with 114,447 patients with extracranial injuries. *Journal of Trauma, 37,* 962–968.

Gentilello, L. M., Jurkovich G. J., Stark, M. S., Hassanstash, S. A., & O'Keefe, G. E. (1997). Is hypothermia in the victim of major trauma protective or harmful? A randomized prospective study. *Annals of Surgery, 226*(4), 439–449.

Ghirnikar, R. S., Lee, Y. L., He, T. R., & Eng, L. F. (1996). Chemokine expression in rat stab wound brain injury. *Journal of Neuroscience, 46,* 727–733.

Giulian, D., Corpuz, M., Chapman, S., Mansouri, M., & Robertson, C. (1993). Reactive mononuclear phagocytes release neurotoxins after ischemic and traumatic injury to the central nervous system. *Journal of Neuroscience Research, 36,* 681–693.

Giulian, D., Vaca, K., & Corpuz, M. (1993). Brain glia release factors with opposing actions upon neuronal survival. *Journal of Neuroscience Research, 13,* 29–37.

Glabinski, A. R., Balasingam, V., Tani, M., Kunkel, S. L., Strieter, R. M., Yong, V. W., & Ransohoff, R. M. (1996). Chemokine monoctye chemoattractant protein-1 is expressed by astrocytes after mechanical injury to the brain. *Journal of Immunology, 156,* 4363–4368.

Gough, D. B., Jordon, A., Mannick, J. A., & Rodrick, M. L. (1992). Impaired cell-mediated immunity in experimental abdominal sepsis. *Archives of Surgery, 127,* 859–863.

Graham, D. I., Adams, J. H., & Gennarelli, T. A. (1993). Pathology of brain damage in head injury. In P. R. Cooper (Ed.), *Head injury* (pp. 91-113). Baltimore: Williams & Wilkins.

Graziano, C., Miller, C. L., & Lim, R. C. (1980). Role of the monocyte function in alteration of the thrombofibrinolytic system after shock. *Surgical Forum, 31,* 25–27.

Green, J. M., & Thompson, C. B. (1994). Modulation of T cell proliferative response by accessory cell interactions. *Immunology Research, 13,* 234–243.

Grum, C. M., Simon, R. H., Dantzker, D., & Fox, I. H. (1985). Evidence for adenosine triphosphate degradation in critically ill patients. *Chest, 88,* 763–767.

Han, J., Thompson, P., & Beutler, B. (1990). Dexamethasone and pentoxifylline inhibit endotoxin-induced cachectin/tumor necrosis factor synthesis at separate points in the signaling pathway. *Journal of Experimental Medicine, 172,* 391–394.

Hara, T., Fu, S. M., & Hansen, J. A. (1985). Human T cell activation, IL: a new T cell activation pathway used by a major T cell population via a disulfide bonded dimer of a 44-kilodalton peptide (9. 3 antigen). *Journal of Experimental Medicine, 161,* 1513–1524.

Harkema, J. M., Singh, G., Wang, P., & Chaudry, I. H. (1992). Pharmacologic agents in the treatment of ischemia, hemorrhagic shock, and sepsis. *Journal of Critical Care, 7,* 189–216.

Harlan, J. M., Vedder, N. B., Winn, R. K., & Rice, C. L. (1991). Mechanisms and consequences of leukocyte-endothelial interaction. *Western Journal of Medicine, 155,* 365–369.

Hartl, R., Medary, M., Ruge, M., Arfors, K. E., & Ghajar, J. (1997). Blood-brain barrier breakdown occurs early after traumatic brain injury and is not related to white blood cell adherence. *Acta Neurochir, 70*(Suppl.), 240–242.

Hartl, W. H., Herndon, D. N., & Wolfe, R. R. (1990). Kinin/prostaglandin system: its therapeutic value in surgical stress. *Critical Care Medicine, 18,* 1167.

Hechtman, H. B., Valeri, C. R., & Shepro, D. (1984). Role of humoral mediators in adult respiratory distress syndrome. *Chest, 86*(4), 623–627.

Hershman, M. J., Pietsch, J. D., Trachtenberg, L., Mooney, T. H. R., Shields, R. E., & Sonnenfeld, G. (1989). Protective effects of recombinant human tumour necrosis factor alpha and interferon against surgically simulated wound infection in mice. *British Journal of Surgery, 76,* 1282–1286.

Hess, M. L., Warner, M. F., Smith, J. M., Manson, N. H., & Greenfield, L. J. (1983). Improved myocardial hemodynamic and cellular function with calcium channel blockade (verapamil) during canine hemorrhagic shock. *Circulatory Shock, 10,* 119–130.

Hibbs, J. B., Taintor, R. R., & Vavrin, Z. (1987). Macrophage cytotoxicity: Role for L-arginine deiminase and imino nitrogen oxidation to nitrite. *Science, 240,* 473–476.

Hill, J., Lindsay, T., Rusche, J., Valeri, C. R., Shepro, D., & Hechtman, H. B. (1992). A Mac-1 antibody reduces liver and lung injury but not neutrophil sequestration after intestinal ischemia-reperfusion. *Surgery, 112,* 166–172.

Hirasawa, H., Sugai, T., & Ohtake, Y. (1990). Energy metabolism and nutritional support in auric multiple organ failure patients. In T. Tanaka & A. Okada (Eds.), *Nutritional Support in Organ Failure* (pp. 439-446). Amsterdam: Elsevier.

Hoffmann, H., Weis, M., Birg, A., Schonharting, M. M., & Jochum, M. (1995). Amelioration of endotoxin-induced acute lung injury in pigs by HWA 138 and A 80 2715: New analogs of pentoxifylline. *Shock, 4,* 166–170.

Holmin, S., Soderlund, J., Biberfeld, P., & Mathiesen, T. (1998). Intracerebral inflammation after human brain confusion. *Neurosurgery, 42,* 291–299.

Homayoun, P., Rodriguez de Turco, E. B., Parkins, N. E., Lane, D. C., Soblosky, J., Carey, M. E., & Bazen, N. G. (1997). Delayed phospholipid degradation in rat brain after traumatic brain injury. *Journal of Neurochemistry, 69,* 199–205.

Homo-Delarche, F., Fitzpatrick, F., Christeff, N., Nunez, E. A., Bach, J. F., & Dardenne, M. (1991). Sex steroids, glucocorticoids, stress and autoimmunity. *Journal of Steroid Biochemisty and Molecular Biology, 40,* 619–637.

Horn, R. G., & Collins, R. D. (1968). Studies on the pathogenesis of the generalized Schwartzman reaction. *Laboratory Investigations, 18,* 101–107.

Hosford, D., Koltai, M., & Braquet, P. (1993). Platelet-activating factor in shock, sepsis, and organ failure. In G. Schlag & H. Redl (Eds.), *Pathophysiology of shock, sepsis, and organ failure* (pp. 502-517). Berlin: Springer-Verlag.

Inoue, T., Saito, H., Fukushima, R., Inaba, T., Lin, M. T., Fukatsu, K., & Muto, T. (1995). Growth hormone and insulin-like growth factor I enhance host defense in a murine sepsis model. *Archives of Surgery, 130,* 1115–1122.

Isaksson, J., Lewen, A., Hillered, L., & Olsson, V. (1997). Up-regulation of intercellular adhesion molecule-1 in cerebral microvessels after cortical contusion trauma in a rat model. *Acta Neuropathology, 94,* 16–20.

Jaeschke, H. (1991). Reactive oxygen and ischemia/reperfusion injury of the liver. *Chemical–Biological Interactions, 79,* 115–136.

Jelkman, W. (1992). Erythropoietn: structure, control of production, and function. *Physiology Review, 72,* 449–489.

Jelkmann, W., Fandrey, J., Frede, S., & Pagel, H. (1994). Inhibition of erythropoietin production by cytokines, implications for the anemia involved in inflammatory states. *Annals of the New York Academy of Sciences, 718,* 300–309.

Jelkmann, W., Pagel, H., Wolff, M., & Fandrey, J. (1992). Monokines inhibiting erythropoietin production in human hepatoma cultures and in isolated perfused rat kidneys. *Life Science, 50,* 301–308.

Jennett, B. (1996). Epidemiology of head injury. *Journal of Neurol Neurosurg Psychiatry, 60,* 362–369.

Johnston, R. B. (1988). Monocytes and macrophages. *New England Journal of Medicine, 318,* 747–752.

Junger, W. G., Hoyt, D. B., Redl, H., Liu, F. C., Loomis, W. H., Davies, J., & Schlag, G. (1995). Tumor necrosis factory antibody treatment of septic baboons reduces the production of sustained T-cell suppressive factors. *Shock, 3,* 173–178.

Kaczorowski, S. L., Schiding, J. K., Toth, C. A., & Kochanek, P. M. (1995). Effect of soluble complement receptor-1 on neutrophil accumulation after traumatic brain injury in rats. *Journal of Cerebral Blood Flow and Metabolism, 15,* 860–864.

Kapur, M. M., Jain, P., & Gidh, M. (1986). The effect of trauma on serum C3 activation and its correlation with Injury Severity Score in man. *Journal of Trauma, 26,* 464–466.

Khansari, D. N., Margo, A. J., & Faith, C. E. (1990). Effects of stress on the immune system. *Immonology Today, 11,* 170–175.

Kinney, J., & Gump, F. (1982). The metabolic response to injury. In S. Dudrick (Ed.), *Manual of preoperative and postoperative care* (pp. 15). Philadelphia: Saunders.

Knapp, W., & Baumgartner, G. (1978). Monocyte-mediated suppression of human B lymphocyte differentiation in vitro. *Journal of Immunology, 121,* 1177–1183.

Knaus, W. A., Draper, E. A., Wagner, D. P., & Zimmerman, J. E. (1985). Prognosis in acute organ system failure. *Annals of Surgery, 202,* 685–693.

Kochanek, P. M. (1993). Pathobiology and cellular mechanisms. *Critical Care Medicine, 21,* S333–S335.

Kochanek, P. M. (1997). Brain damage secondary to hemorrhagic-traumatic shock, sepsis, and traumatic brain injury. In G. Schlag, H. Redl, & D. Traber (Eds.), *Inflammatory process in the pathobiology of secondary damage after traumatic brain injury* (pp. 197–213). Berlin: Springer.

Koga, T., Wand-Wurttenberger, A., DeBruyn, J., Munk, M. E., Schoel, B., & Kaufmann, S. H. (1989). T cells against a common bacterial heat shock protein recognize stressed macrophages. *Science, 245,* 1112–1115.

Koike, K., Moore, E. E., Moore, F. A., Carl, V. S., Pitman, J. M., & Banerjee, A. (1992). Phospholipase A$_2$ inhibition decouples lung injury from gut ischemia reperfusion. *Surgery, (112)* 173–178.

Kossmann, T. (1998). Cytokines in traumatic brain injury. In K. R. H. von Wild (Ed.), *Pathophysiological principles and controversies in neurointensive care* (pp. 26–33). Munich: Zuckerschwerdt.

Kossmann, T., Hans, V., Imhof, H. G., Trentz, O., & Morganti-Kossmann, M. C. (1996). Interleukin-6 released in human cerebrospinal fluid following traumatic brain injury may trigger nerve growth factor production in astrocytes. *Brain Research, 713,* 143–152.

Kossmann, T., Lenzlinger, P. M., Stover, J. F., Stocker, R., Morganti-Kossmann, M. C., & Trentz, O. (1997). Neurochemical alterations and current pharmacological strategies in the treatment of traumatic brain injury. *Unfallchirurg, 100,* 613–622.

Kossmann, T., Stahel, P. F., Lenzlinger, P. M., Redl, H., Dubs, R. W., Trentz, O., Schlag, G., & Morganti-Kossmann, M. C. (1997). Interleukin-8 released into the cerebrospinal fluid after brain injury is associated with blood-brain barrier dysfunction and nerve growth factor production. *Journal of Cerebral Blood Flow and Metabolism, 17,* 280–289.

Kraus, J. F. (1993). Epidemiology of head injury. In P. R. Cooper (Ed.), *Head injury* (pp. 1–25). Baltimore: Williams & Williams.

Kremer, J. M., Bigauoette, J., Michalek, A. V., Timchalk, M. A., Lininger, L., Rynes, R. I., Huyck, C., Zieminski, J., & Bartholomew, L. E. (1985). Effects of manipulation of dietary fatty acids on clinical manifestations of rheumatoid arthritis. *Lancet, 1*(8422), 184–187.

Kupfer, S. R., Underwood, L. E., Baxter, R. C., & Clemmons, D. R. (1993). Enhancement of the anabolic effects of growth hormone and insulin-like growth factor I by use of both agents simultaneously. *Journal of Clinical Investigations, 91,* 391–396.

Kurz, A., Sessler, D. I., & Lenhardt, R. (1996). Perioperative normothermia to reduce the incidence of surgical-wound infection and shorten hospitalization. *New England Journal of Medicine, 334,* 1209–1215.

Leberman, M. D. (1990). Effects of nutrient substrates on immune function. *Journal of Nutrition, 6,* 88–91.

Ledbetter, J. A., Martin, P. J., Spooner, C. E., Wofsy, D., Tsu, T. T., Beatty, P. G., & Gladstone, P. (1985). Antibodies to Tp67 and Tp44 augment and sustain proliferative responses of activated T cells. *Journal of Immunology, 135,* 2331–2336.

Lehmann, V., Benninghoff, B., & Dröge, W. (1988). Tumor necrosis factor-induced activation of peritoneal macrophages is regulated by prostaglandin E$_2$ and cAMP. *Journal of Immunology, 141,* 587–591.

Liebscher, G., Shapiro, M. J., Barner, H., Daake, C., Moskoff, M., Durham, R. M., & Baue, A. E. (1994). ATP-MgCl$_2$ as an afterload reducing agent. [Abstract]. *Critical Care Medicine, 2.*

Lilly, M. P., & Gann, D. S. (1992). The hypothalamic-pituitary-adrenal immune axis. *Archives of Surgery, 127,* 1463–1472.

Linsley, P. S., Greene, J. L., Brady, W., Bajorath, J., Ledbetter, J. A., & Peach, R. (1994). Human B7-1 (CD80) and B7-2 (CD86) bind with similar avidities but distinct kinetics to CD28 and CTLA-4 receptors. *Immunity, 1,* 793–801.

Linsley, P. S., & Ledbetter, J. A. (1993). The role of the CD28 receptor during T cell responses to antigen. *Annual Review of Immunology, 11,* 191–212.

Lopez-Diez, F., Nieto, M. L., Fernandez-Gallardo, S., Gijon, M. A., & Sanchez-Crespo, M. (1989). Occupancy of platelet receptors for platelet activating factor in patients with septicemia. *Journal of Clinical Investigations, 83,* 1733–1740.

Lowry, S. F. (1993). Anticytokine therapies in sepsis. New Horizons: Sepsis: Cellular and physiological alterations. *Critical Care Medicine, 1,* 120–126.

Luer, M. S., Rhoney, D. H., Hughes, M., & Hatton, J. (1996). New pharmacologic strategies for acute neuronal injury. *Journal of Pharmacotherapy, 16,* 830–848.

Luster, M. I., Pfeifer, R. W., & Tucker, A. N. (1985). Influence of sex hormones on immunoregulation with specific reference to natural and environmental estrogens. In J. A. Thomas, K. S. Korach, & J. A. McLachlan (Eds.), *Endocrine toxicology* (pp. 67-83). New York: Raven Press.

Maitra, S. R., & Sayeed, M. M. (1987). Effect of diltiazem on intracellular $Ca^{2+}$ mobilization in hepatocytes during endotoxic shock. *American Journal of Physiology, 253,* R545–R548.

Malangoni, M. A., Livingston, D. H., Sonnenfeld, G., & Polk, H. C. (1990). Interferon gamma and tumor necrosis factor alpha. *Archives of Surgery, 125,* 444–446.

Marion, B. W., Penrod, L. E., Kelsey, S. F., Obrist, W. D., Kochanek, P. M., Palmer, A. M., Wisniewski, S. R., & DeKosky, S. T. (1997). Treatment of traumatic brain injury with moderate hypothemia. *New England Journal of Medicine, 336,* 540–546.

McCullough, J. N., Spillert, C. R., & Lazaro, E. J. (1990). Direct correlation between injury severity and two markers of the functional status of the immune system. *Circulatory Shock, 31,* 309–316.

McGowan, J. E., Barnes, M. W., & Finland, N. (1975). Bacteremia at Boston City Hospital: Occurrence and mortality during 12 selected years (1935–1972) with special reference to hospital-acquired cases. *Journal of Infectious Diseases, 132,* 316–335.

McIntosh, T. K. (1993). Novel pharmacologic therapies in the treatment of experimental traumatic brain injury: A review. *Journal of Neurotrauma, 10,* 215–261.

McIntosh, T. K., Smith, D. H., Meaney, D. F., Kotapka, M. J., Gennarelli, T. A., & Graham, D. I. (1996). Neuropathological sequelae of traumatic brain injury: Relationship to neurochemical and biomechanical mechanisms. *Laboratory Investigations, 74,* 315–342.

McRitchie, D. I., Girotti, M. J., Rotstein, O. D., & Teodorczyk-Injeyan, J. A. (1990). Impaired antibody production in blunt trauma. *Archives of Surgery, 125,* 91–96.

Means, R. T., & Krantz, S. B. (1992). Progress in understanding the pathogenesis of the anemia of chronic disease. *Blood, 80,* 1639–1647.

Meldrum, D. R., Ayala, A., & Chaudry, I. H. (1992). Energetics of defective macrophage antigen presentation following hemorrhage as determined by ultraresolution $^{31}P$ nuclear magnetic resonance spectrometry: Restoration with $ATP$-$MgCl_2$. *Surgery, 112,* 150–158.

Meldrum, D. R., Ayala, A., & Chaudry, I. H. (1994). Energetics of lymphocyte ''burnout'' in late sepsis: Adjuvant treatment with $ATP$-$MgCl_2$ improves energetics and decreases lethality. *Journal of Surgical Research, 56,* 537–542.

Meldrum, D. R., Ayala, A., Perrin, M. M., Ertel, W., & Chaudry, I. H. (1991a). Diltiazem restores IL-2, IL-3, IL-6 and IFN-gamma synthesis and decreases susceptibility to sepsis following hemorrhage. *Journal of Surgical Research, 51,* 158–164.

Meldrum, D. R., Ayala, A., Wang, P., Ertel, W., & Chaudry, I. H. (1991b). Association between decreased splenic ATP levels and immunodepression: Amelioration with $ATP$-$MgCl_2$. *American Journal of Physiology, 261,* R351–R357.

Meyer, M. (1995). Neurotrophins: Aspects of their in vivo action and physiology. In N. J. Rothwell (Ed.), *Immune responses in the nervous system.* (pp. 101–116). Oxford: Bios Scientific.

Mileski, W., Borgstrom, D., Lightfoot, E., Rothlein, R., Faanes, R., Lipsky, P., & Baxter, C. (1992). Inhibition of leukocyte-endothelial adherence following thermal injury. *Journal of Surgical Research, 52,* 334–339.

Miller, J. D. (1993). Traumatic brain swelling and edema. In P. R. Cooper (Ed.), *Head injury* (pp. 331–354). Baltimore: Williams & Wilkins.

Miller-Graziano, C. L., Fink, M., Wu, J. Y., Szabo, G., & Kodys, K. (1988). Mechanisms of altered monocyte prostaglandin $E_2$

production in severely injured patients. *Archives of Surgery, 123,* 293–299.

Milligan, C. E., Webster, L., Piros, E. T., Evans, C. J., Cunningham, T. J., & Levitt, P. (1995). Induction of opioid receptor-mediated macrophage chemotactic activity after neonatal brain injury. *Journal of Immunology, 154,* 6571–6581.

Minnard, E. A., Shou, J., Naama, H., Cech, A., Gallagher, H., & Daly, J. M. (1994). Inhibition of nitric oxide synthesis is detrimental during endotoxemia. *Archives of Surgery, 129,* 142–148.

Molloy, R. G., O'Riordain, M. G., Holzheimer, R., Nestor, M., Collins, K., Mannick, J. A., & Rodrick, M. L. (1993). Mechanism of increased tumor necrosis factor production after thermal injury. Altered sensitivity to $PGE_2$ and immunomodulation with indomethacin. *Journal of Immunology, 151,* 2142–2149.

Moncada, S., Palmer, R. M. J., & Higgs, E. A. (1991). Nitric oxide: Physiology, Pathophysiology and Pharmacology. *Pharmacological Reviews, 43,* 109–142.

Moore, F. A., Peterson, V. M., Moore, E. E., Rundus, C., & Poggett, R. (1990). Inadequate granulopoiesis after major torso trauma: A hematopoietic regulatory paradox. *Surgery, 108,* 667–675.

Morgan, B. P., Gasque, P., Singhrao, S., & Piddlesden, S. J. (1997). Role of complement in inflammation and injury in the nervous system. *Experimental and Clinical Immunogenetics, 14,* 19–23.

Morganti-Kossman, M. C., & Kossman, T. (1995). The immunology of brain injury. In N. J. Rothwell (Ed.), *Immune responses of the nervous system* (pp. 158–187). Oxford: Bios Scientific Publishers.

Morrison, A. M., Wang, P., & Chaudry, I. H. (1996). A novel nonanticoagulant heparin prevents vascular endothelial cell dysfunction during hyperdynamic sepsis. *Shock, 6,* 46–51.

Mullen, P., Windsor, A., Walsh, C., Fisher, B., Blocher, C., Fowler, A., & Sugerman, H. (1992). Effect of monoclonal antibody to tumor necrosis factor-$\alpha$ on neutrophil oxidant generation. *Circulatory Shock, 37,* 21. [Abstract]

Mulligan, M. S., Varani, J., Dame, M. K., Lane, C. L., Smith, C. W., Anderson, D. C., & Ward, P. A. (1991). Role of endothelial-leukocyte adhesion molecule 1 (ELAM-1) in neutrophil-mediated lung injury in rats. *Journal of Clinical Investigations, 88,* 1396–1406.

Nathan, C. F. (1987). Secretory products of macrophages. *Journal of Clinical Investigations, 79,* 319–326.

Nava, E., Palmer, R. M. J., & Moncada, S. (1991). Inhibition of nitric oxide synthesis in septic shock: How much is beneficial? *Lancet, 338,* 1555–1557.

O'Keefe, G. E., Gentilello, L. M., & Maier, R. V. (1998). Incidence of infectuous complications associated with the use of histamine2-receptor antagonists in critically ill trauma patients. *Annals of Surgery, 227*(1), 120–125.

O'Keefe, G. E., Jurkovich, G. J., & Maier, R. V. (1997). 10-Year trends in costs, resource utilization, and survival outcome in an established trauma center. *Surgery Forum, 48,* 595–597.

O'Riordain, M. G., Collins, K. H., Pilz, M., Saporoschetz, I. B., Mannick, J. A., & Rodrick, M. L. (1992). Modulation of macrophage hyperactivity improves survival in a burn-sepsis model. *Archives of Surgery, 127,* 152–158.

Ohlsson, K., Björk, P., Bergenfeldt, M., Hageman, R., & Thompson, R. C. (1990). Interleukin-1 receptor antagonist reduces mortality from endotoxin shock. *Nature, 348,* 550–552.

Ossa, J. C., de la, Malago, M., & Gewertz, B. L. (1992). Neutrophil-endothelial cell binding in neutrophil-mediated tissue injury. *Journal of Surgical Research, 53,* 103–107.

Parratt, J. R. (1994). Nitric oxide and cardiovascular dysfunction in sepsis and endotoxaemia: An introduction and an overview. In

G. Schlag & H. Redl (Eds.), *Shock, sepsis and organ failure—Nitric oxide* (pp. 1–29). Heidelberg: Springer-Verlag.

Parratt, J. R., Stoclet, J. C., & Furman, B. L. (1993). Substances mainly derived from vascular endothelium, endothelium derived relaxing factor, or nitric oxide and endothelin as chemical mediators in sepsis and endotoxaemia. In E. Neugebauer & J. W. Holaday (Eds.), *Handbook of mediators of septic shock* (pp. 381-393). Boca Raton, FL: CRC Press.

Parrillo, J. (1993). Pathogenetic mechanisms of septic shock. *New England Journal of Medicine, 328,* 1471–1477.

Pellicane, J. V., DeMaria, E. J., Leeper-Woodford, S., Lee, R. B., & Fowler, A. A. (1992). Tumor necrosis factor antibody improves survival following hemorrhagic shock in awake rats. *Circulatory Shock, 37,* 54. [Abstract]

Petros, A., Bennett, D., & Vallance, P. (1991). Effect of nitric oxide synthase inhibitors on hypotension in patients with septic shock. *Lancet, 338,* 1557–1558.

Phillips, J. O., Metzler, M. H., Palmieri, M. T., Huckfeldt, R. E., & Dahl, N. G. (1996). A prospective study of simplified omeprazole suspension for the prophylaxis of stress-related mucosal damage. *Critical Care Medicine, 24*(11), 1793–1800.

Pleines, U. E., Stover, J. F., Kossmann, T., Trentz, O., & Morganti-Kossmann, M. C. (1998). Soluble ICAM-1 in CSF coincides with the extent of cerebral damage in patients with severe traumatic brain injury. *Journal of Neurotrauma, 15*(6), 399–409.

Pober, J. S., & Cotran, R. S. (1990). Cytokines and endothelial cell biology. *Physiological Reviews, 70,* 427–451.

Read, R. A., Moore, E. E., Moore, F. A., Carl, V. S., & Banerjee, A. (1993). Platelet-activating factor-induced polymorphonuclear neutrophil priming independent of CD11B adhesion. *Surgery, 114,* 308–313.

Redl, H., Vogl, C., Schiesser, A., Paul, E., Thurnher, M., Bahrami, S., & Schlag, G. (1990). Effect of the PAF antagonist BN 52021 in ovine endotoxin shock. *Journal of Lipid Mediators, 2*(S), 195–201.

Redmond, H. P., Hofmann, K., Shou, J., Leon, P., Kelly, C. J., & Daly, J. M. (1992). Effects of laparatomy on systemic macrophage function. *Surgery, 111,* 647–655.

Regel, G. (1996). Brain damage secondary to hemorrhagic-traumatic shock, sepsis and traumatic brain injury. In G. Schlag, H. Redl, & D. Traber (Eds.), *Pathophysiology, management and outcome after multiple trauma* (pp. 229–262). Berlin: Springer.

Regel, G., Lobenhoffer, P., Grotz, M., Pape, H. C., Lehmann, U., & Tscherne, H. (1995). Treatment results of patients with multiple trauma: An analysis of 3406 cases treated between 1972 and 1991 at a German level I trauma center. *Journal of Trauma, 38*(1), 70–77.

Rink, A., Fung, K. M., Trojanowski, J. Q., Lee, V. M., Neugebauer, E., & McIntosh, T. K. (1995). Evidence of apoptotic cell death after experimental traumatic brain injury in the rat. *American Journal of Pathology, 147,* 1575–1583.

Robinson, D. R., Prickett, J. D., Polisson, R., Steinberg, A. D., & Levine, L. (1985). The protective effect of dietary fish oil on murine lupus. *Journal of Prostaglandins, 30,* 51–75.

Rollo, I. M. (1980). Drugs used in the chemotherapy of malaria. In L. S. Goodman & A. G. Gilman (Eds.), *Pharmacological basis of therapeutics* (pp. 1038-1060). New York: MacMillan.

Rothwell, N. J., & Strijbos, P. J. (1995). Cytokines in neurodegeneration and repair. *International Journal of Developmental Neuroscience, 13,* 179–185.

Ryan, J., & Geczy, C. (1987). Coagulation and the expression of cell mediated immunity. *Immunology and Cell Biology, 65,* 127–139.

Sauaia, A., Moore, F. A., Moore, E. E., Haenel, J. B., Read, R. A., & Lezotte, D. C. (1994). Early predictors of postinjury multiple organ failure. *Archives of Surgery, 129,* 39–45.

Sayeed, M. M., Adler, R. J., Chaudry, I. H., & Baue, A. E. (1981). Effect of hemorrhagic shock on hepatic transmembrane potentials and intracellular electrolytes, in vivo. *American Journal of Physiology, 240,* R211–R219.

Scarborough, D. (1990). Cytokine modulation of pituitary hormone secretion. *Academic Science, 594,* 169–187.

Schirmer, W. J., Schirmer, J. M., Naff, G. B., & Fry, D. E. (1988). Contribution of toxic oxygen intermediates to complement-induced reductions in effective hepatic blood flow. *Journal of Trauma, 28,* 1295–1300.

Schirmer, W. J., Schirmer, J. M., Naff, G. B., & Fry, D. E. (1988). Systemic complement activation produces hemodynamic changes characteristic of sepsis. *Archives of Surgery, 123,* 316–321.

Schlag, G., & Redl, H. (1996). Mediators of injury and inflammation. *World Journal of Surgery, 20,* 406–410.

Schlag, G., Redl, H., Davies, J., & Haller, I. (1994). Anti-tumor necrosis factor antibody treatment of recurrent bacteremia in a baboon model. *Shock, 2,* 10–18.

Schlosshauer, B. (1993). The blood-brain barrier: Morphology, molecules and neurothelin. *BioEssays, 15,* 341–346.

Schroder, J., Kahlke, V., Staubach, K., Zabel, P., & Stuber, F. (1998). Gender differences in human sepsis. *Archives of Surgery, 133,* 1200–1205.

Shackford, S. R., Bourguignon, P. R., Wald, S. L., Rogers, F. B., Osler, T. M., & Clark, D. E. (1998). Hypertonic saline resuscitation of patients with head injury: A prospective, randomized clinical trial. *Journal of Trauma, 44,* 50–58.

Shi, Y., Radvanyi, L. G., Shaw, P., Green, D. R., Miller, R., & Mills, G. B. (1995). CD28-mediated signaling in vivo prevents activation-induced apoptosis in the thymus and alters peripheral lymphocytes homeostasis. *Journal of Immunology, 155,* 1829–1837.

Shires, G. T., Cunningham, J. N., Baker, C. R. F., Reeder, S. F., Illner, H., Wagner, I. Y., & Maher, J. (1972). Alterations in cellular membrane function during hemorrhagic shock in primates. *Annals of Surgery, 176,* 288–294.

Shuman, R. B., Schuster, D. P., & Zuckerman, G. R. (1987). Prophylactic therapy for stress bleeding: A reappraisal. *Annals of Internal Medicine, 106,* 562–567.

Siesjo, B. K. (1993). Basic mechanisms of traumatic brain damage. *Annals of Emergency Medicine, 22,* 959–969.

Soboleva, M. K., & Manakova, T. E. (1993). Plasma erythropoietin activity in infants with sepsis. *Bulletin of Experimental Biology and Medicine, 115,* 545–548.

Solomkin, J. S. (1990). Neutrophil disorders in burn injury: Complement, cytokines, and organ injury. *Journal of Trauma, 30,* 580–585.

Spiegel, K., Emmerling, M. R., & Barnum, S. R. (1997). Strategies for inhibition of complement activation in the treatment of neurodegenerative diseases. In P. L. Wood (Ed.), *Neuroinflammation: Mechanisms and management* (pp. 129–176). Totowa: Humana Press.

Stahel, P. F., & Barnum, S. R. (1997). Bacterial meningitis: Complement gene expression in the central nervous system. *Journal of Immunopharmacology, 38,* 65–72.

Stahel, P. F., Morganti-Kossman, M. C., & Kossmann, T. (1998). The role of the complement system in traumatic brain injury. *Brain Research, 27,* 243–256.

Stahl, G. L., Bitterman, H., Terashita, Z., & Lefer, A. M. (1988). Salutary consequences of blockade of platelet activating factor in hemorrhagic shock. *European Journal of Pharmacology, 149,* 233–240.

Stewart, J. M. (1993). The kinin system in inflammation, in proteases, protease inhibitors, and protease-derived peptides. Agents and actions. *Birkhauser Verlag: Basel,* 145.

Stiletto, R., Bruck, E., & Bittner, G. (1998). Low cost prone positioning of critically ill ARDS patients with the MPS (modular prone positioning system). *Critical Care, 2*, 59.

Stiletto, R. J. (1998). The role of positioning in the prevention of ALI and ARDS in polytrauma patients. *Critical Care, 2*, 58.

Strieter, R. M., Remick, D. G., Ward, P. A., Spengler, R. N., Lynch, J. P. I., Larrick, J., & Kunkel, S. L. (1988). Cellular and molecular regulation of tumor necrosis factor-alpha production by pentoxifylline. *Biochemical Biophysical Research Communications, 155*, 1230–1236.

Sumpio, B. E., Hull, M. J., Baue, A. E., & Chaudry, I. H. (1986). Comparison of effects of ATP-$MgCl_2$ and adenosine-$MgCl_2$ on renal function following ischemia. *American Journal of Physiology, 252*, R388–R393.

Tang, T., Frenette, P. S., Hynes, R. O., Wagner, D. D., & Mayadas, T. N. (1996). Cytokine-induced meningitis is dramatically attenuated in mice deficient in endothelial selectins. *Journal of Clinical Investigations, 97*, 2485–2490.

Teale, D. M., & Atkinson, A. M. (1992). Inhibition of nitric oxide synthesis improves survival in a murine peritonitis model of sepsis that is not cured by antibiotics alone. *Journal of Antimicrobial Chemotherapy, 30*, 839–842.

Thiemermann, C., & Vane, J. (1990). Inhibition of nitric oxide synthesis reduces the hypotension induced by bacterial lipopolysaccharides in the rat in vivo. *European Journal of Pharmacology, 182*, 591–595.

Tornqvist, E., Liu, L., Aldskogius, H., Holst, H. V., & Svensson, M. (1996). Complement and clusterin in the injured nervous system. *Neurobiol Aging, 17*, 695–705.

Tracey, K. J., Beutler, B., Lowry, S. F., Merryweather, J., Wolpe, S., Milsark, I. W., Hariri, R. J., Fahey, T. J.,III, Zentella, A., Albert, J. D., Shires, G. T., & Cerami, A. (1986b). Shock and tissue injury induced by recombinant human cachectin. *Science, 234*, 470–474.

Tracey, K. J., Fong, Y., Hesse, D. G., Manogue, K. R., Lee, A. T., Kuo, G. C., Lowry, S. F., & Cerami, A. (1987). Anti-cachectin/TNF monoclonal antibodies prevent septic shock during lethal bacteremia. *Nature, 330*, 662–664.

Tracey, K. J., Lowry, S. F., Beutler, B., Cerami, A., Albert, J. D., & Shires, G. T. (1986a). Cachectin/TNF mediates changes of skeletal muscle plasma membrane potential. *Journal of Experimental Medicine, 164*, 1368–1373.

Tran, D. D., Cuesta, M. A., van Leeuwen, P. A., Nauta, J. J., & Wesdorp, R. I. (1993). Risk factors for multiple organ system failure and death in critically injured patients. *Surgery, 114*, 21–30.

Tuchschmidt, J., Oblitas, D., & Fried, J. C. (1991). Oxygen consumption in sepsis and septic shock. *Critical Care Medicine, 19*, 664–671.

Unanue, E. R., & Allen, P. M. (1987). The basis for the immunoregulatory role of macrophages and other accessory cells. *Science, 236*, 551–557.

Unanue, E. R., & Benacerraf, B. (1998). *Textbook of immunology.* Baltimore: Williams & Williams.

Vane, J. R., Anggard, E. E., & Botting, R. M. (1990). Regulatory functions of the vascular endothelium. *New England Journal of Medicine, 323*, 27–36.

Verhoef, J., Hustinx, W. M. N., Frasa, H., & Hoepelman, A. I. M. (1996). Issues in the adjunct therapy of severe sepsis. *Antimicrobial Agents and Chemotherapy, 38*, 167–182.

Voerman, H. J., Strack van Schijndel, R. J. M., de Boer, H., van der Veen, E. A., & Thijs, L. G. (1992). Growth hormone: Secretion and administration in catabolic adult patients, with emphasis on the critically ill patient. *Netherlands Journal of Medicine, 41*, 229–244.

Walker, C., Kristensen, F., & Bettens, F., DeWeck, A. L. (1983). Lymphokine regulation of activated ($G_1$) lymphocytes: Prostaglandin $E_2$-induced inhibition of interleukin 2 production. *Journal of Immunology, 130*, 1770–1773.

Wang, P., Ba, Z. F., & Chaudry, I. H. (1994). Nitric oxide. To block or enhance its production during sepsis? *Archives of Surgery, 129*, 1137–1143.

Wang, P., Ba, Z. F., Reich, S. S., Zhou, M., Holme, K. R., & Chaudry, I. H. (1996). Effects of a nonanticoagulant heparin on cardiovascular and hepatocellular function after hemorrhagic shock. *American Journal of Physiology, 270*, H1294–H1302.

Wang, P., Ba, Z. F., Zhou, M., & Chaudry, I. H. (1993). Pentoxifylline restores cardiac output and tissue perfusion following trauma-hemorrhage and decreases susceptibility to sepsis. *Surgery, 114*, 352–359.

Wang, P., & Chaudry, I. H. (1996). Mechanism of hepatocellular dysfunction during hyperdynamic sepsis. *American Journal of Physiology, 270*, R927–R938.

Wang, R., Fang, Q., Zhang, L., Radvany, L., Sharma, A., Noben-Trauth, N., Mills, G. B., & Shi, Y. (1997). CD 28 ligation prevents bacterial toxin-induced septic shock in mice by inducing IL-10 expression. *Journal of Immunology, 158*, 2856–2861.

Ward, P. A., Till, G. O., Kunkel, R., & Beauchamp, C. (1983). Evidence for role of hydroxyl radical in complement and neutorphil-dependent tissue injury. *Journal of Clinical Investigations, 72*, 789–801.

Warden, G. D., Mason, A. D., & Pruitt, B. A. (1974). Evaluation of leukocyte chemotaxis in vitro in thermally injured patients. *Journal of Clinical Investigations, 54*, 1001–1004.

Weigent, D. A., Carr, D. J. J., & Blalock, J. E. (1990). Bi-directional communication between the neuroendocrine and immune system. *Annals of the New York Academy of Sciences, 579*, 17–27.

Westfall, M. V., & Sayeed, M. M. (1989). Effect of diltiazem on skeletal muscle 3-O-methylglucose transport in bacteremic rats. *American Journal of Physiology, 256*, R716–R721.

Wichmann, M. W., Angele, M. K., Ayala, A., Cioffi, W. G., & Chaudry, I. (1997). Flutamide: A novel agent for restoring the depressed cell-mediated immunity following soft-tissue trauma and hemorrhagic shock. *Shock, 8*(4), 1–7.

Wichmann, M. W., Ayala, A., & Chaudry, I. (1997). Male sex steroids are responsible for depressing macrophage immune function after trauma-hemorrhage. *American Journal of Physiology, 273*, C1335–C1340.

Wichmann, M. W., Zellweger, R., DeMaso, C. M., Ayala, A., & Chaudry, I. H. (1996). Enhanced immune responses in females as opposed to decreased responses in males following hemorrhagic shock. *Cytokine, 8*(11), 853–863.

Wichterman, K. A., Baue, A. E., & Chaudry, I. H. (1980). Sepsis and septic shock - A review of laboratory models and a proposal. *Journal of Surgical Research, 29*, 189–201.

Wieloch, T. (1998). Mechanisms of neuronal death. In K. R. H. von Wild (Ed.), *Pathophysiological principles and controversies in neurointensive care* (pp. 3-14). Munich: Zuckschwerdt.

Williams, D. L., Sherwood, E. R., Browder, I. W., McNamee, R. B., Jones, E. L., Rakinic, J., & Di Luzio, N. R. (1988). Effect of glucan on neutrophil dynamics and immune function in Escherichia coll peritonitis. *Journal of Surgical Research, 44*, 54–61.

Williams, J. G., Garcia, I., & Maier, R. V. (1993). Prostaglandin $E_2$ mediates lipopolysaccharide-induced macrophage procoagulant activity by a cyclic adenosine monophosphate-dependent pathway. *Surgery, 114*, 314–323.

Wilmore, D. W., Goodwin, C. W., Aulick, L. H., Powanda, M. C., Mason, Jr., & Pruitt, Jr. (1980). Effect of injury and infection on visceral metabolism and circulation. *Annals of Surgery, 192,* 491–504.

Yakovlev, A. G. (1997). Activation of CPP32-like caspases contributes to neuronal apoptosis and neurological dysfunction after traumatic brain injury. *Journal of Neurosciences, 17,* 7415–7424.

Yang, L., & Hsu, B. (1992). The roles of macrophage and PGE-2 in postburn immunosuppression. *Burns, 18,* 132–136.

Zabel, P., Schade, F. U., & Schlaak, M. (1993). Inhibition of endogenous TNF formation by pentoxifylline. *Journal of Immunobiology, 187*(3–5), 447–463.

Zabel, P., & Schade, F. U. (1994). Pentoxifylline. *Journal of Intensive Care Medicine, 20,* 149–156.

Zapata-Sirvent, R. L., Hansbrough, J. F., Cox, M. C., & Carter, W. H. (1992). Immunologic alterations in a murine model of hemorrhagic shock. *Critical Care Medicine, 20,* 508–517.

Zellweger, R., Ayala, A., DeMaso, C. M., & Chaudry, I. H. (1995a). Trauma-hemorrhage causes prolonged depression in cellular immunity. *Shock, 4,* 149–153.

Zellweger, R., Ayala, A., Schmand, J. F., Morrison, M. H., & Chaudry, I. H. (1995b). PAF-antagonist administration after hemorrhage-resuscitation prevents splenocyte immunodepression. *Journal of Surgical Research, 59,* 366–370.

Zellweger, R., Ayala, A., Stein, S., DeMaso, C. M., & Chaudry, I. H. (1997a). Females in proestrus state tolerate sepsis better than males. *Critical Care Medicine, 25,* 106–110.

Zellweger, R., Ayala, A., Zhu, X. -L., Holme, K. R., DeMaso, C. M., & Chaudry, I. H. (1995c). A novel nonanticoagulant heparin improves splenocyte and peritoneal macrophage immune function after trauma-hemorrhage and resuscitation. *Journal of Surgical Research, 59,* 211–218.

Zellweger, R., Wichmann, M. W., Ayala, A., Stein, S., DeMaso, C. M., & Chaudry, I. H. (1997b). Females in proestrus state maintain splenic immune functions and tolerate sepsis better than males. *Critical Care Medicine, 25*(1), 106–110.

Zellweger, R., Zhu, X. -H., Wichmann, M. W., Ayala, A., DeMaso, C. M., Chaudry, I. H. (1996). Prolactin administration following hemorrhagic shock improves macrophage cytokine release capacity and decreases mortality from subsequent sepsis. *Journal of Immunology, 157,* 5748–5754.

Zhang, R. L., Chopp, M., Li, Y., Zaloga, C., Jiang, N., Jones, M. L., Miyasaka, M., & Ward, P. A. (1994). Anti-ICAM-1 antibody reduces ischemic cell damage after transient middle cerebral artery occlusion in the rat. *Neurology, 44,* 1747–1751.

Zhu, X.-H., Zellweger, R., Wichmann, M. W., Ayala, A., & Chaudry, I. H. (1997). Effects of prolactin and metoclopramide on macrophage cytokine gene expression in late sepsis. *Cytokine, 9,* 437–446.

Zhu, X. -L., Ertel, W., Ayala, A., Morrison, M. H., Perrin, M. M., & Chaudry, I. H. (1993). Chloroquine inhibits macrophage tumour necrosis factor-α mRNA transcription. *Immunology, 80,* 122–126.

Ziegler, E. J., McCutchan, J. A., Fierer, J., Glauser, M. P., Sadoff, J. C., Douglas, H., & Braude, A. I. (1982). Treatment of gram–negative bacteremia and shock with human antiserum to mutant *Escherichia coli. New England Journal of Medicine, 307,* 1225–1230.

Zimmerman, J. E., Knaus, W. A., Wagner, D. P., Sun, X., Hakim, R. B., & Nystrom, P. O., (1996). A comparison of risks and outcomes for patients with organ system failure: 1982–1990. *Critical Care Medicine, 41*(10), 1633–1641.

# 45

# Stress-Induced Autonomic and Immunologic Reactivity

BERT N. UCHINO, GARY G. BERNTSON, JULIANNE HOLT-LUNSTAD, JOHN T. CACIOPPO

## I. INTRODUCTION

### A. Overview

Exposure to acute psychosocial stress is a ubiquitous part of everyday life. Researchers have long suspected that stressful episodes may have implications for both psychological well being and physical health (Ishigami, 1918–1919; Selye, 1956; Solomon & Moos, 1964). However, it is only recently that direct, systematic investigations of the biological plausibility of these claims in humans have been pursued (Cohen, Tyrrell, & Smith, 1991; Kiecolt-Glaser & Glaser, 1995). Much of this research has been conducted under the rubric of the reactivity hypothesis of cardiovascular disease (Manuck, 1994). As viewed from an allostatic perspective, these autonomic changes reflect adjustments that are achieved through multiple, interacting systems (Berntson & Cacioppo, 2000; McEwen, 1998; Sterling & Eyer, 1988). Importantly, these stress-induced changes are coordinated by the central nervous system (CNS) and thus may have cascading effects across multiple physiological processes. As will be reviewed in this chapter, recent research in psychoneuroimmunology (PNI) is consistent with this view and suggests the importance of a more integrated approach to understanding stress processes and outcomes. These data have important implications for the mechanisms linking stress to health outcomes at differing functional levels of analysis.

### B. Autonomic Reactivity and the Immune System

High levels of autonomic activation during stress may facilitate adaptive coping during tasks that require taxing physical responses (e.g., running from a rabid dog). The common types of stressors that accompany everyday life, however, often do not require such excessive physical demands. In fact, the autonomic activation accompanying acute mental stress typically exceeds metabolic demand and thus may have additional adaptive functions, as well as "hidden" costs (Obrist, 1981; Turner, 1989). The potential implications of exaggerated autonomic reactivity for stress has been the focus of intense research and its ramifications for cardiovascular disease are broadly considered from the vantage of the reactivity hypothesis (Krantz & Manuck, 1984; Manuck, 1994).

The reactivity hypothesis suggests that individuals experiencing exaggerated cardiovascular reactivity may be at increased risk for the development and/ or expression of cardiovascular disorders. Although definitive data are needed, the available evidence appears consistent with this reactivity hypothesis

(Manuck, 1994). For instance, animal models suggest that high heart rate reactivity during stress is associated with increased coronary artery atherosclerosis (Manuck, Kaplan, & Clarkson, 1983), an effect that appears mediated by activation of the sympathetic nervous system (Kaplan & Manuck, 1989). In one of the few prospective human studies, Light, Dolan, Davis, and Sherwood (1992) found that high heart rate to acute stress predicted elevations in ambulatory blood pressure 10 to 15 years later. This finding was noteworthy because high and low HR reactors did not differ in resting blood pressure at the initial time of assessment.

An important conceptual bridge between traditional studies of cardiovascular reactivity and PNI is provided by basic research on neuroendocrine–immune interactions. This area of research provides pharmacological evidence for the role of the autonomic nervous system (ANS) in immune function and possibly immune-related disease processes. The lymphocyte subsets commonly examined in such research include helper (CD4+) T cells, suppressor/cytotoxic (CD8+) T cells, and natural killer cells. Helper T cells serve to coordinate the different immune effector responses, whereas suppressor T cells appear to turn off or downregulate the immune response. Both cytotoxic T cells and natural killer cells have the ability to lyse virus-infected and some malignant cells, but cytotoxic T cells perform this process specifically in the context of major histocompatibility complex class I molecules.

Of particular relevance to our discussion is evidence indicating that the sympathetic nervous system (SNS) plays an important role in regulating immune responses (Felton, Ackerman, Wiegand, & Felton, 1987; Felton & Olschowka, 1987). Williams, Snyderman, and Lefkowitz (1976) provided initial evidence that lymphocytes express adrenergic receptors. Subsequent studies have found these adrenergic receptors to be primarily of the $\beta_2$ subtype, although evidence also exists for $\alpha_2$ receptors (Plaut, 1987). In addition, different subsets of lymphocytes appear to have a greater density of adrenergic receptors and hence may be more susceptible to influences from the SNS. For instance, the density of $\beta$-adrenergic receptors is greater on suppressor/cytotoxic T cells and natural killer cells than helper T cells (Khan, Sansoni, Silverman, Engleman, & Melmon, 1986; Maisel, Fowler, Rearden, Motulsky, & Michael, 1989; Maisel, Harris, Rearden, & Michel, 1990; Van Tits et al., 1990). These data are consistent with studies reporting greater increases in suppressor/cytotoxic T cells and natural killer cells in the periphery following exercise or infusions of epinephrine (EPI) (Crary et al.,

1983a, b; Landmann, Durig, Gudat, Wesp, & Harder, 1985; Maisel et al., 1990; Murray et al., 1992; Tvede, Kappel, Halkjoer-Kristensen, Galbo, & Pedersen, 1993; Van Tits et al., 1990).

There may be several mechanisms by which the SNS influences immune function. Felton and colleagues demonstrated that sympathetic nerve fibers innervate both primary and secondary lymphoid organs (Felton et al., 1987), thus providing a relatively direct mechanism by which the SNS may influence aspects of immunity. In fact, Felton and Olschowka (1987) found synaptic-like contacts between SNS fibers and splenic lymphocytes and destruction of lymphoid, sympathetic fibers via treatment with 6-hydroxydopamine potentiated immune responses to antigen. These observations have led some to argue that the SNS exerts a tonic inhibitory influence on lymphoid immune processes.

The SNS may also influence immunity via hormones such as EPI released from the adrenal medulla. In vivo infusions of EPI result in decreases in the proliferative response to mitogens and increases in natural killer cell activity (NKCA), an effect that appears mediated primarily by a $\beta_2$-adrenergic mechanism (Nomoto, Karasawa, & Uehara, 1994; Schedlowski et al., 1993, 1996; Van Tits et al., 1990). One partial explanation for the decreased proliferative response to mitogens and increased NKCA are differences in cell trafficking during SNS activation (Crary et al., 1983b; Tvede et al., 1993). For instance, there may be a lower number of helper T cells and a higher number of natural killer cells following SNS activation that may account, in part, for these findings. A more complicated pattern of data exist for the in vitro NKCA and proliferative response of mitogens following direct incubation with SNS hormones (Hadden, Hadden, & Middleton, 1970; Hatfield, Petersen, & DiMicco, 1986; Hellstrand, Hermodsson, & Strannegard, 1985; Madden & Livnat, 1991).

The evidence linking activation of the parasympathetic nervous system (PNS) to immune function is more limited (Haas & Schauenstein, 1997). Gordon, Cohen, and Wilson (1978) provided evidence that lymphocytes express muscarinic receptors. Subsequent research by Strom, Lane, and George (1981) indicated that muscarinic receptors were primarily found on T-lymphocytes, with an increased number of active binding sites following lymphocyte activation. There also appears to be vagal innervation of lymphoid tissues which may be a source of acetycholine (Najima, 1995; Rinner et al., 1994). In a preliminary study, PNS dennervation resulted in a decreased antibody response to sheep red blood cells in mice (Alito et al., 1987). These data are opposite of those reported following SNS dennervation and suggest that the PNS may potentiate lymphoid immune processes.

Although more data are needed, existing studies suggest that hormones of the PNS tend to potentiate aspects of the cellular immune response. For instance, incubation of cholinergic agonists (i.e., carbamylcholine) with T cells resulted in greater cytotoxic activity (Katz, Zaytoun, & Fauci, 1982; Strom, Sytkowski, Carpenter, & Merrill, 1974). Consistent with a cholinergic mechanism, induction of cellular cGMP resulted in a similar augmentation of NKCA (Katz, Zaytoun, & Fauci, 1982). Activation of muscarinic receptors appears to be responsible for the enhanced cytotoxicity because muscarinic antagonists (i.e., atropine) but not nicotinic antagonists (e.g., *d*-tubocurarine) blocked the effects of PNS agonists on cell-mediated cytotoxicity (Katz et al., 1982; Strom et al., 1974).

In sum, basic research on neuroendocrine–immune interactions provides the impetus for an expanded conceptual role of autonomic reactivity to include stress-induced modulation of immune function, with implications for related disease processes. This position is strengthened by recent research reviewed below modeling cardiovascular, endocrine, and immune responses during acute stress in humans. We should emphasize, however, that there are reciprocal interactions between the CNS and the immune system such that peripheral immune processes may in turn influence the CNS. Maier and Watkins (1998) recently reviewed research suggesting that immune changes during stress may be integrated with basic immune processes that facilitate recovery and recuperation following infection or injury. One important pathway responsible for this bidirectional communication appears to be through vagal autonomic afferents (Bluthe et al., 1994; Bret-Dibat, Bluthe, Kent, Kelly, & Dantzer, 1995; Maier, Goehler, Fleshner, & Watkins, 1998). Therefore, although we will focus on stress-induced autonomic reactivity and immune processes, the reverse pathway is not trivial and critical data are only recently becoming available. We will return to this important issue at several points in this review.

## II. ACUTE PSYCHOSOCIAL STRESS AND IMMUNITY

### A. Laboratory Studies in Humans

Cardiovascular changes during acute laboratory stress are well documented and appear to provide information on an individual's reactions to daily hassles and stressors (Manuck, 1994; Matthews, Owens, Allen, & Stoney, 1992; Pollack, 1991). It is only relatively recently, however, that PNI researchers have examined short-term immune changes using such standardized laboratory paradigms. There have been at least 34 published studies that have examined immune alterations during acute psychosocial stress (e.g., Benschop et al., 1994; Cacioppo et al., 1995; Delahanty et al., 1996; Herbert et al., 1994; Manuck, Cohen, Rabin, Muldoon, & Bachen, 1991; Matthews et al., 1995; Naliboff et al., 1995; Uchino, Cacioppo, Malarkey, & Glaser, 1995). With one exception (Landmann et al., 1984), all of these studies have been published within the past 10 years. The most common stressors utilized in these studies included speech tasks, mental arithmetic, and the Stroop task. The laboratory tasks vary in duration from 4 min (Willemsen et al., Hucklebridge, 1998) to 40 min (Knapp, et al., 1992), with many studies using stressors of approximately 12 to 20 min (e.g., Cacioppo et al., 1995; Manuck et al., 1991).

Most of the studies examining these acute stress paradigms have reported reliable short-term changes in immune function (Kiecolt-Glaser, Cacioppo, Malarkey, & Glaser, 1993; Uchino, Kiecolt-Glaser, & Glaser, 2000). The most common effects include stress-induced increases in suppressor/cytotoxic T cells and natural killer cells (Benschop et al., 1994; Cacioppo et al., 1995; Herbert et al., 1994; Marsland, Manuck, Fazzari, Stewart, & Rabin, 1995; Matthews et al., 1995; Mills, Ziegler, Dimsdale, & Parry, 1995; Sgoutas-Emch et al., 1994), decreases in the proliferative response of peripheral blood leukocytes (PBL) to the mitogens concanavalin A (Con A) and phytohemagglutinin (PHA) (Cacioppo et al., 1995; Delahanty et al., 1996; Herbert et al., 1994; Marsland et al., 1995; Matthews et al., 1995; Sgoutas-Emch et al., 1994; Stone et al., 1993), and increases in NKCA (Benschop et al., 1994; Cacioppo et al., 1995; Delahanty et al., 1996; Matthews et al., 1995; Sgoutas-Emch et al., 1994; Uchino et al., 1995). However, recent studies that have examined NKCA adjusted for the concomitant increase in natural killer cells have suggested little change or even a decrease in NKCA following acute stress (Cacioppo et al., 1998; Naliboff et al., 1995). Together, these studies provide clear evidence that brief psychological stress (as short as 4 to 6 min) may result in reliable changes in lymphocyte trafficking and function (Uchino et al., 2000).

Of course, it is possible that these short-term changes in immune function may be operating independently of autonomic regulatory processes. In one of the first studies to suggest the importance of the ANS on stress-induced immune changes, Manuck and colleagues (1991) classified individuals as high or low SNS reactors. High SNS reactors were above the median on three of the five measures of heart rate, systolic blood pressure (SBP), diastolic blood pressure (DBP), norepinephrine (NE), or EPI. The remaining participants were classified as low SNS reactors. Results revealed that high SNS reactors showed a greater decrease in the proliferative response to mitogens and a greater increase in suppressor/cytotoxic T cells than low SNS reactors (also see Herbert et al., 1994; Matthews et al., 1995; Stone et al., 1993). Interestingly, it was not the case that these individuals were more reactive in general as Manuck and colleagues (1991) did not find any SNS group differences in cortisol reactivity. These data suggest that hormones from the hypothalamo-pituitary-adrenal (HPA) axis were not responsible for the pattern of results reported by these authors.

Recent research from pharmacological blockade studies provides relatively direct evidence that some of these stress-induced immune alterations are mediated by the SNS. Benschop et al. (1994) found that the administration of propanolol, a nonselective $\beta$-adrenergic blocker, eliminated stress-induced increases in natural killer cells and NKCA. Bachen and colleagues (1995) replicated the effects of Benschop et al. (1994) and provided further evidence that general SNS blockade (i.e., labetalol, a nonselective $\alpha$- and $\beta$-adrenergic blocker) eliminated the stress-related decrease in the proliferative response of PBLs to Con A and PHA. Although the effects of SNS blockade on the proliferative response of PBLs to mitogens were not found by Benschop et al. (1994), this discrepancy might be due to the fact that Bachen and colleagues used a nonselective $\alpha$- and $\beta$-adrenergic antagonist, whereas Benschop and colleagues used a more selective $\beta$-adrenergic antagonist. Activation of an $\alpha$-adrenergic mechanism has been linked to a decreased in vitro proliferative response of PBLs to mitogens (Heilig, Irwin, Grewal, & Sercarz, 1993).

Although prior studies suggest that SNS activation may be responsible for aspects of immune changes during acute stress, the general classifications or pharmacological blockades used in prior research did not allow for an examination of relatively specific ANS pathways that may be activated during stress. For instance, heart rate is governed by both the SNS and the PNS and the underlying autonomic substrates of heart rate reactivity may vary in a reciprocal, coupled (e.g., coactivated), or uncoupled fashion (Berntson, Cacioppo, & Quigley, 1993). Ignoring

such specific sources of variability may obscure reliable relationships between the ANS and immune function. In addition, measures of the ANS may differ in their operating characteristics (e.g., threshold, gain, asymptope), which might provide further insight into how the ANS modulates aspects of immune responses during stress (Cacioppo et al., 1992).

Recent research has begun to shed light on the complex autonomic and endocrine pathways potentially responsible for short-term stress-induced changes in immune function. It is clear that the SNS is one mechanism mediating stress-induced changes in immunity (e.g., Bachen et al., 1995; Manuck et al., 1991). Another potential mechanism involves the coactivation of an opioid pathway as immune cells express opiate receptors (Carr, Rogers, & Weber, 1996). Naliboff et al. (1995) specifically investigated the possibility that an opioid mechanism may underlie these stress-induced immune changes. In separate sessions, participants were either given saline or a $\mu$ opiate receptor blocker (i.e., naloxone) and performed a mental arithmetic task. Results revealed that the stressor led to significant increases in suppressor/cytotoxic T cells, natural killer cells, and NKCA. These immune changes were comparable for the saline and naloxone conditions, suggesting that an opioid mechanism was not responsible for acute stress effects on immune function. However, this is the only study to evaluate an opioid mechanism, and multiple opioid receptor populations (i.e., $\varepsilon$, $\sigma$, $\gamma$, $\mu$; Lord, Waterfield, Hughes, & Kosterlitz, 1977; Mehrishi & Mills 1983; see review by Carr et al., 1996) and/or potential interactions caution against overinterpretation of this negative finding.

Hormones of the HPA axis (e.g., cortisol) provide another potential mechanism linking SNS activation and immune changes during acute stress because corticotropin-releasing hormone (CRH) activates both the HPA axis and the ANS (Irwin, Hauger, Brown, & Britton, 1989). Consistent with this position, Lovallo, Pincomb, Brackett, and Wilson (1990) found that high heart rate reactors showed greater increases in plasma cortisol due to stress than low heart rate reactors. Due to the widespread influence of HPA hormones on immune function, we tested whether the HPA could be a second mechanism coordinating stress-induced autonomic–immune changes (Sgoutas-Emch et al., 1994). In this study, we identified individuals as relatively low or high in heart rate reactivity to a speech stressor. Approximately 3 weeks later, we retested these low and high heart rate reactors and examined cardiovascular, endocrine, and immune responses to a mental arithmetic stressor. Consistent with past research, results revealed that the heart rate reactivity classification was stable across sessions and plasma levels of EPI and NE were increased during acute stress. We also replicated prior research on immune changes from acute stress as (a) the number of circulating suppressor/cytotoxic T cells and natural killer cells were increased, (b) the proliferative response to Con A was reduced, and (c) NKCA was increased.

Although nomothetic analyses revealed no significant change in cortisol during stress, considerable interindividual variability existed in stress-induced cortisol responses. Consistent with Lovallo and colleagues (1990), we found that high heart rate reactors had significantly greater cortisol responses during stress than low heart rate reactors. Moreover, high heart rate reactors also showed greater NKCA during stress. Analyses of catecholamine responses did not reveal the same pattern of results suggesting that heart rate reactivity was serving as a relatively specific marker of HPA activation and may be an additional mechanism coordinating aspects of immune changes during acute stress.

Subsequent studies by our laboratories have examined whether the sympathetic or parasympathetic substrates of heart rate reactivity may be responsible for the effects reported above. Prior research suggested that preejection period (PEP) and respiratory sinus arrhythmia (RSA) were good noninvasive indices of sympathetic and parasympathetic influences on the heart, respectively (Berntson et al., 1993; Sherwood et al., 1990). In order to further validate these measures, however, we first conducted a pharmacological blockade study in which participants received on 3 consecutive days either (a) atropine sulfate (muscarinic antagonist), (b) metoprolol ($\beta_1$ antagonist), or (c) saline (Berntson et al., 1994; Cacioppo et al., 1994). Analyses of postinfusion measures revealed that PEP was shortened during sympathetic blockade but not affected by parasympathetic blockade. RSA, in comparison, was not influenced by sympathetic blockade but significantly reduced during parasympathetic blockade.

These data provided evidence for the utility of PEP and RSA as noninvasive indices of sympathetic and parasympathetic influences on the heart. In subsequent studies, we evaluated whether the associations between heart rate reactivity, cortisol reactivity, and immune changes were specifically associated with sympathetic or parasympathetic control of the heart (Cacioppo et al., 1995; Uchino et al., 1995). In one study we examined cardiovascular, endocrine, and immune responses to acute stress in 23 young, healthy women (Uchino et al., 1995). Participants performed a 12-min mental arithmetic task while measures of

cardiovascular reactivity were recorded continuously, and blood was drawn from an indwelling catheter at baseline and immediately following the stressor.

Replicating prior research, results revealed that the stressor led to increases in heart rate, SBP, and DBP. In addition, PEP was shortened and RSA decreased in response to acute stress, suggesting reciprocal activation of the SNS and PNS during stress. Neuroendocrine measures provided converging evidence for sympathetic activation as plasma levels of NE and EPI were increased in response to mental stress. Similar to prior research, acute stress also resulted in greater NKCA. More important, analyses revealed that the sympathetic substrates of heart rate reactivity (i.e., PEP) predicted stress-induced cortisol responses ($r = -.45$, $p < .05$), whereas parasympathetic activation (i.e., RSA) was not related to cortisol responses ($r = -.18$, ns). In addition, PEP reactivity predicted greater NKCA during stress ($r = -.56$, $p < .01$). RSA reactivity was uncorrelated with stress-induced NKCA ($r = -.12$, ns). Consistent with a sympathetic mechanism, SBP was also correlated with increased NKCA during stress ($r = .63$, $p < .01$).

Based on these simple correlational analyses, we used path analyses to directly examine the potential mediators responsible for the association between PEP and NKCA during stress. A conceptual model was tested in which cardiac sympathetic control, as indexed by PEP, was influencing NKCA via stress-induced changes in SBP reactivity. As a noninvasive measure of sympathetic influences on the myocardium, a shortening of PEP should be related to an increase in both the rate and the force of contractility. SBP reactivity, in turn, may influence NKCA via vascular or soluble immune factors (Ottaway & Husband, 1992). For instance, the increased vascular pressure may lead to a migration of lymphoid cells into the circulation with a concomitant increase in the in vitro NKCA. The results of this path model are depicted in Figure 1 and provided mediational evidence as the previously significant relationship between PEP and NKCA was rendered nonsignificant

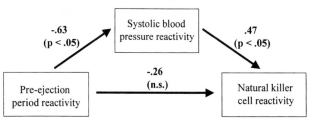

**FIGURE 1** SBP reactivity as a mediator of the stress-induced PEP and NKCA relationship (adapted from Uchino, Cacioppo, Malarkey, & Glaser, 1995).

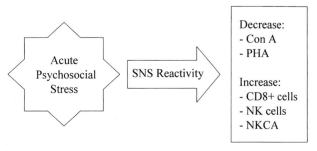

**FIGURE 2** SNS mediation of short-term stress effects on immunity.

when including SBP as a mediator (see Baron & Kenny, 1986).

The association between cardiac sympathetic control and NKCA responses to short-term psychological stress was apparently not mediated by activation of the HPA as suggested by Sgoutas-Emch et al. (1994). As summarized in Figure 2, the likely mechanism for short-term immune changes during acute stress appears to be SNS activation. We should note, however, that the potential role of other hormonal pathways (e.g., opioid, HPA axis) in relatively acute stress should not be ignored. In fact, the coactivation of cortisol in high but not low cardiac sympathetic reactors may be a mechanism with significant implication for longer-term immune alterations in repeatedly stressed individuals (Cacioppo et al., 1998).

## B. Discussion of Laboratory Studies

There are a number of issues raised by the prior research on acute stress and immune function. One limitation of the human studies is that the experimental stressors are necessarily short-term and moderately stressful. Although there is no clear differentiation of when an acute stressor becomes chronic (Baum, O'Keefe, & Davidson, 1990), animal models may be useful to understand how repetitive or chronic exposure to stressors may influence immunity, as well as the central mechanisms responsible for these changes (Chrousos & Gold, 1992; Moynihan & Ader, 1996).

As noted earlier, Maier and Watkins (1998) reviewed research primarily from animals models, suggesting that immune changes during stress may be integrated with basic immune processes that facilitate recovery from antigenic challenges. For instance, activation of the immune system with lipopolysaccharide leads to the release of interleukin-1(IL-1) from macrophages. IL-1 appears to orchestrate much of what has been termed sickness (e.g., fever, reduced food and water intake, increased HPA activation).

One important pathway responsible for this bidirectional communication between the immune system and the CNS appears to be through the PNS afferents as vagotomy blocks much of the sickness effects due to antigenic challenges (Bluthe et al., 1994; Bret-Dibat et al., 1995; Maier et al., 1998). These data highlight the importance of differentiating the afferent and efferent effects of the PNS. For instance, the prior laboratory acute stress studies with humans provide some data on the efferent effects of vagal activity but do not provide a clear test of the role of vagal afference. Studies that examine longer-term stress and track changes in the PNS and immune function during and *following* stress would be necessary to examine this mechanism.

The potential role of vagal efference on immune function during stress deserves some discussion. As reviewed earlier, there is evidence that tonic vagal processes may potentiate immune processes as PNS dennervation resulted in a decreased antibody response to sheep red blood cells in mice (Alito et al., 1987). In vitro studies suggest that situations leading to an increase in cholinergic hormones may result in a potentiation of the immune response (Katz et al., 1982; Strom et al., 1974). However, acute stress usually is associated with vagal withdrawal. It should be noted that there appears to be individual differences in the autonomic substrates of PNS changes during stress, with some individuals showing apparent vagal activation (Berntson et al., 1994). These data suggest that some individuals may be "buffered" from the SNS effects of acute stress due to activation of the PNS.

Consistent with the hypothesis by Maier and Watkins (1998), both infections and stressors result in activation of the HPA axis. In fact, prior studies that have found repetitive stress to inhibit immunity have tended to attribute these differences to activation of the HPA axis. This explanation is consistent with basic PNI research suggesting that the major influence of HPA hormones on immune processes appears inhibitory (Munck, Guyre, & Holbrook, 1984). For instance, glucocorticoids appear to exert part of their effects on the immune response by inhibiting aspects of antigen presentation (Baus, Andris, Dubois, Urbain, & Leo, 1996; Moser et al., 1995). In vitro studies have provided direct evidence for an inhibitory role of HPA hormones as preincubation of PBLs with glucocorticoids tend to decrease the proliferative response to mitogens as well as NKCA (Gatti et al., 1987; Holbrook, Cox, & Horner, 1983; Parrillo & Fauci, 1978; Pedersen & Beyer, 1986; Weigers et al., 1993; Wiegers, Reul, Holsboer, & De Kloet 1994). Many of these effects were blocked by the specific glucocorticoid receptor antagonist RU-486 (Weigers et al., 1993, 1994).

The short-term stressors used in laboratory human studies were probably not ideal for examining the role of cortisol on stress-induced immune changes because the hormonal cascade that ultimately leads to the release of cortisol from the adrenal cortex may take about 20 to 30 min to detect (Krieger & Allen, 1975). However, even for studies examining more chronic stress, an examination of plasma cortisol is complicated by the fact that cortisol is released in a pulsatile fashion and not all cortisol assessed in plasma is biologically active. Thus, plasma assessments could underestimate the role of cortisol in stress-induced immune changes. Moreover, there may be individual differences in the threshold of HPA activation and as reviewed earlier, these changes appear larger in individuals characterized by greater cardiac sympathetic reactivity during stress (Cacioppo et al., 1995; Uchino et al., 1995).

There are important methodological issues raised by prior work examining cortisol as an endocrine mediator of stress-induced changes in immune function. Diurnal variations in cortisol are well documented, with the major secretory episodes appearing during the early morning and subsequent declines appearing during the course of the day (Greenspan & Baxter, 1994; Van Cauter, 1990). Cortisol is also released in response to eating and exercise. Thus, stress studies may need to be designed in consideration of these peaks to avoid potential confoundings or ceiling effects. As noted earlier, the pulsatile release of cortisol also raises the possibility that single plasma assessments may be relatively insensitive and multiple assessments may provide a better characterization of the HPA axis during a given epoch. Of course, multiple assessments may be difficult over a short period of time. The use of salivary cortisol provides a useful alternative as multiple determinations can be made relatively easily. Salivary cortisol is also unbound (biologically active) and correlates well with plasma and urinary assessments across varying assessment contexts (Kirschabaum & Hellhammer, 1994).

Many PNI studies on stress and immunity assess mean levels of cortisol during a particular point in time. The determination of 24-h cortisol profiles may be useful for examining how more naturalistic stressors influence the HPA axis. In such assessments, the nadir and acrophase provide useful indices of the integrity of the HPA axis. For instance, cortisol is typically low during the late night (nadir) but some individuals (e.g., mania patients) show a shift in this pattern that may represent a failure to adequately

suppress nocturnal cortisol responses (Linkowski et al., 1994). Additional measures include the number of pulsatile releases of cortisol that may provide a sensitive measure of environmental influences on the HPA axis (Linkowski et al., 1993).

It should be noted that activation of the HPA axis does not appear to be the sole pathway responsible for immune changes following repetitive stress in animals (Keller et al., 1988; Keller, Weiss, Schleifer, Miller, & Stein, 1983; Sundar, Cierpial, Kilts, Ritchie, & Weiss, 1990). For instance, hypophysectomy eliminated stress-induced changes in lymphocyte trafficking but did not impact on stress-induced decreases in mitogen responsiveness to PHA (Keller et al., 1988). In addition, the effects of HPA hormones on stress-induced decreases in mitogen proliferation were primarily found for PBL but not splenic lymphocytes (Cunnick, Lysle, Kucinski, & Rabin, 1989). These data highlight the complex neuroendocrine pathways involved in stress-induced immune alterations.

One promising integrating mechanism linking repetitive stress to immune alterations may involve the activation and release of central CRH. As reviewed by Dunn and Berridge (1990), central administration of CRH mimics many of the physiological and behavioral states seen during stress. For instance, central CRH activates both the ANS and the HPA axis (Irwin et al., 1989) and stimulates the release of $\beta$-endorphins (Rivier, Brownstein, Speiss, Rivier, & Vale, 1982). Considerable research indicates that increased CRH in brain regions involved in emotional responses (e.g., amygdala, paraventricular nucleus) may mediate many behavioral responses to stress (Dunn & Berridge, 1990). These include freezing behaviors (Kalin & Takahashi, 1990; Swiergiel, Takahashi, & Kalin, 1993), decreased appetitive behavior (Krahn, Gosnell, Grace, & Levine, 1986), decreased sexual behavior (Sirinathsinghji, Rees, Rivier, & Vale, 1983), increased grooming behavior (Holohan, Kalin, & Kelly, 1997), and enhancement of the startle response (Lee & Davis, 1997a, b).

Some potential central pathways involved in stress-induced immunologic changes are depicted in Figure 3. The figure is meant to be illustrative and not exhaustive. CRH containing neurons and receptors are prevalent in the amygdala, hypothalamus, and locus coeruleus (Gray, 1993; Menzaghi, Heinrichs, Pichs, Weiss, & Koob, 1993; Valentino, Foote, & Page, 1993). Subsequent efferent pathways provide one mechanism by which stress may influence immune function. For instance, the amygdala has direct projections to the hypothalamus (Gray, 1993; LeDoux, 1995). Release of CRH from the hypothalamus activates the HPA axis. As reviewed earlier, cortisol

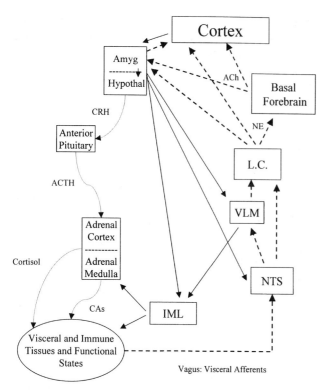

**FIGURE 3**  Illustrative model of the central mechanisms potentially underlying stress-induced immune alterations, including
efferent (solid lines) and afferent projections (broken lines). Ach,
acetylcholine; ACTH, adrenocorticotropic hormone; Amyg, amygdala; CAs, catecholamines; CRH, corticotropin-releasing hormone;
Hypothal, hypothalamus; IML, sympathetic preganglionic neurons
of the intermediolateral cell column; L.C., locus coeruleus; NE,
norepinephrine; NTS, nucleus tractus solitarus; VLM, ventral lateral
medulla.

has been linked to some of the stress-related changes
in immune function, at least during more repetitive
stress. The hypothalamus also has efferent projections
to the ANS via the sympathetic preganglionic neurons of the intermediolateral cell column, the ventral
lateral medulla, and the nucleus tractus solitarus
(Menzaghi et al., 1993; Spyer, 1989). In combination,
the release of HPA hormones and activation of the
ANS may account for many of the stress-induced
changes in immune function detailed earlier in this
review.

Of special note in Figure 3 are the afferent
(ascending) pathways to critical brain structures that
may be activated in stressful circumstances. As
mentioned earlier, vagal afference appears to play
an important role in the immune response to infection
that may have implications for stress processes (Maier
& Watkins, 1998). Berntson, Sarter, and Cacioppo
(1998) also reviewed evidence for the role of these
afferent pathways in modulating anxiety-related
cardiovascular reactivity. According to their model,
the ascending pathways depicted in Figure 3 provide

an opportunity for anxiety- or stress-induced physiological reactions to influence cortical information
processing (e.g., attentional functions). For instance,
activation of the locus coeruleus via afferent pathways
is linked to increased EEG arousal and vigilance to
significant stimuli (Aston-Jones, Rajkowski, Kubiak,
Valentino, & Shipley, 1996). The reciprocal interactions between these central mechanisms may allow
for an orchestrated (and flexible) response to stress
that may be modulated by (a) the type of stressor,
(b) prior experience, and (c) aspects of the social
environment.

## III.  HEALTH IMPLICATIONS

An important issue that requires close examination
is the biological relevance of acute or repetitive stress
effects on health. It is clear from prior research that
this is not a simple relationship. The pattern of
immune changes may have different implications
depending on the specific disease endpoint. For
instance, stress-induced downregulation of immunity
may place an individual at risk for infectious or
malignant diseases, but may be beneficial in the
context of autoimmune disorders (Borysenko, 1987).

The complexity of stress effects on immunity and
health highlights the importance of examining potential mechanisms linking stress to disease processes at
differing functional levels of analysis (e.g., social,
biological; Cacioppo & Berntson, 1992). However, we
first examine if acute stress effects on immunity are
temporally stable across assessments. An examination
of the temporal reliability of these immune changes is
important for at least two reasons. First, these data
bear on the replicability and generalizability of research findings across occasions, people, and places.
Second, if stress-related factors are to influence
disease processes with a long-term etiology, the
physiological assessments should be characterized
by adequate temporal stability.

### A.  Temporal Stability of Acute Stress Changes in Humans

The temporal stability of immunological changes
during acute stress has only recently been examined.
Marsland et al. (1995) reported data on the 3-week
temporal stability of several quantitative and functional immune measures in response to a stressful
speech task. Marsland and colleagues found that most
baseline quantitative measures of immunity (e.g.,
helper T cells, suppressor/cytotoxic T cells) evidenced significant temporal stability ($.22 \leq r \leq .75$).

Moreover, immune responses to acute stress were also associated with significant temporal stability for most quantitative measures ($.25 \leq r \leq .53$), as well as changes in the proliferative response of PBLs to mitogens ($r = .50$, $p < .005$).

In two separate studies of men and women, Mills, Dimsdale, and colleagues (Mills et al. 1995; Mills, Haeri, & Dimsdale, 1995) reported significant 6-week test–retest scores for baseline quantitative measures of helper T cells ($r$'s $= .57$ and $.61$), suppressor/cytotoxic T cells ($r$'s $= .70$ and $.50$), and the ratio of these T cells ($r$'s $= .92$ and $.90$). Residualized change scores for natural killer cells and the ratio of helper T cells to suppressor/cytotoxic T cells ($r$'s $= .55$ and $.60$) in response to acute stress also evidenced significant temporal reliability. In contrast to Marsland and colleagues, the test–retest correlation for suppressor/cytotoxic T cells in response to acute stress was not significant in either study.

According to psychometric theory, several assessments of an individual across times and situations are likely to provide a more accurate individual difference assessment of immune function. Consistent with this possibility, Fletcher, Klimas, Morgan, and Gjerset (1997) found that the proliferative response of PBLs to PHA and pokeweed mitogen and NKCA was characterized by adequate generalizability ($G$) coefficients ($G$s $< .70$) which increased when assessments were aggregated across times ($G \geq .85$). Unfortunately, the high costs of immunological assays make repeated determinations difficult in many circumstances.

Although the data reviewed above suggest that measures of immune response during acute stress may be characterized by adequate to good temporal reliability, additional data are needed to verify such an individual difference assessment. As illustrated in Figure 3 the potential pathways responsible for these changes are complex and as such may limit the reliabilities of these immunologic endpoints unless this complexity is taken into account. These issues highlight the importance of more integrative analyses and suggest that the reliability of immune responses may improve as we gain a greater understanding of the full model depicted in Figure 3.

## B. The Biological Relevance of Stress-Induced Immune Changes

The biological relevance of acute stress assessments on health outcomes is probably one of the most important questions faced by researchers (Cohen & Herbert, 1996). Recall that laboratory assessments are thought to model how individuals respond physiologically to stressors in their daily lives. We have conducted several studies to investigate the biological plausibility of acute stress effects on health-related outcomes. Based on evidence linking activation of the HPA axis to a downregulation of the immune response (Cupps & Fauci, 1982; Schobitz, Reul, & Holsboer, 1994), we examined if the coactivation of cortisol in high but not low cardiac sympathetic reactors may be a mechanism with significant implication for longer-term immune alterations. In this pilot study conducted in collaboration with Janice Kiecolt-Glaser, 22 older adult women participated in a 5-min baseline assessment, 6 min of a mental arithmetic stressor, and 6 min of a speech stressor (Cacioppo et al., 1998). Later in that afternoon, these older adults also received an influenza vaccination. An examination of the immune response to influenza vaccination is important because infectious diseases are the fourth leading cause of death in older adult populations (Center for Disease Control, 1996; Yoshikawa, 1983). In this study, we measured the in vitro virus-specific IL-2 response approximately 2 weeks and 3 months postvaccination. IL-2 is important for the clonal expansion of virus-specific B cells and cytotoxic T cells. IL-2 also augments the cytolytic capacity of activated cytotoxic T cells and natural killer cells. Thus, an impaired IL-2 response has implications for both the humoral and cellular immune responses to vaccination.

Consistent with prior research, results of this study revealed the expected inverted U-shaped in vitro IL-2 response across time, with a decline in the T-cell response 3 months postvaccination. Consistent with the possibility that these laboratory paradigms may provide information on an individual's response to daily hassles and stressor, we found that PEP reactivity to acute psychological stress predicted a decline in the T-cell response 3 months later ($r = .68$, $p < .05$). In contrast, neither heart rate nor parasympathetic reactivity (i.e., RSA) predicted a decline in this T-cell response in older adults (Cacioppo et al., 1998). Recall that we previously found PEP reactivity to be a strong predictor of stress-induced changes in plasma cortisol levels. Given the immunosuppressive effects of HPA hormones, we examined if cortisol responses to acute stress would in turn predict the T-cell response to vaccination. Results revealed that stress-induced changes in cortisol levels predicted a decrease in the T cell response to vaccination ($r = -.56$, $p < .05$), whereas plasma EPI levels did not. Together, these data suggest that the acute stress assessment indexed an individual's reactions to daily hassles during this period and individuals characterized by high cardiac sympathetic reactivity may be more at risk for infectious diseases due to the coactivation of the HPA axis during stress.

More recently, we examined whether PEP reactivity predicts antibody titers to the Epstein–Barr virus (EBV). One of the hallmarks of immunity is memory in which pathogens that have been eradicated from the host are met with a more effective immune response upon subsequent exposure. However, latent herpesviruses (e.g., EBV) avoid elimination by going latent and "hiding," staying relatively inactive in certain cells. The exposed individual is infected for life but the cellular immune response is usually successful at keeping the virus in check. However, individuals with compromised cellular immune responses (e.g., HIV+ populations, patients on immunosuppressive therapies) may experience reactivation of one or more of these latent viruses. In such cases, antibody titers to the virus provide for a measure of the virus-specific cellular immune response. For these measures, increased antibody titers to latent viruses suggest poorer cellular immunity because the cellular immune response is relatively less effective in controlling the steady state expression of latent viruses.

In this next study conducted in collaboration with Ronald Glaser, 54 older adult women participated in a 6-min baseline assessment followed by 6 min of a math stressor and 6 min of a speech stressor (Cacioppo et al., 1998). Participants were divided based on a median split on PEP reactivity scores during these acute stressors. As expected, preliminary analyses revealed that the high PEP reactivity group showed higher heart rate, SBP, and DBP during stress, but no difference in stress-induced parasympathetic reactivity (i.e., RSA reactivity), than the low PEP reactivity group. More important, high PEP reactors showed greater EBV virus capsid antigen (VCA) immunoglobin G (IgG) titers than low PEP reactors. Given the relatively long half-life of IgG (i.e., 20 days), these data likely reflect the cumulative influence of the acute stressors individuals experienced in daily life and not exposure to the acute stressors used in the laboratory paradigm, per se.

In vitro studies suggest that cortisol can reactivate latent EBV (Glaser, Kutz, MacCallum, & Malarkey, 1995). Due to the observed coupling of PEP reactivity with cortisol changes in our studies (Cacioppo et al., 1995, 1998; Uchino et al., 1995), pulsatile changes in cortisol concomitant with changes in cardiac sympathetic control may be an important mechanism responsible for the above results. In collaboration with Ronald Glaser we tested this possibility by incubating latently infected cells in varying concentrations of dexamethasone (DEX) (i.e., $10^{-5}$ M to $10^{-9}$ M every 24 h for 3 days). The different concentrations of DEX were thought to model the in vivo effects of pulsatile cortisol changes that are likely to occur with acute stressors. Control cells were incubated with media only, or a single concentration of DEX for 3 days.

Replicating prior research, we found that the control media alone resulted in only a small percentage (3 to 5%) of EBV antigen-positive cells. In addition, single concentrations of DEX were associated with greater reactivation of EBV as measured by antigen-positive cells after 3 days ($10^{-9}$ M, 7%; $10^{-7}$ M, 8%; $10^{-5}$ M, 12%). However, varying the concentration of DEX over 3 days resulted in an approximate threefold increase in EBV antigen-positive cells (36%). These results are consistent with the notion that changes in HPA hormones, which covary with stress-induced cardiac sympathetic reactivity, may have greater health consequences than tonic levels of these hormones.

The biological relevance of stress-related effects in humans has been documented by a number of other researchers. Glaser et al., (1992) found that medical students higher in perceived stress had lower seroconversion rates to a hepatitus B vaccination. Kiecolt-Glaser and colleagues found that the chronic stress of caregiving for a relative with Alzheimer's disease was associated with a poorer immune response to an influenza vaccination and slower wound healing following a standard punch biopsy (Kiecolt-Glaser, Glaser, Gravenstein, Malarkey, & Sheridan, 1996; Kiecolt-Glaser, Marucha, Malarkey, Mercado, & Glaser, 1995).

In a common cold challenge paradigm, Cohen and colleagues (1991, 1998) exposed participants to various common cold viruses and quarantined them for a period of 5–7 days. In their first report, an index of psychological stress was related in a dose–response manner to increased infections and clinical colds (Cohen et al., 1991). In an additional study using a similar paradigm, these authors reported that only longer-term stressors resulted in increased susceptibility to the common cold virus (Cohen et al., 1998).

Although more research is needed, the studies reviewed above are suggestive of the biological relevance of stress-induced immune changes on infectious and malignant diseases. These studies are also consistent with psychosocial intervention designed to help individuals cope with stress, including chronically stressed populations such as cancer patients (Fawzy et al., 1990a, b; Spiegel, Bloom, Kraemer, & Gottheil, 1989) and HIV+ individuals (LaPerriere et al., 1990). In one of the first studies demonstrating a direct effect of a psychosocial intervention on immunity, Kiecolt-Glaser and colleagues (1985) found that relaxation training increased NKCA and decreased antibody titers to latent herpes simplex virus (HSV) in an older adult population. Fawzy and colleagues (1990a, b) evaluated the effects of a 6-week structured group intervention that consisted of education, problem-solving skills, and stress management such as relaxation and support in stage I or II cancer patients. The structured group intervention was associated with increases in aspects of cellular immunity such as percentage natural killer cells and NKCA 6 months later compared to that seen in the control condition. Importantly, a 6-year follow-up revealed lower mortality rates in individuals assigned to the group intervention than those seen in the control condition.

There are several additional issues in human PNI research that requires discussion in evaluating the biological relevance of stress-related immune changes. One issue relates to the problematic interpretation of any single measure of immune function (e.g., decreases in response of PBLs to Con A, changes in the number of natural killer cells) as representing a downregulation of immune function. To this point, it is possible that a composite of measures of immunity may provide a better overall characterization of an individual's immune status with implications for health. According to this model, the separate measures combine to influence the composite so that changes to one aspect may have cascading consequences. For instance, Kiecolt-Glaser, Dura, Speicher, Trask, and Glaser (1991) found that chronically stressed caregivers of AD patients who showed the largest decrements in immunity on a composite measure conceptually linked to cellular immune responses (i.e., antibody titers to latent EBV, response of PBLs to Con A and PHA) were low in social support. Of course, if one is attempting to model potential mechanisms a conceptual disaggregation of the composite may provide insight into what stage(s) of the immune response is influenced by stress-related processes.

A second important issue in examining the biological relevance of stress-related immune changes relates to the study population. Aging is typically associated with a decline in aspects of immune function (Goodwin, Shearles, & Tung, 1982; Roberts-Thomson, Whittingham, Youngchaiyud, & Mackay, 1974). As a result, the health effects of stress may be more evident in older adult populations (Kiecolt-Glaser et al., 1991, 1996). These observations highlight the importance of carefully choosing the study population depending on the research question of interest.

## C. Potential Pathways Responsible for Stress Effects on Health: An Emphasis on Multilevel Integrative Analyses

A discussion of the pathways linking stress to immune-related health alterations (and vice versa) would need to consider the diverse functional levels in review of the complexity of the potential links outlined earlier. As indicated in Figure 3, the reciprocal neural pathways could be modulated not only by lower level interactions among the SNS, CRH, etc., but by higher level cortical cognitive factors. In addition, although most of the emphasis has been on biological mechanisms, understanding stress effects on disease may require attention to complementary social, personologic, psychological, and behavioral levels of analyses (Anderson, 1998; Cacioppo & Berntson, 1992). These complementary functional levels of analyses are illustrated in Figure 4. An important aspect of Figure 4 is that the different functional levels are embedded and hence processes at more macro levels can influence the more microlevel processes and vice versa. We believe that a multilevel approach provides a useful heuristic to understanding complex phenomena such as the relationship between stress and health and that collecting simultaneous data within and across levels of analyses provides an excellent means by which competing hypotheses can be examined (Cacioppo & Berntson, 1992; Platt, 1964).

Integrative research on the mechanisms linking stress to health across functional levels of analyses is in its infancy. However, the prior literature does provide some data on these mechanisms. At a more macro level of analysis, the present review suggests that social stressors may be particularly important

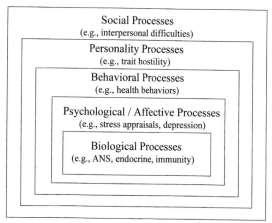

**FIGURE 4**  Levels of analyses potentially involved in the relationship between stress and health.

sources of stress explaining variations in immunologic and health outcomes (e.g., Kiecolt-Glaser et al., 1996; Padgett et al., 1998). For instance, Padgett and colleagues (1998) exposed latently infected HSV rats to either social stress (i.e., social group reorganization) or physical stress (i.e., restraint stress). Results revealed that only social stress was associated with significant reactivation of HSV (i.e., over 40% of socially stressed animals). These findings are consistent with research indicating that social stressors appear to have relatively large and lasting effects on mood (Bolger, DeLongis, Kessler, & Schilling, 1989) and immunity in humans (Herbert & Cohen, 1993) and nonhuman primates (Coe, 1993). Cohen and colleagues (1998) also reported that the effects of longer-term stressors (e.g., 1 to 6 months) on susceptibility to the common cold were associated primarily with interpersonal and work stressors.

There are potential personality factors that may be responsible for the results detailed earlier. Personality factors such as neuroticism are linked to greater subjective stress and hence may be responsible for the results of stress on immunity and health (Bolger & Eckenrode, 1991; Smith & Gallo, in press). Cohen and colleagues (1991, 1998) reported that self-esteem and the big five personality factors could not account for the effects of stress on susceptibility to the common cold. However, a number of additional personality factors, including trait hostility and optimism, appear to influence physiological processes and health outcomes (Scheier & Bridges, 1995; Segerstrom, Taylor, Kemeny, & Fahey, 1998; Smith, 1992; Smith & Gallo, in press). An examination of these personality factors and the extent to which they explain variance in stress outcomes would be a promising avenue for future research.

Stress has been linked to changes in health behaviors (e.g., alcohol consumption, lack of sleep) which in turn may influence immunity (Irwin et al., 1994; Kiecolt-Glaser & Glaser, 1988). Therefore, it is also important to evaluate the effects of health behaviors as pathways responsible for the effects of stress on health outcomes. In most of the human studies detailed earlier, health behaviors including sleep, exercise, and alcohol consumption could not account for the effects of stress on immune function or health outcomes (Cohen et al., 1991, 1998; Kiecolt-Glaser et al., 1995, 1996). As noted by Smith and Ruiz (in press), the measurement of health behaviors is difficult as health behaviors are typically not highly correlated and can be unstable over time. The use of more objective indices of health behaviors (e.g., mean corpuscular volume for alcohol consumption), along with established self-report methods (e.g., Buysse,

Reynolds, Monk, Berman, & Kupfer, 1989) may prove useful for providing a strong test of a health behavior mediation model.

It is often assumed that immune alterations during stress are mediated by neuroendocrine mechanisms. However, Cohen and colleagues reported that plasma cortisol and catecholamines did not account for the effects of stress on susceptibility to the common cold. In our study we found some evidence that cortisol may be a mediator of the effects of stress on immune responses to an influenza vaccination (Cacioppo et al., 1998). As reviewed earlier, single assessments of plasma cortisol levels (or other endocrine hormones) may not be ideal and could explain some of the discrepancies in prior human research. Depending on the model being tested, the measurement of urinary or salivary hormones may be more appropriate as it is more likely to reflect longer-term alterations in hormone levels (Baum & Greenberg, 1995). Elucidating the neuroendocrine mechanisms responsible for stress-induced immune changes in humans is an important area of future research as it provides a direct link to animal models of stress and disease (Moynihan & Ader, 1996).

Although hormones of the HPA axis appear to play an important role in stress and disease, as noted earlier there are other important hormonal pathways that need to be considered. For instance, Sheridan et al. (1998) reported that the effects of restraint stress on lymphocyte trafficking and cytokine responses in virus-infected rats were mediated by activation of the HPA axis as blockade of glucocorticoid receptors by RU-486 eliminated these effects. However, the decreased cytolytic T-cell response to stress was not influenced by treatment with RU-486 but by $\beta$-adrenergic blockade, suggesting a sympathetic mechanism for this effect.

A closer examination of additional or more complex neuroendocrine pathways is further highlighted by the study of Padgett and colleagues (1998). These authors found that both social stress and restraint stress in rats were associated with comparable activation of the HPA axis as indexed by plasma corticosterone levels. However, as detailed earlier, only social stress resulted in significant reactivation of HSV in rats. The authors hypothesized that interactions among the HPA and SNS may be an important pathway responsible for these findings. It is interesting that additional analyses by Padgett and colleagues (1998) revealed that HSV reactivation in socially stressed animals was more likely in dominant than in submissive rats. These data suggest the possibility that pulsatile changes in cortisol associated with repeated attempts at dominance may be a more complex mechanism linking social stress to reactivation of the latent virus (see Cacioppo et al., 1998).

## IV. SUMMARY AND CONCLUSIONS

We have attempted to review the links between stress-induced autonomic and immune responses and their implications for health outcomes. These data indicate significant influences of the ANS on immune function. Acute stress studies in humans suggest the importance of SNS activation as a mediator of subsequent immune changes, although other hormonal pathways might be operating during longer-term or more repetitive stress. Indeed, repetitive stress studies suggest reciprocal interactions between the CNS and immune system and highlight the importance of examining both efferent and afferent pathways. Although we have also reviewed data on the biological plausibility of stress effects in humans, this continues to be an important arena for future research.

We have also attempted to outline in broad strokes the potential mechanisms responsible for health effects of acute or repetitive stress at functional levels of analyses ranging from the social to biological. In a general sense, this literature reviews highlights the importance of an integrative approach to stress processes and outcomes that acknowledges the complexity of these pathways. We believe that the identification of mechanisms at multiple levels of analyses represents the next, critically important phase in human PNI stress research.

## Acknowledgments

Preparation for this chapter was generously supported by National Institute on Aging, Grants 1 R55 AG13968 and PO1-AG11585, and National Institute of Mental Health, Grants 1 RO1MH58690 and T32-MH19728.

## References

Alito, A. E., Romeo, H. E., Baler, R., Chuluyan, H. E., Braun, M., & Cardinali, D. P. (1987). Autonomic nervous system regulation of murine immune responses as assessed by local surgical sympathetic and parasympathetic denervation. *Acta Physiologica et Pharmacologia Latinoamericana, 37,* 305–319.

Anderson, N. B. (1998). Levels of analysis in health science: A framework for integrating sociobehavioral and biomedical research. *Annals of the New York Academy of Sciences, 840,* 563–576.

Aston-Jones, G., Rajkowski, J., Kubiak, P., Valentino, R. J., & Shipley, M. T. (1996). Role of the locus coeruleus in emotional activation. In G. Holstege, R. Bandler, & C. B. Saper (Eds.), *Progress in Brain Research* (pp. 379–402). New York: Elsevier.

Bachen, E. A., Manuck, S. B., Cohen, S., Muldoon, M. F., Raible, R., Herbert, T. B., & Rabin, B. S. (1995). Adrenergic blockade ameliorates cellular immune responses to mental stress in humans. *Psychosomatic Medicine, 57,* 366–372.

Baron, R. M., & Kenny, D. A. (1986). The moderator-mediator distinction in social psychological research: Conceptual, strategic, and statistical considerations. *Journal of Personality and Social Psychology, 51,* 1173–1182.

Baum, A., & Greenberg, N. (1995). Measurement of stress hormones. In S. Cohen, R. C. Kessler, & L. U. Gordon (Eds.), *Measuring stress: A guide for health and social scientists* (pp. 175–192). New York: Oxford University Press.

Baum, A., O'Keefe, M. K., & Davidson, L. M. (1990). Acute stressors and chronic response: The case of traumatic stress. *Journal of Applied Social Psychology, 20,* 1643–1654.

Baus, E., Andris, F., Dubois, P. M., Urbain, J., & Leo, O. (1996). Dexamethasone inhibits the early steps of antigen receptor signaling in activated T lymphocytes. *Journal of Immunology, 156,* 4555–4561.

Benschop, R. J., Nieuwnehuis, E. E. S., Tromp, E. A. M., Godaert, G. L. R., Ballieux, R. E., & van Doornen, L. J. P. (1994). Effects of B-adrenergic blockade on immunologic and cardiovascular changes induced by mental stress. *Circulation, 89,* 762–769.

Berntson, G. G., & Cacioppo, J. T. (2000). From homeostasis to allodynamic regulation. In J. T. Cacioppo, L. G. Tassinary, & G. G. Berntson (Eds.), *Handbook of psychophysiology* (pp. 459–481). New York: Cambridge University Press.

Berntson, G. G., Cacioppo, J. T., Binkley, P. F., Uchino, B. N., Quiqley, K. S., & Fieldstone, A. (1994). Autonomic cardiac control. III. Psychological stress and cardiac response in autonomic space as revealed by pharmacological blockades. *Psychophysiology, 31,* 599–608.

Berntson, G. G., Cacioppo, J. T., & Quigley, K. S. (1993). Cardiac psychophysiology and autonomic space in humans: Empirical perspectives and conceptual implications. *Psychological Bulletin, 114,* 296–322.

Berntson, G. G., Sarter, M., & Cacioppo, J. T. (1998). Anxiety and cardiovascular reactivity: The basal forebrain cholinergic link. *Behavioural Brain Research, 94,* 225–248.

Bluthe, R. M., Walter, V., Parnet, P., Laye, P., Lestage, J., Verrier, D., Poole, S., Stenning, B. E., Kelley, K. W., & Dantzer, R. (1994). Lipopolysaccharide induces sickness behaviour by a vagal mediated mechanism. *Comptes Rendus de l'Academie des Sciences (III), 317,* 499–503.

Bolger, N., DeLongis, A., Kessler, R. C., & Schilling, E. A. (1989). Effects of daily stress on negative mood. *Journal of Personality and Social Psychology, 57,* 808–818.

Bolger, N., & Eckenrode, J. (1991). Social relationships, personality, and anxiety during a major stressful event. *Journal of Personality and Social Psychology, 61,* 440–449.

Borysenko, M. (1987). The immune system: An overview. *Annals of Behavioral Medicine, 9,* 3–10.

Bret-Dibat, J. L., Bluthe, R. M., Kent, S., Kelley, K. W., & Dantzer, R. (1995). Lipopolysaccharide and interleukin-1 depress food motivated behavior in mice by a vagal-mediated mechanism. *Brain, Behavior, and Immunity, 9,* 242–246.

Buysse, D. J., Reynolds, C. F., Monk, T. H., Berman, S. R., & Kupfer, D. J. (1989). Pittsburgh sleep quality index: A new instrument for psychiatric practice and research. *Psychiatry Research, 28,* 193–213.

Cacioppo, J. T., & Berntson, G. G. (1992). Social psychological contributions to the decade of the brain: Doctrine of multilevel analysis. *American Psychologist, 47,* 1019–1028.

Cacioppo, J. T., Berntson, G. G., Binkley, P. F., Quiqley, K. S., Uchino, B. N., & Fieldstone, A. (1994). Autonomic cardiac control. II. Basal response, noninvasive indices, and autonomic space as revealed by autonomic blockade. *Psychophysiology, 31,* 586–598.

Cacioppo, J. T., Berntson, G. G., Malarkey, W. B., Kielcolt-Glaser, K. G., Sheridan, J. F., Poehlmann, K. M., Burleson, M. H., Ernst, J. M., Hawkley, L. C., & Glaser, R. (1998). Autonomic, neuroendocrine, and immune responses to psychological stress: The reactivity hypothesis. *Annals of the New York Academy of Sciences, 840,* 664–673.

Cacioppo, J. T., Malarkey, W. B., Kiecolt-Glaser, K. G., Uchino, B. N., Sgoutas-Emch, S. A., Sheridan, J. F., Berntson, G. G., & Glaser, R. (1995). Heterogeneity in neuroendocrine and immune responses to brief psychological stressors as a function of autonomic cardiac activation. *Psychosomatic Medicine, 57,* 154–164.

Cacioppo, J. T., Uchino, B. N., Crites, S. L., Snydersmith, M. A., Smith, G., Berntson, G. G., & Lang, P. J. (1992). Relationship between facial expressiveness and sympathetic activation in emotion: A critical review, with emphasis on modeling underlying mechanisms and individual differences. *Journal of Personality and Social Psychology, 62,* 110–128.

Carr, D. J. J., Rogers, T. J. & Weber, R. J. (1996). The relevance of opioids and opioid receptors on immunocompetence and immune homeostasis. *Proceedings of the Society for Experimental Biology and Medicine, 213,* 248–257.

Center for Disease Control (1996). Prevention and control of influenza: Recommendations of the advisory committtee on immunization practices (ACIP). *Morbidity and Mortality Weekly Report, 45,* 1–24.

Chrousos, G. P., & Gold, P. W. (1992). The concepts of stress and stress system disorders: Overview of physical and behavioral homeostasis. *Journal of the American Medical Association, 267,* 1244–1252.

Coe, C. L. (1993). Psychosocial factors and immunity in nonhuman primates: A review. *Psychosomatic Medicine, 55,* 298–308.

Cohen, S., Frank, E., Doyle, W. J., Skoner, D. P., Rabin, B. S., & Gwaltney, J. M. (1998). Types of stressors that increase susceptibility to the common cold in healthy adults. *Health Psychology, 17,* 214–223.

Cohen, S., & Herbert, T. B. (1996). Health psychology: Psychological factors and physical disease from the perspective of human psychoneuroimmunology. *Annual Review of Psychology, 47,* 113–142.

Cohen, S., Tyrrell, D. A. J., & Smith, A. P. (1991). Psychological stress and susceptibility to the common cold. *New England Journal of Medicine, 325,* 606–612.

Crary, B., Borysenko, M., Sutherland, D. C., Kutz, I., Borysenko, J. Z., & Benson, H. (1983a). Decrease in mitogen responsiveness of mononuclear cells from peripheral blood after epinephrine administrations in humans. *Journal of Immunology, 130,* 694–697.

Crary, B., Hauser, S. L., Borysenko, M., Kutz, I., Hoban, C., Ault, K. A., Weiner, H. L., & Bensen, H. (1983b). Epinephrine-induced changes in the distribution of lymphocyte subsets in peripheral blood of humans. *Journal of Immunology, 131,* 1178–1181.

Cunnick, J. E., Lysle, D. T., Kucinski, B. J., & Rabin, B. S. (1989). Stress-induced alterations of immune function: Diversity of effects and mechanisms. *Annals of the New York Academy of Sciences, 650,* 283–287.

Cupps, T. R., & Fauci, A. S. (1982). Corticosteroid-mediated immunoregulation in man. *Imunological Reviews, 65,* 133–155.

Delahanty, D. L., Dougall, A. L., Hawken, L., Trakowski, J. H., Schmitz, J. B., Jenkins, F. J., & Baum, A. (1996). Time course of natual killer cell activity and lymphocyte proliferation in response to two acute stressors in healthy men. *Health Psychology, 15,* 48–55.

Dunn, A. J., & Berridge, C. W. (1990). Physiological and behavioral responses to corticotropin-releasing factor administration: Is CRF a mediator of anxiety or stress responses? *Brain Research Reviews, 15,* 71–100.

Fawzy, F. I., Cousins, N., Fawzy, N. W., Kemeny, M. E., Elashoff, R., & Morton, D. (1990a). A structured psychiatric intervention for cancer patients. I. Changes over time in method of coping and affective disturbances. *Archives of General Psychiatry, 47,* 720–725.

Fawzy, F. I., Kemeny, .E., Fawzy, N. W., Elashoff, R., Morton, D., Cousins, N., & Fahey, J. L. (1990b). A structured psychiatric intervention for cancer patients. II. Changes over time in imunological measures. *Archives of General Psychiatry, 47,* 729–735.

Felton, D. L., Ackerman, K. D., Wiegand, S. J., & Felton, S. Y. (1987). Noradrenergic sympathetic innervation of the spleen. I. Nerve fibers associate with lymphocytes and macrophages in specific compartments of the splenic white pulp. *Journal of Neuroscience Research, 18,* 28–36.

Felton, S. Y., & Olschowka, J. (1987). Noradrenergic sympathetic innervation of the spleen. II. Tyrosine hydroxylase (TH)-positive nerve terminals form synapticlike contacts on lymphocytes in the splenic white pulp. *Journal of Neuroscience Research, 18,* 37–48.

Fletcher, M. A., Klimas, N. G., Morgan, R., & Gjerset, G. (1997). Lymphocyte proliferation. In N. Rose (Ed.), *Manual of clinical laboratory immunology* (pp. 313–319). Washington, DC: American Association for Microbiology.

Gatti, G., Masera, R., Cavallo, R., Sartori, M. L., Delponte, D., Carignola, R., Salvadori, A., & Angeli, A. (1987). Studies on the mechanism of cortisol inhibition of human natural killer cell activity: Effects of calcium entry blockers and calmodulin antagonists. *Steroids, 49,* 601–616.

Glaser, R., Kiecolt-Glaser, J. K., Bonneau, R., Malarkey, W., & Hughes, J. (1992). Stress-induced modulation of the immune response to recombinant hepatitis B vaccine. *Psychosomatic Medicine, 54,* 22–29.

Glaser, R., Kutz, L. A., MacCallum, R. C., & Malarkey, W. B. (1995). Hormonal modulation of Epstein–Barr virus replication. *Neuroendocrinology, 62,* 356–361.

Goodwin, J. S., Searles, R. P., & Tung, K. S. K. (1982). Immunological responses of a healthy elderly population. *Clinical and Experimental Immunology, 48,* 403–410.

Gordon, M. A., Cohen, J. J., & Wilson, I. B. (1978). Muscarinic cholinergic receptors in murine lymphocytes: Demonstration by direct binding. *Proceedings of the National Academy of Sciences, 75,* 2902–2904.

Gray, T. S. (1993). Amygdaloid CRF pathways: Role ir. Autonomic, neuroendocrine, and behavioral responses to stress. *Annals of the New York Academy of Sciences, 697,* 53–60.

Greenspan, F. S., & Baxter, J. D. (1994). *Basic and clinical endocrinology.* Norwalk, CT: Appleton and Lange.

Haas, H. S., & Schauenstein, K. (1997). Neuroimmunomodulation via limbic structures—The neuroanatomy of psychoimmunology. *Progress in Neurobiology, 51,* 195–222.

Hadden, J. W., Hadden, E. M., & Middleton, E. (1970). Lymphocyte blast transformation. I. Demonstration of adrenergic receptors in human peripheral lymphocytes. *Cellular Immunology, 1,* 583–595.

Hatfield, S. P., Petersen, B. H., & DiMicco, J. A. (1986). Beta adrenoceptor modulation of the generation of murine cytotoxic T lymphocytes in vitro. *Journal of Pharmacology and Experimental Therapeutics, 239,* 460–466.

Heilig, M., Irwin, M., Grewal, I., & Sercarz, E. (1993). Sympathetic regulation of T-helper cell function. *Brain, Behavior, and Immunity, 7,* 154–163.

Hellstrand, K., Hermodsson, S., & Strannegard, O. (1985). Evidence for a B-adrenoceptor-mediated regulation of human natural killer cells. *Journal of Immunology, 134,* 4095–4099.

Herbert, T. B., & Cohen, S. (1993). Stress and immunity in humans: A meta-analytic review. *Psychosomatic Medicine, 55,* 364–379.

Herbert, T. B., Cohen, S., Marsland, A. L., Bachen, E. A., Rabin, B. S., Muldoon, M. F., & Manuck, S. B. (1994). Cardiovacular reactivity and the course of immune response to an acute psychological stressor. *Psychosomatic Medicine, 56,* 337–344.

Holahan, M. R., Kalin, N. H., & Kelley, A. E. (1997). Microinfusion of corticotropin-releasing factor into the nucleus accumbens shell results in increased behavioral arousal and oral motor activity. *Psychopharmacology, 130,* 189–196.

Holbrook, N. J., Cox, W. I., & Horner, H. C. (1983). Direct suppression of natural killer activity in human peripheral blood leukocyte cultures by glucocorticoids and its modulation by interferon. *Cancer Research, 43,* 4019–4025.

Irwin, M., Hauger, R. L., Brown, M., & Britton, K. T. (1989). CRF activates autonomic nervous system and reduces natural killer cytotoxicity. *American Journal of Physiology, 255,* R744–R747.

Irwin, M., Mascovich, A., Gillin, J. C., Willoughby, R., Pike, J., & Smith, T. L. (1994). Partial sleep deprivation reduces natural killer cell activity in humans. *Psychosomatic Medicine, 56,* 493–498.

Ishigami, T. (1918–1919). The influence of psychic acts on the progress of pulmonary tuberculosis. *American Review of Tuberculosis, 2,* 470–484.

Kalin, N. H., & Takahashi, L. K. (1990). Fear-motivated behavior induced by prior shock experience is mediated by corticotropin-releasing hormone systems. *Brain Research, 509,* 80–84.

Kaplan, J. R., & Manuck, S. B. (1989). The effects of propanolol on behavioral interactions among adult male Cynomolgus monkeys (Macaca fascicularis) housed in disrupted social groupings. *Psychosomatic Medicine, 51,* 449–462.

Katz, P., Zaytoun, A. M., & Fauci, A. S. (1982). Mechanisms of human cell-mediated cytotoxicity. I. Modulation of natural killer cell activity by cyclic nucleotides. *Journal of Immunology, 129,* 287–296.

Keller, S. E., Schleifer, S. J., Liotta, A. S., Bond, R. N., Farhoody, N., & Stein, M. (1988). Stress-induced alterations of immunity in hypophysectomized rats. *Proceedings of the National Academic Sciences of the USA, 85,* 9297–9301.

Keller, S. E., Weiss, J. M., Schleifer, S. J., Miller, N. E., & Stein, M. (1983). Stress-induced suppression of immunity in adrenalectomized rats. *Science, 221,* 1301–1304.

Khan, M. M., Sansoni, P., Silverman, E. D., Engleman, E. G., & Melmon, K. L. (1986). Beta-adrenergic receptors on human suppressor, helper, and cytolytic lymphocytes. *Biochemical Pharmacology, 35,* 1137–1142.

Kiecolt-Glaser, J. K., Cacioppo, J. T., Malarkey, W. B., & Glaser, R. (1993). Acute psychological stressors and short-term immune changes: What, why, for whom, and to what extent? *Psychosomatic Medicine, 54,* 680–685.

Kiecolt-Glaser, J. K., Dura, J. R., Speicher, C. E., Trask, J. O., & Glaser, R. (1991). Spousal caregivers of dementia victims: Longitudinal changes in immunity and health. *Psychosomatic Medicine, 53,* 345–362.

Kiecolt-Glaser, J. K., & Glaser, R. (1995). Psychoneuroimmunology and health consequences: Data and shared mechanisms. *Psychosomatic Medicine, 57,* 269–274.

Kiecolt-Glaser, J. K., & Glaser, R. (1988). Methodological issues in the behavioral immunology research with humans. *Brain, Behavior, and Immunity, 2,* 67–78.

Kiecolt-Glaser, J. K., Glaser, R., Gravenstein, S., Malarkey, W. B., & Sheridan, J. (1996). Chronic stress alters the immune response to influenza virus vaccine in older adults. *Proceedings of the National Academy of Sciences, 93,* 3043–3047.

Kiecolt-Glaser, J. K., Glaser, R., Williger, D., Stout, J., Messick, G., Sheppard, S., Ricker, D., Romisher, S. C., Briner, W., Bonnell, G., & Donnerberg, R. (1985). Psychosocial enhancement of immunocompetence in a geriatric population. *Health Psychology, 4,* 25–41.

Kiecolt-Glaser, J. K., Marucha, P. T., Malarkey, W. B., Mercado, A. M., & Glaser, R. (1995). Slowing of wound healing by psychological stress. *Lancet, 346,* 1194–1196.

Kirschbaum, C., & Hellhammer, D. H. (1994). Salivary cortisol in psychoneuroendocrine research: Recent developments and applications. *Psychoneuroendocrinology, 19,* 313–333.

Knapp, P. H., Levy, E. M., Giorgi, R. G., Black, P. H., Fox, B. H., & Heeren, T. C. (1992). Short-term immunological effects of induced emotion. *Psychosomatic Medicine, 54,* 133–148.

Krahn, D. D., Gosnell, B. A., Grace, M., & Levine, A. S. (1986). CRF antagonist partially reverses CRF- and stress-induced effects on feeding. *Brain Research Bulletin, 17,* 285–289.

Krantz, D. S., & Manuck, S. B. (1984). Acute physiologic reactivity and risk of cardiovascular disease: A review and methodologic critique. *Psychological Bulletin, 96,* 435–464.

Krieger, D. T., & Allen, W. (1975). Relationship of bioassayable and immunoassayable plasma ACTH and cortisol concentrations in normal subjects and in patients with Cushing's disease. *Journal of Clinical Endocrinology and Metabolism, 10,* 675–687.

Landmann, R. M. A., Durig, M., Gudat, F., Wesp, M., & Harder, F. (1985). Beta-adrenergic regulation of the blood lymphocyte phenotype distribution in normal subjects and splenectomized patients. *Advances in Experimental Medicine and Biology, 186,* 1051–1062.

Landmann, R. M. A., Muller, F. B., Perini, C. H., Wesp, M., Erne, P., & Buhler, F. R. (1984). Changes in immunoregulatory cells induced by psychological and physical stress: Relationship to plasma catecholamines. *Clinical Experimental Immunology, 58,* 127–135.

LaPerriere, A. R., Antoni, M. H., Schneiderman, N., Ironson, G., Klimas, N., et al. (1990). Exercise intervention attentuates emotional distress and natural killer cell decrements following notification of positive serologic status for HIV-1. *Biofeedback and Self-Regulation, 15,* 229–242.

LeDoux, J. E. (1995). Emotion: Clues from the brain. *Annual Review of Psychology, 46,* 209–235.

Lee, Y., & Davis, M. (1997a). Role of the septum in the excitatory effect of corticotropin-releasing hormone on the acoustic startle reflex. *Journal of Neuroscience, 17,* 6424–6433.

Lee, Y., & Davis, M. (1997b). Role of the hippocampus, the bed nucleus of the stria terminalis, and the amygdala in the excitotory effect of corticotropin-releasing hormone on the acoustic startle reflex. *Journal of Neuroscience, 17,* 6434–6446.

Light, K. C., Dolan, C. A., Davis, M. R., & Sherwood, A. (1992). Cardiovascular responses to an active coping challenge as predictors of blood pressure patterns 10 to 15 years later. *Psychosomatic Medicine, 54,* 217–230.

Linkowski, P., Kerkhofs, M., Van Onderbergen, A., Hubain, P., Copinschi, G., L'Hermite-Baleriaux, M., Leclercq, R., Brasseur, M., Mendlewicz, J., & Van Cauter, E. (1994). The 24-hour profiles of cortisol, prolactin, and growth hormone secretion in mania. *Archives of General Psychiatry, 51,* 616–624.

Linkowski, P., Van Onderbergen, A., Kerkhofs, M., Bosson, D., Mendlewicz, J., & Van Cauter, E. (1993). Twin study of the 24-h cortisol profile: Evidence for genetic control of the human circadian clock. *American Journal of Physiology, 264,* E173–E181.

Lord, J. A. H., Waterfield, A. A., Hughes, H., & Kosterlitz, H. W. (1977). Endogenous opioid peptides: Multiple agonists and receptors. *Nature, 267,* 495–499.

Lovallo, W. R., Pincomb, G. A., Brackett, D. J., & Wilson, M. F. (1990). Heart rate reactivity as a predictor of neuroendocrine respones to aversive and appetitive challenges. *Psychosomatic Medicine, 52,* 17–26.

Madden, K. S., & Livnat, S. (1991). Catecholamine action and immunologic reactivity. In R. Ader, D. L. Felten, & N. Cohen (Eds.), *Psychoneuroimmunology* (pp. 283–310). New York: Academic Press.

Maier, S. F., Goehler, L. E., Fleshner, M., & Watkins, L. R. (1998). The role of the vagus nerve in cytokine-to-brain communication. *Annals of the New York Academy of Sciences, 840,* 289–300.

Maier, S. F., & Watkins, L. R. (1998). Cytokines for psychologists: Implications of bidirectional immune-to-brain communication for understanding behavior, mood, and cognition. *Psychological Review, 105,* 83–107.

Maisel, A. S., Fowler, P., Rearden, A., Motulsky, H. J., & Michel, M. C. (1989). A new method for isolation of human lymphocyte subsets reveals differential regulation of B-adrenergic receptors by terbutaline treatment. *Clinical Pharmacology and Therapeutics, 46,* 429–439.

Maisel, A. S., Harris, T., Rearden, C. A., & Michel, M. C. (1990). B-adrenergic receptors in lymphocytes subsets after exercise: Alterations in normal individuals and patients with congestive heart failure. *Circulation, 82,* 2003–2010.

Marsland, A. L., Manuck, S. B., Fazzari, T. V., Stewart, C. J., & Rabin, B. S. (1995). Stability and individual differences in cellular immune responses to acute psychological stress. *Psychosomatic Medicine, 57,* 295–298.

Manuck, S. B. (1994). Cardiovascular reactivity in cardiovascular disease: "Once more unto the breach." *International Journal of Behavioral Medicine, 1,* 4–31.

Manuck, S. B., Cohen, S. C, Rabin, B., Muldoon, M. F., & Bachen, E. A. (1991). Individual differences in cellular immune response to stress. *Psychological Science, 2,* 111–115.

Manuck, S. B., Kaplan, J. R., & Clarkson, T. B. (1983). Behavioral induced heart rate reactivity and atherosclerosis in Cynomolus monkeys. *Psychosomatic Medicine, 45,* 95–108.

Matthews, K. A., Caggiula, A. R., McAllister, C. G., Berga, S. L., Owens, J. F., Flory, J. D., & Miller, A. L. (1995). Sympathetic reactivity to acute stress and immune response in women. *Psychosomatic Medicine, 57,* 564–571.

Matthews, K. A., Owens, J. F., Allen, M. T., & Stoney, C. M. (1992). Do cardiovascular responses to laboratory stress relate to ambulatory blood pressure levels?: Yes, in some of the people, some of the time. *Psychosomatic Medicine, 54,* 686–697.

McEwen, B. S. (1998). Stress, adaptation, and disease: Allostasis and allostatic load. *Annals of the New York Academy of Sciences, 840,* 33–44.

Mehrishi, J. N., & Mills, I. H. (1983). Opiate receptors on lymphocytes and platelets in man. *Clinical Immunology and Immunopathology, 27,* 240–249.

Menzaghi, F., Heinrichs, S. C., Pich, E. M., Weiss, F., & Koob, G. F. (1993). The role of limbic and hypothalamic corticotropin-releasing factor in behavioral responses to stress. *Annals of the New York Academy of Sciences, 697,* 142–154.

Mills, P. J., Haeri, S. L., & Dimsdale, J. E. (1995). Temporal stability of acute stressor-induced changes in cellular immunity. *International Journal of Psychophysiology, 19,* 287–290.

Mills, P. J., Ziegler, M. G., Dimsdale, J. E., & Parry, B. L. (1995). Enumerative immune changes following acute stress: Effects of the menstrual cycle. *Brain, Behavior, and Immunity, 9,* 190–195.

Moser, M., De Smedt, T., Sornasse, T., Tielemans, F., Chentoufi, A. A., Muraille, E., Van Mechelen, M., Urbain, J., & Leo, O. (1995). Glucocorticoids down-regulate dendritic cell function in vitro and in vivo. *European Journal of Immunology, 25,* 2818–2824.

Moynihan, J. A., & Ader, R. (1996). Psychoneuroimmunology: Animal models of disease. *Psychosomatic Medicine, 58,* 546–558.

Munck, A., Guyre, P. M., & Holbrook, N. J. (1984). Physiological function of glucocorticoids in stress and their relation to pharmacological actions. *Endocrine Reviews, 5,* 25–44.

Murray, D. R., Irwin, M., Reardon, A., Ziegler, M., Motulsky, H., & Maisel, A. S. (1992). Sympathetic and immune alterations during dynamic exercise: Mediation via a $\beta_2$-adrenergic-dependent mechanism. *Circulation, 86,* 203–213.

Najima, A. (1995). An electrophysiological study of the vagal innervation of the thymus in the rat. *Brain Research Bulletin, 38,* 319–323.

Naliboff, B. D., Solomon, G. F., Gilmore, S. L., Benton, D., Morley, J. E., & Fahey, J. L. (1995). The effects of the opiate antagonist naloxone on measures of cellular immunity during rest and brief psychological stress. *Journal of Psychosomatic Research, 39,* 345–359.

Naliboff, B. D., Solomon, G. F., Gilmore, S. L., Fahey, J. L., Benton, D., & Pine, J. (1995). Rapid changes in cellular immunity following a confrontational role-play stressor. *Brain, Behavior, and Immunity, 9,* 207–219.

Nomoto, Y., Karasawa, S., & Uehara, K. (1994). Effects of hydrocortisone and adrenaline on natural killer cell activity. *British Journal of Anaesthesia, 73,* 318–321.

Obrist, P. A. (1981). *Cardiovascular psychophysiology: A perspective.* New York: Plenum.

Ottaway, C. A., & Husband, A. J. (1992). Central nervous influences in lymphocyte migration. *Brain, Behavior, and Immunity, 6,* 97–116.

Padgett, D. A., Sheridan, J. F., Dorne, J., Berntson, G. G., Candelora, J., & Glaser, R. (1998). Social stress and the reactivation of latent herpes simplex virus type 1. *Proceedings of the National Academy of Sciences, USA, 95,* 7231–7235.

Parrillo, J. E., & Fauci, A. S. (1978), Comparison of the effector cells in human spontaneous cellular cytotoxicity and antibody-dependent cellular cytotoxicity: Differential sensitivity of effecctor cells to in vivo and in vitro corticosteroids. *Scandinavian Journal of Immunology, 8,* 99–107.

Pedersen, B. K., & Beyer, J. M. (1986). Characterization of the in vitro effecs of glucocorticoids on NK cell activity. *Allergy, 41,* 220–224.

Platt, J. R. (1964). Strong inference. *Science, 146,* 347–353.

Plaut, M. (1987). Lymphocyte hormone receptors. *Annual Review of Immunology, 5,* 621–669.

Pollak, M. H. (1991). Heart rate reactivity to laboratory tasks and ambulatory heart rate in daily life. *Psychosomatic Medicine, 53,* 1–12.

Rivier, C., Brownstein, M., Speiss, J., Rivier, J., & Vale, W. (1982). In vivo corticotropin-releasing factor-induced secretion of adrenocorticotropin, $\beta$-endorphin, and corticosterone. *Endocrinology, 110,* 272–278.

Rinner, I., Kukulansky, T., Felsner, P., Skriener, E., Globerson, A., Kasai, M., Hirokawa, K., Korsatko, W., & Schauenstein, K. (1994). Cholinergic stimulation modulates apoptosis and differentiation of murine thymocytes via a nicotinic effect on thymic epithelium. *Biochemical and Biophysical Research Communications, 203,* 1057–1062.

Roberts-Thomson, I. C., Whittingham, S., Youngchaiyud, U., & MacKay, I. R. (1974). *Lancet, ii,* 368–370.

Schedlowski, M., Falk, A., Rohne, A., Wagner, T. O. F., Jacobs, R., Tewes, U., & Schmidt, R. E. (1993). Catecholamines induce alterations of distribution and activity of human natural killer (NK) cells. *Journal of Clinical Immunology, 13,* 344–351.

Schedlowski, M., Hosch, W., Oberbeck, R., Benschop, R. J., Raab, H., & Schmidt, R. E. (1996). Catecholamines modulate human NK cell circulation and function via spleen-independent $\beta_2$-adrenergic mechanisms. *Journal of Immunology, 156,* 93–99.

Scheier, M. F., & Bridges, M. W. (1995). Person variables and health: Personality predispositions and acute psychological states as shared determinants for disease. *Psychosomatic Medicine, 57,* 255–268.

Schobitz, B., Reul, J. M. H. M., & Holsboer, F. (1994). The role of the hypothalamic-pituitary-adrenocorticol system during inflammatory conditions. *Critical Reviews in Neurobiology, 8,* 263–291.

Segerstrom, S. C., Taylor, S. E., Kemeny, M. E., & Fahey, J. L. (1998). Optimism is associated with mood, coping, and immune change in response to stress. *Journal of Personality and Social Psychology, 74,* 1646–1655.

Selye, H. (1956). *The stress of life.* New York: McGraw-Hill.

Sgoutas-Emch, S. A., Cacioppo, J. T., Uchino, B. N., Malarkey, W., Pearl, D., Kiecolt-Glaser, J. K., & Glaser, R. (1994). The effects of an acute psychological stressor on cardiovascular, endocrine, and cellular immune response: A prospective study of individuals high and low in heart rate reactivity. *Psychophysiology, 31,* 264–271.

Sheridan, J. F., Dobbs, C., Jung, J., Chu, X., Konstantinos, A., Padgett, D., & Glaser, R. (1998). Stress-induced neuroendocrine modulation of viral pathogenesis and immunity. *Annals of the New York Academy of Sciences, 840,* 803–808.

Sherwood, A., Allen, M., Fahrenberg, J., Kelsey, R., Lovallo, W., & Van Doornen, L. (1990). Methodological guidelines for impedance cardiography. *Psychophysiology, 27,* 1–23.

Sirinathsinghji, D. J. S., Rees, L. H., Rivier, J., & Vale, W. (1983). Corticotropin-releasing factor is a potent inhibitor of sexual receptivity in the female rat. *Nature, 305,* 232–235.

Smith. T. W. (1992). Hostility and health: Current status of a psychosomatic hypothesis. *Health Psychology, 11,* 139–150.

Smith, T. W., & Gallo, L. C. (in press). Personality traits as risk factors for physical illness. In A. Baum, T. Revenson, & J. Singer (Eds.), *Handbook of health psychology.* Hillsdale, NJ: Lawrence Erlbaum.

Smith, T. W., & Ruiz, J. M. (in press). Methodological issues in adult health psychology. In P. C. Kendall, J. N. Butcher, & G. N. Holmbeck (Eds.), *Handbook of research methods in clinical psychology.* New York: Wiley.

Solomon, G. F., & Moos, R. H. (1964). Emotions, immunity, and disease: A speculative theoretical integration. *Archives of General Psychiatry, 11,* 657–674.

Spiegel, D., Bloom, J. R., Kraemer, H. C., & Gottheil, E. (1989). Effect of psychosocial treatment on survival of patients with metastatic breast cancer. *Lancet, ii,* 888–891.

Spyer, K. M. (1989). Neural mechanisms involved in cardiovascular control during affective behavior. *Trends in Neuroscience, 12,* 506–513.

Sterling, P., & Eyer, J. (1988). Allostasis: A new paradigm to explain arousal pathology. In S. Fisher and J. Reason (Eds.), *Handbook of life stress, cognition, and health* (pp. 629–649). New York: Wiley.

Stone, A. A., Valdimarsdottir, H. B., Katkin, E. S., Burns, J., Cox, D. S., Lee, S., Fine, J., Ingle, D., & Bovbjerg, D. H. (1993). Effects of mental stressors on mitogen-induced lymphocyte responses in the laboratory. *Psychology and Health, 8,* 269–284.

Strom, T. B., Lane, M. A., & George, K. (1981). The parallel, time-dependent, bimodal change in lymphocyte cholinergic binding activity and cholinergic influence upon lymphocyte-mediated cytotoxicity after lymphocyte activation. *Journal of Immunology, 127,* 705–710.

Strom, T. B., Sytkowski, A. J., Carpenter, C. B., & Merrill, J. P. (1974). Cholinergic augmentation of lymphocyte-mediated cytotoxicity. A study of the cholinergic receptor of cytotoxic T lymphocytes. *Proceedings of the National Academy of Sciences, USA, 71,* 1330–1333.

Sundar, S. K., Cierpial, M. A., Kilts, C., Ritchie, J. C., & Weiss, J. M. (1990). Brain IL-1-induced immunosuppression occurs through activation of both pituitary-adrenal axis and sympathetic nervous system by corticotropin-releasing factor. *The Journal of Neuroscience, 10,* 3701–3706.

Swiergiel, A. H., Takahashi, L. K., & Kalin, N. H. (1993). Attenuation of stress-induced behavior by antagonism of corticotropin-releasing factor receptors in the central amygdala in the rat. *Brain Research, 623,* 229–234.

Turner, J. R. (1989). Individual differences in heart rate response during behavioral challenge. *Psychophysiology, 26,* 497–505.

Tvede, N., Kappel, M., Halkjoer-Kristensen, J., Galbo, H., & Pedersen, B. K. (1993). The effects of light, moderate and severe bicycle exercise on lymphocyte subsets, natural and lymphokine activity killer cells, lymphocyte proliferative response and interleukin 2 production. *International Journal of Sports Medicine, 14,* 275–282.

Uchino, B. N., Cacioppo, J. T., Malarkey, W., & Glaser, R. (1995). Individual differences in cardiac sympathetic control predict endocrine and immune responses to acute psychological stress. *Journal of Personality and Social Psychology, 69,* 736–743.

Uchino, B. N., Kiecolt-Glaser, J. K., & Glaser, R. (2000). Psychological modulation of cellular immunity. In J. T. Cacioppo, L. G. Tassinary, & G. G. Berntson (Eds.), *Handbook of Psychophysiology* (pp. 397–424). New York: Cambridge University Press.

Valentino, R. J., Foote, S. L., & Page, M. E. (1993). The locus coeruleus as a site for integrating corticotropin-releasing factor and noradrenergic mediation of stress responses. *Annals of the New York Academy of Sciences, 697,* 173–88.

Van Cauter, E. (1990). Diurnal and ultradian rhythms in human endocrine function: A mini review. *Hormone Research, 34,* 45–53.

Van Tits, L. J., Michel, M. C., Grosse-Wilde, H., Happel, M., Eigler, F. W., Soliman, A., & Brodde, O. E. (1990). Catecholamines increase lymphocyte $B_2$-adrenergic receptors via a $B_2$-adrenergic, spleen-dependent process. *American Journal of Physiology, 258,* E191–E202.

Wiegers, G. J., Croiset, G., Reul, J. M. H. M., Holsboer, F., & De Kloet, E. R. (1993). Differential effects of corticosteroids on rat peripheral blood T-lymphocyte mitogenesis in vivo and in vitro. *American Journal of Physiology, 265,* E825–830.

Wiegers, G. J., Reul, J. M. H. M., Holsboer, F., & De Kloet, E.R. (1994). *Endocrinology, 135,* 2351–2357.

Willemsen, G., Ring, C., Carroll, D., Evans, P., Clow, A., & Hucklebridge, F. (1998). Secretory immunoglobulin A and cardiovascular reactions to mental arithmetic and cold pressor. *Psychophysiology, 35,* 252–259.

Williams, L. T., Snyderman, R., & Lefkowitz, R. J. (1976). Identification of B-adrenergic receptors in human lymphocytes by (-) [$^3$H] alprenolol binding. *Journal of Clinical Investigation, 57,* 149–155.

Yoshikawa, T. T. (1983). Geriatric infectious diseases: An emerging problem. *Journal of the American Geriatrics Society, 31,* 34–39.

# 46

# Neuroendocrine and Immune Alterations Following Natural Disasters and Traumatic Stress

DOUGLAS L. DELAHANTY, ANGELA LIEGEY DOUGALL,
ANDREW BAUM

## I. INTRODUCTION

Following the Ader and Cohen (1975) landmark study demonstrating classical conditioning of immune system activity, the past 25 years have seen dramatic growth in research examining the relationship between stress and immunity. The demonstration of links between the brain and the immune system confirmed the possibility that emotional states like stress could affect immunity, and hundreds of studies have measured the effects of acute and chronic stress in humans and animals. Most of these studies have evaluated the immunomodulating effects of acute stress in the laboratory or more chronic stress in naturalistic settings. Few have examined the relationship between severe, traumatic stress and immunity. In part this reflects the obstacles to studying victims of severe or traumatic stressors; baseline data are rarely available, adequate control groups are difficult to find, identify, and assemble, and a multitude of logistical, practical, and other problems make collecting specimens in a timely fashion in the field very difficult. In some cases, victims' homes may have been destroyed and communication severely disrupted, making sampling and follow-up assessment a challenge. Regardless of the reason, relatively little is known about the effects of extreme stress on persistent biological alterations in humans, including changes in immune system activity. This chapter reviews this small literature, concentrating on possible mechanisms through which immune changes may occur.

### A. Traumatic Stress and Posttraumatic Stress Disorder

Stressors can vary along a number of dimensions and research has begun to show that simply distinguishing between acute and chronic stress experiences may not encompass a number of stressful events and responses. For example, stressful situations can differ in the duration of the actual event, the duration of threat experienced, the duration of responding to the event, whether persistent or chronic stress is ongoing or resolved, how severely disrupting an event is, or whether it introduces life threat, harm, or loss (e.g., Baum, Cohen, & Hall, 1993; Baum, O'Keefe, & Davidson, 1990; Matthews, Gump, Block, & Allen, 1997). Extremely severe stressors that involve life threat and direct bodily harm appear to be qualitatively different than most other stressors.

Natural disasters and other traumatic stressors are unusual in that the duration of the precipitating event is often acute while responding to the event can persist well beyond it. In the present chapter, we will define traumatic stress broadly, with precipitating events that are sudden, powerful, and beyond the realm of normal experience (Baum, 1987). This would include natural disasters such as floods, hurricanes, and tornadoes, human-caused disasters such as plane crashes, technological disasters, and motor vehicle accidents, and more individual traumas such as rape, abuse, or assault. The observation that distress often persists well after the traumatic event is over suggests that responses to these types of events are particularly resistant to adaptation or habituation. Unusually persistent, severe, and disruptive stress can evolve into or cause posttraumatic stress disorder (PTSD), marked by reexperiencing of precipitating events and by arousal, numbing, and avoidance. Perturbations in endocrine activity associated with stressors involving life threat suggest that changes in immune system functions associated with stress may persist as well.

Although PTSD is observed in a substantial number of trauma victims, most people exposed to traumatic stressors do not develop PTSD, leading to some debate over what characterizes a normal response to traumatic stressors (Yehuda, Resnick, Kahana, & Giller, 1993a). Percentages vary according to type of traumatic event studied, but research has suggested that 1–2% of the general population and up to 25% of victims exposed to traumatic stressors develop PTSD (Breslau, Davis, Andreski, & Peterson, 1991; Davidson, Hughes, Blazer, & George, 1991; Helzer, Robins, & McEvoy, 1987). Women appear to be more likely to develop PTSD than men; the U.S. National Comorbidity Study found that women were nearly twice as likely to develop PTSD following a traumatic event (Kessler, Sonnega, Bromet, & Nelson, 1995). The most common causes of PTSD in men were combat and witnessing death or severe injury. Sexual abuse and rape were the most common causes in women, and it is possible that differences in traumatic events account for gender differences in PTSD. A discussion of whether PTSD constitutes a normative or maladaptive response to traumatic stress is beyond the scope of this chapter. It is also unclear whether PTSD represents a diagnostic label for exaggerated stress responses or if it is a distinct syndrome with unusual properties and symptoms. However, we will consider the possibility that biological reactions to traumatic stress differ between those victims who meet PTSD criteria and those who do not.

## B. Traumatic Stress and Immunity

Research examining intense, naturalistic stressors has typically studied one of a heterogenous group of events that differ along a number of dimensions (e.g., human versus natural cause, frequency of occurrence or reported occurrence, number of individuals affected, extent of personal life threat experienced). Because these variables almost certainly affect the degree of distress, arousal, and responses that follow, we review the findings of studies examining different types of traumatic events separately.

Natural and human-caused disasters share a number of commonalities. They typically threaten a large number of individuals, often occur with little, if any, warning, and are characterized by damage, death, loss of belongings, and feelings of loss of control. However, there are a number of important distinctions between natural and humanmade disasters that may influence recovery. Due to the ability to track storms and communicate with large numbers of people quickly, there is typically some warning prior to natural disasters. However, humanmade disasters are generally more unpredictable. In short, because they are never supposed to happen (planes are not supposed to fall from the sky, nuclear power plants are not supposed to fail), they are very unpredictable. In addition, humanmade disasters may be accompanied by greater feelings of loss of control since many of these disasters effect a loss of control over technology, and a causal agent can usually be identified and blamed for the accident. For these and other reasons, the consequences of humanmade disasters appear to be more persistent than those of naturalistic disasters (Baum, 1987; Baum et al., 1993).

### 1. Natural Disasters

We found very few published studies that systematically examined psychological and immunological sequelae of naturalistic disasters. Boyce and colleagues (1993) had an unusual opportunity to examine the impact of the 1989 Loma Prieta earthquake on self-reported respiratory illness in a sample of kindergarten students. These students were enrolled in a study of changes in immunological activity in response to a normative life stressor (starting kindergarten). Prior to kindergarten entry, 20 students gave blood samples and received pneumococcal vaccines. Two weeks after the start of kindergarten, the students provided another blood sample. At each time point, CD4+/CD8+ ratios, lymphocyte responses to pokeweed mitogen, and serum antibody responses to the pneumococcal vaccine were examined. The students were then followed for 12 weeks during which parents recorded instances of respiratory illnesses. After about 6 weeks of monitoring, the Loma Prieta earthquake intervened and a new study design with three respiratory illness assessments before and three after the earthquake was created.

Some data were inconclusive. Six children had increases in respiratory illness episodes following the earthquake, but five had decreases. However, changes in immune measures from before to after school predicted changes in respiratory illness such that greater increases in both CD4+/CD8+ ratios and lymphocyte response to pokeweed mitogen predicted greater incidence of respiratory illness after the earthquake. These results persisted even after controlling for respiratory illness incidence prior to the earthquake. While these results are based on a small sample of young children, they suggest that children who exhibited immunological upregulation in response to a major life event (starting school) were more likely to develop respiratory illnesses following a catastrophic event such as an earthquake. Unfortunately, no immunological measures were taken after the earthquake occurred, making it impossible to discern if these same immunological upregulation patterns existed after it.

The immunological effects of stress associated with disasters have been examined in two other research groups. These studies followed similar methods in evaluating reactions to the 1994 Northridge, California earthquake and the 1992 landfall of Hurricane Andrew (Ironson et al., 1997; Segerstrom, Solomon, Kemeny, & Fahey, 1998; Solomon, Segerstrom, Grohr, Kemeny, & Fahey, 1997, respectively). Immune and psychological variables were collected at repeated time points following the disasters, and both enumerative and functional immune measures were assessed.

Solomon and colleagues (1997) studied 68 (46% male, 54% female) medical center employees at three points after the Northridge earthquake (approximately 2 or 3 weeks and 2 and 4 months after the earthquake), collecting a number of distress and immune measures. The earthquake was a moderate-sized event, registering 6.7 on the Richter scale. However, the epicenter was located less than 2 km from the medical center, which was severely damaged. Employees were also told that the center would not be rebuilt, leading to rumors and worries about layoffs and job security and exacerbating distress. The study was designed to measure the impact of the *aftermath* of the earthquake (e.g., life disruption, loss of utilities at home, unsafe work environment, injuries to self or family, expectation of job loss or change) rather than impact of the earthquake itself. Results

showed that participants experienced distress, including anxiety, confusion, and earthquake-related worry, but that these states decreased significantly over time. Despite this improvement in mood, immune measures such as numbers of CD3+, CD8+, and CD16+56+ cells, proliferative responses to phytohemagglutinin (PHA), and natural killer (NK) cell cytotoxicity all decreased over time. Interaction effects indicated that participants reporting the lowest levels of earthquake-specific distress had higher numbers of CD3+ and CD8+ cells than those reporting more distress. Participants whose levels of distress corresponded with self-report of life disruption exhibited more CD3+ and CD8+ cells, but participants who reported low distress combined with high life disruption, or high distress combined with low life disruption, exhibited significantly lower numbers of these cells. As is the case for most studies of disasters, this study did not have true baseline or predisaster measures of immune status. However, the findings are generally consistent with studies examining the long-term immunological consequences of chronic stress (Calabrese, Kling, & Gold, 1987; Esterling, Kiecolt-Glaser, Bodnar, & Glaser, 1994; Kiecolt-Glaser, Dura, Speicher, Trask, & Glaser, 1991; Kiecolt-Glaser et al., 1987a, b).

One of the better predictors of immune system activity in this sample of earthquake victims was worry (Segerstrom et al., 1998). A subgroup of the medical center sample, including 47 hospital employees who were victims of the earthquake and 25 age-, gender-, and race-matched controls, were studied to evaluate the relationship between trait worry and immune levels. Those victims who scored above the median on self-reported trait worry had fewer NK cells than those victims scoring below the median and controls. This relationship was not mediated by intrusive thoughts, avoidant behaviors, anxiety, or health behaviors, suggesting that worry may independently increase risk of immune system changes following a natural disaster.

Similar results were found in victims of Hurricane Andrew (Ironson et al., 1997). Hurricane Andrew caused more damage than any previous storm recorded in the United States, leaving over 175,000 residents homeless. Researchers studied 180 community volunteers (35% male, 65% female) who lived in damaged neighborhoods that were directly affected by the storm. Victims ranged in degree of damage personally suffered as well as degree of injury, with many left homeless and others with no electricity or telephone for nearly 1 month. Researchers met with victims 1 to 4 months after the hurricane and measured posttraumatic stress symptoms, numbers of

CD8+, CD4+, and CD56+ cells/mm$^3$, and NK cell activity. Approximately 33% of the victims met PTSD criteria. In general, hurricane victims had significantly higher numbers of CD56+ cells/mm$^3$ and significantly lower numbers of CD8+ and CD4+ cells/mm$^3$ than did 72 gender-matched prehurricane laboratory controls. In addition, NK activity was significantly lower in hurricane victims than in controls. PTSD symptoms were negatively associated with NK activity ($r = -.20$, $p < .05$). Greater damage and lost resources were also associated with lower levels of NK activity. Observed NK activity among hurricane victims remained lower than that of laboratory controls 2 years after the hurricane, but returned to the levels of laboratory controls at a 4-year followup (Ironson et al., 1998). Due to difficulties in collecting samples in the acute aftermath of a natural disaster, researchers have typically measured more chronic effects of disaster stress. Overall, the chronic effects of disasters appear to include reductions in immune system activity, but one report has suggested that more acute effects are associated with increases in measures of immune status (Kemeny, cited in Solomon et al., 1997). Kemeny studied both acute and long-term effects of the 1992 Whittier Narrows earthquake on a sample of colleagues and laboratory personnel located about 50 km from the epicenter of the earthquake. Blood samples were collected from 19 participants within 4 h of the earthquake and then again 6 weeks and one year later. Although life threat and disruption experienced by this sample is arguably less than among the victims of the disasters reviewed above, participants had significantly higher numbers of NK and cytotoxic T cells within 4 h of the earthquake than at later time points. Cell numbers did not differ between the 6-week and the 1-year time points. These findings parallel consistent findings of increased numbers and activity of nonspecific immune cells (such as NK cells) during and following acute stress exposure in humans (Delahanty et al., 1996; Naliboff et al., 1991; Schedlowski 1993a, b; Wang, Delahanty, Dougall, & Baum, 1998).

In sum, research findings suggest that chronic disaster stress is associated with fewer immune cells or weaker function in victims of a variety of naturalistic disasters. The lack of published studies examining immunological functioning in the immediate aftermath of disasters makes drawing conclusions concerning acute-phase immune sequelae of disasters difficult. The one study that has been reported found higher numbers of NK and cytotoxic T cells during acute responding immediately after an earthquake, but the small sample size, distance from the earthquake, and other methodological limitations makes it difficult to draw definitive conclusions. None of these studies measured true predisaster baseline levels of function, so determining whether victims exhibited increased activity in the acute phase of trauma responding is impossible. However, laboratory studies also suggest that initial responding to a stressful event may be characterized by heightened immune responses, while more chronic stress is typified by reductions in cell numbers and/or activity.

## 2. Human-Caused Disasters

Despite differences in characteristics of natural and human-caused disasters, studies of the immune sequelae of human-caused disasters report findings similar to those reported above. However, research has suggested that immune alterations following humanmade disasters may be more resistant to recovery and may persist longer than changes following natural disasters (Boscarino & Chang, 1999; Laudenslager et al., 1998; McKinnon, Weisse, Reynolds, Bowles, & Baum, 1989). For instance, more than 6 years after the nuclear accident at Three Mile Island (TMI), some measures of immune status among a sample of residents living within 5 miles of the damaged reactor differed from those living at a control site more than 80 miles from TMI, and differences in immunity were related to the extent of stress reported (McKinnon et al., 1989). As a group, TMI residents exhibited greater numbers of neutrophils, but fewer B lymphocytes, cytotoxic T lymphocytes, and NK cells than did controls. In addition, TMI residents had significantly higher antibody titers to herpes simplex virus (HSV), suggesting disturbance of cellular or molecular functions that permit reactivation of latent viruses. These effects were correlated with elevations in blood pressure and in urinary stress hormones, suggesting an unusually persistent stress response (Baum, Gatchel, & Schaeffer, 1983). Although the subject sample was small (12 TMI residents, 8 controls), the results suggest that stress-related immune changes may persist for years following a technological accident.

Somewhat different results were observed in more acute traumatic stress situations such as the recovery of human remains and cleanup of an air disaster among emergency workers (Delahanty, Dougall, Craig, Jenkins, & Baum, 1997). On September 8, 1994, USAir Flight 427 from Chicago to Pittsburgh crashed, exploding on impact and killing all 132 passengers and crew aboard. Debris and remains were scattered over an isolated hillside, and rescue and emergency workers were responsible for recovering and identifying the remains. We studied 159 rescue workers and 41 controls within 2 months and again 6 months after the crash. Two months after the crash, those workers who reported the highest levels of stress and intrusive thoughts about their work at the crash site also had marginally higher systolic blood pressure, and significantly *greater* NK activity than did other workers and control participants. Whereas heightened NK activity has been consistently reported during and immediately following acute stressors (Delahanty et al., 1996; Delahanty, Dougall, Browning, Hyman, & Baum, 1998; Naliboff et al., 1991; Schedlowski et al., 1993b; Wang et al., 1998), chronic stress has typically been associated with lower levels of NK activity relative to controls (Irwin, Daniels, Smith, Bloom, & Weiner, 1987; Kennedy, Kiecolt-Glaser, & Glaser, 1988; Kiecolt-Glaser, Fisher, Ogrocki, Stout, Speicher, & Glaser, 1987; Kiecolt-Glaser et al., 1987b). As NK activity was highest in the group reporting the greatest distress we hypothesized that *increased* NK activity in these rescue workers was due to acute stress responding triggered by the interview or data collection, which served as a reminder of the stressful event. As experimenters, we may have inadvertently triggered memories or intrusive thoughts about experiences at the site and elicited acute stress responding in those most affected by the crash. It has been hypothesized that extreme stress responses during the event may lead to recurrent thoughts about the event that may maintain distress. Cues that became conditioned to stress during the event may serve as triggers for subsequent intrusive thoughts, prolonging distress (Baum, 1990; Baum et al., 1993). It is possible that physiological changes during the event also may become conditioned to these reminders, resulting in persistent alterations in immune status or reactivity.

Studies examining immune activity in war veterans have typically examined differences between those veterans meeting criteria for PTSD and those without PTSD. Those studies examining NK activity in this population have reported mixed results, with one study finding no differences in NK activity between veterans with and those without PTSD (Mosnaim et al., 1993) and one finding *higher* NK cytotoxicity in veterans with PTSD (Laudenslager et al., 1998). Mosnaim and colleagues examined NK activity and methionine-enkephalin (MET)-stimulated NK activity in 13 male Vietnam veterans with PTSD and a history of substance abuse. Comparison groups of age-comparable males included a group of chronic alcoholics ($n = 11$), a group of chronic nonalcoholic drug abusers ($n = 8$), a group of chronic users of both drugs and alcohol ($n = 8$), and a group of medication-free healthy controls ($n = 22$). The majority (11 of 13)

of the PTSD patients also reported some type of pain (typically backache), and they continued to receive prescribed medication and were allowed non-narcotic analgesics. Nonstimulated NK activity (E:T ratio of 40:1) was similar among all groups, but PTSD patients, as a group, were more likely to show significant inhibition of activity in response to stimulation with $10^{-8}$ and $10^{-6}$ M MET. Inhibition of MET-stimulated NK activity was not consistently observed in all patients, leading the authors to suggest the possible existence of subgroups of PTSD based upon immunological tests. As PTSD patients were also comorbid for alcohol dependence and were taking pain medications, this study did not examine the impact of PTSD alone on immunity. Alcohol and medications that patients were allowed have been shown to have immunomodulating activity.

More recently, Boscarino and Chang (1999) demonstrated that chronic, combat-related PTSD symptomatology was also associated with elevated leukocyte and T-cell counts. Twenty years after military service, immune functioning and PTSD symptoms were assessed in Vietnam theater veterans with ($n = 293$) and without ($n = 2197$) partial PTSD diagnoses (presence of at least one of the diagnostic criteria in the past year and ever having met full diagnostic criteria for PTSD). After controlling for intelligence, race, age, income, education, type of enlistment, Vietnam volunteer status, region of birth, cigarette smoking, illicit drug use, body mass index, and alcohol consumption, those veterans meeting partial PTSD criteria had leukocyte and T-cell counts above the normal range. These counts fell within clinical ranges that are often associated with disease. Veterans with PTSD also had higher white blood cell (WBC), total lymphocyte, T-cell, and CD4-cell counts than veterans without PTSD.

Laudenslager and colleagues (1998) measured a variety of lymphocyte subsets (CD2, −4, −8, −16, −20, and −56), NK activity, and neuroendocrine levels in 10 male Vietnam veterans with long-term PTSD and 9 male veterans without PTSD who were being treated for substance abuse. Results revealed that veterans with PTSD had higher NK activity than veterans without PTSD. There were no differences between groups in enumerative immune measures or resting neuroendocrine levels. However, limitations related to the control group (the control group reported more recent alcohol abuse and more recent drinking than did PTSD patients) suggest viewing the results with caution. As will be noted later, there are endocrine changes that have been identified in some PTSD patients that could explain this heightened NK activity, or the possibility that the study elicited intrusive thoughts and acute distress may apply. Increased numbers of NK cells are typically associated with acute stress experiences, and, as hypothesized in the Flight 427 study, it is possible that this study was actually picking up differences in reactivity to the data collection (Delahanty et al., 1997).

Although this hypothesis may explain higher NK activity in these samples, another measure of immunity that does not appear to be as reactive to intrusive thoughts or acute stress was found to be greater in combat veterans with PTSD than in non-PTSD controls (Burges Watson, Muller, Jones, & Bradley, 1993). These investigators examined immune response to a cutaneous, cell-mediated immunity (CMI) multitest in 25 Vietnam veterans undergoing treatment for PTSD, 20 servicemen without combat experience or PTSD, and 28 civilian controls. All participants were male. The immune multitest involved calculating a compound score of the average response elicited in positive skin reactions to tetanus, diphtheria, streptococcus, tuberculin, *Candida albicans*, trichophyton, and proteus. Veterans with PTSD exhibited greater delayed-type hypersensitivity responses to a battery of antigens than did non-PTSD veterans or controls.

### 3. Summary

Although research linking disasters with immune function has reported mixed results, there are some consistencies in these data. Chronic stress associated with both human-caused and natural disasters appears to be associated with fewer cells and weaker function of a wide range of immune measures. In addition, immune system changes associated with human-caused disasters appears to be very persistent, lasting up to 6 years as shown following the TMI accident. Some evidence suggests that acute-phase responding to disasters is associated with increases in some immune measures, but the lack of published studies on this necessitates viewing this conclusion with caution.

Results are more inconsistent when considering those who do and do not meet PTSD diagnostic criteria. Some studies find evidence of enhanced immune status among PTSD patients or those meeting criteria for PTSD, primarily for chronic combat-related PTSD in war veterans. Several problems characterize this literature, including the possibility of acute responding due to intrusive thoughts. However, perhaps the most important consideration should be the length of time intervening between the traumatic events and assessments of immune status. These victims have typically presented with symptoms of PTSD for decades, and their PTSD is often comorbid with substance abuse, making conclusions about the nature of PTSD-related immune changes difficult. The chronicity of these cases of PTSD is unusual and this may also account for some observed effects. Of these combat veteran studies, one found no effects of PTSD on cell numbers and lower NK activity after stimulation, one found greater NK activity among PTSD patients, and one found greater delayed hypersensitivity. Additional research examining the impact of less chronic PTSD on immune variables in victims of a variety of traumas is needed before concluding with any certainty that PTSD is associated with alterations in immune functioning.

## C. Neuroendocrine Changes in Response to Traumatic Stress

Although relatively few studies have examined immune system reactions following traumatic stressors such as disasters, many more have measured levels of hormones thought to mediate immune system activity during stress (Baum et al., 1983; Baum, Schaeffer, Lake, Fleming, & Collins, 1986; Mason, Kosten, Southwick, & Giller, 1990; Resnick, Yehuda, Pitman, & Foy, 1995; Southwick, Yehuda, & Wang, 1998; Yehuda, Giller, Levengood, Southwick, & Siever, 1995). Catecholamines and cortisol participate in regulation of the immune system (Benschop, Schedlowski, Wienecke, Jacobs, & Schmidt, 1997; Carlson, Brooks, & Roszman, 1989; Crary et al., 1983a, b; Cupps & Fauci, 1982; Jetschmann et al., 1997; O'Leary, Savard, & Miller, 1996; Tonnesen, Christensen, & Brinklov, 1987; Van Tits et al., 1990), and adrenergic blockade by such drugs as propranolol and labetalol attenuate acute stress-related changes in immune activity (Bachen et al., 1995; Benschop et al., 1994; Benschop, Rodriguez-Feuerhahn, & Schedlowski, 1996). Changes in neuroendocrine levels in response to traumatic stress may suggest coincident changes in immune activity.

Studies of neuroendocrine sequelae of traumatic stress are consistent with observed differences in immune system activity. Research at TMI found evidence of elevated levels of urinary catecholamines and cortisol in chronically stressed victims of the disaster (Baum et al., 1983, 1986; Schaeffer & Baum, 1984). These differences persisted for several years after the accident. After more than 6 years, TMI residents still had higher levels of epinephrine (EPI) than did controls (McKinnon et al., 1989). Levels of norepinephrine (NE) and cortisol 6 years postaccident were in the same direction, but were nonsignificant.

Research examining neuroendocrine levels in victims of traumatic stress with PTSD has measured both resting levels of catecholamines and cortisol and changes in neuroendocrine levels in response to stressors that either were or were not reminiscent of the stressful event (for a review, see Orr, 1994). Both types of studies have suggested that PTSD is associated with hyperarousal of the sympathetic nervous system and heightened adrenergic activity. In addition, although mixed results have been reported, several studies have found alterations in the negative feedback system of the hypothalamo-pituitary-adrenal (HPA) axis. More precisely, Yehuda and colleagues have suggested that PTSD patients possess an abnormally sensitive negative feedback loop, resulting in lower than normal resting levels of glucocorticoids (Yehuda et al., 1995; Yehuda, Resnick, Kahana, & Giller, 1993; Yehuda, Southwick, Nussbaum, Giller, & Mason, 1990).

Stress typically stimulates increases in catecholamines and cortisol (Delahunt & Mellsop, 1987; Raggatt & Morrissey, 1997; Rubin, Miller, Clark, Poland, & Arthur, 1970; Schedlowski et al., 1993a). PTSD patients also typically exhibit elevated catecholamines, but some studies suggest that they have lower resting levels of cortisol than do controls (Friedman, 1991; Krystal et al., 1989; Mason et al., 1990; Southwick, Bremner, Krystal, & Charney, 1994; van der Kolk, 1996). As cortisol is generally regarded as an immunosuppressive agent (Balow, Hurley, & Fauci, 1975; Cupps & Fauci, 1982), lower levels of cortisol associated with PTSD may be a mechanism supporting elevated immune activity seen in some of the previously mentioned studies.

## 1. Basal Levels of Catecholamines and Cortisol in PTSD

Studies examining catecholamines in patients with PTSD have reported mixed results. Levels of *plasma* NE and EPI do not appear to differ between PTSD patients and controls (Blanchard, Kolb, Prins, Gates, & McCoy, 1991; McFall, Murburg, Ko, & Veith, 1990; Southwick et al., 1993), but the majority of studies have reported greater *urinary* catecholamine excretion in PTSD patients than in controls (Kosten, Mason, Giller, Ostroff, & Harkness, 1987; Yehuda, Southwick, Giller, Ma, & Mason, 1992; see Pitman & Orr, 1990, for an exception). Urinary catecholamine excretion is more likely to reflect persistent elevation of sympathetic hormones in PTSD than are plasma differences as urinary catecholamine measures average levels across the collection period (usually 24 h). The absence of significant differences in studies of plasma

catecholamines may be due to timing of the blood draws, anxiety about needle sticks in controls reflected as higher catecholamine levels, or the possibility that a general increase in the sympathetic system may not be evident during the acute time frame encompassed by a single blood sample.

As noted earlier, chronic stress is usually associated with elevated HPA activity and cortisol levels. Although one study of combat veterans has reported greater levels of urinary cortisol in PTSD patients (Pitman & Orr, 1990), a number of studies have shown that combat veterans with PTSD have lower 24-h levels of urinary cortisol and greater numbers of glucocorticoid receptors on lymphocytes than veterans without PTSD or than normal controls (Mason, Giller, Kosten, Ostroff, & Harkness, 1986; Yehuda, Boisoneau, Mason, & Giller, 1993; Yehuda et al., 1993; Yehuda, Lowy, Southwick, Shaffer, & Giller, 1991; Yehuda et al., 1990). Decreases in cortisol levels do not appear to habituate, as they have been shown to persist for decades in Holocaust survivors with PTSD (Yehuda 1995). However, extension to other populations has been equivocal. Heim, Ehlert, Hanker, and Hellhammer (1998) reported reduced salivary cortisol levels in response to corticotropin-releasing factor challenge in female abuse-related PTSD patients with chronic pelvic pain. Similarly, adolescent victims of the 1988 Armenian earthquake with the most severe PTSD exhibited significantly lower 8 AM salivary cortisol levels and greater cortisol suppression to dexamethasone administration (Goenjian et al., 1996). However, elevated urinary cortisol levels have been found in women with PTSD related to childhood sexual abuse compared to child sexual abuse victims without PTSD and nonabused controls (Lemieux & Coe, 1995).

Although results are mixed the majority of studies of nonstimulated urinary cortisol in patients with PTSD suggest that they produce and excrete less cortisol than controls. Based on their findings of low cortisol excretion in PTSD patients, Yehuda and colleagues hypothesized that if PTSD patients experienced enhanced cortisol feedback inhibition, then one would expect to observe enhanced suppression of cortisol in response to dexamethasone, rather than the nonsuppression as typified in major depression (Yehuda, Boisoneau, Lowy, & Giller, 1995). Earlier studies examining dexamethasone suppression in PTSD patients used the standard 1-mg dose of dexamethasone; however, this almost completely suppresses cortisol levels in normals. Yehuda, Boisoneau, Lowy, and Giller (1995) used a lower dose (.5 mg), which results in more modest cortisol suppression. Results have supported their hypothesis; PTSD patients showed greater suppression of cortisol in response to dexamethasone than did controls, even in patients with comorbid major depression (Goenjian et al., 1996; Heim et al., 1998; Yehuda, Boisoneau, Lowy, & Giller, 1995).

### 2. Change in Catecholamine and Cortisol Levels in Response to Reminiscent Stimuli

A number of studies have demonstrated that victims of traumatic stress with PTSD demonstrate significantly greater physiological reactivity to stimuli reminiscent of the precipitating stressor than do victims without PTSD (Blanchard et al., 1996; Blanchard, Kolb, & Gerardi, 1986; Pitman, Orr, Forgue, de Jong, & Claiborn, 1987). After viewing a combat film, war veterans with PTSD exhibited greater increases in distress, blood pressure, heart rate, and plasma EPI than controls (McFall et al., 1990). Similarly, veterans with PTSD exposed to reminiscent auditory stimuli had greater heart rate and NE increases that combat veterans without PTSD (Blanchard et al., 1991). These studies suggest that, in victims with PTSD, cues present during exposure to the traumatic stressor may become conditioned to the physiological arousal associated with the stressor such that the cues may come to elicit hyperarousal on their own. Interestingly, these responses do not seem to habituate over time and with repeated exposures, and behavioral sensitization may actually occur.

### 3. Summary

Overall, findings of studies examining neuroendocrine levels of victims of traumatic or disaster stress are consistent with immune findings. Chronically stressed individuals exhibit heightened levels of catecholamines and cortisol relative to controls. However, the pattern of neuroendocrine response to trauma appears to differ if the victim meets PTSD criteria. Whereas chronic stress is associated with heightened catecholamine and cortisol levels, PTSD is associated with elevated catecholamines, but *lower* cortisol levels, apparently due to enhanced sensitivity of the negative feedback loop of the HPA axis. It is difficult to determine whether this enhanced sensitivity is a consequence of PTSD, or whether abnormalities in the HPA axis predispose individuals exposed to traumatic stress to develop PTSD. Overall, PTSD appears to be characterized by heightened catecholamine and attenuated cortisol levels at baseline, and exaggerated catecholaminergic and cortisol responses to acute stress.

## II. CONCLUSIONS AND FUTURE DIRECTIONS

Although several studies have considered the physiological responses to a number of naturalistic and laboratory stressors, relatively few have examined the effects of extreme naturally occurring stress on neuroendocrine and immune activity in humans. Those studies that have examined the psychophysiological sequelae of traumatic stress have differed on a number of dimensions including assessment time (amount of time since traumatic stressor occurred), demographic profiles (studies have typically examined either male veterans or female assault victims without examining gender differences in response to the same stressor), and historical variables (history of previous traumatic stress experience or previous psychopathology). Chronically stressed victims typically exhibited heightened catecholamine and cortisol levels and immunosuppression. On the other hand, some studies of PTSD patients suggest they exhibit heightened catecholamines, lower resting cortisol levels, and greater cellular immunity than similarly exposed, non-PTSD patients. These results are not consistently reported, and examination of a variety of traumatic events across different victim populations is necessary to further explain them.

A number of mechanistic questions also persist, and the complex interrelatedness of physiological processes require concurrent measurement of different physiological systems. The timing of physiological changes following traumatic and disaster stress is unknown. Acute-phase psychophysiological responding to traumatic events may differ from more chronic responses. This has been suggested by pseudoprospective studies of disasters in which immune activity is increased in acute-phase responding, but decreased during chronic distress. In addition, chronic PTSD has been associated with altered HPA axis functioning and consequent lower cortisol levels. At which point does acute responding become chronic, and at what point does enhanced HPA feedback sensitivity develop in PTSD? A diagnosis of PTSD requires a 1-month duration of symptomatology, but at what point do neuroendocrine and immune abnormalities appear? Further, are these changes due to the traumatic experience or are some individuals predisposed to respond in a certain fashion to traumatic events? Prospective examination of immune changes from the time of the event could answer a number of these questions. Understanding the relationship between extreme stress and physiological responses will then lead to a greater understanding of the stress–neuroendocrine–immune–health link.

# References

Ader, R., & Cohen, N. (1975). Behaviorally conditioned immuno-suppression. *Psychosomatic Medicine, 37*, 333–340.

Bachen, E. A., Manuck, S. B., Cohen, S., Muldoon, M. F., Raible, R., Herbert, T. B., & Rabin, B. S. (1995). Adrenergic blockade ameliorates cellular immune responses to mental stress in humans. *Psychosomatic Medicine, 57*, 366–372.

Balow, J. E., Hurley, D. L., & Fauci, A. S. (1975). Immunosuppressive effects of glucocorticosteroids: Differential effects of acute vs chronic administration on cell-mediated immunity. *The Journal of Immunology, 114*, 1072–1076.

Baum, A. (1987). Toxins, technology, and natural disasters. In G. B., VandenBos, & B. K. Bryant (Eds.), *Cataclyzms, crises, and catatrophes: Psychology in actrion* (pp. 7–53). Washington, DC: American Psychological Association.

Baum, A. (1990). Stress, intrusive imagery, and chronic distress. *Health Psychology, 9*, 653–675.

Baum, A., Cohen, L., & Hall, M. (1993). Control and intrusive memories as possible determinants of chronic stress. *Psychosomatic Medicine, 55*, 274–286.

Baum, A., Gatchel, R. J., & Schaeffer, M. A. (1983). Emotional, behavioral, and physiological effects of chronic stress at Three Mile Island. *Journal of Consulting and Clinical Psychology, 51*, 565–572.

Baum, A., O'Keefe, M. K., & Davidson, L. M. (1990). Acute stresors and chronic response: The case of traumatic stress. *Journal of Applied Social Psychology, 20*, 1643–1654.

Baum, A., Schaeffer, M. A., Lake, C. R., Fleming, R., & Collins, D. L. (1986). Psychological and endocrinological correlates of chronic stress at Three Mile Island. In R. William (Ed.), *Perspectives on Behavioral Medicine* (pp. 201–217). New York: Academic Press.

Benschop, R. J., Nieuwenhuis, E. E., Tromp, E. A., Godaert, G. L., Ballieux, R. E., & van Doornen, L. J. (1994). Effects of beta-adrenergic blockade on immunologic and cardiovascular changes induced by mental stress. *Circulation, 89*, 762–769.

Benschop, R. J., Rodriguez-Feuerhahn, M., & Schedlowski, M. (1996). Catecholamine-induced leukocytosis: Early observations, current research, and future directions. *Brain, Behavior, and Immunity, 10*, 77–91.

Benschop, R. J., Schedlowski, M., Wienecke, H., Jacobs, R., & Schmidt, R. E. (1997). Adrenergic control of natural killer cell circulation and adhesion. *Brain, Behavior, and Immunity, 11*, 321–332.

Blanchard, E. B., Hickling, E. J., Buckley, T. C., Taylor, A. E., Vollmer, A., & Loos, W. R. (1996). Psychophysiology of posttraumatic stress disorder related to motor vehicle accidents: Replication and extension. *Journal of Consulting and Clinical Psychology, 64*, 742–751.

Blanchard, E. B., Kolb, L. C., & Gerardi, R. J. (1986). Cardiac response to relevant stimuli as an adjunctive tool for diagnosing post traumatic stress disorder in Vietnam veterans. *Behavior Therapy, 17*, 592–606.

Blanchard, E. B., Kolb, L. C., Prins, A., Gates, S., & McCoy, G. C. (1991). Changes in plasma norepinephrine to combat-related stimuli among Vietnam veterans with post traumatic stress disorder. *Journal of Nervous and Mental Disease, 179*, 371–373.

Boscarino, J. A., & Chang, J. C. (1999). Higher abnormal leukocyte and lymphocyte counts 20 years after exposure to severe stress: Research and clinical implications. *Psychosomatic Medicine, 61*, 378–386.

Boyce, W. T., Chesterman, E. A., Martin, N., Folkman, S. Cohen, F., & Wara, D. (1993). Immunologic changes occurring at kindergarten entry predict respiratory illnesses after the Loma Prieta earthquake. *Journal of Developmental and Behavioral Pediatrics, 14*(5), 296–303.

Breslau, N., Davis, G. C., Andreski, P., & Peterson, E. (1991). Traumatic events and posttraumatic stress disorder in an urban population of young adults. *Archives of General Psychiatry, 48*(3), 216–222.

Burges Watson, I. P., Muller, H. K., Jones, I. H., & Bradley, A. J. (1993). Cell-mediated immunity in combat veterans with post-traumatic stress disorder. *Medical Journal of Australia, 159*, 513–516.

Calabrese, J. R., Kling, M. A., & Gold, P. W. (1987). Alterations in immunocompetence during stress, bereavement, and depression: Focus on neuroendocrine regulation. *American Journal of Psychiatry, 144*, 1123–1134.

Carlson, S. L., Brooks, W. H., Roszman, T. L. (1989). Neurotransmitter-lymphocyte interactions: Dual receptor modulation of lymphocyte proliferation and cAMP production. *Journal of Neuroimmunology, 24*, 155–162.

Crary, B., Borysenko, M., Sutherland, D. C., Kutz, I., Borysenko, J. Z., & Benson, H. (1983a). Decrease in mitogen responsiveness of mononuclear cells from peripheral blood after epinephrine administration in humans. *Journal of Immunology, 130*, 694–697.

Crary, B., Hauser, S. L., Borysenko, M., Kutz, I., Hoban, C., Ault, K. A., Weiner, H. L., & Benson, H. (1983b). Epinephrine-induced changes in the distribution of lymphocyte subsets in peripheral blood of humans. *Journal of Immunology, 131*, 1178–1181.

Cupps, T. R., & Fauci, A. S. (1982). Corticosteroid-mediated immunoregulation in man. *Immunological Reviews, 65*, 133–155.

Davidson, J. R., Hughes, D., Blazer, D. G., & George, L. K. (1991). Post-traumatic stress disorder in the community: An epidemiological study. *Psychological Medicine, 21*, 713–721.

Delahanty, D. L., Dougall, A. L., Browning, L. J., Hyman, K. B., & Baum, A. (1998). Duration of stressor and natural killer cell activity. *Psychology and Health, 13*, 1121–1134.

Delahanty, D. L., Dougall, A. L., Craig, K. J., Jenkins, F. J., & Baum, A. (1997). Chronic stress and natural killer cell activity after exposure to traumatic death. *Psychosomatic Medicine, 59*, 467–476.

Delahanty, D. L., Dougall, A. L., Hawken, L., Trakowski, J. H., Schmitz, J., Jenkins, F. J. & Baum, A. (1996). Time course of natural killer cell activity and lymphocyte proliferation in response to two acute stressors in healthy men. *Health Psychology, 15*, 48–55.

Delahunt, J. W., & Mellsop, G. (1987). Hormone changes in stress. *Stress Medicine, 3*, 123–134.

Esterling, B. A., Kiecolt-Glaser, J. K., Bodnar, J. C., & Glaser, R. (1994). Chronic stress, social support, and persistent alterations in the natural killer cell response to cytokines in older adults. *Health Psychology, 13*, 291–298.

Friedman, M. J. (1991). Biological approaches to the diagnosis and treatment of post-traumatic stress disorder. *Journal of Traumatic Stress, 4*, 67–89.

Goenjian, A. K., Yehuda, R., Pynoos, R. S., Steinberg, A. M., Tashjian, M., Yang, R. K., Najarian, L. M., & Fairbanks, L. A. (1996). Basal cortisol, dexamethasone suppression of cortisol, and MHPG in adolescents after the 1988 earthquake in Armenia. *American Journal of Psychiatry, 153*, 929–934.

Heim, C., Ehlert, U., Hanker, J. P., & Hellhammer, D. H. (1998). Abuse-related posttraumatic stress disorder and alterations of the hypothalamic-pituitary-adrenal axis in women with chronic pelvic pain. *Psychosomatic Medicine, 60*, 309–318.

Helzer, J. E., Robins, L. N., & McEvoy, F. (1987). Post-traumatic stress disorder in the general population: Findings of the Epidemiologic Catchment Area Survey. *New England Journal of Medicine, 317*, 1630–1634.

Ironson, G., Balbin, E., Steffan, P., Cruess, D., Baum, A., Schneiderman, N., & Fletcher, M. A. (1998, November). Changes in PTSD symptoms, intrusive thoughts, and natural killer cell cytotoxicity longitudinally after hurricane. In C. C. Benight (Chair), *The immunologic effects of traumatic stress: A public health issue*. Symposium conducted at the 14th annual meeting of the International Society for Traumatic Stress Studies, Washington, DC.

Ironson, G., Wynings, C., Schneiderman, N., Baum, A., Rodriguez, M., Greenwood, D., Benight, C. C., Antoni, M., LaPerriere, A., Huang, H., Klimas, N., & Fletcher, M. A. (1997). Posttraumatic stress symptoms, intrusive thoughts, loss, and immune function after Hurricane Andrew. *Psychosomatic Medicine, 59*, 128–141.

Irwin, M., Daniels, M., Smith, T. L., Bloom, E., & Weiner, H. (1987). Impaired natural killer cell activity during bereavement. *Brain, Behavior, and Immunity, 1*, 98–104.

Jetschmann, J. U., Benschop, R. J., Jacobs, R., Kemper, A., Oberbeck, R., Schmidt, R. E., & Schedlowski, M. (1997). Expression and in-vivo modulation of alpha- and beta-adrenoceptors on human natural killer (CD16+) cells. *Journal of Neuroimmunology, 74*, 159–164.

Kennedy, S., Kiecolt-Glaser, J. K., & Glaser, R. (1988). Immunological consequences of acute and chronic stressors: Mediating role of interpersonal relationships. *British Journal of Medical Psychology, 61*, 77–85.

Kessler, R., Sonnega, A., Bromet, E., & Nelson, C. B. (1995). Posttraumatic stress disorder in the National Comorbidity Survey. *Archives of General Psychiatry, 52*, 1048–1060.

Kiecolt-Glaser, J. K., Dura, J. R., Speicher, C. E., Trask, J., & Glaser, R. (1991). Spousal caregivers of dementia victims: Longitudinal changes in immunity and health. *Psychosomatic Medicine, 53*, 345–362.

Kiecolt-Glaser, J. K., Fisher, L., Ogrocki, P., Stout, J. C., Speicher, C. E., & Glaser, R. (1987a). Marital quality, marital disruption, and immune function, *Psychosomatic Medicine, 49*, 13–34.

Kiecolt-Glaser, J. K., Glaser, R., Dyer, C., Shuttleworth, E. C., Ogrocki, P., & Speicher, C. E. (1987b). Chronic stress and immunity in family caregivers of Alzheimer's disease victims. *Psychosomatic Medicine, 49*, 523–535.

Kosten, T. R., Mason, J. W., Giller, E. L., Ostroff, R. B., & Harkness, L. (1987). Sustained urinary norepinephrine and epinephrine elevation in post-traumatic stress disorder. *Psychoneuroendocrinology, 12*, 13–20.

Krystal, J. H., Kosten, T. R., Southwick, S., Mason, J. W., Perry, B. D., & Giller, E. L. (1989). Neurobiological aspects of PTSD: Review of clinical and preclinical studies. *Behavior Therapy, 20*, 177–198.

Laudenslager, M. L., Aasal, R., Adler, L., Berger, C. L., Montgomery, P. T., Sandberg, E., Wahlberg, L. J., Wilkins, R. T., Zweig, L., & Reite, M. L. (1998). Elevated cytotoxicity in combat veterans with long-term post-traumatic stress disorder: Preliminary observations. *Brain, Behavior, and Immunity, 12*, 74–79.

Lemieux, A. M., & Coe, C. L. (1995). Abuse-related posttraumatic stress disorder: Evidence for chronic neuroendocrine activation in women. *Psychosomatic Medicine, 57*, 105–115.

Mason, J. W., Giller, E. L., Kosten, T. R., Ostroff, R. B., & Harkness, L. (1986). Urinary free-cortisol levels in post-traumatic stress disorder patients. *Journal of Nervous and Mental Disease, 174*, 145–159.

Mason, J. W., Kosten, T. R., Southwick, S. M., & Giller, E. L. (1990). The use of pscyhoendocrine strategies in post-traumatic stress disorder. *Journal of Applied Social Psychology, 20*, 1822–1846.

Matthews, K. A., Gump, B. B., Block, D. R., & Allen, M. T. (1997). Does background stress heighten or dampen children's cardio-

vascular responses to acute stress? *Psychosomatic Medicine, 59*(5), 488–496.

McFall, M., Murburg, M., Ko, G., & Veith, R. C. (1990). Autonomic response to stress in Vietnam combat veterans with post-traumatic stress disorder. *Biological Psychiatry, 27*, 1165–1175.

McKinnon, W., Weisse, C. S., Reynolds, C. P., Bowles, C. A., & Baum, A. (1989). Chronic stress, leukocyte subpopulations, and humoral response to latent viruses. *Health Psychology, 8*(4), 389–402.

Mosnaim, A. D., Wolf, M. E., Maturana, P., Mosnaim, G., Puente, J., Kucuk, O., & Gilman-Sachs, A. (1993). In vitro studies of natural killer cell activity in post traumatic stress disorder patients. Response to methionine-enkephalin challenge. *Immunopharmacology, 25*, 107–116.

Naliboff, B., Benton, D., Solomon, G., Morley, J., Fahey, J., Bloom, E., Makinodan, T., & Gilmore, S. (1991). Immunological changes in young and old adults during brief laboratory stress. *Psychosomatic Medicine, 53*, 121–132.

O'Leary, A. Savard, J., & Miller, S. M. (1996). Psychoneuroimmunology: Elucidating the process. *Current Opinion in Psychiatry, 9*, 427–432.

Orr, S. P. (1994). An overview of psychophysiological studies of PTSD. *PTSD Research Quarterly, 5*, 1–7.

Pitman, R., & Orr, S. (1990). Twenty-four hour urinary cortisol and catecholamine excretion in combat-related posttraumatic stress disorder. *Biological Psychiatry, 27*, 245–247.

Pitman, R. K., Orr, S. P., Forgue, D. F., de Jong, J., & Claiborn, J. M. (1987). Psychophysiologic assessment of posttraumatic stress disorder imagery in Vietnam combat veterans. *Archives of General Psychiatry, 44*, 970–975.

Raggatt, P. T. F., & Morrissey, S. A. (1997). A field study of stress and fatigue in long-distance bus drivers. *Behavioral Medicine, 23*, 122–129.

Resnick, H. S., Yehuda, R., Pitman, R. K., & Foy, D. W. (1995). Effect of previous trauma on acute plasma cortisol level following rape. *American Journal of Psychiatry, 152*, 1675–1677.

Rubin, R. T., Miller, R. G., Clark, B. R., Poland, R. E., & Arthur, R. J. (1970). The stress of aircraft carrier landings. II. 3-Methoxy-4-hydroxyphenylglycol excretion in naval aviators. *Psychosomatic Medicine, 32*, 589–597.

Schaeffer, M. A., & Baum, A. (1984). Adrenal cortical response to stress at Three Mile Island. *Psychosomatic Medicine, 46*(3), 227–237.

Schedlowski, M., Jacobs, R., Alker, J., Prohl, F., Stratmann, G., Richter, S., Hadicke, A., Wagner, T. O. F., Schmidt, R. E., & Tewes, U. (1993a). Psychophysiological, neuroendocrine and cellular immune reactions under psychological stress. *Neuropsychobiology, 28*, 87–90.

Schedlowski, M., Jacobs, R., Stratmann, G., Richter, S., Hadicke, A., Tewes, U., Wagner, T. O. R., & Schmidt, R. E. (1993b). Changes of natural killer cells during acute psychological stress. *Journal of Clinical Immunology, 13*, 119–126.

Segerstrom, S. C., Solomon, G. F., Kemeny, M. E., & Fahey, J. L. (1998). Relationship of worry to immune sequelae of the Northridge earthquake. *Journal of Behavioral Medicine, 21*, 433–450.

Solomon, G. F., Segerstrom, S. C., Grohr, P., Kemeny, M., & Fahey, J. (1997). Shaking up immunity: Psychological and immunological changes after a natural disaster. *Psychosomatic Medicine, 59*, 114–127.

Southwick, S. M., Bremner, D., Krystal, J. H., & Charney, D. S. (1994). Psychobiologic research in post-traumatic stress disorder. *Psychiatric Clinics of North America, 17*, 251–264.

Southwick, S. M., Krystal, J. H., Morgan, A. C., Johnson, D., Nagy, L., Nicolaou, A. Heninger, G. R., & Charney, D. S. (1993). Abnormal noradrenergic function in post-traumatic stress disorder. *Archives of General Psychiatry, 50,* 266–274.

Southwick, S. M., Yehuda, R., & Wang, S. (1998). Neuroendocrine alterations in posttraumatic stress disorder. *Psychiatric Annals, 28*(8), 436–442.

Tonnesen, E., Christensen, N. J., & Brinklov, M. M. (1987). Natural killer cell activity during cortisol and adrenaline infusion in healthy volunteers. *European Journal of Clinical Investigation, 17,* 497–503.

van der Kolk, B. A. (1996). The body keeps the score: Approaches to the psychobiology of posttraumatic stress disorder. In B. A., van der Kolk, A. C. McFarlane & L. Weisarth (Eds.), *Traumatic stress.* (pp. 214–241). New York: The Guilford Press.

Van Tits, L. J., Michel, M. C., Grosse-Wilde, H., Happel, M., Eigler, F. W., Soliman, A., & Brodde, O. E. (1990). Catecholamines increase lymphocyte beta 2-adrendergic receptors via a beta 2-adrenergic spleen-dependent process. *American Journal of Physiology, 258,* E191–E202.

Wang, T., Delahanty, D. L., Dougall, A. L., & Baum, A. (1998). Responses of natural killer cell activity to acute laboratory stressors at different times of day. *Health Psychology, 17,* 428–435.

Yehuda, R., Boisoneau, D., Mason, J. W., & Giller, E. L. (1993). Glucocorticoid receptor number and cortisol excretion in mood, anxiety, and psychotic disorders. *Biological Psychiatry, 34,* 18–25.

Yehuda, R., Boisoneau, D., Lowy, M. T., & Giller, E. L. (1995). Dose-response changes in plasma cortisol and lymphocyte glucocorticoid receptors following dexamethasone administration in combat veterans with and without posttraumatic stress disorder. *Archives of General Psychiatry, 52,* 583–593.

Yehuda, R., Giller, E. L., Levengood, R. A., Southwick, S. M., & Siever, L. J. (1995). Hypothalamic-pituitary-adrenal functioning in post-traumatic stress disorder. In M. J. Friedman, D. S. Charney, & A. Y. Deutch (Eds.), *Neurobiological and clinical consequences of stress: From normal adaptation to PTSD* (pp. 351–365). Philadelphia: Lippincott-Raven.

Yehuda, R., Kahana, B., Binder-Brynes, K., Southwick, S. M., Mason, J. W., & Giller, E. L. (1995). Low urinary cortisol excretion in Holocaust survivors with posttraumatic stress disorder. *American Journal of Psychiatry, 152,* 982–986.

Yehuda, R., Lowy, M. T., Southwick, S. M., Shaffer, D., & Giller, E. L. (1991). Lymphocyte glucocorticoid receptor number in posttraumatic stress disorder. *American Journal of Psychiatry, 148,* 499–504.

Yehuda, R., Resnick, H., Kahana, B., & Giller, E. L. (1993). Long-lasting hormonal alterations to extreme stress in humans: Normative or maladaptive? *Psychosomatic Medicine, 55,* 287–297.

Yehuda, R., Southwick, S., Giller, E. L., Ma, X., & Mason, J. W. (1992). Urinary catecholamine excretion and severity of PTSD symptons in Vietnam combat veterans. *The Journal of Nervous and Mental Disease, 180* (5), 321–325.

Yehuda, R., Southwick, S. M., Krystal, J. H., Bremner, D., Charney, D. S., & Mason, J. W. (1993). Enhanced suppression of cortisol following dexamethasone administration in posttraumatic stress disorder. *American Journal of Psychiatry, 150,* 83–86.

Yehuda, R., Southwick, S. M., Nussbaum, G., Giller, E. L., & Mason, J. W. (1990). Low urinary cortisol excretion in PTSD. *Journal of Nervous and Mental Disorders, 178,* 366–369.

# PSYCHONEUROIMMUNOLOGY
# AND PATHOPHYSIOLOGY

CHAPTER

# 47

# Impact of Brain Injury on Immune Function

ELISABETH TARKOWSKI

Although there exists within the central nervous system (CNS) an immunosuppressive microenvironment, acute, subacute, and chronic brain injuries may elicit a local inflammatory response. In addition, brain injuries may have an impact on the systemic immune responsiveness. The aim of this chapter is to describe changes in local and systemic immune responses following different types of brain injury, such as acute brain contusion, stroke, tumor, and dementia. In addition, the influence of such changes on the pathophysiology of the brain damage will be discussed.

## I. IMPACT OF BRAIN INJURY ON LOCALIZED INFLAMMATORY RESPONSES

Previously, the brain was considered to be an immunologically privileged site. The brain-blood barrier, with tight junctions between endothelial cells, and the presence of a basement membrane lined by astrocyte feet provided separation between the circulating cells and molecules of the immune system on the one hand and the brain tissues on the other. The lack of lymphatic vessels and the paucity of constitutive expression of major histocompatibility complex (MHC) class I and II molecules in brain tissues lent further support to this hypothesis. However, this concept has now been revised because of the existence of structures with functions similar to those of lymphatic vessels (Prineas, 1979), and evidence has emerged for the existence of lymphocyte trafficking within brain tissue (Hickey, 1991). Furthermore, brain resident cells such as microglia and astrocytes are now considered to play a key role in the immune system of the CNS. The microglia cells, a class of specialized brain mononuclear phagocytes, are distinct from either blood monocytes, spleen macrophages or resident peritoneal macrophages (Giulian, 1987). They are as numerous as neurons and are dispersed throughout the nervous system, being found in the mature brain in a resting, highly ramified state and interacting with neighboring cells. They respond almost instantaneously (within minutes) to disturbances in their microenvironment and become activated. Microglia activation involves changes in shape, enhanced expression of MHC, proliferation, homing to the site of injury, and functional changes, e.g., the release of cytotoxic and inflammatory mediators. Subsequently, activated microglia may transform into phagocytic cells (Gehrmann, Matsumoto, & Kreutzberg, 1995). In addition, activated microglia secrete growth factors (Giulian, 1987) that stimulate the proliferation of astrocytes, which are also among the first cells to respond to CNS injury. The reactive astrocytes become larger, extending thicker and longer processes, and contain an increased amount of glial fibrillary acidic protein, an astrocyte specific intermediary filament (Yong, 1996). By hypertrophy and, to a lesser extent, by proliferation, reactive astrocytes build a gliotic scar. Both astrocytes and microglia exhibit the ability to express MHC molecules when exposed to various cytokines (Fierz, Endler, Reske, Wekerle, & Fontana, 1985; Wong, Bartlett, Clark-Lewis, Battye, & Schrader, 1984) such as interferon-$\gamma$ (IFN-$\gamma$) and tumor necrosis factor-$\alpha$ (TNF-$\alpha$) and, following exposure, to act as antigen-presenting cells for T lymphocytes. Moreover, brain resident cells such as neurons (Ringheim, Burgher, Heroux, 1995; Sawada, Itoh, Suzumura, & Marunouchi, 1993), astrocytes, and microglia have been demonstrated to produce molecules displaying inflammatory properties, e.g., the cytokines interleukin (IL)-1, TNF-$\alpha$, and IL-6 (Frei et al., 1989; Giulian, Baker, Shih, & Lachman, 1986; Lieberman, Pitha, Shin, & Shin, 1989), and to express cytokine receptors. Thus, the prerequisites for defining the brain as an lymphoid organ with immune function are fulfilled.

Supporting this idea of the brain as a site of immunological activity, antigen-specific immune responses in response to infection in the brain have been demonstrated. Furthermore, immune response to brain-specific autoantigens may be elicited and causes an autoimmune response leading to tissue damage and disease. In addition, a growing body of evidence points to the development of inflammatory responses in brain tissues in response to primarily "non-immune" neuronal insult such as brain trauma, stroke, tumor formation, and degenerative processes.

## A. Effect of Experimental Acute Brain Damage on Local Inflammation

Experimental brain injury leads to localized upregulation in production of cytokines such as IL-1$\beta$ (Giulian, & Lachman, 1985; Gourin, & Shackford, 1997), IL-6 (Qu Yan et al., 1992; Woodroofe et al., 1991), TNF (Fan et al., 1996; Gourin, & Shackford, 1997; Holmin et al., 1997; Rostworowski, Balasingam, Chabot, Owens, & Yong, 1997; Taupin, Toulmond, Serrano, Benavides, & Zavala, 1993), and chemokines (Ghirnikar, Lee, He, & Eng, 1996) and to increased expression of cytokine receptors. Cytokines and chemokines contribute to the development of inflam-

mation by stimulating endothelial cells to express adhesion molecules allowing influx and accumulation of leukocytes in the damaged brain tissue (Bevilacqua, Pober, Wheeler, Cotran, & Gimbrone, 1985). Cytokines can also directly affect resident cells in the brain. For example, IL-1, IL-6, and TNF-$\alpha$ induce proliferation of astrocytes (Giulian, & Lachman, 1985; Selmaj, Farooq, Norton, Raine, & Brosnan, 1990) and granulocyte-macrophage colony-stimulating factor (GM-CSF) proliferation of microglia (Giulian, Li, Li, George, & Rutecki, 1994; Lee, Liu, Brosnan, & Dickson, 1994), resulting in the triggering of scar formation with gliosis.

In experimental animal models, cell adhesion molecules such as E-selectin and the intracellular adhesion molecule 1 (ICAM-1), the expression of which is a prerequisite for the influx of leukocytes, are upregulated early on after focal ischemia (Schroeter, Jander, Witte, & Stoll, 1994; Wang, Yue, Barone, & Feuerstein, 1995) and traumatic brain injury (Shibayama, Kuchiwaki, Inao, Yoshida, & Ito, 1996) in rats. Within a few hours of occlusion of the middle cerebral artery and subsequent ischemic brain damage, neutrophils and T lymphocytes accumulation have been observed in the vicinity of the lesion (Schroeter et al., 1994). Subsequently, macrophages invade the damaged brain tissue (Hallenbeck & Dutka, 1990; Kochanek & Hallenbeck, 1992; Schroeter et al., 1994). In contrast, in the rodent model of brain contusion, neutrophils are relatively few in evidence and the cellular inflammatory reaction consists mostly of activated macrophages, CD4- and CD8-expressing T 'cells, and natural killer cells (Holmin, Mathiesen, Shetye, & Biberfeld, 1995). Activation of astrocytes (Clark et al., 1993) and MHC class II-positive microglial cells (Finsen, Jörgensen, Diemer, & Zimmer, 1993; Gehrmann, Bonnekoh, Miyazawa, Hossmann, & Kreutzberg, 1992; Postler, Lehr, Schluesener, Meyermann, 1997) is also observed within the first few days after the onset of stroke or brain contusion (Holmin et al., 1995), providing the prerequisite for an immunological response.

The influx of inflammatory cells might aggravate brain damage by (a) plugging the surrounding capillaries, (b) producing toxic oxygen radicals and enzymes leading to membrane damage, (c) triggering edema and tissue destruction, and (d) increasing the tendency to develop thrombosis in the surrounding blood vessels (Hallenbeck & Dutka, 1990; Kochanek & Hallenbeck, 1992). Treatment modalities, affecting the inflammatory response in experimental animal models of focal ischemia can lead to a reduction of infarct size. For example, the use of cytolytic antibodies specific for neutrophil leukocytes leads to a decreased accumulation of neutrophils (Kochanek & Hallenbeck, 1992), decreased brain edema (Shiga et al., 1991), increased blood flow in the damaged brain area (Kochanek & Hallenbeck, 1992), reduced size of the brain infarct, and decreased neurological deficit (Kochanek & Hallenbeck, 1992). Interaction with ICAM-1, expressing cells has a similar effect, reducing inflammation and brain damage (Connolly et al., 1996). In this regard, ICAM-1-deficient mice showed a threefold increase in blood flow in the infarcted hemisphere, a fourfold reduction in infarct volume, a 35% increase in survival and reduced neurologic deficit compared with wild-type controls (Connolly et al., 1996). Finally, treatment with transforming growth factor-$\beta$ (TGF-$\beta$) and with IL-1 receptor antagonist (IL-1ra), two compounds with immuno-suppressive properties, had beneficial effects in experimental animal models of stroke with reduction in infarct size (Gross et al., 1994; Relton & Rothwell, 1992) or in animal models of fluid percussion injury by inhibiting neuronal damage (Toulmond & Rothwell, 1995).

Interestingly, certain proinflammatory cytokines display protective properties when provided to the CNS. For example, IL-1$\beta$ exhibits neuroprotective effects in ischemia-induced neuronal damage (Brenneman, Schultzberg, Bartfai, & Gozes, 1992). IL-6 acts as a nerve growth factor, being able to induce differentiation of neurites (Satoh et al., 1988). In addition, intracerebral IL-6 exerts neuroprotective properties during permanent focal cerebral ischemia in the rat (Loddick, 1998). Interestingly, TNF-$\alpha$, a powerful cytokine inducing apoptosis in the extra-neural compartments of the body, has been demonstrated to protect rat hippocampal, septal and cortical cells against metabolic–excitotoxic insults (Cheng, Christakos, & Mattson, 1994) and to facilitate regeneration of injured axons (Schwartz et al., 1991). In vitro studies have demonstrated that TNF-$\alpha$ may exert its neuroprotective effect by stimulating the production of a neuroprotective, calcium-binding protein, calbindin, by astrocytes (Mattson et al., 1995). Taken together, these findings argue for an important role for cytokines in the development of inflammation, astroglial scarring, and possibly neuronal plasticity in the brain.

## B. Effect of Acute Brain Damage on Local Inflammation in Humans

In contrast to the abundance of information that exists regarding experimental acute brain damage, scant information is available in the human context. Holmin (1997) has demonstrated the presence of inflammatory cells in acutely contused human brain tissue biopsies, a pattern of inflammatory responses similar to that seen in experimental rodent models. In order to avoid artifacts due to postmortem studies, contused brain tissue biopsies were obtained from 12 patients who were operated on between 3 h and 5 days following brain trauma and analyzed by im-munohistochemistry (Holmin, 1997). Patients under-going brain surgery within 24 h of trauma showed a clear intravascular accumulation of polymorpho-nuclear leukocytes and moderate intravascular de-posits of lymphocytes and monocytes/macrophages. Regions affected by polymorphonuclear leukocyte extravasation showed neuronal damage. The brains of patients operated between 3 and 5 days following trauma showed a strong parenchymal inflammatory response dominated by mononuclear phagocytes but comprising also polymorphonuclear leukocytes and lymphocytes. This delayed parenchymal inflamma-tory reaction has also been described in rodent models of acute brain damage. However, rodent brain tissue was mainly invaded by mononuclear cells during the delayed inflammatory reaction, while the human brain parenchyma contained a sizeable fraction of polymorphonuclear leukocytes. In patients operated on within 24 h of brain trauma, most of the microglia showed intact morphology, whereas in patients operated on 3 to 5 days later, a high density of reactive microglia cells was detected expressing MHC class II. In addition, increased levels of com-plement factors (Kossman, Stahel, Morganti-Koss-mann, Jones, & Barnum, 1997a), inflammatory cyto-kines such as IL-1$\beta$, IL-6, IL-8, and TNF-$\alpha$, and of the anti-inflammatory cytokine IL-10 have been demon-strated in the cerebrospinal fluid (CSF) of patients following a severe head injury (Bell et al., 1997; Goodman, Robertson, Grossman, & Narayan, 1990; Kossman et al., 1997b; McClain, Cohen, Ott, Dinarello, & Young, 1987; Ross, Halliday, Campell, Byrnes, & Rowlands, 1994). Interestingly, the CSF levels of the nerve growth factor (NGF) are also elevated after traumatic brain injury and these levels can be correlated to the levels of IL-6 and IL-8 (Kossman et al., 1997a, b). Moreover, the CSF of patients contain-ing high levels of IL-6 induced in vitro NGF production by astrocytes, whereas control CSF with-out IL-6 had no effect. The induction of NGF was completely abolish by adding anti-IL-6 antibodies (Koss-mann, Hans, Imhof, Trentz, & Morganti-Kossmann, 1996).

We have recently studied the potential role of inflammatory mechanisms in the pathophysiology of

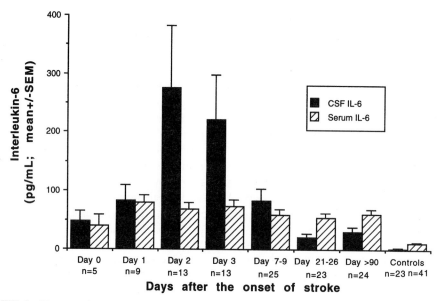

**FIGURE 1**   Kinetics of IL-6 production in cerebrospinal fluid and serum in patients with acute stroke.

ischemic brain damage by analyzing patterns of cytokine release in CSF as a consequence of acute stroke (Tarkowski et al., 1995c, 1997) and by relating cytokine levels to infarct volume, clinical outcome, and intrathecal levels of proteins regulating apoptosis. Significantly increased ($p < .001$) levels of IL-6 in the CSF of stroke patients were observed in virtually all cases studied compared to that seen in healthy controls. These increases were observed during the whole observation period, but were significantly more pronounced within the first days after stroke onset with a peak level on days 2 and 3 (Figure 1). This initial increase was significantly correlated ($r = .65$; $p = .002$) with the volume of infarct measured by magnetic resonance imaging 1 to 2 months later. Serum levels of IL-6 in stroke patients were significantly lower than IL-6 levels in CSF ($p = .013$) and did not display any significant correlation to the size of the brain lesion, suggesting an intrathecal production of IL-6 (Figure 1). Significantly increased CSF levels of IL-1$\beta$, IL-8, GM-CSF, and IL-10 were also observed early during a stroke, with a peak on day 2 for the proinflammatory cytokines IL-1$\beta$, IL-8, and GM-CSF, and on day 3 for the immunoregulatory cytokine IL-10. The levels of TNF-$\alpha$ in CSF of stroke patients did not differ significantly from the TNF-$\alpha$ levels in CSF from healthy controls. However, a high level of intrathecal TNF-$\alpha$ was associated with the occurrence of white matter disease. These studies demonstrate an intrathecal production of proinflammatory and immunoregulatory cytokines in patients with stroke, supporting the notion of localized immune response to the acute brain lesion. In addition, the significant correlation between early intrathecal

production of IL-6 and the subsequent size of the brain lesion in stroke can be used as a prognostic tool for predicting the extent of brain damage before it is possible to accurately visualize it via radiological methods.

IL-1$\beta$, one of the proinflammatory cytokines, is produced intrathecally early after the onset of a stroke and stimulates the production of nitric oxide, a potent mediator of inflammation. We have assessed the intrathecal levels of nitrate, one of the main metabolites of nitric oxide, in acute stroke and related these levels to brain damage in 14 stroke patients followed prospectively on days 0–3, 7–9, and 21–26 and after day 90. Analyses of nitrate were performed by the gas chromatography/mass spectrometry technique. Intrathecal levels of nitrate increased significantly 3 months after the onset of stroke compared with the first 3 days (Tarkowski et al., 2000). Interestingly, the levels of nitrate measured at the onset of a stroke were negatively correlated to the final size of infarct volume measured by MRI. In contrast, the intrathecal levels of nitrate were significantly positively correlated to the neurological deficit and negatively correlated to levels of soluble bcl-2, a protein downregulating neuronal apoptosis, in the late stage of a stroke (unpublished results). Thus, the early nitric oxide production in stroke is associated with a decreased infarct volume, suggesting a protective effect, whereas the late nitric oxide production is associated with more severe neurological deficit, suggesting a neurotoxic effect. Therapeutic regimens which modulate nitric oxide production in stroke should take into consideration the dual effects of nitric oxide on ischemic brain damage.

The neuronal death that accompanies an ischemic stroke has previously been attributed to a necrotic process. However, numerous studies in experimental models of ischemia have recently indicated that programmed cell death, also called apoptosis, may contribute to neuronal death. Cytokines are known to modulate apoptosis. In this respect, Holmin (1997) demonstrated that injection of IL-$\beta$ into rat brains elicited massive nuclear DNA fragmentation (i.e. apoptosis) within 24 h whereas intracerebral injection of TNF-$\alpha$ did not. The IL-1$\beta$ mediated apoptosis was mostly confined to neuronal cells but also applied to invading inflammatory cells. On the other hand, the presence of apoptotic cells is known to modulate the production of cytokines by immunocompetent cells. In this respect, Voll has demonstrated that the presence of apoptotic cells increases the secretion of IL-10 and decreases the secretion of TNF-$\alpha$ by monocytes (Voll, Hermann, Roth, Stach, & Kalden, 1997). Since pro- and anti-inflammatory cytokine production in stroke patients is upregulated, we wanted to determine the intrathecal levels of proteins regulating apoptosis. Analysis of CSF levels of soluble (s)Fas/APO-1 and soluble (s)bcl-2, two proteins downregulating apoptosis was performed at defined time intervals following onset of stroke. Significantly decreased CSF levels of sFas/APO-1 were observed during the whole observation period with a maximal decrease on day 21 after the onset of stroke (Figure 2) (Tarkowski et al., 1998, 1999). The intrathecal levels of sFas/APO-1 were significantly inversely correlated to the volume of brain infarct and to the neurological deficit 3 months after the onset of a stroke. In addition, the intrathecal levels of sFas/APO-1 were

significantly correlated to the levels of IL-1$\beta$, IL-6, IL-10, and GM-CSF 3 weeks after the onset of the disease. Also, the intrathecal levels of sbcl-2 were significantly decreased during the three first days after a stroke debut and, at the same time, positively and significantly correlated to the levels of IL-6 and TNF-$\alpha$ (Tarkowski et al., 1998, 1999). These data suggest that patients with acute stroke display locally a propensity toward apoptosis and imply that factors regulating apoptosis may lead to decreased severity of brain damage in stroke.

## C. Effect of Subacute Brain Damage on Local Inflammation

Primary malignant brain tumors such as glioblastomas elicit an inflammatory response including the influx of lymphocytes and macrophages to the brain tissues surrounding the tumor (Giometto et al., 1996; Sawamura & de Tribolet, 1990; Wood & Morantz, 1979). T lymphocytes (predominantly cytotoxic and suppressor cells) have recently been identified as the major constituent of tumor-infiltrating lymphocytes (Kuppner, Hamou, & de Tribolet, 1988; Sawamura & de Tribolet 1990). However, macrophages, natural killer cells, and B lymphocytes are also found, especially at the tumor periphery. The number of tumor-infiltrating lymphocytes isolated from gliomas is low compared to the number found in metastatic brain tumors or compared to non-CNS tumors (Marioka, Baba, Black, & Streit, 1992). In addition, T cells infiltrating the tumor tissues have been found to be partly anergic (Kuppner, Hamou, Sawamura, Bodmer, & de Tribolet, 1989). These T cells also exhibit a reduced proliferative response to mitogenic and allogeneic stimuli and display low levels of cytolytic activity in comparison with autologous peripheral blood lymphocytes (Bodmer, Siepl, & Fontana, 1989). Similarly, monocytes infiltrating gliomas exhibit decreased expression of MHC class II and decreased production of cytokines such as TNF-$\alpha$, IL-1$\beta$ and IL-10 (Woiciechowsky et al., 1998a). Interestingly, a new immunoregulatory molecule was found in the supernatant of human glioblastoma cells (reviewed by Bodmer et al., 1989). This factor could inhibit the response of mouse thymocytes to concanavalin A and to phytohemagglutinin and inhibit the generation of cytotoxic T cells in a mixed lymphocyte culture. This factor was shown to be a member of the transforming growth factor-$\beta$ (TGF-$\beta$) gene family, structurally identical to TGF-$\beta_2$ (reviewed by Bodmer et al., 1989). Neutralizing experiments with a polyclonal neutralizing antibody to TGF-$\beta$ could completely abolish the inhibitory effect

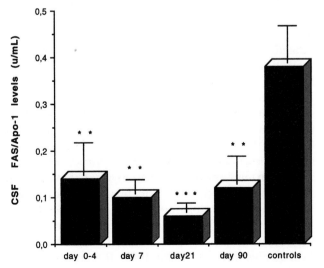

**FIGURE 2**   Kinetics of sFas/APO-1 appearence in cerebrospinal fluid of patients with acute stroke. **$p < .001$; *** $p > .0001$.

of crude supernatant from the glioblastoma cell line on T cell functions. Messenger RNA (mRNA) expression from the TGF-$\beta$ gene has been demonstrated in several glioma cell lines (Yamanaka, Tanaka, Saitoh, & Okoshi, 1994) and in tissues excised from malignant gliomas (Merlo et al., 1993). Elevated TGF-$\beta$ levels were also found in the CSF of patients with malignant gliomas (Tada, Yabu, & Kobayashi, 1993; Weller et al., 1998). In addition, recent studies have demonstrated mRNA expression from the gene of another immunosuppressive cytokine, IL-10, in human gliomas (Huettner, Paulus, & Roggendorf, 1995; Nitta, Hishii, Sato, & Okumura, 1994). IL-10 is an inhibitory cytokine produced by the Th2 subset and downregulates inflammation mediated by the Th1 subset of T-lymphocytes and macrophages (Mossman, 1994). IL-10 has been shown to inhibit the production of IFN-$\gamma$, IL-1$\alpha$, IL-1$\beta$, IL-6, IL-8, granulocyte colony-stimulating factor (G-CSF), and GM-CSF by activated monocytes. IL-10 also inhibits production of TNF-$\alpha$ by both astrocytes and microglial cells, suggesting an important regulatory role for this cytokine within the central nervous system (Frei, Lins, Schwerdel, & Fontana, 1994; Benveniste, Tang, & Law, 1995). Furthermore, IL-10 reduces the antigen (Ag)-specific proliferation of human T cells by diminishing the Ag-presenting capacity of monocytes via downregulation of MHC class II on these cells (Howard & O'Garra, 1992). Human glioma-derived IL-10 inhibits anti-tumoral immune responses in vitro (Hishii et al., 1995). Importantly, several groups (Huettner et al., 1995; Nitta et al., 1994) demonstrated that the levels of IL-10 mRNA expression were significantly higher in highly malignant gliomas and recurrent cases of gliomas than in less malignant tumors. On the other hand, the mRNA transcripts of the proinflammatory cytokines IFN-$\gamma$, IL-6, and GM-CSF were more frequently expressed by tumors from less malignant gliomas (Nitta et al., 1994). In summary, cytokines, which may be directly or indirectly effective in the eradication of glioma cells, for example by stimulating an immune response against tumor cells, are mainly expressed within the less malignant glioma, while IL-10, which may impair the immune response against tumor cells, is expressed mainly within highly malignant gliomas.

## D. Effects of Chronic Brain Damage on Local Inflammation

Recently, it become apparent that chronic brain damage due to neurodegenerative brain diseases such as dementia leads to inflammatory response in the brain. The role of this local inflammation for the pathogenesis of dementias has become the subject of intense investigations.

Dementia is characterized by progressive loss of memory and higher cortical functions. However, dementia is a heterogeneous state caused by a number of different syndromes. Alzheimer's disease and vascular dementia are the two main causes of dementia affecting between 25 and 45% and 15 and 35%, respectively, of all demented patients (Rossor, 1992).

Alzheimer's disease is characterized by atrophy of the brain subsequent to loss of neurons, a decrease in the arborization of the dendrites, and the presence of neurofibrillary tangles and senile plaques. A protein consisting of 42–43 amino acids, with a high tendency to aggregate, called $\beta$-amyloid protein, has been identified as the major component of the senile plaques. $\beta$-Amyloid protein is derived from a 90 to 140-kDa precursor, called amyloid precursor protein, as reviewed by Banati & Beyreuther (1995). Pathological changes in the brain of Alzheimer's disease patients are accompanied by a local inflammatory response. For example, an increased expression of adhesion molecules such as ICAM-1 on the cerebral endothelial cells (Frohman, Frohman, Gupta, de Fougerolles, & van der Noort, 1991) and an increased number of CD4+- and CD8+-T lymphocytes are present in the brain tissue of patients with Alzheimer's disease (McGeer, Akiyama, Itagaki, & McGeer, 1989). In addition, reactive microglial cells have been demonstrated to express MHC class-II molecules and Fc receptors (McGeer, Itagaki, Tago, McGeer, 1987). Thus, all the appropriate components necessary for an immune response are present locally in the brains of patients with Alzheimer's disease. Both activated microglia and T lymphocytes can additionally be a source of cytokine production as reviewed by St. Pierre, Merrill, & Dopp (1996). Indeed, IL-1, IL-2, IL-3, and IL-6 were detected in brain tissues of Alzheimer's disease cases (Araujo & Lapchap, 1994; Bauer et al., 1992; Griffin et al., 1989). These cytokines could be involved in the pathogenesis of Alzheimer's disease, e.g., by promoting inflammatory responses as proposed by Vandenabeele and Fiers (1991). IL-1 has been demonstrated to enhance the synthesis of $\beta$-amyloid protein precursor mRNA in human endothelial cells (Goldgaber et al., 1989), suggesting a direct role for this cytokine in the formation of senile plaque. However, cytokines such as IL-1 and IL-6 also display neuroprotective properties (Brenneman et al., 1992; Hama, Miyamoto, Tsukui, Nishio, & Hatanaka, 1989). IL-6 may stimulate astrocytes to produce nerve growth factor (NGF) and act independently as neurotrophic factor in synergy with NGF (Frei et al., 1989). IL-6 can also induce neuronal differentiation (Satoh et al., 1988). Interestingly, TNF-$\alpha$, a powerful cytokine inducing apoptosis in the extraneural compartments of the body, has been demonstrated to protect rat hippocampal, septal, and cortical cells against metabolic–excitotoxic insults (Cheng et al., 1994) and to facilitate regeneration of injured axons (Schwartz et al., 1991). More importantly, TNF-$\alpha$ and $\beta$ protect neurons against $\beta$-amyloid protein-triggered toxicity (Barger et al., 1995).

In order to study the involvement of proinflammatory cytokines in dementias, we have investigated the intrathecal pattern of proinflammatory cytokine release, by measuring the CSF levels of IL-1$\beta$, IL-6, IL-8, GM-CSF, IFN-$\gamma$, TNF-$\alpha$, and the naturally occurring antagonists of TNF-$\alpha$, soluble TNF receptors I and II. Patients with both Alzheimer's disease and vascular dementia displayed significantly higher intrathecal levels of TNF-$\alpha$ than controls. In addition, patients with Alzheimer's disease showed significantly negative correlations between the intrathecal levels of TNF-$\alpha$ and the levels of sFas/APO-1 as well as of Tau protein. The level of sbcl-2 in the supernatants of TNF-$\alpha$-exposed cultures of human neuronal cells approached three times higher the levels detected in control supernatants. These results suggest that TNF-$\alpha$ may have a neuroprotective role in these neurodegenerative conditions as evidenced by negative correlations between TNF-$\alpha$ and (i) levels of intrathecal Fas/APO-1 and (ii) levels of Tau protein, both of the parameters closely related to brain damage. The in vitro data cited above provide evidence that TNF-$\alpha$ exerts its neuroprotective effect by stimulating neuronal cells to express bcl-2, a molecule which downregulates apoptosis.

An important component of the local inflammation in the brain is the proliferation and the activation of glial cells. Microglia proliferation is observed as an early and long-lasting pathological change in the brains of patients with Alzheimer's disease (Banati & Beyreuther, 1995). Microgliosis is associated with most senile plaques (Itagaki, McGeer, Akiyama, Zhu, & Selkoe, 1989; Mattiace, Davies, Yen, & Dickson, 1990). Furthermore, microglia in Alzheimer's disease have phenotypic features consistent with a state of activation, such as expression of MHC class II (McGeer et al., 1987) and adhesion molecule leukocyte function antigen 1 (Frohman et al., 1991). Activated microglia may thus contribute to the brain tissue damage seen in Alzheimer's disease. The cellular activation of the glial cells is accompanied by an upregulation of amyloid precursor protein expression (Wisniewski, Vorbrodt, Viegel, Morys, & Lossinsky, 1990), possibly

leading to $\beta$-amyloid accumulation, in the chronic stage of the disease. Microglia can also act as cytotoxic effector cells by releasing harmful substances such as proteases, reactive oxygen intermediates, and nitric oxide (Gerhmann et al., 1995) and thereby mediate neuronal cell injury (Chao, Hu, Molitor, Shaskan, & Peterson, 1992). We have recently demonstrated an intrathecal production of GM-CSF, a cytokine stimulating microglial cell growth and exerting inflammatogenic properties, in patients with early Alzheimer's disease and in patients with vascular dementia (unpublished results). Interestingly, there was a highly significant correlation between the levels of GM-CSF and the levels of Fas/APO-1 and between the levels of GM-CSF and the levels of Tau protein in patients with Alzheimer's disease. It is suggested that secreted GM-CSF induces programmed cell death in the brain tissue of patients with dementia.

CSF levels of the other proinflammatory cytokines studied, such as IL-1$\beta$, IL-6, IL-8, and IFN-$\gamma$ are not significantly altered in any of the dementia groups (Tarkowski, unpublished results). However, other studies show conflicting results. Studies by Bessler, Sirota, Hart, and Djadetti (1989) and Pirtilla, Mehta, Frey, and Wisniewski (1994) confirm that IL-1$\beta$ levels, are not elevated in the CSF of demented patients. Similarly, Yamada (1995) showed no increase in intrathecal IL-6 levels in patients with Alzheimer's disease. In contrast, the studies achieved by Blom-Degen et al. (1995) and Cacabelos et al. (1991) demonstrated increased CSF levels of IL-1$\beta$ and IL-6. A possible explanation for these conflicting results is that the three former studies, in analogy with our study, compared patients with Alzheimer's disease with age-matched healthy controls whereas the two latter studies compared patients with Alzheimer's disease with patients with other neurological diseases as controls. It is not possible to exclude a potential impact of other neurological diseases on intrathecal cytokine production.

Interestingly, the CSF levels of the anti-inflammatory cytokines such as IL-4, IL-10 and TGF-$\beta$ were not significantly more elevated in patients with dementia as compared with healthy age-matched controls (unpublished results). The lack of intrathecal IL-4 production, a cytokine able to downregulate astrocyte activation (St. Pierre et al., 1996), may lead to a long-lasting astrocyte reactivity and thus to the high levels of GM-CSF in the brain. In analogy, no detectable CSF levels of IL-10 and TGF-$\beta$ in patients with Alzheimer's disease were found. These two cytokines are able to downregulate microglial activation (Frei et al., 1994; St. Pierre et al., 1996; Benveniste et al., 1995).

These findings could explain why chronic microglial activation is observed in brains of patients with Alzheimer's disease (Banati, & Beyreuter, 1995). In contrast, the microglial activation is time limited after an ischemic brain lesion (Clark et al., 1993). In this respect, we have previously demonstrated (Tarkowski et al., 1997) intrathecal production of IL-10 in stroke patients occurring early after the onset of the disease and lasting throughout the whole observation period (3 months). Thus, one can hypothesize that secretion of IL-10 may counteract the effects of GM-CSF on microglial cells in stroke patients, inhibiting the glial activation, whereas the deficient production of this immunoregulating cytokine in Alzheimer's disease could lead to a chronic microglial proliferation and thereby increased tissue damage.

## II. EFFECT OF BRAIN INJURY ON SYSTEMIC IMMUNE RESPONSES

### A. Animal Models

Experimental studies of neuro-immune interactions have utilized stereotactic lesions of the CNS with subsequent testing of a variety of immune parameters. Stein, Schiavi, and Camerino (1976), Cross, Markesbery, Brooks, and Roszman (1980); Cross, Brooks, Roszman, and Markesbery (1982); Brooks, Cross, Roszman, and Markesbery (1982); Roszman, Cross, Brooks, and Markesbery (1982) have demonstrated that lesions in the preoptic area of the anterior hypothalamus resulted in a decrease in splenocyte and thymocyte numbers and an inhibition of lymphocyte proliferative responses to concanavalin A as well as decreased delayed-type hypersensitivity (DTH) responses in vivo. In a recent study, Mori et al. (1993) have shown that lesions of the anterior hypothalamus in rat decreased significantly the CD4-/CD8-T-cell ratio of peripheral blood lymphocytes and spleen cells, the number of T-cell receptor $\alpha\beta$-expressing thymocytes, and the functional activity of natural killer cells. Mori concluded that the anterior hypothalamus had some influence on the control of cellular immunological functions at the peripheral level, on maturation of T cells at the level of the thymus, and on the antigenic recognition by T cells. Lesions in the limbic system (Brooks et al., 1982; Cross, Brooks, Roszman, & Markesbery, 1982, Devi & Namasivayam, 1991), substantia nigra (Neveu, Deleplanque, Vitiello, Rouge-Pont, & Le Moal, 1992), brain stem (Jankovic & Isakovic, 1973; Kadlecova, Masek, Seifert, & Petrovicky, 1987; Masek, Kadlecova, & Petrovicky, 1983), and cerebral cortex (Neveu, 1992a; Neveu et al., 1989; Renoux, 1988; Renoux, Biziere, Bardos, & Degenne, 1987; Renoux, Biziere, Renoux, Guillaumin, & Degenne, 1983) were all shown to alter immune functions such as T lymphocyte proliferation to mitogens, DTH responses, natural killer cell activity, antibody production, and macrophage functions.

### B. Effect of Acute Brain Damage on Systemic Immune Response

#### 1. Effect of Brain Trauma on the Systemic Immune Responses

Despite progress in the management of the increased intracranial pressure, infections remain the most common complication in patients with brain injuries. The increased rate of infections is due in part to brain injury-related immunosuppression. In this respect, several studies have described decreased T-cell response early after head injury. For example, decreased amount of T cells (Massei et al., 1988), decreased proliferative response of T-cells to mitogenic stimulation (Hoyt, Ozkan, Hansbrough, Marshall, & van Berkum-Clark, 1990), diminished expression of early activation antigens such as IL-2 receptor and transferrin receptor, and late activation antigens such as HLA-DR (Hoyt et al., 1990) have been demonstrated (Hoyt et al., 1990; Massei et al., 1988; Geniez, Millet, Blanchet, Duboin, & Roquefeuil, 1983; Wolach et al., 1993; Quattrocchi et al., 1991). A decreased reactivity in the DTH skin test, suggesting a reduced cell-mediated responsiveness, has been found in head trauma patients both on admission and 20 days later. In addition, there was a significant difference in the number of deaths and episodes of sepsis between anergic and nonanergic patients with head trauma (Geniez et al., 1983). In contrast, the B-lymphocyte function seems to be unaffected by head trauma (Hoyt et al., 1990). Few studies have examined the function of polymorphonuclear leukocytes and those that have been carried out show normal oxidative burst or superoxide anion release by these cells (Hoyt et al., 1990; Wolach et al., 1993). Serum levels of proinflammatory cytokines such as IL-1, IL-6, TNF-$\alpha$, and IL-8 are found to be elevated in humans following head trauma (Bell et al., 1997; McClain et al., 1987; Morganti-Kossmann et al., 1997; Ott, McClain, Gillespie, & Young, 1994; Ross et al., 1994). It has been speculated (Ott et al., 1994) that these cytokines may play a role in metabolic dysfunction and organ failure following head trauma.

## 2. Early Impact of Stroke on Systemic Immune Responses

### a. T- and B-lymphocyte Responses in Acute Stroke

In analogy with patients with head injury, the occurrence of infections is common in stroke patients and may be, in part, due to impaired cell-mediated immunity. Infections are associated with poor outcome in affected patients and constitute the most common cause of death in the subacute phase of stroke (Oppenheimer & Hachinski, 1992). Moreover, the fever which accompanies about 44% of acute stroke cases is in most circumstances due to infection (Oppenheimer & Hachinski, 1992) and also has a negative effect on the clinical outcome. In this respect, Czlonkowska, Cyrta, and Korlak (1979) reported decreased cell-mediated immunity such as decreased blastogenesis, production of the leucocyte migration inhibition factor, and depression of the DTH skin reactivity in the acute phase of stroke. These changes were more evident in patients with severe brain lesions and with high mortality. In addition, all the patients with fatal outcome had clinical signs of bronchopulmonary or/and urinary tract infection.

We also studied the impact of the early stroke on the systemic T-cell response and cytokine production. To analyze the effect of the acute phase of a stroke on the in vitro T-cell reactivity, the responses of peripheral blood mononuclear cells to mitogens and antigens were studied. We observed decreased T-cell proliferative responses to these compounds during the first week after the onset of stroke. In agreement with these results, production of IFN-$\gamma$, a cytokine originating from activated T-cells, in the supernatants from antigen stimulated lymphocytes, was significantly decreased early during the stroke. Moreover, 80 stroke patients were simultaneously tested for DTH response both in the affected side of the body and in the contralateral side. The number of stroke patients exhibiting no DTH response increased successively during the first week after onset of the stroke only to show a decrease after day eight, suggesting an early but profound inhibition of T-cell mediated in vivo responses.

### b. Systemic Cytokine Production in Acute Stroke

In a recent study we showed that the IL-6 levels in serum were significantly higher in stroke patients than in controls during the entire observation period starting on the day of commencement of the stroke and lasting 3 months ( Figure 1 ) (Tarkowski et al., 1995c). However, in contrast to IL-6 levels in the CSF, the stroke patients did not display any distinct time-related variation of the IL-6 levels in serum ( Figure 1).

No significant correlation was found between the serum levels of IL-6 and the volume of the brain infarct. The serum levels of IL-1$\beta$ and IFN-$\gamma$ did not differ significantly from those of controls. These results are in accordance with other studies which found elevated serum levels of IL-6 but not IL-1$\beta$ or TNF-$\alpha$ already within the first hours following the onset of stroke symptoms (Beamer, Coull, Clark, Hazel, & Silberger, 1995; Fassbender et al., 1994a; Kim, Yoon, Kim, & Ryu, 1996). In addition, a systemic increase of IL-8 mRNA-expressing blood polymorphonuclear leukocytes and augmented IL-8 levels in plasma have been demonstrated in patients with ischemic stroke, suggesting that this cytokine could be involved in blood polymorphonuclear leukocytes recruitment to the sites of cerebral ischemia (Kostulas et al., 1998). The serum levels of the anti-inflammatory cytokine, IL-1ra, were also significantly increased in stroke patients as compared to controls (Beamer et al., 1995) whereas the levels of another anti-inflammatory cytokine, TGF-$\beta$, was significantly decreased on days one and three after the onset of stroke (Kim et al., 1996).

## C. Effect of Subacute Brain Damage on Systemic Immune Response

Brain tumor patients demonstrate a general depression of cell-mediated immunity measured by (i) their response to common skin test antigens (Brooks, Netsky, Normansell, & Horwitz, 1972; Brooks, Roszman, & Rogers, 1976; Mahaley et al., 1977) and (ii) a general reduction in both quantity and function of circulating T cells (Brooks et al., 1976, 1981; Kebudi et al., 1995; Roszman, & Brooks, 1980; Young, Sakalas, Kaplan, 1976). One of the possible mechanisms contributing to the decreased T-cell function is a defective IL-2 secretion coupled with a defective expression of high affinity IL-2 receptor chains observed in patients with gliomas (Roszman, Elliott, & Brooks, 1991). These patients also demonstrate an impairment of serological responses to active immunization with tetanus and influenza vaccine (Mahaley et al., 1977; Wickstrand & Bigner, 1980). In addition, Urbani, Maleci, La Sala, Lande, and Ausiello (1995) reported a failure of peripheral blood mononuclear cells from patients with glioma to produce IFN-$\gamma$ upon mitogenic or antigenic stimulation as a result of defective mRNA expression. Defective expression of GM-CSF, TNF-$\alpha$, and IL-6 mRNAs was also observed in activated peripheral blood mononuclear cells of patients with gliomas as well as a decreased production of these cytokines by these cells (Urbani et al., 1995). Interestingly, the immunosuppression observed in glioma patients is partially relieved by the surgical removal of the tumor (Roszman, Brooks, Steele, & Elliot, 1985; Roszman et al., 1991; Woiciechowsky et al., 1998a). These studies support the hypothesis that cellular and biochemical dysfunctions appear to be related to the occurrence of immunosuppressive mediators such as TGF-$\beta$ and IL-10 (see effect of subacute brain damage on local inflammation) produced by glioma cells.

## D. Effect of Chronic Brain Damage on Systemic Immune Response

### 1. Late Impact of Stroke on Systemic Immune Responses

To assess if healing of brain lesion affects systemic immune responses, stroke patients in the early phase of the stroke were tested for their DTH responses and retested in an identical way in the chronic phase of the stroke. All of the patients displayed significantly enhanced DTH responses during the chronic phase of the disease compared to the early phase (Tarkowski, Blomstrand, & Tarkowski, 1995b). In contrast, healthy controls displayed no significant changes in DTH responses between the first and the second challenge. Furthermore, chronic stroke patients showed significantly more frequent positive DTH responses than age-matched healthy controls. Increased DTH responses may indicate a systemic upregulation of T-lymphocyte activity in the chronic phase of the stroke since the prerequisite for such a response is the ability for antigen-specific memory cells to recognize antigen, become activated, proliferate, and produce cytokines. A possible upregulation either in antigen presenting cell function or in effector cell function might even contribute to increased DTH responses. However, there was also a good correlation between the in vivo and in vitro reactivities to the immunogen used for DTH. Consequently, peripheral blood mononuclear cells in 50% of stroke patients but only in 20% of matched controls showed antigen-specific proliferative responses in vitro, indicating increased T-cell function in these patients (Tarkowski, Ekelund, & Tarkowski, 1991b). In contrast, immunization of stroke patients and controls with influenza vaccine, a T-cell-dependent B-cell antigen, raised similar antigen-specific serum IgG, IgA, and IgM antibody responses in both study groups (Tarkowski et al., 1991b). These results suggest that stroke enhances systemic T-lymphocyte responses in the chronic phase of the disease and that systemic B-lymphocyte responses are not affected by stroke.

The systemic upregulation of the immune responsiveness in chronic phase of stroke could be mediated by changes in hormonal status in these patients due to the long-lasting intrathecal cytokine production that occur after the onset of stroke (Tarkowski et al., 1995c, 1997). In this respect, IL-6 stimulates the hypothalamus-pituitary to produce adrenocorticotropin (ACTH), leading to an increased production of corticosteroids in the blood. Åström, Olsson, & Asplund (1993) have reported that 22% of stroke patients have pathological dexamethasone test with high postdexamethasone cortisol levels 3 years after stroke. These high cortisol levels were associated with presence of major mental depression late after stroke. Since increased activity in hypothalamo-pituitary-adrenocortical axis is most likely to be associated with decreased immune responsiveness, it cannot explain the in vivo and in vitro enhancement of T-cell reactivity found in the chronic phase of stroke. However, other hormones secreted by the pituitary gland have been reported to upregulate immune responsiveness. In this respect, both growth hormone and prolactin have been reported to enhance T-lymphocyte growth as reviewed by Carr (1992). Interestingly, IL-6 has been reported to induce release of prolactin from rat pituitary cells (Spangelo et al., 1989; Yamaguchi et al., 1990). Thus, the high IL-6 levels that we observed in the CSF of stroke patients in the chronic phase of the disease could stimulate the pituitary gland to prolactin release. To our knowledge very little is known about the hormonal status of patients in the chronic phase of stroke. It should be tested if increased T-cell reactivity in chronic stroke is associated with increased production of this hormone.

### 2. Impact of Chronic Neurodegenerative Diseases on the Systemic Immune Responses

Previous studies have shown conflicting results regarding T-cell counts and proliferative response to mitogens and antigens (Hu, Walls, Creasey, McCusker, & Broe, 1995; MacDonald, Golstone, Morris, Exton-Smith, & Callard, 1982; Miller, Neighbour, Katzman, Aronson, & Lipkowitz, 1981; Shalit, Sredni, Brodie, Kott, & Huberman, 1995; Singh, Fudenberg, & Brown, 1987), T-cell suppressor activity (Miller et al., 1981; Skias, Bania, Reder, Luchins, & Antel, 1985), and B-lymphocyte function including antibody production (Mayer, Chughtai, & Cape, 1976; McDonald et al., 1982; Miller et al., 1981) in patients with Alzheimer's disease. Decreased DTH response to skin antigens has been reported in patients with Alzheimer's disease compared to age-matched controls (Torack & Gebel, 1982). A possible explanation to these conflicting results is the heterogeneity of patients with

Alzheimer's disease. This group may include Alzheimer patients both with early disease onset and with late onset (Blennow & Wallin, 1992; Wallin, Blennow, & Scheltens, 1994). It is also difficult to delineate patients with pure Alzheimer's disease and patients with vascular dementia (Jellinger, 1996; Kosunen et al., 1996). These different syndromes may influence immune responses in different ways. Furthermore, Shalit et al. (1995) have shown that the immune responses may vary with the duration of the disease. Also, the age of the probants is of importance since it influences the immune responses (Fillit, Meyer, & Bona, 1992). All these variables are not properly defined in most of the studies on impact of dementia on immune responses.

We have extensively studied the cytokine levels in the sera of patients with early Alzheimer's disease, patients with vascular dementia and healthy age-matched controls. The serum levels of the proinflammatory cytokines, IL-6, IL-8, and GM-CSF and those of the anti-inflammatory cytokine TGF-$\beta$ were significantly increased in both groups of demented patients compared to that seen in controls (unpublished results). In contrast, the serum levels of some other proinflammatory cytokines including IL-1$\beta$, TNF-$\alpha$, and IFN-$\gamma$ and anti-inflammatory cytokines IL-4 and IL-10 did not differ between the different groups studied. Similarly, Singh et al. (1987) found increased serum levels of IL-6 but not IL-12, IFN-$\gamma$, and IFN-$\alpha$ in patients with Alzheimer's disease. No difference in serum levels of IL-1$\beta$, IL-6, and IL-2 and in the capacity of peripheral blood mononuclear cells to produce IL-1 and IL-2 was found between patients with Alzheimer's disease and controls (Bessler et al., 1989; Blum-Degen et al., 1995; Pirttila et al., 1994).

## III. LATERALIZATION OF DTH IN STROKE PATIENTS

Besides the effects of stroke on the systemic immune responses, Thompson and Bywaters (1962) reported a sparing effect of paresis due to stroke on arthritis. Surprisingly, Mizushima and Yamamura (1969) demonstrated that in 34 stroke patients DTH induced swelling and induration was more intense on the paretic side than on the contralateral one, in spite of decreased tissue clearance of phenolsulfophthalein from the skin on the paretic side compared to that seen on the contralateral one. In an experimental rat model of adjuvant arthritis, central paresis after unilateral spinal cord injury exacerbated the course of arthritis on the paretic side compared to that on the

contralateral one, whereas peripheral paresis due to unilateral section of the sciatic nerve had a protective effect against arthritis ipsilaterally (Courtright & Kusell, 1965).

In order to study the impact of lesions in the CNS on the lateralization of T-cell-mediated and neurogenic cutaneous inflammatory responses, we have evaluated antigen-specific cutaneous response on both sides of the body in patients with stroke. Assessment of electrically evoked axon reflex vasodilatation was simultaneously used to test for cutaneous sympathetic activity. It was found that DTH responses differed significantly in size on the affected side compared to the contralateral side. Several clinical features including duration of stroke, its course and presence of motor deficit were associated with the lateralisation of DTH responses.

It was shown that: (i) Early stroke leads to lateralization of the DTH responses depending of the course of the disease: minor stroke is associated with smaller DTH on the paretic side than that seen in the contralateral side, whereas major stroke is associated with larger DTH (Figure 3). (ii) Chronic stroke leads to lateralization of DTH responses with enhanced reactivity on the paretic side compared to that seen on the contralateral one. (iii) Patients with minor stroke exhibit a significant shift in lateralization of DTH between the early phase and the chronic phase of the disease (Tarkowski et al., 1995a, b).

It was also demonstrated that: (i) Motor deficit is required for a lateralization of DTH responses in the early phase of the stroke (Tarkowski et al., 1995a). (ii) Initial motor deficit is associated with a significant shift in DTH responses between the early and the

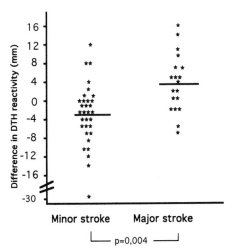

**FIGURE 3**   Differences in DTH responses with regard to clinical outcome of stroke (minor versus major). The horizontal bars represent the mean in each group.

chronic phase of the stroke (Tarkowski et al., 1995b). (iii) motor deficit but not sensory deficit is associated with lateralization of DTH in the chronic phase of the stroke (Tarkowski et al., 1991a).

Patients with early stroke were simultaneously analyzed with respect to side asymmetries of axon reflex vasodilatation and DTH reactivity. A significant correlation ($r = .64$; $p < .0001$) was found between side asymmetries of DTH responses and side asymmetries of axon reflexes in a sympathicus innervated skin area (Figure 4A). Thus, a more intense axon reflex vasodilatation on the paretic side was related to a larger DTH reaction on the ipsilateral side and conversely. Such a relationship was absent in skin areas where cutaneous sympathetic activity had been blocked by regional anesthesia (Figure 4B). These results suggest that the lateralization of cutaneous inflammation in early stroke may be mediated by sympathetic dysfunction (Tarkowski et al., 1995a).

We conclude that stroke lateralizes T-cell-mediated cutaneous inflammation. This effect depends on (1) the duration of the disease, (2) the clinical course of the disease, and (3) the presence of motor deficit and (4) may be mediated by an alteration in the cutaneous sympathetic nerve traffic.

## IV. IMPACT OF THE LOCALIZATION OF BRAIN DAMAGE ON LOCAL AND SYSTEMIC IMMUNE RESPONSE

Despite ample evidence that the central nervous system communicates with the immune system, the specific areas of the CNS that are involved in this interaction are not well characterized in humans. Experimental animals studies of neuro–immune interactions have utilized stereotaxic lesions of the CNS with subsequent testing of a variety of immune parameters. Localization of these lesions are of crucial importance for their impact on the immune responses. For example, lesions in the hypothalamus lead to a decrease in T-cell responses (Brooks et al., 1982; Cross, Markesbery, Brooks, & Roszman, 1980; Cross et al., 1982; Mori et al., 1993; Roszman et al., 1982), whereas lesions in the hippocampus lead to enhanced T-cell responses (Brooks et al., 1982).

In addition, several studies point out specialization of the right and left side of the brain with regard to the modulation of the immune responses. Renoux et al. (1983) and Neveu (1992a) have demonstrated in animal models that ablation of the left fronto-parieto-occipital cortex leads to a decrease in mitogen-induced T-cell proliferation whereas similar ablation of the right side leads to an enhancement of mitogenesis. Neveu et al. (1992b) have shown that right-sided lesions in the substantia nigra enhanced the proliferation of splenic T cells, whereas similar lesions on the left side decreased T-cell proliferation, suggesting an asymmetrical brain modulation of immune responses even at the subcortical level.

### A. Impact of the Localization of Brain Lesions on the Lateralization of DTH

In early stroke, patients with supratentorial brain lesion and minor stroke displayed significantly smaller DTH responses on the paretic side compared with the contralateral one. Among this patient group, only the patients with cortical lesions or cortical lesions involving subcortical areas but not those with isolated subcortical lesions displayed a significant lateralization of DTH responses. In contrast, patients suffering a major stroke displayed no lateralization of DTH responses, neither when the lesions were supratentorial, nor when they were infratentorial.

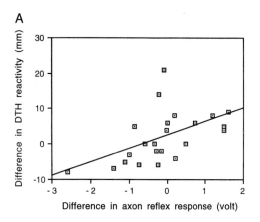

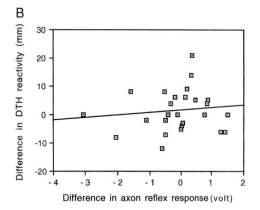

**FIGURE 4** Correlation between differences in DTH responses and in axon reflex responses between paretic and nonparetic sides in patients with stroke. The axon reflex was measured (A) without and (B) with conduction anesthesia.

Stroke patients tested in the chronic phase of the disease showed significantly larger DTH responses on the paretic side than on the contralateral side. Patients with isolated cortical or isolated subcortical brain lesions showed no lateralization of DTH responses. In contrast, patients with large lesion encompassing both the cortical and the subcortical areas exhibited significantly larger DTH responses on the paretic side compared to the contralateral side. Within this group, only patients with lesion in the frontal lobe but not in the posterior lobes displayed a significant lateralization of DTH responses (Figure 5A).

When all the patients with subcortical lesions (i.e. cortical-subcortical and isolated subcortical lesions) were analyzed, lateralization of DTH responses was noted. When analyzed separately, only patients with brain lesions involving putamen displayed a significant lateralization of DTH responses (Figure 5B). Moreover, only patients with the combined lesion of the frontal lobe and putamen but not of the posterior lobes and putamen exhibited significant lateralization of DTH responses.

Patients with lesions on the right side of the brain displayed significantly larger DTH responses on the paretic side than on the contralateral side. In contrast, patients with left-sided lesions or bilateral lesions displayed no significant lateralization of DTH responses.

These results suggest that anatomical localization of the brain lesion affects the lateralization of immune responsiveness. Only lesions in the right brain hemisphere lead to alteration of DTH reactivity, supporting an asymmetrical modulation of the immune response. In addition, the results implicate the frontal cortex and putamen as a putative brain center regulating the magnitude of immune responses (Tarkowski et al., 1998b).

## B. Impact of the Localization of Brain Damage on Systemic Immune Responses

In our studies, the systemic enhancement of DTH responses in the chronic phase of stroke compared to the early phase was associated with a major stroke and a single brain lesion. In contrast, patients with disseminated cerebrovascular disease showed no enhancement of DTH in the chronic stroke phase compared to the early phase. Moreover, in the chronic phase, the size of the DTH response was significantly larger both on the paretic and on the contralateral side in patients with a single brain lesion than in patients with multiple lesions. Patients with lesions in the frontal lobe displayed increased DTH bilaterally compared to patients with lesions in the posterior lobes. The same was true for patients with lesions in the

right hemisphere compared to patients with lesions in the left hemisphere. In conclusion, features of lesions associated with systemic upregulation of DTH response include large size, singularity and localization in the frontal lobe and in the right hemisphere. In contrast, stroke associated with small vessel disease leads to systemic downregulation of DTH responses.

These results are in accordance with those of a previous study demonstrating a relationship between the site of primary intracranial tumors and mitogenic responses of blood lymphocytes (Blomgren, Blom, & Ullen, 1986). It was shown that blood lymphocytes from non-corticosteroid-treated patients with tumors affecting the left cerebral hemisphere exhibited significantly lower proliferative responses to mitogen than those seen in controls, whereas the lymphocytes of patients with tumors in the right hemisphere did not. In addition, patients with tumors affecting central structures of the brain such as the corpus callosum, septum pellucidum and central ganglia, displayed markedly reduced antigen-specific T-cell proliferative responses.

## C. Impact of the Type, Size, and Localization of Brain Damage in Stroke on Local Immune Responsiveness

In our previous studies we have shown that levels of IL-6 and IL-8 in the CSF were in relation to the radiological findings Stroke patients with a large brain lesion displayed significantly increased $(p = .001)$ IL-6 levels in CSF early in the course of stroke (Figure 6A) compared to patients with small brain lesions. Stroke patients with a brain lesion affecting mainly (>50%) the gray matter displayed significantly higher IL-6 levels in CSF but not in serum on days 1 and 7 than stroke patients with mainly white matter lesions ( Figure 6B ). In contrast, patients with small infarct showed higher IL-8 levels than patients with large infarcts and patients with a brain infarct predominantly located (>50%) in the white matter than patients with a brain infarct predominantly located (>50%) in the gray matter (Figures 7A and 7B). These results suggest that brain infarcts elicited different patterns of local cytokine production, possibly reflecting the size and localization of the insult (Tarkowski et al., 1995c, 1997).

## V. CONCLUDING REMARKS

All the types of brain damage depicted in this review, acute, subacute, and chronic, lead to a local inflammation in the brain. This inflammation includes

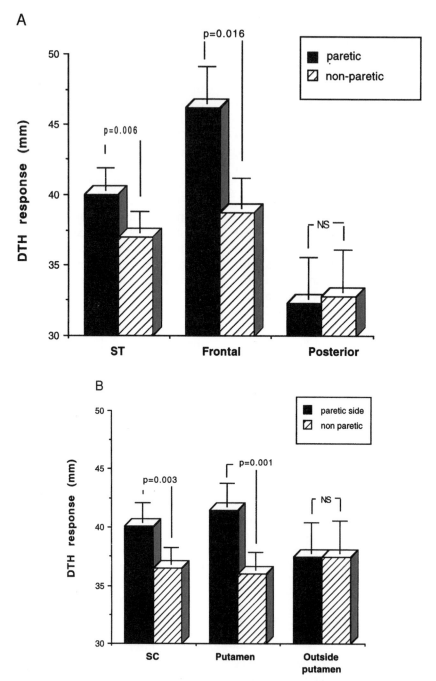

**FIGURE 5** (A) Bar graph showing the size of DTH response (mean±SEM) on the paretic and the nonparetic sides in 42 patients with supratentorial lesion (ST), 11 patients with frontal lobe lesion (frontal), and 8 patients with a posterior lobe lesion (posterior) in the chronic phase of the stroke. (B) Bar graph showing the size of DTH response (mean ± SEM) on the paretic and the nonparetic sides in 35 patients with subcortical lesion (SC), 23 patients with subcortical lesion involving putamen (putamen), and 12 patients with subcortical lesion outside putamen (outside putamen) in the chronic phase of a stroke.

activation of brain resident cells such as astrocytes and microglia, the production of cytokines (Table I) which is probably mediated by these resident brain cells in response to injury, cytokine-mediated upregulation of adhesion molecules on endothelial cells, and the entry of inflammatory leukocytes (such as activated T lymphocytes, polymorphonuclear leukocytes, and monocytes) into damaged brain tissue. As discussed in this review, these local inflammatory responses on the one hand may amplify the brain

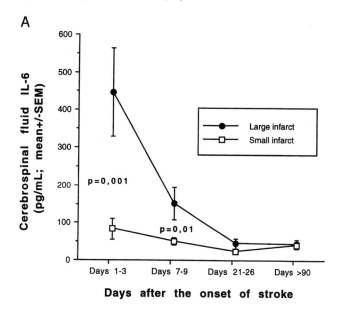

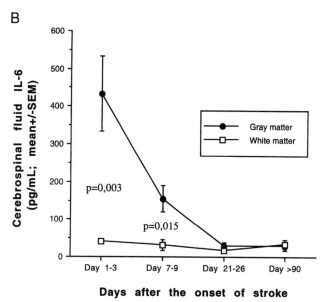

**FIGURE 6**    Kinetics of IL-6 production in cerebrospinal fluid with respect to (A) the size of the subsequent brain lesion (14 stroke patients with large infarcts and 16 stroke patients with small infarcts) and (B) gray versus white matter lesions (14 stroke patients with mainly gray matter lesions and 10 patients with mainly white matter lesions).

damage but, on the other hand, may participate in the healing process and possibly contribute to neuronal plasticity. In Figures 8A and 8B, we propose a possible flow chart of events leading to the development of inflammation and exacerbation of the ischemic brain injury in stroke but also leading to the healing process. In contrast, influx of inflammatory cells could be beneficial following other types of brain injury, such as brain tumor, by eliciting a specific immune response against tumor cells. Inhibition of such inflammatory response by production of anti-inflam-

matory cytokines by glioma cells is associated with increased degree of malignancy. The purpose of various therapeutically trials is to restore the local inflammatory responses against tumor cells (Dietrich, Walker, Saas, & de Tribolet, 1998). Thus, it is of great importance to delineate in detail the characteristics and the role of the local inflammatory responses in different types of brain lesions.

Importantly, the different types of brain injuries studied in this review also affect the systemic immune responsiveness (Tables II and III). Acute brain injuries,

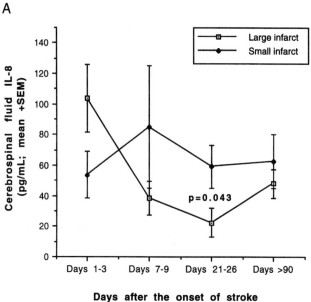

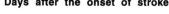

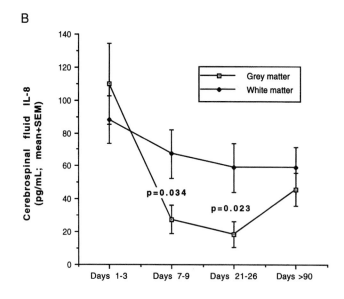

**FIGURE 7** Kinetics of IL-8 production in cerebrospinal fluid with respect to (A) the size of the subsequent brain lesion (13 stroke patients with large infarcts and 17 stroke patients with small infarcts) (pg/mL; mean ± SEM) and (B) gray versus white matter lesions (14 stroke patients with mainly gray matter lesions and 10 patients with mainly white matter lesions) (pg/mL; mean ± SEM).

such as head trauma and stroke, or subacute injuries, such as brain tumor, lead to a downregulation of T-cell-mediated immune responses. This could be due to a general stress reaction following stressful diseases. Also patients with other types of trauma such as burn injuries also display depressed T-cell responses (McIrvine, O'Mahony, Saporoschetz, & Mannick, 1982; Wolfe, Wu, & O'Connor, 1982). In this respect, Woiciechowski et al. (1998b) have

recently demonstrated that the sympathetic activation which follow brain injury may trigger systemic interleukin-10 release. Furthermore, catecholamine-induced release of the immunosuppressive cytokine IL-10 is associated with an increase in infection and sepsis among patients with acute brain injury. Woiciechowski (1998a) speculated that IL-10 could be a mediator of stress-related immunosuppression. In addition, one might discuss a possible direct and

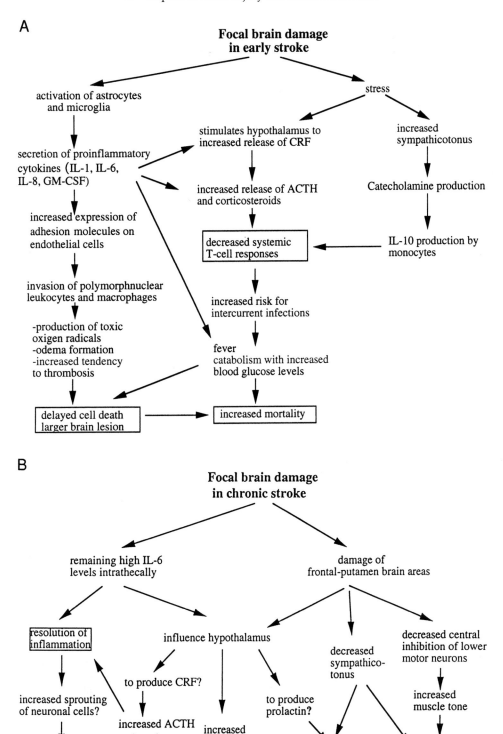

**FIGURE 8**   A hypothetical flow chart of immunological events and interactions during (A) early stroke and (B) chronic stroke.

**TABLE I  Local Cytokine Production Following Brain Injury in Humans**

| Cytokines | Head trauma | Acute stroke | Brain tumor | AD | VD |
|---|---|---|---|---|---|
| Proinflammatory cytokines | | | | | |
| IL-1$\beta$ | Increased | Increased | Increased in glioma grade I–II | Conflicting results | Unchanged |
| IL-6 | Increased | Increased | Increased in glioma grade I–II | Conflicting results | Unchanged |
| IL-8 | Increased | Increased | NA | Unchanged | Unchanged |
| GM-CSF | NA | Increased | Increased in glioma grade I–II | Increased | Increased |
| TNF-$\alpha$ | Increased | Unchanged | NA | Increased | Increased |
| IFN-$\gamma$ | NA | Unchanged | NA | Unchanged | Unchanged |
| Anti-inflammatory cytokines | | | | | |
| IL-4 | NA | NA | NA | Unchanged | Unchanged |
| IL-10 | Increased | Increased | Increased in glioma grade III–IV | Unchanged | Unchanged |
| TGF-$\beta$ | NA | NA | Increased in glioma grade III–IV | Unchanged | Unchanged |
| IL-1ra | NA | NA | NA | Decreased | NA |
| Adhesions molecule | | | | | |
| ICAM-1 | Increased | Increased | NA | Increased | NA |

*Note.* NA, not analyzed; AD, Alzheimer's disease; VD, Vascular dementia; IL, interleukin; GM-CSF, granulocyte-macrophage colony-stimulating factor; TNF, tumor necrosis factor; IFN, interferon; TGF, tumor growth factor.

specific effect of brain damage on systemic immune responses. In favor of this hypothesis is the ablation of the systemic T-cell depression by the surgical removal of brain tumors. Gliomas have been demonstrated to produce locally anti-inflammatory cytokines such as TGF-$\beta$ and IL-10. These cytokines may gain access to the peripheral blood circulation through a disrupted blood-brain barrier and influence the circulating cells of the immune system, acting as neurohormones. However, in other types of brain damage, such as stroke, head injury, or dementia, differences in the patterns of cytokines locally produced in the CSF versus systemically released to the bloodstream are observed (Tables I and III). One possible explanation is that the products of the brain damage and local inflammation may affect systemic immune responses indirectly as depicted in Figure 8A. Some cytokines, such as IL-1 and IL-6 have been shown to act synergistically on the hypothalamus-pituitary to stimulate the release of ACTH in vivo (Perlstein, Mougey, Jackson, & Neta, 1991), leading to increased secretion of corticosteroids in the blood, observed early on during stroke (Olsson et al., 1992; Fassbender, Schmidt, Mössner, Daffertshofer, & Hennerici, 1994b). Increased corticosteroid release in the early phase of stroke could lead to the downregulation of the systemic T-cell responses, as recently reported (Czlonkowska et al., 1979, Tarkowski et al., 1995). In this respect, Johansson, Olsson, Carlberg, Karlsson, and Fagerlund (1997) have demonstrated significant correlation between IL-6 levels and levels of cortisol in the sera of stroke patients. The intrathecal production of several

**TABLE II  Systemic Cytokine Production Following Brain Injury in Humans**

| Cytokines | Head trauma | Acute stroke | Brain tumor | AD | VD |
|---|---|---|---|---|---|
| Proinflammatory cytokines | | | | | |
| IL-1$\beta$ | Increased | Unchanged | NA | Conflicting results | Unchanged |
| IL-6 | Increased | Increased | Decreased production by T-cells | Increased | Increased |
| IL-8 | Increased | Increased | NA | Increased | Increased |
| GM-CSF | NA | NA | Decreased production by T-cells | Increased | Increased |
| TNF-$\alpha$ | Increased | Unchanged | Decreased production by T-cells | Unchanged | Unchanged |
| IFN-$\gamma$ | NA | Unchanged | Decreased production by T-cells | Unchanged | Unchanged |
| Anti-inflammatory cytokines | | | | | |
| IL-4 | NA | NA | NA | Unchanged | Unchanged |
| IL-10 | NA | Increased | Increased | Unchanged | Unchanged |
| TGF-$\beta$ | NA | Decreased | Increased | Increased | Increased |
| IL-1ra | NA | Increased | NA | NA | NA |

*Note.* NA, not done; AD, Alzheimer's disease; VD, vascular dementia; IL, interleukin; GM-CSF, granulocyte-macrophage colony-stimulating factor; TNF, tumor necrosis factor; IFN, interferon; TGF, tumor growth factor.

**TABLE III   Impact of Damage in the Central Nervous System on the Immune Responses**

| Immune responses | Acute brain injury | Acute stroke | Chronic stroke | Brain tumors | Dementia |
|---|---|---|---|---|---|
| Inflammation within the brain | Present | Present | Absent | Decreased | Present |
| Systemic T-cell responses | Decreased | Decreased | Increased | Decreased | Conflicting results |
| Systemic B-cell responses | Unchanged | Unchanged | Unchanged | Unchanged | Conflicting results |
| DTH | Decreased | Decreased | Increased | Decreased | Decreased |

*Note.* Delayed type hypersensitivity.

cytokines, such as IL-6, is long-lasting after the onset of stroke. As discussed in this chapter and depicted in Figure 8B , the intrathecal production of IL-6 could also influence the systemic immune responses during the chronic phase of stroke.

The localization of brain lesions in experimental animal models, in human stroke, and in tumors also has an impact on the systemic immune responses, suggesting that alterations of the systemic immune responses may also be dependent on factors other than the local inflammation occurring in the brain. For example, established stroke leading to brain lesion in the frontal lobe or the right hemisphere is associated with the systemic enhancement of DTH reactivity (Figure 8B). One possibility is that the brain insult may damage certain areas regulating immune responses or efferent nerves supplying the peripheral lymphoid tissues (Felten et al., 1987). Such lesions could affect the autonomic nervous system which mediates the information between the nervous system and the immune system (Felten et al., 1987).

Alteration of the systemic immune responses may in turn influence the outcome of brain injury ( Figure 8A ). For example, decreased immune responsiveness is probably one of the explanations for increased morbidity from infectious diseases early after the stroke (Oppenheimer and Hachinski, 1992). Moreover, fever accompanying infections worsens the brain injury as demonstrated by Ginsberg (1993). In this respect, both locally and systemically produced IL-1 and IL-6 induce fever by a direct effect on the thermoregulatory center in the hypothalamus (Rothwell & Hopkins, 1995), contributing to further cell damage and increased infarct volume. Third, increased release of corticosteroids leads to the hyperglycemia often observed in stroke, even in the absence of diabetes and being correlated with higher mortality (Oppenheimer & Hachinski, 1992).

In conclusion, knowledge about the impact of brain injuries on the local and systemic immune responses will lead to better insight into the pathophysiological mechanisms leading to brain damage and thereby to improved treatment strategies. In addition, understanding the relationship between brain injuries and changes in systemic immune responses may lead to a better insight into the role of the nervous system in the regulation of the immune system and into the cross-talk between the two systems.

## References

Araujo, D. M., & Lapchak, P. A. (1994). Induction of immune system mediators in the hippocampal formation in Alzheimer's and Parkinson's diseases: Selective effects on specific interleukins and interleukin receptors. *Neuroscience, 61*(4), 745–754.

Åström, M., Olsson, T., & Asplund, K. (1993). Different linkage of depression to hypercortisolism early versus late after stroke. A 3-year longitudinal study. *Stroke, 24*, 52–57.

Banati, R. B., & Beyreuther, K. (1995). Alzheimer's disease. In H. Kettenman & B. R. Ransom (Eds.), *Neuroglia* (pp. 1027–1043). New York, Oxford: Oxford University Press.

Barger, S. W., Hörster, D., Furukawa, K., Goodman, Y., Krieglstein, J., & Mattson, M. P. (1995). Tumor necrosis factors $\alpha$ and $\beta$ protect neurons against amyloid $\beta$-peptide toxicity: Evidence for involvement of a $\kappa$B-binding factor and attenuation of peroxide and $Ca^{2+}$ accumulation. *Proceedings of National Academy of Sciences of USA, 92*, 9328–9332.

Bauer, J., Ganter, U., Strauss, S., Stadtmuller, G., Frommberger, U., Bauer, H., Volk, B., & Berger, M. (1992). The participation of interleukin-6 in the pathogenesis of Alzheimer's disease. 45th forum in Immunology. *Research in Immunology, 143*, 650–657.

Beamer, N. B., Coull, B. M., Clark, W. M., Hazel, J. S., & Silberger J. R. (1995). Interleukin-6 and interleukin-1 receptor antagonist in acute stroke. *Annals of Neurology, 37*, 800–804.

Bell, M. J., Kochanek, P. M., Doughty, L. A., Carcillo, J, A., Adelson, P. D., Clarck, R. S., Wisniewski, S. R., Whalen, M. J., & DeKosky, S. T. (1997). Interleukin-6 and interleukin-10 in cerebrospinal fluid after severe traumatic brain injury in children. *Journal of Neurotrauma, 14*(7), 451–457.

Benveniste, E. N., Tang, L. P., & Law, R. M. (1995). Differential regulation of astrocyte TNF-$\alpha$ expression by the cytokines TGF-$\beta$, IL-6 and IL-10. *International Journal of Developmental Neuroscience, 13*, 341–349.

Bessler, H., Sirota, P., Hart, J., & Djadetti, M. (1989). Lymphokine production in patients with Alzheimer's disease. *Age and Ageing, 18*, 21–25.

Bevilacqua, M. P., Pober, J. S., Wheeler, M. E., Cotran, R. S., & Gimbrone, M. A. (1985). Interleukin-1 acts on cultured human vascular endothelium to increase the adhesion of polymorpho-nuclear leukocytes, monocytes, and related leukocyte cell lines. *Journal of Clinical Investigation, 76*, 2003–2011.

Blennow, K., & Wallin, A. (1992). Clinical heterogeneity of probable Alzheimer's disease. *Journal of Geriatric Psychiatry and Neurology, 5*, 106–113.

Blomgren, H., Blom, U., & Ullen, H. (1986). Relation between the site of primary intracranial tumors and mitogenic responses of blood lymphocytes. *Cancer Immunology, Immunotherapy, 21*, 31–38.

Blum-Degen, D., Muller, T., Kuhn, W., Gerlach, M., Przuntek, H., & Riederee, P. (1995). Interleukin-1 beta and interleukin-6 are elevated in the cerebrospinal fluid of Alzheimer's and de novo Parkinson's disease patients. *Neuroscience Letters, 202*(1–2), 17–20.

Bodmer, S., Siepl, C., & Fontana, A. (1989). Immunoregulatory factors secreted by Glioblastoma cells: Glioblastoma-derived T-cell suppressor factor/transforming growth factor-$\beta_2$. In R. Alan (Ed.), *Neuroimmune Networks: Physiology and diseases* pp 73–82. Liss Inc.

Brenneman, D. E., Schultzberg, M., Bartfai, T., & Gozes, I. (1992) Cytokine regulation of neuronal survival. *Journal of Neurochemistry, 58*, 454–460.

Brooks, W. H., Cross, R. J., Roszman, T. L., & Markesbery, W. R. (1982). Neuroimmunomodulation: Neural anatomical basis for impairment and facilitation. *Annals of Neurology, 12*, 56–61.

Brooks, W. H., Latta, R. B., Mahaley, M. S., Roszman, T. L., Dudka, L., & Skaggs A. (1981). Immunobiology of primary intracranial tumors. 5. Correlation of a lymphocyte index and clinical status. *Journal of Neurosurgery, 54*, 331–337.

Brooks, W. H., Netsky, M. G. Normansell D. E., & Horwitz, D. (1972). Depressed cell-mediated immunity in patients with primary intracranial tumors, Characterization of a humoral immunosuppressive factor. *The Journal of Experimental Medicine, 136*, 1631–1647.

Brooks, W. H., Roszman, T. L., & Rogers A. (1976). Impairment of rosette-forming T-lymphocytes in patients with primary intracranial tumors. *Cancer, 37*, 1869–1873.

Cacabelos, R., Barquero, M., Garcia, P., Alvarez, X. A., & Varela de Seijas, E. (1991). Cerebrospinal fluid Interleukin-1 beta (IL-1$\beta$) in Alzheimer's disease and neurological disorders. *Methods and Findings in Experimental and Clinical Pharmacology, 13*(7), 455–458.

Carr, D. J. J. (1992). Neuropeptides receptors on cells of the immune system In J. E. Blalock (Ed.), *Neuroimmunoendocrinology* (2nd ed.) (Vol. 52, pp 84–105). Basel: Karger.

Chao, C. C., Hu, S., Molitor, T. W., Shaskan, E. G., & Peterson, P. K. (1992). Activated microglia mediate neuronal cell injury via a nitric oxide mechanism. *The Journal of Immunology, 149*, 2736–2741.

Cheng, B., Christakos, S., & Mattson, M. P. (1994). Tumor necrosis factors protect neurons against metabolic-excitotoxic insults and promote maintenance of calcium homeostasis. *Neuron, 12*(1), 139–153.

Clark, R. K., Lee, E. V., Fish, C. J., White, R. F., Price, W. J., Jonak, Z. L., Feuerstein, G. Z., & Barone, F. C. (1993). Development of tissue damage, inflammation and resolution following stroke: An immunohistochemical and quantitative planimetric study. *Brain Research Bulletin, 31*, 565–572.

Connolly, E. S., Winfree, C. J., Springer, T. A., Naka, Y., Liai, H., Du Yan, S., Stern, D. M., Solomon, R. A., Gutierrez-Ramos, J-C., & Pinsky, D. J. (1996). Cerebral protection in homozygous null ICAM-1 mice after middle cerebral artery occlusion. Role of neutrophil adhesion in the patogenesis of stroke. *Journal of Clinical Investigation, 97*, 209–216.

Courtright, L. J., & Kusell, K. (1965). Sparing effect of neurological deficit and trauma on the course of adjuvant arthritis in the rat. *Annals of the Rheumatic Diseases, 24*, 360–368.

Cross, R. J., Brooks, W. H., Roszman, T. L., & Markesbery, W. R. (1982). Hypothalamic-immune interactions. Effect of hypophy-sectomi on neuroimmunomodulation. *Journal of the Neurological Sciences, 53*, 557–566.

Cross, R. J., Markesbery, W. R., Brooks, W. H., & Roszman, T. L. (1980). Hypothalamic-immune interactions. I. The acute effect of anterior hypothalamic lesions on the immune response. *Brain Research, 196*, 79–87.

Czlonkowska, A., Cyrta, B., & Korlak, J. (1979). Immunological observations on patients with acute cerebral vascular disease. *Journal of the Neurological Sciences, 43*, 455–464.

Devi, R. S., & Namasivayam, A. (1991). Modulation of the specific immunity by ventral hippocampal formation in albino rats. *Journal of Neuroimmunology, 33*, 1–6.

Dietrich, P.-Y., Walker, P.R, Saas, P, & de Tribolet, N. (1998). Central nervous system tumors and the immune system. In J. Antel, G. Birnbaum, & H-P. Hartung (Eds.), *Clinical neuroimmunology* (pp. 228–253). Oxford: Blackwell Science.

Fan, L., Young, P. R., Barone, F. C., Feuerstein, G. Z., Smith, D. H., & McIntosh, T. K. (1996). Experimental brain injury induces differential expression of tumor necrosis factor-alpha mRNA in the CNS. *Brain Research, Molecular Brain Research, 36*(2), 287–291.

Fassbender, K., Rossol, S., Kammer, T., Daffertshofer, M., Wirth, S., Dollman, M., & Hennerici, M. (1994a). Proinflammatory cyto-kines in serum of patients with acute cerebral ischemia: Kinetics of secretion and relation to the extend of brain damage and outcome of disease. *Journal of the Neurological Sciences, 122*, 135–139.

Fassbender, K., Schmidt, R., Mössner, R., Daffertshofer, M., & Hennerici, M. (1994b). Pattern of activation of the hypothalamic-pituitary-adrenal axis in acute stroke. Relation to acute confu-sional state, extent of brain damage, and clinical outcome. *Stroke, 25*, 1105–1108.

Felten, D. L., Felten, S. Y., Bellinger, D. L., Carlson, S. L., Ackerman, K. D., Madden, K. S., Olschowka, J. A., & Livnat, S. (1987). Noradrenergic sympathetic neural interactions with the immune system: Structure and function. *Immunological Reviews, 100*, 225–260.

Fierz, W., Endler, B., Reske, K., Wekerle, H., & Fontana, A. (1985). Astrocytes as antigen-presenting cells. I. Induction of Ia antigen expression on astrocytes by T cells via immune interferon and its effect on antigen presentation. *The Journal of Immunology, 134*, 3785–3793.

Fillit, H., Meyer, L., & Bona, C. (1992). Immunology of aging. J. C. Brocklehurst, R. C. Tallis, & H. M. Fillit (Eds.), *Textbook of geriatric medicine and gerontology* (4th ed.) (pp. 71–89). London: Churchill Livinstone.

Finsen, B. R., Jörgensen, M. B., Diemer, N. H., & Zimmer, J. (1993). Microglial MHC antigen expression after ischemic and kainic acid lesions of the adult rat hippocampus. *Glia, 7*, 41–49.

Frei, K., Lins, H., Schwerdel, C., & Fontana, A. (1994). Antigen presentation in the central nervous system: The inhibitory effect of IL-10 on MHC class II expression and production of cytokines depends on the inducing signals and the type of cell analyzed. *The Journal of Immunology, 152*, 2720–2728.

Frei, K., Malipiero, U. V., Leist, T. P., Zinckernagel, R. M., Schwab, M. E., & Fontana, A. (1989). On the cellular source and function of interleukin-6 produced in the central nervous system in viral diseases. *European Journal of Immunology, 19*, 689–694.

Frohman, E. M., Frohman, T. C., Gupta, S., de Fougerolles, A., & van der Noort, S. (1991). Expression of intercellular adhesion molecule 1 (ICAM-1) in Alzheimer's disease. *Journal of the Neurological Sciences, 106*(1), 105–111.

Geniez, C., Millet, A., Blanchet, P., Duboin, M. P., & Roquefeuil, B. (1983). La depression immunitaire en traumatologie neurosurgicale. Etude de 1'hypersensibilite cutanee retardee par le multitest. *Agressologie, 24,* 133–137.

Gehrmann, J., Bonnekoh, P., Miyazawa, T., Hossmann, K.-A., & Kreutzberg G. W. (1992). Immunocytochemical study of an early microglial activation in ischemia. *Journal of Cerebral Blood Flow and Metabolism, 12,* 257–269.

Gehrmann, J., Matsumoto, Y., & Kreutzberg, G. W. (1995). Microglia: Intrinsic immuneffector cell of the brain. *Brain Research. Brain Research Reviews, 20,* 269–287.

Ghirnikar, R. S., Lee, Y. L., He, T. R., & Eng, L. F. (1996). Chemokine expression in rat stab wound brain injury. *Journal of Neuroscience Research, 46*(6), 727–733.

Ginsberg, M. D., Globus, M. Y.-T., Dietrich, W. D., & Busto, R. (1993). Temperature modulation of ischemic brain injury-a synthesis of recent advances. In K. Kogure, K. A. Hossman, & B. K. Siesjö (Eds), *Neurobiology of ischemic brain damage* (Vol. 96, pp. 13–22). Amsterdam: Elsevier.

Giometto, B., Bozza, F., Faresin, F., Alessio, L., Mingrino, S., & Tavolato, B. (1996). Immune infiltrat and cytokines in gliomas. *Acta Neurochirurgica (Wien), 138*(1), 50–56.

Giulian, D. (1987). Ameboid microglia as effectors of inflammation in the central nervous system. *Journal of Neuroscience Research, 18,* 155–171.

Giulian, D., Baker, T. J., Shih, L-C. N., & Lachman, L. B. (1986). Interleukin-1 of the central nervous system is produced by ameboid microglia. *The Journal of Experimental Medicine, 164,* 594–604.

Giulian, D., & Lachman, L. B. (1985) Interleukin-1 stimulation of astroglial proliferation after brain injury. *Science, 228,* 497–499.

Giulian, D., Li, J., Li, X., George, J., & Rutecki, P. A. (1994). The impact of microglial-derived cytokines upon gliosis in the CNS. *Developmental Neurosciences, 16,* 128–136.

Goldgaber, D., Harris, H. W., Hla, T., Maciag, T., Donnely, R. J., Jacobsen, J. S., Vitek, M. P., & Gajdusek, D. C. (1989). Interleukin 1 regulates synthesis of amyloid β-protein precursor mRNA in human endothelial cells. *Proceedings of National Academy of Sciences, USA, 86,* 7606–7610.

Goodman, J. C., Robertson, C. S., Grossman, R. G., & Narayan, R. K. (1990). Elevation of tumor necrosis factor in head injury. *Journal of Neuroimmunology, 30,* 213–217.

Gourin, C. G., & Shackford, S. R. (1997). Production of tumor necrosis factor-α and interleukin-1 beta by human cerebral microvascular endothelium after percussive trauma. *The Journal of Trauma, 42*(6), 1101–1107.

Griffin, W. S. T., Stanley, L. C., Ling, C., White, L., MacLeod, V., Perrot, L. J., White, C. L., & Araoz, C. (1989). Brain interleukin-1 and S-100 immunoreactivity are elevated in Down syndrome and Alzheimer disease. *Proceedings of National Academy of Sciences, USA, 86,* 7611–7615.

Gross, C. E., Howard, D. B., Dooley, R. H., Raymond, S. J., Fuller, S., & Bednar, M. M. (1994). TGF-β1 post-treatment in a rabbit model of cerebral ischaemia. *Neurological Research, 16,* 465–470.

Hallenbeck, J. M., & Dutka, A. J. (1990). Background rewiew and current concept of reperfusion injury. *Archives of Neurology, 47,* 1245–1254.

Hama, T., Miyamoto, M., Tsukui, H., Nishio, C., & Hatanaka, H. (1989). Interleukin-6 as a neurotrophic factor for promoting the survival of cultured basal forebrain cholinergic neurons from postnatal rats. *Neuroscience Letters, 104,* 340–344.

Hickey, W. F. (1991). T-lymphocyte entry and antigen recognition in the nervous system. In Ader, Felten, & Cohen (Eds), *Psychoneuroimmunology* (pp. 149–175) (2nd ed). New York: Academic Press.

Hishii, M., Nitta, T., Ishida, H., Ebato, M., Kuroso, A., Yagita, H., Sato, K., & Okumura, K. (1995). Human glioma-derived Interleukin-10 inhibits antitumor immune responses in vitro. *Neurosurgery, 37*(6), 1160–1167.

Holmin, S. (1997). *Inflammation in brain contusion.* Doctoral dissertation, Stockholm University, Sweden.

Holmin, S., Mathiesen, T., Shetye, J., & Biberfeld, P. (1995). Intracerebral inflammatory response to experimental brain contusion. *Acta Neurochirurgica (Wien), 132*(1–3), 110–119.

Holmin, S., Schalling, M., Hojeberg, B., Nordqvist, A. C., Skeftruna, A. K., & Mathiesen, T. (1997). Delayed cytokine expression in the rat following experimental contusion. *Journal of Neurosurgery, 86*(3), 493–504.

Howard, H., & O'Garra, A. (1992). Biological properties of interleukin-10. *Immunology Today, 13*(6), 198–200.

Hoyt, D. B., Ozkan, N. A., Hansbrough, J. F., Marshall, L., & van Berkum-Clark, M. (1990). Head injury: An immunological deficit in T-cell activation. *The Journal of Trauma, 7,* 759–767.

Hu, G. R., Walls, R. S., Creasey, H., McCusker, E., & Broe, G. A. (1995). Peripheral blood lymphocyte subset distribution and function in patients with Alzheimer's disease and other dementias. *Australian and New Zealand Journal of Medicine, 25*(3), 212–217.

Huettner, C., Paulus, W., & Roggendorf, W. (1995). Messenger RNA expression of the immunosuppressive cytokine IL-10 in human glioblastomas. *American Journal of Pathology, 146*(2), 317–322.

Itagaki, S., McGeer, P. L., Akiyama, H., Zhu, S., & Selkoe, D. (1989). Relationship of microglia and astrocytes to amyloid deposit in Alzheimer disease. *Journal of Neuroimmunology, 24,* 173–182.

Jankovic, B. D., & Isakovic, K. (1973). Neuroendocrine correlates of the immune response. II. Changes in the lymphatic organs of brain-lesioned rats. *International Archives of Allergy and Applied Immunology, 45,* 373–384.

Jellinger, K. A. (1996). Diagnostic accuracy of Alzheimer's disease: a clinicopathological study. *Acta Neuropathologica, 91,* 219–220.

Johansson, Å., Olsson, T., Carlberg, B., Karlsson, K., & Fagerlund, M. (1997). Hypercorticolism after stroke-partly cytokine-mediated? *Journal of the Neurological Sciences, 147,* 43–47.

Kadlecova, O., Masek, K., Seifert, J., & Petrovicky, P. (1987). The involvement of some brain structures in the effects of immunomodulators. *Annals of the New York Academy of Sciences, 496,* 394–398.

Kalman, J., Juhasz, A., Laird, G., Dickens P., Jardanhazy, T., Rimanoczy, A., Boncz, I., Parry-Jones, W. L., & Janka, Z. (1997) *Acta Neurologica Scandinavica, 96*(4), 236–240.

Kebudi, R., Ayan, I., Darendeliler, E., Agaogly, L., Ekmekcioglu, S., Yagci, T., Piskin, S., & Bilge, N. (1995). Immunologic status in children with brain tumors and the effect of therapy. *Journal of Neuro-Oncology, 24*(3), 219–227.

Kim, J. S., Yoon, S. S., Kim Y. H., & Ryu, J. S. (1996). Serial measurement of interleukin-6, transforming growth factor-β, and S-100 protein in patients with acute stroke. *Stroke, 27,* 1553–1557.

Kochanek, P. M., & Hallenbeck, J. M. (1992). Polymorphonuclear leukocytes and monocytes/macrophages in the pathogenesis of cerebral ischemia and stroke. *Stroke, 23,* 1367–1379.

Kossmann, T., Hans, V., Imhof, H. G., Trentz, O., & Morganti-Kossmann, M. C. (1996). Interleukin-6 released in human cerebrospinal fluid following traumatic brain injury may trigger nerve growth factor production in astrocytes. *Brain Research, 713*(1–2), 143–152.

Kossmann, T., Stahel, P., Lenzlinger, P., M., Redl, H., Dubs, R. W., Trentz, O., Schlag, G., & Morganti-Kossmann, M. C. (1997b). Interleukin-8 released into the cerebrospinal fluid after brain injury is associated with blood-brain barrier dysfunction and nerve growth factor production. *Journal of Cerebral Blood Flow and Metabolism, 17*(3), 280–289.

Kossmann, T., Stahel, P., Morganti-Kossmann, F., M. C., Jones, J. L., & Barnum, S. R. (1997a). Elevated levels of the complement components C3 and factor B in ventricular cerebrospinal fluid of patients with traumatic brain injury. *Journal of Neuroimmunology, 73*(1–2), 63–69.

Kostulas, N., Kivisäkk, P., Huang, Y., Matusevicius, D., Kostulas, V., & Link, H. (1998). Ischemic stroke is associated with a systemic increase of blood mononuclear cells expressing interleukin-8 mRNA. *Stroke, 29*, 462–466.

Kosunen, O., Soininen, H., Paljärvi, L., Heinonen, O., Talasniemi, S. & Riekkinen, P. J. Sr. (1996). Diagnostic accuracy of Alzheimer's disease: A neuropathological study. *Acta Neuropathologica, 91*, 185–193.

Kuppner, M. C., Hamou, M. F., & de Tribolet, N. (1988). Immunohistological and functional analysis of lymphoid infiltrates in human glioblastomas. *Cancer Research, 48*, 6926–6932.

Kuppner, M. C., Hamou, M. F., Sawamura, Y., Bodmer, S., & de Tribolet N. (1989). Inhibition of lymphocyte function by glioblastoma derived transforming growth factor$\beta_2$. *Journal of Neurosurgery, 71*(2), 211–217.

Lee, S. C., Liu, W., Brosnan, C. F., & Dickson, D. W. (1994). GM-CSF promotes proliferation of human fetal and adult microglia in primary cultures. *Glia, 12*, 309–318.

Levine, J., Goetzl, E., & Basbaum, A. (1987). Contribution of the nervous system to the patophysiology of rheumatoid arthritis and other polyarthritides. *Rheumatic Disease Clinics of North America, 13*, 369–383.

Lieberman, A. P., Pitha, P. M., Shin H. S., & Shin, M. L. (1989) Production of tumor necrosis factor and other cytokines by astrocytes stimulated with lipopolysaccharide or a neurotrop virus. *Proceedings of National Academy of Sciences, USA, 86*, 6348–6352.

Loddick, S. A., Turnbull, A., V., & Rothwell, N., J. (1998). Cerebral interleukin-6 is neuroprotective during permanent focal cerebral ischemia in the rat. *Journal of Cerebral Blood Flow and Metabolism, 18*(2), 176–179.

MacDonald, S. M., Golstone, A. H., Morris, J. E., Exton-Smith, A. N., & Callard, R. E. (1982). Immunological parameters in the aged and in Alzheimer's disease. *Clinical and Experimental Immunology, 49*, 123–128.

Mahaley, M. S., Brooks, W. H., Roszman, T. L., Bigner, D. D., Dudka, L., & Richardson, S. (1977). Immunobiology of primary intracranial tumors. 1. Studies of the cellular and humoral general immune competence of brain-tumor patients. *Journal of Neurosurgery, 46*, 467–476.

Marioka, T., Baba, T., Black, K. L., & Streit, W. J. (1992). Inflammatory cell infiltrates vary in experimental primary and metastatic brain tumors. *Neurosurgery, 30*(6), 891–896.

Masek, K., Kadlecova, O., & Petrovicky, P. (1983). The effect of brain stem lesions on the immune response. In J. W. Hadden, L. Chedid, P. Dukor, F. Spreaficao, & D. Willoughby (Eds.), *Advances in immunopharmacology* (pp. 443–450). New York: Pergamon.

Massei, R., Baratta, P., Mulazzi, D., Tagliabue, M., Somni, F., Ferrero, A. E., Calappi, E., Motti, E. D. F., & Trazzi, R. (1988). Impairment of cell-mediated immunity in severe head injury. *Aggressologie, 29*, 423–426.

Mattiace, L. A., Davies, P., Yen, S. H., & Dickson, D. W. (1990). Microglia in cerebellar plaques in Alzheimer's disease. *Acta Neuropathologica, 80*, 493–498.

Mattson, M. P., Cheng, B., Baldwin, S. A., Smith-Swintosky, V. L., Keller, J, Geddes, J. W., Scheff, S. W., & Christakos, S. (1995). Brain injury and tumor necrosis factors induce calbindin D-28k in astrocytes: Evidence for a cytoprotective response. *Journal of Neuroscience Research, 42*(3), 357–370.

Mayer, P. P., Chughtai, M. A., & Cape, R. T. D. (1976). An immunological approach to dementia in the elderly. *Age and Ageing, 5*, 164–170.

Mc Irvine, A. J., O'Mahony, J. B., Saporoschetz, I., & Mannick, J. A. (1982). Depressed immune response in burn patients: Use of monoclonal antibodies and functional assays to define the role of suppressor cells. *Annals of Surgery, 196*, 297–304.

McClain, C. J., Cohen, D., Ott, L., Dinarello, C. A., & Young, B. (1987). Ventricular fluid interleukin-1 activity in patients with head injury. *Journal of Laboratory and Clinical Medicine, 110*, 48–54.

McGeer, P. L., Akiyama, H., Itagaki, S., & McGeer, E. G. (1989). Immune system response in Alzheimer's disease. *Canadian Journal of Neurological Sciences, 16*, 516–527.

McGeer, P. L., Itagaki, S., Tago, H., & McGeer, E. G. (1987). Reactive microglia in patients with senile dementia of Alzheimer type are positive for the histocompatibility glycoprotein HLA-DR. *Neuroscience Letters, 79*, 195–200.

Merlo, A., Juretic, A., Zuber, M., Filgueira, L., Luscher U., Caetano, V., Ulrich, J., Gratzl, O., Heberer, M., & Spagnoli, G. C. (1993). Cytokine gene expression in primary brain tumors, metastases and meningiomas suggests specific transcription patterns. *European Journal of Cancer, 26A*(15), 2118–2125.

Miller, A. E. Neighbour, P. A., Katzman, R., Aronson, M., & Lipkowitz, R. (1981). Immunological studies in senile dementia of the Alzheimer type: Evidence for enhanced suppressor cell activity. *Annals of Neurology, 10*, 506–510.

Mizushima, Y., & Yamamura, M. (1969). Arthropathy and inflammation reaction in hemiplegic patients. *Acta Rheumatica Scandinavica, 15*, 297–304.

Morganti-Kossmann, M. C, Lenzlinger, P., M., Hans V., Stahel, P., Csuka, E., Ammann, E., Stocker, R., Trentz, O., & Kossmann, T. (1997). Cytokines in the brain. Production of cytokines following brain injury: Beneficial and deleterious for the damage tissue. *Molecular Psychiatry, 2*, 133–136.

Mori, H., Tanaka, R., Yoshida, S., Ono, K., Yamanaka, R., Hara, N., & Takeda, N. (1993). Immunological analysis of the rats with anterior hypothalamic lesions. *Journal of Neuroimmunology, 48*, 45–52.

Mossman, T. R. (1994). Interleukin-10. In A.W. Thomson (Ed.), *The cytokine handbook* (2nd ed.) (pp. 223–237), London: Academic Press.

Neveu, P. J. (1992a). Asymmetrical brain modulation of the immune response. *Brain Research. Brain Research Reviews, 17*, 101–107.

Neveu, P. J., Barneoud, P., Georgiades, O., Vitiello, S., Vincendeau, P., & Le Moal, M. (1989). Brain neocortex modulation of the mononuclear phagocytic system. *Journal of Neuroscience Research, 22*, 392–394.

Neveu, P. J., Deleplanque, B., Vitiello, S., Rouge-Pont, F., & Le Moal, M. (1992b). Hemispheric asymmetry in the effects of substantia nigra lesioning on lymphocyte reactivity in mice. *International Journal of Neuroscience, 64*, 267–273.

Nitta, T., Hishii, M., Sato, K., & Okumura, K. (1994). Selective expression of interleukin-10 gene within glioblastoma multiforme. *Brain Research, 649*, 122–128.

Olsson, T., Marklund, N., Gustafson, Y., & Näsman, B. (1992). Abnormalities at different levels of the hypothalamic-pituitary-adrenocortical axis early after stroke. *Stroke, 23*, 1573–1576.

Oppenheimer, S., & Hachinski, V. (1992). Complication of acute stroke. Stroke octet. *The Lancet, 339*, 721–724.

Ott, L., McClain, C. J., Gillespie, M., & Young, B. (1994). Cytokines and metabolic dysfunction after severe head trauma. *Journal of Neurotrauma, 11*(5), 447–472.

Perlstein, R. S., Mougey, E. H., Jackson, W. E., & Neta, R. (1991). Interleukin-1 and interleukin-6 act synergistically to stimulate the release of adrenocorticotropic hormone in vivo. *Lymphokine and Cytokine Research, 10*, 141–146.

Pirttila, T., Mehta, P. D., Frey, H., & Wisniewski, H. M. (1994). $\alpha_1$-Antichymotrypsin and IL-1$\beta$ are not increased in CSF or serum in Alzheimer's disease. *Neurobiology of Aging, 15*(3), 313–317.

Postler, E., Lehr, A., Schluesener, H., & Meyermann, R. (1997). Expression of the S-100 proteins MRP-8 and -14 in ischemic brain lesions. *Glia, 19*(1), 27–34.

Prineas, J. W. (1979). Multiple sclerosis: presence of lymphatic capillaries and lymphoid tissue in the brain and spinal cord. *Science, 203*, 1123–1125.

Qu Yan, H., Alcaros Banos, M., Herregodts, P., Hooghe, R., & Hooghe-Peters, E. L. (1992). Expression of interleukin (IL)-1$\beta$, IL-6 and their respective receptors in the normal rat brain and after injury. *European Journal of Immunology, 22*, 2963–2971.

Quattrocchi, K. B., Frank, E. H., Miller, C. H., Dull, S. T., Howard, R.R., & Wagner, F. C. Jr. (1991). Severe head injury: Effect upon cellular immune function. *Neurological Research, 13*(1), 13–20.

Relton, J. K., & Rothwell, N. L. (1992). Interleukin-1 receptor antagonist inhibits ischaemic and excitotoxic neuronal damage in the rat. *Brain Research Bulletin, 29*, 243–246.

Renoux, G. (1988). The cortex regulates the immune system and the activities of a T-cell specific immunopotentiator. *International Journal of Neuroscience, 39*, 177–187.

Renoux, G., Biziere, K., Bardos, P., & Degenne, D. (1987). Consequences of bilateral brain neocortical ablation on imuthiol-induced immunostimulation in mice. *Annals of the New York Academy of Sciences, 496*, 346–353.

Renoux, G., Biziere, K., Renoux, M., Guillaumin, J. M., & Degenne, D. A. (1983). Balanced brain asymmetry modulates T-cell-mediated events. *Journal of Neuroimmunology, 5*, 227–238.

Ringheim, G. E., Burgher, K. L., & Heroux, J. A. (1995). Interleukin-6 mRNA expression by cortical neurons in culture: Evidence for neuronal sources of interleukin-6 production in the brain. *Journal of Neuroimmunology, 63*, 113–123.

Ross, S. A., Halliday, M. I., Campell, G. C., Byrnes, D. P., & Rowlands B. J. (1994). The presence of tumor necrosis factor in CSF and plasma after severe head injury. *British Journal of Neurosurgery, 8*, 419–425.

Rossor, M. (1992). Disorders of psychic function. Dementia. In A. K. Asbury, G. M. McKhann, & W. I. McDonald (Eds.), *Disease of the nervous system: clinical Neurobiology* (2nd ed.) (pp. 788–794). Philadelphia: Saunders.

Rostworowski, M., Balasingam, V., Chabot, S. Owens, T., & Yong, V. W. (1997). Astrogliosis in the neonatal and adult murine brain post trauma: Elevation of the inflammatory cytokines and the lack of requirement for endogenous interferon-$\gamma$. *The Journal of Neuroscience, 17*(10), 3664–3674.

Roszman, T. L., & Brooks, W. H. (1980). Immunobiology of primary intracranial tumors. III. Demonstration of a qualitative lymphocyte abnormality in patients with primary brain tumors. *Clinical and Experimental Immunology, 39*, 395–402.

Roszman, T. L., Brooks, W. H., Steele, C., & Elliott, L. H. (1985). Pokeweed mitogen-induced immunoglobulin secretion by peripheral blood lymphocytes from patients with primary intracranial tumors. Characterization of T helper and B cell function. *The Journal of Immunology, 134*, 1545–1550.

Roszman, T. L., Cross, R. J., Brooks, W. H., & Markesbery, W. R. (1982). Hypothalamic–immune interactions. II. The effect of hypothalamic lesions on the ability of adherent spleen cells to limit lymphocyte blastogenesis. *Immunology, 45*, 737–742.

Roszman, T., Elliott, L., & Brooks, W. (1991). Modulation of T-cell function by gliomas. *Immunology Today, 12*(10), 370–374.

Rothwell, N. J., & Hopkins, S. J. (1995). Cytokines and the nervous system. II. actions and mechanisms of action. *Trends in Neurosciences, 18*, 130–136.

Satoh, T., Nakamura, S., Taga, T., Matsuda, T., Hirano, T., Kishimoto, T., & Kasiro, Y. (1988). Induction of neuronal differentiation in PC12 cells by B-cell stimulatory factor 2/interleukin 6. *Molecular and Cellular Biology, 8*, 3546–3549.

Sawada, M., Itoh, Y., Suzumura, A., & Marunouchi, T. (1993). Expression of cytokine receptors in cultured neuronal and glia cells. *Neuroscience Letters, 160*, 131–134.

Sawamura, Y., & de Tribolet, N. (1990). Immunotherapy of brain tumors. *Journal of Neurosurgical Sciences, 34*, 265–278.

Schroeter, M., Jander, S., Witte, O. W., & Stoll, G. (1994). Local immune responses in the rat cerebral cortex after middle cerebral artery occlusion. *Journal of Neuroimmunology, 55*, 195–203.

Schwartz, M., Solomon, A., Lavie, V., Ben, B. S., Belkin, M., & Cohen, A. (1991). Tumor necrosis factor facilitates regeneration of injured central nervous system axons. *Brain Research, 545*, 334–338.

Selmaj, K. W., Farooq, M., Norton, W. T., Raine, C. S., & Brosnan, C. F. (1990). Proliferation of astrocytes in vitro in response to cytokines. A primary role for tumor necrosis factor. *The Journal of Immunology, 144*, 129–135.

Shalit, F., Sredni, B, Brodie C., Kott, E., & Huberman, M. (1995). T lymphocyte subpopulations and activation markers correlate with severity of Alzheimer's disease. *Clinical Immunology and Immunopathology, 75*(3), 246–250.

Shibayama, M., Kuchiwaki, H., Inao, S., Yoshida, K., & Ito, M. (1996). Intercellular adhesion molecule-1 expression on glia following brain injury: Participation of Interleukin-1 beta. *Journal of Neurotrauma, 13*(12), 801–808.

Shiga, Y., Onodera, H., Kogure, K., Yamasaki, Y., Yashima, Y., Syozyhara, H., & Sendo, F. (1991). Neutrophil as mediator of ischemic edema formation in the brain. *Neuroscience Letters, 125*, 110–112.

Singh, V. K., Fudenberg, H. H., & Brown, F. R. (1987). Immunological dysfunction: Simultaneous study of Alzheimer's and old Down's patients. *Mechanism in Ageing and Development, 37*, 257–264.

Skias, D., Bania, M., Reder, A. T., Luchins, D., & Antel, J. P. (1985). Senile dementia of Alzheimer's type (SDAT): Reduced T8+-cell-mediated suppressor activity. *Neurology, 35*, 1635–1638.

Spangelo, B. L., Judd, A. M., Isakson, P. C., & MacLeod, R. M. (1989). Interleukin-6 stimulates anterior pituitary hormone release in vitro. *Endocrinology, 125*(1), 575–577.

St. Pierre, B. A., Merill, J. E., & Dopp, J. M. (1996). Effects of cytokines on the CNS cells: Glia. In R. M. Ransohoff & E. N. Benveniste (Eds.), *Cytokines and the CNS* (pp. 151–168). Boca Raton, FL: CRC Press.

Stein, M., Schiavi, R. C., & Camerino, M. (1976). Influence of brain and behaviour on the immune system. The effect of hypothalamic lesions on immune processes is described. *Science, 191*, 435–440.

Tada, T., Yabu, K., & Kobayashi, S. (1993). Detection of active form of transforming growth factor-$\beta$ in cerebrospinal fluid of patients with glioma. *Japanese Journal of Cancer Research, 84*(5), 544–548.

Tarkowski, E., Blomstrand, & C., Tarkowski, A. (1995b). Stroke induced lateralization of delayed-type hypersensitivity in the early and chronic phase of the disease: a prospective study. *Journal of Laboratory and Clinical Medicine, 46*, 73–83.

Tarkowski, E., Ekelund, P., & Tarkowski, A. (1991a). Enhancement av antigen specific T-cell reactivity on the affected side in stroke patients. *Journal of Neuroimmunology, 34*, 61–67.

Tarkowski, E., Ekelund, P., & Tarkowski, A. (1991b). Increased systemic T-lymphocyte reactivity in patients with established stroke. *Journal of Laboratory and Clinical Medicine, 35*, 171–176.

Tarkowski, E., Naver, H., Wallin, G., Blomstrand, C., & Tarkowski, A. (1995a). Altered T-lymphocyte reactivity in patients with stroke: Effect of sympathetic dysfunction? *Stroke, 26*, 57–62.

Tarkowski, E., Rosengren, L., Blomstrand, C., Wikkelsö, C., Jensen, C., Ekholm, S., & Tarkowski, A. (1995c). Early intrathecal production of interleukin-6 predicts the size of brain lesion in stroke. *Stroke, 26*, 1393–1398.

Tarkowski, E., Rosengren, L., Blomstrand, C., Wikkelsö, C., Jensen, C., Ekholm, S., & Tarkowski, A. (1997). Intrathecal release of pro- and anti-inflammatory cytokines during stroke. *Clinical and Experimental Immunology, 110*, 492–499.

Tarkowski, E., Jensen, C., Ekholm, S., Ekelund, P., Blomstrand, C., & Tarkowski, A. (1998). Localization of the brain lesion affects the lateralization of T-lymphocyte dependent cutaneous inflammation. Evidence for immunoregulatory role of the right frontal cortex-putamen region. *Scandinavian Journal of Immunology, 47*, 30–36.

Tarkowski. E., Rosengren, L., Blomstrand, C., Wikkelsö, C., Jensen, C., Ekholm, S., & Tarkowski. A. (1999). Intrathecal expression of proteins regulating apoptosis in acute stroke. *Stroke, 30*, 321–327.

Tarkowski, E., Rindkvist, Å., Rosengren, L., & Wennmalm Å. (2000). Intrathecal release of nitric oxide in stroke and its relation to final brain injury. *Cerebrovascular Diseases, 10*, 200–206.

Taupin, V., Toulmond, S., Serrano, A., Benavides, J., & Zavala, F. (1993). Increase in IL-6, IL-1 and TNF levels in rat brain following traumatic lesion. Influence of pre- and post-traumatic treatment with Ro5 4864, a peripheral-type (p site) benzodiazepine ligand. *Journal of Neuroimmunology, 42*, 177–186.

Thompson, M., & Bywaters, E. G. L. (1962). Unilateral arthritis following hemiplegia. *Annals of the Rheumatic Diseases, 21*, 370–377.

Torack, R. M., & Gebel, H. M. (1982). Delayed hypersensitivity in Alzheimer's disease following BCG immunostimulation. *Clinical Neuropathology, 1*(4), 169–171.

Toulmond, S., & Rothwell, N. J. (1995). Interleukin-1 receptor antagonist inhibits neuronal damage caused by fluid percussion injury in the rat. *Brain Research, 671*(2), 261–266.

Urbani, F., Maleci, A., La Sala, A, Lande, R., & Ausiello, C-M. (1995). Defective expression of interferon-γ, granulocyte-macrophage colony-stimulating factor, tumor necrosis factor alpha, and interleukin-6 in activated peripheral blood lymphocytes from glioma patients. *Journal of Interferon and Cytokine Research, 15*(5), 421–429.

Vandenabeele, P., & Fiers, W. (1991). Is amyloidogenesis during Alzheimer's disease due to an IL-1-/IL-6-mediated "acute phase response" in the brain? *Immunology Today, 12*, 217–219.

Voll, E. R., Hermann, M., Roth, E. A., Stach, C., & Kalden, J. R. (1997). Immunosuppressive effects of apoptotic cells. *Nature, 390*, 350–351.

Wallin, A., Blennow, K. & Scheltens, P. H. (1994). Research criteria for clinical diagnosis of "pure" Alzheimer's disease. *Drugs of Today, 30*, 265–273.

Wang, X., Yue, T-L., Barone, F. C., & Feuerstein, G. Z. (1995). Demonstration of increased endothelial-leukocyte adhesion molecule-1 mRNA expression in rat ischemic cortex. *Stroke, 26*, 1665–1669.

Weller, M., Bornemann, A., Stander, M., Scabet, M., Dichgans, J., & Meyermann, R. (1998). Humoral immune response to p53 in malignant glioma. *Journal of Neurology, 245*(3), 169–172.

Wikstrand, C. J., & Bigner, D. D. (1980). Immunobiologic aspects of the brain and human gliomas. *American Journal of Pathology, 98*(2), 517–566.

Wisniewski, H. M., Vorbrodt, A. W., Viegel, J., Morys, J., & Lossinsky, A. S. (1990). Ultrastructure of the cells forming amyloid fibers in Alzheimer disease and scrapie. *American Journal of Medical Genetics* (Suppl.), *7*, 287.

Woiciechowsky, C., Asadullah, K., Nestler, D., Eberhardt, B., Platzer, C., Schöning, B., Glöckner, F., Lanksch, W. R., Volk, H-D., & Döcke, W-D. (1998b). Sympathetic activation triggers systemic interleukin-10 release in immunodepression induced by brain injury. *Nature Medicine, 4*, 808–813.

Woiciechowsky, C., Asadullah, K., Nestler, D., Schoning, B., Glockner, F., Docke, W. d., & Volk, H. D. (1998a). Diminished monocytic HLA-DR expression and ex vivo cytokine secretion capacity in patients with glioblastoma: Effect of tumor extirpation. *Journal of Neuroimmunology, 84*(2), 164–171.

Wolach, B., Sazbon, L., Gavrieli, R., Ben Tovim, T., Zagreba, F., & Schlesinger, M. (1993). Some aspect of the humoral and neutrophil functions in postcomatose nawareness patients. *Brain Injury, 7*(5), 401–410.

Wolfe, J. H. N., Wu, V. V. H., & O'Connor, N. E. (1982). Anergy, immunosuppressive serum and impaired lymphocyte blastogenesis in burn patients. *Archives of Surgery, 117*, 1266–1271.

Wong, G. H. W., Bartlett, P. F., Clark-Lewis, I., Battye, F., & Schrader, J. W. (1984). Inducible expression of H-2 and Ia antigens on brain cells. *Nature, 310*, 688–691.

Wood, G. W., & Morantz, R. A. (1979). Immunohistologic evaluation of the lymphoreticular infiltrate of human central nervous system tumors. *Journal of the National Cancer Institute, 62*, 485–491.

Woodroofe, M. N., Sarna, G. S., Wadhwa, M., Hayes, G. M., Loughlin, A. J., Tinker, A., & Cusner, M. L. (1991). Detection of interleukin-1 and interleukin-6 in adult rat following mechanical injury, by in vivo microdialysis: Evidence for a role of microglia in cytokine production. *Journal of Neuroimmunology, 33*, 227–236.

Yamada, K., Kono, K., Umegaki, H., Yamada, K., Iguchi, A., Fukatsu, T., Nakashima, T., Nishiwaki, H., Shimada, Y., Sugita, Y., et al. (1995). Decreased interleukin-6 level in the cerebrospinal fluid of patients with Alzheimer-type dementia. *Neuroscience Letters, 186*(2–3), 219–221.

Yamaguchi, M., Matsuzaki, N., Hirota, K., Miyake, A., & Tanizawa, O. (1990). Interleukin-6 possibly induced by interleukin-1β in the pituitary gland stimulates the release of gonadotropins and prolactin. *Acta Endocrinologica, 122*, 201–205.

Yamanaka, R., Tanaka, R., Saitoh, T., & Okoshi, S. (1994). Cytokine gene expression on glioma cell lines and specimens. *Journal of Neuro-Oncology, 21*(3), 243–247.

Yong, V. W. (1996). Cytokines, astrogliosis, and neutrophism following CNS trauma. In R. M. Ransohoff & E. N. Benveniste (Eds.), *Cytokines and the CNS.* (pp. 151–168). Boca Raton, FL: CRC Press.

Young, H. F., Sakalas, R., & Kaplan, A. M., (1976). Inhibition of cell-mediated immunity in patients with brain tumors. *Surgical Neurology, 5*, 19–23.

CHAPTER

# 48

# Immunological States Associated with Schizophrenia

MARK HYMAN RAPAPORT, NORBERT MÜLLER

## I. INTRODUCTION

In schizophrenia, all the normal mental processes—sensation, perception, language, emotion, interpersonal relationships—appear to go completely awry. People with the disorder, lose touch with the real world. They hear voices that are not there, speak a language that does not exist, laugh for no reason, or sit motionless for hours on end. The entire human personality is laid waste, and the psychological and social building blocks of everyday life are crushed, often beyond recognition.

The National Mental Health Council, 1988

In this chapter we review evidence suggesting that there may be alterations in immune functions associated with schizophrenia. The chapter will be divided into seven major sections: an overview of the history of immune dysfunction in schizophrenia, a

review of the problems and challenges investigating immune dysfunction in schizophrenia, a review of the relationship between systemic illness and the central nervous system, a discussion of the reciprocal relationship between the central nervous system and the cytokine network, a review of recent studies suggesting that immune activation may be a component of schizophrenia, data from our laboratory extending existing work, and a discussion of the limitations of current research and future directions.

## II. THE HISTORY OF IMMUNE DYSFUNCTION IN SCHIZOPHRENIA

Schizophrenia is a heterogeneous syndrome characterized by auditory and visual hallucinations, delusions, ambivalence, paranoid thoughts, a formal thought disorder, and negative symptoms. These negative symptoms manifest themselves as a lack of motivation, problems with grooming, problems with attention, and a paucity of feelings. The hallmark of this syndrome is a decline in social functioning which forces most schizophrenic individuals to isolate themselves from their family and be reliant on public services for financial support. The prevalence of schizophrenia in the United States and throughout the world is approximately 1% and the age of onset of schizophrenia is usually in late adolescence or early adulthood. Certain forms of this syndrome do run in families and some genetic forms of this illness may overlap with bipolar disorder, yet there clearly are sporadic forms of schizophrenia as well. Despite advances in the development of new antipsychotic agents, our current therapies for schizophrenia are palliative.

The first studies demonstrating lymphocytosis and immune dysfunction in schizophrenia were reported both in the United States and in Europe in the early 1900s (Bruce & Peebles, 1903, 1904; Dide, 1905; Ermakov, 1910). Reports in the 1930s continued to find abnormal lymphocytes associated with dementia praecox and dementia paralytica, as well as the possible production of autoantibodies (Dameschek, 1930, 1931; Lehmann-Fauscius, 1937, 1939). Molholm (1942) and Vaughan, Sullivan, and Elmadjian (1949) reported that skin tests of psychotic patients challenged with pertussis toxin and guinea pig serum revealed markedly blunted wheals of induration when compared with normal volunteers. Therefore, prior to the advent of modern pharmacotherapy with antipsychotic medications, investigators found evidence of immune dysfunction associated with the syndrome we currently call schizophrenia. A second line of work has been the investigation of sera from schizophrenic patients for antibodies that are directed against the brain (Fessel, 1962; Heath & Krupp, 1967). Enthusiasm for investigating immunological etiologies for schizophrenia diminished as it became clear that antipsychotic agents which blocked type 2 dopamine receptors decreased positive symptoms of schizophrenia. Research efforts in schizophrenia became increasingly focused on the dopamine hypothesis of schizophrenia (Carlsson & Lindquist, 1963). Interest in immune etiologies for schizophrenia was further diminished when it was found that phenothiazines could stimulate the production of atypical lymphocytes and autoantibodies (Fieve, Blumenthal, & Little, 1966; Zarrabi et al., 1979). There was only sporadic interest in the investigation of the immune system in schizophrenia until the mid-1980s.

## III. PROBLEMS AND CHALLENGES INVESTIGATING IMMUNE DYSFUNCTION AND SCHIZOPHRENIA

The study of immune dysfunction in schizophrenia is challenging because it represents an area of interface between two rapidly evolving disciplines. Schizophrenia, as we currently define it, is a syndrome which will probably have a variety of different processes responsible for its etiology. The definition of schizophrenia has also changed dramatically with time from the older classifications of Blueler and Kreplin to the recent editions of the *Diagnostics and the Statistics Manual* and the *International Classification of Diseases*. Therefore, the types of individuals who have been categorized as schizophrenic have varied greatly over the past several generations. A wide variety of individuals with quite different presentations and prognoses are subsumed within our current definition of schizophrenia. These individuals may vary in age of onset, the types and intensity of symptoms—some being more prone to more positive symptoms and others more prone to negative symptoms—and the presence of family history for schizophrenia. Some individuals have family histories where schizophrenia affects multiple generations, others have family histories with both schizophrenia and bipolar disorder, and some individuals do not have a family history of any psychiatric illness.

The field of immunology has rapidly changed over the past 20 years. Knowledge in immunology has been greatly enhanced by the development of more sophisticated biological techniques from flow cytometry to Western blotting to advances in cell culture and animal modeling. These techniques have helped us identify the presence of immune system modulators and facilitated our understanding of the sophisticated, dynamic interplay that occurs within the immune system. We now understand that the body's defense system is far more complicated than the mere production of antibodies or the actions of macrophages. We realize that the immune system is a complex interdependent network that involves an array of different cell types, with many different functions. It is clear that certain cytokines serve as general activators of inflammation and early phase immune responses, such as interleukin (IL)-6 and IL-1. IL-6 has been associated with the release of positive acute phase proteins (Maes et al., 1993a; Maes, Meltzer, & Bosmans, 1994). We also know that there is a complex relationship between the production of specific cytokines and different types of immune responses: cellular immune responses usually require the IL-2 and interferon-$\gamma$ (IFN-$\gamma$), whereas humeral immune responses usually require IL-4, IL-5, and IL-10 cytokine responses. These cytokines seem to have reciprocal effects on the immune system: IFN-$\gamma$ stimulates cellular responses while inhibiting humoral responses, whereas IL-4 and IL-10 stimulate humoral responses while inhibiting cellular immune activity. (Please review other chapters in this text for elaboration of this concept.) Thus, work at the interface between two rapidly changing fields, schizophrenia and immunology, is difficult, yet the development of both fields is at such a point that we can pursue testable hypotheses.

It is important to acknowledge historical and existing points of concern with research investigating immune function and schizophrenia in order to place contemporary investigations within a proper context. As previously alluded to, one of the major limitations of investigations in this area is the heterogeneity of the syndrome. Any condition with a worldwide prevalence rate of 1 in 100 is more likely to be a variety of different disorders than a single disease entity. This heterogeneity helps to explain why treatment responses are so variable and why it is so difficult to determine consistent biological findings in schizophrenia. A second factor which has increased the heterogeneity of samples in studies has been our reliance on descriptive nosologies to define the syndrome. In order to meet criteria for schizophrenia, one needs to have an arbitrarily proscribed number of symptoms from a diverse and eclectic group of signs and symptoms. Therefore, many individuals who are phenomenologically very different fall under the rubric of schizophrenia. For many years, research in this area was further complicated because different groups of investigators employed competing diagnostic systems that overlapped but were far from identical. This has greatly diminished with the development of similar criteria sets for mental disorders in the *Diagnostics and Statistics Manual IV* and the *International Classification of Diseases X*. A final covariate that limits the homogeneity of these samples is the challenge of gathering reliable data of sufficient quantity and adequate duration from acutely psychotic individuals in order to make an accurate diagnosis. Cross-sectional diagnoses, particularly for new onset psychotic individuals, are notoriously inaccurate.

Statistical limitations pose another challenge for individuals interested in evaluating data from this area of research. The design of many studies calls into question the validity of the inferential statistics reported. A number of studies do not articulate hypotheses, while others test so many variables that it is impossible to be assured that the purported positive finding is anything other than a result of happenstance. A third rarely discussed problem in the field is that many studies, particularly replication studies, employ samples that are too small to detect small to moderate effect size differences. This greatly diminishes the value of the study, yet frequently these studies have been thought to call into question previously reported positive findings. Differences in the methodologies applied to investigate the same immune phenomena have frequently led to disparate findings. These methodological differences have made reports of differences in results difficult to reconcile. An additional source of concern in many of these studies has been the control of confounding biological variables. Schizophrenic patients frequently smoke tobacco, drink alcohol, and abuse illicit drugs; all of these products can perturb immune function. Furthermore, schizophrenic patients usually are prescribed a variety of medications and many of them profoundly alter immune function. The potential confounding effects of malnutrition and chronic stress must always be controlled for with this patient group. At the time that many of the older studies were performed the important immunomodulatory actions of these variables had not been recognized and therefore were not controlled for in the analyses. One last pragmatic limitation to research in this field has been the scarcity of funds necessary to carry out systematic longitudinal work in well-described cohorts of patients. Without support for such studies, it will be difficult to determine whether findings of immune activation in schizophrenia are an epiphenomenon or an intrinsic part of the syndrome.

## IV. SYSTEMIC ILLNESS AND THE CENTRAL NERVOUS SYSTEM DISTURBANCE

There are considerable data suggesting that systemic illness may cause significant neuropsychiatric dysfunction. Tertiary syphilis is an historical example of a systemic illness that has profound neuropsychiatric effects. Although rare today, it was once common to see patients with dementia, poor impulse control, and paranoid behavior secondary to syphilis. Sydenham's Chorea and AIDS are two contemporary examples of infectious diseases that may cause significant neuropsychiatric symptoms (Swedo et al., 1989; Sindic & Laterre, 1991; van Dam, 1991; Rapaport & McAllister, 1991). Sydenham's Chorea is a relatively infrequent sequela of streptococcal infection and is associated with the production of cross-reactive antibodies that bind preferentially to brain tissue (Swedo et al., 1989; Rapaport & McAllister, 1991). Patients with Sydenham's Chorea have abnormal involuntary movements, mood instability, and frequently manifest symptoms of obsessive compulsive disorder (Swedo et al., 1989). On rare occasions, these patients can present with psychotic symptoms. Neuroleptics are the treatment of choice for Sydenham's Chorea and the illness seems to recede simultaneously with the decrease in autoantibody titers (Swedo et al., 1989). Certain autoimmune disorders such as multiple sclerosis and systemic lupus erythematosus (SLE) may also have central nervous system complications. Patients with multiple sclerosis frequently complain of symptoms of anxiety and depression. Oligoclonal antibodies have also been reported in the cerebrospinal fluid of some of these patients (Sindic & Laterre, 1991). Extension of SLE into the central nervous system has been reported to cause symptoms of both depression and psychosis (van Dam, 1991). It is estimated that anywhere from 12 to 27% of individuals with central nervous involvement may become psychotic when they are lupus symptomatic. These episodes of psychosis are indistinguishable from the acute signs and symptoms of schizophrenia. These examples clearly demonstrate that when the brain is challenged by either infectious agents or the body's own immune system, it may respond by producing neuropsychiatric symptoms similar to what is seen in classical psychiatric disorders. It is unclear whether these examples suggest that autoimmune processes might be involved in the etiology of psychiatric disorders or rather that the symptomatology associated with major psychiatric syndromes really represents more generalized global responses to massive alterations in brain homeostasis rather than signs and symptoms that are unique for specific syndromes. However, one clear extrapolation from these findings from clinical medicine is that the immune system can perturb and influence the brain. It is important to understand the relationship between the central nervous system and the immune system.

## V. THE RELATIONSHIP BETWEEN THE CENTRAL NERVOUS SYSTEM AND THE IMMUNE SYSTEM

The advent of sophisticated technologies such as monoclonal antibodies, ELISAs, and molecular techniques greatly facilitated the identification of cytokines and more complex interactions now generally associated with the immune system. Investigations of the interactions between the central nervous system and the immune system include studies demonstrating that systemic stimulation of the immune system can produce behavioral changes and that these behavioral changes are due to cytokines and neurotransmitters, the behavioral effects of cytokines introduced into the brain, the biochemical interactions caused by the cytokines, the presence of cytokines and cytokine receptors in specific brain regions, the localization of cytokines to specific cell types within the brain, and the modulatory effects of CNS on the immune system. A detailed discussion of all the known interactions between the CNS and the cytokine network is beyond the scope of this chapter and so we

will use IL-1, IL-2, and IL-6 to highlight the interactions described above. Animal work clearly shows that exogenous cytokines introduced either directly through intrathecal injection or indirectly by stimulating IL-1 production with endotoxin can stimulate the production of CRH, activate the cascade of adrenocortical hormones, and alter physiological and behavioral parameters (Besedovsky, Del Rey, Sorkin, & Dinarello, 1986; Dunn, 1992, 1994). Denicoff et al. (1987) found that there were profound neuropsychiatric effects associated with the infusion of IL-2 as a treatment for cancer patients. These patients experienced problems with memory, agitation, and, at times, became frankly psychotic. This clinical observation supports animal experiments demonstrating that cytokines have profound effects on neurotransmitters when introduced either in the periphery or in the CNS (Dunn, 1992; Shintani et al., 1993; Dunn, 1994; Zalcman et al., 1994; Banks & Kastin, 1992; Banks, Kastin, & Gutierrez, 1993; Ransohoff & Benveniste, 1996; Benveniste, 1992). Intraventricular injection of IL-1 causes marked increases in noradrenaline, serotonin, noradrenaline and serotonin metabolites, and dopamine (Dunn, 1994). IL-2 in physiological concentrations stimulates dopamine release in a dose-dependent fashion (Lapchak, 1992; Alonso et al., 1993). Peripheral activation of IL-2 increases noradrenergic metabolism in the hippocampus, dopaminergic metabolism in the prefrontal cortex, and cholinergic activity (Zalcman et al., 1994; Awatsuji, Furukawa, Nakajima, Furukawa, & Hayashi, 1993; Hanisch, Seto, & Quirion, 1993). Such findings are intriguing because large numbers of IL-2 receptors are present in the pyramidal cell layer of the hippocampus (Plata-Salaman & French-Mullen, 1993). Nemni et al. (1992) found that chronic administration of IL-2 causes marked reduction in mnestic ability and loss of neurons in the hippocampus. This suggests that IL-2's stimulatory effects on dopamine and serotonin can lead to structural changes, the destruction of hippocampal cells, profound behavioral change, and deterioration in mnestic functioning. IL-2 has been implicated in the modulation of dopamine function in the striatum and may effect motor funtioning through its actions on the locus coeruleus and the nucleus caudatus (Lapcheck 1992; Nistico & DeSarro, 1991).

The intrathecal application of IL-6 in animal models enhanced dopamine and serotonin turnover in the hippocampus and frontal cortex without altering noradrenergic activity (Zalcman et al., 1994). Application of noradrenaline to astrocytes can stimulate the release of IL-6 (Dunn, 1992). TNF-$\beta$ acutely stimulates catecholamine activity, while it chronically tends to desensitize catecholamine release (Soliven & Albert, 1992). Thus, there is unequivocal evidence from animal and human research that cytokines can influence neurotransmitters, releasing factors, hormones, and behavior (Besedovsky et al., 1986; Berkenbosch, Van Oers, Del Ray, Tiders, & Besedovsky, 1987; Zalcman et al., 1994; Benveniste, 1992; Denicoff et al., 1987; Alonso et al., 1993; Lapchak, 1992). Conversely, neurotransmitters can stimulate the release of cytokines (Dunn, 1992).

It is clear that inflammatory responses and responses that activate the immune system in the periphery can affect the central nervous system. Data from in vitro animal models suggest that certain cytokines can be actively transported across the blood-brain barrier (Banks & Kastin 1992; Banks et al., 1993; Gutierrez, Banks, & Kastin, 1993). It is also possible that some cytokines in the periphery may influence the release of cytokines in the CNS via circumventricular organelles: IL-1 receptors have been isolated in glial cells around arterioles and the choroid plexus (Licinio & Wong, 1994; Saper & Breder, 1994). Cytokines also are produced by a variety of cells present within the central nervous system, including neurons, astrocytes, and microglial cells. Both astrocytes and microglia can be stimulated by neurotransmitters and exogenous stimuli to produce cytokines and also adhesion molecules, like I-CAM-1 and V-CAM-1 (Müller & Ackenheil, 1998). Thus a variety of different cells found in the CNS can produce brisk and varied cytokine production in response to peripheral stimulation. These cytokines may not only elicit changes in neurotransmitter levels in specific areas in the brain, but may cause temporary alterations in the blood-brain barrier as well (Frei et al., 1989; Muraguchi et al., 1988). Such alteration may increase the permeability of the head-brain barrier to substances from the periphery.

In closing the discussion of the interactions between the central nervous system and the immune system, it is important to acknowledge material that is extensively covered in other portions of this book. In vivo studies demonstrate that stress may decrease immune function and exacerbate chronic viral illnesses (Kiecolt-Glaser & Glaser 1987; Laudenslager 1987; Bartrop, Lazarus, Luckhurst, Kilch, & Penny, 1977; Zisook et al., 1994). There is also a large body of data suggesting that depressive disorders are associated with alterations of immune function (Müller, Ackenheil, Hofschuster, Mempel, & Eckstein, 1993a; Maes et al., 1993a, b). Data from animal models of depression, and human psychiatric conditions clearly show that the CNS can affect immune function. Thus, there is bidirectional communication between the immune system and the brain that is clearly important to intact homeostasis in humans (Reichlin, 1993).

## VI. RECENT STUDIES INVESTIGATING IMMUNE FUNCTION IN SCHIZOPHRENIA

Three lines of investigation suggest that alterations in immune function may somehow be associated with schizophrenia. First, epidemiological data demonstrate associations between prenatal viral infection and subsequent onset of schizophrenia in offspring years later. Second, studies demonstrate that immune dysfunction is associated with acute exacerbation of schizophrenia. Finally, research suggests that immune activation may be present in chronically ill individuals with schizophrenia. The most convincing indirect evidence which implicates a possible viral mechanism in schizophrenia continues to be epidemiological data. As early as 1977, Torrey, Torrey, and Petersen (1997) demonstrated that there was a bias in the seasonality of birth for schizophrenic patients. A disproportionate number of patients were born in the late winter and early spring and the majority of episodes initial onset of psychotic symptoms occurred in the early summer (Torrey et al., 1997). It has been postulated that this pattern of birth and illness is consistent with prenatal exposure to viral infection, which then predisposes individuals toward the development of schizophrenia in late adolescence or early adulthood. Mednick, Machon, Huttenen, and Bonnett (1988) performed an elegant study investigating the outcome of a birth cohort from Finland, whose fetal development overlapped with the influenza A2 epidemic of 1957. They found that there was an increased risk of schizophrenia for children whose mothers had this neurotrophic form of influenza during the second trimester of their pregnancy. This finding has been replicated by some other groups. A related line of intriguing epidemiological evidence has been the published association between location of birth in northern geographic areas and a greater risk of both schizophrenia and multiple sclerosis (Templer, Regier, & Corgiat, 1985; Templer, Cappellety, & Kauffman, 1988). In summary, epidemiological evidence suggests an association between maternal infection with neurotropic viruses and development of schizophrenia in their progeny and an association between northern latitudes, possible viral exposure, and schizophrenia. For an in-depth review of the viral hypothesis and its newer elaborations, please see the review by Yolken and Torrey (1995).

There has been a variety of disparate findings of immune stigmata in patients with schizophrenia. When evaluated as isolated independent studies, this literature may seem scattered and unconnected. One way of reconciling the majority of these findings, inspite of differences in methodology, is to hypothesize that acute psychiatric decompensation, and in this case, acute psychosis, may be associated with immune activation. It is described elsewhere in this text that the initiation of immune activation requires production of IL-6 and/or IL-1. This usually produces at least transient increases in IL-2, which is an important factor in the initiation of both TH-1 and TH-2 responses. Inferential data from a number of groups suggest an association between acute psychosis and the production of proinflammatory cytokines (particularly IL-6) (Ganguli et al., 1994; Maes et al., 1994), IL-2 and soluble IL-2 receptors (SIL-2Rs), in the serum of schizophrenic patients (Ganguli & Rabin, 1989; Rapaport, McAllister, Pickar, Nelson, & Paul, 1989; Hornberg, Arolt, Wilke, Kruse, & Kirchner, 1995; Müller & Ackenheil, 1995). Additional evidence that would be supportive of this hypothesis are the ex vivo studies which report blunted mitogen-stimulated lymphocyte IL-2 production in acutely decompensated schizophrenic patients (Ganguli et al., 1995; Hornberg et al., 1995; Villemain et al., 1989). Müller et al. (1997) also reported higher soluble IL-6 receptors in both the serum and the cerebrospinal fluid (CSF) of schizophrenic patients. Increased levels of proinflammatory cytokines would be consistent with findings from the 1980s and the early 1990s investigating the numbers and percentages of circulating lymphocytes in schizophrenic patients. These studies reported increases in CD-4+ T cells (DeLisi, Goodman, Neckers, & Wyatt, 1982; Ganguli, Rabin, Kelly, Lyte, & Ragu, 1987; Rabin, Ganguli, Cunnick, & Lysle, 1988; Henneberg, Riedl, Dumke, & Kornhuber, 1990; Müller, Ackenheil, Hofschuster, Mempel, & Eckstein, 1993b, c), increased numbers of total T cells (DeLisi et al., 1982; Müller et al., 1993c), and the increased presence of CD-5+ B cells (McAllister et al., 1989). Therefore, a panoply of studies in acutely ill schizophrenic patients suggest that mild immune activation may be a state marker of recent psychotic decompensation. In an extension of this work, Maes et al. (1996) and Müller, Empl, Riedel, Schwarz, and Ackenheil (1997b) found that effective neuroleptic treatment and symptomatic improvement was associated with resolution of this mild systemic immune activation. Such findings of mild immune activation which resolves with effective treatment are similar to what has been reported by a number of European groups for major depression (Maes, Bosmans, &

Meltzer, 1995; Müller et al., 1993a). Therefore, one may be observing a generalized response to extreme psychopathologic states rather than a syndrome-specific response.

A third line of investigation of the immunology of schizophrenia has been based on the hypothesis that immune activation may be a trait marker for a minority of patients with schizophrenia. Our group has been one of the major proponents of this hypothesis. We deliberately have used serum measurements of the SIL-2R as our primary biological correlate for this work because of the following properties: (1) the tremendous stability of the SIL-2R in the blood; (2) the stability of SIL-2Rs in fresh and frozen serum and plasma samples; (3) the assay is carefully elaborated, very sensitive and specific, and well-accepted; and (4) increased serum SIL-2R levels are reliably reported in a variety of medical conditions where immune activation occurs including transplant rejection, response to acute infection, and the active phase of autoimmune diseases (Rubin & Nelson, 1990). Our path of investigation is derived from the initial finding in 1989 that a significant number of patients with schizophrenia had serum SIL-2Rs to standard deviations beyond the mean of their matched controls (Rapaport et al., 1989). This suggested to us that the study of immunological outliers within this heterogeneous group of individuals with the syndrome called schizophrenia might be a mechanism for identifying a biologically distinct cohort of patients. In order to pursue this line of investigation we had to demonstrate that these tremendous elevations (compared to matched controls) seen in serum SIL-2Rs were not were not a neuroleptic effect (Rapaport, McAllister, Kirch, & Pickar, 1990; Rapaport et al., 1991; Rapaport & Lohr, 1994). We also needed to demonstrate that this finding could be consistently replicated in schizophrenic patients (Rapaport et al., 1993; Rapaport, 1994b) and was present across different ethnic groups (Rapaport et al., 1994). An additional concern was the specificity of this finding for schizophrenia; our group determined that these markedly high levels of serum SIL-2Rs were not present in euthymic bipolar patients, symptomatic patients with panic disorder, symptomatic patients with social phobia, or symptomatic patients with depression (Rapaport, 1994; Rapaport & Stein 1994a, b; Rapaport & Irwin, 1996). Our current investigations focus on two issues: determining if there is a relationship between clinical variables and patients with markedly increased serum SIL-2Rs, and investigating the longitudinal stability of increased serum SIL-2Rs in patients with schizophrenia. We had previously found that very high levels of serum

SIL-2Rs were associated with tardive dyskinesia (Rapaport & Lohr, 1994). In follow-up studies, we confirmed this finding and demonstrated that increased levels of serum SIL-2Rs were also associated with the prodromal symptoms of tardive dyskinesia, disturbance in muscle force (Rapaport, Caligiuri, & Lohr, 1997). Preliminary data from our longitudinal studies suggest that greater than 65% of patients initially identify with markedly elevated serum SIL-2Rs maintain those elevations over time. Interim analysis of these data confirm our previous findings that such increases in SIL-2Rs are not associated with age of onset of illness, neuroleptic exposure, comorbid diagnosis, use of alcohol, or use of cigarettes. Preliminary statistical review of data from our longitudinal study suggests that summary measures of psychopathology were significantly higher for patients with markedly elevated serum SIL-2Rs, as compared to patients with normal serum levels. So, although these patients were not acutely exacerbated, patients with marked elevations of serum SIL-2Rs were more ill. However, longitudinal data confirming the presence of immune activation in these individuals across a variety of serum cytokine measures and determining what, if any, relationship there is between immune activation and clinical variables is essential in order to validate work related to this hypothesis.

This section demonstrates that currently there are at least three viable and coherent areas of research investigating the relationship between schizophrenia and the immune system. Review of studies investigating prenatal viral infections and risk of schizophrenia, acute exacerbations of psychosis and immune activation, and some studies of immune outliers and schizophrenia all suggest that these are three areas of research that merit further study. However, we would be remiss not to acknowledge that we deliberately did not devote a great deal of time to the investigation of neuroleptic effects and schizophrenia, investigation of cytokine levels in the CSF, or investigations of antibody production in the serum or the CSF. Findings in these areas are controversial and, in general, do not significantly add to a coherent discussion of immune findings and schizophrenia. Review of these important areas of data can be found in other publications (Müller & Ackenheil, 1998; Rapaport & McAllister, 1991).

## VII. FUTURE DIRECTIONS

The investigation of immune dysfunction in schizophrenia is challenging because of the rapid evolution of the two fields. However, one of the major constraints to working in this area has been the lack of funding sufficient for investigators to identify, and longitudinally track, large cohorts of patients. Even the recent studies in this field tend to be of smaller size and relatively short duration. There is a need, particularly when dealing with such a heterogeneous syndrome, for carefully done, very large sample size studies. Ideally, individuals in such a cohort could be monitored for several years in order to determine both the relationship between acute variations in psychotic symptoms and immune parameters as well as the relationship between immune activation and longitudinal prognosis. A second area where it is important to direct research efforts is the continued elaboration of the location, structure, function, behavioral effects, and physiological effects of cytokines and other immunomodulators within the CNS. This requires redoubled efforts employing animal models. A further welcome addition to work in this field would be the application of newer molecular biology techniques to this research area. There is a need to encourage more extensive collaborations between clinicians, who have been responsible for most of the clinical research in this area of endeavor, and basic immunologists. For example, our group has been engaged in pilot work investigating modulation of the promoter region of the alpha chain of the soluble IL-2 receptor as part of our ongoing evaluation why SIL-2Rs may be increased in some patients. We also have begun to use cDNA cloning to ascertain whether there are autoantibodies unique to schizophrenia, which might be reacting with, as of yet, uncharacterized proteins. Although endeavors such as these are high risk, they are essential if this area of investigation is to move forward in a fashion comparable to other areas of psychoneuroimmunology.

## References

Alonso, R., Chaudieu, I., Diorio, J., Krishnamurthy, A., Quirion, R., & Boksa, P. (1993). Interleukin-2 modulates evoked release of [3H]dopamine in rat cultured mesencephalic cells. *Journal of Neurochemistry, 61,* 1284–1290.

Awatsuji, H., Furukawa, Y., Nakajima, M., Furukawa, S., & Hayashi, K. (1993). Interleukin-2 as a neurotrophic factor for supporting the survival of neurons cultured from various regions of fetal rat brain. *Journal of Neuroscience Research, 35,* 305–311.

Banks, W. A., & Kastin, A. J. (1992). The interleukins-1 alpha, -1 beta, and -2 do not acutely disrupt the murine blood-brain barrier. *International Journal of Immunopharmacology, 14,* 629–636.

Banks, W. A., Kastin, A. J., & Gutierrez, E. G. (1993). Interleukin-1 alpha in blood has direct access to cortical brain cells. *Neuroscience Letters, 163,* 41–44.

Bartrop, R. W., Lazarus, L., Luckhurst, E., Kilch, L. G., & Penny, R. (1977). Depressed lymphocyte function after bereavement. *Lancet*, *I*, 834–836.

Berkenbosch, F., Van Oers, J., Del Ray, A., Tiders, F., & Besedovsky, H. O. (1987). Corticotropin-releasing factor-producing neurons in the rat activated by interleukin-1. *Science*, *238*, 524–526.

Benveniste, E. N. (1992). Inflammatory cytokines within the central nervous system: sources, function, and mechanism of action. *American Journal of Physiology*, *263* (Cell Physiology 32), C1–C16.

Besedovsky, H. O., Del Rey, A., Sorkin, E., & Dinarello, C. A. (1986). Immunregulatory feedback between interleukin-1 and glucocorticoid hormones. *Science*, *233*, 652–654.

Bruce, L. C., & Peebles, A. M. S. (1903). Clinical and experimental observations on catatonia. *Journal of Mental Science*, *49*, 614–628.

Bruce, L. C., & Peebles, A. M. S. (1904). Quantitative and qualitative leukocyte counts in various forms of mental disease. *Journal of Mental Science*, *50*, 409–417.

Carlsson, A., & Lindquist, M. (1963). Effect of chlorpromazine and haloperidole on the formation of 3-methoxytyramine and normetanophrine in mouse brain. *Acta Pharmacologica*, *20*, 140–144.

Dameschek, W. (1930). The white blood cells in dementia praecox and dementia paralytica. *Archives of Neurological Psychiatry*, *24*, 855.

Dameschek, W. (1931). White blood cells in general paresis. *Massachusetts Department of Mental Diseases Bulletin*, *15*, 26–39.

Delisi, L. E., Goodman, S., Neckers, L. M., & Wyatt, R. J. (1982). An analysis of lymphocyte subpopulations in schizophrenic patients. *Biological Psychiatry*, *17*, 1003–1009.

Denicoff, K. D., Rubinoff, D. R., Papa, M. Z., Simpson, C., Seipp, C. A., Lotze, M. T., Chang, A. E., Rosenstein, D., & Rosenberg, S. A. (1987). The neuropsychiatric effects of treatment with interleukin-2 and lymphokine-activated killer cells. *Annals of Internal Medicine*, *107*, 293–300.

Dide, M. (1905). La demence precoce est un syndrome mental toxi-infectieux subaigu ou chronique. *Revue Neurologique*, *13*, 381–386.

Dunn, A. J. (1992). Endotoxin-induced activation of cerebral catecholamine and serotonin metabolism: Comparison with interleukin-1. *Journal of Pharmacology and Experimental Therapy*, *261*, 964–969.

Dunn, A. J. (1994). Pituitary-adrenal activation and behavioral activity of interleukin-1. *Neuropsychopharmacology*, *10*(1), 833.

Ermakov, J. (1910). Investigation of the blood in some forms of mental disorder. *Archives of Internal Neurology*, *2*, 369.

Fessel, W. (1962). Autoimmunity and mental illness: preliminary report. *Archives of General Psychiatry*, *6*, 320–323.

Fieve, R., Blumenthal, B., & Little, B. (1966). The relationship of atypical lymphocytes, phenothiazines, and schizophrenia. *Archives of General Psychiatry*, *15*, 539–534.

Frei, K., Malipiero, U. V., Leist, T. P., Zinkernagel, R. M., Schwab, M. E., & Fontana, A. (1989). On the cellular source and function of interleukin 6 produced in the central nervous system in viral diseases. *European Journal of Immunology*, *19*, 689–694.

Ganguli, R., & Rabin, B. S. (1989). Increased serum interleukin 2 receptor levels in schizophrenic and brain damaged subjects. *Archives of General Psychiatry*, *46*, 292.

Ganguli, R., Rabin, B. S., Kelly, R. H., Lyte, M., & Ragu, U. (1987). Clinical and laboratory evidence of autoimmunity in acute schizophrenia. *Annals of the New York Academy of Sciences*, *496*, 676–685.

Ganguli, R., Brar, J. S., Chengappa, K. R., Deleo, M., Yang, Z. W., Shurin, G., & Rabin, B. (1995). Mitogen-stimulated interleukin 2 production in never-medicated. First episode schizophrenics—

the influence of age of onset and negative symptoms. *Archives of General Psychiatry*, *52*, 668–672.

Ganguli, R., Yang, A., Shurin, G., Chengappa, R., Brar, J. S., Gubbi, A. V., & Rabin, B. S. (1994). Serum interleukin-6 concentration in schizophrenia elevation associated with duration of illness. *Psychiatry Research*, *51*, 1–10.

Gutierrez, E. G., Banks, W. A., & Kastin, A. J. (1993). Murine tumor necrosis factor alpha is transported from blood to brain in the mouse. *Journal of Neuroimmunology*, *47*, 169–176.

Hanisch, U. K., Seto, D., & Quirion, R. (1993). Modulation of hippocampal acetylcholine release: A potent central action of interleukin-2. *Journal of Neuroscience*, *13*, 3368–3374.

Heath, R., & Krupp, I. (1967). Schizophrenia as an immunological disorder. I. demonstration of antibrain globulins by flourescent antibody techniques. *Archives of General Psychiatry*, *16*, 1–9.

Henneberg, A., Riedl, B., Dumke, H. O., & Kornhuber, H. H. (1990). T-lymphocyte subpopulations in schizophrenic patients. *European Archives of Psychiatry and Neurological Sciences*, *239*, 283–284.

Hornberg, M., Arolt, V., Wilke, I., Kruse, A., & Kirchner, H. (1995). Production of interferons and lymphokines in leukocyte cultures of patients with schizophrenia. *Schizophrenia Research*, *15*, 237–242.

Kent, S., Bluthe, R. M., Kelley, K. W., & Dantzer, R. (1992). Sickness behavior and drug development. *Trends in Pharmacological Sciences*, *13*, 24–28.

Kiecolt-Glaser, J. K., & Glaser, R. (1987). Psychosocial influences on herpes virus latency. In E. Kursak, E. J. Lipowski, & P. V. Morozov (Eds.), *Viruses, immunity, and mental disorders* (pp. 403–412). London, New York: Plenum.

Lapchak, P. A. (1992). A role for Interleukin-2 in the regulation of striatal dopaminergic function. *Neuroreport*, *3*, 165–168.

Lapchak, P. A., Araujo, D. M., Quirion, R., & Beaudet, A. (1991). Immunoradiographic localization of interleukin 2-like immunoreactivity and interleukin 2 receptors (Tac antigen-like immunoreactivity) in the rat brain. *Neuroscience*, *44*, 173–184.

Laudenslager, M. L. (1987). Psychosocial stress and susceptibility to infections disease. In E. Kurstak, E. J. Lipowski, & P. V. Morozov (Eds.), *Viruses, immunity, and mental disorders* (pp. 391–402). London, New York: Plenum.

Lehmann-Facius, H. (1937). Uber die liquordiagnose der schizophrenien. *Klinische Wochenschrift*, *16*, 1646–1648.

Lehmann-Facius, H. (1939). Serologisch-analytische versuche mit liquoren und seren von schizophrenien. *Allgemeine Zeitschrist für Psychiatrie*, *110*, 232–343.

Licinio, J., & Wong, M. L. (1994). Localizations of interleukin-1 and interleukin-1 mRNA in brain: pathophysiological implications. *Neuropsychopharmacology*, *10*(1), 834.

Maes, M., Bosmans, E., & Meltzer, H. Y. (1995). Immunoendocrine aspects of major depression: Relationships between plasma interleukin-6 and soluble interleukin-2 receptor, prolactin and cortisol. *European Archives of Psychiatry and Clinical Neuroscience*, *245*, 172–178.

Maes, M., Bosmans, E., Ranjan, R., Vandoolaeghe, B., Meltzer, H. Y., DeLey, M., Berghmans, R., Stans, G., & Desnyder, R. (1996). Lower plasma CC16, a natural anti-inflammatory protein and increased plasma interleukin-1 receptor antagonist in schizophrenia: Effects of antipsychotic drugs. *Schizophrenia Research*, *21*, 39–50.

Maes, M., Meltzer, H. Y., & Bosmans, E. (1994). Immune-inflammatory markers in schizophrenia: Comparison to normal controls and effects of clozapine. *Acta Psychiatrica Scandinavica*, *89*, 346–351.

Maes, M., Meltzer, H. Y., Scharpé, S., Bosmans, E., Suy, E., De Meester, I., Calabrese, J., & Cosyns, P. (1993a). Relationships between interleukin-6 activity, acute phase proteins, and function of the hypothalamic-pituitary-adrenal axis in sever depression. *Psychiatry Research, 49,* 11–27.

Maes, M., Scharpé, S., Meltzer, H. Y., Bosmans, E., Suy, E., Calabrese, J., & Cosyns, P. (1993b). Relationships between lower plasma L-Tryptophan levels and immune-inflammatory variables in depression. *Psychiatry Research, 49,* 151–165.

McAllister, C. G., Rapaport, M. H., Pickar, D., Podruchny, T.A., Christison, G., Alphs, L.D., & Paul, S. M. (1989). Increased number of CD5[+] B-lymphocytes in schizophrenic patients. *Archives of General Psychiatry, 46,* 890–894.

Mednick, S., Machon, R., Huttenen, M., & Bonnett, D. (1988). Adult schizophrenia following prenatal exposure to an influenza epidemic. *Archives of General Psychiatry, 45,* 189–192.

Molholm, H. B. (1942). Hyposensitivity to foreign protein in schizophrenic patients. *Psychiatric Quarterly, 16,* 565.

Müller, N., & Ackenheil, M. (1995). The immune system and schizophrenia. In B. E. Leonard & K. Miller (Eds.), *Stress, the immune system and psychiatry* (pp. 137–164). Chichester, NY: Wiley.

Müller, N., & Ackenheil, M. (1998). Psychoneuroimmunology and the cytokine action in the CN8: Implications for psychiatric disorders. *Progress in Neuro-psychopharmacology and Biological Psychiatry, 22,* 1–33.

Müller, N., Ackenheil, M., Hofschuster, E., Mempel, W., & Eckstein, R. (1993a). Investigations of the cellular immunity during depression and the free interval: Evidence for an immune activation in affective psychosis. *Progress in Neuro-psychopharmacology and Biological Psychiatry, 17,* 713–730.

Müller, N., Ackenheil, M., Hofschuster, E., Mempel, W., & Eckstein, R. (1993b). Cellular immunity, HLA-class I antigens, and family history of psychiatric disorder in endogenous psychoses. *Psychiatry Research, 48,* 201–217.

Müller, N., Ackenheil, M., Hofschuster, E., Mempel, W., & Eckstein, R. (1993c). T-cells and psychopathology in schizophrenia: Relationship to the outcome of neuroleptic therapy. *Acta Psychiatrica Scandinavica, 87,* 66–71.

Müller, N., Dobmeier, P., Empl, M., Riedel, M., Schwarz, M., & Ackenheil, M. (1997a). Soluble IL-6 receptors in the serum and cerebrospinal fluid of paranoid schizophrenic patients. *European Psychiatry* (in press).

Müller, N., Empl, M., Riedel, M., Schwarz, M., & Ackenheil, M. (1997b). Decrease of soluble IL-6 receptor and increase of soluble IL-2 receptor serum levels in schizophrenic patients reflect the immunomodulatory effect of neuroleptics. *European Archives of Psychiatry and Clinical Neuroscience* (submitted).

Muraguchi, A., Hirano, R., Tang, B., Matsuda, T., Horii, Y., Nakajima, K., & Kishimoto, T. (1988). The essential role of B-cell stimulating factor 2 (BSF-2/IL-6) for the terminal differentiation of B cells. *Journal of Experimental Medicine, 167,* 332–344.

Nemni, R., Iannaccone, S., Quattrini, A., Smirne, S., Sessa, M., Lodi, M., Erminio, C., & Canal N. (1992). Effect of chronic treatment with recombinant interleukin-2 on the central nervous system of adult and old mice. *Brain Research, 591,* 248–252.

Nistico, G., & De Sarro, G. (1991). Is interleukin 2 a neuromodulator in the brain? *Trends in Neuroscience, 14,* 146–150.

Plata-Salaman, C. R., & French-Mullen, J. M. (1993). Interleukin-2 modulates calcium currents in dissociated hippocampal CA1 neurons. *Neuroreport, 4,* 579–581.

Rabin, B. S., Ganguli, R., Cunnick, J. E., & Lysle, D. T. (1988). The central nervous system-immune system relationship. *Clinics in Laboratory Medicine, 8,* 253–268.

Ransohoff, R. M., & Benveniste, E. N. (1996). *Cytokines in the CNS.* Boca Raton, FL: CRC Press.

Rapaport, M. H. (1994). Immune parameters in euthymic bipolar patients and normal volunteers. *Journal of Affective Disorders, 32,* 149–156.

Rapaport, M. H., Caligiuri, M. P., & Lohr, J. B. (1997). An association between increased serum-soluble interleukin-2 receptors and a disturbance in muscle force in schizophrenic patients. *Progress in Neuro-psychopharmacology and Biological Psychiatry, 21,* 817–827.

Rapaport, M. H., Doran, A. R., Nelson, D. M., McAllister, C. G., Magliozzi, J. R., & Paul, S. M. (1991). Haloperidol and soluble interleukin-2 receptors. *Biological Psychiatry, 30,* 1063–1065.

Rapaport, M. H., & Irwin, M. (1996). Serum soluble interleukin-2 receptors and natural killer cell function in major depression. *Research Communications in Biological Psychology and Psychiatry, 21(1,2),* 73–78.

Rapaport, M. H., & Lohr, J. B. (1994). Serum interleukin-2 receptors in neuroleptic have schizophrenic subjects and in medicated schizophrenic subjects with and without tardive dyskinesia. *Acta Psychiatrica Scandinavica, 90,* 311–5.

Rapaport, M. H., & McAllister, C. G. (1991). Neuroimmunologic factors in schizophrenia. In Gorman & Kertzner (Eds.), *Psychoimmunology update* (pp. 31–47). Washington, DC: American Psychiatric Press.

Rapaport, M. H., McAllister, C. G., Kim, Y. S., Han, J. H., Pickar, D., Nelson, D. M., Kirch, D. G., & Paul, S. M. (1994). Increased soluble interleukin-2 receptors in Caucasian and Korean schizophrenic patients. *Biological Psychiatry, 35,* 767–771.

Rapaport, M. H., McAllister, C. G., Kirch, D. G., & Pickar, D. (1990). The effects of typical and atypical neuroleptics on mitroten-induced T lymphocyte responsiveness. *Biological Psychiatry, 29,* 715–717.

Rapaport, M. H., McAllister, C. G., Pickar, D., Nelson, D. M., & Paul, S. M. (1989). Elevated levels of soluble interleukin 2 receptors in schizophrenia. *Archives of General Psychiatry, 46,* 292.

Rapaport, M. H., & Stein, M. B. (1994a). Serum interleukin-2 and soluble interleukin-2 receptor levels in generalized social phobia. *Anxiety, 1(2),* 50–53.

Rapaport, M. H., & Stein, M. B. (1994b). Serum cytokine and soluble interleukin-2 receptors in patients with panic disorder. *Anxiety, 1(1),* 22–25.

Rapaport, M. H., Torrey, E. F., McAllister, C. G., Nelson, D. M., Pickar, D., & Paul, S. M. (1993). Increased serum soluble interleukin-2 receptors in schizophrenic monozygotic twins. *European Archives of Psychiatry and Clinical Neuroscience, 243,* 7–10.

Reichlin, S. (1993). Neuroendocrine-immune interactions. *New England Journal of Medicine, 329,* 1246–1253.

Rubin, L. A., & Nelson, D. L. (1990). The soluble interleukin-2 receptor biology, function and clinical application. *Annals of Internal Medicine, 113,* 619–627.

Saper, C. B., & Breder, C. D. (1994). The neurologic basis of fever. *New England Journal of Medicine, 330(26),* 1880–1886.

Shintani, F., Kanba, S., Nakaki, T., Nibuya, M., Kinoshita, N., Suzuki, E., Yagi, G., Kato, R., & Asai, M. (1993). Interleukin-1 beta augments release of norepinephrine, dopamine, and serotonin in the rat anterior hypothalamus. *Journal of Neuroscience, 13,* 3574–3581.

Sindic, C. J., & Laterre, E. C. (1991). Oligoclonal free kappa and lambda bands in the cerebrospinal fluid of patients with mulitple sclerosis and other neurological diseases: an immunoaffinity-mediated capillary blot study. *Journal of Neuroimmunology, 33*, 63–72.

Soliven, B., & Albert, J. (1992). Tumor necrosis factor modulates the inactivation of catecholamine secretion in cultured sympathetic neurons. *Journal of Neurochemistry, 58*, 1073–1078.

Swedo, S., Rapoport, J., Cheslow, D. L., Leonard, H. L., Ayoub, E. M., Hosier, D. M., & Wald, E. R. (1989). High prevalence of obsessive-compulsive symptoms in patients with Sydenham's Chorea. *American Journal of Psychiatry, 146*, 246–249.

Templer, D., Cappelletty, G., & Kauffman, I. (1988). Schizophrenia and multiple sclerosis: Distribution in Italy. *British Journal of Psychiatry, 153*, 389–390.

Templer, D. I., Regier, M. W., & Corgiat, M. D. (1985). Similar distribution of schizophrenia and multiple sclerosis. *Journal of Clinical Psychiatry, 46*, 73.

Torrey, E. F., Torrey, B. B., & Petersen, M. R. (1977). Seasonality of schizophrenic births in the United States. *Archives of General Psychiatry, 34*, 1065–1070.

van Dam, A. P. (1991). Diagnosis and pathogenesis of CNS lupus. *Rheumatology Investigation, 11*, 1–11.

Vaughn, W. T., Sullivan, J. C., & Elmadjian, F. (1949). Immunity and schizophrenia. *Psychosomatic Medicine, 11*, 327.

Villemain, F., Chatenoud, L., Galinowski, A., Homo-Delarache, F., Genestet, D., Loo, H., Zarifarain, E., & Bach, J. F. (1989). Aberrant T-cell-medicated immunity in untreated schizophrenic patients: Deficient interleukin-2 production. *American Journal of Psychiatry, 146*, 609–616.

Yolken, R. H., & Torrey, E. F. (1995). Viruses, schizophrenia, and bipolar disorder. *Clinical Microbiology Review, 8*, 131–145.

Zalcman, S., Green-Johnson, J. M., Murray, L., Nance, D. M., Dyck, D., Anisman, H., & Greenberg, A. H. (1994). Cytokine-specific central monoamine alterations induced by interleukin-1, -2, and -6. *Brain Research, 643*, 40–49.

Zarrabi, M., Zucker, S., Miller, F., Derman, R. M., Romano, G. S., Hartnett, J. A., & Varma, A. O. (1979). Immunologic and co-agulation disorders in chlorpromazine-treated patients. *Annals of Internal Medicine, 91*, 194–199.

Zisook, S., Shuchter, S. R., Irwin, M., Darko, D. F., Sledge, P., & Resovsky, K. (1994). Bereavement, depression, and immune function. *Psychiatry Research, 52*, 1–10.

# Depression and Immunity

MICHAEL IRWIN

## I. INTRODUCTION

Substantial evidence has shown that major depression is associated with immune variations. In a meta-analytic review of over 35 independent study samples conducted through 1991, depression was found to be associated with reliable alterations in several enumerative measures and in functional assays such as mitogen-induced lymphocyte proliferation and natural killer (NK) cell activity (Herbert & Cohen, 1993a). Since 1991, many additional studies on the relationship between depression and immune measures have been published which in general have supported the conclusions that depression is associated with changes in several immune measures such as major immune cell classes, lymphocyte proliferation, and NK activity. Nevertheless, conflicting results have been obtained for many other measures, suggesting an enormous heterogeneity in the findings.

The role of several moderating factors that might contribute to variability in the link between depression and immunity has been explored in a series of separate studies as will be reviewed below. While several moderator variables including age, gender, ambulatory status, and depressive symptom severity clearly have a role, only part of the heterogeneity can be explained by these factors. Further investigations are clearly needed to understand what variables correlate with immune alterations in depression and whether there are subgroups of depressed subjects who are at risk for immune alterations.

The present chapter will review and summarize results of studies on immune alterations in depression. In view of the complexity and heterogeneity of the immunological findings in depression, we will also consider the possible characteristics related to depressed subjects or to the nature of their depressive disorder which might moderate the association between depression and immune alterations. Identification of such moderators are particularly important as converging evidence suggests that immune alterations in major depressive disorder are not specific correlates of this disorder. Rather, similar kinds of changes in natural and cellular immunity occur in association with stress and other psychiatric disorders which supports the possibility that certain shared behavioral or biological characteristics underlie and/or mediate the immune changes. An additional challenge of immune studies in depression is to move beyond a description of immune variations and to evaluate whether alterations of the immune system in depression have clinical implications. A third and final section of this chapter will review ongoing investigations of specific immune responses in depression that are related to outcome.

## II. IMMUNE RESULTS IN DEPRESSION

Three general domains of immune measures have been examined in studies of depressed subjects: enumerative measures, functional measures, and markers of immune activation. Each domain will be briefly described with a review of the respective immune findings in depressive disorder.

### A. Enumerative Measures

Enumerative measures provide a measure of the total number of circulating immune cells and quantify the absolute and relative numbers of the major immune cell classes such as neutrophils, lymphocytes, and monocytes. In addition, enumerative measures provide an assessment of the number and percentage of cells expressing cell surface markers related to B cells and T-lymphocyte subset phenotypes.

One of the first immunological findings identified in the study of depressed subjects was change in the total number of white blood cells and numbers and percentages of neutrophils and lymphocytes (Albrecht, Helderman Schlesser, & Rush, 1985; Irwin et al., 1990a, b; et al., 1990b; Irwin, Smith & Gillin, 1987; Kronfol & House, 1989; Kronfol, Turner, Nasrallah, & Winokur, 1984; Maes et al., 1992a; Schleifer, Keller, Bond, Cohen, & Stein, 1989; Schleifer, Keller, Siris, Davis & Stein, 1985; Schleifer et al., 1984; Sengar , Waters, Dunne, & Bover, 1982). Along with an increase in the total number of white blood cells, increases in the number of neutrophils and decreases in the number of lymphocytes have been reliably demonstrated (Herbert & Cohen, 1993a). In regards to numbers of monocytes, a relative increase in the number of monocytes has been found in many studies of depressed subjects (Maes et al., 1992a), whereas other depression samples have shown decreases or no differences in the absolute or relative numbers of monocytes (Irwin et al., 1987, 1990a, b).

Cellular enumeration of lymphocyte subsets by the quantification of phenotypic specific cell surface markers has been widely used to evaluate alterations of the immune system in relation to diagnostic depression. Depression is negatively related to the number and percentages of lymphocytes that are B cells, T cells, T helper cells, and T suppressor/cytotoxic cells (Herbert Cohen, 1993a). A decrease in circulating number of cells that express the NK phenotype has also been reported which in part is moderated by gender; a decline of NK cell numbers is found in male but not female depressed subjects as compared to that seen in gender matched controls (Evans et al., 1992). However, multiple discrepant findings have also been reported and, in one of the largest study samples of depressed subjects, no difference in the number of peripheral blood lymphocytes or T lymphocyte subsets was found between depressed patients and controls (Schleifer et al., 1989). Indeed, with accumulation of studies, it is questionable as to whether there are consistent changes in the number of circulating B, T, or NK cells in depression.

### B. Functional Measures

Function of the immune system has been typically evaluated in depressed subjects by assay of nonspecific mitogen-induced lymphocyte proliferation, mitogen-stimulated cytokine production, and NK cytotoxicity. Lymphocyte proliferation assays examine how well lymphocytes divide in response to a nonspecific mitogen. This assay along with the release of cytokines assumes that with more proliferation and more cytokine release, the lymphocytes are functioning more effectively. The purpose of the third functional assay, NK-cell cytotoxicity, is to determine the ability of NK cells to lyse tumor cells in culture.

#### 1. Mitogen-Induced Lymphocyte Proliferation

A reliable association between depression and lower proliferative responses to the mitogens phytohemaglutinin (PHA), concanavalin A (Con A), and pokeweed has been found (Herbert & Cohen, 1993a). Some of the first observations evaluating depression and mitogen responses showed reduced proliferation in depressed subjects as compared to that seen in controls (Kronfol & House, 1985; Kronfol et al., 1983; Schleifer et al., 1984). However, subsequent studies failed to replicate these observations, raising questions about the reliability of this immune alteration in depression (Schleifer et al., 1989). Nevertheless, with over a dozen studies now conducted on lymphocyte proliferation in depression (Albrecht et al., 1985; Altshuler, Plaeger-Marshall, Richeimer, Daniels, & Baxter, 1989; Bartoloni et al., 1990; Birmaher et al., 1994; Calabrese et al., 1986; Cosyns, Maes, Vandewoude, Stevens, DeClerck & Schotte, 1989; Darko et al., 1989; Kronfol & House, 1989; Kronfol, House, Silva, Greden, & Carroll, 1986; Lowy, Reder, Gormley, & Meltzer, 1988; Maes, Bosman, Suy, Minner, & Raus, 1989; McAdams & Leonard, 1993; Schleifer et al., 1985; Syvalahti, Eskola, Ruuskanen, & Laine, 1985), it appears that an impairment in the response of lymphocytes to all three nonspecific mitogens predominates in studies of depressed subjects.

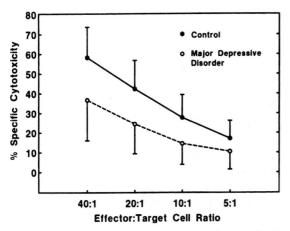

**FIGURE 1** Natural killer cell cytotoxicity in depressed subjects and controls. Each point represents the mean (±SD) of the percentage specific cytoxicity for each group across the four effector to target cell ratios. (Irwin et al., 1987).

### 2. Natural Killer Cytotoxicity

A reduction of NK activity is considered to be one of the most reliable and reproducible alterations of ex vivo immune function in depression (Stein, Miller & Trestman, 1991). Irwin and colleagues first reported a decline of NK activity in depressed patients as compared to that seen in age- and gender-matched comparison controls, (Irwin et al., 1987) (Figure 1), and 10 subsequent independent samples have replicated this observation. (Bartoloni et al., 1990; Birmaher et al., 1994; Caldwell, Irwin, & Lohr, 1991; Evans et al., 1992; Irwin, Lacher, & Caldwell, 1992a; Irwin et al., 1990a, b; Kronfol et al., 1989; Maes et al., 1992c; Nerozzi et al., 1989; Shain et al., 1991;). Although there are some discrepant findings (Mohl et al., 1987; Schleifer et al., 1989), Herbert and Cohen (1993a) found a fixed effect size of (-0.266 to −0.254). The factors that might moderate and/or mediate the effects of depression on NK activity will be discussed below.

### C. Markers of Immune Activation

Most previous studies have suggested that depression results in reductions of nonspecifc cellular and natural immunity. However, Maes has argued that major depression is associated with immune activation reminiscent of an acute phase response (Maes, Smith, & Scharpe, 1995). Evidence has been accumulated showing increases in levels of cells bearing activation markers such as HLA-DR+, CD25+ (interleukin-2 receptor) (Maes et al., 1992a), and increases in humoral factors or plasma proteins associated with the acute phase of the immune response ($\alpha$1-acid glycoprotein, $\alpha$1-antitrypsin, and haptoglobin) (Maes

et al., 1992b). In addition, cytokines such as interleukin-6 (IL-6), which are typically associated with an inflammatory process are reportedly elevated in depression and there are also reported increases in the circulating concentration of the soluble IL-2 receptor that is released with immune activation (Maes et al., 1995).

While these findings that an inflammatory process may occur in association with depression primarily emanate from one research group, there are additional preclinical data that suggest that macrophage activation might occur in depressed subjects and could be a key factor in the observed impairments of T-cell proliferation (Maier, Watkins, & Fleshner, 1994). In a putative animal model of depression (uncontrollable shock), concomitant monokine release occurs, and this macrophage activation produces an impairment in T-cell-mediated proliferation.

Replication of clinical data concerning immune activation in depression is clearly needed, but there have been few independent studies separate from the work of Maes. Importantly, correlations have been found between cigarette smoking and increases in haptoglobin, $\alpha$1-acid glycoprotein, and $\alpha$1-antitypsin, suggesting the possibility that increased prevalence of tobacco consumption in depressed and other psychiatric populations may underlie the relationship between depression and markers of immune activation.

### D. Summary of Results

The relationship between clinical depression and measures of immunological function shows considerable variability with a predominance of heterogeneous findings for many of the immune parameters. However, it appears that depressed patients are likely to show an increase in total white blood cell counts with a relative neutrophilia and a relative lymphopenia. In addition, depressed subjects are likely to show impairments in functional assays of mitogen-induced lymphocyte proliferation and NK cytotoxicity. Further research is needed to characterize immune activation in depression.

## III.  MODERATORS OF THE DEPRESSION–IMMUNE LINK

It is not known what accounts for the studywise heterogeneity in the relationship between depression and immunity. Stein, Miller, and Trestman (1991) proposed that alterations in the immune system in major depression are not specific biologic correlates of this disorder, but rather occur in association with other variables that characterize depressed subjects such as age, hospitalization stress, and severity of depressive symptoms. Indeed, subject characteristics such as age, gender, and symptom severity have been evaluated as possible moderators of the relationship between depression and immunity (Herbert & Cohen, 1993a), but have been found to explain only partially the heterogeneity observed.

The role of other factors in moderating the effects of depression on the immune system has not been systematically explored. However, several exploratory studies have been conducted that indicate the possibility that additional subject characteristics and/or depression status variables may moderate the relation between depression and immunity.

In the present chapter, the role of several moderator variables will be considered in addition to age, gender, and symptom severity. For example, life stressors have been found to be associated with changes in the immune system (Herbert & Cohen, 1993b), and such stress-induced immune alterations are similar to the kinds of changes found in depressed subjects. Thus, we will discuss whether the subacute stress of hospitalization and/or chronic life stress often reported in depressed patients contribute to the immune changes found in diagnostic depression (Caldwell et al., 1991; Irwin et al., 1990b).

Second, symptom severity has been suggested as an important correlate of immune changes in depressed subjects, but what specific symptoms account for this relation requires further study to know whether there are certain subgroups or subtypes of depressed subjects who are most at risk for immune changes. Some evidence suggests that depressed patients with neurovegetative symptoms are more likely to show immune changes (Cover & Irwin, 1994), and a number of observations implicate sleep in the regulation of some aspects of immune function (Irwin et al., 1994, 1996; Irwin, Smith, & Gillin, 1992b).

Finally, comorbidity in depression has emerged as a major concern in biologic research in psychiatry with recent epidemiological data showing, for example, that as many as 50% of depressed patients are comorbid for an anxiety disorder such as panic (Stein & Uhde, 1988; Murphy, Oliver, Sobol, Monson, & Leighton, 1986). Moreover, the prevalence of alcohol and tobacco dependence is high in depressed subjects (Breslau, Peterson, Schultz, Chilcoat, & Andreski, 1998; Schuckit, 1986), but few studies have examined the contribution of alcohol intake or cigarette smoking on alterations of immune function in depressed subjects despite the well-recognized effects of these substances on immune parameters. The following will also consider the effects of comorbidity for anxiety and/or substance dependence in the relation between depression and immunity.

## A. Subject Characteristics

### 1. Age

Age has been proposed as a key moderator in the association between depression and immunity. In three reviews (Weisse, 1992; Stein et al., 1991; Herbert & Cohen, 1993a) it was concluded that older depressed patients are more likely to show immune differences than younger depressed subjects. The findings of Schleifer and colleagues (1989) (Figure 2) are most representative of this conclusion; controls showed an age-related increase in CD4 numbers and mitogen responses, whereas depressed patients did not show such changes in either T-cell numbers or lymphocyte proliferation with advancing age. However, specific age group comparisons of depressives vs. controls have not been conducted and it is not known, for example, whether elderly depressed

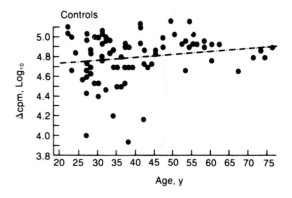

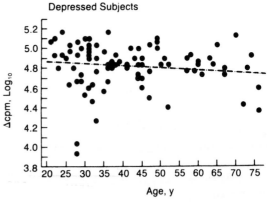

**FIGURE 2**   Scatterplots of raw data of controls and depressed patients for PHA-induced lymphocyte stimulation vs. age. Each point represents mean of three replicates of stimulated cultures minus unstimulated cultures (Δ cpm [counts per minute]). Lines are fitted regression of relation between adjusted data and age (Schleifer et al., 1989, with permission. Copyright © 1989, American Medical Association.)

subgroups show greater immune differences than adolescent or young adult samples. Furthermore, in studies of depressed patients, age and hospitalization status are correlated and, as cautioned by Herbert and Cohen, (1993a), the separate effects of age and hospitalization status on depression–immunity associations cannot be determined without carefully matching depressed inpatients and outpatients with controls on both age and hospitalization status. Of course, another strategy would be to design a study that was restricted to either inpatient or outpatient depressed subjects and then to evaluate the effects of age within that hospitalization status subgroup. For example, Irwin and his associates (1990b) focused on inpatient depressed subjects and found that these subjects had lower NK activity than controls. However, within the inpatient depressed subjects, there was no effect of age or an age by depressive symptom interaction on NK activity (Irwin et al., 1990b).

## 2. Gender

The stability of the depression immune relationship across gender also deserves further attention due to the well-recognized effects of reproductive hormones such as progesterone to antagonize the suppressive effects of glucocorticoids on cellular immune function (Dietrich, Chasserot-Golaz, Beck, & Bauer, 1986). Many studies have included only male depressed subjects and eliminated the possible contribution of gender (Irwin et al., 1990a, b). Other studies have included male and female depressives and evaluated effects of gender using correlational analyses (Schleifer et al., 1989). The latter have typically not found any effects of gender on either enumerative or functional immune measures in depression, a finding consistent with the conclusion reached by Herbert and Cohen (1993a). However, only a few studies have stratified the sample and made direct comparisons between depressives and controls matched on the basis of gender. Miller, Asnis, Lackner, Halbreich, and Norin (1991) found, in outpatient depressives, that female subjects had higher NK activity than controls, whereas male depressives were similar to controls. In contrast, Evans and his colleagues (1992). (Figure 3) studied both inpatient and outpatient depressed subjects and found that men with major depression had a marked reduction in number of NK cells (Leu-11) and in NK activity compared with controls. By contrast, depressed women did not differ significantly on any of these immune measures. Similar comparisons on the basis of gender have not been conducted for other immune measures.

## 3. Stress

Both life stress and depression have been associated with similar changes of immune measures

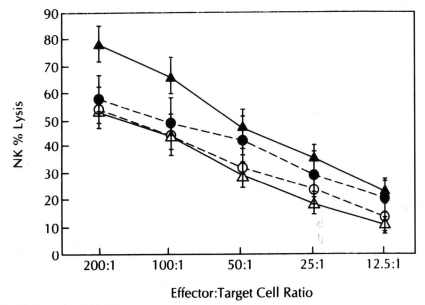

**FIGURE 3**  Natural killer cytotoxicity in depressed subjects and controls stratified on the basis of gender. Each point represents the mean (±SEM) of the percentage specific cytotoxicity for each group across the five effector to target cell ratios. Solid triangles indicate male controls ($n = 10$); solid circles, female controls ($n = 9$); open triangles, men with major depression ($n = 17$); and open circles, women with major depression ($n = 13$) (Evans et al., 1992 with permission. Copyright © 1992, American Medical Association.)

(Herbert & Cohen, 1993a, b), and it is possible that these two conditions together might interact and influence immunity more than the presence of life stress or depression alone. Depressed subjects are more likely to experience severe life events during their depressive episode due in part to the functional impairments associated with depression (Brown, Harris, & Hepworth, 1994). For example, a depressive episode may be associated with deterioration in work performance such that the person loses his/her job. Likewise, impairment in social interactions during depression may affect a spousal relationship, leading to threatened divorce or separation. To our knowledge, the joint contribution of threatening life events and depression on immune function has only preliminarily been examined in one study.

In a sample of 36 subject pairs of depressed patients and comparison controls, the presence of severe threatening life stress was assessed using the objective methods of Brown and Harris (1978). Subjects in both groups were classified as having low or high stress and NK activity was measured. Findings demonstrate a reduction of NK activity in subjects with major depression as compared with that seen in persons who are neither stressed nor depressed. Second, individuals who are undergoing severe life stress show a similar reduction of NK activity even though they do not have clinically significant depressive symptoms. The combination of severe stress and depression did not result in any further reduction of NK activity. Thus, the immune changes found in life stress parallel those found in depression. However, the changes found in depressed subjects can not be explained simply by the occurrence of severe life stress (Irwin et al., 1990b). In other words, life stress influences cellular immunity, but it does not appear to moderate the association between depression and immunity. Similar conclusions were also reached in the evaluation of the effects of acute hospitalization stress on depression-related impairments of NK activity (Caldwell et al., 1991).

## B. Depression Status

### 1. Ambulatory Status

A decrease of mitogen responses in hospitalized patients with major depression but not in ambulatory patients with depression suggests that alterations of immunity in depression are related to hospitalization status or to severity of depressive symptoms (Schleifer et al., 1984, 1985). While subsequent study of both inpatient and outpatient depressed subjects failed to identify an effect for hospitalization status

(Schleifer et al., 1989), the meta-analyses conducted by Herbert and Cohen (1993a) showed that hospitalization status indeed moderated the effects of depression on mitogen responses but had no effect on other immune measures. Suppression of mitogen-induced lymphocyte proliferation in depressed subjects tends to be greater in inpatient than in outpatient samples. However this meta-analytic result requires caution. The set of studies that was used included hospitalized subjects who were more severely depressed than the ambulatory subjects. Thus, the meta-analytic effect of ambulatory status may be better explained by the moderating effects of depressive symptom severity than by hospitalization status per se.

### 2. Depression Severity

To examine the contribution of depressive symptom severity on immune measures, Schleifer and his colleagues (1989) measured severity of depressive symptoms (total HDRS scores) and assessed B, T, and T-cell subset numbers, mitogen-induced lymphocyte stimulation, and NK activity in a sample of 30 inpatient and 61 outpatient depressed subjects. Severity of depressive symptoms was found to be associated with a decline of Con A and PHA lymphocyte responses independent of the effects of gender, age, and hospitalization status. However, neither the enumerative measures nor NK activity was correlated with severity of depressive symptoms in this large sample. Evans and colleagues also found that neither NK-cell numbers nor NK activity correlated with severity of depressive symptoms, even though diagnostic depression was associated with a decline in numbers of NK cells and NK activity as compared to levels found in comparison controls (Evans et al., 1992). While these negative findings contrast with those of Irwin and colleagues, who found that severity of depressive symptoms is a distinct correlate of NK activity in three independent samples (Irwin et al., 1987, 1990a, b), it appears that the moderating effect of severity of depressive symptoms on NK activity is small. Correlations between severity of depressive symptoms and other immune measures such as total white blood cell count or percentages of neutrophils and lymphocytes are also not consistently supported.

The lack of relationship between depressive symptom severity and measures of lymphocyte proliferation and NK activity is surprising considering the robust association between these immune measures and diagnostic depression. However, the discrepancy between these two observations raises an important question concerning the link between depression and

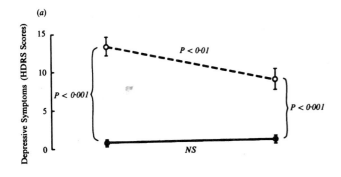

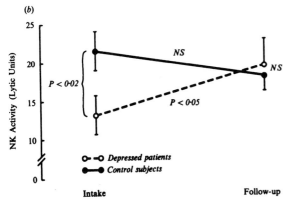

**FIGURE 4**   Change in severity of depressive symptoms from intake to 6 months follow-up in the depressed patients and control subjects. Results are depicted as means (±SEM) for Hamilton scores. For NK activity, there were a significant increase from intake to follow-up in the depressives, but no change in the controls (Irwin et al., 1992a).

immune changes. If there is no association between depressive symptom severity and immune alterations in depressed subjects, then it is possible that immune alterations might persist even into remission and be indicative of a trait rather than a state marker of depression.

To our knowledge, only one longitudinal case-control study has been conducted to examine state vs. trait issues in the depression-immune link (Irwin et al., 1992a) (Figure 4). This longitudinal design also provided an opportunity to test the temporal relationship between symptom severity and immunity beyond the prior correlational analyses conducted in cross-sectional samples. Assessment of NK activity was obtained in the second week of hospitalization and repeated at 6 months after discharge from the hospital in 20 depressed subjects. Matched comparison controls were studied at the same interval and on the same day as their depressed subject pair. The depressed subjects showed a decrease in HDRS and an increase of NK activity from intake to follow-up. There was no change in either depression scores or NK activity in the controls.

The temporal relationship between depressive symptom severity and reduced NK activity contrasts with the findings showing no association between depressive symptom severity and NK activity. It might be that the state of current depression is actually a higher order variable. In other words, depression correlates with symptom severity, but the association between acute diagnostic depression and altered immunity might relate to an interaction and/or combination of depressive symptom severity with other correlates of the state of depression.

### 3. Depression Subtype

That a constellation of subject characteristics and depressive symptoms explains the decline of cellular immunity in depression is also consistent with findings generated in the study of immune alterations in melancholic depression. Melancholic depressed patients are typically older, hospitalized, and have more severe depressive symptoms (Mitchell, Hickie, & Eyers, 1990; Parker et al., 1990). While none of these characteristics alone has been found to moderate the association between depression and immunity, these characteristics together with the diagnosis of melancholia have considerable predictive significance in determining impaired cell mediated immunity in depression. Melancholic depressed subjects are reported to be at increased risk for immune alterations and to show lower levels of mitogen-induced lymphocyte proliferation and of NK activity than depressed subjects without melancholia (Cosyns et al., 1989; Maes et al., 1989, 1991, 1995). In addition, patients with melancholia show impaired in vivo immune responses measured by delayed type hypersensitivity skin responses whereas nonmelancholic depressed subjects have responses similar to controls (Hickie, Hickie, Lloyd, Silove & Wakefield, 1993). Moreover, the decrement of delayed type hypersensitivity responses was predicted by the diagnosis of melancholia independent of the separate effects of age, hospitalization status, and depression severity.

### 4. Neurovegetative Symptoms

Rather than the sum of depressive symptoms as reflected in total HDRS scores, certain symptoms may be relatively more important in moderating the association between diagnostic depression and immunity. Indeed, the association between melancholic depression and impaired cellular immunity may be due in part to these patients' increased prevalence of neurovegetative symptoms such as sleep disturbance, appetite disturbance with associated nutritional impairments and weight loss, and/or increased psychomotor retardation. Thus, to examine whether certain depressive symptoms account for some of the immune changes in depression, Cover and Irwin (1994) extended previous analyses that examined the relationship between depressive symptoms and immunity by evaluating the contribution of clusters of depressive symptoms.

Six symptom clusters, defined by factor analysis of items from the HDRS, were identified: anxiety/somatization, weight loss, cognitive disturbance, diurnal variation, retardation, and sleep disturbance (Cleary & Guy, 1977). In a sample of depressed inpatients, no correlation was found between total HDRS scores and NK activity. Likewise, there was no correlation between four symptom clusters (anxiety/somatization, weight loss, cognitive disturbance, or diurnal variation) and NK activity. However, two symptom clusters, retardation and sleep disturbance, were correlated with NK activity, and together these two symptom variables accounted for over 16% of the variance in NK activity (Cover & Irwin, 1994).

### 5. Nutritional Status

In regards to the lack of relationship between weight loss and NK activity as described above, Schleifer and colleagues (1989) also found that statistical control for weight and recent weight loss was not associated with depression-related declines in lymphocyte proliferation. However, further investigation of the potential effects of nutritional factors in the depression-immune relation is clearly needed before excluding nutritional status as a variable that might account for immune alterations in depressed subjects.

### 6. Sleep Disturbance

Insomnia is one of the most common complaints of depressed subjects, but its role in moderating and/or mediating immune alterations in depression has been relatively unexplored. However, with evidence that subjective insomnia correlates with NK activity in depression (Cover & Irwin, 1994), the hypothesis emerged that disordered sleep may be a distinct factor accounting for some of the observed immune alterations found in depression. Consequently, a series of studies has now been conducted to test more carefully the role of sleep in the modulation of multiple aspects of the immune system and to determine the moderating effects of sleep disturbance on immune measures in depressed subjects.

First, observations regarding subjective complaints of insomnia and immunity were extended by assessment of disordered sleep by EEG (Irwin et al., 1992b). Many aspects or parameters of sleep are assessed during all-night EEG studies; thus the initial approach was to identify those measures of EEG that are altered in association with insomnia or subjective sleep disturbance and then to characterize the relationship of these EEG measures to immunity. Self-report of sleep disturbance or insomnia is characterized by disturbances of EEG sleep continuity measures with increases of sleep latency (the interval from lights out to onset of sleep) and decreases in total sleep time and sleep efficiency (the ratio of sleep to the amount of time in bed) (Benca, Obermeyer, Thisted, & Gillin, 1992). Considering the relation between subjective sleep disturbance and NK activity, we hypothesized that measures of sleep continuity would correlate with NK activity in depressed subjects. In addition, if sleep has a distinct role in the modulation of immune function independent of diagnostic depression and other depressive symptoms, then similar correlations between sleep and NK activity should also be identified in control subjects who differ in the amount and quality of their sleep. Indeed, both total sleep time and sleep efficiency were positively correlated with NK activity in separate groups of depressed subjects and controls who underwent all-night EEG study with assessment of NK activity in the morning upon awakening (Irwin et al., 1992b). These data were some of the first to indicate that sleep amounts are associated with immune function and to suggest that disordered sleep may be a key variable in understanding the behavioral mechanisms underlying the link between depression and immune alterations. Recent studies in bereaved subjects have replicated this correlation between EEG sleep and immunity and shown by way of causal statistical analyses that disordered sleep also mediates the relationship between severe life stress and a decline of NK responses (Hall et al., 1998).

A second line of studies to investigate the contribution of sleep on immune function has focused on the immunological assessment of a group of insomniac subjects who report disordered sleep but who are not depressed or suffering from some other psychiatric disorder. Primary insomnia is diagnostically characterized by the presence of subjective sleep difficulties that persist unrelated to another mental disorder or a known organic factor, such as a physical condition, psychoactive substance use disorder, or a medication (American Psychiatric Association, 1994). In a recent study of such primary insomniac patients who have no current or lifetime history of another mental disorder, EEG sleep and immune measures (NK activity, NK-cell numbers, and lymphokine activated killer (LAK) cell activity) were compared with sleep and immune measures obtained from depressed subjects and controls. Both psychiatric groups, insomniac and depressed subjects, showed significant disturbances in sleep continuity with prolonged sleep latency and decreases in total sleep time and sleep efficiency as compared to the controls. Furthermore, the insomniac and depressed groups showed similar alterations in NK and LAK responses. The insomniac subjects showed a reduction of NK activity and LAK activity as compared to levels in controls. The declines of NK and LAK responses in insomniac subjects were similar to those observed in depressed subjects (Irwin & Gillin, 1998).

A third strategy used to evaluate the relationship between disordered sleep and immunity has involved an experimental approach, sleep deprivation. In an effort to mimic the kind of disordered sleep found in depressed subjects, the effect of partial night sleep loss on lymphocyte function and NK and LAK responses has been tested. Depressed subjects often report symptoms of early or late insomnia with loss of sleep during only parts of the night. Thus, it was thought that a partial night sleep deprivation paradigm would parallel the kinds of sleep continuity disturbance reported in depression. In contrast, previous studies linking sleep and immunity have examined the effects of prolonged, total sleep deprivation (Dinges et al., 1994; Moldofsky, Lue, Davidson, & Gorczynski, 1989; Palmblad, Petrini, Wasserman, & Akerstedt, 1979).

In two separate studies, one that examined sleep loss during the late part of the night (i.e., awake from 3 AM to 7 AM) (Irwin et al., 1994) and the other that tested the effects of sleep loss during the early part of

the night (i.e., awake from 11 PM to 3 AM) (Irwin et al., 1996), substantial alterations of functional immune measures occurred in association with partial sleep deprivation. This modest sleep loss, typical of depressed subjects and other psychiatric and non-psychiatric groups who report sleep disturbance, was associated with declines of NK activity and LAK activity and stimulated IL-2 production. The reduction of NK and LAK responses appeared to be due to impairments in the activity of these cells, rather than a selective redistribution of circulating populations of NK cells and LAK precursors. For example, calculation of NK lytic activity per number of NK cells (CD16,56) and of LAK cytotoxicity per number of LAK precursors (CD16,56 + CD25) revealed impairments of individual effector cell function. Furthermore, partial night sleep loss induced a marked decline in the stimulated production of IL-2 by peripheral blood mononuclear cells. Interestingly, this effect of sleep loss on the release and/or utilization of IL-2 was due to effects on both lymphocyte and adherent, antigen-presenting cell populations. In experiments that involved mixing adherent and nonadherent cells obtained after baseline and partial sleep deprivation nights, sleep loss was found to alter either cell type with an associated decrement of stimulated IL-2 production (Figure 5) Others have also shown that sleep is critical in the regulation of IL-2 production. Sleep onset is associated with a marked enhancement in the production of IL-2 by T cells (Born, Lange, Hansen, Mölle, & Fehm, 1997; Uthgenannt, Schoolmann, Pietrowsky, Fehm, & Born, 1995).

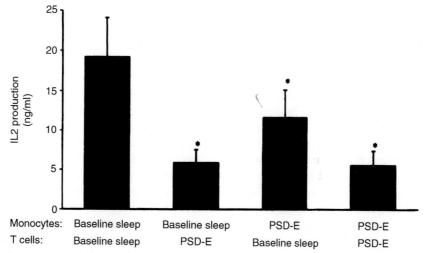

**FIGURE 5**   Effects of mixing adherent (monocyte) and nonadherent (lymphocyte) cell populations from the baseline and PSD-E conditions on mean (±SEM) interleukin-2 production. As compared to monocyte baseline–lymphocyte baseline values, mixtures of monocyte PSD-E-lymphocyte PSD-E, monocyte PSD-E-lymphocyte baseline, and monocyte PSD-E-lymphocyte PSD-E were lower (Irwin et al., 1996).

## 7. Circadian Phase Shift

Circadian rhythms are often disrupted in major depression (Steiger & Holsboer, 1997), but the possible effects of abnormal diurnal variation on immune measures obtained in depressed subjects has received little attention. Most studies examining immune measures in depression have standardized the time of blood sampling in the depressed subjects and controls. However, this strategy with typically only one assessment of immune numbers and/or function does not consider the possibility of a phase shift between the two groups. Thus, immunological differences between the depressed subjects and controls may not be related to changes in either enumerative or functional measures, but rather may be an experimental artifact of a phase difference between the groups.

There is now considerable evidence that counts of all major immune cell classes and lymphocyte subsets show circadian rhythmicity. Kronfol and colleagues found that the absolute number of lymphocytes and lymphocyte subsets (CD3, CD4, and CD8) peaked around midnight with a nadir about 10 AM. (Kronfol, Nair, Zhang, Hill, & Brown, 1997) (Figure 6). Moreover, there is a diurnal rhythmicity of human cytokine production (Petrovsky & Harrison, 1997), and Born and his associates (1997) have shown that this rhythmicity is preserved during conditions of sustained wakefulness. NK activity also shows a circadian rhythm with peak activity around noon and a nadir around midnight (Kronfol et al., 1997).

The diurnal variation of NK cell and B-lymphocyte measures appears to be disrupted in patients with major depression (Pettito, Folds, Ozer, Quade, & Evans, 1992; Pettito, Folds, & Evans, 1993). In contrast to the diurnal rhythm found in controls, depressed patients show blunted diurnal variation in levels of NK cells, NK cytotoxic activity, and B-cell numbers. However, despite these findings absolute mean levels of the immune measures were not statistically different between patients with major depression and comparison controls at either the morning or the evening time of assessment. Thus, it does not appear that a phase shift accounts for the observed changes in immune measures between depressed subjects and controls. Nevertheless, conclusions from these data remain limited, as it is not possible to determine chronobiological rhythms in studies which have used only two time points to assess diurnal variation in immunity. Additional studies are needed to fully address the effects of circadian phase or phase shifts on immunity in depressed individuals. Such future investigations should include multiple and frequent

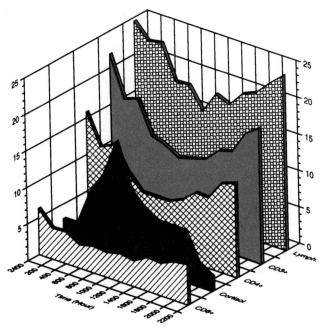

**FIGURE 6**   Temporal relationship between the circadian rhythms of cortisol and the absolute numbers of total lymphocytes, CD3+ cells, CD4+ cells, and CD8+ cells. The rhythms of the different biologic measures are plotted over the same 24-h time period. Plasma cortisol values are expressed in pg/dL. Lymphocytes are expressed in $1 \times 100$ cells/mm$^3$. Significant negative cross-correlations between cortisol on the one hand and different lymphocyte subsets on the other are seen, with a lag period for the lymphocytes of 2 h (Kronfol et al., 1997, with permission).

assessments of immune function across the 24-h period, using a time series analysis of the resulting data to evaluate for possible chronobiological differences in circadian cycle between depressed patients and nondepressed controls.

## C. Comorbidity

### 1. Anxiety Disorder

Few psychoneuroimmunology studies of depression have considered the possibility of immunological differences between diagnostic subtypes of major depression. There are even fewer studies that have evaluated immunological differences between major depressed patients who differ in diagnostic comorbidity. One exception is the work of Andreoli and colleagues who compared 51 pairs of major depressed subjects and age- and gender-matched controls on immune measures of T-cell numbers and function (Andreoli et al., 1992). The depressed subjects were further stratified on the basis of comorbid panic disorder to determine whether this additional diagnosis contributed to immune variability. Depressed subjects with panic disorder (*n*=28) were found to have greater numbers of T cells and lymphocyte proliferation in response to PHA than depressed subjects without panic disorder. These comorbid depressed subjects also showed increased PHA- and Con A-induced lymphocyte proliferation compared to controls. In contrast, depressed subjects without panic disorder showed similar levels of T cells and lymphocyte proliferation as controls. While replication of these findings is an important next step, these data suggest that a diagnostically distinct subgroup of depressed subjects may correspondingly show differences in psychobiology. Whether identification of other subgroups of depressed subjects may explain some of the heterogeneity of the depression–immune link is not known.

## 2. Alcohol Dependence

Alcohol use and alcohol dependence are associated with alterations in cell-mediated immune function (Chiappelli & Gottesfeld, 1995). However, in most clinical depression–immune studies, the possible moderating effects of alcohol have not been assessed. Moreover, in many studies, it is often not known whether the depressed subjects are free of current alcohol abuse or dependence, although it is presumed with the diagnosis of a major depressive disorder that the depressive symptoms are not due to the physiological effects of alcohol abuse. Data regarding the influence of prior alcohol dependence on immune function in acutely depressed subjects are even more limited, despite epidemiological data showing that as many as 30% of depressed patients are comorbid for alcohol dependence (Cadoret, 1981).

To test the possible joint contribution of alcoholism and depression on immune parameters in depressed subjects, we compared white blood cell counts and NK cell activity in depressed patients with and without histories of alcohol abuse or dependence, alcoholics with and without secondary depression, and controls (Irwin et al., 1990a). The presence of the dual diagnoses of alcoholism and depression produced a further decrease of NK activity compared to the separate effects of alcoholism and depression alone (Figure 7). Depressed subjects with histories of alcoholism had lower NK activity compared with depressed subjects without such histories. In addition, alcoholics who have secondary depression showed a further decrease in cytotoxicity compared with alcoholics who are not clinically depressed.

The influence of alcohol abuse on these immune measures is particularly striking considering that this result reflects the effects of past consumption of

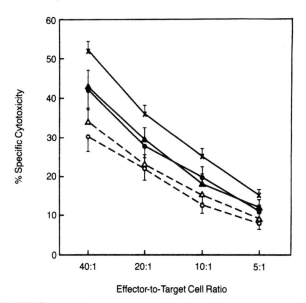

**FIGURE 7** NK activity across the four effector-to-target cell ratios in controls subjects (x), primary alcoholics (closed circles), primary alcoholics with secondary depression (open circles), depressed patients (closed triangles), and depressed patients with histories of alcohol abuse (open triangles) (Irwin et al., 1990a).

alcohol. Both the depressed and the alcoholic subjects were free of alcohol for a minimum of 2 weeks, and thus the decline of NK activity was not due to a direct pharmacological effect of alcohol. Consequently, in studies of depressed subjects, it may not be reasonable to assume that the influence of alcohol abuse on the immune parameter has dissipated simply due to a washout period lasting days to weeks. Rather, more systematic and careful assessment of current alcohol use along with dependence histories is needed in future studies of the relation between depression and immunity in order to reveal the effects of depression independent of variations in alcohol consumption.

## 3. Tobacco Dependence

In view of the prevalence of tobacco dependence in depressed subjects (Breslau et al., 1998) and the possible influence of cigarette smoking on immune function (Ferson, Edwards, Lind, Milton & Hersey, 1979), it is also important to examine whether cigarette smoking moderates the relationship between depression and immunity. However, only a few studies concerned with immune alterations in depressed subjects have assessed smoking histories (Andreoli et al., 1993; Irwin et al., 1990b). While neither study found that smoking histories correlated with immune function in depressed subjects, the lack of a relationship between quantity of cigarette use and NK activity is not surprising due to a rather restricted range of cigarette use in the depressed subjects with most reporting moderate (one to two packs per day) consumption. To our knowledge, no study has evaluated whether there is a possible interaction between depression and smoking on enumerative and functional measures of immunity.

Jung and Irwin (1999) recently examined the influence of current cigarette smoking on total white blood cells, numbers of major immune cell classes, and NK activity in depressed subjects and in controls. In a large series of previously described subjects ($n = 245$), depressed subjects and controls were stratified on the basis of nonsmoking and current smoking status. Values of total white blood cell counts and differential and of NK activity were compared in the four groups. For total white blood cell count, depressed subjects showed on the average higher numbers of total cells than controls, and smokers had elevated total white blood cell counts compared to nonsmokers. In addition, there was a significant interaction between depression and smoking on total cell counts. Depressed smokers had higher numbers of white blood cells than depressed nonsmokers and control nonsmokers and smokers. No effect for smoking or interaction between depression and smoking was found for percentages of neutrophils, lymphocytes, or monocytes.

For NK activity, there was a significant effect for depression. Depressed subjects showed on the average lower values of NK activity than controls. However, pairwise comparisons demonstrated that the difference between depressed subjects and controls was due to the marked reduction of NK activity in the depressed smokers compared to that seen in the depressed nonsmokers.

The immunologic changes found in depressed smokers were not due to the simple effects of smoking. Controls who were current smokers showed white blood cell counts and levels of NK activity that were similar to those found in control nonsmokers. Furthermore, there was no correlation between amount of smoking and NK activity in either the control or the depressed smokers, a finding consistent with previous studies of smoking populations (Meliska, Stunkard, Gilbert, Jensen, & Martinko, 1995).

These data have several implications. First, smoking status is a critical variable to assess in studies examining the relationship between depression and immunity. The combined effects of depression and smoking appear to predict changes in numbers of white blood cells and NK activity independent of the effects of depression and smoking alone. Due to the interaction between depression and smoking on total

white blood cell counts and NK activity, inconsistent findings are likely to be reported if different studies have samples of depressed subjects who differ in the prevalence of smoking. Cigarette use alone and/or in combination with depression might also contribute to the suppression of other nonspecific measures of immune function such as mitogen-induced lymphocyte proliferation. Moreover, cigarette smoking is associated with immune activation (Mendall et al., 1997), and it is important to address whether smoking status alters the reported the relationship between depression and increases in serum levels of interleukin-6 and acute phase proteins.

The health implications of reduced NK activity in depressed smokers are uncertain. However, there is evidence that depression might interact with other characteristics such as cigarette smoking to impact health, rather than there being a unitary link between depression and cancer. In a 12-year follow-up of 2264 adult men and women, depressed mood was found to interact with cigarette smoking, and together depressed mood and cigarette smoking were associated with a marked increase in the relative risk of cancer (Linkins & Comstock, 1990). As compared to the risk seen in never smokers who were without depressed mood, smokers with depressed mood as measured by elevated scores on the Center for Epidemiological Studies of Depression (CES-D) Scale had a relative risk of 18.6 for cancers at sites associated with smoking and a relative risk of 2.9 for cancers at sites *not* associated with smoking. In contrast, smokers who were without depressed mood showed only a relative risk of 4.2 for cancers at sites associated with smoking and no increase in relative risk of cancers at sites not associated with smoking.

## IV. POSSIBLE CLINICAL IMPLICATIONS OF IMMUNE CHANGES IN DEPRESSION

The immunologic consequences of major depression and their possible clinical relevance to infectious diseases have not been delineated (Stein et al., 1991). Major depression has been associated with alterations in the distribution of T-cell subsets and with declines in nonspecific measures of immune function, such as NK activity and mitogen-induced lymphocyte proliferation. The clinical significance of these immunologic findings is uncertain because the in vitro assays employed were nonspecific and thus not directly relevant to specific disease endpoints.

To address these issues, the effect of major depression on varicella zoster virus (VZV)-specific cellular immunity has recently been examined (Irwin et al., 1998). The frequency of cells in the peripheral blood capable of proliferating in response to VZV antigen (VZV-responder cell frequency, VZV-RCF) was determined in patients with major depression and in age- and gender-matched normal controls. In addition, we evaluated VZV-RCF in a group of older adults to determine whether the decline in VZV-RCF observed in major depression was comparable in magnitude to that typically found in older persons who are known to be at increased risk of developing HZ. As shown in Figure 8, VZV-specific responder cell frequency was significantly lower in the subjects with major depression than in matched normal controls.

To assess the possible clinical significance of the reduced VZV-RCF observed in the depressed subjects, VZV-RCF values in the depressed subjects were compared to those in the normal older subjects. As reported previously (Hayward & Herberger, 1987), VZV-RCF values decline with increasing age. Furthermore, depressed subjects had a level of VZV-RCF comparable to that of normal subjects more than 20 years their senior.

These findings suggest that major depression is associated with a marked decline in VZV-specific cellular immunity, as measured by the frequency of peripheral blood mononuclear cells capable of proliferating in response to VZV antigens. Furthermore,

consistent with prior observations, the present study documents an age-related decline in VZV-specific cellular immunity in normal adults. While the results reported here do not directly link depression with an increase in VZV reactivation and in the incidence of HZ, comparable declines in VZV-specific cellular immunity observed in older adults have been correlated with a significant increase in the incidence of HZ and its complications (Oxman & Alani, 1993). The levels of VZV-RCF observed in these depressed subjects were similar to those observed in normal adults over the age of 60, in whom the incidence of HZ is more than double that in younger normal adults.

Animal models have yielded compelling evidence that behavioral stressors may impact viral diseases, such as herpes simplex, influenza, and coxsackie virus infections, via alterations in immune function (Sheridan, Dobbs, Brown, & Zwilling, 1994). In contrast, there is a paucity of clinical data addressing the confluence of behavioral, immunologic, and outcome variables in the same individual at the same time (Kiecolt-Glaser & Glaser, 1995). Psychosocial stress appears to be associated with reduced immunologic control of latent herpesviruses (Epstein–Barr virus, herpes simplex virus, and cytomegalovirus) as evidenced by elevated antibody titers (Kiecolt-Glaser & Glaser, 1995). Cohen and colleagues have found

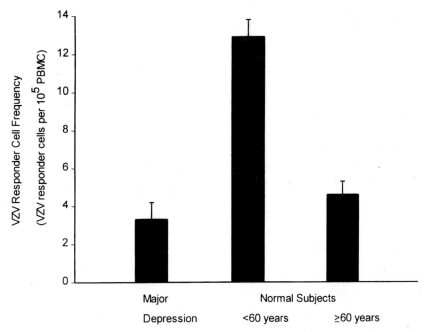

**FIGURE 8**  VZV responder cell frequency (mean +SEM) in subjects with major depression and in normal subjects < 60 and ≥ 60 years of age. Mean age for depressed subjects ($n = 11$) was 51. 3 ± 15. 7 years (range, 32–77). Mean age for normal controls < 60 years old ($n = 7$) was 40. 1 ± 9. 3 years (range, 28–57) and for those ≥ 60 years old ($n = 35$), it was 71. 2 ± 6. 7 years (range, 60–80). PBMC, peripheral blood mononuclear cells (Irwin et al., 1998).

that psychological stress is associated with increased rates of respiratory infection after experimental inoculation of common cold viruses (Cohen, Tyrrell, & Smith, 1991; Cohen, Doyle, Skoner, Rabin, & Gwaltney, 1997), and Glaser and colleagues have reported that psychological stress is associated with decreased immune responses to hepatitis B and influenza vaccinations (Glaser et al., 1992; Kiecolt-Glaser, Glaser, Gravenstein, & Malarkey, 1996). Whether these observations generated in psychologically stressed persons will generalize to depressed subjects is not yet known.

## V. SUMMARY AND CONCLUSIONS

The relation of depression to immunological assays is complex and variable. However, meta-analyses have demonstrated that depressed subjects are likely to show changes in several immune assays. Depressed subjects are likely to have changes in major immune cell classes with an increase in total white blood cell counts and a relative increase in numbers of neutrophils. The relative number of lymphocytes is likely to be reduced in depressed subjects. Depression also appears to be associated with increases in at least one measure of immune activation, although further investigations are clearly needed to replicate these interesting observations. Finally, depression is reliably associated with a suppression of mitogen-induced lymphocyte proliferation and with a reduction of NK activity. Despite the heterogeneity of findings, the effect sizes in the relationship between depression and lymphocyte proliferation and NK activity are large as compared to those observed in other areas of psychological and medical research.

Several moderating factors may explain and account for the heterogeneity that has been found in the depression–immune results. Future immunologic studies in depressed subjects are needed to clarify the effects of gender and reproductive hormones on the relation between depression and immunity. Severity of melancholic symptoms and sleep disturbance appear to moderate the immune changes in depression but the biological mechanisms that account for the link between these neurovegetative symptoms and depression are not yet known. Finally, assessment of comorbidity in depressed subjects deserves an increased focus. Data generated from our laboratory clearly show that assessment of alcohol and tobacco dependence is critical in the interpretation of immune changes in depressed subjects.

The clinical significance of changes in immune responses in depressed subjects remains an unanswered question. Studies that use immune measures with disease specific endpoints, as has been recently conducted in the study of VZV immune responses, would help identify the possible link between depression, immune system alterations, and health outcomes.

## Acknowledgments

The work reported in this chapter was supported by Grants NIMH-5-T32-18399, NIH-2-P50-30914, NIH-2M01-RR00827, and NIAAA-10215.

## References

Albrecht, J., Helderman, J., Schlesser, M., & Rush, J. (1985). A controlled study of cellular immune function in affective disorders before and during somatic therapy. *Psychiatry Research, 15,* 185–193.

Altshuler, L. L., Plaeger-Marshall, S., Richeimer, S., Daniels, M., & Baxter, L. R., Jr. (1989). Lymphocyte function in major depression. *Acta Psychiatrica Scandinavica, 80,* 132–136.

American Psychiatric Association (1994). *Diagnostic and statistical manual of mental disorders: DSM-IV.* Washington, DC: American Psychiatric Press.

Andreoli, A. V., Keller, S. E., Rabaeus, M., Marin, P., Bartlett, J. A., & Taban, C. (1993). Depression and immunity: Age, severity, and clinical course. *Brain, Behavior, and Immunity, 7,* 279–292.

Andreoli, A., Keller, S. E., Rabaeus, M., Zaugg, L., Garrone, G., & Taban, C. (1992). Immunity, major depression, and panic disorder comorbidity. *Biological Psychiatry, 31,* 896–908.

Bartoloni, C., Guidi, L., Antico, L., Pili, R., Cursi, F., Carbonin, P., Gambassi, G., Rumi, C., Di Giovanni, A., Menichella, G., et al. (1990). Psychological status of institutionalized aged: Influences on immune parameters and endocrinological correlates. *International Journal of Neuroscience, 51,* 279–281.

Benca, R. M., Obermeyer, W. H., Thisted, R. A., & Gillin, J. C. (1992). Sleep and psychiatric disorders: A meta analysis. *Archives of General Psychiatry, 49,* 651–668.

Birmaher, B., Rabin, B. S., Garcia, M. R., Jain, U., Whiteside, T. L., Williamson, D. E., al-Shabbout, M., Nelson, B. C., Dahl, R. E., & Ryan, N. D. (1994). Cellular immunity in depressed, conduct disorder, and normal adolescents: Role of adverse life events. *Journal of American Academy of Child and Adolescent Psychiatry, 33,* 671–678.

Born, J., Lange, T., Hansen, K., Molle, M., & Fehm, H. L. (1997). Effects of sleep and circadian rhythm on human circulating immune cells. *Journal of Immunology, 158,* 4454–4464.

Breslau, N., Peterson, E. L., Schultz, L. R., Chilcoat, H. D., & Andreski, P. (1998). Major depression and stages of smoking. A longitudinal investigation. *Archives of General Psychiatry, 55,* 161–166.

Brown, G. W., & Harris, T. (1978). *Social origins of depression: A study of psychiatric disorders in women.* New York: The Free Press.

Brown, G. W., Harris, T. O., & Hepworth, C. (1994). Life events and endogenous depression. *Archives of General Psychiatry, 51,* 525–534.

Cadoret, R. J. (1981). Depression and alcoholism. In R. E. Meyer, B. C. Glueck, & J. E. OBrien (Eds. ), *Evaluation of the alcoholic.* Rockville, MD: Nat Institute on Alcohol Abuse and Alcoholism.

Calabrese, J. R., Skwerer, R. G., Barna, B., Gulledge, A. D., Valenzuela, R., Butkus, A., Subichin, S., & Krupp, N. E. (1986).

Depression, immunocompetence, and prostaglandins of the E series. *Psychiatry Research, 17*, 41–47.

Caldwell, C. L., Irwin, M., & Lohr, J. (1991). Reduced natural killer cell cytotoxicity in depression but not in schizophrenia. *Biological Psychiatry, 30*, 1131–1138.

Chiappelli, F., & Gottesfeld, Z. (1995). Introduction to the symposium on alcohol and T-cell immunity. *Alcoholism: Clinical and Experimental Research, 19*, 535–538. [comment]

Cleary, P., & Guy, W. (1977). Factor analysis of the Hamilton Depression Scale. *Drugs Experimental Clinical Research, 1*, 115–120.

Cohen, S., Doyle, W. J., Skoner, D. P., Rabin, B. S., & Gwaltney, J. M. (1997). Social ties and susceptibility to the common cold. *Journal of the American Medical Association, 277*, 1940–1944.

Cohen, S., Tyrrell, D. A., & Smith, A. P. (1991). Psychological stress and susceptibility to the common cold. *New England Journal of Medicine, 325*(9), 606–656.

Cosyns, P., Maes, M., Vandewoude, M., Stevens, W. J., DeClerck, L. S., & Schotte, C. (1989). Impaired mitogen-induced lymphocyte responses and the hypothalamic-pituitary-adrenal axis in depressive disorders. *Journal of Affective Disorders, 16*, 41–48.

Cover, H., & Irwin, M. (1994). Immunity and depression: Insomnia, retardation and reduction of natural killer cell activity. *Journal of Behavioral Medicine, 17*, 217–223.

Darko, D. F., Gillin, J. C., Risch, S. C., Bulloch, K., Golshan, S., Tasevska, Z., & Hamburger, R. N. (1989). Mitogen-stimulated lymphocyte proliferation and pituitary hormones in major depression. *Biological Psychiatry, 26*, 145–155.

Dietrich, J. B., Chasserot-Golaz, S., Beck, G., & Bauer, G. (1986). Antagonism of glucocorticoid induction of Epstein-Barr virus early antigens by different steriods in Daudi lymphoma cells. *Journal of Steroid Biochemistry, 24*, 417–421.

Dinges, D. F., Douglas, S. D., Zaugg, L., Campbell, D. E., McMann, J. M., Whitehouse, W. G., Orne, E. C., Kapoor, S. C., Icaza, E., & Orne, M. T. (1994). Leukocytosis and natural killer cell function parallel neurobehavioral fatigue induced by 64 hours of sleep deprivation. *Journal of Clinical Investigation, 93*, 1930–1939.

Evans, D. L., Folds, J. D., Petitto, J. M., Golden, R. N., Pedersen, C. A., Corrigan, M., Gilmore, J. H., Silva, S. G., Quade, D., & Ozer, H. (1992). Circulating natural killer cell phenotypes in men and women with major depression. *Archives of General Psychiatry, 49*, 388–395.

Ferson, I., Edwards, A., Lind, A., Milton, G. W., & Hersey, P. (1979). Low natural killer-cell activity and immunoglobulin levels associated with smoking in human subjects. *British Journal of Cancer, 23*, 603–609.

Glaser, R., Kiecolt-Glaser, J. K., Bonneau, R. H., Malarkey, W., Kennedy, S., & Hughes, J. (1992). Stress-induced modulation of the immune response to recombinant hepatitis B vaccine. *Psychosomatic Medicine, 54*, 22–29.

Hall, M., Baum, A., Buysse, D. J., Prigerson, H. G., Kupfer, D. J., & Reynolds, C. F. (1998). Sleep as a mediator of the stress-immune relationship. *Psychosomatic Medicine, 60*, 48–51.

Hayward, A. R., & Herberger, M. (1987). Lymphocyte responses to varicella zoster virus in the elderly. *Journal of Clinical Immunology, 7*, 174–178.

Herbert, T. B., & Cohen, S. (1993a). Depression and immunity—A meta-analytic review. *Psychological Bulletin, 113*, 472–486.

Herbert, T. B., & Cohen, S. (1993b). Stress and immunity in humans: A meta-analytic review. *Psychosomatic Medicine, 55*, 364–379.

Hickie, I., Hickie, C., Lloyd, A., Silove, D., & Wakefield, D. (1993). Impaired in vivo immune responses in patients with melancholia. *British Journal of Psychiatry, 162*, 651–657.

Irwin, M., Caldwell, C., Smith, T. L., Brown, S., Schuckit, M. A., & Gillin, J. C. (1990a). Major depressive disorder, alcoholism, and reduced natural killer cell cytotoxicity: Role of severity of depressive symptoms and alcohol consumption. *Archives of General Psychiatry, 47*, 713–719.

Irwin, M., Costlow, C., Williams, H., Artin, K. H., Levin, M. J., Hayward, A. R., & Oxman, M. N. (1998). Cellular immunity to varicella–zoster virus in depression. *Journal of Infectious Disease, 178*(S), 104–108.

Irwin, M., & Gillin, J. C. (1998). The neuroimmunology of normal and disturbed sleep. *European Sleep Research Society, 1998*. [abstract]

Irwin, M., Lacher, U., & Caldwell, C. (1992a). Depression and reduced natural killer cytotoxicity: A longitudinal study of depressed patients and control subjects. *Psychological Medicine, 22*, 1045–1050.

Irwin, M., Mascovich, A., Gillin, J. C., Willoughby, R., Pike, J., & Smith, T. L. (1994). Partial sleep deprivation reduces natural killer cell activity in humans. *Psychosomatic Medicine, 56*, 493–498.

Irwin, M., McClintick, J., Costlow, C., Fortner, M., White, J., & Gillin, J. C. (1996). Partial night sleep deprivation reduces natural killer and cellular immune responses in humans. *The FASEB Journal, 10*, 643–653.

Irwin, M. R., Patterson, T. L., Smith, T. L., Caldwell, C., Brown, S. A., Gillin, J. C., & Grant, I. (1990b). Reduction of immune function in life stress and depression. *Biological Psychiatry, 27*, 22–30.

Irwin, M., Smith, T. L., & Gillin, J. C. (1987). Low natural killer cytotoxicity in major depression. *Life Sciences, 41*, 2127–2133.

Irwin, M., Smith, T. L., & Gillin, J. C. (1992b). Electroencephalographic sleep and natural killer activity in depressed patients and control subjects. *Psychosomatic Medicine, 54*, 107–126.

Jung, W., & Irwin, M. (1999). Reduction of natural killer cytotoxic activity in major depression. *Psychosomatic Medicine* (In press).

Kiecolt-Glaser, J. K., & Glaser, R. (1995). Psychoneuroimmunology and health consequences: Data and shared mechanisms. *Psychosomatic Medicine, 57*, 269–274.

Kiecolt-Glaser, J. K., Glaser, R., Gravenstein, S., & Malarkey, W. B. (1996). Chronic stress alters the immune response to influenza virus vaccine in older adults. *Proceedings of the National Academy of Sciences, 93*, 3043–3047.

Kronfol, Z., & House, J. D. (1985). Depression, hypothalamic-pituitary adrenocortical activity and lymphocyte function. *Psychopharmacology Bulletin, 21*, 476–478.

Kronfol, Z., & House, J. D. (1989). Lymphocyte mitogenesis, immunoglobulin and complement levels in depressed patients and normal controls. *Acta Psychiatrica Scandinavica, 80*, 142–147.

Kronfol, Z., House, J. D., Silva, J., Greden, J., & Carroll, B. J. (1986). Depression, urinary free cortisol excretion, and lymphocyte function. *British Journal of Psychiatry, 148*, 70–73.

Kronfol, Z., Turner, R., Nasrallah, H., & Winokur, G. (1984). Leukocyte regulation in depression and schizophrenia. *Psychiatry Research, 13*, 13–18.

Kronfol, Z., Nair, M., Goodson, J., Goel, K., Haskett, R., & Schwartz, S. (1989). Natural killer cell activity in depressive illness: A preliminary report. *Biological Psychiatry, 26*, 753–756.

Kronfol, Z., Nair, M., Zhang, Q., Hill, E. E., & Brown, M. B. (1997). Circadian immune measures in healthy volunteers: Relationship to hypothalamic-pituitary-adrenal axis hormones and sympathetic neurotransmitters. *Psychosomatic Medicine, 59*, 42–50.

Kronfol, Z., Silva, J., Greden, J., Dembinski, S., Gardner, R., & Carroll, B. (1983). Impaired lymphocyte function in depressive illness. *Life Sciences, 33*, 241–247.

Linkins, R. W., & Comstock, G. W. (1990). Depressed mood and development of cancer. *American Journal of Epidemiology, 132*(5), 962–972.

Lowy, M. T., Reder, A. T., Gormley, G. J., & Meltzer, H. Y. (1988). Comparison of in vivo and in vitro glucocorticoid sensitivity in depression: relationship to the dexamethasone suppression test. *Biological Psychiatry, 24,* 619–630.

Maes, M., Bosmans, E., Suy, E., Minner, B., & Raus, J. (1989). Impaired lymphocyte stimulation by mitogens in severely depressed patients. A complex interface with HPA-axis hyperfunction, noradrenergic activity and the ageing process. *British Journal of Psychiatry, 155,* 793–798.

Maes, M., Lambrechts, J., Bosmans, E., Jacobs, J., Suy, E., Vandervorst, C., deJonckheere, C., Minner, B., & Raus, J. (1992a). Evidence for a systemic immune activation during depression: Results of leukocyte enumeration by flow cytometry in conjunction with monoclonal antibody staining. *Psychological Medicine, 22,* 45–53.

Maes, M., Scharpe, S., Van Grootel, L., Uyttenbroeck, W., Cooreman, W., Cosyns, P., & Suy, E. (1992b). Higher alpha 1-antitrypsin, haptoglobin, ceruloplasmin and lower retinol binding protein plasma levels during depression: Further evidence for the existence of an inflammatory respose during that illness. *Journal of Affective Disorders, 24,* 183–192.

Maes, M., Smith, R., & Scharpe, S. (1995). The monocyte-T-lymphocyte hypothesis of major depression. *Psychoneuroendocrinology, 20,* 111–116.

Maes, M., Stevens, W., Peeters, D., DeClerk, L., Scharpe, S., Bridts, C., Schotte, C., & Cosyns, P. (1992c). A study of the blunted natural killer cell activity in severely depressed patients. *Life Science, 50,* 505–513.

Maier, S. F., Watkins, L. R., & Fleshner, M. (1994). Psychoneuroimmunology: The interface between behavior, brain, and immunity. *American Journal of Psychology, 49,* 1004–1017.

McAdams, C., & Leonard, B. E. (1993). Neutrophil and monocyte phagocytosis in depressed patients. *Progess in Neuro-Psychopharmacology and Biological Psychiatry, 17,* 971–984.

Meliska, C. J., Stunkard, M. E., Gilbert, D. G., Jensen, R. A., & Martinko, J. M. (1995). Immune function in cigarette smokers who quit smoking for 31 days. *Journal of Allergy & Clinical Immunology, 95,* 901–910.

Mendall, M. A., Patel, P., Asante, M., Ballam, L., Morris, J., Strachan, D. P., Camm, A. J., & Northfield, T. C. (1997). Relation of serum cytokine concentrations to cardiovascular risk factors and coronary heart disease. *Heart, 78,* 273–277.

Miller, A. H., Asnis, G. M., Lackner, C., Halbreich, U., & Norin, A. J. (1991). Depression, natural killer cell activity, and cortisol secretion. *Biological Psychiatry, 29,* 878–886.

Mohl, P. C., Huang, L., Bowden, C., Fischbach, M., Vogtsberer, K., & Talal, N. (1987). Natural killer cell activity in major depression. *American Journal of Psychiatry, 144,* 1619. [letter]

Moldofsky, H., Lue, F. A., Davidson, J. R., & Gorczynski, R. (1989). Effects of sleep deprivation on human immune function. *The FASEB Journal, 3,* 1972–1977.

Murphy, J. M., Oliver, D. C., Sobol, A. M., Monson, R. R., & Leighton, A. H. (1986). Diagnosis and outcome: Depression and anxiety in a general population. *Psychological Medicine, 16,* 117–26.

Nerozzi, D., Santoni, A., Bersani, G., Magnani, A., Bressan, A., Pasini, A., Antonozzi, I., & Frajese, G. (1989). Reduced natural killer cell activity in major depression: Neuroendocrine implications. *Psychoneuroendocrinology, 14,* 295–302.

Oxman, M. N., & Alani, R. (1993). Varicella and herpes zoster. In T. B. Fitzpatrick et al. (Eds. ), *Dermatology in general medicine* (pp. 2543–2572). New York: McGraw-Hill.

Palmblad, J., Petrini, B., Wasserman, J., & Akerstedt, T. (1979). Lymphocyte and granulocyte reactions during sleep deprivation. *Psychosomatic Medicine, 41*(4), 273–278.

Parker, G., Hadzi-Pavlovic, D., Boyce, P., Wilhelm, K., Brodaty, H., Mitchell, P., Hickie, I., & Eyers, K. (1990). Classifying depression by mental state signs. *British Journal of Psychiatry, 157,* 55–65.

Petitto, J. M., Folds, J. D., Ozer, H., Quade, D., & Evans, D. L. (1992). Abnormal diurnal variation in circulating natural killer cell phenotypes and cytotoxic activity in major depression. *American Journal of Psychiatry, 149,* 694–696.

Petitto, J. M., Folds, J. D., & Evans, D. L. (1993). Abnormal diurnal variation of B lymphocyte circulation patterns in major depression. *Biological Psychiatry, 34,* 268–267.

Petrovsky, N., & Harrison, L. C. (1997). Diurnal rhythmicity of human cytokine production. *Journal of Immunology, 158,* 5163–5168.

Rapaport, M. H., & Irwin, M. (1996). Serum soluble interleukin-2 receptors and natural killer cell function in major depression. *Communications in Biological Psychiatry, 21,* 73–78.

Schleifer, S. J., Keller, S. E., Bond, R. N., Cohen, J., & Stein, M. (1989). Major depressive disorder and immunity: Role of age, sex, severity, and hospitalization. *Archives of General Psychiatry, 46,* 81–87.

Schleifer, S. J., Keller, S. E., Meyerson, A. T., Raskin, M. J., Davis, K. L., & Stein, M. (1984). Lymphocyte function in major depressive disorder. *Archives of General Psychiatry, 41,* 484–486.

Schleifer, S. J., Keller, S. E., Siris, S. G., Davis, K. L., & Stein, M. (1985). Depression and immunity: Lymphocyte function in ambulatory depressed patients, hospitalized schizophrenic patients, and patients hospitalized for herniorrhaphy. *Archives of General Psychiatry, 42,* 129–133.

Schuckit, M. A. (1986). Genetic and clinical implications of alcoholism and affective disorder. *American Journal of Psychiatry, 143,* 140–147.

Sengar, D. P., Waters, B. G., Dunne, J. V., & Bover, I. M. (1982). Lymphocyte subpopulations and mitogenic responses of lymphocytes in manic-depressive disorders. *Biological Psychiatry, 17,* 1017–1022.

Shain, B. N., Kronfol, Z., Naylor, M., Goel, K., Evans, T., & Schaefer, S. (1991). Natural killer cell activity in adolescents with major depression. *Biological Psychiatry, 29,* 481–484.

Sheridan, J. F., Dobbs, C., Brown, D., & Zwilling, B. (1994). Psychoneuroimmunology: Stress effects on pathogenesis and immunity during infection. *Clinical Microbiological Reviews 7,* 200–212.

Steiger, A., & Holsboer, F. (1997). Nocturnal secretion of prolactin and cortisol and the sleep EEG in patients with major endogenous depression during an acuted episode and after full remission. *Psychiatry Research, 72,* 81–88.

Stein, M. B., & Uhde, T. W. (1988). Panic disorder and major Depression. A tale of two syndromes. *Psychiatry Clinics of North America, 11,* 441–461.

Stein, M., Miller, A. H., & Trestman, R. L. (1991). Depression, the immune system, and health and illness. *Archives of General Psychiatry, 48,* 171–177.

Syvalahti, E., Eskola, J., Ruuskanen, O., & Laine, T. (1985). Nonsuppression of cortisol and immune function in depression. *Proceedings in Neuropsychopharmacology and Biological Psychiatry, 9*(4), 413–422.

Uthgenannt, D., Schoolmann, D., Pietrowsky, R., Fehm, H. L., & Born, J. (1995). Effects of sleep on the production of cytokines in humans. *Psychosomatic Medicine, 57,* 97–104.

Weisse, C. S. (1992). Depression and immunocompetence: A review of the literature. *Psychological Bulletin, 111*(3), 475–489.

# Psychosocial Influences, Immune Function, and the Progression of Autoimmune Disease

MALCOLM P. ROGERS, ELIZABETH B. BROOKS

## I. INTRODUCTION

The field of psychoneuroimmunology was sparked by probing questions about the role of psychological factors in the onset and course of diseases like rheumatoid arthritis. As knowledge of the underlying immunological mechanisms in autoimmune disorders grew, more attention was directed at the possible links between the immune system and psychological states, as well as the immune and central nervous system. There have been many recent excellent reviews of this field (Ader, Felten, & Cohen, 1991; Kiecolt-Glaser & Glaser, 1995; Reichlin, 1993; Stein, Miller, & Trustman, 1991). In several reviews, particular attention has focused on the role of the macrophage (Perry, 1992; Adams, 1994) because of its secretion of inflammatory cytokines.

Recently, the study of the response of immune cells in certain clinical conditions associated with a stress response has helped to unravel the neuroendocrine–neuroimmune stress response system. Chrousos and Gold (1992) defined stress as a state of disharmony or threatened homeostasis. Vogel and Bower (1991) suggested that various concomitants of stress may comediate a disease response. These concomitants include biochemical (neurotransmitters, steroids, peptides), physiological (heart rate, blood pressure), and behavioral elements (anxiety, depression). Fricchione and Stefano (1994) have proposed a bidirectional neuroimmune hypothesis, drawing on a variety of previous work (Chrousos & Gold, 1992; Evans et al., 1992; Perkins, Leserman, Gilmore, Petitto, & Evans, 1991; Stefano, 1989, 1994). Hormones and neurotransmitters can modulate immune function through specific lymphocyte receptors. In turn, cytokines produced by these immune cell activations influence endocrine function by modulating the hypothalamo-pituitary-adrenal axis. Bidirectional communication between the brain and the immune system may be of critical importance in the development and perpetuation of various diseases and especially autoimmune diseases.

The two major stress response systems are the limbic-hypothalamo-pituitary-adrenal axis and the sympathetic nervous system (see Figure 1). Both psychological stress and physical stress in the form of fever, ultraviolet light, and infection may trigger the stress response or the inflammatory response, which are closely linked. Evidence indicates that

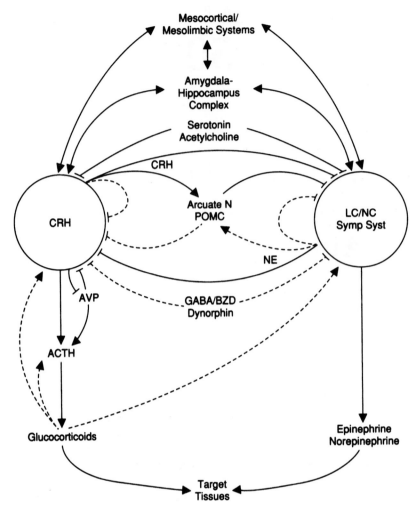

**FIGURE 1**   A simplified, heuristic representation of the central and peripheral components of the stress system, their functional interrelations, and their relationships to other central nervous system systems involved in the stress responses. The hypothalamic corticotropin-releasing hormone (CRH) neuron in the paraventricular nucleus and the centers of the arousal and autonomic systems in the brain stem represent major centers of this system connected anatomically and functionally to each other (see text). POMC indicates proopiomelanocortin; LC/NE Symp Syst, locus ceruleus-norepinephrine/sympathetic system; AVP, arginine, vasopressin; GABA, γ-aminobutyric acid; BZD, benzodiazepine; and ACTH, corticotropin. (Reprinted, with permission, from Chrousos & Gold, (1992). Stress and Stress Disorders. *Journal of the American Medical Association, 267,* 1244–1252.

both stress response systems stimulate one other (Chrousos, 1992). There are similar neurotransmitter effects on both the sympathetic and hypothalamo-pituitary-adrenal (HPA) systems. Serotonin and acetylcholine stimulate both systems, while GABAergic, opioid, and glucocorticoid substances inhibit them. Animal studies have shown that the immune response is affected by lesions in key brain areas, which may influence neurotransmitter physiology.

Immune activation resulting in the secretion of corticotropin releasing hormone (CRH) leads to a series of events with effects on inflammatory processes mediated by a range of factors. These factors include mediators of inflammation such as eicosanoids and platelet-activating factor, serotonin, and cytokines such as interleukin-1, interleukin-6, and tumor necrosis factor (Chrousos, 1992; Plata-Salaman, 1989).

The psychoneuroendocrine–immune response proposed by Evans et al. (1992) emphasizes the concept that depression and stress can result in altered endocrine and immune system function. Significantly, for the focus of this chapter, Chrousos and Gold (1992) have suggested that hypofunctioning of CRH contributes to the onset of an animal model of autoimmune disease, namely rheumatoid arthritis (RA).

A hypofunctional CRH neuron in this Lewis rat model allows for the development of a rheumatoid-arthritis-like syndrome and other autoimmune inflammatory phenomena. A generalized CRH neuron gene defect in Lewis rats makes them CRH-hyporesponsive to noxious stimuli. They also display behavioral hypoarousal and a hyperimmune profile.

A stress system marked by CRH hyporeactivity is associated with autoimmune diseases such as rheumatoid arthritis and other diseases such as chronic fatigue syndrome and posttraumatic stress disorder. On the other hand, a stress system marked by CRH hyperactivity can be predicted to lead to melancholic depression and immunosuppression.

If such linkages can be clearly established, we will be better able to understand the pathogenesis of diseases which involve both the nervous and immune systems. Treatment and even prevention of these diseases might then be fostered.

## II. AUTOIMMUNITY: HISTORY AND CONCEPTS

Autoimmunity is a disorder of the immune system in which self-generated humoral (auto) antibodies and cell mediated immune processes are directed against one's own body tissues.

If reactions between autoantibodies or immunocompetent cells and their corresponding autoantigens result in tissue injury, the process is considered autohypersensitivity. Tissue damage or chemical abnormality resulting from such reactions, or tissue or cell injury associated with identifiable autoantibodies or self-injurious cells is considered presumptive evidence of autoimmune disease (Cohen, 1998).

Autoimmune disorders are divided into organ-specific and nonspecific diseases (see Table I). The organ-specific diseases include Hashimoto's thyroiditis, multiple sclerosis, autoimmune gastritis, pernicious anemia, and insulin-dependent diabetes mellitus, which selectively attacks the islet cells of the pancreas. The nonspecific conditions, with multiple organ system involvement, include systemic lupus erythematosus (SLE) and rheumatoid arthritis.

Although the fundamental mechanisms of autoimmune diseases remain a mystery, certain facts have emerged. It is clear that T cells play a central role in causing autoimmune reactions. The way in which dormant self-reactive T cells become activated in response to self-antigens is not entirely clear, but genetic and environmental factors appear to play a significant role. In some experimental models, for example, infection may trigger autoimmune disease.

**TABLE I  Autoimmune Disorders**

| Nonspecific | Organ-specific |
|---|---|
| Rheumatoid arthritis | Multiple sclerosis |
| Systemic lupus erythematosus | Diabetes mellitus |
| Juvenile rheumatoid arthritis | Psychogenic purpura |
| Systemic sclerosis (scleroderma) | Hashimoto's thyroiditis |
| Autoimmune spondyloarthropathy<br>  Psoriatic arthritis | Grave's disease |
|   Reiter's Reactive arthritis | Myasthenia gravis |
|   Ankylosing spondylitis | Ulcerative colitis and<br>  Crohn's disease |
| | Pernicious anemia |
| | Autoimmune hemolytic<br>  anemia |
| | Addison's disease |
| | Relapsing polychondritis |
| | Dermatositis/polymyositis |
| | Goodpasture's syndrome |
| | Pemphigus vulgaris |
| | Autoimmune Hepatitis |
| | Autoimmune bullous<br>  diseases |

There are also interactions between different molecules involved in antigen binding to the T-cell receptor. Even in normal individuals, autoreactive B and T cells are present, but tolerance exists which silences the activation of those cells. Only small numbers of self-proteins are able to act as autoantigens. Autoantibodies are found normally, and are not necessarily associated with the development of autoimmune disease. The autoreactive T cells are generally inhibited by the presence of antigen, lack of costimulating factors, and active peripheral suppression. In autoimmune diseases, there is felt to be a breakdown in the usual regulatory responses of the immune system and an abnormal autoreactive T- and B-cell collaboration.

There appears to be a common genetic link for many autoimmune disorders. For example, the first degree relatives of patients with idiopathic inflammatory myopathy (IIM) have a higher frequency of autoimmune disease in general. Women are more often affected and the frequency of disease increases with age—a pattern also noted in the general population (Ginn et al., 1998).

Many specific disorders, such as myasthenia gravis (MG), are considered part of a generalized autoimmune disorder (AID) because 7% of patients have other AIDs and more than one autoimmune antibody is detected in 52.5% of patients with MG (Xu et al., 1996). Anti-neutrophil cytoplasmic antibody is associated with many different autoimmune diseases, especially the vasculitides (Schnabel, Hauuschild, & Gross, 1996). There is also an animal model of generalized autoimmune disease (Sadlock et al., 1995). Interleukin-2-deficient mice crossed to a BALB/c genetic background develop a lymphoproliferative syndrome with severe hemolytic anemia and inflammatory lesions in multiple organs associated with a variety of autoantibodies and a proliferation of activated CD4+ T cells. This model suggests that an essential role of IL-2 is the maintenance of self-tolerance.

Females are far more likely to develop some autoimmune disorders, such as RA and SLE. Pregnancy also alters the activity of some autoimmune disorders. These observations suggest an effect not only of sex hormones, but also of prolactin and growth hormone, which are different in males and females. Hypoprolactinemia, for example, impairs immune function, while excessive prolactin secretion exacerbates a number of autoimmune disorders (Chikanza, 1999). It is clear that the immune responses of males and females are not identical, with females generally exhibiting a stronger response in both humoral and cell-mediated immune responses (Grossman, Roselle, & Mendenhall, 1991).

Given the genetic predisposition, what actually triggers the onset of an autoimmune disease? Although the answer is unknown, there is evidence that cytokines play a large role in the pathogenesis (Anisman et al., 1996). During an acute febrile illness, immune-derived cytokines initiate an acute phase response, characterized by fever, inactivity, fatigue, anorexia, and catabolism. Extensive metabolic and neuroendocrine changes occur. Acute-phase proteins are produced in the liver and bone marrow. The metabolic activity of leukocytes is greatly increased, and specific immune reactivity is suppressed.

The so-called stress proteins or heat shock proteins (Hsp) are also felt to play a significant role in inflammation and autoimmunity (Polla, Bachelet, Elia, and Santoro, 1998) (see Figure 2). Autologous stress proteins, especially conserved peptides of Hsp60, provide an important initial line of defense against infection (Winfield & Jarjour, 1991). These stress proteins are presented to T cells bearing $\gamma/\delta$ receptors by relatively nonpleomorphic class 1B

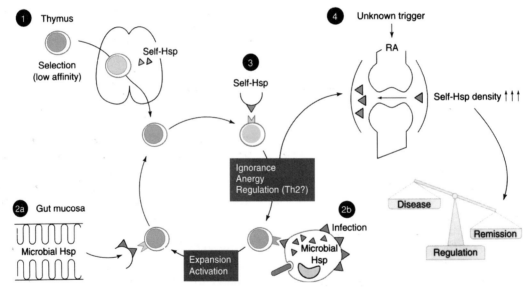

**FIGURE 2**   How heat shock proteins (Hsps) control the balance of T-cell regulation in inflammatory diseases. Thymic selection (step 1) leads to a T-cell repertoire of Hsp-reactive T cells. The mechanisms that contribute to the maintenance and safe containment of such self-reactive T cells are schematically represented. Conserved microbial Hsp epitopes as present in the periphery of the immune system in the "tolerizing gut mucosal environment" (step 2a) or transiently during infection (step 2b) will expand and/or activate self-Hsp-reactive T cells. Low-level expression of self-Hsp epitopes on (nonprofessional) APCs (step 3) will lead to ignorance, anergy, or a regulatory phenotype in self-Hsp-reactive T cells. These latter mechanisms, activated by stress-induced overexpressed self-Hsp molecules, are thought to lead to active regulatory control of inflammation in autoimmunity such as in RA joints (step 4). Conserved Hsp epitopes are represented by colored triangles; red indicates self- (host origin) Hsp epitopes; green indicates microbial Hsp epitopes. APC, antigen-presenting cell; RA, rheumatoid arthritis;Th2, T helper 2 cell. (Reprinted from van Eden et al. (1998) Do heat shock proteins control the balance of T-cell regulation in inflammatory diseases? *Immunology Today*, 19, 303–307, with permission from Elsevier Science.)

molecules. Natural antibodies may represent a parallel mechanism for B cells. B- and T-cell repertoires expand throughout the life cycle of the organism through an evolving process of gene rearrangement and major histocompatibility gene pleomorphism. The fact that stress proteins of bacteria are homologous to stress proteins in the host puts the host at risk for autoimmune reactions and disease. There is a growing body of evidence which suggests that autoreactivity in chronic inflammatory arthritis involves, at least initially, $\gamma/\delta$ cells which recognize stress protein Hsp60. Autoantibodies to stress proteins have been identified in RA and SLE and may also play a role in ulcerative colitis and Lyme disease (Jarjour et al., 1991).

On the other hand, the presence alone of autoantibodies to human stress proteins does not necessarily lead to autoimmune disease (Feige & van Eden, 1996). Further, in a study of Crohn's disease patients, no statistically significant pattern or frequency of antibodies against a combination of mycobacterial and human stress proteins was found (Markesich, Sawai, Butel, & Graham, 1991).

One hypothesis suggests a possible role for $\beta$-endorphins (Morch & Pederson, 1995). The increased cytokine production in immunoinflammatory disorders induces production of $\beta$-endorphins from the pituitary gland and lymphocytes. $\beta$-Endorphins themselves may directly inhibit antibody production. In addition, $\beta$-endorphin enhancement of natural killer cell activity suppresses B-cell function. $\beta$-endorphins also cause inhibition of human T helper cell function, which, in turn, downregulates antibody production. Thus, enhanced cytokine levels, by stimulating $\beta$-endorphin production, may diminish antibody production through a variety of mechanisms. $\beta$-Endorphin concentrations are decreased in several animal models of autoimmune disease (Sacerdote, Lechner, Sidman, Wick, & Panerai, 1999).

Different doses of certain stressors can have differential and even opposite effects on peripheral blood lymphocytes (Schauenstein, Rinner, Felsner, & Mangge, 1992). Stress effects also appear to be dependent on the tissue origin of the lymphocytes. The balance between sympathetic and parasympathetic stimulation is important to extrinsic immunoregulation. For example, increased levels of catecholamines induced experimentally seems to protect lymphocytes from the immunosuppressive effects of other endogenous stress hormones. In a variety of ways, defects in immune–neuroendocrine cross-talk may contribute to the onset of autoimmunity.

## A. The Hypothalamo-Pituitary-Adrenal Axis in Autoimmunity

The concept of an integrated bidirectionally regulated neuroendocrine–immune system adaptive response to stress has been well established (Wilder, 1995). The level of the coordinated response to stress varies greatly according to the nature of the external stressors and characteristics of the host such as age, gender, reproductive status, and other genetic factors. The combination of these factors and a dysfunctional communication between the nervous, endocrine, and immune systems contributes to the development of autoimmune diseases, both in animal models and in human diseases.

Genetic differences in the magnitude of the glucocorticoid response to stress in rats can determine the susceptibility to autoimmune diseases such as experimental allergic encephalomyelitis (Mason, 1991). Defects in the hypothalamo-pituitary-adrenal axis have been observed in autoimmune and rheumatic diseases (Cutolo et al., 1999) and, as described above, appear to have an important role in a rat model of RA (Chrousos, 1992). Prolactin levels are often elevated in patients with SLE and other autoimmune diseases. Levels of sex hormones and thyroid hormone are decreased during severe inflammatory disease (Anisman et al., 1996).

Chronic inflammation and acute immune challenge activate the HPA axis. Alteration in the hypothalamic control mechanism in chronic stress models, in which CRH is no longer the major hormone, has been described (Harbuz, Conde, Marti, & Lightman, 1997). These models include experimental allergic encephalomyelitis, eosinophilia myalgia syndrome, SLE, and leishmaniasis. Changes in the HPA axis occur in both mouse and rat models, which suggests that this may be a common denominator of chronic immune activation. In some cases arginine vasopressin (AVP) appears to take over as the major stimulator of the axis. Central neurotransmitter systems are able to influence the severity of peripheral inflammation. Depletion of serotonin at the time of the development of an inflammatory episode reduces the severity of inflammation.

Another example of neuroendocrine dysregulation in autoimmune disease is that the circadian pattern of cortisol and natural killer (NK) cell activity is altered in patients with systemic rheumatic diseases such as rheumatoid arthritis, scleroderma, and other connective tissue diseases (Masera et al., 1994).

Overall, there is clear evidence for impaired regulation of neuroendocrine and immunologic systems in autoimmune diseases. Animal models of autoimmune disorders have been particularly helpful in elucidating these complex relationships (Moynihan & Ader, 1996).

## III. DISEASE-RELATED STUDIES

Immune system dysfunction is central to the etiology of autoimmune disorders. This fact becomes even more interesting when taken together with evidence of the role of psychological states in the onset of these disorders (e.g., RA), and in mental changes which result from the disorder (e.g., SLE, MS). Accordingly, we will discuss these and other autoimmune disorders in detail.

### A. Autoimmune Disorders

#### 1. Rheumatoid Arthritis

For centuries, clinicians have been impressed by the role of psychological and emotional factors on RA. In the 1950s and 1960s, RA came to be viewed as one of the classical psychosomatic diseases, one of the "holy seven." Over time, however, the view that RA was caused or triggered by a unique and specific conflict or personality style has not held up. There are continuing observations about personality features common to patients with RA and other autoimmune disorders (Dupond et al., 1990), such as hyperconformability and excessive kindness, although it seems more plausible that these are the result rather than the cause of these chronic diseases. Instead, the construct of pathogenesis has shifted to a nonspecific stressor which might trigger or exacerbate the course of RA, at least in a subset of patients.

The principal methodological difficulty of most of the efforts to link onset or exacerbation of disease to stressful events has been the retrospective nature of the analysis. Patients also tend to attribute the cause of their arthritis or flare-ups to psychological stress, excessive physical activity, or fluctuations in the weather (Affleck, Pfeiffer, Tennen, & Fifield, 1987). Not surprisingly, patients have difficulty with the uncertainty and sense of helplessness often associated with this disease and look for reasons to explain their disease, a process which often distorts retrospective memory of stress.

Nevertheless, some interesting data does lend support to the role of stress in RA. Meyerowitz and his co-investigators (Meyerowitz, Jacox, & Hess, 1968) studied eight sets of twins discordant for RA. They found convincing evidence in the majority of the twin sets that the arthritic twin experienced an increase in life stress prior to the onset of arthritis. One example was a twin who remained home to care for a psychotic stepfather (and became ill) while the other left home and remained healthy.

Two studies used a quantitative measure of stress by having subjects list life events over the 6 months prior to the onset of RA. Both found an increase in such events compared to the controls prior to the onset of arthritis (Heisel, 1972; Baker, 1982). However, another study (Hendrie, Paraskevas, Baragar, & Adamson, 1971) did not support these later observations. More recently, Wallace and Metzger (1994) suggested that flare-ups in RA and lupus were triggered by the stress of the San Francisco earthquake.

A few investigators have attempted to measure fluctuations in disease activity over the course of weeks in relation to fluctuations in immune and psychological measures. Rimon and his colleagues (Rimon, Viukari, & Halonen, 1979) looked for changes in viral antibody levels in patients with juvenile rheumatoid arthritis in relationship to life stress. They divided patients into a low conflict group and high conflict group. Patients in the high conflict group tended to have higher antibody titers, although this was not statistically significant. Parker's group (Parker et al., 1992) attempted to correlate immunologic factors with psychological factors and disease activity in 80 male patients with RA. Severity of joint involvement was related to measures of depression, and a sense of helplessness was associated with changes in certain subsets of lymphocytes. Harrington and co-workers (1993) found that changes in soluble interleukin-2 receptor levels co-varied with joint inflammation and mood disturbances, although the mood changes may well have been the result not the cause of IL-2 changes.

To this point, there have been studies of coping styles in RA (van Lankveld, van't Pad Bosch, van de Putte, Narring, & van der Staak, 1994) but no studies which combine measures of coping with immune measures. This may happen in the near future as there is an accumulating literature on the effects of induced emotions—positive and negative—on immune function (Esterling, Antoni, Fletcher, Margullies, & Schneiderman, 1994; Futterman, Kemeny, Shapiro, & Fahey, 1994; Knapp et al., 1992).

Some studies have attempted to examine the role of stress in a more prospective, longitudinal approach. In one study (Urrows, Affleck, Tennen, & Higgins, 1994) 67 RA patients completed questionnaires daily for 75 days concerning mood, emotionally significant events, and symptoms. They also underwent joint and tender point examinations every 2 weeks. Controlling for joint tenderness, point tenderness correlated significantly with degree of daily stress.

Both Crown (Crown, Crown, & Fleming, 1975) and Rimon (Rimon, 1969) proposed that the importance of stress in RA might vary according to different subtypes of patients. They suggested that patients without rheumatoid factor (and perhaps a lower genetic predisposition to the disease) might have a greater degree of stress preceding the onset, a more acute onset, and a greater tendency for course exacerbation due to stress. Rimon's view has received support from work by Stewart and colleagues (Stewart, Knight, Palmer, & Highton, 1994) which finds a greater role for stress effects on disease onset and continuing activity in the seronegative subgroup of RA patients.

Both the rate of disease progression (Feigenbaum, Masi, & Kaplan, 1979) and the level of functional limitation disproportionate to objective measures of disease activity (Moos & Solomon, 1964) have been associated with maladaptive defenses. A 15-year follow-up (Rimon & Laakso, 1985) of Rimon's earlier study (Rimon, 1969) confirmed the importance of psychological stress on disease course over time. As in the original study, the so-called "major conflict group" characterized by acute onset, absence of family history, and a lower incidence of rheumatoid factor was more vulnerable to these stress effects. Slightly more than half of the 74 patients in the follow-up were in this major conflict group. Subsequent studies have supported the concept that interpersonal stress may exacerbate the RA disease activity in at least a significant portion of RA patients (Zautra, Hamilton, Potter, & Smith, 1999).

When McFarlane and his associates (McFarlane, Kalucy, & Brooks, 1987) followed a group of 30 patients with RA over a 3-year period, they were surprised to find that symptoms of depression and anxiety actually predicted a better outcome, whereas externalized hostility predicted a poorer outcome. Moreover, patients who denied the emotional significance of their illness seemed to fare worse over time. In evaluating patients' course, it also needs to be kept in mind that the degree of disability cannot be explained fully by the severity of RA (Hagglund, Haley, Reveille, Alarcon, 1989).

Intervention studies have included stress management and support groups. One such study (Shearn & Fireman, 1985) in which 105 RA patients were randomly assigned to either stress management, support groups, or control showed that patients in the intervention groups had greater improvement in joint tenderness.

The evidence that altered immunity is at the root of RA and other autoimmune disorders is convincing (Trentham et al., 1981). The extravascular immune complex hypothesis holds that an interaction between antigens and antibodies occurs in the synovial tissues and in the synovial fluid around the cartilage. These antigens are thought to be constituents of articular tissue or by-products of the inflammatory process, such as collagen, cartilage, fibrinogen, and fibrin. The antigen–antibody interaction in the joint tissues mediated by the macrophage in turn activates the complement sequence, increases vascular permeability, and causes an accumulation of cellular blood elements. Polymorphonuclear leukocytes, attracted by complement-derived chemotactic factors, then release enzymes that cause synovial inflammation and joint damage.

An alternative hypothesis focuses on the cellular arm of the immune system (Trentham et al., 1981). The presence of activated T lymphocytes in rheumatoid synovium and of soluble factors derived from T cells (lymphokines or cytokines) in the synovial fluid supports this hypothesis. In addition the removal of T lymphocytes by thoracic duct drainage (Pearson, Paulus, & Machleder, 1975) and total nodal irradiation are both associated with clinical improvement. Some investigators have proposed an imbalance in the immune system, consisting of a relative lack of suppressor T lymphocytes able to control helper T lymphocytes, as a mechanism in this and other autoimmune diseases (Reinherz et al., 1979).

Solomon (Solomon, 1969) was one of the pioneers in suggesting that psychological factors might influence the immune system, which, in turn, could mediate the pathophysiology of RA and other diseases causes by altered immune reactions. He found that experimental stress could alter the level of antibody response to immunization in rats. Other work (Amkraut, Solomon, & Kraemer, 1971; Rogers et al., 1980) has demonstrated that stress can effect the level of joint inflammation in animal models of arthritis. Various inbred strains of rat are highly susceptible to an autoimmune arthritis induced by the injection of adjuvant together with either mycobacterium tuberculosis, streptococcal cell wall, or collagen. Exposure of rats to a cat or simply the stress of transportation and handling at the time of collagen induction reduced the incidence of arthritis (Rogers et al., 1980). In contrast, the stress of loud noise exacerbated arthritic symptoms. Amkraut's group (Amkraut et al., 1971), using a handling and crowding stress in another model of adjuvant-induced arthritis in male Fischer rats, found that crowding increased susceptibility but handling had no effect. It is clear from these studies that environmental stress can alter disease onset and course in animal models of autoimmune disease. It is equally clear that the specific nature of the stress, together with the specific model, and strain of rat may influence the outcome.

Subsequent work has demonstrated that behavioral conditioning can also influence the severity of arthritis. Klosterhalfen and Klosterhalfen (Klosterhalfen & Klosterhalfen, 1983, 1990) noted that a conditioned stimulus, previously paired with an immunosuppressive drug, could inhibit the development of swollen joints in Wistar rats. Lysle and colleagues (Lysle, Luecken, & Maslonek, 1992) found that a conditioned stimulus paired with electric shock reduced the severity of arthritis. Moreover, this conditioning effect was abrogated by injection of propranolol, a $\beta$-adrenergic receptor antagonist.

Local factors also effect the degree of inflammation in the joint. For example, the more substance P available, the greater is the inflammation. Inflammation does not occur in a joint in a limb previously paralyzed by a CNS lesion (Levine et al., 1984).

Other investigators have focused on the role of glucocorticoids and other neuroendocrine responses in rat models of autoimmune arthritis (Aksentijevich et al., 1992; Sternberg et al., 1992; Sternberg & Wilder, 1989; Zelazowski et al., 1993). In the Lewis rat, hypofunctional corticotropin-releasing hormone (CRH) neurons, associated with lower levels of plasma adrenocorticotropic hormone, are associated with the development of a rheumatoid-arthritis-like syndrome and other autoimmune inflammatory phenomena. On the other hand, Fischer rats, which show normal adrenocorticotropic hormones, manifest only a mild, transient form of arthritis. A generalized CRH neuron gene defect in Lewis rats make them CRH-hyporesponsive to noxious stimuli. They also display behavioral hypoarousal and a hyperimmune profile.

These phenomena are of particular interest in contrast to the CRH-hyperarousal evident in major depression. In any event, Sternberg (1992) and Aksentijevich et al. (1992) both hypothesized that the decreased HPA axis of the Lewis rats rendered them susceptible to inflammatory and autoimmune stimuli. Although the precise way in which glucocorticoids affect the development of arthritis in these animal models is unclear, adrenal responses do have differential effects on the release of Th1 and Th2 cytokines (Meikle, Daynes, & Araneo, 1991).

## 2. Insulin-Dependent Diabetes Mellitus

Insulin-dependent diabetes mellitus is caused by $\beta$-cell destruction which probably results from a cell-mediated autoimmune process in genetically susceptible individuals. A variety of triggering mechanisms have been suggested, including psychological stress (Surwit & Schneider, 1993), fetal viral exposure, early exposure to cows' milk proteins, and a high exposure level to nitrosamines (Dahlquist, 1993). Factors such as high rate of growth, infection, or psychological stress may increase the demand for insulin and thus accelerate or highlight $\beta$-cell destruction. One group of investigators followed up this hypothesis by looking at changes in T-cell subsets in relation to reexperiencing grief at the loss of a loved one (McClelland, Patel, Brown, & Kelner, 1991). Diabetics who experienced a recent loss had a marked increase in helper T-cell percentages after viewing a film about the loss of a love affair, presumably resonating with their own earlier loss. The recruitment of additional helper T cells could augment the ongoing immune attack on $\beta$ cells.

One of the strongest bits of evidence, however, comes from observations about the effect of stress on an animal model of diabetes (Carter, Herrman, Stokes, & Cox, 1987; Lehman, Rodin, McEwen, & Brinton, 1991). In the Lehman et al. (1991) study of biobreeding (BB) rats, which serves as an animal model for autoimmune insulin-dependent diabetes mellitus, a significantly higher rate of disease developed in the rats exposed to a chronic moderate stress over a 14-week period. Eighty percent of male rats and 70% of female rats exposed to the stress developed diabetes, compared with 50% of both control groups. Carter (Carter et al., 1987) showed that a variety of stresses, including restraint, overcrowding, rotation, and random rehousing, promoted the earlier onset of disease in susceptible BB Wistar rats.

Durant and co-investigators (Durant et al., 1993) have also noted the variable effect of environmental stress and adrenalectomy in modulating the expression of autoimmune type 1 diabetes in the nonobese diabetic (NOD) mouse. Long-term chronic restraint or overcrowding stress tended to protect animals against the development of diabetes, while short-term stress had no effect, and adrenalectomy resulted in the accelerated development of disease. Other hormonal manipulation, such as castration, modulates the incidence of diabetes (Homo-Delarche et al., 1991). It also appears that Th1 and Th2 cells play a significant role in this animal model of IDDM. For example, transfer of Th2 cells can prevent the development of diabetes in adult thymectomized and irradiated BB rats (Powrie & Coffman, 1993), and anti-interferon-$\gamma$ or IL-4 can prevent the development of diabetes in NOD mice (Liblau, Singer, & McDevitt, 1995).

## 3. Thyroiditis

Both Graves' disease and Hashimoto's thyroiditis are thought to be autoimmune disorders. Both cell-mediated and humoral immunity appear to play a role. There seems to be a genetic defect in suppressor T lymphocytes, which in turn permits the survival and expansion of a random "forbidden" clone of thyroid-directed, organ-specific, helper T lymphocytes.

An increased incidence of Graves' disease has been noted in times of stress. For example, in each major war of this century, the incidence of Graves' has increased. During World War II in Scandinavia, Graves' disease was reported to be five times more frequent, returning quickly to normal levels after the war (Kracht & Kracht, 1952; Rosch, 1992). Hetzel (Hetzel, 1970) has identified that stress may play a significant role in the pathogenesis of thyrotoxicosis, and Winsa (Winsa, Karlsson, Adami, & Bergstrom, 1991) also noted an association between stressful life events and Graves' disease. Others (Hidaka & Amino, 1998) have noted that delivery and allergic rhinitis can induce the onset of Graves' disease, perhaps as a result of the overproduction of Th2 (type 2 helper T cells).

Obese strain (OS) chickens spontaneously develop autoimmune thyroiditis and hypothyroidism. As in models of arthritis, there is evidence that abnormalities in the HPA axis play a role in susceptibility to this disease (Wick et al., 1993). For example, OS chickens, compared to control strains, show elevated corticosteroid-binding proteins, decreased free corticosteroids, and a blunted response to IL-1 and other stimulants, reminiscent of the defect in the Lewis rat.

## 4. Atherosclerosis

There is even some evidence that atherosclerosis may in part be mediated by immune activity. Decades of evidence support a role for certain kinds of stress and personality style in the pathogenesis of coronary artery disease. Sympathetic activation undoubtedly plays a role in this pathogenic process. Within atherosclerotic lesions one finds evidence of many immune components: immunoglobulins, complement, mononuclear phagocytes, activated T cells, and numerous cytokines. Wick (1995) and others have postulated that such immune elements, in conjunction with increased sympathetic activity, may play a role in atherosclerosis.

## 5. Other Autoimmune Diseases

Dilated cardiomyopathy (DCM) is also felt to have an autoimmune etiology (Portig, Pankuwit, & Maisch, 1997). Antibodies to Hsp60, Hsp70, and heat shock cognate protein (Hsc) 70 were all detected in the sera of patients with this disease, suggesting that an earlier infection might have triggered this disease.

There has long been speculation that psychological factors play a role in the onset and course of Crohn's disease and ulcerative colitis (Knoflach, 1986).

Psychogenic purpura (autoerythrocyte sensitization) is a condition of inflammatory bruises primarily in adult women thought to be caused by sensitization of patients to the stroma of their own erythrocytes. One investigator has noted that most cases occur within a short period of time after severe emotional stress (Ratnoff, 1989). Injury and surgical procedures were also noted to be probable precipitating events.

There is no current evidence about the role of stress or psychoneuroendocrine factors in autoimmune bullous diseases (Rye & Webb, 1997), experimental autoimmune orchiitis (EAO) (Sakamoto, Matsumoto, & Kumazawa, 1998), vitiligo (Le Poole et al., 1993), or a model of experimental autoimmune prostatitis (Orsilles & Depiante-Depaoli, 1998), but that may be simply from a lack of attention to the issue. Oxidative stress, produced by an increased metabolic rate, combined with a decrease in antioxidant capacity, was noted in this rat model of autoimmune prostatitis.

## B. Autoimmune Diseases That Affect the Central Nervous System

### 1. Systemic Lupus Erythematosus (SLE)

A few earlier uncontrolled and retrospective studies suggested that high levels of life stress preceded disease flare-ups in patients with SLE (Kreindler & Cancro, 1970). One prospective study utilized prolonged 2-h neuropsychological testing as a convenient induced stress (Hinrichsen, Barth, Ruckemann, Ferstl, & Kirch, 1992). They observed that SLE patients had reduced CD19+ T-cell mobilization compared to normal controls, despite normal catecholamine responses. A similar attenuation of cell mobilization was noted after physical stress (bicycle ergometry) (Hutt, Kirch, Kreuzfelder, Scheiermann, & Ohnhaus, 1986) and a shorter term psychological stress (Hinrichsen et al., 1989). The physiological importance of cell mobilization, however, remains unclear. These investigators concluded that the attenuated cell mobilization was not the result of diminished catecholamine secretion but rather a reduced response of lymphocyte subpopulations due to sympathetic stimulation.

In another careful prospective study of the relationship between daily stress and lupus activity, Adams and colleagues (Adams, Dammers, Saia, Brantly, & Gaydos, 1994) studied 41 patients with lupus erythematosus. Much like Rimon's (Rimon, 1989) work with RA patients, Adams and his team found that some individuals appeared to be stress responders, while others did not. Although there was no clear evidence that in these susceptible individuals stress exacerbated underlying disease activity, stress, anxiety, depression, and anger were all associated with self-reported symptomatology. Another group of investigators (Wekking, Vingerhoets, van Dam, Nossent, & Swaak, 1991) compared prospectively groups of patients with SLE and RA in terms of the relationship between disease activity and daily stress. Wekking and her co-investigators found that there was a stronger correlation between level of daily stress and physical and psychosocial status in SLE patients.

More than half of patients with systemic lupus experience some form of neuropsychiatric symptomatology, ranging from seizures, headaches, psychosis, mood disorders, and cognitive impairment (Kelly & Rogers, 1995). Psychosis occurs in about 10% and seizures in about 20% of patients. A recent study (Glanz, Schur, & Khoshbin, 1998) reported that the typical electroencephalographic (EEG) abnormalities, which consist of $\theta$ and $\delta$ slowing and sharp wave activity, occur predominately in the left side, in the temporal area. These findings suggest damage to the left temporolimbic region. The authors noted that other studies have supported the concept of a particular vulnerability of hippocampal and hypothalamic cells in immune processes, including paraneoplastic limbic encephalopathy (PLE) (Felten & Felten, 1987), herpes simplex virus encephalitis (HSVE) (Hierons, Janota, & Corsellis, 1978; Kapur et al., 1994), and Lyme disease encephalopathy (Kaplan, Meadows, Vincent, Logigian, & Steere, 1992). The symptoms of memory impairment, language difficulties, confusion, and hallucinations are consistent with damage to the left temporolimbic area. Why this area is particularly vulnerable is less clear. It may be that cytokines have a predilection for this region of the brain. The presence of IL-1 has been demonstrated in regions of the hypothalamus and thalamus in humans (Breder, Dinarello, & Saper, 1988) and in the rat hippocampus and olfactory tubercle (Lechan et al., 1990).

Cognitive and affective changes are probably the most prevalent neuropsychiatric symptoms (Denburg, Carbotte, & Denburg, 1997; Denburg, Denburg, Carbotte, Fisk, & Hanly 1993), occurring in over 50% of patients. These cognitive changes have been demonstrated by neuropsychological testing even in SLE patients who have not had manifest neuropsychiatric events or subjective symptoms. Typical deficits involve attention and concentration, verbal and nonverbal memory, verbal fluency, visuospatial skills, psychomotor speed, and cognitive flexibility. These cognitive changes have been noted to occur independently of generalized disease activity, corticosteroid use, or emotional distress.

Most observers agree that cognitive change and psychosis are generally secondary to a more diffuse process involving both alterations in small blood vessels in the brain and antibodies and cytokines directed to neuronal tissue (Denburg, Carbotte, & Denburg, 1987). There is some evidence that different antibodies are associated with different patterns of neuropsychiatric symptoms. For example, elevated titers of lymphocytotoxic antibody (LCA) are associated with specific visuospatial cognitive impairment (Denburg, Behmann, Carbotte, & Denburg, 1994).

Animal models of lupus have also been informative. Ader first identified the phenomenon of conditioned immunosuppression (Ader, Felten, & Cohen, 1975). He applied this approach to the New Zealand hybrid mice, an animal model of lupus (Ader, 1989). The use of a flavored solution as a conditioned stimulus, when paired with an immunosuppressive drug, delayed the development and mortality of lupus. In one study, lupus-prone Mrl–lpr/lpr mice with manifest disease voluntarily consumed more of the flavored solution, suggesting that they had somehow learned that the solution alleviated symptoms of their disease and immune dysregulation (Ader, Grota, Moynihan, & Cohen, 1991b). His group of investigators (Grota, Ader, & Cohen, 1987) and others (Sakic, Szechtman, Keffer, Talangbayan, Stead & Denburg, 1992) have also utilized this mouse lupus model, in which disease develops quickly from 3 to 16 weeks of age, to investigate immune-mediated CNS and behavioral changes. Grota observed that the learning capacity of mice was diminished after they developed clinical signs of disease. Sakic (Sakic et al., 1994) and others (Szechtma, Sakic, & Denburg, 1997) made similar observations, noting decreases not only in learning but also in spontaneous activity and responses to a novel environment. These mice were hesitant to explore a new environment showing significantly less sniffing or touching of new objects. They also were unable to find a platform in a water maze from which to escape, instead assuming a more helpless response, reminiscent of learned helplessness seen when animals are exposed to a repeated noxious stress from which they cannot escape. In addition, they also developed abnormalities in their learning skills. All of these changes were noted early, after only a few weeks of illness, when autoantibodies are just forming, and other manifestations such as arthritis, anemia, and nephropathy are not yet apparent. Others have noted that the brains of these MRL–lpr mice show CNS inflammation and perivascular deposition of IgG antibodies as early as 8 weeks of age (Vogelweid, Johnson, Besch-Williford, Basler, & Walker, 1991). Furthermore, treatment of the MRL–lpr mice with cyclophosphamide, a potent immunosuppressive drug used in human SLE patients to control renal disease, tended to reverse many of the depressive-like behaviors.

One of the earliest immune abnormalities in MRL-lpr mice is overproduction of the cytokine IL–6, associated with the stimulation of autoantibody production. Sakic and colleagues hypothesized that the elevated IL–6 production was associated with the withdrawn and helpless behavior of the mice.

These findings have interesting connections to the manifestations of SLE in humans. Increased levels of certain cytokines have been observed in major depression. Maes and co-investigators (Maes et al., 1991) found that antinuclear antibodies (ANA) and circulating soluble interleukin-2 (IL-2)receptors were found more frequently in depressed patients than in normal volunteers. Such discoveries may help to explain the fact that neuropsychiatric lupus can present with major depression or schizophrenia-like symptoms. In further investigations, Maes and colleagues (Maes et al., 1995a; Maes, 1995b) found that plasma concentrations of interleukin-6 (IL-6), soluble interleukin-6 receptor (sIL-6R), soluble interleukin-2 receptor (sIL-2R), and transferrin receptor (TfR) were all elevated in major depression, whether active or in remission, suggesting that the coordinated and upregulated production of these cytokines may be a trait marker for major depression. Interestingly, in more severe, melancholic depression, the same authors (Maes et al., 1993) noted that IL-6 production was actually increased, in conjunction with a failure to suppress cortisol production in response to dexamethasone, itself a well-described, though nonspecific, marker for severe depression (APA Task Force 1987).

There is also evidence that the interleukins increase the activation of the HPA axis and that, in depression, glucocorticoid receptors both on lymphocytes (Lowry, Gormley, Reder, & Meltzer, 1989) and in the hippocampus (Saplolsky, Krey, & McEwen, 1986) are diminished. Hans Selye (Selye, 1970) was the first to suggest that severe chronic stress would lead to depression, loss of weight, reduced gonadal function, ulcer disease, and immunosuppression, producing many of the physiological changes known to occur with depression. Prolonged and elevated CRH pro-

duction may be at the core of the physiology of depression. Licinio and his colleagues (Licinio, Gold, & Wang, 1995) have proposed a mechanism by which prolonged elevations in CRH might lead to medical diseases as well. They proposed that CRH might prompt the production of proopiomelanocortin (POMC) transcription factors which might bind to intracellular targets. If the target was a viral genome, it might predispose to infection; if it was an oncogene, it might predispose to cancer; or if it was an inflammatory mediator gene it might predispose to an inflammatory disease.

Elevations in serum IL-6 have been observed in a subset of human patients with depression (Song et al., 1998), specifically those patients who tend to be unresponsive to antidepressant therapy (Sluzewska et al., 1995). Sakic and his coinvestigators (Sakic, Szechtman, Talangbayan, Denburg, Carbotte, & Denburg, 1994) were able to increase the production of IL-6 in nonlupus MRL mice by administration of an adenovirus vector carrying cDNA. The increase in IL-6 was associated with lowered preference for sucrose solution and other manifestations of learned helplessness and the behavioral abnormalities which had previously occurred only in the spontaneously lupus developing mice (Sakic, Szechtman, Braciak, Richards, Gauldie, & Denburg, 1997). These investigators are beginning to explore the impact of antidepressants on this model of IL-6-induced depressive-like syndrome.

Depression is common in SLE and in some cases appears to be a manifestation of immune processes involving the brain, in part based on its cooccurrence with identifiable neurologic events (Utset et al., 1994) or antibodies such as antiribosomal P (Schneebaum et al., 1991). Although some depressions may be more reactive, based on the disruptive and life-change impact of SLE, at least a subset of depression may in fact by triggered by IL-6 or other cytokines as postulated by Szechtman and his colleagues (1997).

### 2. Multiple Sclerosis and Experimental Allergic Encephalomyelitis

Multiple sclerosis is an inflammatory, immune-mediated disorder of the nervous system, which results in loss of myelin and multifocal pathological changes called plaques. Its mean age of onset is 30 and women account for 70% of those affected. The course is variable, with only 15% having a progressive course from the outset and 85% showing a relapsing/remitting course. However, of the latter group, 40–65% will experience slow progression (Coyle, 1996). Clinicians and researchers have long been interested in the possible connections between stress and the course of MS (Warren, Warren, Greenhill, & Patterson, 1982). In a recent study (Ackerman, Martino, Heyman, Moyna, & Rabin, 1996), the stress of public speaking was associated with a variety of autonomic, neuroendocrine, and immunologic responses, no different in healthy subjects than in MS patients. These changes included increases in neutrophils, monocytes, CD8+ suppressor/cytotoxic T lymphocytes and NK cells, along with parallel changes in NK-cell activity. The investigators speculated that these intact stress-induced immune alterations may contribute to immune changes associated with disease activity. However, the relationship between stress and disease activity is less clear than in other autoimmune disorders like RA, perhaps because of the time lag between immune changes and neurologic symptom manifestation and because most studies have been retrospective (Grant et al., 1989; Sibley, Bamford, Clark, Smith, & Lagma, et al., 1991). Grant et al. (1989) found a higher proportion of patients with early MS to be experiencing marked life adversity than a control group of health volunteers. The Sibley et al., study (1991) did not find a correlation between exacerbation and stress.

There have been a few prospective studies. Franklin's study (Franklin et al., 1992) followed 55 relapsing/remitting MS patients over 20 months. Those who reported significant stressful events were significantly more likely to experience relapse. Another prospective study (Nisipeanu & Korczyn, 1993) followed a group of MS patients who were exposed to the stress of missile attacks on Israel during the Persian Gulf War of 1991. Thirty-two patients with relapsing/remitting disease were identified. They found fewer exacerbations and relapses than during the 2 prior years. Only 3 patients experienced exacerbations of more than 24 h, confirmed by examination. One occurred during the war and two occurred afterward. All later remitted completely. The authors of this study speculated that the severe stressor may have protected the patients, perhaps by activating the hypothalamo-pituitary and sympathetic nervous system-adrenal axes. A subcommittee of the American Academy of Neurology also made a comprehensive review of the relationship of MS to psychological stress and physical trauma (Goodin et al., 1999). This report concluded that although such a relationship was plausible from a biological viewpoint, the actual evidence was mixed, some for and some against the hypothesis that stress could trigger or exacerbate MS.

Depression in MS patients occurs at a rate varying between 27 and 54%, higher than in other neurologic disorders (Minden & Schiffer, 1990). Foley and colleagues (Foley et al., 1992) looked at the relationship between various immune measures and depression in patients with chronic-progressive multiple sclerosis. They found that periods of greater depression were correlated with lower CD8+ cell numbers and percentage and a higher CD4/CD8 cell ratio.

Although the etiology of MS remains unclear, there is evidence that viral infections may exacerbate it (Panitch, Hirsch, Schindler, & Johnson, 1987) and stress is well known to affect susceptibility to infection (Kort, 1994; Stone & Bovberg, 1994). This provides some further indirect evidence for the effect of stress on the course of MS.

The understanding of the role of oligodendrocytes, lymphocytes, endothelial cells, and the cytokine network in the pathogenesis of MS has increased dramatically (Coyle, 1996). MS is understood to be a demyelinating disease in which an autoimmune reaction is directed against oligodendrocytes (Boccaccio & Steinman, 1996). Once triggered, the immune system attacks and destroys myelin and myelin forming cells. Under attack, the oligodendrocyte responds to the attack through modulation of its metabolism and gene expression. Heat shock and other protective molecules are induced.

Experimental allergic encephalomyelitis (EAE) is widely used as an animal model for multiple sclerosis. About 10 days after the injection of adjuvants and myelin basic protein (MBP), susceptible rats develop a progressive paralysis associated with demyelinization. The transfer of MBP-specific CD4+ T cells alone can produce the disease in recipient rats (Kennedy, Torrance, Picha, Mohler, 1992). There are data to suggest that stressful experiences can suppress the clinical expression of this disorder in rats and that it does so by altering immune responses (Buklica et al., 1991; Griffin, Lo, Wolny, & Whitacre, 1993; Kuroda, Mori, & Hori, 1994; Levine, Strebel, Wenk, & Harman, 1962). In the early 1960s Levine (Levine et al., 1962) had observed that the stress of physical restraint diminished the incidence and severity of EAE. Later, he and his coinvestigators also demonstrated that such stress could prevent relapses (Levine & Saltzman, 1987). Griffin and co-investigators (Griffin et al., 1993) had noted that female Lewis rats exhibited significantly higher basal circadian levels of corticosterone than their male counterparts. They then explored the possible differential effects of restraint stress on male and female expression of EAE. Indeed, they found that both clinical and histopathological changes of EAE were more suppressed in female than male Lewis rats. Stress seemed to effect presentation or processing of the myelin basic protein

(MBP) and to decrease interleukin-2 and interferon $\gamma$ production.

Early neonatal experiences, such as maternal deprivation and weaning, also influence the timing and severity of EAE in adult Dark August rats (Laban, Markovic, & Dimitrijevic, & Jankovic, 1995). Elevated glucocorticoid levels suppress the clinical severity of the disease (Levine & Strebel, 1969; MacPhee, Antoni, & Mason, 1989). Stress may act not only through glucocorticoid but also opioid receptors, which have been found on some lymphoid cells (Bidlack, Saripalli, & Lawrence, 1992). The $\kappa$-opioid receptor appears to play a role in this disease. High doses of the opioid methionine-enkephalin inhibited EAE, while low doses produced the opposite effect (Jankovic & Maric, 1987). In later work, repeated injections of the opioid receptor agonist, MR 2034, produced a profound suppression of EAE signs and symptoms, as well as suppression of histologic lesions and anti-myelin basic protein antibody production (Radulovic, Djergovic, Miljevic, & Jankovic, 1994).

EAE appears to be mediated via T helper cells subtype 1 (Th1) cells involving at least one of its cytokines, IL-2, the production of which can be reduced by stress (Griffin et al., 1993). Cytokines, including IL-2, interferon-$\gamma$, and tumor necrosis factor (TNF), have also been implicated in the myelin damage, which is the hallmark of MS (Hartung, 1993; Khoury, Hancock, & Weiner, 1992). Recovery, on the other hand, appears to be associated with IL-10 messenger RNA (mRNA) (Kennedy et al., 1992) and the production of MBP-specific antibodies (MacPhee, Day, & Mason, 1992) (see Figure 3).

The heat shock protein, $\alpha$-B-crystallin, has also been identified as the critical myelin antigen involved in the inflammatory process affecting myelin (van Noort, 1996). Another cytokine, insulin-like growth factor (IGF)-1, promotes oligodendrocyte development and myelin production. In the murine model of EAE, administration of this cytokine delayed the onset of disease. However, once signs of the disease were present, administration resulted in severe relapse (Lovett-Racke, Bittner, Cross, Carlino, & Racke, 1998).

Overall, there is clear evidence in this animal model of MS that stress acting via glucocorticoid or

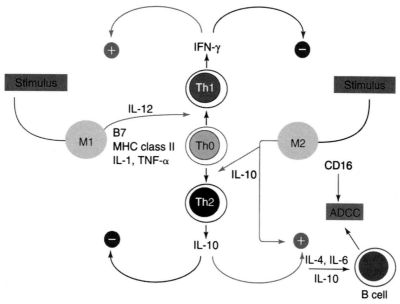

**FIGURE 3**  Two distinct macrophage populations regulate the function of CD4- T cells. In this model, M1 cells represent the prototypical antigen-presenting cells. They express MHC class II for the presentation of antigenic peptides and express B7 molecules for the costimulation of T cells. M2 cells lack the tools for antigen-specific T-cell activation but express FcRs, which enable them to destroy antibody-reactive target cells. M1 and M2 cells exert opposite effects on Th-cell development. M1 cells generate IL-12, which facilitates the development of Th1 cells, whereas M2 cells generate IL-10, which facilitates the generation of Th2 cells. Th1 cells release IFN-$\gamma$, which stimulates M1 cells and inhibits M2 cells, whereas Th-2-produced IL-10 inhibits M1 cells and promotes the generation of M2 cells. Through the release of IL-1 and TNF-$\alpha$, M1 functions as a proinflammatory macrophage, whereas M2 cells, by virtue of IL-10 production, act as anti-inflammatory macrophages. ADCC, antibody-dependent cell-mediated cytotoxicity; IFN-$\gamma$, interferon-$\gamma$, IL-1, interleukin 1; MHC, major histocompatibility complex; Th, T helper cell; TNF-$\alpha$, tumor necrosis factor $\alpha$. (Reprinted from Kummerle-Deschner, H. et al. (1998) Pediatric rheumatology: autoimmune mechanisms and therapeutic strategies. *Immunology Today, 19*, 250–253, with permission from Elsevier Science.)

opioid receptors can alter the clinical and histologic severity of disease. An important mediator of disease severity, IL-2, a cytokine produced by Th1 cells, is also effected by stress.

### 3. Other Autoimmune Disorder That Affect the Central Nervous System

There are numerous other autoimmune disorders in which cognitive status may change, including animal models of autoimmune dementia (Michaelson, Alroy, Goldstein, Chapman, & Feldon, 1991), developmental learning disabilities (Schrott et al., 1992), reading disabilities, and left-handedness (Geschwind, 1984; Gilger, Pennington, Green, Smith, & Smith, 1992). Investigators have also speculated about autoimmunity as the etiology of schizophrenia (Knight, Knight, & Ungvari, 1992; Kornhuber & Kornhuber, 1987; Yang et al., 1994), autism (Van Gent, Heijnen, & Treffers, 1997) and, as we have discussed, certain types of major depression (Maes et al., 1991). Maes and co-investigators found that antinuclear antibodies and circulating soluble interleukin-2 receptors were found more frequently in depressed patients than in normal volunteers. The latter speculations are made more plausible by the fact that neuropsychiatric lupus can present with major depression or schizophrenia-like symptoms.

Following up on Geschwind's (1984) hypothesis about autoimmunity and left-handedness, Searleman and Fugagli (1987) found a significantly higher incidence of left-handedness in males with Type I diabetes mellitus, as well as patients with two other autoimmune disorders, Crohn's disease and ulcerative colitis. This finding is of particular interest in light of the apparent predilection of left temporolimbic involvement in SLE (Glanz et al., 1998). In another study (Hassler & Gupta, 1993) left-handedness, musical talent, and anomalous dominance were related. Female musicians, male left-handers, and those with reversed dominance for language functions were all associated with immune vulnerability.

Trichotillomania, compulsive hair-pulling, and Sydenhams chorea, an involuntary movement disorder, have also been linked with an autoimmune process. Swedo (Swedo et al., 1997) has noted that patients with Sydenham's chorea often have obsessive–compulsive disorder (OCD) and that OCD symptoms may be exacerbated by streptococcal infection. Further, patients with OCD have a higher frequency of the D8/17 lymphocyte marker of susceptibility to streptococcal infections (Murphy et al., 1997). Stein (Stein et al., 1997) has published a case report of a patient with Sydenham's chorea who developed trichotillomania. Thus, there is an emerging hypothesis that cases of OCD, Tourette's, and other movement disorders developing in childhood may be the result of an autoimmune process triggered by repeated streptococcal infections, in the same fashion as has been established in rheumatic fever and heart disease (Swedo et al., 1997).

Paraneoplastic neurologic disorders (PNDs) (Darnell, 1996) (which include most prominently paraneoplastic limbic encephalopathy or PLE) are thought to be autoimmune neuronal degenerations that develop in some patients with systemic cancer. PLE is associated with a variety of symptoms associated with limbic disturbance such as language and memory difficulties, confusion, hallucinations, agitation, and seizures (Posner, 1991).

Psychosis has been described in three cases of myasthenia gravis and thymoma (Musha, Tanaka, & Ohuti, 1993).

Finally eosinophilia–myalgia syndrome (EMS) (Krupp, Masur, & Kaufman, 1993) also has neurocognitive manifestations. Chronic fatigue syndrome does as well, although its pathogenesis and even its validity is uncertain, some investigators have noted changes in immune function and postulated a role for cytokines.

## C. Pregnancy and Autoimmunity

There are abundant clinical observations that pregnancy and the postpartum period can be associated with fluctuations in autoimmune diseases. Typically, RA remits during pregnancy and flares in the postpartum period (Ostensen, 1999). SLE and, in particular, its renal manifestations tend to flare during pregnancy (Ostensen, 1999). Pregnancy is associated with a suppression of cell-mediated immune function and the preservation of humoral immunity, presumably protecting the fetus and placenta against cell-mediated attack by the mother. In early pregnancy, several cytokines increase but, in later pregnancy, Th1 cytokines, interferon-$\gamma$ and IL-2 decline, whereas the Th2 cytokines, especially IL-4, increase. Concurrent hormonal changes occur, including marked increases in corticosteroid, estrogen, and progesterone levels. Both corticosteroids and estrogens suppress cell-mediated immune function and enhance humoral immune function.

Following delivery, these hormone levels drop precipitously, triggering an increase in T-cell immunity associated with exacerbation of disease. Increased production of prolactin during the postpartum period, especially in conjunction with nursing, may also contribute to the development or exacerbation of autoimmune disease (Berczi, 1993; Brennan & Silman, 1994).

## IV. IMPLICATIONS OF PSYCHONEUROIMMUNOLGY ON MOOD DISORDERS

As we have seen earlier, there is evidence for the dysregulation and hyperactivity of the CRF-HPAS axis in major depression. There is also accumulating evidence for dysregulation of the immune system during major depression, much of it presumably related to the underlying neurotransmitter abnormalities. In ex vivo tests, NK-cell activity and lymphocyte response to mitogen stimulation are diminished. Simultaneously, there is an activation of in vivo measures, with an increase in the ratio of helper to suppressor T lymphocytes, increased autoantibody titers, and increased secretion of monocytic interleukins.

Special attention has been focused on the cytokines because of their wide-ranging effects on the nervous system. Maes and colleagues (Maes et al., 1992) have proposed a complex sequential activation of the immune system during different degrees of depression severity. Monocytosis and increased IL production is followed by activation of resting mature T cells. During the second phase these activated T cells acquire IL-2 receptors; and in the most severe stages of depression, these activated IL-2-producing cells may promote proliferation of their own clones and other T-cell and B-cell subsets and an expression of surface Ig receptors.

These cytokines may well have causative effects on some of the neurovegetative symptoms of major depression. Indeed, Smith (1991) was among the first to suggest that excessive secretion of cytokines, such as IL-1 from activated cells of the monocyte/macrophage lineage might trigger depression. IL-1 affects the sleep cycle, and appetite as well. Anergia, somnolence, fearfulness, and changes in activity level may also be related to the effects of IL-1. Cytokines are also thought to play a role in the symptoms of chronic fatigue syndrome, a mysterious disorder which has significant overlap with depression. The exogenous administration of interleukins in the treatment of cancer has a variety of systemic side effects, including fever, fatigue, and cognitive impairment. Other investigators have noted a correlation between some but not all symptoms of depression, such as sleep deprivation and psychomotor retardation, and decreases in NK cell activity (Cover & Irwin, 1994). At the same time, sleep deprivation by itself can have immunosuppressive effects. Palmblad (Palmblad, Petrini, Wasserman, & Ackerstedt, 1979) noted that sleep deprivation could alter cell-mediated immunity.

When the depression is treated, the impact on immune function is not entirely clear both in patients with seasonal (Skwerer et al., 1988) and nonseasonal depression (Albrecht, Helderman, Schlesser, & Rush, 1985).

There have also been efforts to explain other mental and psychological symptoms on the basis of immunologic mediators. For example, some have attributed the etiology of schizophrenia to neuroimmunologic changes, either related to viral infection or to autoimmunity. The findings, although interesting, have often been inconsistent.

## V. CONCLUSION

Taken as a whole, these studies provide strong evidence for the role of psychological factors in the regulation of immune functions and in the clinical expression of autoimmune disorders. Multiple sclerosis and systemic lupus erythematosus provide the most compelling examples of immunological factors influencing cognitive, affective, and behavioral states. In rheumatoid arthritis, on the other hand, the evidence for the reverse pathway—psychological factors effecting immune function and clinical activity—is strongest. Observations about the effect of stress on the onset and course of autoimmune disorders in humans were among the first clues to our understanding of psychoneuroimmunological interactions. We now know that these interactions are bidirectional, both in terms of immune-mediated disturbances in the brain and in terms of the brain's modulating effect on immune cell activity. Autoimmune diseases and, in particular, related animal models, provide exciting opportunities to explore bidirectional neuroimmunological connections. There is clear evidence that the HPA axis and the endocrine system influences susceptibility to autoimmune diseases, and that immune products, in turn, influence the central nervous system in a wide variety of ways. These interactions between the immune system, the neuroendocrine system, and psychological states are abundant and relevant to our understanding of the pathophysiology of autoimmune diseases.

Research at a molecular level is also expanding rapidly and has thrown considerable light on the intricacies of immune and brain interactions and their cytokine mediators. Animal models of autoimmune diseases have provided a particularly useful window on these complex psycho-neuroimmunological interactions. Exploring the role of various neurotransmitters, neuromodulators, and cytokines in the stress response may also have important implications for autoimmune disorders, not only in the circumstances of their onset and course but on the way in which they influence the affective and cognitive capacities of the central nervous system.

# References

Ackerman, K. D., Martino, M., Heyman, R., Moyna, N. M., & Rabin, B. S. (1996). Immunologic response to acute psychological stress in MS patients and controls. *Journal of Neuroimmunology, 68,* 85–94.

Adams, D. O. (1994). Molecular biology of macrophage activation: A pathway whereby psychosocial factors can potentially affect health. *Psychosomatic Medicine, 56,* 316–327.

Adams, S. G., Jr., Dammers, P. M., Saia, T. L., Brantly, P. J., & Gaydos, G. R. (1994). Stress, depression, and anxiety predict average symptom severity and daily symptom fluctuation in lupus erythematosus. *Journal of Behavioral Medicine, 17,* 459–477.

Ader, R. (1989). Conditioned immune responses and pharmacotherapy. *Arthritis Care and Research, 2,* S58–S64.

Ader, R., Felten, D. L., & Cohen, N. (1975). Behaviorally conditioned immunosuppression. *Psychosomatic Medicine, 37,* 333–340.

Ader, R., Felten, D. L., & Cohen, N. (Eds.) (1991). *Psychoneuroimmunology* (2nd ed.). San Diego, CA: Academic Press.

Ader, R., Grota, L. J., Moynihan, J. A., & Cohen, N. (1991b). Behavioral adaptations in autoimmune disease-susceptible mice. In R. Ader, D. L. Felten, & N. Cohen (Eds.), *Psychoneuroimmunology* (2nd ed.) (pp. 685–708). San Diego, CA: Academic Press.

Affleck, G., Pfeiffer, C., Tennen, H., & Fifield, J. (1987). Attributional processes in rheumatoid arthritis patients. *Arthritis and Rheumatism, 30,* 927–931.

Aksentijevich, S., Whitfield, H. J., Young, W. S. 3d., Wilder, R. L., Chrousos, G. P., Gold, P. W., & Sternberg, E. M. (1992). Arthritis-susceptible Lewis rats fail to emerge from the stress hyporesponsive period. *Brain Research. Developmental Brain Research, 65,* 115–118.

Albrecht, J., Helderman, J. H., Schlesser, M. A., & Rush, A. J. (1985). A controlled study of cellular immune function in affective disorders before and during somatic therapy. *Psychiatry Research, 15,* 185–193.

APA Task Force on Laboratory Tests in Psychiatry, (1987). The dexamethasone suppression test: An overview of its current status in psychiatry. *American Journal of Psychiatry, 144,* 1253–1262.

Amkraut, A. A., Solomon, G. F., & Kraemer, H. C. (1971). Stress, early experience, and adjuvant-induced arthritis in the rat. *Psychosomatic Medicine, 33,* 203–214.

Anisman, H., Baines, M. G., Berczi, I., Bernstein, C. N., Blennerhassett, M. G., Gorczynski, R. M., Greenberg, A. H., Kisil, F. T., Mathison, R. D., Nagy, E., Nance, D. M., Perdue, M. H., Pomerantz, D. K., Sabbadini, E. R., Stanisz, A., & Warrington, R. J. (1996). Neuroimmune mechanisms in health and disease. 2. Disease. *CMAJ, 155,* 1075–1082.

Baker, G. B. (1982). Life events before the onset of rheumatoid arthritis. *Psychotherapy and Psychosomatics, 381,* 173–177.

Berczi, I. (1993). Prolactin, pregnancy, and autoimmune disease. (Editorial). *Journal of Rheumatology, 20,* 1095–1100.

Bidlack, J. M., Saripalli, L. D., & Lawrence, D. M. P. (1992). k-Opioid binding sites on a murine lymphoma cell line. *European Journal of Pharmacology, 227,* 257–265.

Boccaccio, G. L., & Steinman, L. (1996). Multiple sclerosis: From a myelin point of view. *Journal of Neuroscience Research, 45,* 647–654.

Breder, C. D., Dinarello, C. A., & Saper, C. B. (1988). Interleukin-1 immunoreactive innervation of the human hypothalamus. *Science, 240,* 321–324.

Brennan, P., & Silman, A. (1994). Breast-feed and the onset of rheumatoid arthritis. *Arthritis and Rheumatism, 37,* 808–813.

Bukilica, M., Djordjevic, S., Maric, I., Dimitrijevic, M., Markovic, B. M., & Jankovic, B. D. (1991). Stress-induced suppression of experimental allergic encephalomyelitis in the rat. *International Journal of Neuroscience, 59,* 167–175.

Carter, W. R., Herrman, J. M., Stokes, K., & Cox, D. J. (1987). Promotion of diabetes onset by stress in the BB rat. *Diabetologia, 30,* 674–675.

Chikanza, I. C. (1999). Prolactin and neuroimmunomodulation: In vitro and in vivo observations. *Annals of the New York Academy of Sciences, 876,* 119–130.

Chrousos, G. P., & Gold, P. W. (1992). The concepts of stress and stress system disorders: Overview of physical and behavioral homeostasis. *Journal of the American Medical Association, 267,* 1244–1252.

Cohen, S. D. (1998). From immunity to autoimmune disease: A historical trail. In *Allergy and asthma proceedings.* Oceanside, CA: Oceanside Publications.

Cover, H., & Irwin, M. (1994). Immunity and depression: Insomnia, retardation, and reduction of natural killer cell activity. *Journal of Behavioral Medicine, 17,* 217–223.

Coyle, P. K. (1996). The neuroimmunology of multiple sclerosis. *Advances in Neuroimmunology, 6,* 143–154.

Crown, S. & Crown, J. M., & Fleming, A. (1975). Aspects of the psychology and epidemiology of rheumatoid arthritis. *Psychological Medicine, 5,* 291–299.

Cutolo, M., Masi, T., Bijlsma, J. W. J., Chikanza, I. C., Bradlow, H. L., & Castagnetta, J. (Eds.) (1999). Neuroendocrine immune basis of rheumatic diseases. *Annals of the New York Academy of Sciences, 876.*

Dahlquist, G. (1993). Etiological aspects of insulin-dependent diabetes mellitus: An epidemiological perspective. *Autoimmunity, 15,* 61–65.

Darnell, R. B. (1996). Onconeural antigens and the paraneoplastic neurologic disorders: At the intersection of cancer, immunity, and the brain. *Proceedings of the National Academy of Sciences, USA, 93,* 4529–4539.

Denburg, S. D., Behmann, S. A., Carbotte, R. M., & Denburg, J. A. (1994). Lymphocyte antigens in neuropsychiatric systemic lupus erythematosus: Relationship of lymphocyte antibody specificities to clinical disease. *Arthritis and Rheumatism, 37,* 369–375.

Denburg, J. A., Carbotte, R. M., & Denburg, S. D. (1987). Neuronal antibodies and cognitive function in systemic lupus erythematosus. *Neurology, 37,* 464–467.

Denburg, S. D., Carbotte, R. M., & Denburg J. A. (1997). Cognition and mood in systemic lupus erythematosus. *Annals of the New York Academy of Sciences, 823,* 44–58.

Denburg, S. D., Denburg, J. A., Carbotte, R. M., Fisk, J. D., & Hanly, J. G. (1993). Cognitive deficits in systemic lupus erythematosus. *Rheumatic Diseases Clinics of North America, 19,* 815–831.

Dupond, J. L., Humbert, P., Taillard, C., de Wazieres, B., & Vuitton, D. (1990). Relationship between autoimmune diseases and personality traits in women. *Presse Medicale, 19,* 2019–2022.

Durant, S., Coulaud, J., Amrani, A., el Hasnaoui, A., Dardenne, M., & Homo-Delarche, F. (1993). Effects of various environmental stress paradigms and adrenalectomy on the expression of autoimmune type 1 diabetes in the non-obese diabetic (NOD) mouse. *Journal of Autoimmunity, 6,* 735–751.

Esterling, B. A., Antoni, M. H., Fletcher, M. A., Margullies, S., & Schneiderman, N. (1994). Emotional disclosure through writing or speaking modulates latent Epstein-Barr virus antibody titers. *Journal of Consulting and Clinical Psychology, 62,* 130–140.

Evans, D. L., Folds, J. D., Petitto, J. M., Golden, R. N., Pedersen, C. A., & Corrigan, M. (1992). Circulatory natural killer cell phenotypes in men and women with major depression. *Archives of General Psychiatry, 44,* 388–395.

Feige, U., & van Eden, W. (1996). Infection, autoimmunity and autoimmune disease. *EXS, 77,* 359–373.

Feigenbaum, S. L., Masi, A. T., & Kaplan, S. B. (1979). Prognosis in rheumatoid arthritis: A longitudinal study of newly diagnosed younger adult patients. *American Journal of Medicine, 66,* 377–384.

Felten, D. L., & Felten, S. Y. (1987). Immune interactions with specific neural structures. *Brain, Behavior, and Immunity, 1,* 279–283.

Foley, F. W., Traugott, U., LaRocca, N. G., Smith, C. R., Perlman, K. R., Caruso, L. S., & Scheinberg, L. C. (1992). A prospective study of depression and immune dysregulation in multiple sclerosis. *Archives of Neurology, 49,* 238–244.

Franklin, G., Nelson, L., Heaton, R., et al. (1992). Stress and its relationship to acute exacerbations in multiple sclerosis. *Journal of Neurological Rehabilitation, 49,* 238–244.

Fricchione, G. L., & Stefano, G. B. (1994). The stress response and autoimmunoregulation. *Advances in Neuroimmunology, 4,* 13–27.

Futterman, A. D., Kemeny, M. E., Shapiro, D., & Fahey, J. L. (1994). Immunological and physiological changes associated with induced positive and negative mood. *Psychosomatic Medicine, 56,* 499–511.

Geschwind, N. (1984). The biology of cerebral dominance: Implications for cognition. *Cognition, 17,* 193–208.

Gilger, J. W., Pennington, B. F., Green, P., Smith, S. M., & Smith, S. D. (1992). Reading disability, immune disorders and non-right-handedness: Twin and family studies of their relations. *Neuropsychologia, 30,* 209–227.

Ginn, L. R., Lin, J. P., Plotz, P. H., Bale, S. J., Wilder, R. L., Mbauya, A., & Miller, F. W. (1998). Familial autoimmunity in pedigrees of idiopathic inflammatory myopathy patients suggests common genetic risk factors for many autoimmune diseases. *Arthritis and Rheumatism, 41,* 400–405.

Glanz, B. J., Schur, P. H., & Khoshbin, S. (1998). EEG abnormalities in systemic lupus erythematosus. *Clinical Electroencephalography, 29,* 128–131.

Goodin, D. S., Ebers, G. C., Johnson, K. P., Rodriguez, M., Sibley, W. A., & Wolinsky, J. S. (1999). The relationship of MS to physical trauma and psychological stress: Report of the Therapeutics and Technology Assessment Subcommittee of the American Academy of Neurology. *Neurology, 52,* 1737–1745.

Grant, I., Brown, G., Harris, T., McDonald, W. I., Patterson, T., & Trimble, M. R. (1989). Severely threatening events and marked life difficulties preceding onset or exacerbation of multiple sclerosis. *Journal of Neurology, Neurosurgery and Psychiatry. 52,* 8–13.

Griffin, A. C., Lo, W. D., Wolny, A. C., & Whitacre, C. C. (1993). Suppression of experimental autoimmune encephalomyelitis by restraint stress: Sex differences. *Journal of Neuroimmunology, 44,* 103–116.

Grossman, C. J., Roselle, G. A., & Mendenhall, C. L. (1991). Sex steroid regulation of autoimmunity. *Journal of Steroid Biochemistry and Molecular Biology, 40,* 649–659.

Grota, L. J., Ader, R., & Cohen, N. (1987). Taste aversion learning in autoimmune Mrl-lpr/lpr and Mrl +/+ mice. *Brain, Behavior, and Immunity, 1,* 238–250.

Hagglund, K. J., Haley, W. E., Reveille, J. D., & Alarcon, G. S. (1989). Predicting individual differences in pain and functional impairment among patients with rheumatoid arthritis. *Arthritis and Rheumatism, 32,* 851–858.

Harbuz, M. S., Conde, G. L., Marti, O., & Lightman, S. L. (1997). The hypothalamic-pituitary-adrenal axis in autoimmunity. *Annals of the New York Academy of Sciences, 823,* 214–224.

Hartung, H. (1993). Immune-mediated demyelination. *Annals of Neurology, 33,* 563–567.

Harrington, L., Affleck, G., Urrows, S., Tennen, H., Higgins, P., Zautra, A., & Hoffman, S. (1993). Temporal covariation of soluble interleukin-2 receptor levels, daily stress, and disease activity in rheumatoid arthritis. *Arthritis and Rheumatism, 36,* 199–203.

Hassler, M., & Gupta, D. (1993). Functional brain organization, handedness, and immune vulnerability in musicians and non-musicians. *Neuropsychologia, 31,* 655–660.

Heisel, J. S. (1972). Life changes as etiologic factors in juvenile arthritis. *Journal of Psychosomatic Research, 16,* 411–420.

Hendrie, H. C., Paraskevas, F., Baragar, F. D., & Adamson, J. D. (1971). Stress, immunoglobulin levels and early polyarthritis. *Journal of Psychosomatic Research, 15,* 337–342.

Hetzel, B. S. (1970). The pathogenesis of thyrotoxicosis. *Medical Journal of Australia, 2,* 663–667.

Hidaka, Y., & Amino, N. (1998). Stress, endocrine, and immune system: Stress induces the onset of autoimmune diseases. *Rinsho Byori. Japanese Journal of Clinical Pathology, 46,* 581–586.

Hierons, R., Janota, I., & Corsellis, J. A. N. (1978). The late effects of necrotizing encephalitis of the temporal lobes and limbic areas: A clinic-pathological study of ten cases. *Psychological Medicine, 8,* 21–42.

Hinrichsen, H., Barth, J., Ferstl, R., & Kirch, W. (1989). Changes of immunoregulatory cells induced by acoustic stress in patients with systemic lupus erythematosus, sarcoidosis, and in healthy controls. *European Journal of Clinical Investigation, 19,* 372–377.

Hinrichsen, H., Barth, J., Ruckemann, M., Ferstl, R., & Kirch, W. (1992). Influence of prolonged neuropsychological testing on immunoregulatory cells and hormonal parameters in patients with systemic lupus erythematosus. *Rheumatology International, 12,* 47–51.

Homo-Delarche, F., Fitzpatrick, F., Christeff, N., Nunez, E. A., Bach, J. F., & Dardenne, M. (1991). Sex steroids, glucocorticoids, stress and immunity. *Journal of Steroid Biochemistry and Molecular Biology, 40,* 619–637.

Hutt, H. T., Kirch, W., Kreuzfelder, E., Scheiermann, N., & Ohnhaus, E. E. (1986). Changes of lymphocyte subpopulations induced by physical stress in normal subjects and patients with systemic lupus erythematosus (SLE). *European Journal of Clinical Investigation, 16,* A35. [abstract 193]

Jankovic, B. D., & Maric, D. (1987). Enkephalins and autoimmunity: Differential effect of methionine-enkephalin on experimental allergic encephalitis in Wistar and Lewis rats. *Journal of Neuroscience Research, 18,* 88–94.

Jarjour, W. N., Jeffries, B. D., Davis, J. S., 4th, Welch, W. J., Mimura, T., & Winfield, J. B. (1991). Autoantibodies to human stress proteins. A survey of various rheumatic and other inflammatory diseases. *Arthritis and Rheumatism, 34,* 1133–1138.

Kaplan, R. F., Meadows, M. E., Vincent, L. C., Logigian, E. L., & Steere, A. C. (1992). Memory impairment and depression in patients with Lyme encephalopathy: Comparison with fibromyalgia and non-psychotically depressed patients. *Neurology, 42,* 1263–1267.

Kapur, N., Barker, S., Burrows, E. H., Ellison, D., Brice, J., Illis, L. S., Scholey, K., Colbourn, C., Wilson, B., & Loates, M. (1994).

Herpes simplex encephalitis: Long term magnetic resonance imaging and neuropsychological profile. *Journal of Neurology, Neurosurgery, and Psychiatry, 57,* 1334–1342.

Kelly, M. J., & Rogers, M. P. (1995). Neuropsychiatric aspects of systemic lupus erythematosus. In A. Stoudemire & B. S. Fogel (Eds.), *Medical-Psychiatric Practice* (Vol. 3).

Kennedy, M. K., Torrance, D. S., Picha, K. S., & Mohler, K. M. (1992). Analysis of cytokine mRNA expression in the central nervous system of mice with experimental autoimmune encephalomyelitis reveals that IL-10 mRNA expression correlates with recovery. *Journal of Immunology, 149,* 2496–2505.

Khoury, S. J., Hancock, W. W., & Weiner, H. L. (1992). Oral tolerance to myelin basic protein and natural recovery from experimental autoimmune encephalomyelitis are associated with down-regulation of inflammatory cytokines and differential up-regulation of transforming growth factor B, interleukin 4, and prostaglandin E expression in the brain. *Journal of Experimental Medicine, 176,* 1355–1364.

Kiecolt-Glaser, J. K., & Glaser, R. (1995). Psychoneuroimmunology and health consequences: Data and shared mechanisms. *Psychosomatic Medicine, 57,* 269–274.

Klosterhalfen, W., & Klosterhalfen, S. (1983). Pavlovian conditioning of immunosuppression modified adjuvant arthritis in rats. *Behavioral Neuroscience, 97,* 663–666.

Klosterhalfen, S., & Klosterhalfen, W. (1990). Conditioned cyclosporin effects but not conditioned taste aversion in immunized rats. *Behavioral Neuroscience, 104,* 716–724.

Knapp, P. H., Levy, E. M., Giorgi, R. G., Black, P. H., Fox, B. H., & Heeren, T. C. (1992). Short-term immunological effects of induced emotion. *Psychosomatic Medicine, 54,* 133–148.

Knight, J., Knight, A., & Ungvari, G. (1992). Can autoimmune mechanisms account for the genetic predisposition to schizophrenia? *British Journal of Psychiatry, 160,* 533–540.

Knoflach, P. (1986). Etiology and pathogenesis of Crohn's disease and ulcerative colitis. *Wiener Klinische Wochenschrift, 98,* 754–758.

Kornhuber, H. H., & Kornhuber, J. (1987). A neuroimmunological challenge: Schizophrenia as an autoimmune disease. *Archives of Italian Biology, 125,* 271–272.

Kort, W. J. (1994). The effect of chronic stress on the immune response. *Advances in Neuroimmunology, 4,* 1–11.

Kracht, J., & Kracht, U. (1952). Zur histopathologic und therapie de schreckthyotoxicosis der wildkaminchens. *Virchows Archiv, 321,* 238–274.

Kreindler, S., & Cancro, R. (1970). An ego psychological approach to psychiatric manifestations in systemic lupus erythematosus. *Diseases of the Nervous System, 31,* 102–107.

Krupp, L. B., Masur, D. M., & Kaufman, L. D. (1993). Neurocognitive dysfunction in the eosinophilia-myalgia syndrome. *Neurology, 43,* 931–936.

Kummerle-Deschner, J. B., Hoffman, M. K., Niethammer, D., & Dannecker, G. E. (1998). Pediatric rheumatology: Autoimmune mechanisms and therapeutic strategies. *Immunology Today, 19,* 250–253.

Laban, O., Markovic, B. M., Dimitrijevic, M., & Jankovic, B. D. (1995). Maternal deprivation and early weaning modulate experimental allergic encephalomyelitis in the rat. *Brain, Behavior, and Immunity, 9,* 9–19.

Lechan, R. M., Toni, R., Clark, B. D., Cannon, J. G., Shaw, A. R., Dinarello, C. A., & Reichlin, S. (1990). Immunoreactive interleukin-1B localization in the rat forebrain. *Brain Research, 514,* 135–140.

Lehman, C. D., Rodin, J., McEwen, B., & Brinton, R. (1991). Impact of environmental stress on the expression of insulin-dependent diabetes mellitus. *Behavioral Neuroscience, 105,* 241–245.

Le Poole, C., Breder, I. C., Das, P. K., van den Wijngaard, R. M., Bos, J. D., & Westerhof, W. (1993). Review of the etiopathomechanism of vitiligo: A convergence theory. *Experimental Dermatology, 2,* 145–153.

Levine, J. D., Clark, R., Devor, M., Helms, C., Moskowitz, M. A., & Basbaum, A. I. (1984). Intraneuronal substance P contributes to the severity of experimental arthritis. *Science, 226,* 547–549.

Levine, S., & Saltzman, A. (1987). Nonspecific stress prevents relapses in experimental allergic encephalomyelitis in rats. *Brain, Behavior, and Immunity, 1,* 336–341.

Levine, S., & Strebel, R. (1969). Allergic encephalomyelitis: Inhibition of passive cellular transfer by exogenous and endogenous steroids. *Experientia, 25,* 189–190.

Levine, S., Strebel, R., Wenk, E. J., & Harman, P. J. (1962). Suppression of experimental allergic encephalomyelitis by stress. *Proceedings of the Society for Experimental Biology and Medicine, 109,* 294–298.

Liblau, R. S., Singer, S. M., & McDevitt, H. O. (1995). Th1 and Th2 CD4+ T cells in the pathogenesis of organ-specific autoimmune diseases. *Immunology Today, 16,* 34–38.

Licinio, J., Gold, P. W., & Wang, M. L. (1995). A molecular mechanism for stress-induced alterations in susceptibility to disease. *Lancet, 346,* 104–106.

Lovett-Racke, E. A., Bittner, P., Cross, A. H., Carlino, J. A., & Racke, M. K. (1998). Regulation of experimental autoimmune encephalomyelitis with insulin-like growth factor (IGF-1) and IGF-1/IGF-binding protein-3 complex (IGF-1/IGFBP3). *Journal of Clinical Investigation, 101,* 1794–1804.

Lowry, M. T., Gormley, G. J., Reder, A. T., & Meltzer H. Y. (1989). Immune function, glucocorticoid receptor regulation, and depression. In A. H. Miller (Ed.), *Depressive disorders and immunity* (pp. 105–134). Washington, DC: American Psychiatric Press.

Lysle, D. L., Luecken, L. J., & Maslonek, K. A. (1992). Suppression of the development of adjuvant arthritis by a conditioned aversive stimulus. *Brain, Behavior, and Immunity, 6,* 64–73.

MacPhee, I. A. M., Antoni, F. A., & Mason, D. W. (1989). Spontaneous recovery of rats from experimental allergic encephalomyelitis is dependent on regulation of the immune system by endogenous adrenal corticosteroids. *Journal of Experimental Medicine, 169,* 431–445.

MacPhee, I. A. M., Day, N. J., & Mason, D. W. (1992). The role of serum factors in the suppression of experimental allergic encephalomyelitis: Evidence for immunoregulation by antibody to the encephalitogenic peptide. *Immunology, 70,* 527–534.

Maes, M. (1995b). Evidence for an immune response in major depression: A review an hypothesis. *Progress in Neuro-Psychopharmacology and Biological Psychiatry, 19,* 11–38.

Maes, M., Bosmans, E., Suy, E., Vandervorst, C., Dejonckheere, C., & Raus, J. (1991). Antiphospholipid, antinuclear, Epstein-Barr and cytomegalovirus antibodies, and soluble interleukin-2 receptors in depressive patients. *Journal of Affective Disorders, 21,* 133–140.

Maes, M., Meltzer, H. Y., Bosmans, E., Bergmans, R., Vandoolaeghe, E., Ranjan, R., & Desnyder, R. (1995a). Increased plasma concentrations of interleukin-6, soluble interleukin-6, soluble interleukin-2 and transferrin receptor in major depression. *Journal of Affective Disorders, 34,* 301–309.

Maes, M., Scharpe, S., Meltzer, H. Y., Bosmans, E., Calabrese, J., & Cosyns, P. (1993). Relationships between interleukin-6 activity, acute phase proteins, and function of the hypothalamic-pituitary-adrenal axis in severe depression. *Psychiatry Research, 49,* 11–27.

Maes, M., Stevens, W., DeClerck, L., Bridts, C., Peeters, D., Schotte, C., & Cosyns, P. (1992). Immune disorders in depression: Higher

T helper/T suppressor-cytotoxic cell ratio. *Acta Psychiatrica Scandinavica, 86,* 423–431.

Markesich, D. C., Sawai, E. T., Butel, J. S., & Graham, D. Y. (1991). Investigations on etiology of Crohn's disease. Humoral immune response to stress (heat shock) proteins. *Digestive Disease Science, 36,* 454–460.

Masera, R. G., Carignola, R., Staurenghi, A. H., Sartori, M. L., Lazzero, A., Griot, G., & Angeli, A. (1994). Altered circadian rhythms of natural killer (NK) cell activity in patients with autoimmune rheumatic diseases. *Chronobiologia, 21,* 127–132.

Mason, D. (1991). Genetic variation in the stress response: Susceptibility to experimental allergic encephalomyelitis and implications for human inflammatory disease. *Immunology Today, 12,* 57–60.

McClelland, D. C., Patel, V., Brown, D., & Kelner, S. P., Jr. (1991). The role of affiliative loss in the recruitment of helper cells among insulin-dependent diabetics. *Behavioral Medicine, 17,* 5–17.

McFarlane, A. C., Kalucy, R. S., & Brooks, P. M. (1987). Psychological predictors of disease course in rheumatoid arthritis. *Journal of Psychosomatic Research, 31,* 757–764.

Meikle, A. W., Daynes, R. A., & Araneo, B. A. (1991). Adrenal androgen secretion and biologic effects. *Endocrinology and Metabolism Clinics of North America, 20,* 381–400.

Meyerowitz, S., Jacox, R. R., & Hess, D. W. (1968). Monozygotic twins discordant for rheumatoid arthritis: A genetic, clinical, and psychological study of 8 sets. *Arthritis and Rheumatism, 11,* 1–21.

Michaelson, D. M., Alroy, G., Goldstein, D., Chapman, J., & Feldon, J. (1991). Characterization of an experimental autoimmune dementia model in the rat. *Annals of the New York Academy of Sciences, 640,* 290–294.

Minden, S. L., & Schiffer, R. B. (1990). Affective disorders in multiple sclerosis: Review and recommendations for clinical research. *Archives of Neurology, 47,* 98–104.

Moos, R. H., & Solomon, G. F. (1964). Minnesota Multiphasic Personality Inventory response patterns in patients with rheumatoid arthritis. *Journal of Psychosomatic Research, 26,* 17–28.

Morch, H., & Pederson, B. K. (1995). Beta-endorphin and the immune system—Possible role in autoimmune disorders. *Autoimmunity, 21,* 161–171.

Moynihan, J. A., & Ader, R. (1996). Psychoneuroimmunology: Animal models of disease. *Psychosomatic Medicine, 58,* 546–558.

Murphy, T. K., Goodman, W. K., Fudge, M. W., Williams, R. C., Jr., Ayoub, E. M., Dalal, M., Lewis, M. H., & Zabriskie, J. B. (1997). B-lymphocyte antigen D8/17: A peripheral marker for childhood-onset obsessive-compulsive disorder and Tourette's syndrome? *American Journal of Psychiatry, 154,* 402–407.

Musha, M., Tanaka, F., & Ohuti. M. (1993). Psychoses in three cases with myasthenia gravis and thymoma—Proposal of a paraneoplastic autoimmune neuropsychiatric syndrome. *Tohoku Journal of Experimental Medicine, 169,* 335–344.

Nisipeanu, P., & Korczyn, A. D. (1993). Psychological stress as risk factor for exacerbations in multiple sclerosis. *Neurology, 43,* 1311–1312.

Orsilles, M. A., & Depiante-Depaoli, M. (1998). Oxidative stress-related parameters in prostate of rats with experimental autoimmune prostatitis. *Prostate, 34,* 270–274.

Ostensen, M. (1999). Sex hormones and pregnancy in rheumatoid arthritis and systemic lupus erythematosus. *Annals of the New York Academy of Sciences, 876,* 131–144.

Palmblad, J., Petrini, B., Wasserman, J., & Ackerstedt, T. (1979). Lymphocyte and granulocyte reactions during sleep deprivation. *Psychosomatic Medicine, 41,* 273–278.

Panitch, H. S., Hirsch, R. L., Schindler, J., & Johnson, K. P. (1987). Treatment of multiple sclerosis with gamma interferon: Exacerbations associated with activation of the immune system. *Neurology, 37,* 1097–1102.

Parker, J. C., Smarr, K. L., Angelone, E. O., Mothersead, P. K., Lee, B. S., Walker, S. E., Bridges, A. J., & Caldwell, C. W. (1992). Psychological factors, immunologic activation, and disease activity in rheumatoid arthritis. *Arthritis Care and Research, 5,* 196–201.

Pearson, C. M., Paulus, H. E., & Machleder, H. I. (1975). The role of the lymphocyte and its products in the propagation of joint disease. *Annals of the New York Academy of Sciences, 256,* 150–168.

Perkins, D. O., Leserman, J., Gilmore, J. H., Petitto, J. M., & Evans, D. L. (1991). Stress, depression, and immunity: Research findings and clinical implications. In N. P. Plotkinoff, A. J. Margo, R. E. Faith, & J. Wybran (Eds.), *Stress and immunity* (pp. 167–188). Boca Raton, FL: CRC Press.

Perry, V. H. (1992). The role of macrophages in models of neurological and psychiatric disorder. *Psychological Medicine, 22,* 551–553.

Plata-Salaman, C. R. (1989). Immunomodulators and feeding regulation: A humoral link between the immune and nervous systems. *Brain, Behavior, and Immunity, 3,* 193–213.

Polla, B. S., Bachelet, M., Elia, G., & Santoro, M. G. (1998). Stress proteins in inflammation. *Annals of the New York Academy of Sciences, 851,* 75–85.

Portig, I., Pankuwit, S., & Maisch, B. (1997). Antibodies against stress proteins in sera of patients with dilated cardiomyopathy. *Journal of Molecular and Cellular Cardiology, 29,* 2245–2251.

Posner, J. B. (1991). Paraneoplastic syndromes. *Neurology Clinics, 9,* 919–936.

Powrie, F., & Coffman, R. L. (1993). Cytokine regulation of T-cell function: Potential for therapeutic intervention. *Immunology Today, 14,* 270–274.

Radulovic, J., Djergovic, D., Miljevic, C., & Jankovic, B. D. (1994). Kappa-Opioid receptor functions: Possible relevance to experimental allergic encephalomyelitis. *Neuroimmunomodulation, 1,* 236–241.

Ratnoff, O. D. (1989). Psychogenic purpura (autoerythrocyte sensitization): An unsolved dilemma. *American Journal of Medicine, 87*(3N), 16N–21N.

Reichlin, S. L. (1993). Neuroendocrine–immune interactions. *New England Journal of Medicine, 329,* 1246–1248.

Reinherz, E. L., Rubenstein, A., Geha, R. S., Strelkauskas, A. J., Rosen, F. S., & Schlossman, S. F. (1979). Abnormalities of immunoregulatory T cells in disorders of immune function. *New England Journal of Medicine, 301,* 1018–1022.

Rimon, R. H. (1969). A psychosomatic approach to rheumatoid arthritis: A clinical study of 100 female patients. *Acta Rheumatology Scandinavica, 13*(Suppl.), 1–154.

Rimon, R. H. (1989). Connective tissue diseases. In S. Cheren (Ed.), *Psychosomatic medicine: Theory, physiology, and practice* (Vol. 2), (pp. 565–609). Madison, CT: International Universities Press.

Rimon, R. H., & Laakso, R. (1985). Life stress and rheumatoid arthritis: A 15-year follow-up study. *Psychotherapy and Psychosomatics, 43,* 38–43.

Rimon, R. H., Viukari, M., & Halonen, P. (1979). Relationship between life stress factors and viral antibody levels in patients with juvenile rheumatoid arthritis. *Scandinavian Journal of Rheumatology, 8,* 62–64.

Rogers, M. P., Trentham, D. E., McCune, W. J., Ginsberg, B. I., Rennke, H. G., Reich, P., & David, J. R. (1980). Effect of psychological stress on the induction of arthritis in rats. *Arthritis and Rheumatism, 23,* 1337–1342.

Rosch, P. J. (1992). Stress and Graves' disease. *Lancet, i* 428.

Rye, B., & Webb, J. M., (1997). Autoimmune bullous diseases. *American Family Physician, 55,* 2709–2718.

Sacerdote, P., Lechner, O., Sidman, C., Wick, G., & Panerai, A. E. (1999). Hypothalamic B-endorphin concentrations are decreased in animal models of autoimmune disease. *Journal of Neuroimmunology, 97,* 129–133.

Sadlock, B., Lohler, J., Scharle, H., Klebb, G., Haber, H., Sickel, E., Noelle, R. J., & Horak, I. (1995). Generalized autoimmune disease in interleukin-2-deficient mice is triggered by an uncontrolled activation and proliferation of CD4+ T cells. *European Journal of Immunology, 25,* 3053–3059.

Sakamoto, Y., Matsumoto, T., & Kumazawa, J. (1998). Cell-mediated autoimmune response to testis induced by bilateral testicular injury can be suppressed by cyclosporin A. *Journal of Urology, 159,* 1735–1740.

Sakic, B., Szechtman, H., Braciak, T., Richards, C., Gauldie, J., & Denburg, J. A. (1997). Reduced preference for sucrosed in autoimmune mice: A possible role of interleukin-6. *Brain Research Bulletin, 44,* 155–165.

Sakic, B., Szechtman, H., Keffer, M., Talangbayan, H., Stead, R., & Denburg, J. A. (1992). A behavioral profile of autoimmune lupus-prone MRL mice. *Brain, Behavior, and Immunity, 6,* 265–285.

Sakic, B., Szechtman, H., Talangbayan, H., Denburg, S. D., Carbotte, R. M., & Denburg, J. A. (1994). Disturbed emotionality in autoimmune MRL-lpr mice. *Physiology and Behavior, 56,* 609–617.

Saplolsky, R. M., Krey, L. C., & McEwen, B. S. (1986). The neuroendocrinology of stress and aging: The glucocorticoid cascade hypothesis. *Endocrinology Review, 7,* 284–301.

Scharrer, B., & Stefano, G. B. (1994). Neuropeptides and auto-regulatory immune processes. In B. Scharrer, E. M. Smith, & G. B. Stefano (Eds.), *Neuropeptides and immunoregulation.* New York, NY: Springer-Verlag.

Schauenstein, K., Rinner, I., Felsner, P., & Mangge, H. (1992). Bidirectional interaction between immune and neuroendocrine systems. An experimental approach. *Padiatr Padol, 27,* 81–85.

Schnabel, A., Hauuschild, S., & Gross, W. L. (1996). Anti-neutrophil cytoplasmic antibodies in generalized autoimmune diseases. *International Archives of Allergy and Immunology, 109,* 201–206.

Schneebaum, A. B., Singleton, J. D., West, S. G., Blodgett, J. K., Allen, L. G., Cheronis, J. C., & Kotzin, B. L. (1991). Association of psychiatric manifestations with antibodies to ribosomal P proteins in systemic lupus erythematosus. *American Journal of Medicine, 90,* 54–62.

Schrott, L. M., Denenberg, V. H., Sherman, G. F., Waters, N. S., Rosen, G. D., & Galaburda, A. M. (1992). Environmental enrichment, neocortical ectopias, and behavior in the auto-immune NZB mice. *Brain Research. Developmental Brain Research, 67,* 85–93.

Searleman, A., & Fugagli, A. K. (1987). Suspected autoimmune disorders and left-handedness: Evidence from individuals with diabetes, Crohn's disease, and ulcerative colitis. *Neuropsychologia, 25,* 367–374.

Selye, H. (1970). The evolution of the stress concept. *American Journal of Cardiology, 26,* 289–299.

Shearn, M. A., & Fireman, B. H. (1985). Stress management and mutual support groups in rheumatoid arthritis. *American Journal of Medicine, 78,* 771–775.

Sibley, W., Bamford, C., Clark, K., Smith, M. S., & Laguna, J. F. (1991). A prospective study of physical trauma and multiple sclerosis. *Journal of Neurology, Neurosurgery, and Psychiatry, 54,* 584–589.

Skwerer, R. G., Jacobson, F. M., Duncan, C. C., Kelly, K. A., Sack, D. A., Tamarkin, L., Gaist, P. A., Kasper, S., & Rosenthal, N. E. (1988). Neurobiology of seasonal affective disorder and photo-therapy. *Journal of Biological Rhythms, 3,* 135–154.

Sluzewska, A., Rybakowski, J. K., Sobieska, M., Bosmans, E., Pollet, H., & Wiktorowicz, K. (1995). Increased levels of alpha-1-acid glycoprotein and interleukin-6 in refractory depression. *Depression, 3,* 170.

Smith, R. S. (1991). The macrophage theory of depression. *Medical Hypotheses, 35,* 298–306.

Solomon, G. F. (1969). Stress and antibody response in rats. *International Archives of Allergy, 35,* 97–104.

Song, C., Lin, A., Bonaccorso, S., Heide, C., Verkerk, R., Kenis, G., Bosmans, E., Scharpe, S., Whelan, A., Cosyns, P., de Jongh, R., & Maes, M. (1998). The inflammatory response system and the availability of plasma tryptophan in patients with primary sleep disorders and major depression. *Journal of Affective Disorders, 49,* 211–219.

Stefano, G. B. (1989). Role of opioid neuropeptides in immunor-egulation. *Progress in Neurobiology, 33,* 149–159.

Stefano, G. B. (1994). Pharmacological and binding evidence for opioid receptors on vertebrate and invertebrate blood cells. In B. Scharrer, E. M. Smith, & G. B. Stefano (Eds.), *Neuropeptides and immunoregulation.* New York, NY: Springer-Verlag.

Stefano, G. B., Cadet, P., Dokun, A., & Scharrer, B. (1991). A neuroimmunoregulatory like mechanism responding to electri-cal shock in the marine bivalve Mytilus edulis. *Brain, Behavior, and Immunity, 4,* 323–329.

Stein, M., Miller, A. H., & Trustman, R. L. (1991). Depression, the immune system, and health and illness. *Archives of General Psychiatry, 48,* 171–177.

Stein, D. J., Wessels, C., Carr, J., Hawkridge, S., Bouwer, C., & Kalis, N. (1997). Hair-pulling in a patient with Sydenhams chorea. *American Journal of Psychiatry, 154;* 1320.

Sternberg, E. M., Glowa, J. R., Smith, M. A., Calogero, A. E., Listwak, S, J., Aksentijevich, S., Chrousos, G. P., Wilder, R. L., & Gold, P. W. (1992). Corticotropin-releasing hormone related to behavioral and neuroendocrine response to stress in Lewis and Fischer rats. *Brain Research, 570,* 54–60.

Sternberg, E. M., Young, W. S., 3rd, Bernardini, R., Calogero, A. E., Chrousos, G. P., Gold, P. W., & Wilder, R. L. (1989). A central nervous system defect in biosynthesis of corticotropin-releasing hormone is associated with susceptibility to streptococcal cell wall-induced arthritis in Lewis rats. *Proceedings of the National Academy of Sciences USA, 86,* 4771–4775.

Stewart, M. W., Knight, R. G., Palmer, D. G., & Highton, J. (1994). Differential relationships between stress and disease activity for immunologically distinct subgroups of people with rheumatoid arthritis. *Journal of Abnormal Psychology, 103,* 251–258.

Stone, A. A., & Bovberg, D. H. (1994). Stress and humoral immunity: A review of the human studies. *Advances in Neuroimmunology, 4,* 49–56.

Surwit, R. S., & Schneider, M. S. (1993). The role of stress in the etiology and treatment of diabetes mellitus. *Psychosomatic Medicine, 55,* 380–393.

Swedo, S. E., Leonard, H. L., Mittleman, B. B., Allen, A. J., Rapoport, J. L., Dow, S. P., Kanter, M. E., Chapman, F., & Zabriskie, J. (1997). Identification of children with pediatric autoimmune neuropsychiatric disorders associated with streptococcal infec-tions (PANDAS) as a marker associated with rheumatic fever. *American Journal of Psychiatry, 154,* 110–112.

Szechtman, H., Sakic, B., & Denburg, J. A. (1997). Behavior of MRL mice: An animal model of disturbed behavior in systemic autoimmune disease. *Lupus, 6,* 223–229.

Trentham, D. E., Belli, J. A., Anderson, R. J., Buckley, J. A., Goetzl, E. J., David, J. R., & Austen, K. F. (1981). Clinical and immunologic effects of total lymphoid irradiation in refractory rheumatoid arthritis. *New England Journal of Medicine, 305,* 976–982.

Urrows, S., Affleck, G., Tennen, H., & Higgins, P. (1994). Unique clinical and psychological correlates of fibromyalgia tender points and joint tenderness in rheumatoid arthritis. *Arthritis and Rheumatism, 3,* 1513–1520.

Utset, T. O., Golden, M., Siberry, G., . Kiri, N., Crum, R. M., & Petri, M. (1994). Depressive symptoms in patients with systemic lupus erythematosus: Association with central nervous system lupus and Sjogren's syndrome. *Journal of Rheumatology, 21,* 2039–2045.

van Eden, W., van der Zee, R., Paul, A. G. A., Prakken, B. J., Wendling, U., Anderton, S. M., & Wauben, M. H. M. (1998). Do heat shock proteins control the balance of T-cell regulation in inflammatory diseases? *Immunology Today, 19,* 303–307.

Van Gent, T., Heijnen, C. J., & Treffers, P. D. (1997). Autism and the immune system. *Journal of Child Psychology and Psychiatry, 38,* 337–349.

van Lankveld, W., van't Pad Bosch, P., van de Putte, L., Narring, G., & van der Staak, C. (1994). Disease-specific stressors in rheumatoid arthritis: Coping and well-being. *British Journal of Rheumatology, 33,* 1067–1073.

Van Noort, J. M. (1996). Multiple sclerosis: An altered immune response or an altered stress response? *Journal of Molecular Medicine, 74,* 285–296.

Vogel, W. H., & Bower, D. B. (1991). Stress, immunity, and cancer. In N. P. Plotkinoff, A. J. Margo, R. E. Faith, & J. Wybran (Eds.), *Stress and immunity* (pp. 493–507). Boca Raton, FL: CRC Press.

Vogelweid, C. M., Johnson, G. C., Besch-Williford, C. L., Basler, J., & Walker, S. E. (1991). Inflammatory central nervous system disease in lupus-prone MRL/lpr mice: Comparative histologic and immunohistochemical findings. *Journal of Neuroimmunology, 35,* 89–99.

Wallace, D. J., & Metzger, A. L. (1994). Can an earthquake cause flares of rheumatoid arthritis or lupus nephritis? *Arthritis and Rheumatism, 37,* 1826–1828.

Warren, S. A., Warren, K. G., Greenhill, S., & Patterson, M. (1982). How multiple sclerosis is related to animal illness, stress, and diabetes. *Canadian Medical Association Journal, 126,* 377–382.

Wekking, E. M., Vingerhoets, A. J., van Dam, A. P., Nossent, J. C., & Swaak, A. J. (1991). Daily stressors and systemic lupus erythematosus: A longitudinal analysis—first findings. *Psychotherapy and Psychosomatics, 55,* 108–113.

Wick, G., Hu, Y., Gruber, J., Kuehr, T., Wozak, E., & Hala, K. (1993). The role of modulatory factors in the multifaceted pathogenesis of autoimmune thyroiditis. *International Review of Immunology, 9,* 77–89.

Wilder, R. L. (1995). Neuroendocrine–immune system interactions and autoimmunity. *Annual Review of Immunology, 13,* 307–338.

Winfield, J. B., & Jarjour, W. N. (1991). Stress proteins, autoimmunity, and autoimmune disease. *Current Topics in Microbiology and Immunology, 167,* 161–189.

Winsa, B., Karlsson, A., Adami, H. O., & Bergstrom, R. (1991). Stressful life events and Graves' disease. *Lancet ii,* 1475–1479.

Xu, X., Zhang, H., Guo, H., Wang, X., Sun, H., Han, X., Li, B., Pang, F., Wang, H., Wen, S. G., Jiang, Y., & Tan, M. (1996). Clinical neuroimmunology. *Advances in Neuroimmunology, 6,* 249–257.

Yang, Z. W., Chengappa, K. N., Shurin, G., Brar, J. S., Rabin, B. S., Gubbi, A. V., & Ganguli, R. (1994). An association between anti-hippocampal antibody concentration and lymphocyte production of IL-2 in patients with schizophrenia. *Psychological Medicine, 24,* 449–455.

Zautra, A. J., Hamilton, N. A., Potter, P., & Smith, B. (1999). Field Research on the relationship between stress and disease activity in rheumatoid arthritis. *Annals of the New York Academy of Sciences, 876,* 397–412.

Zelazowski, P., Patchev, V. K., Zelazowksi, E. B., Chrousos, G. P., Gold, P. W., & Stemberg, E. M. (1993). Release of hypothalamic corticotropin-releasing hormone and arginine-vasopressin by interleukin 1 beta and alpha MSH: Studies in rats with different susceptibility to inflammatory diseases. *Brain Research, 631,* 22–26.

# 51

# Ovarian and Sympathoadrenal Hormones, Pregnancy, and Autoimmune Diseases

RONALD L. WILDER, ILIA J. ELENKOV

## I. INTRODUCTION

Pregnancy and the postpartum periods are associated with significant changes in the levels of several hormones, such as cortisol, estrogen, progesterone, and possibly catecholamines (Chrousos, Torpy, & Gold, 1998). Moreover, the expression of several autoimmune diseases frequently change in the context of pregnancy and the postpartum periods. For example,

rheumatoid arthritis (RA), multiple sclerosis (MS), and autoimmune thyroid disease (ATD) tend to improve during pregnancy but commonly flare up or develop initially in the postpartum period (Buyon, 1998; Confavreux, Hutchinson, Hours, Cortinovis-Tourniaire, & Moreau, 1998; Hazes, 1991; Silman, Kay, & Brennan, 1992; Wilder, 1995, 1998). In apparent contrast, autoimmune diseases that present with symptoms associated predominantly with antibody-mediated damage, such as systemic lupus erythematosus (SLE) and specifically the immune complex-mediated glomerulonephritis, tend to develop or flare during pregnancy (Buyon, 1998; Khamashta, Ruiz-Irastorza, & Hughes, 1997; Petri, 1997; Petri, Howard, & Repke, 1991). RA, MS, and ATD appear to be driven by excessive and sustained production by activated macrophages of proinflammatory cytokines such as interleukin (IL)-12 and tumor necrosis factor (TNF)-$\alpha$. Production of IL-10, an anti-inflammatory cytokine that antagonizes the effects of IL-12 and TNF-$\alpha$, appears to be deficient in these autoimmune states (Feldmann, Brennan & Maini, 1996; Kotake et al., 1997). On the other hand, SLE appears to be associated with excessive production of IL-10, while IL-12 and TNF-$\alpha$ production appears deficient in SLE (Horwitz et al., 1998; Mitamura et al., 1991). Although an understanding of mechanisms underlying these observation is clearly incomplete, there are sufficient data available to suggest that one of the mechanisms through which pregnancy and postpartum periods modulate autoimmune disease activity is through a differential regulatory control of ovarian and sympathoadrenal hormones on IL-12, TNF-α versus IL-10 production. It is our intention to review these evolving concepts.

## II. ROLE OF IL-12, TNF-α, AND IL-10 IN IMMUNOREGULATION

Immune responses are regulated by monocytes/macrophages, and other phagocytic or antigen presenting cells, which are components of innate or natural immune system, and by the T helper (Th) lymphocyte subsets Th1 and Th2, which are components of the acquired (adaptive) immune system (Fearon & Locksley, 1996; Mosmann & Sad, 1996). In general, Th1 responses promote cellular immunity, while Th2 responses facilitate humoral immunity (see Figure 1). Among the factors currently known to influence patterns of Th cell development, cytokines produced by cells of the innate immune system are the most important. The production of IL-12 by monocytes/macrophages and dendritic cells results in Th1 differentiation, whereas the production of IL-10 by monocytes/macrophages and a subset of lymphocytes antagonizes the activities of IL-12. IL-12 acts at three stages during innate/adaptive immune responses. First, it induces interferon (IFN)-γ production from NK and T cells, which contributes to phagocytic cell activation and inflammation; second, IL-12 and IL-12-induced IFN-γ favor Th1 cell differentiation by priming CD4+ T cells for high IFN-γ production; and third, IL-12 contributes to optimal IFN-γ production and to the proliferation of differentiated Th1 cells in response to antigen. Thus, IL-12 represents a functional bridge between early nonspecific innate and subsequent antigen-specific adaptive immunity (Trinchieri, 1995). In addition, both IL-12 and TNF-α are potent stimulators of the activity of natural killers (NK) cells, T cytotoxic (Tc) lymphocytes, and activated macrophages. Overproduction of IL-12 and TNF-α drives chronic inflammatory responses, and thus, these two cytokines are considered major proinflammatory cytokines. In contrast to IL-12 and TNF-α, IL-10 inhibits several macrophage functions. Together with IL-4, this cytokine stimulates the development, proliferation, and function of antibody-producing B cells and promotes humoral immunity (Fearon & Locksley, 1996; Mosmann & Sad, 1996). IL-10 also prevents antigenspecific T-cell proliferation and inhibits the production of the principal proinflammatory cytokines IL-12, TNF-α, and IFN-γ. Thus, IL-10 is considered a major anti-inflammatory cytokine.

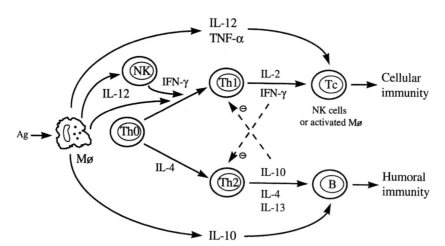

**FIGURE 1**  Role of cytokines in regulation of cellular and humoral immunity. IL-12 and IFN-γ are central inducers of cell-mediated immunity. Th1 cells secrete IL-2 and IFN-γ. These cytokines, in concert with IL-12 and TNF-α, activate macrophages, NK and Tc cells, the primary components of cellular immunity. Th2 cells secrete IL-4, IL-10, and IL-13. These cytokines, together with monocyte/macrophage-derived IL-10, provide optimal help for B-cell development and antibody production. Cytokines that orchestrate the actions of Th1 and Th2 poles of the immune system tend to be mutually inhibitory. Thus, IFN-γ inhibits the proliferation of Th2 cells, while IL-10 is a potent inhibitor of Th1-type cytokine synthesis. Ag, antigen; NK, natural killer cell; Mø, monocyte/macrophage; T, T cell; B, B cell; Th, T helper cell, Tc, T cytotoxic cell; IL, interleukin; TNF, tumor necrosis factor; IFN, interferon.

# III. AUTOIMMUNE DISEASES ARE CHARACTERIZED BY IL-12/TNF-α OR IL-10 DOMINANT CYTOKINE PROFILES

## A. Animal Models of Autoimmune Diseases

Although IL-12 is essential for the clearance of certain intracellular pathogens such as *Mycobacterium tuberculosis*, an increasing body of evidence suggests that excessive production of IL-12 plays a central role in inducing proinflammatory cytokine profiles and Th1-related cellular immune responses that mediate tissue damage typical of organ-specific autoimmunity. In this context, animals models of autoimmune diseases have provided a particularly useful window on the complex pathogenesis of autoimmunity. For example, recent studies indicate that stimulation of IL-12 secretion by microbial products is essential for the generation of the pathogenic autoreactive Th1 effector cells that induce experimental allergic encephalomyelitis (EAE), both in the presence and absence of IFN-γ (Segal, Dwyer, & Shevach, 1998; Segal, Klinman, & Shevach, 1997). The disease-promoting effects of IL-12 are antagonized by IL-10 produced by antigen nonspecific CD4+ T cells. IL-12 also promotes activation of effector cells that induce a severe destructive granulomatous form of murine experimental autoimmune thyroiditis (Braley-Mullen et al., 1998), as well as tissue- or organ-specific inflammatory responses resulting in insulin-dependent diabetes mellitus (IDDM) in NOD mice (Rabinovitch, Suarez-Pinzon, & Sorensen, 1996), and type II collagen-induced arthritis in DBA/1 mice (Germann et al., 1995).

Animal studies also provide evidence for an inverse bias of pro-/anti-inflammatory cytokine balance in SLE. In the NZB/W $F_1$ mouse a genetic polymorphism of an allele of the TNF-α gene correlates with the production of low levels of TNF-α. Regular administration of TNF-α by systemic injection from birth correlates with retardation of onset and reduced severity of immune complex nephritis in NZB/W mice (Jacob & McDevitt, 1988), while anti-IL-10 antibodies injected into NZB/W $F_1$ mice provide disease protection (Ishida et al., 1994). Thus, TNF-α deficiency and/or IL-10 overproduction has been implicated in the pathogenesis of SLE.

## B. Human Studies

Data from different human studies point to a critical role of alteration of IL-12, TNF-α/IL-10 balance in the development of organ-specific and systemic autoimmune diseases (see Table I). Most myelin antigen-specific T-cell clones derived from peripheral blood or cerebrospinal fluid of MS patients during active disease show a Th1-type cytokine profile (Brod, Benjamin, & Hafler, 1991) characterized by increased IFN-γ and TNF-αβ secretion, while during remission, IL-4 and IL-10-producing Th2-like cells emerge. A recent study indicated that IL-12 is responsible for increased IFN-γ secretion in MS, as anti-IL-12 antibodies reverse increased anti-CD3-induced IFN-γ production in MS patients to normal. Furthermore, a marked increase in T-cell receptor mediated IL-12 secretion in progressive MS patients versus controls levels is found (Balashov, Smith, Khoury, Haffer, & Weiner, 1997). In addition, IL-12 expression is augmented in blood mononuclear cells in MS (Matusevicius et al., 1998), while increased production of TNF-α precedes disease activity (van Oosten et al., 1998). CD4+ T-cell clones isolated from lymphocytic infiltrates of patients with ATD exhibit a clear-cut Th1 phenotype, with a high production of TNF-α and IFN-γ. This includes IFN-γ-induced upregulation of major histocompatibility complex (MHC) II protein on thyroid cells, as well as their consequent destruction via cytotoxic T cells (De Carli, D'Elios, Zancuogli, Romagnani, & del Prete, 1994). In addition, cartilage and bone destruction, characteristic of RA, is widely believed to be driven by proinflammatory cytokines. Thus, cytokine profiles of synovial tissues in patients with RA in their early stages are skewed toward proinflammatory macrophage-derived and type 1 cytokines, such as TNF-α, IL-1αβ, and IFN-γ (Feldmann et al., 1996; Kotake et al., 1997). Current evidence suggests that IL-12, produced mainly by macrophage-lineage cells, induces the IFN-γ-dominant cytokine production by infiltrating T cells in joints with chronic RA (Morita et al., 1998). Although most authors frequently detect IL-10 production in active RA joints, the amount of IL-10 produced in the joints appears to be insufficient to exert its maximal inhibitory effect on TNF-α and IL-12 overproduction (Feldmann et al., 1996; Kotake et al., 1997). A high prevalence of IFN-γ-containing lymphocytes has also been shown to be involved in islet cell destruction in patients with insulin-dependent diabetes mellitus (IDDM), and interestingly, increa-sed IL-12 production by peripheral blood mononuclear cells was recently reported in high-risk IDDM first-degree relatives (Szelachowska, Kretowski, & Kinalska, 1997), suggesting that high IL-12 production is involved in the pathogenesis of human IDDM.

A major feature in SLE is IL-10 overproduction that appears to be combined with deficiency of IL-12 and TNF-α secretion. In patients with recent-onset SLE,

TABLE I   Changes in Pro- and Anti-inflammatory Cytokine Production in Autoimmune Diseases and Pregnancy; Effect of Ovarian and Sympathoadrenal Hormones

| Disease/state or hormone | IL-12 | TNF-α | IL-10 | Comments |
|---|---|---|---|---|
| MS | ↑ | ↑ | ↓ | IL-12 appears to drive proinflammatory cytokine profiles and Th1-related autoreactive cellular immune responses in MS, RA, IDDM, and ATD[a] |
| RA | ↑ | ↑ | ↓ | |
| IDDM | ↑ | ↑ | ↓ | |
| ATD | ↑ | ↑ | ND | |
| SLE | ↓ | ↓ | ↑↑↑ | |
| Pregnancy | ↓ | ↓ | ↑↑↑ | Opposite changes in recurrent abortions |
| Cortisol | ↓↓ | ↓↓ | No effect | Lymphocyte-derived IL-10 is enhanced |
| Epinephrine | ↓↓↓ | ↓↓↓ | ↑↑↑ | Epinephrine is the most potent modulator of the production of these cytokines ex vivo; β-adrenoreceptor-mediated effect |
| Norepinephrine | ↓↓ | ↓↓ | ↑↑ | β-Adrenoreceptor-mediated effect |
| Estrogen | No effect | ↓ | No effect | Estrogen potentiates TNF-α production at low concentrations; it increases IL-10 production by antigen-specific T-lymphocyte clones |
| Progesterone | ND | ↓ | No effect | The effects of estrogen and progesterone, as shown here, are at high concentrations that are achievable during pregnancy |

Note. ATD, autoimmune thyroid disease; IDDM, insulin-dependent diabetes mellitus; MS, multiple sclerosis; RA, rheumatoid arthritis; SLE, systemic lupus erythematosus; IL, interleukin, TNF, tumor necrosis factor; ND, not determined.

[a]For details and references, see text.

prior to the initiation of treatment with corticosteroids, monocyte-enriched cells constitutively produce increased amounts of IL-10 and decreased amounts of IL-12 following stimulation. Lymphocyte-enriched cells in these patients also produce decreased amounts of IFN-γ and TNF-α following stimulation. In "rested" cells, these defects are accentuated, and a defect in IL-12 production was suggested (Horwitz et al., 1998). This is consistent with two other studies, showing that peripheral blood mononuclear cells and particularly monocytes from patients with active SLE produce significantly lower amounts of both IL-12 and TNF-α than controls (Liu & Jones, 1998a; Mitamura et al., 1991). In addition, spontaneous production of IL-10 by monocytes and B cells from lupus patients is increased 3.1- to 6-fold, respectively, compared to controls (Mongan, Ramdahin, & Warrington, 1997), and serum IL-10 levels in SLE patients also appear to be higher than those of controls (Liu & Jones, 1998b). Whether the deficiency of IL-12 and TNF-α production is a primary defect or secondary to the excessive production of IL-10 remains to be determined. Nevertheless, the immune complex-mediated glomerulonephritis, the most common manifestation of SLE, autoimmune thrombocytopenic purpura (ATP), and autoimmune hemolytic anemia (AHA), which may be initial manifestations of SLE, in large part, are suspected to be antibody-mediated conditions dependent upon Th2-type cytokines, particularly IL-10.

## IV. PREGNANCY IS ASSOCIATED WITH SUPPRESSED PRODUCTION OF PROINFLAMMATORY CYTOKINES AND A SHIFT TO IL-10 CYTOKINE DOMINANCE

### A. Animal Studies

An example of a physiologic, rather than a pathologic, state in which cytokine biases appear to occur is that of mammalian pregnancy. Evidence has accumulated to indicate that pregnancy is associated with enhanced humoral and reduced cellular immune activity. This, in fact, is consistent with recent data from animal studies suggesting that the cytokine expression associated with pregnancy polarizes toward a Th2-type dominant cytokine profile. Early murine pregnancy is associated with increases in several cytokines, but as pregnancy progresses the Th1-type cytokines, IL-2 and IFN-γ, decline, and the Th2-type cytokines, particularly IL-4 and IL-10, increase (Wegmann, Lin, Guilbert, & Mosmann, 1993). In addition, the constitutive production of Th2-associated cytokines (IL-4, IL-5, and IL-10) has been demonstrated at the maternal–fetal interface

(Lin, Mosmann, Guilbert, Tuntipopipat, & Wegmann, 1993). IL-4 mRNA expression by murine placenta is 5- to 10-fold higher than in the peripheral blood (Delassus, Coutinho, Saucier, Darche, & Kourilsky, 1994). Most significantly, the inflammatory cytokines, TNF-$\alpha$ and IFN-$\gamma$, terminate normal pregnancy when injected into pregnant mice (Raghupathy, 1997). In addition, TNF-$\alpha$ mRNA expression is increased in the placentae of mice with pregnancy loss, and more specifically, TNF-$\alpha$ messages are localized to the uterine epithelium and stroma, as well as to the giant and spongiotrophoblast cells of the placenta (Gorivodsky et al., 1998). These proinflammatory cytokines may damage the placenta directly or indirectly via activation of cytotoxic and NK cells. In fact, strong evidence indicates that increased NK activity is linked with spontaneous fetal resorption in mice (Raghupathy, 1997).

## B. Human Studies

The human embryo and subsequent fetus is a semiallograft and immunologically foreign to the mother. A recent study by Lim et al. (1998) showed a lack of expression of mRNA of Th1 type cytokines such as IL-2, IL-12, and IFN-$\gamma$ and the presence of mRNA of IL-4 and IL-6 in the peri-implantation endometrium of fertile, multiparous women. These data suggest that local Th2 shift may facilitate successful embryonic implantation and maintenance of pregnancy. A decrease in the production of IL-2 and IFN-$\gamma$ by antigen- and mitogen-stimulated peripheral blood mononuclear cells, accompanied by an increase in the production of IL-4 and IL-10, is observed in normal pregnancy, with the lowest quantities of IL-2 and IFN-$\gamma$ and the highest quantities of IL-4 and IL-10 are present in the third trimester of pregnancy (Marzi et al., 1996). Placental tissues from mothers at term express high levels of IL-10 (Cadet, Rady, Tyring, Yandell, & Hughes, 1995), while IL-10 is present in the amniotic fluid of the majority of pregnancies, with higher concentrations found at term than during the second trimester (Greig, Herbert, Robinette, & Teot, 1995). Thus, these studies suggest that proinflammatory cytokine production and cellular immunity are suppressed, and there is a shift in cytokine balance toward IL-10 dominance during normal pregnancy (see Table I).

This is further substantiated by recent studies in women with recurrent abortions where cytokine balance appears to be skewed toward dominance of proinflammatory cytokines. Thus, the expression of IL-12 in peripheral blood mononuclear cells is increased, while IL-10 expression is decreased in women at risk for premature pregnancy termination, while high expression of IL-10 was observed in cells from healthy pregnant women (Szereday, Varga, & Szekeres-Bartho, 1997). Similarly, serum levels of IL-12 are significantly elevated in pregnant women with a history of recurrent miscarriage compared to normal pregnant women (Wilson, McInnes, Leung, McKillop, & Walker, 1997). The production of IL-4 and IL-10 by decidual T cells is decreased in women with unexplained recurrent abortions in comparison with that of women with normal gestation (Piccinni, Beloni, Maggi, Scarselli, & Romagnani, 1998). Furthermore, spontaneous recurrent abortion (SRA) has often been treated by means of immunization with paternal white blood cells. Recently Gafter, Sredni, Segal, and Kalechman (1997) reported that in women with SRA that were immunized with paternal mononuclear cells, and who became pregnant and gave birth to live newborns, the secretion of IL-12, IL-2, and IFN-$\gamma$ by patients mononuclear cells decreased, while production of IL-10 increased.

## V. IL-12, TNF-$\alpha$/IL-10 BALANCE IS DIFFERENTIALLY AFFECTED BY ADRENAL AND OVARIAN HORMONES

The neuroendocrine axis affects the innate and acquired immune systems through an extensive array of mediators and diverse targets (Chrousos, 1995; Vizi, Orso, Osipenko, Hasko, & Elenkov, 1995; Wilder, 1995). A complete discussion of these neuroendocrine regulatory effects is beyond the scope of this chapter. Nevertheless, the available data on the regulatory actions of cortisol, epinephrine, norepinephrine, estrogen, and progesterone on macrophage production of IL-12, TNF-$\alpha$, and IL-10 are sufficient to illustrate the relevant concepts. As already mentioned, excessive and sustained production of IL-12 and TNF-$\alpha$ relative to IL-10 are characteristic of RA, MS, IDDM, and ATD, whereas excessive production of IL-10 appears to be a central abnormality in SLE. A summary of the known effects of the major sympathoadrenal (cortisol, epinephrine and norepinephrine) and ovarian (estrogen and progesterone) hormones on macrophage production of TNF-$\alpha$, IL-12, and IL-10 is shown in Table I.

## A. Effect of Sympathoadrenal Hormones

Norepinephrine, the principal neurotransmitter released by the sympathetic nervous system, has actions similar to those of epinephrine, the principal hormone released by the adrenal medulla. Cortisol production by the adrenal cortex generally correlates with the production of the sympathoadrenomedullary mediators, epinephrine and norepinephrine. These hormones represent the major end products of the stress system, i.e., the hypothalamo-pituitary-adrenal (HPA) axis and the autonomic sympathetic nervous system that constitute the stress system (Chrousos & Gold 1992; Wilder 1995). Cortisol, epinephrine, and norepinephrine are clearly the most potent inhibitors of macrophage TNF-$\alpha$ production (Beutler, Krochin, Milsark, Luedke, & Cerami, 1986; Severn, Rapson, Hunter, & Liew, 1992; Elenkov, Hasko, Kovacs, & Vizi, 1995), (see Table I). In addition, we have shown that the principal sympathoadrenal stress hormones through stimulation of glucocortcoid and $\beta$-adrenoreceptors on monocytes are also potent inhibitors of IL-12 production, which may explain their striking effects in suppressing cell-mediated immune mechanisms (Elenkov, Papanicolaou, Wilder, & Chrousos, 1996). These results have been confirmed and extended by others. Thus, Blotta, DeKruyff, and Umetsu (1997) have demonstrated that the synthetic glucocorticoid dexamethasone suppresses the production of IL-12 from human monocytes that subsequently results in decreased capacity of the monocytes to induce IFN-$\gamma$ and an increased ability to induce IL-4 in T cells. Moreover, in vivo, the administration of therapeutic doses of the $\beta_2$-adrenoreceptor agonist, salbutamol, in humans results in inhibition of IL-12 production by whole blood cultures stimulated with LPS. In conjunction with their ability to suppress IL-12 production, $\beta_2$-adrenoreceptor agonists inhibit the development of Th1-type cells, while promoting Th2 cell differentiation (Panina-Bordignon et al., 1997). It is particularly noteworthy that cortisol, in contrast to its potent suppressive effects on TNF-$\alpha$ and IL-12, has no effects on IL-10 production from human monocytes (Elenkov et al., 1996). This is consistent with a recent report that in RA patients corticosteroid therapy depresses proinflammatory cytokine mRNA but has minimal effects on anti-inflammatory IL-10 mRNA production (Kotake et al., 1997). Interestingly, lymphocyte-derived IL-10 production appears to be even upregulated by glucocorticoids. Thus, rat CD4+ T cells pretreated with dexamethasone exhibit increased levels of mRNA for IL-10, IL-4, and IL-13 (Ramierz, Fowell, Puklavec, Simmonds, & Mason, 1996). The effects of epinephrine and norepinephrine are even more striking. Through stimulation of $\beta$-adrenergic receptors on monocytes, they strongly stimulate IL-10 production (Elenkov et al., 1996). Importantly this also operates in vivo. Thus, a recent study indicates that acute brain trauma is followed by massive release of catecholamines, which triggers

secretion of substantial amounts of systemic IL-10 (Woiciechowsky et al., 1998). Considered together, these data indicate that glucocorticoids and catecholamines strongly influence the cytokine response in a way that suppresses Th1 responses and favors Th2-type reactions. Thus, disorders driven by IL-10, such as SLE, may flare in high cortisol and catecholamine output states, i.e., acute stress or pregnancy. Conversely, clinical situations associated with relative sympathoadrenal insufficiency are expected to be dominated by excessive macrophage IL-12 and TNF-$\alpha$ production relative to IL-10.

## B. Effect of Ovarian Hormones

Progesterone is a steroid hormone which typically increases during pregnancy and is essential for the maintenance of pregnancy. Progesterone decreases steady state levels of TNF-$\alpha$ mRNA in LPS-activated mouse macrophages. In addition, the production of intracellular and secreted TNF-$\alpha$ is also decreased by progesterone (Miller & Hunt, 1998). Importantly, progesterone when present in bulk human peripheral blood mononuclear cells, at concentrations comparable to those present at the maternal–fetal interface, induces the development of Ag-specific CD4+ T cells lines and clones that show enhanced ability to produce IL-4. Moreover, progesterone also induces the expression of IL-4 mRNA and production in established human Th1 clones (Piccinni et al., 1995). This observation was confirmed recently by Correale, Arias, and Gilmore (1998), who showed that progesterone enhances the secretion of IL-4 from antigen-specific human T-cell clones without affecting the secretion of IL-10.

The ovarian hormone estradiol is also increased during pregnancy. Recent studies involving neuroantigen-specific human T-cell clones and murine splenic macrophages in vitro indicate that estradiol (E2) has biphasic effects on secretion of TNF-$\alpha$, with enhancement occurring at low doses of E2 and inhibition at high concentrations (Chao, van Alten, Greager, & Walter, 1995; Deshpande, Khalili, Pergolizzi, Michael, & Chang, 1997; Gilmore, Winer, & Correale, 1997). In another study, estrone (E1) and estriol (E3), like E2 had a biphasic effect on TNF-$\alpha$ secretion, with low concentrations stimulatory and high doses inhibitory (Correale et al., 1998). Importantly, in the presence of high doses of E1, E2, and E3 the majority of the antigen-specific T-cell clones, however, show enhancement of antigen- and anti-CD3-stimulated human IL-10 production (Correale et al., 1998; Gilmore et al., 1997). Interestingly, estradiol does not affect the production of IL-12 and IL-10 by murine splenic macrophages (Deshpande et al., 1997). Estrogens and progesterone are most likely to drive a Th2 shift only at concentrations associated with pregnancy (up to 35,000 pg/mL) (Correale et al., 1998). Thus, at these doses and higher, in the above-mentioned studies, IL-4 and IL-10 secretion are stimulated and TNF-$\alpha$ inhibited. Since steroid hormones accumulate at higher concentrations in target or source tissues than in the peripheral circulation, a localized Th2-like environment with potential for an impact on immunity is more likely to occur at concentrations achieved during pregnancy.

However, it should be pointed out that most of the actions of ovarian hormones, and specifically of estrogens, might be indirect rather than direct on cytokine-producing cells. Estrogen enhances the activity of the stress system; i.e., it enhances cortisol and catecholamine production (Chrousos et al., 1998). The secretion of the hypothalamic corticotropin releasing hormone (CRH) is essential for activation of the peripheral arms of the stress system, i.e., the hypothalamo-pituitary-adrenal axis and systemic sympathoadrenal system (Chrousos & Gold, 1992). The CRH gene contains a functional estrogen-responsive element (Vamvakopoulos & Chrousos, 1993), which may explain higher levels of CRH in the CRH neurons of female rats, and higher HPA axis responsiveness of women (Bohler et al., 1990) and individuals (Lindholm & Schultz-Moller, 1973). Estradiol also decreases corticosteroid receptor levels in the hypothalamus, the anterior pituitary, and the hippocampus, resulting in decreased corticosteroid feedback and increased stress system activation (Chrousos et al., 1998). Conversely, estrogen deficiency, such as observed in the postpartum period and at menopause, is expected to result in a hyporesponsive HPA axis and suboptimal cortisol and catecholamine production. In addition, estrogens are potent inhibitors of the extraneuronal uptake of norepinephrine (uptake-2) (Salt, 1972). Through this mechanism, estrogens, via an increase of local levels of catecholamines are probably able to amplify the effects of catecholamines on pro-/anti-inflammatory cytokine balance.

In other words, the interactions between the stress system and estrogens have the potential to significantly modulate the production and actions of cortisol and catecholamines. Thus, it appears likely that the combined direct and indirect effects of estrogens on TNF-$\alpha$, IL-12 production relative to IL-10 production are possibly very large. The interaction between estrogens and the stress system hormones probably contribute to the dramatic changes in autoimmune disease in the context of changing reproductive status.

Declining estrogen levels may facilitate the development of cell-mediated autoimmune diseases such as RA, whereas high estrogen levels may promote autoimmune diseases associated with humoral immunity such as SLE. Progesterone appears to magnify these effects.

## VI. DIFFERENTIAL HORMONAL CONTROL OF IL-12, TNF-$\alpha$/IL-10 BALANCE MAY CONTRIBUTE TO THE EXPRESSION OF AUTOIMMUNE DISEASES IN PREGNANCY AND THE POSTPARTUM PERIODS

About 70–75% of RA patients experience remission during pregnancy (Buyon, 1998; Østensen & Husby, 1983). Moreover, the risk of developing new onset RA during pregnancy, compared to other periods, is decreased by about 70%. In contrast, RA onset risk is markedly increased in the postpartum period, particularly in the first 3 months (odds ratio of 5.6 overall and 10.8 after first pregnancy) (Silman, 1992, 1994; Silman et al., 1992; Spector, Roman, & Silman, 1990). Breast-feeding further increases risk of disease onset or flare (Brennan & Silman 1994). In women with MS, the rate of relapse declines during pregnancy, especially in the third trimester, and increases during the first 3 months postpartum before returning to the prepregnancy rate (Confavreux et al., 1998). As already mentioned, SLE tends to develop or flare during pregnancy. Similarly, ATP is the most common autoimmune disease that originates in pregnancy (Wilder, 1995). Clinical features of AHA are also worsened during pregnancy. ATP and AHA often are the initial manifestations of SLE and can improve in the postpartum period.

Pregnancy is associated with marked increases in the plasma levels of estrogen, progesterone, cortisol, and possibly catecholamines. The antithesis of this is the postpartum period. Plasma levels of CRH, cortisol, progesterone, and estrogens increase progressively throughout pregnancy and reach maximal levels around labor and delivery (Chrousos et al., 1998; Magiakou et al., 1996a). The last trimester of human pregnancy is characterized by mild hypercortisolism, with total and free plasma cortisol concentrations and 24-h urinary free cortisol excretion increased to levels similar to those seen in mild Cushing syndrome (Magiakou et al., 1996a). During this period, cortisol continues to be secreted in a pulsatile and circadian fashion, while the levels of cortisol-binding globulin in plasma are elevated. It should be noted that during pregnancy the placenta produces CRH, but this production terminates at labor and delivery (Chrousos et al., 1998). It appears that the placenta secretes sufficient CRH to be responsible for the hypercortisolism observed in the last trimester of pregnancy. This hypercortisolism in the last trimester of pregnancy induces mild hypothalamic CRH suppression similar to that observed in patients treated with glucocorticoids or suffering from endogenous hypercortisolism. Animal studies suggest that catecholamine levels also change during pregnancy. In rats, 24-h urinary excretion of norepinephrine during pregnancy is significantly higher than seen in the controls and shows a progressive increase during the last third of pregnancy. At term the excretion rate is 2.6-fold greater than that of controls. Excretion of epinephrine and dopamine do not differ between pregnant and nonpregnant animals. This is consistent with increased sympathetic activity during late gestation, with no change in adrenal medullary function (Cohen, Galen, Vega-Rich, & Young, 1988). Following parturition, the recovery from the state of hypothalamic CRH suppression most likely includes a period of hypocortisolemia. After labor and delivery, plasma levels of all of these hormones decline precipitously. Thus, the postpartum period is associated with suppressed hypothalamic CRH neuron responsiveness, hypoactivity of the pituitary adrenal axis, elevated corticosteroid binding globulin, and decreased free cortisol. Estrogen and progesterone are also decreased in the postpartum period.

Minimum levels are reached about 2 weeks postpartum. Depressed hormone levels, particularly estradiol, can, however, be detected for up to 1 year postpartum. Furthermore, CRH-induced adrenocorticotropin hormone (ACTH) responses are severely depressed for up to 3 months postpartum, implying that hypothalamic CRH priming of the pituitary and pituitary-adrenal axis responsiveness is severely deficient (Chrousos et al., 1998; Magiakou et al., 1996b). Breast-feeding increases plasma prolactin and oxytocin levels, which further attenuates cortisol production in the postpartum period (Amico & Finley, 1986; Amico, Johnston, & Vagnucci, 1994). Thus, the postpartum period, in sharp contrast with pregnancy, is characterized by deficient production of both adrenal and ovarian hormones and, notably, a substantial fraction (20–30%) of premenopausal onset RA develops within 1 year of a pregnancy (Pritchard, 1992; R. Wilder, unpublished observations). These data suggest that premenopausal onset of RA may be influenced by the same factors that influence perimenopausal/menopausal onset of RA, i.e., deficient adrenal and ovarian steroid hormone production.

Some investigators have been less impressed with the role of hormones in pregnancy-associated remissions of certain autoimmune diseases such as RA and have focused on the role of fetal–maternal MHC disparity (Nelson et al., 1993). We, however, should note that hormones and effects of fetal–maternal MHC disparity are not incompatible mechanisms in explaining the changes in RA disease activity in the context of pregnancy. The survival of a histoincompatible fetus is dependent upon deviation/inhibition of the maternal cell-mediated immune response to the fetus (Formby, 1995; Marzi et al., 1996).

Similar mechanisms are probably involved in the reported therapeutic effects of allogeneic cell immunization in RA patients (Smith & Fort, 1996). Both pregnancy and allogeneic immunization undoubtedly involve hormonal changes. Cortisol is a potent inhibitor (Table I) of the production of proinflammatory cytokines such as IL-12 and TNF-$\alpha$ (Beutler et al., 1986; Elenkov et al., 1996). These cytokines play key roles in the rejection of allogeneic tissues and in the pathogenesis of RA. Since cortisol is produced during the third trimester of pregnancy at levels similar to those observed in patients with untreated Cushing syndrome, its potential to modify immune responsiveness cannot be ignored (Chrousos et al., 1998). Estrogen and progesterone, which, like cortisol, are produced at supraphysiologic concentrations during pregnancy, as mentioned above, also have the capacity to skew the immune response toward humoral immunity (see Table I). Thus, a key point is that effects overall of the sympathoadrenal and ovarian hormones on TNF-$\alpha$ and IL-12 differ from the effects on IL-10; i.e., adrenal and ovarian hormonal excess during pregnancy versus deficiency during the postpartum period has the potential to shift proinflammatory/anti-inflammatory cytokine balance in opposite directions (Elenkov, Hoffman & Wilder, 1997; Wilder, 1995, 1996a,b, 1998).

The strongest evidence, however, in support of the importance of cortisol and progesterone to fetal survival is the effect of RU486, a cortisol and progesterone receptor antagonist. RU486 is also a potent enhancer of proinflammatory cytokine production and cell-mediated immune function in the setting of an appropriate antigenic challenge and is a powerful abortifacient. RU486 has also been demonstrated to powerfully upregulate Th1 cytokine production in response to proinflammatory stimuli such as bacterial cell walls (Sternberg et al., 1989; Wilder, 1995). The induction of the production of TNF-$\alpha$ and IFN-$\gamma$ is probably one of the mechanisms of the powerful abortifacient effect of RU486.

# VII. CONCLUSIONS

The data reviewed here are consistent with the view that the increased levels of cortisol, estrogens, progesterone, and possibly catecholamines in the third trimester of pregnancy might orchestrate the improvement in autoimmune diseases, such as RA, MS, IDDM, and ATD, via suppression of proinflammatory (IL-12 and TNF-$\alpha$) and potentiation of anti-inflammatory (IL-4 and IL-10) cytokine production. Conversely, this particular type of hormonal control of pro-/anti-inflammatory cytokine balance might contribute to the flares up of ATP, AHA, and SLE observed during pregnancy. Postpartum, the hormonal state abruptly shifts. The deficit in hormones that inhibit Th1-type cytokines and cell-mediated immunity might permit autoimmune diseases such as RA to first develop or established disease to flare up. Clearly these hypotheses require further investigation, but the answers should provide critical insights into mechanisms underlying a variety of autoimmune diseases. For example, during menopause there is a decline of cortisol and estrogen levels, and, through mechanisms similar to those in the postpartum period, the neuroendocrine milieu may orchestrate the high incidence of RA and ATD developing in women at menopause. The converse of this hormonal imbalance might explain the high incidence of SLE in women in the reproductive years and its decline around menopause.

# References

Amico, J. A., & Finley, B. E. (1986). Breast stimulation in cycling women, pregnant women and a woman with induced lactation, pattern of release of oxytocin, prolactin and luteinizing hormone. *Clinical Endocrinology (Oxford), 25,* 97–106.

Amico, J. A., Johnston, J. M., & Vagnucci, A. H. (1994). Suckling-induced attenuation of plasma cortisol concentrations in postpartum lactating women. *Endocrine Research, 20,* 79–87.

Balashov, K. E., Smith, D. R., Khoury, S. J., Haffer, D. A., & Weiner, H. L. (1997). Increased interleukin 12 production in progressive multiple scelrosis: Induction by activated CD4+ T cells via CD40 ligand. *Proceedings of the National Academy of Sciences, USA, 94,* 599–603.

Beutler, B., Krochin, N., Milsark, I. W., Luedke, C., & Cerami, A. (1986). Control of cachectin (tumor necrosis factor) synthesis, mechanisms of endotoxin resistance. *Science, 232,* 977–980.

Blotta, M. H., DeKruyff, R. H., & Umetsu, D. T. (1997). Corticosteroids inhibit IL-12 production in human monocytes and enhance their capacity to induce IL-4 synthesis in CD4+ lymphocytes. *Journal of Immunology, 158,* 5589–5595.

Bohler, H. C., Jr., Zoeller, R. T., King J. C., Rubin B. S., Weber, R., & Merriam, G. R. (1990). Corticotropin releasing hormone mRNA is elevated on the afternoon of proestrus in the parvocellular paraventricular nuclei of the female rat. *Brain Research, Molecular Brain Research, 8,* 259–262.

Braley-Mullen, H., Sharp G. C., Tang, H., Chen., K., Kyriakos, M., & Bickel, J. T. (1998). Interleukin-12 promotes activation of effector cells that induce a severe destructive granulomatous form of murine experimental autoimmune thyroiditis. *American Journal of Pathology, 152,* 1347–1358.

Brennan, P., & Silman, A. (1994). Breast-feeding and the onset of rheumatoid arthritis. *Arthritis and Rheumatism, 37,* 808–813.

Brod, S. A., Benjamin, D., & Hafler, D. A. (1991). Restricted T cell expression of IL-2/IFN-gamma mRNA in human inflammatory disease. *Journal of Immunology, 147,* 810–815.

Buyon, J. P. (1998). The effects of pregnancy on autoimmune diseases. *Journal of Leukocyte Biology, 63,* 281–287.

Cadet, P., Rady, P. L., Tyring, S. K., Yandell, R. B., & Hughes, T. K. (1995). Interleukin-10 messenger ribonucleic acid in human placenta: implications for a role for interleukin-10 in fetal allograft protection. *American Journal of Obstetrics and Gynecology, 173,* 25–29.

Chao, T. C., van Alten, P. J., Greager, J. A., & Walter, R. J. (1995). Steroid sex hormones regulate the release of tumor necrosis factor by macrophages. *Cellular Immunology, 160,* 43–49.

Chrousos, G. P. (1995). The hypothalamic-pituitary-adrenal axis and immune-mediated inflammation. *New England Journal of Medicine, 332,* 1351–1362.

Chrousos, G. P., & Gold, P. W. (1992). The concepts of stress and stress system disorders. Overview of physical and behavioral homeostasis. *Journal of the American Medical Association, 267,* 1244–1252.

Chrousos, G. P., Torpy, D. J., & Gold, P. W. (1998). Interactions between the hypothalamic-pituitary-adrenal axis and the female reproductive system, clinical implications. *Annals of Internal Medicine, 129,* 229–240.

Cohen, W. R., Galen, L. H., Vega-Rich, & Young, J. B. (1988). Cardiac sympathetic activity during rat pregnancy. *Metabolism, 37,* 771–777.

Confavreux, C., Hutchinson, M., Hours, M. M., Cortinovis-Tourniaire, P., & Moreau, T. (1998). Rate of pregnancy-related relapse in multiple sclerosis. Pregnancy in Multiple Sclerosis Group. *New England Journal of Medicine, 339,* 285–291.

Correale, J., Arias, M., & Gilmore, W. (1998). Steroid hormone regulation of cytokine secretion by proteolipid protein-specific CD4+ T cell clones isolated from multiple sclerosis patients and normal control subjects. *Journal of Immunology, 161,* 3365–3374.

De Carli, M., D'Elios, M. M., Zancuogli, G., Romagnani, S., & del Prete, G. (1994). Human TH1 and TH2 cells, functional properties, regulation of development and role in autoimmunity. *Autoimmunity, 18,* 301–308.

Delassus, S., Coutinho, G. C., Saucier, C., Darche, S., Kourilsky, P. (1994). Differential cytokine expression in maternal blood and placenta during murine gestation. *Journal of Immunology, 152,* 2411–2420.

Deshpande, R., Khalili, H., Pergolizzi, R. G., Michael, S. D., & Chang, M. D. (1997). Estradiol down-regulates LPS-induced cytokine production and NF$\kappa$B activation in murine macrophages. *American Journal of Reproductive Immunology, 38,* 46–54.

Elenkov, I. J., Hasko, G., Kovacs, K. J., & Vizi, E. S. (1995). Modulation of lipopolysaccharide-induced tumor necrosis factor-$\alpha$ production by selective $\alpha$- and $\beta$-adrenergic drugs in mice. *Journal of Neuroimmunology, 61,* 123–131.

Elenkov, I. J., Hoffman, J., & Wilder, R. L. (1997). Does differential neuroendocrine control of cytokine production govern the expression of autoimmune diseases in pregnancy and the postpartum period? *Molecular Medicine Today, 3,* 379–383.

Elenkov, I. J., Papanicolaou, D. A., Wilder, R. L., & Chrousos, G. P. (1996). Modulatory effects of glucocorticoids and catecholamines on human interleukin-12 and interleukin-10 production: Clinical implications. *Proceedings of the Association of American Physicians*, 108, 374–381.

Fearon, D. T., & Locksley, R. M. (1996). The instructive role of innate immunity in the acquired immune response. *Science*, 272, 50–54.

Feldmann, M., Brennan, F. M., & Maini, R. N. (1996). Role of cytokines in rheumatoid arthritis. *Annual Reviews of Immunology*, 14, 397–440.

Formby, B. (1995). Immunologic response in pregnancy: Its role in endocrine disorders of pregnancy and influence on the course of maternal autoimmune diseases. *Endocrinology and Metabolism Clinics of North America*, 24, 187–205.

Gafter, U., Sredni, B., Segal, J., & Kalechman, Y. (1997). Suppressed cell-mediated immunity and monocyte and natural killer cell activity following allogeneic immunization of women with spontaneous recurrent abortion. *Journal of Clinical Immunology*, 17, 408–419.

Gallucci, W. T., Baum, A., Laue, L., Rabin, D. S., Chrousos, G. P., Gold, P. W., & Kling, M. A. (1993). Sex differences in sensitivity of the hypothalamic-pituitary-adrenal axis. *Health Psychology*, 12, 420–425.

Germann, T., Szeliga, J., Hess, H., Storkel, S., Podlaski, F. J., Gately, M. K., Schmitt., E., & Rude, E., (1995). Administration of interleukin-12 in combination with type II collagen induces severe arthritis in DBA/1 mice. *Proceedings of the National Academy of Sciences, USA*, 92, 4823–4830.

Gilmore, W., Winer, L. P., & Correale, J. (1997). The effect of estradiol on cytokine secretion by PLP-specific T cell clones isolated from MS patients and normal control subfjects. *Journal of Immonology*, 158, 446–452.

Gorivodsky, M., Zemlyak, I., Orenstein, H., Savion, S., Fein, A., Torchinsky, A., & Toder, V. (1998). TNF-alpha messenger RNA and protein expression in the uteroplacental unit of mice with pregnancy loss. *Journal of Immunology*, 160, 4280–4288.

Greig, P. C., Herbert, W. N., Robinette, B. L., & Teot, L. A. (1995). Amniotic fluid interleukin-10 concentrations increase through pregnancy and are elevated in patients with preterm labor associated with intrauterine infection. *American Journal of Obstetrics and Gynecology*, 173, 1223–1227.

Haas, D. A., & George, S. R. (1989). Estradiol or ovariectomy decreases CRF synthesis in hypothalamus. *Brain Research Bulletin*, 23, 215–218.

Hazes, J. M. (1991). Pregnancy and its effect on the risk of developing rheumatoid arthritis. *Annals of Rheumatic Diseases*, 50, 71–74.

Horwitz, D. A., Gray, J. D., Behrendsen, S. C., Kubin, M., Rengaraju, M., Ohtsuka, K., & Trinchieri, G. (1998). Decreased production of interleukin-12 and other Th1-type cytokines in patients with recent-onset systemic lupus erythematosus. *Arthritis and Rheumatism*, 41, 838–844.

Ishida, H., Muchamuel, T., Sakaguchi, S., Andrade. S., Menon, & Howard (1994). Continuous administration of anti-interleukin 10 antibodies delays onset of autoimmunity in NZB/W F1 mice. *Journal of Experimental Medicine*, 179, 305–311.

Jacob, C. H., & McDevitt (1988). Tumor necrosis factor-$\alpha$ in murine autoimmune lupus nephritis. *Nature*, 331, 356–359.

Khamashta, M. A., Ruiz-Irastorza, G., & Hughes, G. R. (1997). Systemic lupus erythematosus flares during pregnancy. *Rheumatic Diseases Clinics of North America*, 23, 15–30.

Kotake, S., Schumacher, H. R., Jr., Yarboro, C. H., Arayssi, T. K., Pando, J. A., Kanik, K. S., Gourley, M. F., Klippel, J. H., & Wilder, R. L. (1997). In vivo gene expression of type 1 and type 2 cytokines in synovial tissues from patients in early stages of rheumatoid, reactive, and undifferentiated arthritis. *Proceedings of the Association of American Physicians*, 109, 286–301.

Lim, K. J., Odukoya, O. A., Ajjan, R. A., Li, T. C., Weetman, A. P., & Cooke, I. D. (1998). Profile of cytokine mRNA expression in peri-implantation human endometrium. *Molecular Human Reproduction*, 4, 77–81.

Lin, H., Mosmann, T. R., Guilbert, L., Tuntipopipat, S., & Wegmann, T. G. (1993). Synthesis of T helper 2-type cytokines at the maternal–fetal interface. *Journal of Immunology*, 151, 4562–4573.

Lindholm, J., & Schultz-Moller, N. (1973). Plasma and urinary cortisol in pregnancy and during estrogen-gestagen treatment. *Scandinavian Journal of Clinical and Laboratory Investigation*, 31, 119–122.

Liu, T. F., & Jones, B. M. (1998a). Impaired production of IL-12 in systemic lupus erythematosus. I. Excessive production of IL-10 suppresses production of IL-12 by monocytes. *Cytokine*, 10, 140–147.

Liu, T. F., & Jones, B. M. (1998b). Impaired production of IL-12 in systemic lupus erythematosus. II. IL-12 production in vitro is correlated negatively with serum IL-10, positively with serum IFN-gamma and negatively with disease activity in SLE. *Cytokine*, 10, 148–153.

Magiakou, M. A., Mastorakos, G., Rabin, D., Margioris, A. N., Dubbert, B., Calogero, A. E., Tsigos, C., Munson, P. J., & Chrousos, G. P. (1996a). The maternal hypothalamic-pituitary-adrenal axis in the third trimester of human pregnancy. *Clinical Endocrinology (Oxford)*, 44, 419–428.

Magiakou, M. A., Mastorakos, G., Rabin, D., Dubbert, B., Gold, P. W., & Chrousos, G. P. (1996b). Hypothalamic corticotropin-releasing hormone suppression during the postpartum period, implications for the increase in psychiatric manifestations at this time. *Journal of Clinical Endocrinology and Metabolism*, 81, 1912–1917.

Marzi, M., Vigano, A., Trabattoni, D., Villa, M. L., Salvaggio, A., Clerici, E., & Clerici, M. (1996). Characterization of type 1 and type 2 cytokine production profile in physiologic and pathologic human pregnancy. *Clinical and Experimental Immunology*, 106, 127–133.

Matusevicius, D., Kivisakk., P., Navikas., V., Soderstrom, M., Fredrikson, S., & Link, H. (1998). Innterleukin-12 and perforin mRNA expression is augmented in blood mononuclear cells in multiple sclerosis. *Scandinavian Journal of Immunology*, 47, 582–590.

Miller, L., & Hunt, J. S. (1998). Regulation of TNF-$\alpha$ production in activated mouse macrophages by progesterone. *Journal of Immunology*, 160, 5098–5104.

Mitamura, K., Kang, H., Tomita, Y., Hashimoto, H., Sawada, S., & Horie, T. (1991). Impaired tumour necrosis factor-$\alpha$ (TNF-$\alpha$) production and abnormal B cell response to TNF-$\alpha$ in patients with systemic lupus erythematosus (SLE). *Clinical and Experimental Immunology*, 85, 386–391.

Mongan, A. E., Ramdahin, S., & Warrington, R. J. (1997). Interleukin-10 response abnormalities in systemic lupus erythematosus. *Scandinavian Journal of Immunology*, 46, 406–412.

Morita, Y., Yamamura, M., Nishida, K., Harada, S., Okamoto, H., Inoue, H., Ohmoto, Y., Modlin, R. L., & Makino, H. (1998). Expression of interleukin-12 in synovial tissue from patients with rheumatoid arthritis. *Arthritis and Rheumatism*, 41, 306–314.

Mosmann, T. R., & Sad, S. (1996). The expanding universe of T-cell subsets, Th1, Th2 and more. *Immunology Today*, 17, 138–146.

Nelson, J. L., Hughes, K. A., Smith, A. G., Nisperos, B. B., Branchaud, A. M., & Hansen, J. A. (1993). Maternal-fetal disparity in HLA class II alloantigens and the pregnancy-induced amelioration of rheumatoid arthritis. *New England Journal of Medicine*, 329, 466–471.

Østensen, M., & Husby, F. (1983). A prospective clinical study of the effect of pregnancy on rheumatoid arthritis and ankylosing spondylitis. *Arthritis and Rheumatism, 26,* 1155–1160.

Panina-Bordignon, P., Mazzeo, D., Lucia, P. D., D'Ambrosio, D., Lang, R., Fabbri, L., Self, C., & Sinigaglia, F. (1997). β2-Agonists prevent Th1 development by selective inhibition of interleukin 12. *Journal of Clinical Investigation, 100,* 1513–1519.

Petri, M. (1997). Hopkins Lupus Pregnancy Center, 1987 to 1996. *Rheumatic Diseases Clinics of North America, 23,* 1–13.

Petri, M., Howard, D., & Repke, J. (1991). Frequency of lupus flare in pregnancy. The Hopkins Lupus Pregnancy Center experience. *Arthritis and Rheumatism, 34,* 1538–1545.

Piccinni, M. P., Beloni, L., Maggi, E., Scarselli, G., & Romagnani, S. (1998). Defective production of both leukemia inhibitory factor and type 2 T-helper cytokines by decidual T cells in unexplained recurrent abortions. *Nature Medicine, 4,* 1020–1024.

Piccinni, M. P., Giudizi, M. G., Biagiotti, R., Beloni, L., Giannarini, L., Sampognaro, S., Parronchi, P., Manetti, R., Annunziato, F., Livi, C., Romagnani, S., & Maggi, E. (1995). Progesterone favors the development of human T helper cells producing Th2-type cytokines and promotes both IL-4 production and membrane CD30 expression in established Th1 cell clones. *Journal of Immunology, 155,* 128–133.

Pritchard, M. H. (1992). An examination of the role of female hormones and pregnancy as risk factors for rheumatoid arthritis, using a male population as control group. *British Journal of Rheumatology, 31,* 395–399.

Rabinovitch, A., Suarez-Pinzon, W. L., & Sorensen, O. (1996). Interleukin 12 mRNA expression in islets correletes with beta-cell destruction in NOD mice. *Journal of Autoimmunity, 9,* 645–652.

Raghupathy, R. (1997). Th1-type immunity is incompatible with successful pregnancy. *Immunology Today, 18,* 478–482.

Ramierz, F., Fowell, D. J., Puklavec, M., Simmonds, S., & Mason, D. (1996). Glucocorticoids promote a TH2 cytokine response by CD4+ T cells in vitro. *Journal of Immunology, 156,* 2406–2412.

Salt, P. J. (1972). Inhibition of noradrenaline uptake-2 in the isolated rat heart by steroids, clonidine and methoxylated phenylethylamines, *European. Journal of Pharmacology, 20,* 329–340.

Segal, B. M., Dwyer, B. K., & Shevach, E. M. (1998). An interleukin (IL)-10/IL-12 immunoregulatory circuit controls susceptibility to autoimmune disease. *Journal of Experimental Medicine, 187,* 537–546.

Segal, B. M., Klinman, D. M., & Shevach, E. M. (1997). Microbial products induce autoimmune disease by an IL-12-dependent pathway. *Journal of Immunology, 158,* 5087–5092.

Severn, A., Rapson, N. T., Hunter, C. A., & Liew, F. Y. (1992). Regulation of tumor necrosis factor production by adrenaline and β-adrenergic agonists. *Journal of Immunology, 148,* 3441–3445.

Silman, A. J. (1992). Parity status and the development of rheumatoid arthritis. *American Journal of Reproductive Immunology, 28,* 228–230.

Silman, A. J. (1994). Epidemiology of rheumatoid arthritis. *APMIS, 102*(10), 721–728.

Silman, A., Kay, A., & Brennan, P. (1992). Timing of pregnancy in relation to the onset of rheumatoid arthritis. *Arthritis and Rheumatism, 35,* 152–155.

Smith, J. B., & Fort, J. G. (1996). Treatment of rheumatoid arthritis by immunization with mononuclear white blood cells, results of a preliminary trial. *Journal of Rheumatology, 23,* 220–205.

Spector, T. D., Roman, E., & Silman, A. J. (1990). The pill, parity, and rheumatoid arthritis. *Arthritis and Rheumatism, 33,* 782–789.

Sternberg, E. M., Hill, J. M., Chrousos, G. P., Kamilaris, T., Listwak, S. J., Gold, P. W., & Wilder, R. L. (1989). Inflammatory mediator-induced hypothalamic-pituitary-adrenal axis activation is defective in streptococcal cell wall arthritis-susceptible Lewis rats. *Proceeding of the National Academy of Sciences, USA, 86,* 2374–2378.

Szelachowska, M., Kretowski, A., & Kinalska, I. (1997). Increased in vitro interleukin-12 production by peripheral blood in high-risk IDDM first degree relatives. *Hormone and Metabolic Research, 29,* 168–171.

Szereday, L., Varga, P., & Szekeres-Bartho, J. (1997). Cytokine production by lymphocytes in pregnancy. *American Journal of Reproductive Immunology, 38,* 418–422.

Trinchieri, G. (1995). Interleukin-12, a proinflammatory cytokine with immunoregulatory functions that bridge innate resistance and antigen-specific adaptive immunity. *Annual Reviews of Immunology, 13,* 251–262.

Vamvakopoulos, N. C., & Chrousos, G. P. (1993). Evidence of direct estrogenic regulation of human corticotropin-releasing hormone gene expression. Potential implications for the sexual dimorphism of the stress response and immune/inflammatory reaction. *Journal of Clinical Investigation, 92,* 1896–1902.

van Oosten, B. W., Barkhof, F., Scholten, P. E., von Blomberg, B. M., Ader, H. J., & Polman, C. H. (1998). Increased production of tumor necrosis factor alpha, and not of interferon gamma, preceding disease activity in patients with multiple sclerosis. *Archives in Neurology, 55,* 793–798.

Vizi, E. S., Orso, E., Osipenko, O. N., Hasko, G., & Elenkov, I. J. (1995). Neurochemical, electrophysiological and immunocyto-chemical evidence for a noradrenergic link between the sympathetic nervous system and thymocytes. *Neuroscience, 68,* 1263–1276.

Wegmann, T. G., Lin, H., Guilbert, L., & Mosmann, T. R. (1993). Bidirectional cytokine interactions in the maternal–fetal relationship, is successful pregnancy a TH2 phenomenon? *Immunology Today, 14,* 353–356.

Wilder, R. L. (1995). Neuroendocrine–immune interactions and autoimmunity. *Annual Reviews of Immunology, 13,* 307–338.

Wilder, R. L. (1996a). Adrenal and ovarian steroid hormone deficiency in the pathogenesis of rheumatoid arthritis. *Journal of Rheumatology Supplement, 44,* 10–12.

Wilder, R. L. (1996b). Hormones and autoimmunity: animal models of arthritis. *Baillière's Clinical Rheumatology, 10,* 259–271.

Wilder, R. L. (1998). Hormones, pregnancy, and autoimmune diseases. *Annals of New York Academy of Sciences, 840,* 45–50.

Wilson, R., McInnes, I., Leung, B., McKillop, H., & Walker, J. J. (1997). Altered interleukin 12 and nitric oxide levels in recurrent miscarriage. *European Journal of Obstetrics and Gynecology and Reproductive Biology, 75,* 211–214.

Woiciechowsky, C., Asadullah, K., Nestler, D., Eberhardt, B., Platzer, C., Schoning, B., Glockner, F., Lanksch, W. R., Volk, H. D., & Docke, W. D. (1998). Sympathetic activation triggers systemic interleukin-10 release in immunodepression induced by brain injury. *Nature Medicine, 4,* 808–813.

CHAPTER

# 52

# Neuroendocrine Influences on Autoimmune Disease: Multiple Sclerosis

ALEXANDRE PRAT, JACK P. ANTEL

Multiple sclerosis (MS) is considered an immune-mediated disorder dependent on recruitment of lymphocytes from the systemic compartment into the central nervous system (CNS). Given that the disease effects are restricted to the CNS, the working postulate is that an initial phase in the immune response involves development of antigen-specific T cells directed at determinants present within the CNS. Most attention has focused on the oligodendrocytes and myelin proteins as being the apparent primary disease targets. The demonstration that an inflammatory demyelinating disease of the CNS can result from systemic immunization of either humans, as occurs with neural tissue containing vaccines (acute disseminated encephalomyelitis), or animals (experimental autoimmune encephalomyelitis (EAE)), with myelin components, indicates that the CNS is capable of being the target of a T-cell-dependent autoimmune disorder. Furthermore, such T cells when isolated from the CNS are found to be polarized toward a proinflammatory (Th1) phenotype, i.e., produce the cytokines interferon (IFN)-$\gamma$ and tumor necrosis factor

(TNF)-$\alpha$. The predominance of a Th1 polarized immune response in the CNS in autoimmune disease could reflect preferential attraction of such cells to this compartment, preferential migration across the blood-brain barrier (BBB), or preferential survival or expansion of this phenotype within the tissue. Other animal models of immune dependent CNS demyelination, such as that associated with Theiler murine encephalomyelitis virus (TMEV) infection, indicate that persistent CNS viral infection can also initiate such a process. In this chapter, we will consider the cascade of immunologic events that occur within the systemic immune compartment, at the interface of the systemic and CNS compartments (BBB), and within the CNS which likely contribute to the immune pathogenesis of the MS disease process. We will further consider how the disease process may be subject to neural regulation mediated by specific neurohormones and neurotransmitters.

MS is a disease which has an uneven geographic distribution being highest overall in European-derived populations and lower in Asian and African populations. The small but definite increased incidence rate within families and the 35% concordance rate in identical twins suggest a genetic contribution. An association between MS incidence and HLA genotype has long been established but this trait alone is insufficient to account for the genetic susceptibility to the disease. Ongoing molecular genetic studies of large numbers of familial MS cases will establish the contribution of other gene loci including those which regulate the immune response and its interaction with the nervous system. MS has its peak age of onset in young adulthood, with a greater prevalence in females than males. Typically the disease follows a relapsing course, although up to 50% of cases will convert to a secondary progressive form over time. Cases with later age of onset more frequently follow a progressive disease course. Whether these age-related differences relate to properties of the immune system or other modulating factors remains to be defined.

## I. SYSTEMIC IMMUNE SYSTEM AND MS

We will consider the systemic immune response in terms of antigen-specific T cells, which are essential for initiating the disease process and in terms of the overall state of immune activation which is a major variable in determining whether immune cells will exit the circulation and access the target tissues. Extensive studies have been conducted on lymphocytes derived from peripheral blood (PB) of patients with MS, aimed at determining whether specific properties that underlie disease development and progression can be found. Such studies form a basis for determining how the immune response in the disease is modulated either by therapy or in the context of this chapter by mediators of neural regulation of the immune response.

Descriptions of the molecular mechanisms by which T cells recognize antigen complexed to MHC molecules expressed by antigen-presenting cells (APCs) are available in many immunology texts. Amongst Caucasian MS patients, there is an increase in the proportion of individuals who bear the HLA-DR2 phenotype. There is no apparent specific T-cell receptor (TcR) genotype associated with MS susceptibility. T-cell populations reactive with a number of myelin antigens can be recovered from the blood of MS patients; however, similar cells, albeit at probably a lesser frequency, can also be found in nonaffected individuals. Although there do appear to be immunodominant peptide sequences of different myelin proteins recognized by T cells, the responding cells appear to express a broad repertoire of TcRs. A continuing challenge in establishing the disease relevance of a particular T-cell population identified in human peripheral blood is that, due to interspecies histocompatibility restrictions, direct disease transfer experiments cannot be performed. Thus, one is limited to use of clinical-laboratory correlative studies. In the EAE model of MS, the myelin antigen-

specific T cells used to adoptively transfer the disease are usually characterized as being of the Th1 phenotype. The myelin-reactive T cells generated in vitro from MS patients early in the disease course do not appear to differ markedly in cytokine phenotype from those derived from controls. Myelin-reactive T-cell lines derived from progressive MS patients were found in one study to acquire a Th2 phenotype, i.e., produce the anti-inflammatory cytokines IL-10 and IL-4, an effect possibly attributable to repeated steroid administration (Correale, Arias, & Gilmore, 1998). In general, T cells from humans are more likely to be of a mixed cytokine phenotype (Th0) than are murine T cells.

A large number of studies support the concept that the systemic immune system is in a relative state of activation in MS patients compared to controls, but with an as-yet imperfect correlation with clinical- or MRI-defined disease activity. Evidence for immune activation is derived by detection of increased levels of an array of immune regulatory and effector molecules whose production is known to be linked with the activation process. Peripheral blood-derived monocytes are the potential antigen-presenting cells (APC) most readily available for study in MS patients. These cells express increased amounts of TNF-$\alpha$ when the disease is active. In progressive MS patients, there is increased production of IL-12 by monocytes, a cytokine shown to polarize T cells into a proinflammatory Th1 phenotype. Monocytes are inconsistently reported to have upregulated expression of MHC class II molecules and of the crucial costimulatory molecules B7-1 and CD40, needed for complete T-cell activation to occur.

As regards the properties of PB-derived T cells in MS, there are reports of disease activity being linked to upregulated expression of cell adhesion molecules (see section on BBB) and of cytokines which contribute to the effector arm of the immune response. Some of the adhesion molecules, such as intercellular adhesion molecules (ICAM), are cleaved from the cell surface, enabling one to conveniently assay the soluble forms of these molecules using biological samples. Detection of cytokines at the protein level remains a technical challenge in immediately ex vivo lymphocytes. Assays involving short-term stimulation such as ELISspot and intracellular cytokine staining show increased IFN-$\gamma$ production in patients with progressive disease consistent with the previously mentioned increase in IL-12 production by monocytes; patients with the relapsing disease do not show this change. The state of immune activation is subject to being modulated by an array of exogenous and endogenous factors including the cytokine IFN-$\beta$, the currently approved therapy for MS.

In the context of this chapter, the effects of neuro-transmitters and neurohormones which are known to be physiologic modulators of the immune response, as discussed in other chapters, also need to be considered as modulators of the MS disease process. Epidemiological studies have looked for relationships between the activity of MS and stress. Warren and colleagues, based on a retrospective study, reported that MS patients in exacerbation had encountered greater stress in the preceding 3 months than had stable MS patients (Warren, Greenhill, & Warren, 1982). However, Nisipeanu and Korczyn (1993) found, in a prospective study, that the number of disease relapses in MS patients was reduced during the time of threat of missile attack in Israel during the 1991 Persian Gulf War. These data might be considered consistent with the observation that daily cycles of restraint stress resulted in a significant suppression of EAE (Whitacre, Dowdell, & Griffin, 1998). A link between susceptibility to MS and bipolar disease has been suggested but remains to be established.

The status of the autonomic system in MS patients has been investigated by Arnason and co-workers (Karaszewski, Reder, Maselli, Brown, & Arnason, 1990). This group reported that the psychogalvanic skin response was lacking in MS patients with rapidly progressive disease, providing evidence of central sympathetic denervation. This finding was consistent with their results that $\beta$-adrenergic receptors were upregulated on CD8 T lymphocytes in this patient group (Karaszewski, Reder, Anlar, & Arnason, 1993). Progressive MS patients also showed evidence of parasympathetic denervation as determined by the increased density of muscarinic cholinergic receptors expressed on their peripheral blood lymphocytes (Anlar, Karaszewski, Reder, & Arnason, 1992).

Corticosteroids continue to be a mainstay therapy for acute exacerbations of MS. In an early study using the dexamethasone suppression test (Reder, Lowy, Meltzer, & Antel, 1987), we had found that patients who failed to suppress appeared to respond less well to ACTH, then used as a standard therapy for disease relapses. The nonsuppressors had lower levels of serum dexamethasone than did the suppressors, likely reflecting decreased absorption and/or enhanced metabolism. These lower levels would result in less pronounced negative feedback on the HPA axis and higher serum cortisol (i.e., DST nonsuppression). Michelson and colleagues (Michelson et al., 1994), based on their analysis of the HPA axis in MS patients, concluded that these patients showed evidence of mild activation of the axis, consistent with data derived from animals that were exposed to chronic inflammatory stress. The adrenal glands of

MS patients are also increased in size compared to those of controls (Reder, Makowiec, & Lowy, 1994). Lymphocytes themselves can produce immuno-reactive ACTH material in response to CRH stimulation (Reder, 1992). Experience with EAE indicates that corticosteroids can suppress this disease but rapid withdrawal can result in disease recurrence (Reder, Thapar, & Jensen, 1994). As mentioned earlier, prolonged corticosteroid therapy may be one factor accounting for the apparent cytokine shift toward a Th2 profile of myelin-reactive T cells derived from secondary progressive MS patients (Correale & colleagues, 1998). These cells are also found to be resistant to development of apoptosis.

More recently, we have considered the potential role of neuropeptide-mediated signaling on lymphocyte function in MS. Neuropeptides are small molecular weight peptides synthesised by neurones of the peripheral and central nervous system. They are usually colocalized with "classical" neurotransmitters (noradrenaline, acetylcholine) in nerve terminal vesicles close to the synaptic cleft and potentiate the effect of neurotransmitters on the dendrite. Ultrastructural studies have revealed that a fine distribution of substance P (SP), vasoactive intestinal polypeptide (VIP), and calcitonin gene-related peptide (CGRP)-positive neurones can be found in nerve terminal associated with the basal lamina of most blood vessels of the brain, indicating sites of potential contact with immune cells. The expected expression of these neuropeptides by autonomic nerves supplying lymphoid organs provide a further potential site for neural regulation of the immune response. Monocytes and T lymphocytes have also previously been shown to express SP (NK-1), CGRP, and VIP receptors (Payan, Brewster, & Goetzl, 1983, 1984; Hartung, Wolters, & Toyka, 1986; Ganea, 1996; Martinez, Delgado, Gomariz, & Ganea, 1996; Wang, Xin, Tang, & Ganea, 1996; Lotz, Vaughan, & Carson, 1988; Ho, Lai, Zhu, Uvaydova, & Douglas, 1997; Kavelaars et al., 1994). NK-1 receptor activation by endogenous and selective ligands has been linked to proinflammatory cytokine production by immune cells (IL-1, IL-2, TNF-$\alpha$) and VIP receptor activation can inhibit IL-4 and IL-10 secretion by PB immune cells at least in mouse (Laurenzi, Persson, Dalsgaard, & Haegerstrand, 1990; Martin, Anton, Gombein, Shanahan, & Merrill, 1993; Martin, Charles, Sanderson, & Merrill, 1992; Martinez and colleagues, 1996; Wang and colleagues, 1996). All these neuropeptides can modulate the migration of T lymphocytes in a Boyden chamber assay (Schratzberger, Reinisch, & Prodinger, 1997). Very little is known regarding whether expression of neuropeptides or their receptors is modulated in the periphery or in the CNS during the course of inflammatory disease.

Bradykinin, a member of the blood-derived kinin family, is also produced and stored by neurones. Bradykinin can act on two different kinin receptors; the inducible $B_1$ and the constitutive $B_2$ receptors. The $B_1$ receptor is not expressed under physiological conditions but is upregulated during inflammation in animals (reviewed by Marceau, 1995; Marceau, Hess, & Bachvarov, 1998). Our studies have involved analysis of expression and function of the bradykinin $B_1$ receptor on peripheral blood lymphocytes in MS (Prat et al., 1998; Prat and co-workers 1999). We found that this receptor is selectively upregulated in patients with actively relapsing or progressive disease, less readily detected on stable MS patients' cells, and not detected in normal controls. We had previously established that lymphocytes from active MS patients showed higher rates of migration through a fibronectin-coated membrane in a Boyden chamber assay. A selective $B_1$ agonist inhibited such migration. Furthermore we showed that $B_1$ receptor activation on the surface of MS T cells with highly selective $B_1$ ligands induced a rapid and transient increase in the production of IL-10 and a decrease in IFN-$\gamma$. This shows that a neuropeptide receptor can correlate with inflammatory disease activity and modulate functions of highly specialized immune cells, suggesting a certain form of control by the nervous system on the immune system. The studies cited in this section provide precedents that neurohormones and neuropeptides for which lymphocytes have receptors may, via their effects on the systemic immune system, influence the natural history of MS and/or might be used therapeutically to modulate the course of the disease.

## II. BLOOD-BRAIN BARRIER AND MS

This structure represents the initial site of immune: CNS interaction. The dynamic properties of the cells that comprise this structure are important variables in determining the magnitude of the inflammatory response that will infiltrate the CNS under disease conditions. In MS, sequential MRI studies which show gadolinium uptake into new lesions document that increased BBB permeability is an early event in lesion development. In this section we will consider the basic properties of the blood-brain barrier, its properties during inflammatory disease, and the influence of neurohormones and neurotransmitters on these properties.

## A. Anatomy and Histology of the BBB

Although credit for the term blood-brain barrier is often ascribed to Lewandowsky, it is almost impossible to clearly attribute the paternity of the BBB concept to a specific author. At the end of the 19th century, Paul Erlich clearly demonstrated that not all blood substances enter the brain. Goldman also demonstrated, in 1913, that while intrathecal injection of trypan blue stained brain and spinal cord tissues, intravenous injection did not.

The BBB appears early during development, E14 in mouse (Risau, Hallmenn, Albrecht, & Henke-Falhe, 1986), suggesting that the CNS needs to be isolated from the periphery to initiate and complete a normal neural maturation. Brain endothelium forms a primary vascular complex which surrounds the neuroectoderm (Bar, 1980). Migratory angioblasts, which display some endothelial and immunological characteristics, invade the brain during early embryogenesis (day 10 in rat and day 3 in chick). Endothelial cell proliferation is maximal during embryogenesis and early postnatal life; in the adult CNS, the turnover of endothelial cells is quite limited. Bone marrow-derived cells can enter and colonize the brain, both in the perivascular regions and to a lesser extent, the parenchyma, even after the CNS has gained full protection from the BBB (Hickey & Kimura, 1988). There is increasing evidence of continual immune surveillance ongoing within the CNS by lymphocytes which are able to traffic in and out of this compartment.

### 1. Endothelial Cells of the BBB

The functional events which define the BBB occur at the level of capillaries. Brain capillaries are composed of a fine network of tightly adherent endothelial cells, surrounded by a very narrow basal lamina (or extracellular matrix) which covers the abluminal surface of the endothelial cells (Robertson, Dubois, Bowman, & Goldstein, 1985). Reese and Karnowsky (1967) and Reese (1969) using peroxidase, demonstrated the essential role of tight junction between brain endothelial cells to restrict permeability of the BBB. At the microscopic level, these endothelial cells show a typical continuous cobblestone appearance and a high mitochondria content (8–11% of the total endothelial cell volume) which is thought to provide enough energy to develop the high-resistance tight junctions (Oldendorf, Cornford, & Brown, 1977), a unique way to control the trafficking of molecules, cells, and viruses to brain. These tight junctions consist of strongly anastomosed plasma membrane of one or several endothelial cells which fuse and form a complex surface of ridges and grooves as seen by freeze–fracture images of interendothelia *zonula occludentes* (Shivers, Edmonds, & Del Maestro, 1984; Nagy, Peters, & Huttner, 1984). Tightness of these intercellular junctions can be monitored in vitro using several techniques: the transmembrane recording of electrical resistance and the diffusion of dyes or labeled macromolecules across an endothelial cell monolayer. These features of the BBB endothelium differ from the fenestrated and "leaky" endothelial cells with pinocytic vesicles which are found in peripheral organs and which allow almost a free access of either lipophilic or hydrophilic blood substances to enter organs by mean of para- or transcellular passive diffusion or active transfer.

Not all capillary endothelial cells of the brain provide active protection. Endothelial cells of the circumventricular organs, namely the hypothalamic median eminence, the pituitary, the choroid plexus, the pineal gland, the subfornical organs, the area postrema and the organosum of the lamina terminalis have fenestrations that allow direct contact between neurons and the blood (Dermietzel & Leibstein, 1978). This is very important in the context of immune signaling of the nervous system since the above-cited unprotected neural regions are important regulatory sites of the autonomic nervous system and of pituitary-derived hormones including gonadotrophic, thyroid, and adrenocorticotrophic factors.

A number of molecular markers are now in use to identify brain (microvascular) endothelial cells in vivo or in vitro. However, their expression is either not restricted to brain endothelial cells, as they can be found on either peripheral organ endothelial cells or they can be expressed by other endogenous cells of the CNS (i.e., resident microglia, pericytes, or astrocytes). Factor VIII and von Willebrand Factor (vWF) are probably the most well characterized and frequently used markers for endothelial cells. Brain endothelial cells can de novo synthesize vWF, a factor VIII-related antigen, but do not produce the procoagulant factor VIII. vWF factor serves a dual function in homeostasis: during deendothelialization of the vascular wall it facilitates adhesion of the platelets to the subendothelial extracellular matrix (basal lamina) and also serves as the plasma carrier of the procoagulant factor VIII. Studies on the expression of vWF immunoreactivity by brain endothelial cells also show a fine, vesicular, and perinuclear staining in large and medium-size vessels (Miyagami, Tsubokawa, Smith, & Kornblith, 1984). Dorovini-Zis and colleagues (Dorovini-Zis & Huynh, 1992) reported that such

staining can be increased by the proinflammatory cytokine IFN-$\gamma$.

The lectin *Ulex europaeus agglutinin I* (UEA-I) is a suitable reagent for staining small vessel-derived endothelial cells. Comparative studies using UEA-1 and vWF have shown that while endothelial cells from large brain vessels equally express both antigens, endothelial cells derived from capillaries and microvessels of normal-appearing white matter are more intensely stained for UEA-1 than for vWF (Weber, Seitz, Liebert, Gallasch, & Wechsler, 1985). Our experience with UAE-1 staining is similar. Using UEA-1 lectin covalently bound to the fluorescent molecule FITC, we have shown that human brain microvessel-derived endothelial cells express a much more intense staining for UEA-1-FITC than they do for vWF and that the intensity of the staining is dependent on the dose of UEA-1-FITC used (Figures 1 and 2).

The enzyme $\gamma$-glutamyltranspeptidase ($\gamma$GT) (EC 2.3.2.2) catalyzes the transfer of $\gamma$-glutamyl residue of gluthatione to amino acids and is the key enzyme in the Orlowski cycle (Orlowski & Meister, 1970). This transpeptidase can be detected in brain microvessel ECs (DeBault & Cancilla, 1980a) and is inducible upon stimulation by unknown glial factors (DeBault & Cancilla, 1980b). De Bault (1981) demonstrated that a single glial foot process could induce $\gamma$GT-negative brain endothelial cells to produce de novo high levels of $\gamma$GT, whereas glial cell conditioned media did not. A further example of an astrocyte-inducible brain endothelial cell marker is the Ig-like glycoprotein detected by HT7 monoclonal antibody (Risau, Hallmenn, & Albrecht, 1986a; Risau et al., 1986b). This molecule, located on the luminal surface of the chick brain endothelium in vivo and in vitro, is named Ox-47 in rat and neurothelin, basigin, and gp42 in mouse (Seulberger, Lottspeich, & Risau, 1990; Seulberger, Unger, and Risau, 1992). Little information, however, has been published on the expression of HT7 by the human BBB. ZO-1 is the name of a monoclonal antibody directed against a 225-kDa protein expressed along tight junctions of BBB endothelial cells including human. In vitro, a similar pattern was observed by Rubin and co-workers (Rubin et al., 1991), but ZO-1 staining did not correlate with the electrical resistance in their artificial BBB model.

## 2. Endothelial Cell–Astrocyte Interaction: A Necessary Step for the BBB

Function of the BBB is dependent on contributions from a number of cell constituents in addition to the endothelial cells. Astrocytes cast large processes or

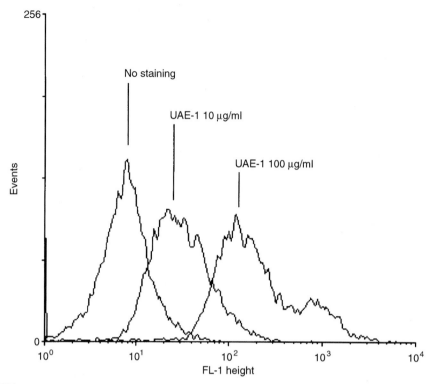

**FIGURE 1**   Cytofluorometric analysis of a primary culture of human brain microvascular endothelial cells stained with the lectin UAE-1 conjugated to FITC. The scan shows a homogenous cell population and a dose dependant staining with the endothelial cell-specific lectin.

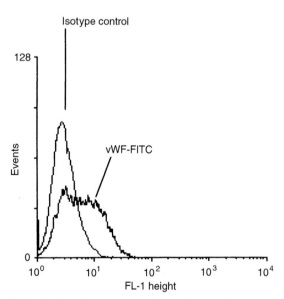

**FIGURE 2**   Cytofluorometric analysis of permeabilized human brain microvascular endothelial cells stained with a monoclonal antibody raised against vWF. The homogenous endothelial cell population express a much lower level of vWF compared to the UAE-1 staining (Figure 1).

end feet which ensheath the endothelial cells (Peters, Josephson, & Vincent, 1991) and cover the entire abluminal surface of brain capillaries. Tao-Cheng and Brightman (1988) were the first to suggest that astrocytic end feet contribute to the functional integrity of the BBB. Brain microvascular endothelial cells need constant input from the neuroglia in order to maintain their BBB-related properties. Immediately ex vivo intact brain microvessels and animal and human brain endothelial cells in culture soon lose their functional BBB capacity as measured by their electrical resistance (Rubin and co-workers, 1991). Although a direct contact between the endothelial cells and astrocytes was initially thought to be needed to generate a BBB, Rubin and colleagues, (1991) have shown that a high transendothelial resistance can be reinduced on human and bovine endothelial cell monolayer when cultured in astrocyte-conditioned media, suggesting that an astrocytic-derived soluble factor may be responsible for the endothelial cell to mature into BBB. A similar experiment by Neuhaus and co-workers (Neuhaus, Risau, & Wolburg, 1991) demonstrated that transwell coculture of endothelial cells with astrocytes is sufficient to induce BBB characteristics by the endothelial cells. Following culture of human brain endothelial cell in astrocyte-conditioned media, Stanimirovic and co-workers (Stanimirovic, Ball, & Durkin, 1995) showed an increased activity of protein kinase C (PKC), suggesting a membrane receptor-mediated action of this astrocytic derived factor. Recently, Kakinuma and colleagues (Kakinuma, Hama, Sugyama, Yagami, Goto, Murakmi, & Fukamizu, 1998) showed that, following brain damage and BBB disruption, angiotensinogen production by reactive astrocytes is needed to reinduce BBB function by brain microvascular endothelial cell, in vivo. They used angiotensinogen knockout mice to demonstrate that expression by astrocytes of angiotensinogen and its active metabolites angiotensin I and IV are not only needed but sufficient to reinduce functional and molecular characteristics of the BBB.

### 3. Pericytes and Perivascular Microglia of the BBB

Pericytes and perivascular microglia, which may act both as contractile and phagocytic cells, are widely distributed at the level of the BBB microcapillaries. Although some authors seem to consider perivascular microglia and pericytes to be the same (Dermietzel & Krause, 1991), Hickey and Kimura (1988) clearly demonstrated that perivascular microglia are bone marrow derived and apparently migrate into the brain. Pericytes are thought to originate from perivascular fibroblasts in the periphery. The findings that perivascular microglia and pericytes serve as phagocytic and professional antigen-presenting cells (Hickey & Kimura, 1988) fits well with the paradigm regarding the BBB that endothelial cells form a dynamic barrier for molecules and cells, whereas perivascular microglia and pericytes assume the responsibility of carrying immunological signals from one side to the other (see later section on immune properties of BBB).

### 4. The Basement Membrane

At the level of the BBB, the basement membrane is a heterogeneous and complex mixture of high-molecular-weight glycoproteins synthesized by adjacent perivascular cells. The perivascular space around tight brain microvessels is small, in contrast to leaky brain vessels, and it can be subclassified at the electro-microscopic level into the inner *lamina densa* and the outer *lamina rarae* (Palotie et al., 1983; Dermietzel & Krause, 1991). The major molecular components of this basement membrane are: laminin, a complex glycoprotein; collagen type IV, which acts as a microfibrillary support apparatus; proteoglycans, mainly heparan sulfate which is more prominent in the outer *lamina rarae* and fibronectin, which is enriched in the developing basal membrane and is thought to promote the proliferation of endothelial cells. Later, during development, levels of fibronectin in the basement membrane decrease and those of laminin increase. Although these molecules provide a fibrillary and elastic support to brain microvessels, they are also involved in the selective transport of highly charged molecules through the BBB (for review see (Dermietzel & Krause, 1991)) and they can be degraded by a family of enzymes called matrix-metalloproteinase (Yong, Krekosky, Forsyth, Bell, & Edwards, 1998). Using an artificial migration chamber, Stuve and colleagues demonstrated that migration of activated PB lymphocytes through a fibronectin membrane was dependent on the secretion of matrix metalloproteinase-9 (Stuve et al., 1996). This promigratory behavior of T lymphocytes is upregulated during MS attacks and can be modulated through neuropeptide receptor engagement (Prat et al., 1999).

### 5. Neuropeptide Effect on the BBB

The effects of neural-derived mediators on BBB permeability have been explored in experimental and clinical settings. An array of neuropeptides are well established to contribute to the local inflammatory response in a variety of organs such as the skin and bowel indicating a relation between the autonomic nervous system and the inflammatory response. Sympathetic, parasympathetic, and c-sensory fibers innervate cerebral blood vessels in various mammalian species. These nerve fibers, which release classical neurotransmitters (noradrenaline and acetylcholine), have colocalized neuropeptides. Some reports also suggest that many of the CGRP, SP, and VIP immunoreactive fibers do not contain noradrenaline or acetylcholine, suggesting a pure neuropeptidergic innervation of mammalian cerebrovessels (Chedotal, Cozzari, Faure, Hartman, & Hamel, 1994). These nerve fibers originate from the ophthalmic division of the trigeminal nerve and bilaterally from dorsal root ganglia of the first three cervical nerves (Nozaki, Uemura, Okamoto, Kikuchi, & Mizumo, 1990). CGRP, VIP, substance P, and neurokinin A immunoreactivity has been described not only in nerve fibers running along CNS blood vessels but also within cerebrovascular endothelial cells, suggesting that brain endothelial cells may also release neuroactive peptide to modulate cerebral blood flow (Linnik & Moskowitz, 1989; Ozaka, Kayashima, & Fujimoto, 1997; Dikranian, Loesch, and Burnstock, 1994).

The presence of functional substance P (NK1), bradykinin (B$_2$), and VIP-specific binding sites has been shown on brain endothelium: their activation increases inositol phosphate accumulation, prostacyclin release and intracellular free calcium concentration (Xu, Qu, Moore, Hsu, & Hogan, 1992; Thorin, Shatos, Shreeve, Walters, & Bevan, 1997). Ligation of the SP (NK-1), bradykinin B2, CGRP, and VIP receptor with endogenous as well as with synthetic agonists exerts a dose-dependent vasorelaxation, which is dependent on the production of nitric oxide by endothelial cells. These neuropeptides are thus potent cerebrovascular vasodilators. This is the scientific rationale underlying the clinical trial of the RMP-7 bradykinin $B_2$ agonist for the adjuvant treatment of brain tumor. This B2 agonist is thought to "open" the BBB, thereby facilitating the delivery of chemotherapeutic agents and viruses used for the treatment of brain tumors.

## B. Immune Properties of BBB

The initial notion that the brain is an immune-privileged organ, not physiologically accessible to peripheral immune cells (Barker & Billingham, 1977), requires revision (Selmaj, 1996; Cross, Cannella, Brosnan, & Raine, 1991). The questions in the field of autoimmune CNS disorders now are *why* and *how* immune cells cross the BBB. Studies of the EAE model have shown that animals with an intact BBB can develop clinically significant perivascular mononuclear cell infiltrates when injected in the periphery with T cells primed with a CNS autoantigen. This occurrence confirms that brain microvascular endothelial cells are not absolutely impermeable to peripheral T cells and that cells of the BBB may actively regulate the entry of immune cells into the brain. The molecular mechanisms responsible for lymphoid cell recruitment and infiltration to form inflammatory foci in the CNS are detailed in other chapters and are summarized in this presentation in the context of their contribution to development of autoimmune CNS disease and specifically MS. We have focused the next part of this chapter on the following topics relevant to immune properties of the BBB: (1) cytokine and chemokine production, (2) adhesion molecules and immune cell trafficking, and (3) antigen presentation at the BBB.

### 1. Cytokine and Chemokine Production at the BBB

Cytokines were initially defined as soluble glycoproteins produced and released by immune cells and which acted as intercellular messengers within the immune system. Subsequently, many of these molecules were shown to interact with and be produced by other cell types including endothelial cells and glial cells. Individual cytokines are often categorized into those considered to be pro- or anti-inflammatory. Among proinflammatory cytokines produced and secreted by brain microvascular endothelial cells are IL-1$\alpha$ and $\beta$, IL-6, and GM-CSF (Fabry, Raine, & Hart, 1994). Cytokines considered to downregulate the cellular immune response and produced by endothelial cells include IFN-$\beta$, the most commonly used therapy in MS and transforming growth factor $\beta$ (TGF-$\beta$). Perivascular microglia are sources of the proinflammatory cytokines IL-12, TNF, and IL-1 and the anti-inflammatory cytokines IL-10 and TGF$\beta$.

Chemokines are a subgroup of small cytokines (8–10 kDa), produced within a target tissue and which provide a mechanism whereby specific populations of inflammatory cells including Th1 and Th2 T cells and monocytes are attracted to the target tissue. (Bonecchi et al., 1998; Borges et al., 1997; Boring et al., 1997; del Pozo, Sanchez-Mateos, & Sanchez-Madrid, 1996; Eng, Ghirnikar, & Lee, 1996; Meeusen, Premier, & Brandon, 1996; Morikawa, Tohya, Ishida, Matsuura, & Kakudo, 1995; Smeltz & Swanborg, 1998; Jourdan et al., 1998). The number of known chemokines and chemokine receptors continues to expand rapidly. At least three classes of chemokines have been defined by the arrangement of the conserved cysteine (C) residues of the mature proteins: the CXC or $\alpha$-chemokines that have one amino acid residue separating the first two conserved cysteine residues; the CC or $\beta$-chemokines in which the first two conserved cysteine residues are adjacent; and the C or $\gamma$-chemokines which lack two (the first and third) of the four conserved cysteine residues. Production of chemokines within the CNS is well documented; cellular sources include glial and endothelial cells (Zach et al., 1997; McManus et al., 1998). High levels of IL-8 can be found in primary cultures of human brain microvascular endothelial cells and IL-8 binding sites are expressed by endothelial cells in vivo, suggesting that IL-8 can be presented to immune cells on their luminal surface. Expression of chemokines is a dynamic process dependent on the activation state of the cells which produce or express them. This issue is most relevant for MS in which the state of activation of glial cells varies in concert with disease activity. The $\beta$-chemokines MIP-1$\alpha$, MCP-1, and RANTES have been demonstrated to be expressed by glial cells, macrophages, and endothelial cells in active MS lesions.

### 2. Adhesion Molecules and Cell Trafficking through the BBB: Relevance to MS

An early and necessary step for immune cell invasion of the CNS is the adhesion of immune cells

and the nervous system, with neurotransmitters and neurohormones being key mediators. To be resolved is the magnitude of effects that fluctuations in these responses can have on the course of autoimmune disease of the nervous system and whether pharmacological manipulation of the mediators of these immune:neural interactions can provide an approach to disease therapy.

# References

Anlar, B., Karaszewski, J. W., Reder, A. T., & Arnason, G. W. (1992). Increased muscarinic cholinergic receptor density on CD4 lymphocytes in progressive multiple sclerosis. *Journal of Neuroimmunology, 36*(2–3), 171–177.

Antel, J. P., & Becher, B. (1998). Central nervous system–immune interactions: contribution to neurologic disease and recovery. In J. Antel, G. Birnbaum, & H. P. Hartung (Eds.), *Clinical Neuroimmunology* (pp. 26–39). Malden: Blackwell Science.

Archelos, J. J., & Hartung, H. P. (1997). The role of adhesion molecules in multiple sclerosis: Biology, pathogenesis and therapeutic implications. *Molecular Medicine Today, 3*(7), 310–321. [review]

Bar, T. (1980). The vascular system of the cerebral cortex. *Advances in Anatomy Embryology and Cell Biology, 59*, I–VI. [review]

Barker, C. F., & Billingham, R. E. (1977). Immunologically privileged sites. *Advances in Immunology, 25*, 1–54. [review]

Bo, L., Peterson, J. W., Mork, S., Hoffman, P. A., Gallatin, W. M., Ransohoff, R. M., & Trapp, B. D. (1996). Distribution of immunoglobulin superfamily members ICAM-1, -2, -3, and the beta 2 integrin LFA-1 in multiple sclerosis lesions. *Journal of Neuropathology and Experimental Neurology, 55*(10), 1060–1072.

Bonecchi, R., Bianchi, G., Bordignon, P. P., D'Ambrosio, D., Lang, R., Borsatti, A., Sozzani, S., Allavena, P., Gray, P. A., Mantovani, A., & Sinigaglia, F. (1998). Differential expression of chemokine receptors and chemotactic responsiveness of type 1 T helper cells (Th1s) and Th2s. *Journal of Experimental Medicine, 187*(1), 129–134.

Borges, E., Tietz, W., Steegmaier, M., Moll, T., Hallmann, R., Hamann, A., & Vestweber, D. (1997). P-selectin glycoprotein ligand-1 (PSGL-1) on T helper 1 but not on T helper 2 cells binds to P–selectin and supports migration into inflamed skin. *Journal of Experimental Medicine, 185*(3), 573–578.

Boring, L., Gosling, J., Chensue, S. W., Kunkel, S. L., Farese, R. V. J., Broxmeyer, H. E., & Charo, I. F. (1997). Impaired monocyte migration and reduced type 1 (Th1) cytokine responses in C–C chemokine receptor 2 knockout mice. *Journal of Clinical Investigation, 100*(10), 2552–2561.

Brosnan, C. F., Cannella, B., Battistini, L., & Raine, C. S. (1995). Cytokine localization in multiple sclerosis lesions: Correlation with adhesion molecule expression and reactive nitrogen species. *Neurology, 45*(Suppl. 6), 21. [review]

Cannella, B., & Raine, C. S. (1995). The adhesion molecule and cytokine profile of multiple sclerosis lesions. *Annals of Neurology, 37*(4), 424–435.

Chedotal, A., Cozzari, C., Faure, M. P., Hartman, B. K., & Hamel, E. (1994). Distinct choline acetyltransferase (ChAT) and vasoactive intestinal polypeptide (VIP) bipolar neurons project to local blood vessels in the rat cerebral cortex. *Brain Research, 646*(2), 181–193.

Correale, J., Arias, M., & Gilmore, W. (1998). Steroid hormone regulation of cytokine secretion by proteolipid protein–specific CD4+ T cell clones isolated from multiple sclerosis patients and normal control subjects. *Journal of Immunology, 161*(7), 3365–3374.

Corsini, E., Gelati, M., Dufour, A., Massa, G., Nespolo, A., Ciusani, E., Milanese, C., La Mantia, L., & Salmaggi, A. (1997). Effects of beta-IFN-1b treatment in MS patients on adhesion between PBMNCs, HUVECs and MS-HBECs: An in vivo and in vitro study. *Journal of Neuroimmunology, 79*(1), 76–83.

Cross, A. H., Cannella, B., Brosnan, C. F., & Raine, C. S. (1990). Homing to CNS vasculature by antigen specific lymphocytes. I. Localisation of C14-labelled cells during acute, chronic and relapsing experimental allergic encephalomyelitis. *Laboratory Investigation, 63*(2), 162–170.

Cross, A. H., Cannella, B., Brosnan, C. F., & Raine, C. S. (1991). Hypothesis: Antigen-specific T cells prime central nervous system endothelium for recruitment of nonspecific inflammatory cells to effect autoimmune demyelination. *Journal of Neuroimmunology, 33*(3), 237–244.

DeBault, L. E. (1981). gamma-Glutamyltranspeptidase induction mediated by glial foot process-to endothelium contact in co-culture. *Brain Research, 220*(2), 432–435.

DeBault, L. E., & Cancilla, P. A. (1980a). gamma-Glutamyl transpeptidase in isolated brain endothelial cells: Induction by glial cells in vitro. *Science, 207*(4431), 653–655.

DeBault, L. E., & Cancilla, P. A. (1980b). Induction of gamma-glutamyl transpeptidase in isolated cerebral endothelial cells. *Advances in Experimental and Medical Biology, 131*, 79–88.

del Pozo, M. A., Sanchez–Mateos, P., & Sanchez-Madrid, F. (1996). Cellular polarization induced by chemokines: A mechanism for leukocyte recruitment? *Immunology Today, 17*(3), 127–131. [review]

Dermietzel, R., & Krause, D. (1991). Molecular anatomy of the blood–brain barrier as defined by immunocytochemistry. *International Review in Cytology, 127*, 57–109.

Dermietzel, R., & Leibstein, A. G. (1978). The microvascular pattern and perivascular linings of the area postrema. A combined freeze-etching and ultrathin section study. *Cell and Tissue Research, 186*(1), 97–110.

Dhib-Jalbut, S., Jiang, H., & Williams, G. J. (1996). The effect of interferon beta-1b on lymphocyte-endothelial cell adhesion. *Journal of Neuroimmunology, 71*(1–2), 215–222.

Dikranian, K., Loesch, A., & Burnstock, G. (1994). Localisation of nitric oxide syntase and its colocalisation with vasoactive peptides in coronary and cerebral arteries. An electron microscope study. *Journal of Anatomy, 184*(3), 583–590.

Dorovini-Zis, K., & Huynh, H. K. (1992). Ultrastructural localization of factor VIII-related antigen in cultured human brain microvessel endothelial cells. *Journal of Histochemistry and. Cytochemistry, 40*(5), 689–696.

Eng, L. F., Ghirnikar, R. S., & Lee, Y. L. (1996). Inflammation in EAE: Role of chemokine/cytokine expression by resident and infiltrating cells. *Neurochemical Research, 21*(4), 511–525. [review]

Fabry, Z., Raine, C. S., & Hart, M. N. (1994). Nervous tissue as an immune compartment: The dialect of the immune response in the CNS. *Immunology Today, 15*(5), 218–224.

Ganea, D. (1996). Regulatory effects of vasoactive intestinal peptide on cytokine production in central and peripheral lymphoid organs. *Advances in Neuroimmunology, 6*(1), 61–74.

Girvin, A. D., Gordon, K. B., Tan, L., & Miller, S. D. (1998). Expression of MHC class II and co-stimulatory molecules by endothelial cells of the Blood Brain barrier: Effect on antigen presentation. *Journal of Neuroimmunology, 90*, 21. [abstract]

Hartung, H. P., Wolters, K., & Toyka, K. V. (1986). Substance P: Binding properties and studies on cellular responses in guinea pig macrophages. *Journal of Immunology, 136*,(10), 3856–3863.

Hickey, W. F., & Kimura, H. (1988). Perivascular microglial cells of the CNS are bone marrow-derived and present antigen in vivo. *Science, 239*(4837), 290–292.

Ho, W. Z., Lai, J. P., Zhu, X. H., Uvaydova, M., & Douglas, S. D. (1997). Human monocytes and macrophages express substance P and neurokinin-1 receptor. *Journal of Immunology, 159*, 5654–5660.

Jemison, L. M., Williams, S. K., Lublin, F. D., Knobler, R. L., & Korngold, R. (1993). Interferon-gamma-inducible endothelial cell class II major histocompatibility complex expression correlates with strain- and site-specific susceptibility to experimental allergic encephalomyelitis. *Journal of Neuroimmunology, 47*(1), 15–22.

Jourdan, P., Abbal, C., Nora, N., Hori, T., Uchiyama, T., Vendrell, J. P., Bousquet, J., Taylor, N., Pene, J., & Yssel, H. (1998). IL-4 induces functional cell-surface expression of CXCR4 on human T cells. *Journal Immunology, 160*(9), 4153–4157.

Kakinuma, Y., Hama, H., Sugyama, F., Yagami, K., Goto, K., Murakami, K., & Fukamizu, K. (1998). Impaired blood–brain barrier function in angiotensinogen-deficient mice. *Nature Medicine, 4*(9), 1078–1080.

Karaszewski, J. W., Reder, A. T., Anlar, B., & Arnason, G. W. (1993). Increased high affinity beta-adrenergic receptor densities and cyclic AMP responses of CD8 cells in multiple sclerosis. *Journal Neuroimmunology, 43*(1–2), 1–7.

Karaszewski, J. W., Reder, A. T., Maselli, R., Brown, M., & Arnason, B. W. (1990). Sympathetic skin responses are decreased and lymphocyte beta-adrenergic receptors are increased in progressive multiple sclerosis. *Annals of Neurology, 27*(4), 366–372.

Kavelaars, A., Broeke, D., Jeurissen, F., Kardux, J., Meijer, A., Franklin, R., Gelfand, E. W., & Heijnen, C. B. (1994). Activation of human monocytes via a non-neurokinin substance P receptor that is coupled to Gi protein, calcium, Phospholipase D, MAP kinase, and IL–6 production. *Journal Immunology, 153*(3691), 3699

Keszthelyi, E., Karlik, S., Hyduk, S. J., Rice, G. P., Gordon, G., Yednock, T., & Horner, H. (1996). Evidence for a prolonged role of alpha 4 integrin throughout active experimental allergic encephalomyelitis. *Neurology, 47*(4), 1053–1059.

Laurenzi, M. A., Persson, M. A. A. Dalsgaard, C. J., & Haegerstrand, A. (1990). The neuropeptide substance P stimulates production of IL-1 in human blood monocytes: Activated cells are preferentially influenced by the neuropeptide. *Scandinavian Journal Immunology, 31*, 529–533.

Linnik, M. D., & Moskowitz, M. A. (1989). Identification of immunoreactive substance P in human and other mammalian endothelial cells. *Peptides, 10*(5), 957–962.

Lotz, M., Vaughan, J. H., & Carson, D. A. (1988). Effect of neuropeptides on production of inflammatory cytokines by human monocytes. *Science, 241*(1218), 1221

Lou, J., Dayer, J. M., Grau, G. E., & Burger, D. (1996). Direct cell/cell contact with stimulated T lymphocytes induces the expression of cell adhesion molecules and cytokines by human brain microvascular endothelial cells. *European Journal of Immunology, 26*(12), 3107–3113.

Marceau, F. (1995). Kinin B1 receptor: A review. *Immunopharmacology, 30*(1), 1–26.

Marceau, F., Hess, J. F., & Bachvarov, D. R. (1998). The B1 receptors for kinins. *Pharmacological Review, 50*(3), 357–386.

Martin, F. C., Anton, P. A., Gombein, J. A., Shanahan, F., & Merrill, J. E. (1993). Production of interleukin-1 by microglia in response to substance P: Role for a non–classical NK-1 receptor. *Journal of Neuroimmunology, 42*(53), 60.

Martin, F. C., Charles, A. C., Sanderson, M. J., & Merrill, J. E. (1992). Substance P stimulates IL-1 production by astrocytes via intracellular calcium. *Brain Research, 599*, 13–18.

Martinez, C., Delgado, M., Gomariz, R. P., & Ganea, D. (1996). Vasoactive intestinal peptide and pituitary adenylate cyclase-activating polypeptide-38 inhibit IL-10 production in murine T lymphocytes. *Journal of Immunology, 156*(11), 4128–4136.

McCarron, R. M., Wang, l., Stanimirovic, D. B., & Spatz, M. (1995). Differential regulation of adhesion molecule expression by human cerebrovacular and umbilical vein endothelial cells. *Endothelium, 2*, 339–346.

McDonnell, G. V., McMillan, S. A., Douglas, J. P., Droogan, A. G., & Hawkins, S. A. (1998). Raised CSF levels of soluble adhesion molecules across the clinical spectrum of multiple sclerosis. *Journal of Neuroimmunology, 85*(2), 186–192.

McManus, C., Berman, J. W., Brett, F. M., Staunton, H., Farrell, M., & Brosnan, C. F. (1998). MCP-1, MCP-2 and MCP-3 expression in multiple sclerosis lesions: An immunohistochemical and in situ hybridization study. *Journal of Neuroimmunology, 86*(1), 20–29.

Meeusen, E. N., Premier, R. R., & Brandon, M. R. (1996). Tissue-specific migration of lymphocytes: A key role for Th1 and Th2 cells? *Immunology Today, 17*(9), 421–424.

Michelson, D., Stone, L., Galliven, E., Magiakou, M. A., Chrousos, G. P., Sternberg, E. M., & Gold, P. W. (1994). Multiple sclerosis is associated with alterations in hypothalamic-pituitary-adrenal axis function. *Journal of Clinical Endocrinology and Metabolism, 79*(3), 848–853.

Miyagami, M., Tsubokawa, T., Smith, B. H., & Kornblith, P. L. (1984). [Immunocytochemical localization of factor VIII-related antigen in blood vessels of the human central nervous system]. *NoTo Shinkei, 36*(8), 755–765. [Japanese]

Morikawa, Y., Tohya, K., Ishida, H., Matsuura, N., & Kakudo, K. (1995). Different migration patterns of antigen-presenting cells correlate with Th1/Th2-type responses in mice. *Immunology, 85*(4), 575–581.

Mossner, R., Fassbender, K., Kuhnen, J., Schwartz, A., & Hennerici, M. (1996). Vascular cell adhesion molecule—A new approach to detect endothelial cell activation in MS and encephalitis in vivo. *Acta Neurolologica Scandinavica, 93*(2–3), 118–122.

Nagy, Z., Peters, H., & Huttner, I. (1984). Fracture faces of cell junctions in cerebral endothelium during normal and hyperosmotic conditions. *Laboratory Investigation, 50*(3), 313–322.

Neuhaus, J., Risau, W., & Wolburg, H. (1991). Induction of blood–brain barrier characteristics in bovine brain endothelial cells by rat astroglial cells in transfilter coculture. *Annals of the New York Academy of Sciences, 633*, 578–580.

Nikcevich, K. M., Welsh, J., & Ting, J. P. Y. (1998). Molecular control of class II by CIITA in CNS endothelial cells. *Journal of Neuroimmunology, 90*, 23. [abstract]

Nisipeanu, P., & Korczyn, A. D. (1993). Psychological stress as risk factor for exacerbations in multiple sclerosis. *Neurology, 43*(7), 1311–1312.

Nozaki, K., Uemura, Y., Okamoto, S., Kikuchi, H., & Mizumo, N. (1990). Origins and distribution of cerebrovascular nerve fibers showing calcitonin gene–related peptide-like immunoreactivity in the major cerebral artery of the dog. *Journal of Comparative Neurology, 297*(2), 219–226.

Oldendorf, W. H., Cornford, M. E., & Brown, W. J. (1977). The large apparent work capability of the blood-brain barrier: A study of the mitochondrial content of capillary endothelial cells in brain and other tissues of the rat. *Annals of Neurology, 1*(5), 409–417.

Omari, K., & Dorovini-Zis, K. (1998). Expression of the costimulatory molecules B7 and LFA-3 by cerebral endothelium is important for effective T-cell proliferation. *Journal of Neuroimmunology, 90*, 23. [abstract]

Orlowski, M., & Meister, A. (1970). The gamma-glutamyl cycle: a possible transport system for amino acids. *Proceedings of the National Academy of Sciences, USA, 67*(3), 1248–1255.

Ozaka, T., Kayashima, K., & Fujimoto, S. (1997). Weibel-Palade bodies as a storage site of calcitonin gene-related peptide and endothelin-1 in blood vessels of the rat carotid body. *Anatomical Research, 247*(3), 388–394.

Palotie, A., Tryggvason, K., Peltonen, L., & Seppa, H. (1983). Components of subendothelial aorta basement membrane. Immunohistochemical localization and role in cell attachment. *Laboratory Investigation, 49*(3), 362–370.

Payan, D. G., Brewster, D. R., & Goetzl, E. J. (1983). Specific stimulation of human T lymphocytes by substance P. *Journal of Immunology, 131*(4), 1613–1615.

Payan, D. G., Brewster, D. R., & Goetzl, E. J. (1984). Stereospecific receptors for substance P on cultured human IM-9 lymphoblasts. *Journal of Immunology, 133*(6), 3260–3265.

Peters, A., Josephson, K., & Vincent, S. L. (1991). Effects of aging on the neuroglial cells and pericytes within area 17 of the rhesus monkey cerebral cortex. *Anatomical Research, 299*(3), 384–398.

Prat, A., Becher, B., Blain, M., & Antel, J. P. (1998). Induction of B7. 1 and B7. 2 co-stimulatory molecules on the surface of human brain endothelial cells. *Journal of Neuroimmunology, 90*, 24. [abstract]

Prat, A., Biernacki, K., Becher, B., & Antel, J. P. (2000). B7 expression and antigen presentation by human brain endothelial cells: Requirement of pro-inflammatory cytokines. *Journal of Neuropathology and Experimental Neurology, 59*, 129–136.

Prat, A., Weinrib, L., Becher, B., Duquette, P., Couture, R., & Antel, J. P. (1998). Expression of bradykinin B1 receptor on lymphocytes from MS patients. *Neurology, 50*, A151. [abstract]

Prat, A., Weinrib, L., Becher, B., Poirier, J., Duquette, P., Couture, R., & Antel, J. P. (1999). Bradykinin B1 receptor expression and function on T lymphocytes in active multiple sclerosis. *Neurology, 53*, 2087–2092.

Prineas, J. W. (1979). Multiple sclerosis: Presence of lymphatic capillaries and lymphoid tissue in the brain and spinal cord. *Science, 203*(4385), 1123–1125.

Reder, A. T. (1992). Regulation of production of adrenocorticotropin-like proteins in human mononuclear cells. *Immunology, 77*(3), 436–442.

Reder, A. T., Lowy, M. T., Meltzer, H. Y., & Antel, J. (1987). Dexamethasone suppression test abnormalities in multiple sclerosis: Relation to ACTH therapy. *Neurology, 37*(5), 849–853.

Reder, A. T., Makowiec, R. L., & Lowy, M. T. (1994). Adrenal size is increased in multiple sclerosis. *Archives of Neurology, 51*(2), 151–154.

Reder, A. T., Thapar, A., & Jensen, M. A. (1994). A reduction in serum glucocorticoids provokes experimental allergic encephalomyelitis: Implications for treatment of inflammatory brain disease. *Neurology, 44*(12), 2289–2294.

Reese, T. S. (1969). Junctions between intimately apposed cell membranes in the vertebrate brain. *Journal of Cell Biology, 40*(3), 648–677.

Reese, T. S., & Karnovsky, M. J. (1967). Fine structural localization of a blood-brain barrier to exogenous peroxidase. *Journal of Cell Biology, 34*(1), 207–217.

Rieckmann, P., Michel, U., Albrecht, M., Bruck, W., Wockel, L., & Felgenhauer, K. (1995). Cerebral endothelial cells are a major source for soluble intercellular adhesion molecule-1 in the human central nervous system. *Neuroscience Letters, 186*(1), 61–64.

Risau, W., Engelhardt, B., & Wekerle, H. (1990). Immune function of the blood-brain barrier: Incomplete presentation of protein (auto-) antigen by rat brain microvascular endothelium in vitro. *Journal of Cell Biology, 110*(5), 1757–1766.

Risau, W., Hallmenn, R., & Albrecht, U. (1986a). Differentiation dependent expression of proteins in brain endothelium during development of the blood-brain barrier. *Developmental Biology, 117*(2), 537–545.

Risau, W., Hallmenn, R., Albrecht, U., & Henke-Falhe, S. (1986b). Brain induces the expression of an early cell surface marker for blood-brain barrier-specific endothelium. *EMBO Journal, 5*(12), 3179–3183.

Robertson, P. L., Dubois, M., Bowman, P. D., & Goldstein, G. W. (1985). Angiogenesis in the developing rat brain: An in vivo and in vitro study. *Brain Research, 355*(2), 219–223.

Rubin, L. L., Barbu, K., Bard, F., Cannon, C., Hall, D. E., Horner, H., Janatpour, M., Liaw, C., Manning, K., & Morales, J. (1991). Differentiation of brain endothelial cells in cell culture. *Annals of the New York Academy Sciences, 633*, 420–425.

Schratzberger, P., Reinisch, N., & Prodinger, W. M. (1997). Differential chemotactic activities of sensory neuropeptides for human peripheral blood mononuclear cells. *Journal of Immunology, 158*, 3895–3901.

Selmaj, K. (1996). Pathophysiology of the blood-brain barrier. *Springer Seminars in Immunopathology, 18*, 57–73.

Seulberger, H., Lottspeich, F., & Risau, W. (1990). The inducible bloodbrain barrier specific molecule HT7 is a novel immunoglobulin-like cell surface glycoprotein. *EMBO Journal, 9*(7), 2151–2158.

Seulberger, H., Unger, C. M., & Risau, W. (1992). HT7, Neurothelin, Basigin, gp42 and OX-47—Many names for one developmentally regulated immuno-globulin-like surface glycoprotein on blood-brain barrier endothelium, epithelial tissue barriers and neurons. *Neuroscience Letters, 140*(1), 93–97.

Shivers, R. R., Edmonds, C. L., & Del Maestro, R. F. (1984). Microvascular permeability in induced astrocytomas and peritumor neuropil of rat brain. A high-voltage electron microscope-protein tracer study. *Acta Neuropathologica (Berlin), 64*(3), 192–202.

Smeltz, R. B., & Swanborg, R. H. (1998). Concordance and contradiction concerning cytokines and chemokines in experimental demyelinating disease. *Journal of Neuroscience Research, 51*(2), 147–153. [review]

Sobel, R. A., Blanchette, B. W., Bhan, A. K., & Colvin, R. B. (1984). The immunopathology of experimental allergic encephalomyelitis. II. Endothelial cell Ia increases prior to inflammatory cell infiltration. *Journal of Immunology, 132*(5), 2402–2407.

Stanimirovic, D., Shapiro, A., Wong, J., Hutchison, J., & Durkin, J. (1997). The induction of ICAM-1 in human cerebromicrovascular endothelial cells (HCEC) by ischemia-like conditions promotes enhanced neutrophil/HCEC adhesion. *Journal of Neuroimmunology, 76*(1–2), 193–205.

Stanimirovic, D. B., Ball, R., & Durkin, J. P. (1995). Evidence for the role of protein kinase C in astrocyte-induced proliferation of rat cerebromicrovascular endothelial cells. *Neuroscience Letters, 197*(3), 219–222.

Stins, M. F., Gilles, F., & Kim, K. S. (1997). Selective expression of adhesion molecules on human brain microvascular endothelial cells. *Journal of Neuroimmunology, 76*(1–2), 81–90.

Stuve, O., Dooley, N. P., Uhm, J. H., Antel, J., Francis, G. S., Williams, G., & Yong, V. W. (1996). Interferon beta-1b decreases the migration of T lymphocytes in vitro: Effects on matrix metalloproteinase-9. *Annals of Neurology, 40*(6), 853–863.

Tao-Cheng, J. H., & Brightman, M. W. (1988). Development of membrane interactions between brain endothelial cells and astrocytes in vitro. *International Journal of Developmental Neuroscience, 6*(1), 25–37.

Thorin, E., Shatos, M. A., Shreeve, S. M., Walters, C. L., & Bevan, J. A. (1997). Human vascular endothelium heterogeneity. A comparative study of cerebral and peripheral cultured vascular endothelial cells. *Stroke, 28*(2), 375–381.

Verbeek, M. M., Westphal, J. R., Ruiter, D. J., & de Waal, R. M. (1995). T lymphocyte adhesion to human brain pericytes is mediated via very late antigen-4/vascular cell adhesion molecule-1 interactions. *Journal of Immunology, 154*(11), 5876–5884.

Wang, H. Y., Xin, Z., Tang, H., & Ganea, D. (1996). Vasoactive intestinal polypeptide inhibits IL-4 production in murine T cells by a post–transcriptional mechanism. *Journal of Immunology, 156*(9), 3243–3253.

Warren, S., Greenhill, S., & Warren, K. G. (1982). Emotional stress and the development of multiple sclerosis:Case–control evidence of a relationship. *Journal of Chronic Diseases, 35*(11), 821–831.

Weber, T., Seitz, R. J., Liebert, U. G., Gallasch, E., & Wechsler, W. (1985). Affinity cytochemistry of vascular endothelia in brain tumors by biotinylated Ulex europaeus type I lectin (UEA I). *Acta Neuropathologica (Berlin), 67*(1–2), 128–135.

Whitacre, C. C., Dowdell, K., & Griffin, A. C. (1998). Neuroendocrine influences on experimental autoimmune encephalomyelitis. *Annals of the New York Academy of Sciences, 840*(705), 716.

Wong, D., & Dorovini-Zis, K. (1992). Upregulation of intercellular adhesion molecule-1 (ICAM-1) expression in primary cultures of human brain microvessel endothelial cells by cytokines and lipopolysaccharide. *Journal of Neuroimmunology, 39*(1–2), 11–21.

Wong, D., & Dorovini-Zis, K. (1995). Expression of vascular cell adhesion molecule-1 (VCAM-1) by human brain microvessel endothelial cells in primary culture. *Microvascular Research, 49*(3), 325–339.

Xu, J., Qu, Z. X., Moore, S. A., Hsu, C. Y., & Hogan, E. L. (1992). Receptor-linked hydrolysis of phosphoinositides and production of prostacyclin in cerebral endothelial cells. *Journal of Neurochemistry, 58*(5), 1930–1935.

Yong, V. W., Krekosky, C. A., Forsyth, P. A., Bell, R., & Edwards, D. R. (1998). Matrix metalloproteinases and diseases of the CNS. *Trends in Neuroscience, 21*(2), 75–80.

Zach, O., Bauer, H. C., Richter, K., Webersinke, G., Tontsch, S., & Bauer, H. (1997). Expression of a chemotactic cytokine (MCP-1) in cerebral capillary endothelial cells in vitro. *Endothelium, 5*(3), 143–153.

# 53

# The Neuroendocrine System and Rheumatoid Arthritis: Focus on the Hypothalamo-Pituitary-Adrenal Axis

SOPHIE LIGIER, ESTHER M. STERNBERG

## I. INTRODUCTION

Rheumatoid arthritis (RA) is a chronic inflammatory disease affecting an estimated 1% of the American population (Lawrence et al., 1998). Its peak incidence rate is in the middle-aged subgroup, with a female to male ratio of approximately 2.5:1. Although it usually initially presents as a symmetrical polyarticular synovitis with prominent hand involvement, RA has multiple potential systemic manifestations (Klippel & Dieppe, 1997). Fever, weight loss, and cachexia can be part of the first symptoms. Articular and bony destruction and chronic pain result in progressive loss of function, though cartilage damage and subchondral erosions can be found fairly early on in the course of the illness. Vasculitis, neutropenia, splenomegaly, pulmonary fibrosis, amyloidosis, and

scleromalacia are some of the disease's complications which tend to occur in patients with long-standing disease. Laboratory testing usually reveals nonspecific evidence of ongoing inflammatory activity (elevated sedimentation rate and C-reactive protein) and indices of chronic disease (normochromic normocytic anemia). Rheumatoid factor autoantibodies directed against the Fc portion of IgG molecules were detected in approximately 70% of patients.

The pathophysiology of RA remains unclear. Although no putative antigenic trigger has clearly been identified, it is regarded as a T-cell-driven autoimmune process associated with the production of autoantibodies. In addition to the rheumatoid factor, anti-collagen antibodies have been identified (Terato, DeArmey, Ye, Griffiths, & Cremer, 1996). Moreover, RA is frequently accompanied by a variety of other known autoimmune or autoimmune-associated disorders (Sjögren's syndrome, Raynaud's phenomenon, systemic lupus erythematosus, and Hashimoto's thyroiditis) that are themselves characterized by autoantibody production. This suggests a generalized autoimmune susceptibility in affected individuals. Also regarded as supporting an autoimmune etiology for RA is the fact that treatment regimens usually include drugs that directly target the immune system (Barrera, Boerbooms, van de Putte, & van der Meer, 1996). Agents such as low-dose methotrexate have been studied for their impact on

**449**

cytokine production and their ability to modulate the immune response. Others are regarded as being more nonspecific immunosuppressors (azathioprine, cyclophosphamide). More recently, biologic therapies such as tumor necrosis factor-$\alpha$ (TNF-$\alpha$) antagonists (Moreland et al., 1997) have shown great promise in altering the natural disease course by targeting specific steps of the immune effector cascade. Low-dose corticosteroids are also widely used in the treatment of RA, both as immunosuppressors and as immunomodulators. Finally, certain class II DR molecules have been strongly linked to poor disease prognosis, reinforcing the idea that the initiating events of the disease involve immune dysregulation (Klippel & Dieppe, 1997). It should be remembered that both genetic and environmental factors are likely to play a role in the pathogenesis of RA, as monozygotic twin studies show at best a 15% disease concordance rate (Ollier & MacGregor, 1995).

The potential role of disturbances in endogenous glucocorticoid secretion in the pathogenesis of RA has been questioned almost ever since exogenous corticosteroid administration was first discovered to have a dramatic effect on disease symptoms in the 1940s (Hench, Kendall, Slocumb, & Polley, 1949). One of the defining features of RA is the circadian rhythm of its symptoms, with pain and stiffness typically worse at night and in the early morning (Harkness et al., 1982). This worsening occurs a few hours after plasma cortisol levels are at their lowest. Exacerbation of the illness has also been noted in the setting of the administration of the metyrapone test (Pal, 1970) (Saldanha, Tougas, & Grace, 1986), which decreases cortisol production by blocking 11$\beta$-hydroxylase. Interestingly, pan-hypopituitarism has been linked to the development of arthritis (Sugar, 1953), and there are reports of autoimmune diseases such as thyroiditis developing in patients with Cushing's disease shortly after the removal of pituitary adenomas and consequent drop in circulating cortisol levels (Takasu, Ohara, Yamada, & Komiya, 1993). In response to these observations, multiple studies have subsequently attempted to characterize corticosteroid production in RA patients and to examine more comprehensively the hypothalamo-pituitary-adrenal (HPA) axis response. As we will see, perhaps some of the more compelling evidence supporting the importance of the neuroendocrine system in RA comes from animal models of chronic arthritis, where inflammatory susceptibility has been linked to a deficient HPA axis response.

Our discussion will focus on findings linking the HPA axis to the inflammatory processes in RA, with emphasis on both animal models of erosive arthritis and studies in humans. We will only briefly touch upon the potential role of the hypothalamo-pituitary-gonadal axis in RA, as this is comprehensively addressed elsewhere in this volume. We will attempt to put these findings in perspective with respect to the complex multifactorial nature of this disease. Evidence supporting a role for the neuroendocrine system in the development and course of rheumatoid arthritis is increasing, indicating that it may constitute one more piece of the puzzle in understanding this disease.

Before addressing more specifically the relationship between RA and the neuroendocrine system, we will briefly review some basic notions about neural–immune interactions.

## II. GENERAL CONCEPTS OF NEURAL–IMMUNE INTERACTIONS

### A. Defining Stress and the Stress Response

Part of the difficulty with the notion that stress might contribute to disease arises from the vague definition that is often associated with the word "stress." The popular definition, and early studies, often did not distinguish between the stressful stimulus and the organism's physiological response to that stimulus. It is now known that a range of physical or psychological or immune/inflammatory stimuli can activate a series of neuroendocrine and neuronal responses which produce a characteristic set of physiological responses (for review, see (Chrousos & Gold, 1992)). These include activation of the HPA axis and of the sympathetic nervous system. Sympathetic nervous system activation leads to increased heart rate, muscle blood flow, and sweating. Activation of central corticotropin-releasing hormone (CRH) and of the locus coeruleus produce behavioral effects of increased focused attention. Together these early behavioral and physiological responses comprise the fight-or-flight response.

The HPA axis becomes rapidly activated, in as short a time as 3–5 min, after exposure of the organism to a range of stressors, including physical (exercise), chemical, psychological (performance tasks), thermal and infectious/immune stimuli. When the neuroendocrine stress response is activated, the hypothalamus secretes CRH and arginine vasopressin (AVP). These neuropeptides stimulate the pituitary gland to secrete corticotropin (ACTH) which triggers glucocorticoid production by the adrenal glands (see

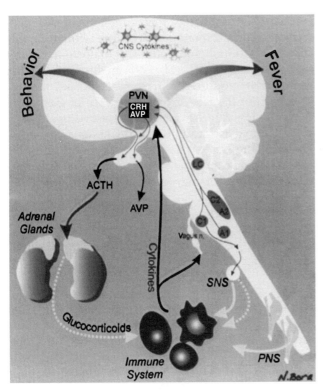

**FIGURE 1** Neural–immune interactions. Adapted with permission from Sternberg, E. M. (1997). Neural–immune interactions in health and disease. *Journal of Clinical Investigation, 100*(11), 2641–2647. See text for details.

Figure 1). Glucocorticoids feed back and suppress this HPA axis cascade at every level.

In addition to the HPA axis, stressful stimuli activate brain-stem adrenergic pathways and the sympathetic nervous system outflow from the brain stem to the periphery. Several neuronal pathways connect the hypothalamus to noradrenergic areas in the brain stem, such as the locus coeruleus and A2 and C2 regions (Sawchenko et al., 1996). Thus activation of hypothalamic CRH can stimulate these noradrenergic regions and sympathetic outflow to the periphery. In turn, adrenergic outflow from the brain stem can activate the hypothalamus to secrete CRH.

## B. Interactions between the Immune and Neuroendocrine Systems: Bidirectional Communication Pathways

### 1. Inflammatory Stress: The HPA Axis Response to Peripheral Immune System Activation

There are many mechanisms by which the immune and central nervous system (CNS) communicate. Interruptions or perturbations at a variety of levels

in these pathways produce different effects on expression and susceptibility to inflammatory and autoimmune disease (for review, see Sternberg (1997), Sternberg, Chrousos, Wilder, & Gold (1992), Chrousos (1995)). Peripheral inflammation results in the production of a variety of inflammatory mediators including cytokines, which can signal the brain via several routes. Cytokines can cross the blood-brain barrier at leaky points (the circumventricular organs) or via specific active transport mechanisms (Banks & Kastin, 1997). One of the most important mechanisms by which peripheral cytokines signal the brain is through second messenger systems, such as the nitric oxide synthase (NOS)/nitric oxide (NO) and the cyclooxygenase/prostaglandin system (Karanth, Lyson, & McCann, 1993). Inflammatory stimuli can also induce the CNS stress response through afferent peripheral neural signaling. Thus, cytokines from the peritoneum can cause early rapid activation of the nucleus of the tractus solitarius (NTS) in the brain stem (Bluthe et al., 1994; Watkins et al., 1995) via the vagus nerve. RA is characterized by increased local synovial and systemic levels of proinflammatory cytokines which are directly involved in the disease's pathophysiology (Brennan, Maini, & Feldmann, 1995). Such increased cytokine production plays a key role in neuroendocrine activation pathways in this chronic inflammatory disease.

### 2. CNS Stress Response Effects on the Immune Response: the HPA Axis and Peripheral Nervous System Activation

The nervous system in turn regulates the immune system systemically, regionally, and locally (Sternberg, 1997). Systemically the HPA axis hormonal response plays immunosuppressive and immunomodulatory roles. A large part of the impact of the neuroendocrine stress response on the immune system is mediated through the effects of glucocorticoids on both acute phase innate and later phase specific immunity.

Exogenous corticosteroids have been used for several decades in humans to suppress overactive immune responses, and they are clearly potent agents. However, although early studies of glucocorticoids' anti-inflammatory actions were interpreted as pharmacological rather than physiological, more recent studies indicate that more physiological concentrations of glucocorticoids play an important role in keeping the immune system in check (McEwen et al., 1997). It is important to remember that glucocorticoids are not only anti-inflammatory and immunosuppressive agents; part of their actions are as immunomodulators. At lower concentrations, they cause a shift in immune responses, with relatively greater suppression of the proinflammatory cytokines TNF-$\alpha$, interleukin (IL)-1 (DeRijk et al., 1997; DeRijk, Petrides, Deuster, Gold, & Sternberg, 1996) and less suppression of the anti-inflammatory cytokine IL-10 (Elenkov, Papanicolaou, Wilder, & Chrousos, 1996). Thus glucocorticoids cause a shift from a T helper 1 (Th1) to a T helper 2 (Th2) type response, and favor humoral over cellular immune response patterns. In large concentrations, the ultimate effect of HPA axis suppression of immune responses through adrenal glucocorticoids is to suppress immune/inflammatory responses to stimulus-appropriate levels and prevent the immune response from continuing unchecked.

Activation of the stress response also results in increased neural output to peripheral tissues. Both the sympathetic and peripheral nervous systems play a role in regulating the immune response. The sympathetic nervous system plays an important role in modulating inflammatory responses through regional innervation of immune organs including the spleen, thymus, and lymph nodes (Felten & Felten, 1991). In animal studies, sympathetic denervation can have different effects on regional inflammation depending on the site and mode of denervation (Madden, Felten, Felten, Hardy, & Livnat, 1994a; Madden et al., 1994b). Natural sympathetic denervation of the spleen that occurs with aging may play a role in some of the immunosuppression seen in aging (Madden, Thyagarajan, & Felten, 1998). Recent studies have shown that reconstitution of splenic innervation with treatment with drugs such as deprenyl are associated with reconstitution of splenic immune cell responsiveness in aged or denervated animals (ThyagaRajan, Felten, & Felten, 1998).

At sites of peripheral inflammation, peripheral nerves regulate local inflammatory responses through release of neuropeptides that are largely proinflammatory. Previous studies have also shown that both peripheral sympathetic noradrenergic (NA) nerves and substance P-containing nerves play a role in joint inflammation (Goetzl, Chernov, Renold, & Payan, 1985). The peripheral nervous system affects inflammation through neuropeptides, such as substance P (SP) or vasoactive intestinal polypeptide (VIP). These may be released from nerve endings or synapses at sites of inflammation, or they can be synthesized and released by immune cells depending on the type of inflammation involved. Some peripheral neuropeptides can be pro- or anti-inflammatory, depending on the component and time point of inflammation measured. For example, peripheral CRH is present in higher concentrations in inflamed joints in Lewis

compared to Fischer rats; it is proinflammatory and its immunoneutralization is associated with decreased cellular infiltration and volume of exudate in chronic inflammation (Karalis et al., 1991). In this context, while central CRH suppresses immune responses through activation of the HPA axis and release of glucocorticoids, peripheral CRH released at nerve terminals is proinflammatory. Additionally, sympathetic postganglionic neurons are also key in regulating the fluid extravasation component of the early inflammatory response (Green, Janig, & Levine, 1997; Green et al., 1998).

### 3. Relationship between the Nature of the Stressor and the HPA Axis Response: Psychological versus Physical Stress, Acute versus Chronic Stress

The components of the stress response achieved will vary with the type of the stimulus that is used. Stressors can be categorized as being primarily physical in nature (illness, inflammation, exercise) or psychological (performance tasks). Each stressor may yield a different HPA axis activation pattern. The response to psychological stressors appears to be particularly dependent on the individual's critical perception of the event (Ehlert & Straub, 1998). Additionally, even within the category of primarily physical stressors, the HPA axis response differs depending on the type of stressor used. Thus, intermittent electrical footshock in rats will not activate the same stress-responsive neurotransmitter pathways within the brain as a systemic cytokine (IL-1) challenge (Li, Ericsson, & Sawchenko, 1996). With regards to inflammatory stressors, the nature of the immune challenge also determines the degree of the HPA axis response (Stenzel-Poore, Vale, & Rivier, 1993).

The duration of the stressful stimulus is also an important qualitative and quantitative determinant of the elicited HPA axis response. When studying the HPA axis in chronic inflammatory conditions such as RA or erosive arthritis in animal models, it is critical to consider the neuroendocrine consequences of any long-standing peripheral immune activation process. Chronic stressor stimulation results in readjustments of the neurotransmitter and neuroendocrine responses that are activated during acute stress. These physiological changes complicate data interpretation and make it difficult to establish a causal relationship between HPA axis hyporeactivity and predisposition to inflammatory disease in the context of already established chronic inflammation. Any observed differences between affected and diseased subjects may be the direct reflection of the illness. Harbuz et al.

have shown that the control of ACTH secretion is shifted from CRH to AVP (Chowdrey et al., 1995; Harbuz, Conde, Marti, Lightman, & Jessop, 1997), but that this is not a uniform pattern throughout all rat species (Harbuz et al., 1992). This shift may be related to differential sensitivity of CRH and AVP secretion to negative feedback by corticosterone (Makino, Smith, & Gold, 1995). In the setting of repeated acute stress, hypothalamic paraventricular nucleus gluco-corticoid receptor (GR) mRNA decreases, which could potentially explain the shift in the control of ACTH secretion from CRH to AVP. CRH and AVP appear to have a synergistic action as ACTH secretagogues, AVP significantly potentiating the stimulatory action of CRH on ACTH production. Chronic conditions in humans are also associated with this shift in ACTH production control from CRH to AVP. Patients with multiple sclerosis, with significant baseline hypercortisolemia, have been found to have a blunted ACTH response to AVP with normal ACTH response to CRH. Of note, subjects in this study did not exhibit indication of increased peripheral inflammation, as plasma sedimentation rates, IL-6, and IL-1$\beta$ levels were not increased (Michelson et al., 1994).

Thus the neuroendocrine response pattern changes seen in chronic stress may represent central adaptation to a continuous exposure. It is also possible that the peripheral signaling to the CNS evolves during the course of chronic inflammation and that the resulting HPA axis response will also be modified. Indeed, it has been noted that peripheral blood mononuclear cells from patients with early versus chronic RA will have different patterns of cytokine secretion (Kanik et al., 1998).

In addition to a shift in the stress hormonal response pattern, there is a dampening of the response to acute stimulation in animals with chronic inflammation (Shanks et al., 1998) which varies with the type of acute stressor studied. Aguilera et al. (Aguilera, Jessop, Harbuz, Kiss, & Lightman, 1997) have examined the changes in hypothalamic CRH mRNA expression in response to acute restraint stress in rats developing adjuvant arthritis. Their results showed that this response changes between days 7 and 14, when the arthritis begins to appear: while immobilization produced a rise in CRH mRNA at 7 days postinjection, it failed to do so 14 days postinjection. However, this blunted response was not observed when the nature of the acute stressor was inflammatory (Harbuz et al., 1997). Conversely, it is interesting that a preexisting stressor may dampen the inflammatory response to an immune challenge. Thus the severity of adjuvant arthritis in previously

bile-duct-resected cholestatic Sprague–Dawley rats is decreased compared to that seen in sham operated rats (Swain & Maric, 1994), and this is associated with increased plasma free corticosterone levels. Similarly, repeated psychological stress is associated with a decreased severity in collagen-induced arthritis in female Lewis (LEW/N) rats (Miller, Rapier, Holtsclaw, & Turner, 1995).

## III. ANIMAL MODELS OF HPA AXIS HYPOFUNCTION AND INFLAMMATORY DISEASES

### A. Lewis and Fischer Rats: Models of Resistance and Susceptibility to Chronic Erosive Arthritis

Lewis (LEW/N) and Fischer (F344/N) rats are major histocompatible inbred rat strains differing at a single minor histocompatibility locus, the Neu-1 locus. These strains have been repeatedly used to study a variety of inflammatory disorders. LEW/N rats have been recognized as being particularly susceptible to a variety of inflammatory conditions which vary depending on the antigenic stimulus to which they are exposed (Sternberg, 1997). It has made them an ideal animal model to study diseases categorized as being autoimmune in nature, such as autoimmune thyroiditis and experimental allergic encephalomyelitis (EAE). Female Lewis (LEW/N) rats develop an arthritis in response to group A streptococcal cell wall peptidoglycan polysaccharide (SCW) which mimics human RA clinically, radiologically, and histologically (Sternberg et al., 1989a). Inflammation-resistant F344/N rats represent the other end of the inflammatory phenotype spectrum, developing little pathology with exposure to inflammatory triggers (Sternberg et al., 1989a). Outbred Harlan Sprague–Dawley (HSD) rats exhibit an inflammatory susceptibility intermediate to that of the LEW/N and F344/N rats (Sternberg et al., 1989a).

The mechanisms underlying this differential inflammatory susceptibility are strongly linked to the HPA axis activation response. Importantly, these mechanisms also appear to be particularly important in the control of early inflammation, as female athymic LEW/N rats will still develop the acute response to SCW administration but do not progress to chronic arthritis (Wilder, Allen, & Hansen, 1987). We examined the function of the HPA axis and its ability to modulate the development of the inflammatory response in LEW/N and F344/N rats

(Sternberg et al., 1989a,b). These studies indicated that, in contrast to F344/N rats, LEW/N rats had markedly impaired plasma ACTH and corticosterone responses to SCW, recombinant human IL-1α, the serotonin agonist quipazine, and synthetic rat/human CRH. LEW/N rats also had smaller adrenal glands and larger thymuses than F344/N rats. Replacement doses of dexamethasone decreased the severity of LEW/N rats' SCW-induced arthritis. Conversely, treatment of F344/N rats with the glucocorticoid receptor antagonist RU 486 or the serotonin antagonist LY53857 was associated with development of severe inflammatory disease, including arthritis, in response to SCW. These findings support the concept that susceptibility of LEW/N rats to SCW arthritis is related to defective HPA axis responsiveness to inflammatory and other stress mediators, and that resistance of F344/N rats to SCW arthritis is regulated by an intact HPA axis–immune system feedback loop.

The key role of the HPA axis in controlling inflammation is further supported by the demonstration of axis hypofunction in other species and strains susceptible to autoimmune diseases such as obese strain chickens (Schauenstein et al., 1987), which spontaneously develop thyroiditis, and lupus-prone MRL/MP-*lpr* and NZB/NZW mice (Lechner et al., 1996).

## B. Early Nonspecific Inflammation and Neuroendocrine Activation

Two key points can be made based on the impact of acute dexamethasone administration in abrogating the chronic arthritic process in animals with a deficient stress response. First, it underscores the role of the HPA axis and of corticosteroids in controlling the acute nonspecific innate immune response to antigenic challenge. Second, it suggests that attenuation of the early inflammatory response may significantly reduce the risk of progression to a chronic illness. These findings have relevance to RA at two levels. From the point of view of disease pathophysiology, it suggests that a hypoactive HPA stress response to acute antigenic exposure is one of the many factors predisposing subjects to the development of a chronic inflammatory process. It also underscores the potential importance of the role of corticosteroids in disease treatment, particularly early in the illness. In order to better understand the impact of neuroendocrine functional abnormalities on the development of chronic inflammation, it is thus important to review the acute inflammatory response and its relationship with the HPA axis.

### 1. The Acute Inflammatory Response: A Brief Review

The early innate immune response occurs quickly after tissue injury and contact with foreign antigen. Its two main components are vascular and cellular, both involving a number of mediators. The regulatory mechanisms controlling early inflammation include local factors which, beyond their direct pro- and anti-inflammatory roles, can also activate the neuroendocrine system. In turn, the HPA axis and peripheral neural activation play key roles in the regulation of the early inflammatory response.

The initial physiological response to a peripheral inflammatory trigger is one of vasoconstriction. It is followed by vasodilation and increased vessel wall permeability, responsible for the locally increased blood flow and tissue swelling (calor and turgor), and redness (rubor) clinically observable at the sight of injury (Klippel & Dieppe, 1997). Local release of inflammatory mediators, including neuropeptides such as substance P and CRH, activates neural fibers mediating painful stimuli (dolor). Cellular infiltration follows the initial vascular changes and is at first primarily composed of polymorphonuclear cells, with later recruitment of macrophages, lymphocytes, and plasma cells.

### 2. Subcutaneous Carrageenan: A Model of Nonspecific Acute Inflammation

Multiple mediators are involved in inflammation. One of the most useful experimental models used to study innate immunity and its principal players is the injection of carrageenan into into rats, whether this is in the paw, pleura, or into a subcutaneous air pouch. Carrageenan (or carrageenin) is a polysaccharide derived from the alga *Chondrus crispus* (Di Rosa, 1972), which has been used as an activator of the acute nonspecific inflammatory response in animal models, primarily in rats but also in mice. It produces a protein-rich exudate containing mostly polymorphonuclear cells. Other substances such as dextrans (Dawson, Sedgwick, Edwards, & Lees, 1991; Lo, Almeida & Beaven, 1982), turpentine (Di Rosa, Giroud, & Willoughby, 1971), and zymosan (Dawson et al., 1991) have been most widely used to trigger and study innate immune reactions. However, because of the intensity of the response and its suppression by nonsteroidal anti-inflammatory drugs (NSAIDs) (Almeida, Bayer, Horakova, & Beaven, 1980; Lo, Almeida, & Beaven, 1984; Lo et al., 1982), carrageenan has been widely used to study the relative potencies of anti-inflammatory agents. Cell content, vascular permeability, and exudate volume are the main parameters used to quantitate this inflammatory response.

While the vascular component of this inflammatory response is likely closely linked to the cellular infiltration of polymorphonuclear cells, it has been noted that the time course and both quantitative and qualitative characteristics of an inflammatory exudate will depend on the irritant used (Dawson et al., 1991) (Lo et al., 1982). Each of these characteristics may be under the control of different factors. It is likely that, depending on the mediators released peripherally, the activation response of the HPA axis will be different.

The reaction to subcutaneous injection of carrageenan in the paw occurs quickly, and edema can be detected within a few hours (Di Rosa, 1972). Infiltration by polymorphonuclear cells accompanies the fluid extravasation, lagging slightly behind. Both appear to occur maximally by 6 h following the injection. The response can be divided into separate phases, based on the different mediators involved. Several mediators have been studied in this inflammatory model, all known to be involved in the early nonspecific inflammatory response. Not surprisingly, histamine (Hirasawa, Watanabe, Mue, Tsurufuji, & Ohuchi, 1991; Di Rosa, 1972), bradykinin, prostaglandins, elements of the complement cascade (Di Rosa, 1972), NO (Salvemini et al., 1995, 1996b; Wei et al.,

1995), and IL-8 (Nakagawa et al., 1992) have all been implicated as key players (see Table I). Histamine, 5-hydroxytryptamine (5-HT), and bradykinin appear to be important primarily in the first few hours of the process, while prostaglandins have a key role between 3 and 6 h after injection of carrageenan (Di Rosa, 1972; Di Rosa et al., 1971). Complement fragments (Di Rosa et al., 1971) and IL-8 (Nakagawa et al., 1992) are important chemotactic factors during the first 6–8 h of acute inflammation.

Nitric oxide appears increasingly to be critical in innate immunity. Thus, mice lacking the gene for the inducible form of nitric oxide synthetase (iNOS) show a decreased response to carrageenan injection (Wei et al., 1995). NO has definite proinflammatory actions as a vasodilator and as an activator of prostaglandin E2 (PGE2). Additionally, it can result in cellular damage by combining with superoxide to produce peroxynitrite, a strong oxidizing molecule (Beckman & Koppenol, 1996). Using both the subcutaneous and the paw carrageenan injection approaches, Salvemini et al. have investigated the role of nitric oxide as a potential final common mediator in the inflammatory response (Salvemini et al., 1995; 1996a, b). The constitutive form of nitric oxide synthetase (cNOS) appears to be important very early on (the first hour post-

**TABLE I   Mediators of the Early Inflammatory Response**

| | Effect on the inflammatory process | Predicted effect of glucocorticoids on mediator activity |
|---|---|---|
| LTB4 | —Increased vascular permeability<br>—Increases IL-1 production | Decrease |
| Prostaglandins | —Increased vascular permeability<br>—Increased white blood cell chemotaxis | Decrease |
| Bradykinin | —Increased vascular permeability | Decrease |
| C5a | —Increases white blood cell chemotaxis<br>—Increased vascular permeability | No effect |
| Nitric oxide | —Increased vascular permeability | Decrease |
| IL-8 | —Increased white blood cell chemotaxis<br>—Adhesion molecule upregulation<br>—Increased white blood cell oxygen respiratory burst | Decrease (?)[a] |
| IL-6 | —Lymphocyte activation<br>—Increased antibody production<br>—Systemic effects: fever, induction of acute phase protein production | Decrease (?)[a] |
| IL-1 | —Vascular endothelium activation with adhesion molecule upregulation<br>—Lymphocyte activation<br>—Increases IL-6 | Decrease (?)[a] |
| TNF-$\alpha$ | —Increased vascular permeability<br>—Increased IL-1 and IL-6 production<br>—Increased white blood cell oxygen respiratory burst<br>—Adhesion molecule induction<br>—Systemic effects: fever, induction of acute phase protein production | Decrease (?)[a] |

[a]Based on ex vivo effects of dexamethasone on lipopolysaccharide-stimulated white blood cell cytokine production.

injection), while the inducible form of nitric oxide synthase (iNOS) is responsible for the increased production of NO between 4 and 10 h after carrageenan challenge (Salvemini et al., 1996b). Importantly, iNOS is suppressed by glucocorticoids (Radomski, Palmer & Moncada, 1990).

Table I provides a nonexhaustive list of mediators involved in the early inflammatory response. In addition to the ones discussed above are the major proinflammatory cytokines: IL-1, IL-6, and TNF-$\alpha$. While they play a role in the chronic immune response and can be specific treatment targets in RA (Moreland et al., 1997), they also act synergistically to create the acute-phase response. Locally, TNF-$\alpha$ increases vascular permeability. IL-1 and IL-6 can both be measured early on in inflammatory pleural exudate following carrageenan injection (Utsunomiya, Nagai, & Oh-ishi, 1991). Interestingly, NOS inhibitors can decrease the production of IL-1, IL-6, IL-2, and interferon-$\gamma$ (IFN-$\gamma$) in the local paw inflammation response to carrageenan, while an increase in IL-10 is noted (Ianaro, O'Donnell, Di Rosa, & Liew, 1994). There again, NO appears to be a key mediator, acting to potentially increase the production of inflammatory cytokines and to decrease that of the anti-inflammatory IL-10.

### 3. Impact of the Peripheral Nervous System on Acute Inflammation

The interactions between the nervous system and immunity are discussed extensively elsewhere in this textbook. While efferent neural output clearly affects immune tissue function and the specific immune response, it also has a definite role in modulating the innate immune response, and in particular the accumulation of fluid at the site of inflammation. Levine and his co-workers have investigated the mechanisms by which bradykinin causes plasma extravasation in rats. They have shown that its actions are partially dependent on the presence of postganglionic sympathetic neuron terminals (SPGN) (Green et al., 1998; Miao, Janig, & Levine, 1996b), but that this effect does not require the actual transmission of electrical activity. Corticosteroids inhibit the SPGN-dependent actions of bradykinin on fluid accumulation (Green et al., 1997), illustrating how activation of the HPA axis and the resulting levels of circulating corticosteroid can indirectly decrease inflammation by modulating the effects of the peripheral nervous system. In support of this closely linked relationship, they studied the inhibitory actions of intrathecal nicotine on bradykinin-induced synovial plasma extravasation (Miao, Janig, Green, & Levine, 1996a);

hypophysectomy and glucocorticoid blockade greatly reduced the beneficial effects of nicotine on volume accumulation.

### 4. Impact of Corticosteroids on the Early Inflammatory Response: Surgical and Pharmacological Manipulations of the HPA Axis

In vivo, the severity of the inflammatory response has repeatedly been found to be downregulated by circulating corticosteroids. Corticosteroids affect both the cellular and the vascular components of innate immunity by altering the production of inflammatory mediators, and potentially by acting directly on endothelial cells to modify vessel permeability (Schleimer, 1993). Thus the potency of topical corticosteroids is often assessed based on their blanching or vasoconstritive effect (Smith, 1995), which can be blocked by the glucocorticoid receptor antagonist RU 486 (Gaillard, Poffet, Riondel, & Saurat, 1985). The impact of corticosteroids on inflammatory mediators are reflected by changes in both the volume of fluid accumulation and in the cellular infiltration. The production of all the inflammatory factors discussed above has been found to be decreased by glucocorticoids to varying degrees (see Table I), underscoring the neuroendocrine system's role in the early inflammatory response (DeRijk et al., 1996, 1997; Green et al., 1997; Laue et al., 1988; Miyamasu et al., 1998; Radomski et al., 1990; Samuelsson, 1987; van der Poll & Lowry, 1997).

It would thus not be surprising to find an increased inflammatory susceptibility in animals with a blunted HPA axis activation response to stress and decreased corticosterone production. Simple association between HPA axis hyporesponsiveness and susceptibility to inflammatory disease does not, however, prove a cause and effect relationship between the endocrine and inflammatory disease traits. Evidence that such blunted neuroendocrine responses are causally related to inflammatory susceptibility is derived from manipulations of the HPA in animal models. Interruptions of the HPA axis at various levels, surgically through adrenalectomy or hypophysectomy or pharmacologically with agents such RU486 or the serotonin (5-HT2) receptor antagonist LY53857, render animal strains otherwise resistant to inflammation, so highly susceptible that early mortality is greatly increased following exposure to infectious antigen. Studies in hypophysectomized rats suggest that this mortality may be secondary to septic shock, as occurs in hypophysectomized rats which develop septic shock after exposure to salmonella (Edwards, Yunger, Lorence, Dantzer, & Kelley,

1991). Surviving animals develop autoimmune disease according to the proinflammatory stimulus to which they were exposed, such as EAE (MacPhee, Antoni, & Mason, 1989) after myelin basic protein, or arthritis after exposure to SCW (Sternberg et al., 1989a). These studies suggest that the HPA axis plays a physiologic role in regulating the immune system through the anti-inflammatory and immunosuppressive effects of the glucocorticoids.

It is thus not surprising that adrenalectomized rats will develop a greater volume of a more cellular exudate in response to intrapleural carrageenan injection and will have increased fluid eicosanoid levels (Flower, Parente, Persico, & Salmon, 1986). F344/N rats, as discussed previously, show enhanced HPA axis activation and corticosterone production in response to stress when compared to LEW/N and to a lesser degree Sprague–Dawley rats. Just as they are resistant to the development of chronic erosive arthritis, F344/N rats are also resistant to the development of acute inflammation when compared to LEW/N rats. When examined at 7 h after injection of carrageenan into a subcutaneous air pouch, 6-week-old female LEW/N rats develop exudates with a volume and cellular content that is statistically significantly less than the F344/N strain (Karalis, Crofford, Wilder, & Chrousos, 1995). Similarly, we have found differences between these two rat strains in both cell content and volume. These differences are most striking at 10 days post-injection (Misiewicz, Zelazowska, Raybourne, Cizza, & Sternberg, 1996b), and were particularly significant in 6-week-old vs. 3-month-old animals. Interestingly, only the female LEW/N rats showed any volume or cell content differences when compared to the F344/N animals. The administration of corticosteroids altered the inflammatory response of LEW/N so that it resembled that of the F344/N strain, whereas administration of the glucocorticoid receptor antagonist RU 486 to F344/N rats increased their inflammatory response so that its intensity was similar to that of the LEW/N rats (Karalis et al., 1995). Interestingly, the effect of glucocorticoid administration on the cellular content of the exudate was more marked than its effect on exudate volume; while RU486 had a limited effect on exudate volume in F344/N rats, it had a significant effect on the cellular content (Karalis et al., 1995). As with SCW-induced arthritis, the differing ACTH and corticosterone responses in the two strains and the effects of glucocorticoid and glucocorticoid antagonist administration support the importance of the HPA axis in downregulating acute inflammatory events.

Conversely, reconstitution of the HPA axis in inflammatory susceptible rats can reverse these animals' inflammatory susceptibility. Treatment with low dose dexamethasone prevents expression of SCW-induced arthritis (Sternberg et al., 1989a) and partially or completely prevents, in a dose-related manner, EAE in response to MBP (MacPhee et al., 1989). Transplantation of fetal hypothalamic tissue intracerebroventricularly from inflammatory resistant F344/N rats into inflammatory susceptible LEW/N rats decreases subcutaneous carrageenan inflammation in LEW/N rats by over 85% (Misiewicz et al., 1997). This effect occurs at least in part through reconstitution of the HPA axis, as transplanted rats show a plasma corticosterone and hypothalamic CRH response equal to that of F344/N rats. The graft tissue in these animals only variably expresses CRH, suggesting that the main effects of the transplants on the HPA axis may occur through stimulation of the host hypothalamic CRH expression, possibly by fetal hypothalamic growth factors. Of note, hypothalamic tissue transplantation decreased exudate volume to a greater extent than cellular content (Misiewicz et al., 1996a) and had no effect on the percentage of circulating naive versus memory cells, the latter being known to be increased in the LEW/N strain. This again suggests that different elements of the innate inflammatory response are controlled by separate factors.

## IV. HPA AXIS FUNCTION FINDINGS IN RHEUMATOID ARTHRITIS PATIENTS

As the evidence in animal models continues to accumulate to support a link between the neuroendocrine system and the development of autoimmune diseases, there are a growing number of studies investigating the HPA axis in a variety of chronic inflammatory diseases including RA. As we will see, the interpretation of the generated data is rendered difficult by the presence of a variety of confounding factors, and by methodological differences between the studies.

### A. Human HPA Axis Activation Response Assessment

Most of the studies discussed below use a combination of direct plasma measurements of ACTH and cortisol, and of dynamic testing of the HPA axis with anterior pituitary stimulation. Plasma hormone measurements taken at regular intervals over 24 h can provide a broad quantitative estimate of hormonal secretion, as well as insight into potential disturbances in the circadian rhythm of secretion. Direct pituitary stimulation with CRH is felt to be a good screening test for the assessment of pituitary reserve.

### 1. Ovine CRH (oCRH) Infusion

Ovine CRH is as potent as the human product but has a longer half-life. A standard dose is administered after a period of fasting, and plasma ACTH and cortisol levels are measured at regular intervals over the subsequent 2 h. In the setting of decreased anterior pituitary function, one would expect blunted ACTH and cortisol responses. In the setting of a primary hypothalamic pathology, oCRH should still result in ACTH secretion (Williams, Wilson & Foster, 1992). It is a test which has been useful to differentiate Cushing's disease from major depression, both being associated with circulating hypercortisolemia (Gold et al., 1986). Subjects with depression show a blunted response of ACTH to CRH, appropriate for their degree of circulating hypercortisolemia. This is not the case in subjects with Cushing's disease, who lack the negative feedback effect of cortisol on the ACTH response. This test is often performed in conjunction with the infusion of the other main anterior pituitary hormone secretagogues to provide a global assessment of anterior pituitary functional reserves: luteinizing hormone releasing hormone (LHRH), growth hormone releasing hormone (GHRH), and thyrotropin releasing hormone (TRH).

One of the things which makes the study of the HPA axis particularly difficult is the fact that it is subject to many influences, some of which are intrinsic to the subjects studied, and many which are related to environmental exposures (Table II). Age (Raskind, Peskind, & Wilkinson, 1994), gender (Dorn et al., 1996), ethnic background (Yanovski, Yanovski, Harrington, Gold, & Chrousos, 1995), weight, smoking, psychiatric disorders (Abelson & Curtis, 1996; Adinoff et al., 1990), acute and chronic disease, and chronic pain syndromes all have effects on HPA axis activation patterns. Of particular relevance in the study of RA is the impact of pharmacological agents on HPA axis function, as these patients are invariably receiving several medications for disease management and pain control. Especially important are drugs which are either neurotransmitter agonists or antagonists, as several neurotransmitter systems down or upregulate hypothalamic CRH secretion and can therefore decrease or increase HPA axis activity (Chrousos & Gold, 1992). Acetylcholine, norepinephrine, and serotonin are all known to increase hypothalamic CRH. Drugs targeting these systems, such as tricyclic antidepressants and serotonin reuptake inhibitors, could thus alter neuroendocrine responses. Opiates

**TABLE II**  Factors Known to Modify the HPA Axis Stress Response: What to Keep in Mind When Analyzing Human Data

**Known or suspected modifiers of the HPA axis response**

*Fixed subject characteristics*
- Age
- Gender
- Ethnicity

*Menstrual cycle timing*

*Body mass index*

*Smoking*

*Stress*
- Physical stress (exercise)
- Psychological stress

*Disturbed circadian rhythm (night shift work, long-distance traveling)*

*Acute illness*
- Infection, sepsis
- Surgery

*Chronic illness (other than RA)*
- Chronic osteomyelitis
- Asthma

*Psychiatric illnesses*
- Depression
- Seasonal affective disorder
- Alcoholism
- Panic disorder

*Chronic pain syndromes*
- Fibromyalgia
- Chronic fatigue syndrome

*Medications*
- Corticosteroids
- Non-steroidal anti-inflammatories
- Antidepressants: tricyclics and serotonin reuptake inhibitors
- Benzodiazepines
- Dopaminergic agents, sympathomimetics
- Opiates
- Oral contraceptives, hormonal replacement

and benzodiazepines blunt HPA axis activation. However, the precise effects in vivo of individual drugs cannot be predicted and have not been explored. Future studies should address these issues in in vivo clinical situations. Table II provides a nonexhaustive list of factors known or suspected to have an impact on the functioning of the HPA axis. While it is difficult to control for such factors when studying rheumatoid patients, it is useful to keep these variables in mind when interpreting data. These patients will usually have several characteristics known to be associated with an altered HPA axis response.

## B. Studies of HPA Axis Function in Rheumatoid Arthritis

### 1. HPA Axis Activation Patterns

The question of the role of deficient corticosteroid production in the pathogenesis of RA is not new (Harkness et al., 1982; Pal, 1970; Saldanha et al., 1986). Whereas the initial findings resulted from simply measuring plasma and urinary cortisol and corticosteroid metabolism products, more recent studies (Table III) have used a variety of methods to stimulate the HPA axis in order to bring out more subtle defects in the neuroendocrine activation response. As it has previously been noted (Masi & Chrousos, 1996),

**TABLE III** Summary of HPA Axis Studies in Patients with Rheumatoid Arthritis

| Study | Study population | HPA axis assessment methods | Results |
|---|---|---|---|
| **Crofford et al., 1997** | Early RA, controls<br>*NSAIDs allowed* | 1. Hourly ACTH, cortisol, and IL-6 × 24 h<br>2. CRH stimulation test | 1. Disturbed circadian rhythm<br>2. Overall quantitative hormonal response similar between control and RA groups, at baseline, and post-CRH |
| **Templ et al., 1996** | Newly diagnosed RA, controls<br>*NSAIDs allowed* | CRH, TRH, GnRH, and GHRH stimulation test | Reponses similar in controls and RA subjects, except for a blunted GH to GHRH |
| **Neeck et al., 1990** | Well-established RA, divided into three groups according to disease activity<br>*No clear information on NSAID use* | ACTH and cortisol levels every 2 h × 24 h | Disturbed circadian rhythm in high disease activity group<br>Correlation between ESR and mean of individual cortisol values |
| **Gudbjörnsson et al., 1996** | Well-established RA, controls<br>*NSAIDs stopped for 3 days before testing* | CRH, TRH, GnRH, and GHRH stimulation test; repeated after 1 week on prednisolone 15–20 mg/day | Baseline decreased cortisol ACTH ratio, increased with exogenous glucocorticoid treatment |
| **Hall et al., 1994** | Well-established RA, controls<br>*~50% patients on NSAIDs* | Hourly plasma ACTH and cortisol × 4 h in the morning, 24-h urinary cortisol | Higher ACTH integrated area in untreated RA, no difference between NSAID treated RA and controls |
| **Cash et al., 1992** | Well-established RA, controls<br>*NASIDs and disease modifying agents allowed, prednisone (mean dose 5 mg/day)* | CRH stimulation test: 12h after last prednisone dose and 36h after holding prednisone | 1. Baseline ACTH and cortisol levels elevated in RA<br>2. Responses to CRH blunted at 12h postprednisone, normalizing at 36h postprednisone; high peak ACTH levels at 36h |
| **Chikanza et al., 1992** | Well-established RA, OA, OM undergoing surgery<br>*NSAIDs and disease modifying agents allowed* | 1. Plasma ACTH and cortisol every 2h for 24h<br>2. Daily plasma cortisol levels × 4 days postsurgery<br>3. CRH stimulation test | 1. Basal cortisol levels lower in RA than osteomyelitis, despite comparable ESR values<br>2. Post-op, no peaking of cortisol in RA group, with elevated IL-6 and IL-1β levels<br>3. Similar ACTH and cortisol responses to CRH in RA and OA |
| **Jorgensen et al., 1995** | Well-established RA, controls | CRH and TRH stimulation tests with ACTH, cortisol, β-endorphin, and prolactin measurements | 1. Similar ACTH and cortisol responses to CRH between RA and controls<br>2. Increased baseline and CRH-stimulated β-endorphin response<br>3. Increased TRH-stimulated prolactin response |

overall, these studies show a somewhat hypofunctional HPA axis response in RA, but data interpretation is rendered difficult by the presence of an ongoing inflammatory process.

Neeck et al. studied 26 RA patients with a disease duration varying from 0.3 to 15 years (Neeck, Federlin, Graef, Rusch, & Schmidt, 1990). They compared them to 8 healthy controls who were significantly younger than the arthritis group. Patients had never been on exogenous corticosteroids or disease modifying agents such as gold or D-penicillamine. Plasma ACTH and cortisol were measured every 2 h for 24 h. By separating patients into three groups according to their disease activity, as defined by their erythrocyte sedimentation rate (ESR), these authors were able to show a significant correlation between the arithmetic mean values of cortisol and the ESR levels. Though the circadian rhythm in the low and moderate disease activity groups only showed a somewhat earlier peaking of plasma cortisol, high disease activity was associated with noticeable blunting of ACTH and cortisol circadian rhythms. Similarly, Hall et al. (1994) measured plasma ACTH and cortisol levels hourly for 4 h starting at 9 AM in a total of 15 patients with well-established RA, 8 untreated and 7 on NSAIDs only. Compared with the 13 controls matched for body mass index, age and gender, the untreated RA subjects showed a greater ACTH area under the curve. ACTH values in the NSAID treated subjects were similar to those seen on the controls. This study underscores the impact of these medications on the HPA axis, whether it occurs directly or through peripheral inhibition of prostaglandin production. Plasma and 24-h urinary cortisol levels were not significantly different between patients and controls. This study did not look at a 24-h time span, and thus no conclusion could be made about the circadian rhythm. Additionally, subjects were not separated according to varying inflammatory indices. The authors interpreted these results as possibly indicative of an impaired adrenal response to ACTH, either through the presence of circulating ACTH inhibitors, or due to altered pre- or post-ACTH-receptor-binding events.

Other studies have questioned whether RA is actually associated with an abnormal adrenal response to ACTH. Using the administration of a cocktail of anterior pituitary stimulatory hormones, one can assess the integrity of pituitary functional reserve. Overall, infusion of oCRH to RA patients has failed to demonstrate any significant difference compared to healthy controls. Crofford et al. (1997) found peak levels and time-integrated values of ACTH and cortisol to be similar in 5 RA patients, 4 with disease onset of less than months, compared to healthy controls. Gudbjörnsson, Skogseid, Oberg, Wide, and Hallgren (1996) looked at 18 patients with well established disease and found no difference between their cortisol response to oCRH and that of controls; the ACTH response, however, was significantly blunted in the later part of the study (time points 45, 60, and 90 min). These patients had untreated, moderately active arthritis, and had been taken off their NSAIDs for at least 3 days before testing; there was no information on prior corticosteroid treatment, except that they had not been used in the previous 3 months. Following 1 week of low dose oral prednisolone, the cortisol response to CRH was decreased. Interestingly, the baseline cortisol to ACTH ratio was lowered in the RA group, possibly secondary to adrenal insensitivity to ACTH and in accordance with the findings of Hall et al. (1994). There was no correlation between inflammatory indices such as the erythrocyte sedimentation rate (ESR) and C-reactive protein (CRP) and the baseline and stimulated ACTH responses to CRH. Jorgensen, Bressot, Bologna, and Sany, (1995) found no significant difference between 10 RA patients (6 with active disease) and 5 controls in ACTH and cortisol response to CRH, but an increased response of β-endorphin to CRH and of prolactin to TRH. Finally, Templ et al. (1996) found no difference in ACTH and cortisol responses between 10 RA patients with early disease (onset of symptoms 6–24 weeks) on NSAIDs and controls. Of note, the CRH dose administered and the infusion timing (4 PM as opposed to the 8 PM) were slightly different from those in the studies described above.

One of the recurrent key points of discussion surrounding the results described above is that normal circulating ACTH and cortisol levels in the setting of ongoing systemic inflammation does not necessarily indicate an intact hypothalamo-pituitary-adrenal axis. Though most results point to intact anterior pituitary and adrenal responses to CRH, it is also possible that the hypothalamus in RA is unable to appropriately react to peripheral inflammation and the stimulatory neural and cytokine signals this generates. Chikanza, Petrou, Kingsley, Chrousos, and Panayi (1992) addressed this issue by studying two patient groups with chronic inflammatory conditions: RA and chronic osteomyelitis (OM). They compared their plasma ACTH and cortisol levels, drawn every 2 h for 24 h. Both groups had similarly elevated levels of ESR. The RA patients had well-established disease and were diverse in their previous medication history and disease activity. A third

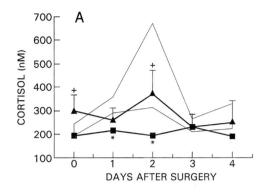

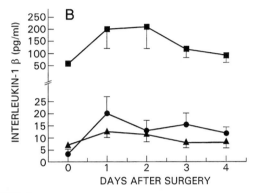

**FIGURE 2**   (A) Plasma cortisol levels following surgery in 10 patients with osteomyelitis (OM) (triangles) and 10 patients with rheumatoid arthritis (RA) (squares). Shaded area shows the mean $\pm 1$ SEM for 10 control patients with osteoarthritis (OA). $^+p < .05$ OM. RA patients and $^*p < .05$ RA vs. OA by student's $t$ test. (B) Plasma IL-1$\beta$ levels following surgery in nine patients with OA, 9 with OM, and 10 with RA. RA patient values were significantly different ($p = .0001$ by Student $t$ test) compared with those of the OM patients and those of the OA patients at all time points. Differences between OM and OA patients were not significant. Values are the, mean and SEM. Adapted with permission from Chikanza, I. C., Petrou, P., Kingsley, G., Chrousos, G., & Panayi, G. S. (1992). Defective hypothalamic response to immune and inflammatory stimuli in patients with rheumatoid arthritis [see comments]. *Arthritis and Rheumatism, 35*(11), 1281–1288.

control group of subjects with noninflammatory rheumatic conditions such as osteoarthritis (OA) and low back pain was also studied. While the RA patients maintained a circadian rhythm of cortisol secretion, their levels were at the lower end of those observed in controls, and lower than those seen on the OM group. Morning plasma cortisol levels were then measured prior to surgery and daily for 4 days postoperatively in subjects with active RA, OA, and OM. Despite elevated plasma IL-1$\beta$ (Figure 2) and IL-6 levels, RA patients failed to show the increase in cortisol seen the OM group and even more so in the OA group at day 2. CRH stimulation revealed similar ACTH and cortisol responses in the RA and OA groups. Taken

together, these results suggest that RA is associated with an abnormal hypothalamic response to peripheral inflammatory cytokines and to the surgical model of physiological stress.

## 2. Peripheral Tissue Sensitivity to Corticosteroids in RA

The ultimate impact of a hypofunctional HPA axis on the inflammatory process will depend on the peripheral tissue's response to circulating glucocorticoids. While it would make sense physiologically for the HPA axis and cortisol levels to be directly related to tissue sensitivity to corticosteroids, the factors controlling tissue response to circulating glucocorticoids are not entirely clear. While there is some evidence that GR numbers decrease with increasing levels of cortisolemia (Kalinyak, Dorin, Hoffman, & Perlman, 1987; Rosewicz et al., 1988), peripheral lymphocyte GR numbers in patients with Cushing's disease have not been found to be significantly different from those in controls (Nawata, Higuchi, Higashizima, Kato, & Ibayashi, 1984). It may be that circulating cortisol feeds back on tissue glucocorticoid responsiveness by affecting postreceptor binding events and not simply the actual number of GRs. We have designed a whole blood assay which enables a global assessment of peripheral white blood cell response to corticosteroids (DeRijk et al., 1996, 1997). Based on stimulated cellular cytokine production in the presence of increasing concentrations of dexamethasone, we determined that peripheral corticosteroid sensitivity is dynamic and decreases with strenuous exercise (DeRijk et al., 1996). Interestingly, there was no correlation between the pre- or postexercise plasma cortisol levels, the change in cortisol level, or the white blood cell glucocorticoid sensitivity as measured by our assay. Catecholamines have been questioned as potential regulators of tissue sensitivity, and there is a known relationship between the adrenergic and the HPA axis responses (Sawchenko et al., 1993, 1996). This may be an indirect way by which the HPA axis impacts on tissue glucocorticoid sensitivity. Other factors such as local cytokine concentrations may impact on tissue steroid sensitivity (Sher et al., 1994).

Schlaghecke, Kornely, Wollenhaupt, and Specker (1992) studied glucocorticoid receptor (GR) affinity and density in patients with active RA who had been off corticosteroids for at least 6 months. They found a decreased number of peripheral lymphocyte GRs when compared to controls, with no significant difference in binding affinity. There was no correlation between GR density and simultaneously obtained plasma cortisol levels. There were no significant differences between control and RA patient isolated plasma cortisol levels. The same group went on to look at the functional significance of this finding (Schlaghecke, Beuscher, Kornely, & Specker, 1994). Looking at peripheral lymphocyte cytokine production and proliferation responses in the presence of glucocorticoids, they found no difference between RA patients and controls. It is not clear whether these findings can be generalized to all tissues, in particular to the synovium.

Taken together, these studies show that studying the HPA axis in a well established chronic inflammatory process such as RA is challenging, even when the disease is still in its early stages. The use of multiple medications including NSAIDs and exogenous corticosteroids (oral, intramuscular, intraarticular) at different doses for variable durations, the study of subjects with different degrees of ongoing inflammation, the methodological differences in the studies, all contribute to the variability and difficulties in the interpretation of the results. A potential solution to these problems would be to assess the HPA axis response in monozygotic twins where one sibling carries a diagnosis of RA. Studying the unaffected twin and comparing their results to healthy controls could provide insight into the role of the HPA axis in predisposing subjects to RA.

## C. Potential Implications for Treatment

Following initial enthusiasm, physicians became more cautious in their use of exogenous corticosteroids in the treatment of RA due to the long list of associated side-effects. These agents, while they provide definite relief of symptoms, were not felt to modify the course of the illness. However, there is now evidence that these agents do have an impact on disease progression. Kirwan (1995) assessed the radiological progression of erosions in 106 RA patients that had been randomized to receive placebo or low-dose daily prednisone (7.5 mg per day) over a 2-year period. The progression of erosions was significantly less in the treated group. Of particular interest is the relatively low doses of glucocorticoids that were used, and the fact that the patients all had relatively new onset disease of less than 2 years duration. Increasingly, early aggressive treatment of RA is being advocated to prevent articular damage before it results in permanent disability. Certainly, as discussed above, the evidence in animal models of inflammation suggests that endogenously produced corticosteroids and their exogenous administration are key elements in curtailing acute inflammation and can prevent the development of experimental chronic inflammatory processes (Sternberg et al., 1989a).

## D. Questioning the Link between Depression and RA

It remains unclear whether or not the blunting in HPA axis response observed in human clinical RA actually precedes disease onset and constitutes a factor in its pathogenesis or whether it is secondary to inflammation. Animal models in which HPA axis responses are genetically blunted, or surgically or pharmacologically interrupted, suggest that blunted HPA axis responses do constitute a factor in the pathogenesis of chronic inflammatory arthritis. These findings also raise interesting questions regarding the potential link between chronic inflammatory illnesses such as RA and affective disorders associated with dysregulation of the HPA axis. Indeed, inbred strains of rats, such as the LEW/N and the F344/N, with differential HPA axis responsiveness, also show differential behavioral responses to stress (Glowa, Geyer, Gold, & Sternberg, 1992).

Disturbances of the HPA axis activation response have been found in subjects with clinical depression. A spectrum of clinical symptoms can be found in major depression. The melancholic subtype of the disease is characterized by a generalized state of hyperarousal, with anxiety, insomnia, decreased appetite, and weight loss as its prominent features. These subjects are hypercortisolemic, with increased CRH levels in the CSF, etc. Subjects with predominantly atypical symptoms represent the other end of the clinical spectrum, with prominent hyperphagia, weight gain and hypersomnia (Gold, Licinio, Wong, & Chrousos, 1995; Gold et al., 1986). Although atypical depression has not been studied as extensively as the melancholic subgroup, studies of diseases with atypical symptoms of depression as part of their clinical presentation have shed light on this class of affective disorders. Indeed, physiological studies of patients with chronic fatigue syndrome, fibromyalgia, and seasonal affective disorder have all revealed a hypoactivity of the HPA axis activation response to oCRH infusion (Crofford et al., 1994; Demitrack et al., 1991; Joseph-Vanderpool et al., 1991).

Some studies have suggested an increased prevalence of clinical depression or depressive symptoms in rheumatoid arthritis patients when compared to controls (Abdel-Nasser et al., 1998; Pincus, Griffith, Pearce, & Isenberg, 1996), with reported rates varying from 14 to 46%. Although the diagnosis of depression in RA can be difficult because standard measurement and diagnostic scales for depression are contaminated by items that reflect RA severity (Peck, Smith, Ward, & Milano, 1989), it would not be unexpected to find an elevated proportion of patients with depressive symptoms. Depression, like RA, is a multifactorial disease. Subjects suffering from RA have many risk factors for depression. Although the association between disease severity and the presence of depression is not clear cut (Bishop, 1988; Hawley & Wolfe, 1988; McFarlane & Brooks, 1988), the presence of an essentially incurable debilitating disease, chronic pain, and the use of potentially mood-altering medications could all contribute to the development of depression. Better clinical characterization of the depressive features found in RA patients could help clarify to what extent these psychiatric complaints are related to a hypofunctional HPA axis, as one might expect in the presence of prominent atypical symptoms. Whether chronic inflammation results in the observed blunted stress response, or whether this physiological state precedes the onset of RA, the altered HPA axis response and central CRH levels could be partially responsible for the mood and behavioral changes observed in RA, through the same mechanisms by which any alteration in HPA axis function leads to such affective symptomatology.

## V. OTHER NEUROENDOCRINE FACTORS IMPLICATED IN RA PATHOGENESIS

### A. Sex Hormones

In general, autoimmune diseases affect women close to three times as often as men (Jacobson, Gange, Rose, & Graham, 1997). RA is no exception, with a female to male prevalence ratio of approximately 2:1. Also in support of the key role of gender and sex hormones in RA pathogenesis is the frequently noted improvement of disease symptomatology during pregnancy, which is almost inevitably followed by clinical worsening in the postpartum period (Da Silva & Spector, 1992). Additionally, it has been noted that the risk of new RA increases in the postpartum period. Some of the rat models for erosive arthritis also demonstrate increased susceptibility and a worse outcome in females. This is particularly true in the LEW/N strain, where females exhibit greater severity of both acute inflammation and chronic erosive arthritis (Allen, Blatter, Calandra, & Wilder, 1983; Misiewicz et al., 1996a, b; Wilder, Calandra, Garvin, Wright, & Hansen, 1982).

Part of the explanation for this phenomenon may lie in the role the hypothalamo-pituitary-gonadal axis and sex hormones play in modulating the immune response. Although the separation is not always entirely clear cut, lymphocyte population in both humans and animal models can be divided into two subsets based on their cytokine production: Th1, characterized by interferon-$\gamma$ and IL-12 production, and Th2 lymphocytes linked to IL-4 production. Th1 cells are primarily involved in promoting cell-mediated immunity, while Th2 cells encourage a humoral immune response (Mosmann & Sad, 1996). The immune response found in RA is characterized by a predominantly Th1 lymphocyte and cytokine pattern. The factors pushing lymphocyte differentiation toward a Th1 versus a Th2 predominance are not entirely clear, but estrogens appear to favor a Th2 response, thus potentially improving the course of RA (Wilder, 1998). It could provide part of the explanation for the clinical improvement observed during pregnancy.

### B. Peripheral Nervous System Activation in RA

As discussed earlier and elsewhere in this textbook, the peripheral nervous system has a definite impact on the immune response which is modulated by the degree of activation of the HPA axis. There have been studies in inflammatory arthritis, in particular in juvenile rheumatoid arthritis (JRA), showing altered sympathetic system responsiveness in these subjects as measured using orthostatic stress (Kavelaars, de Jong-de Vos van Steenwijk, Kuis, & Heijnen, 1998). This may be related to an increase in basal sympathetic tone. Additionally, the peripheral mononuclear white blood cells in JRA show reduced response to $\beta$-2 adrenergic stimulation, which could potentially result in changes of T cell and monocyte function. These changes could further contribute to differential inflammatory responses.

### C. Prolactin

Prolactin is increasingly recognized as having effects on the immune response, primarily stimulatory (Jara et al., 1991; Reber, 1993). It has perhaps been implicated more in the pathogenesis of systemic lupus erythematosus where clinical trials using bromocriptine to block prolactin effects have had variable success in altering the course of the disease (Alvarez-Nemegyei et al., 1998; Walker et al., 1998). There are, however, some data pointing to increased levels of the hormone in RA patients (Chikanza, Petrou, Chrousos, Kingsley, & Panayi, 1993; Jorgensen et al., 1995).

## VI. SUMMARY

When Hench et al. initially reported the dramatic effect of exogenous glucocorticoid administration on the symptoms of RA, they asked a question that has proven to be quite complex, perhaps much more so than the authors could have anticipated: "To what extent could rheumatoid arthritis be merely a syndrome produced by any factor which causes a deficiency of adrenal hormone?" (Hench et al., 1949). Thus, the notion that the stress response plays a role in autoimmune disease is not new, but it is only recently that technology has advanced sufficiently in both neurobiology and immunology, and in clinical psychiatry, psychology and rheumatology, to define the molecular, biochemical and neuroanatomical pathways by which the immune system and the CNS communicate. We now know more about the control of adrenal corticosteroid production and about the multidirectional communication pathways existing between the HPA axis and peripheral inflammatory responses. Rather than a simple cause and effect relationship, it is likely that HPA axis disturbances identified in RA subjects result from a combination of peripheral tissue effects on the HPA axis and from HPA axis effects on peripheral disease.

Human and animal model data indicate that there are definite interactions between the neuroendocrine and immune systems that likely contribute to the development of rheumatoid arthritis and to its clinical course. Impaired and hyperactive HPA axis stress responses in LEW/N and F344/N rats, respectively, are key in explaining their differing inflammatory phenotypes. Despite methodological differences, findings in humans point to downregulated HPA axis activation patterns. Unfortunately, the interpretation of these studies is limited by the presence of a well-established chronic inflammatory process in the study population. It is therefore impossible at this point to definitively prove a causal relationship between a hypoactive HPA axis and the development of RA in humans.

Beyond the findings we have discussed, the HPA axis has an important characteristic that makes it a good potential candidate as a contributor to this multifactorial disease: its activation response appears to be heavily modulated by environmental factors. The currently most widely accepted hypothesis explaining RA pathogenesis involves the exposure of genetically susceptible individuals to environmental factors that will trigger an autoimmune reaction that results in a chronic disease. Much of the attention recently has focused on the class II major histocompatibility complex (MHC), as certain haplotypes confer an increased risk for severe disease. Increasingly emerging, however, is the potential role of non-MHC-related genetic loci in disease predisposition (Becker et al., 1998; Listwak et al., 1999; Wilder et al., 1996). RA, like many common human illnesses, is likely a polygenic disease. The environmental triggers are still unknown. However, monozygotic twin studies showing concordance rates of 15% (Jarvinen & Aho, 1994; Reveille, 1998) indicate that they contribute importantly to the disease pathogenesis. Future studies of the role of HPA axis responses in the pathogenesis of RA should take into account both environmental and genetic variables which could impact on the neuroendocrine responsiveness in the setting of disease.

## References

Abdel-Nasser, A. M., Abd El-Azim, S., Taal, E., El-Badawy, S. A., Rasker, J. J., & Valkenburg, H. A. (1998). Depression and depressive symptoms in rheumatoid arthritis patients: An analysis of their occurrence and determinants. *British Journal of Rheumatology, 37*, 391–397.

Abelson, J. L., & Curtis, G. C. (1996). Hypothalamic-pituitary-adrenal axis activity in panic disorder: Prediction of long-term outcome by pretreatment cortisol levels. *American Journal of Psychiatry, 153*, 69–73.

Adinoff, B., Martin, P. R., Bone, G. H., Eckardt, M. J., Roehrich, L., George, D. T., Moss, H. B., Eskay, R., Linnoila, M., & Gold, P. W. (1990). Hypothalamic-pituitary-adrenal axis functioning and cerebrospinal fluid corticotropin releasing hormone and corticotropin levels in alcoholics after recent and long-term abstinence. *Archives of General Psychiatry, 47*, 325–330.

Aguilera, G., Jessop, D. S., Harbuz, M. S., Kiss, A., & Lightman, S. L. (1997). Differential regulation of hypothalamic pituitary corticotropin releasing hormone receptors during development of adjuvant-induced arthritis in the rat. *Journal of Endocrinology, 153*, 185–191.

Allen, J. B., Blatter, D., Calandra, G. B., & Wilder, R. L. (1983). Sex hormonal effects on the severity of streptococcal cell wall-induced polyarthritis in the rat. *Arthritis and Rheumatism, 26*, 560–563.

Almeida, A. P., Bayer, B. M., Horakova, Z., & Beaven, M. A. (1980). Influence of indomethacin and other anti-inflammatory drugs on mobilization and production of neutrophils: Studies with carrageenan-induced inflammation in rats. *Journal of Pharmacology and Experimental Therapeutics, 214*, 74–79.

Alvarez-Nemegyei, J., Cobarrubias-Cobos, A., Escalante-Triay, F., Sosa-Munoz, J., Miranda, J. M., & Jara, L. J. (1998). Bromocriptine in systemic lupus erythematosus: A double-blind, randomized, placebo-controlled study. *Lupus, 7*, 414–419. [in process citation].

Banks, W. A., & Kastin, A. J. (1997). Relative contributions of peripheral and central sources to levels of IL-1 alpha in the cerebral cortex of mice: Assessment with species-specific enzyme immunoassays. *Journal of Neuroimmunology, 79*, 22–28.

Barrera, P., Boerbooms, A. M., van de Putte, L. B., & van der Meer, J. W. (1996). Effects of antirheumatic agents on cytokines. *Seminars in Arthritis and Rheumatis, 25*, 234–253.

Becker, K. G., Simon, R. M., Bailey-Wilson, J. E., Biddison, W. E., McFarland, H. F., & Trent, J. M. (1998). Clustering of non-MHC susceptibility candidate loci in human autoimmune disease. *Proceedings of the National Academy of Sciences, USA, 95,* 9979–9984.

Beckman, J. S., & Koppenol, W. H. (1996). Nitric oxide, superoxide, and peroxynitrite: The good, the bad, and ugly. *American Journal of Physiology, 271,* C1424–C1437.

Bishop, D. S. (1988). Depression and rheumatoid arthritis. *Journal of Rheumatology, 15,* 888–889. [editorial]

Bluthe, R. M., Walter, V., Parnet, P., Laye, S., Lestage, J., Verrier, D., Poole, S., Stenning, B. E., Kelley, K. W., & Dantzer, R. (1994). Lipopolysaccharide induces sickness behaviour in rats by a vagal mediated mechanism. *Comptes Rendus de l'Académie des Sciences. Série III, Sciences de la Vie, 317,* 499–503.

Brennan, F. M., Maini, R. N., & Feldmann, M. (1995). Cytokine expression in chronic inflammatory disease. *British Medical Bulletin, 51,* 368–384.

Chikanza, I. C., Petrou, P., Chrousos, G., Kingsley, G., & Panayi, G. S. (1993). Excessive and dysregulated secretion of prolactin in rheumatoid arthritis: Immunopathogenetic and therapeutic implications. *British Journal of Rheumatology, 32,* 445–448.

Chikanza, I. C., Petrou, P., Kingsley, G., Chrousos, G., & Panayi, G. S. (1992). Defective hypothalamic response to immune and inflammatory stimuli in patients with rheumatoid arthritis. *Arthritis and Rheumatism, 35,* 1281–1288. [see comments]

Chowdrey, H. S., Larsen, P. J., Harbuz, M. S., Jessop, D. S., Aguilera, G., Eckland, D. J., & Lightman, S. L. (1995). Evidence for arginine vasopressin as the primary activator of the HPA axis during adjuvant-induced arthritis. *British Journal of Pharmacology, 116,* 2417–2424.

Chrousos, G. P. (1995). The hypothalamic-pituitary-adrenal axis and immune-mediated inflammation. *New England Journal of Medicine, 332,* 1351–1362.

Chrousos, G. P., & Gold, P. W. (1992). The concepts of stress and stress system disorders. *Journal of the American Medical Association, 267,* 1244–1252.

Crofford, L. J., Kalogeras, K. T., Mastorakos, G., Magiakou, M. A., Wells, J., Kanik, K. S., Gold, P. W., Chrousos, G. P., & Wilder, R. L. (1997). Circadian relationships between interleukin (IL)-6 and hypothalamic- pituitary-adrenal axis hormones: Failure of IL-6 to cause sustained hypercortisolism in patients with early untreated rheumatoid arthritis. *Journal of Clinical Endocrinology and Metabolism, 82,* 1279–1283.

Crofford, L. J., Pillemer, S. R., Kalogeras, K. T., Cash, J. M., Michelson, D., Kling, M. A., Sternberg, E. M., Gold, P. W., Chrousos, G. P., & Wilder, R. L. (1994). Hypothalamic-pituitary-adrenal axis perturbations in patients with fibromyalgia. *Arthritis and Rheumatism, 37,* 1583–1592.

Da Silva, J. A., & Spector, T. D. (1992). The role of pregnancy in the course and aetiology of rheumatoid arthritis. *Clinical Rheumatology, 11,* 189–194.

Dawson, J., Sedgwick, A. D., Edwards, J. C., & Lees, P. (1991). A comparative study of the cellular, exudative and histological responses to carrageenan, dextran and zymosan in the mouse. *International Journal of Tissue Reactions, 13,* 171–185.

Demitrack, M. A., Dale, J. K., Straus, S. E., Laue, L., Listwak, S. J., Kruesi, M. J., Chrousos, G. P., & Gold, P. W. (1991). Evidence for impaired activation of the hypothalamic-pituitary-adrenal axis in patients with chronic fatigue syndrome. *Journal of Clinical Endocrinology and Metabolism, 73,* 1224–1234.

DeRijk, R., Michelson, D., Karp, B., Petrides, J., Galliven, E., Deuster, P., Paciotti, G., Gold, P. W., & Sternberg, E. M. (1997). Exercise and circadian rhythm-induced variations in plasma cortisol differentially regulate interleukin-1 beta (IL-1 beta), IL-6, and tumor necrosis factor-alpha (TNF alpha) production in humans: High sensitivity of TNF alpha and resistance of IL-6. *Journal of Clinical Endocrinology and Metabolism, 82,* 2182–2191.

DeRijk, R. H., Petrides, J., Deuster, P., Gold, P. W., & Sternberg, E. M. (1996). Changes in corticosteroid sensitivity of peripheral blood lymphocytes after strenuous exercise in humans. *Journal of Clinical Endocrinology and Metabolism, 81,* 228–235.

Di Rosa, M. (1972). Biological properties of carrageenan. *Journal of Pharmacy and Pharmacology, 24,* 89–102.

Di Rosa, M., Giroud, J. P., & Willoughby, D. A. (1971). Studies on the mediators of the acute inflammatory response induced in rats in different sites by carrageenan and turpentine. *Journal of Pathology, 104,* 15–29.

Dorn, L. D., Burgess, E. S., Susman, E. J., von Eye, A., DeBellis, M. D., Gold, P. W., & Chrousos, G. P. (1996). Response to oCRH in depressed and nondepressed adolescents: Does gender make a difference? *Journal of the American Academy of Child and Adolescent Psychiatry, 35,* 764–773.

Edwards, C. K. I., Yunger, L. M., Lorence, R. M., Dantzer, R., & Kelley, K. W. (1991). The pituitary gland is required for protection against lethal effects of Salmonella typhimurium. *Proceedings of the National Academy of Sciences, USA, 88,* 2274–2277.

Ehlert, U., & Straub, R. (1998). Physiological and emotional response to psychological stressors in psychiatric and psychosomatic disorders. *Annals of New York Academy of Sciences, 851,* 477–486.

Elenkov, I. J., Papanicolaou, D. A., Wilder, R. L., & Chrousos, G. P. (1996). Modulatory effects of glucocorticoids and catecholamines on human interleukin-12 and interleukin-10 production: Clinical implications. *Proceedings of the Association of American Physicians, 108,* 374–381.

Felten, S. Y., & Felten, D. L. (1991). Innervation of lymphoid tissue. In R. Ader, D. L. Felten, & N. Cohen (Eds.), *Psychoneuroimmunology* (2nd ed.) (pp. 27–61). Academic Press: San Diego.

Flower, R. J., Parente, L., Persico, P., & Salmon, J. A. (1986). A comparison of the acute inflammatory response in adrenalectomised and sham-operated rats. *British Journal of Pharmacology, 87,* 57–62.

Gaillard, R. C., Poffet, D., Riondel, A. M., & Saurat, J. H. (1985). RU 486 inhibits peripheral effects of glucocorticoids in humans. *Journal of Clinical Endocrinology and Metabolism, 61,* 1009–1011.

Glowa, J. R., Geyer, M. A., Gold, P. W., & Sternberg, E. M. (1992). Differential startle amplitude and corticosterone response in rats. *Neuroendocrinology, 56,* 719–723.

Goetzl, E. J., Chernov, T., Renold, F., & Payan, D. G. (1985). Neuropeptide regulation of the expression of immediate hypersensitivity. *Journal of Immunology, 135.*

Gold, P. W., Licinio, J., Wong, M. L., & Chrousos, G. P. (1995). Corticotropin releasing hormone in the pathophysiology of melancholic and atypical depression and in the mechanism of action of antidepressant drugs. *Annals of New York Academy of Sciences, 771,* 716–729.

Gold, P. W., Loriaux, D. L., Roy, A., Kling, M. A., Calabrese, J. R., Kellner, C. H., Nieman, L. K., Post, R. M., Pickar, D., Gallucci, W., et al. (1986). Responses to corticotropin-releasing hormone in the hypercortisolism of depression and Cushing's disease. Pathophysiologic and diagnostic implications. *New England Journal of Medicine, 314,* 1329–1335.

Green, P. G., Janig, W., & Levine, J. D. (1997). Negative feedback neuroendocrine control of inflammatory response in the rat is dependent on the sympathetic postganglionic neuron. *Journal of Neuroscience, 17,* 3234–3238.

Green, P. G., Miao, F. J., Strausbaugh, H., Heller, P., Janig, W., & Levine, J. D. (1998). Endocrine and vagal controls of sympathetically dependent neurogenic inflammation. *Annals of New York Academy of Sciences, 840,* 282–288.

Gudbjornsson, B., Skogseid, B., Oberg, K., Wide, L., & Hallgren, R. (1996). Intact adrenocorticotropic hormone secretion but impaired cortisol response in patients with active rheumatoid arthritis: Effect of glucocorticoids. *Journal of Rheumatology, 23,* 596–602. [see comments]

Hall, J., Morand, E. F., Medbak, S., Zaman, M., Perry, L., Goulding, N. J., Maddison, P. J., & O'Hare, J. P. (1994). Abnormal hypothalamic-pituitary-adrenal axis function in rheumatoid arthritis. Effects of nonsteroidal antiinflammatory drugs and water immersion. *Arthritis and Rheumatism, 37,* 1132–1137. [see comments]

Harbuz, M. S., Conde, G. L., Marti, O., Lightman, S. L., & Jessop, D. S. (1997). The hypothalamic-pituitary-adrenal axis in autoimmunity. *Annals of New York Academy of Sciences, 823,* 214–224.

Harbuz, M. S., Rees, R. G., Eckland, D., Jessop, D. S., Brewerton, D., & Lightman, S. L. (1992). Paradoxical responses of hypothalamic corticotropin-releasing factor (CRF) messenger ribonucleic acid (mRNA) and CRF-41 peptide and adenohypophysial proopiomelanocortin mRNA during chronic inflammatory stress. *Endocrinology, 130,* 1394–1400.

Harkness, J. A., Richter, M. B., Panayi, G. S., Van de Pette, K., Unger, A., Pownall, R., & Geddawi, M. (1982). Circadian variation in disease activity in rheumatoid arthritis. *British Medical Journal (Clinical Research Edition), 284,* 551–554.

Hawley, D. J., & Wolfe, F. (1988). Anxiety and depression in patients with rheumatoid arthritis: A prospective study of 400 patients. *Journal of Rheumatology, 15,* 932–941.

Hench, P. S., Kendall, E. C., Slocumb, C. H., & Polley, H. F. (1949). The effect of a hormone of the adrenal cortex (17-hydroxy-11-dehydrocorticosterone: compound E) and of pituitary adrenocorticotrophic hormone on rheumatoid arthritis: Preliminary report. *Proceedings of the Staff Meeting of Mayo Clinic, 24,* 181–197.

Hirasawa, N., Watanabe, M., Mue, S., Tsurufuji, S., & Ohuchi, K. (1991). Downward regulation of neutrophil infiltration by endogenous histamine without affecting vascular permeability responses in air-pouch-type carrageenin inflammation in rats. *Inflammation, 15,* 117–126.

Ianaro, A., O'Donnell, C. A., Di Rosa, M., & Liew, F. Y. (1994). A nitric oxide synthase inhibitor reduces inflammation, downregulates inflammatory cytokines and enhances interleukin-10 production in carrageenin-induced oedema in mice. *Immunology, 82,* 370–375.

Jacobson, D. L., Gange, S. J., Rose, N. R., & Graham, N. M. (1997). Epidemiology and estimated population burden of selected autoimmune diseases in the United States. *Clinical Immunology and Immunopathology, 84,* 223–243.

Jara, L. J., Lavalle, C., Fraga, A., Gomez-Sanchez, C., Silveira, L. H., Martinez-Osuna, P., Germain, B. F., & Espinoza, L. R. (1991). Prolactin, immunoregulation, and autoimmune diseases. *Seminars in Arthritis and Rheumatism, 20,* 273–284.

Jarvinen, P., & Aho, K. (1994). Twin studies in rheumatic diseases. *Seminars in Arthritis and Rheumatism, 24,* 19–28.

Jorgensen, C., Bressot, N., Bologna, C., & Sany, J. (1995). Dysregulation of the hypothalamo-pituitary axis in rheumatoid arthritis. *Journal of Rheumatology, 22,* 1829–1833.

Joseph-Venderpool, J. R., Rosenthal, N.E., Chrousos, G. P., Wehr, T. A., Skwerer, R., Kasper, S., & Gold, P.W. (1991). Abnormal pituitary-adrenal responses to corticotropin-releasing hormone in patients with seasonal affective disorder: Clinical and pathophysiological implications. *Journal of Clinical Endocrinology and Metabolism, 72,* 1382–1387.

Kalinyak, J. E., Dorin, R. I., Hoffman, A. R., & Perlman, A. J. (1987). Tissue-specific regulation of glucocorticoid receptor mRNA by dexamethasone. *Journal of Biological Chemistry, 262,* 10441–10444.

Kanik, K. S., Hagiwara, E., Yarboro, C. H., Schumacher, H. R., Wilder, R. L., & Klinman, D. M. (1998). Distinct patterns of cytokine secretion characterize new onset synovitis versus chronic rheumatoid arthritis. *Journal of Rheumatology, 25,* 16–22. [see comments]

Karalis, K., Crofford, L., Wilder, R. L., & Chrousos, G. P. (1995). Glucocorticoid and/or glucocorticoid antagonist effects in inflammatory disease-susceptible Lewis rats and inflammatory disease-resistant Fischer rats. *Endocrinology, 136,* 3107–3112.

Karalis, K., Sano, H., Redwine, J., Listwak, S., Wilder, R. L., & Chrousos, G. P. (1991). Autocrine or paracrine inflammatory actions of corticotropin-releasing hormone in vivo. *Science, 254,* 421–423.

Karanth, S., Lyson, K., & McCann, S. M. (1993). Role of nitric oxide in interleukin 2-induced corticotropin-releasing factor release from incubated hypothalami. *Proceedings of the National Academy of Sciences, USA, 90,* 3383–3387.

Kavelaars, A., de Jong-de Vos van Steenwijk, T., Kuis, W., & Heijnen, C. J. (1998). The reactivity of the cardiovascular system and immunomodulation by catecholamines in juvenile chronic arthritis. *Annals of New York Academy of Sciences, 840,* 698–704.

Kirwan, J. R. (1995). The effect of glucocorticoids on joint destruction in rheumatoid arthritis. The Arthritis and Rheumatism Council Low-Dose Glucocorticoid Study Group. *New England Journal of Medicine, 333,* 142–146. [see comments]

Klippel, J. H., & Dieppe, P. (1997). *Rheumatology* (2nd ed.). London, St. Louis: Mosby.

Laue, L., Kawai, S., Brandon, D. D., Brightwell, D., Barnes, K., Knazek, R. A., Loriaux, D. L., & Chrousos, G. P. (1988). Receptor-mediated effects of glucocorticoids on inflammation: Enhancement of the inflammatory response with a glucocorticoid antagonist. *Journal of Steroid Biochemistry, 29,* 591–598.

Lawrence, R. C., Helmick, C. G., Arnett, F. C., Deyo, R. A., Felson, D. T., Giannini, E. H., Heyse, S. P., Hirsch, R., Hochberg, M. C., Hunder, G. G., Liang, M. H., Pillemer, S. R., Steen, V. D., & Wolfe, F. (1998). Estimates of the prevalence of arthritis and selected musculoskeletal disorders in the United States. *Arthritis and Rheumatism, 41,* 778–799.

Lechner, O., Hu, Y., Jafarian-Tehrani, M., Dietrich, H., Schwarz, S., Herold, M., Haour, F., & Wick, G. (1996). Disturbed immunoendocrine communication via the hypothalamo-pituitary- adrenal axis in murine lupus. *Brain, Behavior, and Immunity, 10,* 337–350.

Li, H. Y., Ericsson, A., & Sawchenko, P. E. (1996). Distinct mechanisms underlie activation of hypothalamic neurosecretory neurons and their medullary catecholaminergic afferents in categorically different stress paradigms. *Proceedings of the National Academy of Sciences, USA, 93,* 2359–2364.

Listwak, S., Barrientos, R. M., Koike, G., Ghosh, S., Gomez, M., Misiewicz, B., & Sternberg, E. M. (1999). Identification of a novel inflammation-protective locus in the fischer rat. *Mammalian Genome, 10,* 362–365. [in process citation]

Lo, T. N., Almeida, A. P., & Beaven, M. A. (1982). Dextran and carrageenan evoke different inflammatory responses in rat with respect to composition of infiltrates and effect of indomethacin. *Journal of Pharmacology and Experimental Therapeutics, 221,* 261–267.

Lo, T. N., Almeida, A. P., & Beaven, M. A. (1984). Effect of indomethacin on generation of chemotactic activity in inflammatory exudates induced by carrageenan. *European Journal of Pharmacology, 99*, 31–43.

MacPhee, I. A. M., Antoni, F. A., & Mason, D. W. (1989). Spontaneous recovery of rats from experimental allergic encephalomyelitis is dependent on regulation of the immune system by endogenous adrenal corticosteroids. *Journal of Experimental Medicine, 169*, 431–445.

Madden, K. S., Felten, S. Y., Felten, D. L., Hardy, C. A., & Livnat, S. (1994a). Sympathetic nervous system modulation of the immune system. II. Induction of lymphocyte proliferation and migration in vivo by chemical sympathectomy. *Journal of Neuroimmunology, 49*, 67–75.

Madden, K. S., Moynihan, J. A., Brenner, G. J., Felten, S. Y., Felten, D. L., & Livnat, S. (1994b). Sympathetic nervous system modulation of the immune system. III. Alterations in T and B cell proliferation and differentiation in vitro following chemical sympathectomy. *Journal of Neuroimmunology, 49*, 77–87.

Madden, K. S., Thyagarajan, S., & Felten, D. L. (1998). Alterations in sympathetic noradrenergic innervation in lymphoid organs with age. *Annals of New York Academy of Sciences, 840*, 262–268.

Makino, S., Smith, M. A., & Gold, P. W. (1995). Increased expression of corticotropin-releasing hormone and vasopressin messenger ribonucleic acid (mRNA) in the hypothalamic paraventricular nucleus during repeated stress: Association with reduction in glucocorticoid receptor mRNA levels. *Endocrinology, 136*, 3299–3309.

Masi, A. T., & Chrousos, G. P. (1996). Hypothalamic-pituitary-adrenal-glucocorticoid axis function in rheumatoid arthritis. *Journal of Rheumatology, 23*, 577–581. [editorial; comment]

McEwen, B. S., Biron, C. A., Brunson, K. W., Bulloch, K., Chambers, W. H., Dhabhar, F. S., Goldfarb, R. H., Kitson, R. P., Miller, A. H., Spencer, R. L., & Weiss, J. M. (1997). The role of adrenocorticoids as modulators of immune function in health and disease: Neural, endocrine and immune interactions. *Brain Research. Brain Research Reviews, 23*, 79–133.

McFarlane, A. C., & Brooks, P. M. (1988). An analysis of the relationship between psychological morbidity and disease activity in rheumatoid arthritis. *Journal of Rheumatology, 15*, 926–931.

Miao, F. J., Janig, W., Green, P. G., & Levine, J. D. (1996a). Inhibition of bradykinin-induced synovial plasma extravasation produced by intrathecal nicotine is mediated by the hypothalamopituitary adrenal axis. *Journal of Neurophysiology, 76*, 2813–2821.

Miao, F. J., Janig, W., & Levine, J. (1996b). Role of sympathetic postganglionic neurons in synovial plasma extravasation induced by bradykinin. *Journal of Neurophysiology, 75*, 715–724.

Michelson, D., Stone, L., Galliven, E., Magiakou, M. A., Chrousos, G. P., Sternberg, E. M., & Gold, P. W. (1994). Multiple sclerosis is associated with alterations in hypothalamic-pituitary-adrenal axis function. *Journal of Clinical Endocrinology and Metabolism, 79*, 848–853.

Miller, S. C., Rapier, S. H., Holtsclaw, L. I., & Turner, B. B. (1995). Effects of psychological stress on joint inflammation and adrenal function during induction of arthritis in the Lewis rat. *Neuroimmunomodulation, 2*, 329–338.

Misiewicz, B., Poltorak, M., Gomez, M., Glowa, J. R., Gold, P. W., & Sternberg, E. M. (1996a). Intracerebroventricularly transplanted embryonic neuronal tissue from inflammatory-resistant F344/N rats decreases acoustic startle responses in inflammatory-susceptible LEW/N rats. *Cell Transplantation, 5*, 287–291.

Misiewicz, B., Poltorak, M., Raybourne, R. B., Gomez, M., Listwak, S., & Sternberg, E. M. (1997). Intracerebroventricular transplantation of embryonic neuronal tissue from inflammatory resistant into inflammatory susceptible rats suppresses specific components of inflammation. *Experimental Neurology, 146*, 305–314.

Misiewicz, B., Zelazowska, E., Raybourne, R. B., Cizza, G., & Sternberg, E. M. (1996b). Inflammatory responses to carrageenan injection in LEW/N and F344/N rats: LEW/N rats show sex- and age-dependent changes in inflammatory reactions. *Neuroimmunomodulation, 3*, 93–101.

Miyamasu, M., Misaki, Y., Izumi, S., Takaishi, T., Morita, Y., Nakamura, H., Matsushima, K., Kasahara, T., & Hirai, K. (1998). Glucocorticoids inhibit chemokine generation by human eosinophils. *Journal of Allergy Clinical Immunology, 101*, 75–83.

Moreland, L. W., Baumgartner, S. W., Schiff, M. H., Tindall, E. A., Fleischmann, R. M., Weaver, A. L., Ettlinger, R. E., Cohen, S., Koopman, W. J., Mohler, K., Widmer, M. B., & Blosch, C. M. (1997). Treatment of rheumatoid arthritis with a recombinant human tumor necrosis factor receptor (p75)-Fc fusion protein. *New England Journal of Medicine, 337*, 141–147. [see comments]

Mosmann, T. R., & Sad, S. (1996). The expanding universe of T-cell subsets: Th1, Th2 and more. *Immunol Today, 17*, 138–146. [see comments]

Nakagawa, H., Ikesue, A., Kato, H., Debuchi, H., Watanabe, K., Tsurufuji, S., Naganawa, M., & Mitamura, M. (1992). Changes in the levels of rat interleukin 8/CINC and gelatinase in the exudate of carrageenin-induced inflammation in rats. *Journal of Pharmacobio-dynamics, 15*, 461–466.

Nawata, H., Higuchi, K., Higashizima, M., Kato, K., & Ibayashi, H. (1984). Glucocorticoid receptors in cultured skin fibroblasts of normal and adrenocorticoid disorders. *Endocrinologica Japonica, 31*, 109–116.

Neeck, G., Federlin, K., Graef, V., Rusch, D., & Schmidt, K. L. (1990). Adrenal secretion of cortisol in patients with rheumatoid arthritis. *Journal of Rheumatology, 17*, 24–29.

Ollier, W. E., & MacGregor, A. (1995). Genetic epidemiology of rheumatoid disease. *British Medical Bulletin, 51*, 267–285.

Pal, S. B. (1970). The secretion rate of cortisol in patients with rheumatoid arthritis. *Clinica Chimica Acta, 29*, 129–137.

Peck, J. R., Smith, T. W., Ward, J. R., & Milano, R. (1989). Disability and depression in rheumatoid arthritis. A multi-trait, multi-method investigation. *Arthritis and Rheumatism, 32*, 1100–1106.

Pincus, T., Griffith, J., Pearce, S., & Isenberg, D. (1996). Prevalence of self-reported depression in patients with rheumatoid arthritis. *British Journal of Rheumatology, 35*, 879–883.

Radomski, M. W., Palmer, R. M., & Moncada, S. (1990). Glucocorticoids inhibit the expression of an inducible, but not the constitutive, nitric oxide synthase in vascular endothelial cells. *Proceedings of the National Academy of Sciences, USA, 87*, 10043–10047.

Raskind, M. A., Peskind, E. R., & Wilkinson, C. W. (1994). Hypothalamic-pituitary-adrenal axis regulation and human aging. *Annals of New York Academy of Sciences, 746*, 327–335.

Reber, P. M. (1993). Prolactin and immunomodulation. *American Journal of Medicine, 95*, 637–644.

Reveille, J. D. (1998). The genetic contribution to the pathogenesis of rheumatoid arthritis. *Current Opinion in Rheumatology, 10*, 187–200.

Rosewicz, S., McDonald, A. R., Maddux, B. A., Goldfine, I. D., Miesfeld, R. L., & Logsdon, C. D. (1988). Mechanism of glucocorticoid receptor down-regulation by glucocorticoids. *Journal of Biological Chemistry, 263*, 2581–2584.

Saldanha, C., Tougas, G., & Grace, E. (1986). Evidence for anti-inflammatory effect of normal circulating plasma cortisol. *Clinical and Experimental Rheumatology, 4*, 365–366.

Salvemini, D., Manning, P. T., Zweifel, B. S., Seibert, K., Connor, J., Currie, M. G., Needleman, P., & Masferrer, J. L. (1995). Dual inhibition of nitric oxide and prostaglandin production contributes to the antiinflammatory properties of nitric oxide synthase inhibitors. *Journal of Clinical Investigation, 96,* 301–308.

Salvemini, D., Wang, Z. Q., Bourdon, D. M., Stern, M. K., Currie, M. G., & Manning, P. T. (1996a). Evidence of peroxynitrite involvement in the carrageenan-induced rat paw edema. *European Journal of Pharmacology, 303,* 217–220.

Salvemini, D., Wang, Z. Q., Wyatt, P. S., Bourdon, D. M., Marino, M. H., Manning, P. T., & Currie, M. G. (1996b). Nitric oxide: A key mediator in the early and late phase of carrageenan- induced rat paw inflammation. *British Journal of Pharmacology, 118,* 829–838.

Samuelsson, B. (1987). An elucidation of the arachidonic acid cascade. Discovery of prostaglandins, thromboxane and leukotrienes. *Drugs, 33,* 2–9.

Sawchenko, P. E., Brown, E. R., Chan, R. K., Ericsson, A., Li, H. Y., Roland, B. L., & Kovacs, K. J. (1996). The paraventricular nucleus of the hypothalamus and the functional neuroanatomy of visceromotor responses to stress. *Progress in Brain Research, 107,* 201–222.

Sawchenko, P. E., Imaki, T., Potter, E., Kovacs, K., Imaki, J., & Vale, W. (1993). The functional neuroanatomy of corticotropin-releasing factor. *Ciba Foundation Symposium, 172,* 5–21, 21–29.

Schauenstein, K., Fassler, R., Dietrich, H., Schwarz, S., Kromer, G., & Wick, G. (1987). Disturbed immune-endocrine communication in autoimmune disease. Lack of corticosterone response to immune signals in obese strain chickens with spontaneous autoimmune thyroiditis. *Journal of Immunology, 139,* 1830–1833.

Schlaghecke, R., Beuscher, D., Kornely, E., & Specker, C. (1994). Effects of glucocorticoids in rheumatoid arthritis. Diminished glucocorticoid receptors do not result in glucocorticoid resistance. *Arthritis and Rheumatism, 37,* 1127–1131.

Schlaghecke, R., Kornely, E., Wollenhaupt, J., & Specker, C. (1992). Glucocorticoid receptors in rheumatoid arthritis. *Arthritis and Rheumatism, 35,* 740–744.

Schleimer, R. P. (1993). An overview of glucocorticoid anti-inflammatory actions. *European Journal of Clinical Pharmacology, 45,* S3-7; discussion S43–4.

Shanks, N., Harbuz, M. S., Jessop, D. S., Perks, P., Moore, P. M., & Lightman, S. L. (1998). Inflammatory disease as chronic stress. *Annals of New York Academy of Sciences, 840,* 599–607.

Sher, E. R., Leung, D. Y., Surs, W., Kam, J. C., Zieg, G., Kamada, A. K., & Szefler, S. J. (1994). Steroid-resistant asthma. Cellular mechanisms contributing to inadequate response to glucocorticoid therapy. *Journal of Clinical Investigation. 93,* 33–39.

Smith, E. W. (1995). Four decades of topical corticosteroid assessment. *Current Problems in Dermatology, 22,* 124–131.

Stenzel-Poore, M., Vale, W. W., & Rivier, C. (1993). Relationship between antigen-induced immune stimulation and activation of the hypothalamic-pituitary-adrenal axis in the rat. *Endocrinology, 132,* 1313–1318.

Sternberg, E. M. (1997). Neural–immune interactions in health and disease. *Journal of Clinical Investigation, 100,* 2641–2647.

Sternberg, E. M., Chrousos, G. P., Wilder, R. L., & Gold, P. W. (1992). The stress response and the regulation of inflammatory disease. *Annals of Internal Medicine, 117,* 854–866.

Sternberg, E. M., Hill, J. M., Chrousos, G. P., Kamilaris, T., Listwak, S. J., Gold, P. W., & Wilder, R. L. (1989a). Inflammatory mediator-induced hypothalamic-pituitary-adrenal axis activation is defective in streptococcal cell wall arthritis- susceptible Lewis rats. *Proceedings of the National Academy of Sciences, USA, 86,* 2374–2378.

Sternberg, E. M., Young, W. S. d., Bernardini, R., Calogero, A. E., Chrousos, G. P., Gold, P. W., & Wilder, R. L. (1989b). A central nervous system defect in biosynthesis of corticotropin- releasing hormone is associated with susceptibility to streptococcal cell wall-induced arthritis in Lewis rats. *Proceedings of the National Academy of Sciences, USA, 86,* 4771–4775.

Sugar, M. (1953). Arthritis and panhypopituitarism. *Journal of Clinical Endocrinology and Metabolism, 13,* 1118–1121.

Swain, M. G., & Maric, M. (1994). Prevention of immune-mediated arthritis in cholestatic rats: Involvement of endogenous glucocorticoids. *Gastroenterology, 107,* 1469–1474.

Takasu, N., Ohara, N., Yamada, T., & Komiya, I. (1993). Development of autoimmune thyroid dysfunction after bilateral adrenalectomy in a patient with Carney's complex and after removal of ACTH-producing pituitary adenoma in a patient with Cushing's disease. *Journal of Endocrinological Investigation, 16,* 697–702. [see comments]

Templ, E., Koeller, M., Riedl, M., Wagner, O., Graninger, W., & Luger, A. (1996). Anterior pituitary function in patients with newly diagnosed rheumatoid arthritis. *British Journal of Rheumatology, 35,* 350–356.

Terato, K., DeArmey, D. A., Ye, X. J., Griffiths, M. M., & Cremer, M. A. (1996). The mechanism of autoantibody formation to cartilage in rheumatoid arthritis: Possible cross-reaction of antibodies to dietary collagens with autologous type II collagen. *Clinical Immunology and Immunopathology, 79,* 142–154.

ThyagaRajan, S., Felten, S. Y., & Felten, D. L. (1998). Restoration of sympathetic noradrenergic nerve fibers in the spleen by low doses of L-deprenyl treatment in young sympathectomized and old Fischer 344 rats. *Journal of Neuroimmunology, 81,* 144–157.

Utsunomiya, I., Nagai, S., & Oh-ishi, S. (1991). Sequential appearance of IL-1 and IL-6 activities in rat carrageenin-induced pleurisy. *Journal of Immunology, 147,* 1803–1809.

van der Poll, T., & Lowry, S. F. (1997). Lipopolysaccharide-induced interleukin 8 production by human whole blood is enhanced by epinephrine and inhibited by hydrocortisone. *Infection and Immunity, 65,* 2378–2381.

Walker, S. E., McMurray, R. W., Houri, J. M., Allen, S. H., Keisler, D., Sharp, G. C., & Schlechte, J. A. (1998). Effects of prolactin in stimulating disease activity in systemic lupus erythematosus. *Annals of New York Academy of Sciences, 840,* 762–772.

Watkins, L. R., Goehler, L. E., Relton, J. K., Tartaglia, N., Silbert, L., Martin, D., & Maier, S. F. (1995). Blockade of interleukin-1 induced hyperthermia by subdiaphragmatic vagotomy: Evidence for vagal mediation of immune-brain communication. *Neuroscience Letters, 183,* 27–31.

Wei, X. Q., Charles, I. G., Smith, A., Ure, J., Feng, G. J., Huang, F. P., Xu, D., Muller, W., Moncada, S., & Liew, F. Y. (1995). Altered immune responses in mice lacking inducible nitric oxide synthase. *Nature, 375,* 408–411.

Wilder, R., Remmers, E., Longman, R., Du, Y., O'Hare, A., Cannon, G., & Griffiths, M. (1996). A genome scan localizes five non-MHC loci controlling collagen-induced arthritis in rats. *Nature Genetics, 14,* 82–85.

Wilder, R. L. (1998). Hormones, pregnancy, and autoimmune diseases. *Annals of New York Academy of Sciences, 840,* 45–50.

Wilder, R. L., Allen, J. B., & Hansen, C. (1987). Thymus-dependent and -independent regulation of Ia antigen expression in situ by cells in the synovium of rats with streptococcal cell wall-induced arthritis. Differences in site and intensity of expression in euthymic, athymic, and cyclosporin A-treated LEW and F344 rats. *Journal of Clinical Investigation, 79,* 1160–1171.

Wilder, R. L., Calandra, G. B., Garvin, A. J., Wright, K. D., & Hansen, C. T. (1982). Strain and sex variation in the susceptibility to streptococcal cell wall-induced polyarthritis in the rat. *Arthritis and Rheumatism, 25,* 1064–1072.

Williams, R. H., Wilson, J. D., & Foster, D. W. (1992). *Williams' textbook of endocrinology* (8th ed.). Philadelphia: Saunders.

Yanovski, J. A., Yanovski, S. Z., Harrington, L., Gold, P. W., & Chrousos, G. P. (1995). Differences in the hypothalamic-pituitary-adrenal axis of black and white men. *Hormone Research, 44,* 208–212.

# Neuroendocrine Influences on the Pathogenesis of Psoriasis

SIBA PRASAD RAYCHAUDHURI, EUGENE M. FARBER

## I. INTRODUCTION

The effects of emotional stress on human physiology are enormous. The skin is the largest organ of the body. During periods of emotional stress it responds in variegated ways. Some of the characteristic responses of cutaneous tissue during stressful situations are flushing/pallor, increased perspiration, and increased activity of the sebaceous glands. We are familiar with the deleterious effects of stress on the natural history of various inflammatory diseases like asthma, rheumatoid arthritis, multiple sclerosis, and ulcerative colitis. Similarly, a number of skin disorders are exacerbated during periods of stress such as psoriasis, eczema, acne, urticaria, and many others. Among these inflammatory dermatoses, psoriasis is the most extensively studied condition in relation to the contributing role of psychoneuroimmunology.

Psoriasis is a relatively common chronic inflammatory skin disease, affecting 2% of populations worldwide (Farber & Peterson, 1961; Lomeholt, 1963). The lesions of psoriasis are characterized by erythema, scaling, and infiltration. In the majority of patients, the psoriatic plaques are distributed over the elbows, knees and scalp. Psoriasis is a nonfatal disease and usually requires life-long treatment but on occasion, psoriasis can be a source of significant morbidity. Generalized involvement of the body (erythroderma), extensive pustular lesions, and an associated mutilating arthritis are severe forms of psoriasis. As of now, there is no cure for psoriasis.

Cytokines, chemokines, growth factors, adhesion molecules, neuropeptides, and T-cell receptors act in integrated ways to evolve in unique inflammatory and proliferative processes typical of psoriasis. The concept of neuroimmunology as it relates to psoriasis is relatively new. Farber, Nickoloff, Recht, and Fraki in 1986 first proposed a possible role of neuropeptides in the pathogenesis of psoriasis (Farber et al., 1986). Subsequently several other investigators also have reported a marked proliferation of terminal cutaneous nerves and an upregulation of neuropeptide positive fibers in psoriatic lesions (Al'Abadie, Senior, Bleehen, & Gawkrodger, 1992; Naukkarinen, Harvima, Aalto, Harvima, & Horsmanheimo 1991; Naukkarinen, Nickoloff & Farber, 1989). On the other hand, there is substantial evidence that activated T lymphocytes play a key role in the pathogenesis of psoriasis. It is essential to understand the relationships between neurogenic factors and activation of the T cells. In this chapter we will present the neuroendocrine factors that influence the inflammatory and proliferative processes of psoriasis.

## II. NEUROGENIC INFLAMMATION AND THE SKIN

The cutaneous sensory nervous system, in addition to conduction of sensory impulses, can also induce a local inflammatory response. Thomas Lewis (1930) clarified the concept of the "triple response" that is observed in human skin in response to an injury. The triple response relates to the morphological changes manifested by wheal, local erythema, and flare in response to an external stimulus. Lewis (1930) suggested that injury to the skin leads to stimulation of sensory nerves, resulting in transmission of impulses to the spinal cord, as well as antidromic stimulation of connecting fibers which innervate the adjacent skin. Jancso, Jancso-Gabor, and Szolcsanyi in the 1960s showed that the inflammatory responses in the skin secondary to stimulation of sensory nerves could be abolished by denervation, and they postulated that the inflammatory response was due to release of neurohormones (Jancso et al., 1967). This process of antidromic stimulation of dorsal roots resulting in vasodilatation, exudation of plasma, and migration of leukocytes is refered to as neurogenic inflammation.

In the past 30 years, extensive research has been carried out to identify the neurohormones as predicted by Lewis and Jancso. Now we know that the neurogenic inflammaation is due to elease of neuropeptides from the unmyelinated sensory nerve ending, and this process afects a variety of immune cells

**TABLE I   Neuropeptide Positive Fibres Identified in Human Skin**

Substance P

Vasoactive intestinal polypeptide

Calcitonin gene-related peptide

Neuropeptide Y

Neurokinin A

Somatostatin

Neurotensin

Galanin

Atrial natriuretic peptide

Peptide histidine methionine

y-Melanocyte stimulating hormone

**TABLE II   Biological Actions of Substance P**

| Keratinocyte | Stimulation of IL-1, GM-CSF synthesis and secretion, comitogen with CGRP, LTB 4 |
|---|---|
| Fibroblasts | Stimulates proliferation |
| Endothelial cells | Stimulates proliferation, increases permeability, upregulation of ELAM-1 |
| Neutrophil | Stimulates chemotaxis, phagocytosis |
| Mast cell | Degranulation, stimulates proliferation and survival in culture |
| Lymphocytes | Stimulates proliferation and IL-2 synthesis, increases IgA, IgM and heavy chain mRNA production |
| Macrophage | Stimulates IL-1, IL-6, TNF secretion |
| Monocyte | Increases chemotaxis, phagocytosis, and arachadonic acid synthesis |

through specific neuropeptide receptors (Blalock, Bost, & Smith, 1985; Weihe & Hartschuh, 1988; Wiedermann, 1987).

A large number of neuropeptides with immunohistochemical staining and/or radioimmunoassay have been identified in the skin (Table I). Among these, substance P (SP), vasoactive intestinal peptide (VIP), and calcitonin gene-related peptide (CGRP) have been most extensively studied in relation to a cutaneous inflammatory reaction. The biological effects of these neuropeptides on various components of cutaneous tissue are listed in Tables II, III, and IV.

In normal human skin, substance P-positive nerve fibers are present in the dermis, epidermis, Meissners corpuscles, and around the sweat glands (Bloom & Polak, 1983; Tainio, Vaalasti, & Rechardt, 1987). The flare component of the triple response can be inhibited by the H-1 receptor antagonist (Hagermark, Hokfelt, & Pernow, 1978). This suggests that the flare response is due to the actions of histamine released by mast cells. Substance P increases permeability of the vessels by activation of the NK-1 receptors on postcapillary venules and by releasing histamine from the mast cells (Devillier et al., 1986).

**TABLE III   Biological Actions of Calcitonin Gene-Related Peptide**

| Keratinocyte | Proliferation in association with SP |
|---|---|
| Endothelial cell | Proliferation upregulation of ELAM-1 |
| Mast cell | Degranulation |
| Langerhans cell | Inhibit antigen presentation |
| T lymphocytes | Chemotactic T-cell proliferation |

**TABLE IV  Biological Actions of Vasoactive Intestinal Polypeptide**

| Keratinocytes | Proliferation increased adenylate cyclase activity |
|---|---|
| Mast cell | Degranulation |
| Endothelial cell | Proliferation |
| Neutrophil | Chemotaxis |
| | Inhibit proliferation |
| Lymphocyte | Inhibit nk cell activity |

CGRP is widely distributed in the skin and is one of the most abundant neuropeptides. It is commonly colocalized with substance P (Gibbins, Wattchow, & Conventry, 1987). Distribution of CGRP-positive nerve fibers in the skin is similar to substance P nerve fibers. Intradermal injection of CGRP induces a local erythema which can be observed for several hours.

Vasoactive intestinal peptide is mainly found in nerve fibers around the arteriolar walls and acini of sweat glands (Bloom & Polak, 1983). Intradermal injection of VIP causes a wheal and flare response. As the axon-reflex flare response fades, a local area of erythema appears due to increased blood flow (Anand, Bloom, & Mcgregor, 1983).

## III. STRESS, PSORIASIS, AND PSYCHONEUROIMMUNOLOGY

Over decades of observations, physicians and patients have learned that stressful life events and psychosocial factors are important in the onset or exacerbation of psoriasis. In several studies of large groups of patients, it has been observed that stress plays an important role in the onset and course of psoriasis. Farber and Nall reported that 33% of 5600 patients noticed the appearance of new lesions at the time of worry (Farber & Nall, 1974). In a series of 536 patients, Braun-falco reported that, in 42%, worry precipitated an exacerbation of psoriasis (Braun-Falco, Burg, & Farber, 1972). Fava, Perini, Santonastaso, and Fornasa (1980) correlated the appearance or exacerbation of psoriasis with stressful events in 80% of patients. Seville (1977) investigated the appearance of psoriasis in a follow-up study consisting of 132 patients for 3 years. In this study he observed that a specific stress occurred within 1 month before the appearance of psoriasis in 39% of subjects (Seville, 1977). Recently, we have reported that patients with higher levels of distress had a greater surface area involvement with psoriasis as compared to the patients who were relatively emotionally stable (Raychaudhuri & Gross, 2000). In the same study, we observed that, in distressed patients, remissions were less frequent.

Understanding regarding the interactions between the hypothalamo-pituitary-adrenal axis and immune-mediated inflammatory reactions has expanded enormously. The field of science which investigates this complex bidirectional interactions between the nervous system and immune system is known as psychoneuroimmunology (Ader, 1981; Felten, Cohen, Ader, Felten, & Carlson, 1991; Jankovic, Markovic, & Spector, 1987). The nervous system and the immune system have been found to share recognition molecules originating from both systems. This bidirectional communication between the nervous system and the immune system is often mediated by the endocrine system. There is now ample evidence that immunocompetent cells express receptors for various neurohormones and neuropeptides. Receptors for neuropeptides like VIP and somatostatin have been found on lymphocytes (Goetzl, Turck, & Sreedharan, 1991). Receptors for glucocorticoids, estrogens, androgens, $\beta$-adrenergic catecholamines, and neurotensin have been found on T cells (Gorman & Locke, 1989; Motulsky & Insel, 1982). Receptors for the cytokines IL-1 and IL-3 have been demonstrated in the brain (Farrar, Hill, Harel-Bellan, & Vinocour, 1987).

How stress influences the inflammatory and the proliferative processes of psoriasis is not clearly understood. Among the cardinal features of psoriasis, in addition to stress as a trigger, are symmetry, exacerbations and remissions, and exogenous and endogenous Koebner phenomenon. Correlating the clinical observation that stress exacerbates psoriasis and the symmetric distribution, Farber proposed a role for neuropeptides in its pathogenesis (Farber et al., 1986). The theory suggests that the release of substance P (SP) and other neuropeptides from unmyelinated terminations of sensory nerve fibers in the skin causes local neurogenic inflammatory responses that trigger psoriasis in a genetically predisposed person.

Stressful events can alter the substance P level in the CNS and in the periphery. In an animal model, it has been reported that stress can increase levels of substance P in the adrenal glands by activating the descending autonomic fibers (Vaupel, Jarry, Schlomer, & Wuttke, 1988). Local release of neuropeptides from sensory nerves in the skin, however, has not been measured after stressful stimuli in either animals or humans. Some of the descending autonomic fibers innervate opiod interneurons in the dorsal horn and, as interneurons exists in the spinal cord for the substance P-containing nerves, it is possible that descending autonomic paths can cause release of cutaneous neuropeptides (Farber, Rein, & Lanigan, 1991).

Stressful conditions stimulate the hypothalamic-pituitary-adrenal axis, resulting in increased blood levels of ACTH, corticosteroids and adrenaline. Recent results suggest that, in addition to these known conventional endocrine changes, there is significant elevation in the levels of nerve growth factor (NGF) during various stressful conditions (Luppi et al., 1993; Maestripieri, De Simone, Aloe, & Alleva, 1990). NGF can influence an inflammatory reaction in a number of ways. It is involved with the mechanisms of T-lymphocyte proliferation and activation and mast cell degranulation (Table V) (Aloe & Levi-Mantalcini, 1977; Pearce & Thrompson, 1986). Thus, in psoriatic patients stress-induced neurohormonal agents like SP and NGF can contribute significantly to the inflammatory processes of psoriasis.

## IV. ROLE OF CUTANEOUS NERVES AND NEUROPEPTIDES IN THE PATHOGENESIS OF PSORIASIS

A functional role for cutaneous nerves and neuropeptides in the pathogenesis of psoriasis is supported by increasing numbers of biochemical and clinical studies. An increased number of neural filaments in both lesional and symptomless psoriatic skin have been reported by Weddell, Cowan, Palmer, and Ramaswamy (1965). With the development of immunohistochemical staining, it is much easier to stain cutaneous nerves and neuropeptides. We were the first to report that there are an increased number of substance P-containing nerves in psoriatic epidermis (Naukkarinen et al., 1989). Other investigators have published similar findings and also demonstrated VIP

containing nerves in psoriatic plaques (Al'Abadie et al., 1992; Naukkarinen et al., 1991). Recently, we performed a double-labeled immunofluorescence study to identify the nerves and neuropeptides in psoriatic tissues (Jiang, Raychaudhuri, & Farber, 1998). Results of our study showed that SP- and CGRP-containing neuropeptide nerve fibers are denser in the psoriatic epidermis. Direct measurement of neuropeptides by radioimmunoassay from the lesional psoriatic biopsies in a majority of studies have shown increased levels of substance P and/or VIP (Anand et al., 1991; Eedy, Johnston, Shaw, & Buchanan, 1991; Pincelli et al., 1992; Wallengren, Ekman, & Sunder, 1987). However, there are other reports that differ. Wallengreen reported reduced VIP level in a suction blister raised from psoriatic plaques (Wallengren et al., 1987), Pincelli et al. (1992) reported reduced levels of substance P in chronic psoriatic plaques, and Anand et al., (1991) found no difference in SP levels in the psoriatic plaques compared to that seen in normal skin. The conflicting results obtained in these studies may be due to several factors. It is unknown when SP and VIP appear and where they are located in the developing lesion. As well, neuropeptide levels are difficult to measure because they are readily metabolized. In a relatively new study, Naukkarinen, Harvima, Paukkonen, Aalto, and Horsmanheimo (1993) studied the dynamics of neuropeptides in tape-strip-induced evolving psoriatic lesions and mature psoriatic plaques. The authors reported that very few nerves contained SP, VIP, or CGRP in control skin, nonlesional skin, and Koebner-negative psoriatic skin. In the evolving Koebner-positive lesions, at the end of 1 week, SP-positive fibers were found in the papillary dermis in all the lesions, and VIP-positive fibers were observed around the capillaries in 66% of the lesions (Naukkarinen et al., 1993). SP fibers were more abundant in mature psoriatic plaques. We conducted a study in 28 patients with psoriasis to identify SP, VIP, and CGRP in the skin biopsies and observed an increase in the number of SP-positive intraepidermal nerve fibers in lesional psoriatic skin specimens (2.8 nerves/ mm biopsy) compared with nonlesional psoriatic skin (.01 nerves/mm biopsy) and normal skin (.04 nerves/ mm biopsy). Increased intraepidermal VIP- and CGRP-positive fibers were also observed in the psoriatic lesions (Chan, Smoller, Raychauduri, Jiang, & Farber, 1997).

The actions of neuropeptides such as SP, VIP, and CGRP can be of great significance in the inflammatory and proliferative process in psoriasis. Keratinocyte hyperproliferation, the hallmark of psoriasis, can be triggered by VIP (Haegerstrand, Jonzon, Dalsgaard, &

**TABLE V  Expression of NGF in the Keratinocytes of Lesional and Nonlesional Psoriatic Skin, Lichen Planus, and Normal Skin**

| Biopsies | Numbers | No. of NGF positive keratinocytes (KC) ($x \pm SD$) | |
| --- | --- | --- | --- |
| | | GF$^+$ KC (mm) | NGF$^+$ KC (mm$^2$) |
| Psoriatic skin | 8 | $12.11 \pm 7.15$ | $84.68 \pm 46.35$ |
| Nonlesional skin | 8 | $2.55 \pm 1.71$ | $44.80 \pm 29.96$ |
| Normal skin | 5 | $0.64 \pm 0.40$ | $18.88 \pm 11.76$ |
| Lichen Planus | 5 | $0.59 \pm 1.31$ | $7.54 \pm 16.86$ |

Nilsson, 1989). CGRP acts synergistically with SP to stimulate keratinocyte proliferation (Wilkinson, 1989), and both SP and VIP can enhance the mitogenic effect of leukotrine B4 on human keratinocyte (Rabier, & Wilkinson, 1991). Degranulation (Brody, 1984) and increased number of mast cells (Cox, 1976) seen in early lesions of psoriasis can be induced by substance P (Erjavec et al., 1981). CGRP, a potent mitogenic factor for endothelial cells (Haegerstrand, Dalsgaard, Jonzon, Larsson, & Nilsson, 1990), might explain angiogenesis observed in the developing lesions of psoriasis (Pinkus & Mehregan, 1966). One of the earliest histologic changes occurring in the psoriatic lesion is infiltration by leukocytes (Ragaz & Ackerman, 1979). Increased adhesion of peripheral blood lymphocytes to endothelium has been observed in psoriasis (Le Roy, Brown, & Graes, 1991; Sackstein, Falanga, Streilein, & Chin, 1988). Both SP and CGRP have been reported to enhance adhesion of lymphomononuclear cells (Rein & Karasek, 1992; Sung et al., 1992). Further, it has been shown that substance P can induce the expression of endothelial leukocyte adhesion molecules (ELAM-1) on postcapillary dermal vessels (Matis, Lavker, & Murphy, 1990). Substance P can cause chemotaxis of neutrophils (Tomoe, Iwamoto, Tomioka, & Yoshida, 1992), stimulate IL-2 synthesis (Calvo, Chavanel, & Senica, 1992) in T cells, and induce IL-1 secretion from keratinocytes (Ansel et al., 1990). All of these functions can contribute significantly to the pathogenesis of psoriasis. Intradermal injection of SP, VIP, and CGRP in normal human skin has been reported to induce rapid time dependent neutrophil infiltration (Smith, Barker, Morris, MacDonald, & Lee, 1993). The same authors also observed that SP induced marked upregulation of E-selectin expression.

Krogstad, Swanbeck, and Wallin (1995) observed that local infiltration of the psoriatic plaques with mepivacaine caused a 40% reduction of blood flow in the lesions. Surface anesthesia of UVB-induced erythema did not affect regional blood flow. It is known that cutaneous anesthesia can prevent vasodilatation induced by the axon reflex (Wardell, Naver, Nilsson, & Wallin, 1993). This observation supports the idea that a local neurogenic mechanism is active in the psoriatic plaque. Striking evidence for the role of neurogenic inflammation in psoriasis comes from studies where peripheral nerve sectioning resulted in clearing of psoriatic plaques. We have reported a number of patients where psoriatic lesions resolved at the site of anesthesia subsequent to damage of sensory nerves (Farber, Lanigan, & Boer, 1990; Raychaudhuri & Farber, 1993). In one patient, it was very interesting to observe that psoriasis resolved at

the anesthetic area over the knee and, with the return of sensation, psoriasis reappeared at the same site (Farber et al., 1990).

These findings encouraged us to look for the cause of neural proliferation and upregulation of neuropeptides in psoriatic tissues. Because nerve growth factor (NGF) plays a role in regulating innervation (Wyatt, Shooeter, & Davies, 1990) and upregulating neuropeptides (Lindsay & Harmar, 1989; Schwartz, Pearson, & Johnson, 1982), we decided to investigate the role of NGF in the lesional and nonlesional psoriatic skin, normal skin, and in other inflammatory skin diseases.

We found that keratinocytes in lesional and nonlesional psoriatic tissue express high levels of NGF compared to that seen in the controls (Table V) (Raychaudhuri, Jiang, & Farber, 1998). In a separate publication, we reported a marked upregulation of NGF-R (nerve growth factor-recptor) in psoriatic lesions (Farber, Chan, Raychaudhuri, & Smoller, 1996).

Nerve growth factor is mitogenic to keratinocytes and protects keratinocytes from apoptosis (Pincelli et al., 1997; Wilkinson, Theeuwes, & Farber, 1994). NGF recruits mast cells and promotes their degranulation, both early events in a developing lesion of psoriasis (Aloe & Levi-Mantalcini, 1977; Pearce & Thrompson, 1986). In addition, NGF activates T lymphocytes and recruits inflammatory cellular infiltrates (Bischoff & Dahinden, 1992; Lambiase et al., 1997; Thorpe, Werrbach-Perez, & Perez-Polo, 1987). Recently, we observed that NGF induces expression of a potent chemokine, RANTES, in the keratinocytes. RANTES is chemotactic for resting CD4+ memory T cells and activated naive and memory T cells (Schall, 1991). It is likely that overexpression of NGF precedes the influx of mast cells and lymphocytes which, in turn, initiates an inflammatory reaction contributing to the pathogenesis of psoriasis.

## V. IS PSORIASIS A NEUROIMMUNOLOGIC DISEASE?

Many authors view psoriasis as an autoimmune disease induced by an unidentified antigen (Chang et al., 1997; Valdimarsson, Baker, Jonsdottir, & Fry, 1986). However, T-cell activation alone fails to clarify various salient features of psoriasis. It does not explain the Koebner phenomenon, the symmetrical distribution of psoriasis lesions, proliferation of cutaneous nerves, and the upregulation of neuropeptides in psoriatic tissue (Al'Abadie et al., 1992; Farber et al., 1986; Naukkarinen et al., 1989, 1991). Also, it does not have an explanation for the striking clinical observation that psoriasis resolves at sites of anesthesia (Farber et al., 1990; Raychaudhuri & Farber, 1993).

It is well known that psoriasis frequently appears at sites of trauma. A wound induces a reaction characterized by proliferation of keratinocytes, fibroblasts, vascular elements, and nerves and an accumulation of inflammatory cells. Recent reports suggest that NGF produced by the keratinocytes plays a role in wound healing (Ansel et al., 1995; Diamond, Holmes, & Coughin, 1992). NGF promotes axonal regeneration and reinnervation of terminal cutaneous nerves. In nonpsoriatics, healing stops after a finite time, depending on the nature of the wound. In psoriatics, a wound frequently results in papulosquamous lesions.

Histologically, a psoriatic lesion is characterized by hyperkeratosis, parakeratosis, acanthosis, angiogenesis, neutrophilic microabscesses, and lymphomononuclear cell infiltrates. In addition, in the past decade another characteristic histological feature of psoriasis has been reported: hyperproliferation of cutaneous nerves (Al'Abadie et al., 1992; Naukkarinen et al., 1989). Figures 1A and 1B represent histological sections from a psoriatic lesion and normal control skin.

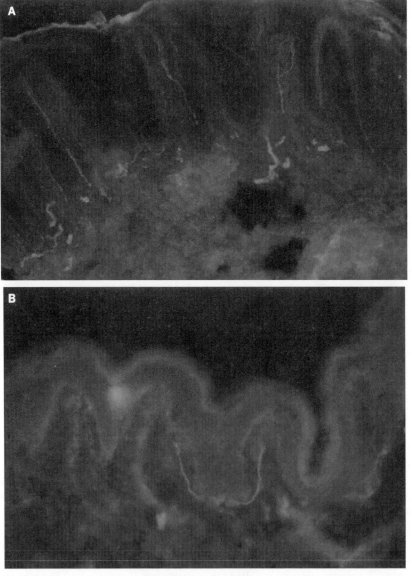

**FIGURE 1** (A) Psoriasis lesion stained with NGF-R antibody. Note: significant proliferation of the terminal cutaneous nerve fibers in the papillary dermis. (B) A healed lesion stained with the same antibody shows only few nerve fibers (magnification X200).

Marked proliferation of terminal cutaneous nerves in the active psoriatic plaque is evident.

It is worth noting that we observed marked upregulation of NGF in nonlesional psoriatic skin as well (Table V). In another study in which we investigated NGF-R expression, we found similar results (Farber et al., 1996). We also studied the expression of NGF and NGF-R in lichen planus, which is also an inflammatory skin disease. No upregulation of NGF in the keratinocytes or increased expression of NGF-R in the cutaneous nerves of lichen planus lesions was noticed (Farber et al., 1996; Raychaudhuri et al., 1998).

These findings suggest that the increased expression of NGF in the keratinocytes of lesional and nonlesional psoriatic tissue may be an early event in the pathogenesis of psoriasis. Proliferation of keratinocytes induced by a wound will result in significantly higher levels of NGF in lesion-free skin compared to control skin. Elevated levels of NGF induce an inflammatory response (Table VI), proliferation of nerves, and upregulation of neuropeptides such as SP and CGRP. Increased levels of neuropeptides and NGF, in addition to their proinflammatory effects, will induce keratinocyte proliferation (Haegerstrand et al., 1989; Pincelli et al., 1997;

**TABLE VI   Inflammogenic Properties of NGF**

1. Degranulates mast cells
2. Upregulates expression of SP, CGRP
3. Activates T cells
4. Upregulates expression of RANTES in keratinocytes
5. Recruits inflammatory cellular infiltrates

Wilkinson, 1989; Wilkinson et al., 1994), which, in turn, will result in increased expression of NGF. Thus, a vicious cycle of a proliferative and inflammatory process is established in one who is genetically psoriatic (Figure 2). In subjects without psoriasis, the expression of NGF is three to four times less per square millimeter of epidermis than that seen in nonlesional psoriatic skin (Table V). The healing events therefore do not generate the critical levels of NGF and neuropeptides to initiate or maintain cascades essential for a chronic inflammatory reaction.

Studies have reported that psychosocial stressful events result in increased levels of NGF in blood and NGF mRNA synthesis in the hypothalamus (Aloe, Alleva, and De Simone, 1990; Luppi et al., 1993;

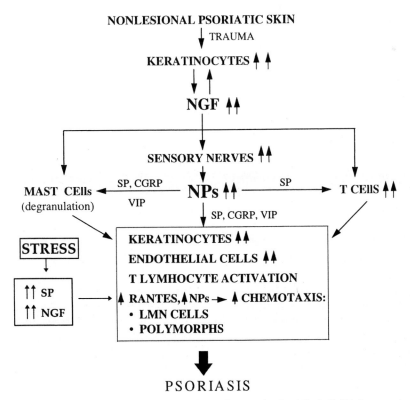

**FIGURE 2**   Role of neurogenic inflammation in the pathogenesis of psoriasis (↑/↑↑, increase in amount/number; LMN, lymphomononuclear cells; NPs, neuropeptides).

Maestripieri et al., 1990). Thus, it is likely that a similar cascade of events as mentioned in the preceding paragraph occurs in distressed psoriatic patients. Therefore, NGF plays a crucial role in the development of an isomorphic lesion and is also responsible for exacerbation of psoriasis during stressful life events.

Currently the alleged role of an antigen in psoriasis is hypothetical; no antigen has yet been discovered for psoriasis. Wrone-Smith and Nickoloff (1996) have reported that, in severe combined immune deficiency (SCID) mice, transplanted nonlesional psoriatic skin converts to a psoriatic plaque subsequent to intradermal delivery of activated T cells. In this model, T cells which induced psoriasis in the nonlesional psoriatic skin were artificially activated with an antigen cocktail. Since an artificial antigen cocktail does not exist in psoriatic skin, we think it is possible that local epidermal and dermal factors such as NGF and SP may be responsible for lesional T lymphocyte activation. Recently, we have identified increased levels of RANTES, a chemokine in psoriatic keratinocytes (Raychaudhuri et al., 1998). RANTES in addition to its chemotactic property, also activates T cells (Schall, 1991).

## VI. PSYCHONEUROIMMUNOLOGY— A NEW APPROACH TO THE TREATMENT OF PSORIASIS

Elucidation of the role of neurogenic inflammation in the pathogenesis of psoriasis has opened a new chapter for the treatment of psoriasis. Currently extensive research is ongoing to design drugs which counter the inflammatory events induced by the neuropeptides.

Neuropeptide receptor analogues have been reported to block the inflammatory effects of neuropeptides, such as plasma extravasation (Xu et al., 1991), nociceptor flexor reflexes (Wiesenfeld-Hallin, Xu, Hakanson, Feng, & Folkers, 1990), and erythematous responses (Wallengren & Moller, 1988). In vitro effects of neuropeptides on lymphocytes (Gozes, Brenneman, Fridkin, Asofsky, & Gozes, 1991), keratinocytes (Rabier & Wilkinson, 1991), and mast cells (Krumins & Broomfield, 1992) can be modulated by neuropeptide receptor antagonists as well. These results indicate that neuropeptide analogues can be applied for inhibiting the inflammatory and vascular changes associated with psoriasis.

Peptide T, a synthetic octapeptide, is a protease-resistant analogue of VIP (Ruff, 1989). The first report of the efficacy of peptide T in psoriasis arose from an anecdotal case report where psoriasis in an AIDS patient significantly improved following the intravenous infusion of peptide T (Wetterberg et al., 1987). Subsequently, IV use of peptide T has been reported to improve psoriasis (Marcusson et al., 1989; Talme et al., 1994). Farber, Cohen, Trozak, and Wilkinson (1991) evaluated the efficacy of peptide T by a direct administration into psoriatic lesion by miniosmotic pump. In a double blind, placebo-controlled study the authors reported that infusion of peptide T in nanogram amounts improved psoriatic lesions both clinically and histopathologically. The mechanism of action of peptide T in ameliorating psoriasis is not clear; possibilities suggested are antagonizing the action of VIP, upregulation of somatostatin in the psoriatic lesions, and immunomodulation (Farber et al., 1991; Johansson 1993, 1994).

Somatostatin analogue (Sandostatin) is the other neuropeptide analogue reported to be efficacious in psoriasis (Camisa et al., 1990). However, a high frequency of gall stones was noted among these patients. Somatostatin is a well known SP inhibitor (Manthya, 1991). Another neuropeptide modulating agent used as a therapeutic agent in psoriasis is Capsaicin (trans-8methyl-N-vanillyl-G-nonenamide), the extract of the hot pepper which depletes SP from the sensory C nerve fibers (Fitzgerald, 1983). Topical use of Capsaicin has been reported to be effective in psoriasis (Bernstein, Parish, Rapaport, Rosenbaum, & Roenigk, 1986), but it is unsuitable because it causes significant burning of the skin.

Substance P antagonists may also be useful therapeutic agents for psoriasis. Spantide, a structural analogue of SP, has been reported to inhibit delayed type cutaneous hypersensitivity reactions in healthy human volunteers (Wallengren, 1991). Spantide can also inhibit SP-induced keratinocyte proliferation in vitro (Rabier & Wilkinson, 1991). Peptide antagonists are metabolically unstable and can cause hypersensitivity reactions. The discovery of CP-96,345, a synthetic nonpeptide SP receptor (NK-1 receptor) antagonist has opened avenues to evaluate the effects of NK-1 receptor antagonism in man (Snider et al., 1991). In animal models, CP-96,345 has been found to inhibit plasma exudation induced by SP and can block nociceptor responses to noxious cutaneous stimuli (Lei, Barnes, & Rogers, 1992; Radhakrishna & Henry, 1991). These results indicate the applicability of SP antagonists in various inflammatory conditions, including psoriasis. Currently, various synthetic Substance P antagonists are being evaluated in psoriasis and other inflammatory diseases.

Peptidase-like neutral endopeptidase (NEP), angiotensin-converting enzyme (ACE), and dipeptidyl amino peptidase IV (DAP IV) are responsible for degradation of neuropeptides (Erdos & Skidgel, 1989). Glucocorticoids can induce NEP (Borson & Gruenert, 1991). This provides another explanation for the efficacy of glucocorticoids in the treatment of psoriasis. Neurogenic inflammation induced by substance P can be suppressed with exogenous human recombinant NEP (Nadel, 1991).

Understanding the factors that increases the morbidity of psoriasis is essential to providing effective care. A treatment regimen that does not control the exogenous and endogenous factors responsible for the increased severity of psoriasis is only partially effective. There is unequivocal evidence that stress is a triggering factor for the appearance or exacerbation of psoriasis (Braun-Falco et al., 1972; Farber & Nall, 1974; Fava, Perini, Santonastaso, & Fornasa, 1980; Seville, 1999; Raychaudhuri & Gross, 2000). This indicates that, in addition to the standard therapies available to dermatologists, it is advisable to consider stress relaxation measures. Psychological evaluation is a sine qua non for the management of psoriasis. This provides information on whether a patient has a primary emotional disorder or an emotional instability secondary to the psychosocial impact of psoriasis. In selected patients, antidepressants or anxiolytics may be appropriate. The other aspect of psychological evaluation is to identify underlying physical and emotional stresses, personality factors, and the way the patient reacts to stressful situations. Analysis of these factors will indicate the desirability of various stress relaxation modalities like hypnosis, biofeedback, meditation, visual imagery, and cognitive organization. A change in lifestyle or attitude can have a significant effect on the course of psoriasis. Studies have demonstrated that psychologic interventions such as hypnosis (Waxman, 1973) and biofeedback (Hughes, England, & Goldsmith, 1981; Polenghi et al., 1994; Winchell & Watts, 1988) are helpful in the treatment of psoriasis. At the Psoriasis Research Institute, we have initiated a total care program. By total care of psoriasis we mean exemplary skin care along with control of the associated factors that affect the morbidity of psoriasis. Total care encompasses the following: complete physical evaluation, evaluation of the type and extent of psoriasis, the personal wellness questionnaire analysis to measure patient's current health status, psychological examination, teaching stress reduction techniques, and patient education (self-help/mutual aid group). We expect that patients adhering to a total care program will require less medications and have longer periods of remission.

To elucidate the molecular and cellular events in the pathogenesis of psoriasis, it is essential to pay close attention to the neuroimmunologic events as mentioned in this chapter. Clearance of psoriatic lesions at sites of anesthesia following nerve injury and exacerbation of psoriasis due to emotional trauma suggest an indisputable role for neurogenic inflammation in the inflammatory and proliferative reactions of psoriasis.

## References

Ader, R. (Ed.) (1981). *Psychoneuroimmunology*. San Diego: Academic Press.

Al'Abadie, M. S. K., Senior, H. J., Bleehen, S. S., & Gawkrodger, D. J. (1992). Neurogenic changes in psoriasis. An imunohistochemical study. *Journal of Investigative Dermatology, 98*, 535. [abstract]

Aloe, L., & Levi-Montalcini, R. (1977). Mast cells increase in tissues of neonatal rats injected with the nerve growth factor. *Brain Research, 133*, 358–366.

Aloe, L., Alleva, E., & De Simone, R. (1990). Changes of NGF level in mouse hypothalamus following intermale aggressive behavior: Biological and immunohistochemical evidence. *Behavioural Research, 39*, 53–61.

Anand, A., Bloom, S. R., & Mcgregor, G. P. (1983). Topical capsaicin pretreatment inhibits axon reflex vasodilation caused by somatostatin and vasoactive intestinal polypeptide in human skin. *British Journal of Pharmacology, 78*, 665–669.

Anand, P., Springall, D. R., Blank, M. A., Sellu, D., Polak, J. M., & Bloom, S. R. (1991). Neuropeptides in skin disease: Increased VIP in eczema and psoriasis but not axillary hyperhidrosis. *British Journal of Dermatology, 124*, 547–549.

Ansel, J. C., Kaynard, A. H., Armstrong, C. A., Olerud, J., Bunnett, N., & Payan, D. (1995). Skin-nervous system interactions. *Dermatology Foundation, 29*(1), 1–12.

Ansel, J., Perry, P., Brown, J., Damm, D., Phan, T., Hart, C., Luger, T., & Hefeneider, S. (1990). Cytokine modulation of keratinocyte cytokines. *Journal of Investigative Dermatology, 94*, 101S–107S.

Bernstein, J. E., Parish, L. C., Rapaport, M., Rosenbaum, M. M., & Roenigk, H. H., Jr. (1986). Effects of topically applied Capsaicin on moderate and severe psoriasis vulgaris. *Journal of American Academy of Dermatology, 15*, 504–507.

Bischoff, S. C., & Dahinden, C. A. (1992). Effect of nerve growth factor on the release of inflammatory mediators by mature human basophils. *Blood, 79*, 2662–2669.

Blalock, J. E., Bost, K. L., & Smith, M. E. (1985) Neuroendocrine peptide hormones and their receptors in the immune system production, processing and action. *Journal of Neuroimmunology, 10*, 31–40.

Bloom, S. R., & Polak, J. M. (1983). Regulatory peptides and the skin. *Clinical Experimental Dermatology, 8*, 3–18.

Borson, D. B., & Gruenert, D. C. (1991). Glucocorticoids induce neutral endopeptidase in transformed human tracheal epithelial cells. *American Journal of Physiology, 260*, L83–L89.

Braun-Falco, O., Burg, G., & Farber, E. M. (1972). Psoriasis: Eine Fragebogen—Studie bei 536 Patienten. *Munch Medicine Wochenshr, 114*, 1–15.

Brody, I. (1984). Mast cell degranulation in the evolution of acute eruptive guttate psoriasis vulgaris. *Journal of Investigative Dermatology, 82*, 460–464.

Calvo, C. F., Chavanel, G., & Senica, A. (1992). Substance P enhances interleukin-2 expression in activated human T cells. *Journal of Immunology, 148*, 3498–3504.

Camisa, C., O'Dorisio., T. M., Maceyko, R. F., Schacht, G. E., Mekhjian, H. S., & Howe B. A. (1990). Treatment of psoriasis with chronic subcutaneous administration of somatostatin analog 201–295 (sandostatin). I. An openlable pilot study. *Clevland Clinic Journal of Medicine, 57,* 71–76.

Chan, J., Smoller, B. R., Raychauduri, S. P., Jiang, W. Y., & Farber, E. M. (1997). Intraepidermal nerve fiber expression of calcitonin-gene related peptide, vasoactive intestinal peptide and substance P in psoriasis. *Archive of Dermatology Research, 289,* 611–616.

Chang, J. C. C., Smith, L. R., Froning, K. J., Kurland, H. H., Schwabe, B. J. Blumeyer, K. K., Karasek, M. A., Wilkinson, D. I., Farber, E. M., Carlo, D. J., & Borstoff, S. W. (1997). Persistance of T-Cell Clones in psoriatic lesions. *Archive of Dermatology, 133,* 703–708.

Cox, A. J. (1976). Mast cells in psoriasis. In E. M. Farber & A. J. Cox (Eds.), *Psoriasis. Proceedings of the Second International Symposium* (pp. 36–37). New York: York Medical Books.

Devillier, P., Regoli, D., Asseraf, A., Descours, B., Marsac, J., & Renoux, M. (1986). Histamine release and local responses of rat and human skin to substance P and other mammalian tachykinins. *Pharmacology, 32,* 340–347.

Diamond, J., Holmes, M., & Coughin, M. (1992). Endogenous NGF and nerve impulses regulate the collateral sprouting of sensory axons in the skin of the adult rat. *Journal of Neuroscience, 12,* 1454–1466.

Eedy, D. J., Johnston, C. F., Shaw, C., & Buchanan, K. D. (1991). Neuropeptides in psoriasis: An immunocytochemical and radio-immunoassay study. *Journal of Investigative Dermatology, 96,* 434–438.

Erdos, E. G., & Skidgel, R. A. (1989). Neutral endopeptidase and related regulators of peptide hormones. *Fedaration of American Society of Experimental Biology Journal, 3,* 145–151.

Erjavec, F., Lembeck, F., Florjanc-Irman, T., Skofitsch, G., Donnerer, J., Saria, A., & Holzer, P. (1981). Release of histamine by substance P. *Archive of Pharmacology, 317,* 67–70.

Farber, E. M., Nickoloff, B. J., Recht, B., & Fraki J. E. (1986). Stress, Symmetry, and Psoriasis: Possible role of neuropeptides. *Journal of American Academy of Dermatology, 14,* 305–311.

Farber, E. M., & Nall, M. L. (1974). The national history of psoriasis in 5,600 patients. *Dermatologica, 148,* 1–18.

Farber, E. M., & Peterson, J. B. (1961). Variations in the natural history of psoriasis. *California Medicine, 95,* 6–11.

Farber, E. M., Chan, J., Raychaudhuri, S. P., & Smoller, B. R. (1996). Increased Nerve Growth Factor Receptor (NGF-R) in papillary dermis of lesional psoriatic skin: Further evidence for a role of the sensory nervous systems in the pathogenesis of psoriasis. *British Journal of Dermatology, 135,* 841.

Farber, E. M., Cohen, E. N., Trozak, D. J., & Wilkinson, D. I. (1991). Peptide T improves psoriasis when infused into lesions in nanogram amounts. *Journal of American Academy of Dermatology, 25,* 658–664.

Farber, E. M., Lanigan, S. W., & Boer, J. (1990). The role of cutaneous sensory nerves in the maintenance of psoriasis. *International Journal of Dermatology, 29,* 418–420.

Farber, E. M., Rein, G., & Lanigan, S. W. (1991). Stress and psoriasis—Psychoneuroimmunologic mechanisms. *International Journal of Dermatology, 30,* 8–12.

Farrar, W. L., Hill, J. M., Harel-Bellan, A., & Vinocour, M. (1987). The immune logical brain. *Immunology Review, 100,* 361–378.

Fava, G. A., Perini, G. I., Santonastaso, P., & Fornasa, C. V. (1980). Life events and psychological distress in dermatological disorders: Psoriasis, chronic urticaria, and fungal infections. *British Journal of Medical Psychology, 53,* 277–282.

Felten, D. L., Cohen, N., Ader, R., Felten, S. Y., & Carlson, S. L. (1991). Central neural circuits involved in neural immune interaction. In R. Ader, D. L. Felten, & N. Cohn (Eds.), *Psychoneuroimmunology (II)* (pp. 3–25). San Diego, CA: Academic Press.

Fitzgerald, M. (1983). Capsaicin and sensory neurons: A review. *Pain, 15,* 109–130.

Gibbins, I. L., Wattchow, D., & Conventry, G. (1987). Two immunohistochemically identified populations of calcitonin gene-related peptide (CGRP)-immunoreactive axons in human skin. *Brain Research, 414,* 143–148.

Goetzl, E. J., Turck, C. W., & Sreedharan, S. P. (1991). Production and recognition of neuropeptides by cells of the immune system. In R. Ader, D. L. Felten, & N. Cohen (Eds.), *Psychoneuroimmunology (II)* (pp. 263–282). San Diego, CA: Academic Press.

Gorman, J. R., & Locke, S. E. (1989). Neural, endocrine and immune interactions. In H. I. Kaplan & B. J. Sadock (Eds.), *The comprehensive textbook of psychiatry* (pp. 111–125). Baltimore, Williams and Wilkinson.

Gozes, Y., Brenneman, D. E., Fridkin, M., Asofsky, R., & Gozes, I. (1991). A VIP antagonist distinguishes spinal cord receptors on spinal cord cells and lymphocytes. *Brain Research, 540,* 319–320.

Haegerstrand, A., Dalsgaard, C. J., Jonzon, B., Larsson, O., & Nilsson, J. (1990). Calcitonin gene-related peptide stimulates proliferation of human endothelial cells. *Proceedings of the National Academy of Sciences, USA, 87,* 3299–3303.

Haegerstrand, A., Jonzon, B., Dalsgaard, C. J., & Nilsson, J. (1989). Vasoactive intestinal polypeptide stimulates cell proliferation and adenylate cyclase activity of cultured human keratinocytes. *Proceedings of the National Academy of Sciences, USA, 86,* 5993–5996.

Hagermark, O., Hokfelt, T., & Pernow, B. (1978). Flare and itch induced by substance P in human skin. *Journal of Investigative Dermatology, 71,* 233–225.

Hughes, H. H., England, R., & Goldsmith, D. A. (1981). Biofeedback and psychotherapeutic treatment of psoriasis: A brief report. *Psychology Reports, 48,* 99–102.

Jancso, N., Jancso-Gabor, A., & Szolcsanyi, J. (1967). Direct evidence for neurogenic inflammation and its prevention by denervation and by pretreatment with capsaicin. *British Journal of Pharmacology, 31,* 138–151.

Jankovic, B. D., Markovic, B. M., & Spector, N. H. (1987). Neuroendocrine correlates of neuroimmunomodulation. *Annals of New York Academy of Sciences, 496,* 3–107.

Jiang, W.-Y., Raychaudhuri, S. P., & Farber, E. M. (1988). Double labeled immunofluorescence study of cutaneous nerves in psoriasis. *International Journal of Dermatology, 37,* 572–574.

Johansson, O., Hilliges, M., Talme, T., Marcusson, J. A., & Wetterberg, L. (1994). Somatostatin immunoreactive cells in lesional psoriatic human skin during peptide T treatment. *Acta Dermatology and Venereoelogy (Stockholm), 74,* 106–109.

Johansson, O., Hilliges, M., Talme, T., Marcusson, J. A., & Wetterberg, L. (1993). Speculation around the mechanism behind the action of peptide T in the healing of psoriasis. *Acta Dermatology and Venereology (Stockholm) 73,* 401–403.

Krogstad, A. L., Swanbeck, G., & Wallin, G. (1995). Axon—Reflex mediated vasodilatation in the psoriatic plaque? *Journal of Investigative Dermatology, 104,* 872–876.

Krumins, S. A., & Broomfield, C. (1992). Evidence of NK 1 and NK 2 tachykinin receptors and their involvement in histamine release in a murine mast cell line. *Neuropeptides, 21,* 65–72.

Lambiase, A., Bracci-Laudiero, L., Bonini, S., Bonini, S., Starace, G., D'Elios, M. M., De Carli, M., & Aloe, L. (1997). Human CD4+ T cell clones produce and release nerve growth factor and express high-affinity nerve growth factor receptors. *Journal of Allergy and Clinical Immunology, 100,* 408–414.

Le Roy, F., Brown, K. A., & Graes, M. W. (1991). Blood mononuclear cells from patients with psoriasis exhibit an enhanced adherence to cultured vascular endothelium. *Journal of Investigative Dermatology, 97*, 511–516.

Lei, Y. H., Barnes, P. J., & Rogers, D. F. (1992). Inhibition of neurogenic plasma exudation in guinea-pig airways by CP-96,345, a new nonpeptide NK1 receptor antagonist. *British Journal of Pharmacology, 105*, 261–262.

Lewis, T. (1930). Observation upon reaction of vessels in human skin to cold. *Heart 15*, 177.

Lindsay, R. M., & Harmar, A. J. (1989). Nerve growth factor regulates expression of neuropeptides genes in adult sensory neurons. *Nature, 337*, 362–364.

Lomeholt, G. (1963). *Psoriasis: Prevalence, spontaneous course and genetics: A census study on the prevalance of skin disease in the Faroe Islands.* Copenhagen, GEC Gad. 1–30.

Luppi, P., Levi-Montalcini, R., Bracci-Laudiero, L., Bertolini, A., Arletti, R., Tavernari, D., Vigneti, E., & Aloe, L. (1993). NGF is released into plasma during human preganancy: An oxytocin-mediated response? *Neuroreport, 4*, 1063–1065.

Maestripieri, D., De Simone, R., Aloe, L., & Alleva, E. (1990). Social status and nerve growth factor serum levels after agonistic encounters in mice. *Physiology and Behavior, 47*, 161–164.

Manthya, P. W. (1991). Supstance P and the inflammatory and Immune response. In S. E. Leeman, J. E. Krause, & F. Lembeck (Eds). Substance P and related peptides: Cellular and molecular physiology. *Annals of New York Academy of Sciences, 632*, 263–271.

Marcusson, J. A., Lazega, D., Pert, C. B., Ruff, M. R., Sundquist, K. G., & Wetterberg L. (1989). Peptide T and psoriasis. *Acta Dermatology and Venereology, Supplement (Stockholm), 146*, 117–121.

Matis, W. L., Lavker, R. M., & Murphy, G. F. (1990). Substance P induces the expression of an endothelial-leukocyte adhesion molecule by microvascular endothelium. *Journal of Investigative Dermatology, 94*, 492–495.

Motulsky, H. J., & Insel, P. A. (1982). Adrenergic receptors in man: direct identification, physiological regulation, and clinical alterations. *New England Journal of Medicine, 307*, 18–29.

Nadel, J. A. (1991). Neutral endopeptide modulates neurogenic inflammation. *European Respiratory Journal, 4*, 745–754.

Naukkarinen, A., Harvima, I., Paukkonen, K., Aalto, M. L., & Horsmanheimo, M. (1993). Immunohistochemical analysis of sensory nerves and neuropeptides and their contacts with mast cells in developing and mature psoriatic lesions. *Archive of Dermatology Research, 285*, 341–346.

Naukkarinen, A., Harvima, I. T., Aalto, M. L., Harvima, R. J., & Horsmanheimo, M. (1991). Quantitative analysis of contact sites between mast cells and sensory nerves in cutaneous psoriasis and lichen planus based on histochemical double staining technique. *Archeive of Dermatology Research, 283*, 433–437.

Naukkarinen, A., Nickoloff, B. J., & Farber, E. M. (1989). Quantification of cutaneous sensory nerves and their substance P content in psoriasis. *Journal of Investigative Dermatology, 92*, 126–129.

Pearce, F. L., & Thrompson, H. L. (1986). Some characteristics of histamine secretion from rat peritoneal mast cells stimulated with nerve growth factor. *Journal of Physiology, 372*, 379–393.

Pincelli, C., Fantini, F., Romualdi, P., Sevignani, C., Lesa, G., Benassi, L., & Giannetti, A. (1992). Substance P is diminished and VIP is augmented in psoriatic lesions and these peptides exert diparate effects on the proliferation of cultured human keratinocytes. *Journal of Investigative Dermatology, 98*, 421–427.

Pincelli, C., Haake, A. R., Benassi, L., Grassilli, E., Magnoni, C., Ottani, D., Polakowska, R., Franceschi, C., & Giannetti, A. (1997).

Autocrine nerve growth factor protects human keratinocytes from apoptosis through its high affinity receptor (TRK): A role for BCL-2. *Journal of Investigative Dermatology, 109*, 757–764.

Pinkus, H., & Mehregan, A. M. (1966). The Primary histologic lesion of seborrheic dermatitis and psoriasis. *Journal of Investigative Dermatology, 46*, 109–116.

Polenghi, M. M., Molinari, E., Gala, C., Guzzi, R., Garutti, C., & Finzi, A. F. (1994). Experience with psoriasis in a psychosomatic dermatology clinic. *Acta Dermato-Venereologica, 186*(Suppl.), 65–66.

Rabier, M., & Wilkinson, D. I. (1991). Neuropeptides modulate leukotrine B 4 mitogenicity toward cultured keratinocytes. *Clinical Research, 39*, 536a.

Radhakrishna, V., & Henry, J. L. (1991). Novel substance P antagonist, CP-96,345, blocks responses of cat spinal dorsal horn neurons to noxious cutaneous stimulation and substance P. *Neuroscience Letters, 132*, 39–43.

Ragaz, A., & Ackerman, B. (1979). Evolution, motivation and regression of lesions of psoriasis. *American Journal of Dermatopathology, 1*, 199–214.

Raychaudhuri, S. P., & Farber, E. M. (1993). Are sensory nerves essential for the pathogenesis of psoriasis? *Journal of American Academy of Dermatology, 28*, 488–489.

Raychaudhuri, S. P., & Gross, J. (2000). Psoriasis risk factors: Role of lifestyle practices. *Cutis* (in press).

Raychaudhuri, S. P., Jiang, W.-Y., & Farber, E. M. (1998). Psoriatic keratinocytes express high levels of nerve growth factor. *Acta Dermatology and Venereology, 78*, 84–86.

Raychaudhuri, S. P., Jiang, W.-Y., Eugene, E. M., Schall, T. J., Ruff, M. R., & Pert, C. B. (1998). Upregulation of RANTES in psoriatic keratinocytes: A possible pathogenic mechanism for psoriasis. *Acta Dermatology and Venereology, 79*, 9–11.

Rein, G., & Karasek, M. (1992). Effect of substance P on adhesion of a human monocyte cell line to fibronectin. *Clinical Research, 40*, 45a.

Ruff, M. R. (1989). Peptide T. *Drugs of the Future, 14*, 1049–1051.

Sackstein, R., Falanga, V., Streilein, J. W., & Chin, Y. H. (1988). Lymphocyte adheision to psoriatic dermal endothelium is medicated by a tissue-specific receptor/ligand interaction. *Journal of Investigative Dermatology, 91*, 423–428.

Schall, T. J. (1991). Biology of the RANTES/SIS cytokine family. *Cytokine, 3*, 165–183.

Schwartz, J., Pearson, J., & Johnson, E. (1982). Effect of exposure to anti-NGF on sensory neurons of adult rats and guinea pigs. *Brain Research, 244*, 378–381.

Seville, R. H. (1977). Psoriasis and stress. *British Journal of Dermatology, 97*, 297–302.

Smith, C. H., Barker, J. N., Morris, R. W., MacDonald, D. M., & Lee, T. H. (1993). Neuropeptides induce rapid expression of endothelial cell adhesion molecules and elicit granulocytic infiltration in human skin. *Journal of Immunology, 151*, 3274–3282.

Snider, R. M., Constantine, J. W., Lowe, J. A. 3rd, Longo, K. P., Lebel, W. S., Woody, H. A., Drozda, S. E., Desai, M. C., Vinick, F. J., Spencer, R. W., et al. (1991). A potent nonpeptide antagonist of the substance P (NK1) receptor. *Science, 25*, 1435–1437.

Sung, C. P., Arleth, A. J., Aiyar, N., Bhatnagar, P. K., Lysko, P. G., & Feuerstein, G. (1992). CGRP stimulates the adhesion of leukocytes to vascular endothelial cells. *Peptides, 13*, 429–434.

Tainio, H., Vaalasti, A., & Rechardt, L. (1987). The distribution of substance P-, CGRP-, galanin and ANP-like immunoreactive nerves in human sweat glands. *Histochemistry Journal, 19*, 375–380.

Talme, T., Lund-Rosell, B., Sundquist, K. G., Hilliges, M., Johansson, O., Wetterberg, L., & Marcusson, J. A. (1994). Peptide T: A new treatment for psoriasis? A review of our experiences. *Acta Dermatology and Venereology, supplement. (Stockholm)*, 186, 76–78.

Thorpe, L. W., Werrbach-Perez, K., & Perez-Polo, J. R. (1987). Effects of nerve growth factor on the expression of IL-2 receptors on cultured human lymphocytes. *Annals of New York Academy of Sciences*, 496, 310–311.

Tomoe, S., Iwamoto, I., Tomioka, H., & Yoshida, S. (1992). Comparison of substance P-induced and compound 48/80 induced neutrophil infiltrations in mouse skin. *International Archive of Allergy and Immunology*, 97, 237–242.

Valdimarsson, H., Baker, B. S., Jonsdottir, I., & Fry, L. (1986). Psoriasis: A disease of abnormal keratinocyte proliferation induced by T lymphocytes. *Immunology Today*, 7, 256–259.

Vaupel, R., Jarry, H., Schlomer, H. T., & Wuttke, W. (1988). Differential response of substance P containing subtypes of adrenomedullary cells to different stressors. *Endocrinology*, 123, 2140–2145.

Wallengren, J. (1991). Substance P antagonist inhibits immediate and delayed type cutaneous hypersensitivity reactions. *British Journal of Dermatology*, 124, 324–328.

Wallengren, J., & Moller, H. (1988). Some neuropeptides as modulators of experimental contact allergy. *Contact Dermatitis*, 19, 351–354.

Wallengren, J., Ekman, R., & Sunder, F. (1987). Occurrence and distribution of nueropeptides in human skin. An immunochemical study of normal skin and blister fluid from inflamed skin. *Acta Dermatologica and Venereologica (Stockholm)*, 67, 185–192.

Wardell, K., Naver, H. K., Nilsson, G. E., & Wallin, B. G. (1993). The cutaneous vascular axon reflex in humans characterized by laser doppler perfusion imaging. *Journal of Physiology (London)*, 460, 185–199.

Waxman, D. (1973). Behavior therapy of psoriasis—A hypnoanalytic and counter conditioning technique. *Postgraduate Medical Journal*, 49, 591–595.

Weddell, G., Cowan, M. A., Palmer, E., & Ramaswamy, S. (1965). Psoriatic skin. *Archive of Dermatology*, 91, 252–266.

Weihe, E., & Hartschuh, W. (1988). Multiple peptides in cutaneous nerves: Regulator under physiological conditions and a pathogenetic role in skin disease? *Seminars in Dermatology*, 7, 284–300.

Wetterberg, L., Alexius, B., Saaf, J., Sonnerborg, A., Britton, S., & Pert, C. (1987). Peptide T in treatment of AIDS. *Lancet*, 1, 159. [letter]

Wiedermann, C. J. (1987). Shared recognition molecules in the brain and lymphoid tissues: The poly peptide mediator network of psychoneuroimmunology. *Immunology Letters*, 16, 371–378.

Wiesenfeld-Hallin, Z., Xu, X. J., Hakanson, R., Feng, D. M., & Folkers, K. (1990). The specific antagonistic effect of intrathecal spantide II on substance P stimulation-induced facilitation of the nociceptive flexor reflex in rat. *Brain Research*, 526, 284–290.

Wilkinson, D. I. (1989). Mitogenic effect of substance P and CGRP on keratinocytes. *Journal of Cell Biology*, 107, 509a.

Wilkinson, D. I., Theeuwes, M. I., & Farber, E. M. (1994). Nerve growth factor increases the mitogenicity of certain growth factors for cultured human keratinocytes: A comparison with epidermal growth factor. *Experimental Dermatology*, 3, 239–245.

Winchell, S. A., & Watts, R. A. (1988). Relaxation therapies in the treatment of psoriasis and possible pathophysiologic mechanisms. *Journal of the American Academy of Dermatology*, 18, 101–104.

Wrone-Smith, T., & Nickoloff, B. J. (1996). Dermal injection of immunocytes induces psoriasis. *Journal of Clinical Investigation*, 98, 878–887.

Wyatt, S., Shooeter, E. M., & Davies, A. M. (1990). Expression of the NGF receptor gene in sensory neurons and their cutaneous targets prior to and during innervation. *Neuron*, 421–427.

Xu, X. J., Hao, J. X., Wiesenfeld-Hallin, Z., Hakanson, R., Folkers, K., & Hokfelt, T. (1991). Spantide II, a novel tachykinin antagonist inhibits plasma extravasation induced by antidromic C-fober stimulation in rat hind paw. *Neuroscience*, 42, 731–737.

# 55

# Psychoneuroimmune Interactions in Infectious Disease: Studies in Animals

ROBERT H. BONNEAU, DAVID A. PADGETT, JOHN F. SHERIDAN

## I. INTRODUCTION

The realization of bidirectional communication among the nervous, endocrine, and immune systems through shared receptors and ligands has led to a major research emphasis on immunoregulation by hormones, neuropeptides, and neurotransmitters. The immune system is responsive to many hormones in the body, and both primary and secondary lymphoid organs are richly innervated by sympathetic, parasympathetic, and sensory fibers. As we have long suspected that mind–body interactions influence the ability of the immune system to respond to infectious challenge, the rebirth of integrative physiology in the context of behavior and molecular biology has led to the development of the fields of neuroendocrine immunology and psychoneuroimmunology (which

encompasses behavior in the mix of disciplines). At the same time, immunologists have isolated, purified, and cloned the "hormones" of the immune system, the cytokines and chemokines; and with these advances it has become ever more important to understand how the immune system functions in the context of the whole body and its complex physiological makeup (Johnson, Arkins, Dantzer, & Kelley, 1997; Miller, 1998).

As the immune system's primary function is to protect the host from infectious and malignant challenges, our laboratories, along with many others, have been conducting studies of immune function in states of stress-induced neuroendocrine activation. We have examined the effects of various experimental stressors on the pathophysiology of both acute and latent viral infections so that we can determine the health consequences of stress-induced immunomodulation. The focus of much of the work has been on determining which stress-induced neuroendocrine products modulate specific components of either natural resistance or adaptive immune responses induced by infectious challenge. This corpus of research also explores how neuroendocrine modulation of immunity affects the host–parasite relationship, resulting in changes in microbial pathogenesis.

Stress can be defined as a state of altered homeostasis resulting from either an external or an internal stimulus. The host's response to stress is designed to restore homeostasis through a variety of adaptive neuroendocrine mechanisms (Ramsey, 1982). While this response to stress is directed toward restoration of health, chronic stress may actually increase our susceptibility to, and the severity of, infectious diseases (Hermann, Tovar, Beck, Allen, & Sheridan, 1993; Dobbs, Vasquez, Glaser, and Sheridan, 1993; Cohen, Tyrrell, & Smith, 1991). The response to stress is initiated in the central nervous system, and is translated into action by the hypothalamo-pituitary-adrenal axis and the autonomic nervous system. The products of nervous and endocrine pathways can modulate natural resistance and adaptive immunity. This conceptual framework has led us to hypothesize that stress and infection may induce a bodywide set of physiologic adaptations, mediated through the activation of neuroendocrine pathways, that intersect and modulate inflammatory and immune responses, thus altering physiological processes such as immunity to infection.

## II. ANIMAL MODELS—ADVANTAGES AND LIMITATIONS

The use of animal models to delineate psychoneuroendocrine effects (i.e., the physiologic changes that arise due to alterations in behavior) on the immune response to infectious agents has a long and diverse history (Ader & Cohen, 1982; Jensen & Rasmussen, 1963; Johnsson & Rasmussen, 1965; Rasmussen, Marsh, & Brill, 1957). Such models allow one the flexibility to investigate an array of infectious pathogens administered at a variety of anatomical sites. More importantly, the use of animal models provides the opportunity to assess the immune response to pathogens in an assortment of tissues and organs. These studies are unlike human subject studies in which stringent limitations exist with respect to the use of pathogens and the sites at which immune responses can be assessed (typically restricted to the serum and peripheral blood cells in humans). Such limitations make it difficult to thoroughly evaluate the neuroendocrine–immune interactions that contribute to an immune defense against a given pathogen. Thus, animal models are able to provide the tools to conduct a comprehensive analysis of neuroendocrine–immune interactions under a variety of experimental conditions.

Most studies which have investigated psychoneuroendocrine effects on immune function have utilized rodent models. The fact that mice and rats are relatively inexpensive, easily manipulated, and have immune systems that compare favorably to that of humans has made the rodent ideal for studying the immune response to specific pathogens. Specifically, inbred strains of mice and rats, whose immune

systems have been typically well-characterized, provide excellent models for conducting such studies since an array of immunological reagents, such as monoclonal antibodies, are readily available.

The use of laboratory rodents in studies in psychoneuroimmunology has a number of other advantages. For example, the mouse is typically the first species in which new knowledge regarding the mechanisms underlying the functioning of the immune system is reported. Thus, the impact of components of the neuroendocrine system on these mechanisms can be readily determined using mouse models. The mouse has also been a valuable resource for understanding neuroendocrine–immune interactions due to the widespread availability of mouse lines with either neurological, endocrinological, or hematological defects. Also, the availability of knockout, transgenic, and recombinant inbred strains of mice, coupled with the use of quantitative trait loci (QTL) analysis, provide a powerful tool for assessing impact of genetics on both susceptibility to infectious disease and the expression of well-defined behavioral traits.

Animal models provide effective tools for the investigation of neuroendocrine immune interactions at multiple levels of analysis. However, in choosing such models, it is important to realize that there are limitations. For example, when studying an infectious disease it is important to ask if the chosen animal is a natural host for the pathogen. If not, how does the pathology in the model compare to pathology in the human host? How well characterized is the immune system of the chosen species, and does the immune response that develops to a particular pathogen mimic that in humans both quantitatively and qualitatively? Are there significant differences in the susceptibility among strains of the species chosen? Last, are comprehensive studies using a particular species cost prohibitive? These are but a few of the relevant question that need to be asked when developing an animal model. Nevertheless, the use of rodent models has been instrumental in providing a better and more detailed understanding of neuroendocrine–immune interactions.

## III. PSYCHONEUROENDOCRINE EFFECTS ON THE IMMUNE SYSTEM: EXPERIMENTAL PARADIGMS

Animal models have been invaluable in investigating neuroendocrine–immune interactions and the impact of these interactions on host defenses against infectious pathogens. As outlined below, such models have provided the opportunity to use a variety of experimental approaches to modulate neuroendocrine activity and assess numerous components of the immune response to a wide range of pathogens. As a result, animal models have been useful in delineating the cellular and the molecular mechanisms that underlie neuroendocrine effects on natural resistance and adaptive immune responses.

Studies of the impact of psychoneuroendocrine–immune interactions on the pathogenesis of infectious diseases have focused on the effects of neuroendocrine products that are elicited following the application of a stressor. A variety of paradigms have been used to stress rodents. The most common have included physical restraint (Bonneau, Sheridan, Feng, & Glaser, 1991a, 1991b, 1993; Bonneau, 1996; Bonneau, Brehm, & Kern, 1997; Bonneau, Zimmerman, Ikeda, & Jones, 1998; Dobbs, Feng, Beck, & Sheridan, 1996; Dobbs, et al., 1993; Feng et al., 1991; Hermann, Beck, & Sheridan, 1995; Hermann et al., 1993, 1994; Hermann, Tovar, Beck, & Sheridan, 1994; Padgett, MacCallum, & Sheridan, 1998a; Rasmussen et al., 1957; Sheridan et al., 1991), footshock (Brenner & Moynihan, 1997; Kusnecov et al., 1992), hyperthermia (Gebhart & Kaufman, 1995; Kriesel et al., 1997; Noisakran, Halford, Veress, & Carr, 1998; Sawtell & Thompson, 1992a,b), auditory stimulation (Freire-Garabal, Balboa, Fernandez-Rial, Nunez, & Belmonte, 1993; Jensen & Rasmussen, 1963), and social disruption (Padgett et al., 1998b).

While many studies have focused on the immunoregulatory roles of the hypothalamo-pituitary-adrenal (HPA) axis and sympathetic nervous system (SNS), other soluble factors such as the opiates and numerous neuropeptides have been shown to affect immune function (reviewed in Eisenstein & Hilburger, 1998; Hall, Suo, & Weber, 1998; Maestroni & Conti, 1996; Sharp, Roy, & Bidlack, 1998; Stevens-Felten & Bellinger, 1997). The synthesis of each of these neuroendocrine products is under the control of multiple environmental as well as physiological factors. Thus, there are numerous and varied means by which immune function can be modulated by the nervous and endocrine systems.

Although the type and magnitude of the neuroendocrine response may vary significantly with a particular stimulus, each of these responses may be effective in mediating changes in a component of the immune response. For example, restraint stress activates the HPA axis, resulting in elevated plasma corticosterone levels, which significantly affects the trafficking of mononuclear cells to sites of inflammation (Hermann et al., 1994, 1995; Sheridan et al., 1998). In addition, sympathetic activity in secondary lymphoid tissues leads to high levels of catecholamines in draining lymph nodes and the spleen which suppresses the activation of antigen-specific cytotoxic T lymphocytes (Dobbs et al., 1993). Through the use of surgical procedures (e.g., adrenalectomy, hypophysectomy) and pharmacologic approaches (treatment with agonists and antagonists), it has been possible to delineate the effects of specific components of the neuroendocrine system on the immune response. The effects of these components can also be determined through the exogenous administration of the individual factors. However, interpretations arising from of these approaches should be guarded as the removal or addition of a substance may disrupt feedforward and/or feedback pathways that are important for regulating the synthesis of other neuroendocrine products.

## IV. NEUROENDOCRINE PATHWAYS AND MODULATION OF IMMUNE RESPONSES TO INFECTIOUS MICROBES

In 1936, Hans Selye noted that in response to a "stressor," the body would activate a specific and predictable set of core stress responses (Selye, 1998). He proposed that this set of physiologic alterations were invoked for adaptation to serious challenges to homeostasis. In general terms, according to Selye, internal or external stressors would activate pathways in the central nervous system and alter hormonal outflow from the endocrine system.

It is thought that physiologic responses to stressors are mediated primarily by two neuroendocrine systems: the SNS and the HPA axis; however, other physiologic systems are undoubtedly involved.

### A. Sympathetic Nervous System and Catecholamines

Elevated tissue and plasma catecholamines result from increased SNS activity induced by a variety of stressors. SNS activation results in the release of norepinephrine from sympathetic nerve terminals and in the secretion of epinephrine from chromaffin cells of the adrenal medulla. Originally, it was thought that through interactions with $\alpha$- and $\beta$-adrenergic receptors, catecholamines mediated adaptive cardiovascular and metabolic effects. However, the discovery that immune cells possess adrenergic receptors has implicated the SNS in modulation of the immune response (Abrass, O'Connor, Scarpace & Abrass, 1985; Fuchs, Albright, & Albright, 1988; Galant, Durisetti, Underwood, & Insel, 1978; Hahn,

Yoo, Ba, Chaudry, & Wang, 1998; Landmann, Burgisser, West, & Buhler, 1985; Loveland, Jarrot, & McKenzie, 1981; Motulsky & Insel, 1982; Sanders, 1998). In addition, it has been demonstrated that both primary and secondary lymphoid organs are directly innervated by noradrenergic postganglionic sympathetic neurons (Felten & Felten, 1991). The distribution of nerve fibers in these organs suggests that immune effector cells contained within them are direct targets of the innervation (Felten & Olschowka, 1987).

## B. Hypothalmo-Pituitary-Adrenal Axis and Glucocorticoids

Stressful stimuli also activate the HPA axis, leading to elevation of plasma glucocorticoids (GC). Although under normal diurnal conditions, GC play an important regulatory role in glucose metabolism and energy conservation, under conditions of stress GC mediate a multitude of additional adaptive metabolic, cardiovascular, and immunologic effects—many of them suppressive.

GC are potent, naturally occurring anti-inflammatory molecules and many cells of the immune system, including macrophages, lymphocytes, neutrophils, and natural killer cells possess glucocorticoid receptors. From in vivo animal models, a number of studies show that corticosterone (or cortisol in humans) at both physiologic and pharmacologic levels effectively depresses inflammatory and cellular immune responses (Kohut et al., 1998). GC inhibit interleukin-2 (IL-2) and interferon (IFN)-$\gamma$ production by lymphocytes, and IL-1 and tumor necrosis factor (TNF)-$\alpha$ expression by macrophages (Kern et al., 1988; Lee et al., 1988; Lew, Oppenheim, & Matsushima, 1988; Northrop, Crabtree, & Mattila, 1992; Vacca et al., 1990). In addition, GC have been shown to inhibit MHC class II antigen expression by antigen-presenting cells (Snyder & Unanue, 1992; Zwilling, Brown, & Pearl, 1992). Furthermore, GC also inhibit lymphocyte trafficking and T-cell binding to endothelial cells by modulating expression of proinflammatory/chemotactic cytokines and adhesion molecules such as intercellular adhesion molecule-1 (ICAM-1) and lymphocyte function-associated antigen-1 (LFA-1) (Pitzalis, Sharrack, Gray, Lee, & Hughes, 1997; van de Stolpe & van der Saag, 1996; Wissink, van de Stolpe, Caldenhoven, Koenderman, & van der Saag, 1997). In the mouse, it has been shown that GC mediate a potent anti-inflammatory effect and a diminished CD4+ T-cell response by modulating cytokine secretion from macrophages (IL-1 and TNF-$\alpha$) and lymphocytes (IL-2 and IFN-$\gamma$) (Bendrups, Hilton,

Meager, & Hamilton, 1993; Dobbs et al., 1996; Russo-Marie, 1992; Snyder & Unanue, 1992).

Recently, the immunomodulatory capabilities of other products of the HPA axis have been recognized. Functional receptors for corticotrophin releasing hormone (CRH) have been demonstrated on macrophages (Webster, Battaglia, & De Souza, 1989; Webster, Tracey, Jutila, Wolfe, & De Souza, 1990). CRH has also been shown to alter NK cell activity (Carr, DeCosta, Jacobsen, Rice, & Blalock, 1990; Irwin, Hauger, Brown, & Britton, 1988; Irwin, Vale, & Britton, 1987), but this effect is thought to be centrally mediated and not due to a direct effect of CRH on NK cells (Irwin & Hauger, 1988). There is evidence, however, for direct effects of CRH on mast cells. Chrousos showed, in a carrageenin-induced aseptic inflammation model in Spraque–Dawley rats, that mast cells are the principal immune target for CRH (Webster, Torpy, Elenkov, & Chrousos, 1998). As CRH has been shown to increase vascular permeability and mast cell degranulation, the production of CRH from postganglionic sympathetic neurons may be responsible for stress-mediated activation of allergic/autoimmune phenomena such as asthma and eczema.

Direct effects of adrenocorticotrophic hormone (ACTH) have been documented on several different types of immune cells, and ACTH receptors have been demonstrated throughout the immune system (Bost, Smith, Wear, & Blalock, 1987; Johnson, Blalock, & Smith, 1988; Smith, Bronsan, Meyer, & Blalock, 1987). ACTH has been shown to inhibit antibody production (Johnson, Smith, Torres, & Blalock, 1982) and to enhance proliferation by B lymphocytes (Brooks, 1990; Alvarez-Mon, Kehrl, & Fauci, 1985). ACTH has also been shown to inhibit T-lymphocyte IFN-$\gamma$ production (Johnson, Torres, Smith, Dion, & Blalock, 1984) and IFN-$\gamma$-induced macrophage activation (Koff & Dunegan, 1985) and MHC class II expression (Zwilling et al., 1992).

The potential immunomodulatory effects of the opioid peptides have also been recently recognized (Mellon & Bayer, 1999). Opioid binding sites have been demonstrated on lymphocytes, polymorphonuclear leukocytes, and platelets (Ausiello & Roda, 1984; Mehrishi & Mills, 1983; Sacerdote, di San Secondo, Sirchia, Manfredi, & Panerai, 1998). $\beta$-Endorphin and met-enkephalin have been shown to enhance the generation of CTLs (Carr & Klimpel, 1986) and NK cell cytotoxicity (Faith, Liang, Murgo, & Plotnikoff, 1984; Matthews, Froelich, Sibbitt, and Bankhurst, 1983) in vitro. However, in vivo, restraint stress-induced release of opioid peptides has been found to depress NK activity. In addition, opioid peptides have been shown to enhance IL-2 production by lymphocytes (Gilmore & Weiner, 1989) and IFN-$\gamma$ production by lymphocytes and NK cells (Brown & Van Epps, 1986; Mandler, Biddison, Mandler, & Serrate, 1986). Opioid peptides have been reported to enhance (Gilman, Schwartz, Milner, Bloom, & Feldman, 1982; Gilmore & Weiner, 1988) or depress (McCain, Lamster, & Bilotta, 1986; McCain, Lamster, Bozzone, & Grbic, 1982) mitogen-induced lymphocyte proliferation. In the context of disease, Coussons-Read showed that treatment of influenza-infected rats with morphine reduced the inflammatory response, and slowed viral clearance (Coussons-Read, Daniels, & Gilmour, 1998).

## V. PSYCHONEUROIMMUNE EFFECTS ON SELECTED INFECTIOUS DISEASES IN EXPERIMENTAL ANIMAL MODELS

### A. Herpes Simplex Virus Infection

Herpes simplex virus (HSV) is a natural pathogen of humans characterized by its ability to cause an acute infection at a peripheral site and establish a latent infection in the local sensory ganglia (reviewed in Blyth & Hill, 1984; Miller, Danaher, & Jacob, 1998; Steiner, 1996; Wagner & Bloom, 1997). The hallmark of infection with HSV is its ability to spontaneously reactivate from this quiescent, noninfectious latent state and cause a recurrent infection in the periphery at or near the original site of infection (Hill, 1985). HSV reactivation and recurrent infections typically occur spontaneously, however, correlations have been made between reactivation and physical or emotional stress, fever, exposure to ultraviolet light, tissue damage, and immune suppression (Hill, 1985; Stevens, 1975). Of particular interest has been the role of psychological stress, and its associated neuroendocrine components, in the development of recurrent HSV infection.

The effects of stress on susceptibility to HSV infections have been known for over 40 years (Rasmussen et al., 1957). While these studies were important in establishing an association between stress and viral infection, they were unable to identify specific anti-viral immune defense mechanisms that were modulated by stress as these were unknown at the time. However, in the past 10 years, murine models have been used to decipher the effects of psychological stress and other psychosocial/neuroendocrine factors on the specific components of the primary immune response to HSV infection (Bonneau et al., 1991a, 1993, 1997; Dobbs et al., 1993; Kusnecov

et al., 1992; Karp, Moynihan, & Ader, 1997; Leo, Callahan, & Bonneau, 1998) and memory (Bonneau et al., 1991b, 1993, 1996, 1998; Leo et al., 1998). More recently, mouse models have been used to determine the impact of neuroendocrine activity on HSV reactivation and define the role of immunity in the reactivation process (Carr et al., 1998; Noisakran et al., 1998; Padgett et al., 1998b).

### 1. Primary HSV Immune Responses

Initial studies of the effect of restraint stress on the primary immune response to HSV infection demonstrated that stress suppresses the lymphoproliferative response in the popliteal lymph nodes following footpad infection with HSV (Bonneau et al., 1991a; Dobbs et al., 1993). Using this model it was also shown that stress suppresses the magnitude of HSV-specific cytotoxic T lymphocyte (CTL) and natural killer (NK) cell responses generated in local HSV infection (Bonneau et al., 1991a). Suppression of the generation of CTL was shown to occur early in the sequence of events involved in the differentiation and maturation HSV-specific precursor CTL (CTLp) to a phenotypically lytic state (Bonneau et al., 1991a). Stress-induced suppression of lymphoproliferation and HSV-specific CTL activity was also seen in studies in which a footshock model of stress was employed (Kusnecov et al., 1992). By using a combination of surgical (adrenalectomy) and pharmacological approaches ($\beta$-adrenergic and glucocorticoid receptor antagonists and corticosterone pellets) a role for both adrenal-dependent and catecholamine-mediated mechanisms in stress-induced suppression of the primary cellular immune response to HSV infection was defined (Dobbs et al., 1993; Bonneau et al., 1993).

A limited number of studies have also examined psychosocial effects on the humoral immune response to HSV infection. For example, differential housing was shown to alter the magnitude, but not the kinetics, of some cytokines that are produced in response to HSV-1 infection. However, such conditions did not alter the levels of circulating IgM or IgG antibodies (Karp et al., 1997). There have also been studies on the effect of stress on different strains of mice during infection. For example, using a footshock model, it was shown that there are strain differences with respect to the production of cytokines in response to HSV infection (Brenner & Moynihan, 1997).

### 2. Memory HSV Immune Responses

Immunological memory is a key component of the overall immune response and is important in reducing the severity of recurrent HSV infection. Because recovery from recrudescent HSV infection is largely controlled by T cells, the ability to generate a population of HSV-specific CTLm during the initial infection with HSV is thought to be critical for the long-term defense against recurrent HSV infection. The psychological stress that is often associated with the primary episode of infection, as well as the development of recurrent disease, emphasizes the potential significance of the effect of stress in modulating the development of HSV-specific T-cell-mediated immunity. In studies to date, restraint stress has been shown not to suppress the generation of memory CTL (CTLm) in response to systemic HSV infection. However, such a stressor has been shown to be effective at inhibiting the activation of CTLm (Bonneau et al., 1991b; Bonneau, 1996; Leo et al., 1998) and their migration to the site of recurrent HSV infection (Bonneau et al., 1991). Further studies into the mechanisms underlying the suppression of CTLm activation revealed that stress does not suppress the expression of the T-cell receptor, IL-2 receptor, nor other accessory molecules required for T-lymphocyte activation. However, it does suppress the production of cytokines involved in CTLm activation, which is likely to be the mechanism underlying stress-induced suppression of CTLm activation (Bonneau, 1996). These studies were extended to show that stress-induced adrenal function is responsible for suppression of cytokine production and the development of lytic activity (Bonneau et al., 1997). As in the studies of the primary immune response, adrenal-dependent mechanisms do not appear to be solely responsible for stress-induced suppression of immunity to HSV infection.

### 3. HSV Reactivation and Recurrent Infection

It has long been known that psychological stress is strongly associated with HSV recrudescence. However, only recently has such a relationship been demonstrated in mice. The immunological and neuroendocrine mechanisms underlying virus reactivation and recrudescent infection have been investigated in the murine model. For years, it was known that local trauma (e.g., hair plucking, tape stripping, chemical-induced trauma, or ultraviolet irradiation) administered to a previously infected area would result in HSV reactivation, but the ability of each of these methods to consistently induce recurrent disease was quite low (Harbour, Hill, & Blyth, 1983; Hill, Blyth, & Harbour, 1978; Hurd & Robinson, 1977). More recently, two stress models have been shown to be effective in inducing HSV reactivation, and both

may be useful in investigating the neuroendocrine mechanisms that underlie behaviorally mediated reactivation of latent HSV infection. For example, the use of a hyperthermic stress model (Sawtell & Thompson; 1992; Thompson & Sawtell, 1997; Sawtell, 1998) has shown that HPA axis activation plays an important role in HSV-1 reactivation in the trigeminal ganglion and reactivation may be associated with an increase in IL-6 expression in the ganglia itself (Noisakran et al., 1998). In addition, the development of a social stress model in mice has been shown to be effective in causing recurrent HSV infection in mice (Padgett et al., 1998b).

### 4. Neuroendocrine Effects on HSV Pathogenesis in Mouse Models

The ultimate impact of suppression of immune function is on viral pathogenesis. Studies in humans have indicated that stress can affect the frequency, severity, and duration of HSV infection. These findings have been substantiated in mouse models in which both restraint (Bonneau et al., 1991a) and footshock (Kusnecov et al., 1992) were shown to result in increased HSV titers at a site of local HSV infection. In subsequent studies, it was shown that stress suppresses the ability of adoptively transferred lymphocytes with HSV-specific lytic activity to confer protection against lethal HSV infection in an immunocompromised host as well as inhibiting the restoration of immune responsiveness to HSV infection following sublethal gamma irradiation (Bonneau et al., 1997). These findings are important since adoptive immunotherapy represents a potentially effective approach by which to control the extent of viral infections in an immunocompromised host. In other studies, the functional glucocorticoid antagonist androstenediol (AED) has been shown to significantly improve the survival of mice with HSV-1-induced encephalitis (Loria & Padgett, 1992). Moreover, it was shown that increased protection was mediated by an augmentation of a type I interferon response (Daigle & Carr, 1998).

## B. Influenza A Viral Infection

Infection with the influenza viruses causes significant morbidity and mortality worldwide (for a brief review, see Laver, Bischofberger, & Webster, 1999). Respiratory infections caused by members of this virus group remain a leading cause of morbidity in the elderly. Why does infection with this virus remain a major public health problem? While influenza viral vaccines have been commercially available for decades, and vaccine application to the general population has been highly recommended by public health experts, the influenza viruses have evolved a number of genetic mechanisms that lead to the development of new strains which may be resistant to current vaccines. In addition, anti-viral vaccine responses may be affected by the state of the individual's health. In a recent study of immunity in a population of individuals giving care to subjects with Alzheimer's dementia, chronic stress was demonstrated to reduce the anti-viral response to vaccination (Kiecolt-Glaser, Glaser, Gravenstein, Malarkey, & Sheridan, 1996). Other studies by Cohen (1991) have demonstrated that the probability of developing a clinically symptomatic infection following experimental exposure to a variety of respiratory viral pathogens, including influenza virus, was negatively correlated with social support. Thus, stress may be a significant variable in resistance to influenza infection.

As in humans, influenza A virus causes an acute, lytic infection of the respiratory tract of mice. Inoculation of influenza virus by nasal instillation results in simultaneous infection of the upper and lower respiratory tract of mice. Influenza viruses infect the epithelial cells throughout the respiratory tract and can replicate in the specialized epithelial cells, called pneumocytes, that line the alveoli sacs and facilitate gas exchange. Viral infection may be limited to the respiratory tract, and generally there is no viremia, or spread through circulation to other tissues. Severe infection destroys the epithelial layer causing significant tissue damage, and lung function diminishes as pneumocytes are lysed. Infection of mice with the highly virulent A/PR8 strain of virus can lead to mortality when mice are infected with a low number of hemagglutinating units (HAU) of the virus (Hermann et al., 1993).

## 1. Stress Modulates Innate Resistance Mechanisms

Influenza viral-induced tissue damage in the lung induces an inflammatory response that is characterized by the trafficking of mononuclear cells to the sites of viral replication. Cellular trafficking is regulated by a number of different genes expressed in the local milieu in response to the cellular damage caused by replication of the virus. Among the key genes are those coding for the proinflammatory cytokines (IL-1 and IL-6), which are pleiomorphic. At the site of antigenic replication, the roles of the proinflammatory cytokines are multiple and include the activation of chemokine genes whose products are associated with directed recruitment of inflammatory cells. In concert with one another, the chemokine and proinflamma-

tory cytokine responses promote the accumulation of cells at the inflammatory site. Subsequent to cytokine production, a high degree of cellular accumulation occurs, causing histological changes that are characterized by local, patchy tissue consolidation. In severe infections, hemorrhagic foci develop. An additional component of natural resistance is the trafficking of NK cells and monocytes to the site of viral replication. This entire set of innate responses functions together to limit viral replication during the early phases of the infection prior to activation of virus-specific T- and B-cell adaptive immune responses.

However, activation of the HPA axis leading to elevated levels of corticosterone affects the trafficking of inflammatory cells to the site of infection and to the lymph nodes that drain them. In the mouse A/PR8 viral model of infection, it has been shown previously that restraint stress (RST) suppressed lymphadenopathy in the draining mediastinal lymph nodes and diminished accumulation of mononuclear cells in the lungs (Hermann et al., 1995). Additional studies showed that the proinflammatory cytokine response was also affected by RST. Interleukin-1$\alpha$ levels in lungs of infected unstressed animals were significantly elevated at 48 h postinfection (p.i.), while lung IL-1$\alpha$ levels in RST mice were not different from those seen in the uninfected controls. However, unlike the lung IL-1$\alpha$ response, the IL-6 response to A/PR8 infection was not suppressed by RST. Lung IL-6 levels in infected, food- and water-deprived, and restrained mice were all elevated significantly over uninfected controls by 24 h p.i. and further elevated 48 h p.i. RST did not suppress the magnitude or kinetics of the lung IL-6 response during the early stages of an influenza viral infection (Konstantinos, 1995). Subsequent studies by Dobbs et al. (1996), showed that elevated serum glucocorticoid levels due to RST promoted the expression of IL-6 in the lung and draining lymph nodes.

As the production of the proinflammatory cytokines leads to the trafficking of innate cellular responses, it was not surprising to observe that RST affected NK-cell activity as well. During an experimental influenza A/PR8 viral infection in C57BL/6 mice, NK-cell activity in the lungs was enhanced 3 days p.i.; however, when RST was used to stress these mice, NK-activity in the lungs was suppressed (Miller, 1995). Thus, a key innate cellular inflammatory response was diminished by the host's response to the stressor.

It is interesting to note that in addition to their inflammatory nature, cytokines are also potent inducers of physiological systems such as the HPA axis. HPA activation results in elevation of plasma corticosterone levels (Hermann et al., 1994). As such, infection by influenza virus can, itself, be perceived as a stressor (Swiergiel, Smagin, Johnson, & Dunn, 1997). Thus, an infection in a peripheral site such as the lung can signal the CNS through cytokines acting as transmitters. In fact, infection of C57BL/6 mice with influenza A/PR8 virus results in a biphasic elevation of plasma corticosterone. A first peak occurs 48 to 72 h after infection at the peak of the proinflammatory cytokine response (Hermann et al., 1994). A second peak occurs at the time of maximal cellular accumulation in the lungs (5–7 days p.i.) when respiration becomes difficult due to cellular infiltration in the lungs. It is thought that this biphasic GC response may provide a level of control over excessive accumulation of cells within the architecturally dependent lung parenchyma. However, pathological perturbation of this negative feedback loop by RST may prevent even the initial recruitment of immune cells to the lung where their presence is required to control viral replication.

## 2. Stress Modulates Adaptive, Virus-Specific Immune Responses

Stress also suppresses the adaptive immune response during viral infection (Sheridan et al., 1991; Bonneau et al., 1991; Dobbs, et al., 1996). Studies of the neuroendocrine pathways involved in stress-induced immunoregulation have shown that sustained, elevated levels of corticosterone, induced by repeated cycles of restraint, suppress T-cell cytokine responses, reduce the accumulation of T cells in the draining lymph nodes, and alter the trafficking of T cells to lungs of viral-infected animals. Suppression of these cellular responses is mediated by corticosterone as blockade of the type II steroid receptors (with the drug RU486) restores lymphadenopathy, cell trafficking to the lungs, and the expression of T-cell cytokine genes. Virus-specific cytolytic T-cell responses, however, remain suppressed. Restoration of CD8+ cytolytic activity requires blocking $\beta$-adrenergic receptors (with nadolol), thus providing evidence for a role of the sympathetic nervous system in virus-specific regulation of cellular immunity (Dobbs et al., 1993).

Stress also affects the kinetics of virus-specific B-cell antibody responses. Delayed seroconversion is observed in A/PR8 virus-infected mice subjected to repeated cycles of restraint, and isotype class switching from antigen-specific IgM to IgG to IgA is prolonged. Following resolution of infection, virus-specific antibody titers are similar in stressed and control infected mice (Feng et al., 1991).

The mouse influenza viral infection model has been used successfully to identify the biochemical pathways by which stress-induced activation of the neuroendocrine response affects the immune response to a respiratory viral infection.

## C. West Nile Virus

West Nile virus (WNV) is an arbovirus that causes a potentially fatal encephalitis. Arbovirus (short for arthropod-borne) infections are caused by any number of viruses transmitted by arthropods such as mosquitoes and ticks. Symptoms of the various types of virus infections transmitted by mosquitoes and ticks are usually similar, but differ in severity. Most infections do not result in any symptoms. Mild cases may occur with only a slight fever and or headache. Severe infections are marked by a rapid onset of headache, high fever, disorientation, coma, tremors, convulsions, paralysis, or death.

Ben-Nathan and Feuerstein (1990) have shown that exposure of mice for 5 min per day to cold water (approx 1°C) for 8–10 days resulted in significantly higher mortality from WNV infection than seen in unstressed mice. In addition, isolation stress similarly increased mortality of infected animals. The data showed that both cold and isolation stress increased blood, brain, and spleen virus titers (Ben-Nathan, Lustig, & Danenberg, 1991; Ben-Nathan, Lustig, & Kobiler, 1996). These data suggest that stress enhanced WNV encephalitis by accelerating virus proliferation or by limiting the immune response necessary to control infection. These findings were extended to show that stress not only enhanced WNV encephalitis, but that stress also altered the virulence of the virus. For example, an attenuated strain of West Nile virus (WN-25), which showed no signs of viremia or tropism for the central nervous system in ICR outbred mice, became virulent and caused encephalitis in ICR animals exposed to cold or isolation stress. Exposure of inoculated mice to cold water 5 min a day for 8 days resulted in 60% mortality, while no mortality was observed in the nonstressed animals. No virus was detected in the brain, blood, or spleens of the nonstressed animals, while infectious virus was isolated from these tissues in the cold-stressed animals. Furthermore, the isolated virus had mutated and become highly virulent (subsequent inoculation of this virus resulted in encephalitis and death of normal, nonstressed animals). These observations suggest that stress can suppress the immune response required to control viral replication, and stress can alter host pressure upon the pathogen, thus altering its virulence.

## D. Mycobacterial Infection and Stress

Even though worldwide eradication of tuberculosis has been a major goal of the World Health Organization (Kochi, 1991), and control of this disease looked very promising in the 1970s and 1980s, the incidence of mycobacterial disease has increased significantly during the past 15 years. While part of the increase in tuberculosis has been observed in patients infected with the human immunodeficiency virus (HIV), the incidence of tuberculosis has also increased in this country in individuals not infected with HIV. Thus, tuberculosis remains one of the most significant public health problems worldwide (Collins, 1989; Kochi, 1991; Pitchenik & Fertel, 1992).

The first scientific observation that a stressful event could alter the host–parasite relationship may have been made in tuberculosis. Ishigami (1919) found that the incidence of tuberculosis correlated with a decrease in opsonic index of the sera (neutralizing antibody) obtained from Japanese school children and attributed it to the stressful environment found in the schools. This observation may have been the foundation for the generally held belief that stressful conditions serve as a cofactor in the development of active tuberculosis infections (Collins, 1989; Wiegeshaus, Balasubramanian, & Smith, 1989).

Most healthy individuals who are infected with *Mycobacterium tuberculosis* develop a protective cell-mediated immune response that controls the growth of the microorganism (Dannenberg, 1993). Upon infection, usually via the respiratory tract, the bacilli grow within alveolar macrophages, but soon thereafter T-cell immunity (e.g., mycobacterial Ag-specific cytotoxic T cells) develops. Activation of CTLs and the associated delayed-type hypersensitivity response results in the destruction of infected macrophages, the formation of caseous necrosis, and the creation of an environment that inhibits further mycobacterial growth. Most infectious foci are eventually sterilized. However, lesions within the apical to subapical regions of the lung escape sterilization and remain as dormant, mycobacterial reservoirs until cell-mediated immunity is compromised perhaps decades later. Reactivation leading to the reappearance and dissemination of replicating bacilli has been attributed to any one of several factors that compromise the cell-mediated immune response including HIV infection, immunosuppressive cancer chemotherapy, age-associated immunosenescence, chronic alcoholism, protein malnutrition, and stress.

Injection of mice with mycobacteria results in two distinct patterns of growth, and strains of mice can be classified as resistant or susceptible based on those patterns of mycobacterial growth (Forget, Skamene, Gros, Miailke & Turcotte, 1981; Gros, Skamene, & Forget, 1981). Studies by Johnson and Zwilling (1985), as well as by Denis, Forget, Pelletier, and Skamene (1988a, 1988b), have indicated that the differences in the growth patterns of the mycobacteria are due to differences in macrophage activation. Given the differences in the ability of macrophages from resistant and susceptible mice to control mycobacterial growth, and the possibility that stress may alter the interaction between the host and the parasite, Zwilling et al. (Brown, Sheridan, Pearl, & Zwilling, 1993; Brown, Lafuse & Zwilling, 1998) extended these studies to include an assessment of the role of the HPA axis activation on mycobacterial growth. Mice were stressed by restraint immediately following the intravenous injection with *Mycobacterium avium*. Activation of the HPA axis by RST suppressed MHC class II (I-A) expression in susceptible mouse strains but not in resistant animals (Zwilling et al., 1990, 1992) Furthermore, suppression of I-A expression by HPA activation correlated with increased mycobacterial growth within macrophages of susceptible mice. Adrenalectomy or treatment of animals with the glucocorticoid receptor antagonist, RU 486, abrogated the effect. In contrast, corticosterone administration in the form of time-release pellets mimicked the effect of HPA activation. These differences in the effects of stress on the growth of mycobacteria in vivo may have important implications for human tuberculosis. Several reports have indicated that humans, like mice, differ in their susceptibility to mycobacterial diseases (Bellamy & Hill, 1998; Hill, 1998; McNerney, 1999). Therefore, these results suggest that HPA activation could contribute to increased susceptibility of individuals to increased mycobacterial growth during primary infection.

Although the primary growth of mycobacteria can determine the severity of the initial infection, other factors may determine reactivation of latent or dormant infections. Because latent disease in mice is reminiscent of the disease in humans, the mouse again provides a good model to assess the influence of stress and the HPA axis on mycobacterial reactivation. Again, from Zwilling et al. (1993), observations show that restraint stress resulted in growth of *M. tuberculosis* in latently infected mice. Furthermore, Cox, Knight, and Ivanyi, (1989) showed that the HPA axis played an important role in regrowth of the bacteria, as treatment of mice with corticosterone also resulted in reactivation of *M. bovis*. These results suggest HPA activation was the cause of suppression of antigen-specific T-cell immunity leading to reactivation. Along these lines, Cox et al. (1989)

showed that injection of mice with anti-CD4 antibody also resulted in reactivation.

### E. Listeria Monocytogenes Infection

Host defense mechanisms against intraperitoneal bacterial infections have also been shown to be suppressed by RST. Repeated cycles of restraint (Zhang et al., 1998) suppressed the trafficking of leukocytes into the peritoneal cavity after intraperitoneal inoculation of *Listeria monocytogenes*. The reduced peritoneal cellularity was modulated by the HPA axis as treatment with RU 486 restored the response. In addition to its effects on cell trafficking, RST also suppressed gene expression of the Th1 type cytokines (while enhancing type II cytokine gene expression), reduced MHC class II molecules on B cells and macrophages, and inhibited the clearance of the bacteria in the spleen. Blockade of the corticosterone receptor restored these immune responses.

### F. Other Microbial Infections

Some of the earliest studies in psychoneuroimmunology showed that adrenal cortical preparations increased the susceptibility of experimental animals (primarily mice and rats) to pneumococcal infection (Vollmer, 1951), growth of *Plasmodium berghei* (Jackson, 1955; Singer, 1954), *Yersinia (Pasteurella) pestis* (Payne, Larson, Walker, Foster, & Meyer, 1955), and susceptibility to *Trichinella spiralis* (Bell, 1987; Coker, 1956a, b). In addition, several different stress paradigms have also been shown to adversely affect the survival of infected animals. For example, Friedman, Ader, and Grota (1973) showed that crowding stress altered the resistance of mice to malarial infection. In another study, crowding stress was shown to result in a marked increase in the susceptibility of mice to *Salmonella typhimurium* (Edwards & Dean, 1977). Hamilton reported that predator stress (cat) reduced the resistance of immune mice to reinfection by the cestode *Hymenolepis nana* (Hamilton, 1974), and cold stress was shown to inhibit the clearance of *Staphylococcus albus* and *Proteus mirabilis* from the lungs of mice (Green & Kass, 1965). Studies of the effects of stress on the resistance of farm animals to experimental infection have also been done. Recently, Gross showed that social stress increased the susceptibility of chickens to aerosol challenge with *Escherichia coli* or to challenge with *M. avium* (Gross, 1984, 1988; Gross, Falkinham, & Payeur, 1989). Holt found that food deprivation increased the susceptibility of chickens to *Salmonella enteritidis*

infection and resulted in a more severe infection (Holt & Porter, 1992). Zamri-Saad et al. (Zamri-Saad, Jasni, Naridi, & Sheikh-Omar, 1991) found that transport stress was associated with an increased susceptibility of goats to infection with *Pasteurella haemolytica*. In this case, transport served as a cofactor to previous injection with dexamethasone. Animals injected with dexamethasone alone did not become infected with the bacteria.

## VI. CONCLUSIONS

The bidirectional communication among the nervous, endocrine, and immune systems that is stimulated by peripheral tissue damage is a key element in protection of the host against infectious challenge. Significant advances in our knowledge of natural resistance and adaptive immune responses have provided us with the opportunity to dissect the impact of nervous and endocrine responses on various stages of an anti-microbial immune response. In some instances, stress-induced reduction in the synthesis of a single cytokine, or the expression of a specific receptor, may have a significant effect on the ability of the host to successfully respond to an infectious challenge. Understanding the mechanisms by which products of the nervous and endocrine systems affect the immune system may allow for the design of intervention strategies that are effective in counteracting or enhancing the effects of psychosocial factors on immune function.

### Acknowledgments

This work was supported by research grants from the National Institutes of Health, RO1-MH46801 (J.F.S.), PO1-AG11585 (J.F.S.), R29-MH56899 (D.A.P.), R29-MH49616 (R.H.B.), and the John D. and Catherine T. MacArthur Foundation Mind-Body Network (J.F.S.).

### References

Abrass, C. K., O'Connor, S. W., Scarpace, P. J., & Abrass, I. B. (1985). Characterization of the $\beta$-adrenergic receptor of the rat peritoneal macrophage. *Journal of Immunology, 135,* 1338–1341.

Ader, R., & Cohen, N. (1982). Behaviorally conditioned immunosuppression and murine systemic lupus erythematosus. *Science, 215,* 1534–1536.

Alvarez-Mon, M., Kehrl, J. H., & Fauci, A. S. (1985). A potential role for adrenocorticotropin in regulating human B lymphocyte functions. *Journal of Immunology, 135,* 3823–3826.

Ausiello, C. M., & Roda, L. G. (1984). Leuenkephalin binding to cultured human T-lymphocytes. *Cell Biology International Reports, 8,* 353–362.

Bell, R. G. (1987). Trichinella spiralis: Differences between "early" and "late" rapid expulsion evident from inhibition studies using cortisone and irradiation. *Experimental Parasitology, 64,* 385–392.

Bellamy, R., & Hill, A. V. (1998). Genetic susceptibility to mycobacteria and other infectious pathogens in humans. *Current Opinions in Immunology, 10*(4), 483–487.

Ben-Nathan, D., & Feuerstein, G. (1990). The influence of cold or isolation stress on resistance of mice to West Nile virus encephalitis. *Experientia, 46,* 285–290.

Ben-Nathan, D., Lustig, S., & Danenberg, H. D. (1991). Stress-induced neuroinvasiveness of a neurovirulent noninvasive Sindbis virus in cold or isolation subjected mice. *Life Sciences, 48,* 1493–1500.

Ben-Nathan, D., Lustig, S., & Kobiler, D. (1996). Cold stress-induced neuroinvasiveness of attenuated arboviruses is not solely mediated by corticosterone. *Archives of Virology, 141,* 1221–1229.

Bendrups A., Hilton, A., Meager, A., & Hamilton, J. A. (1993). Reduction of tumor necrosis factor alpha and interleukin-1beta levels in human synovial tissue by interleukin-4 and glucocorticoids. *Rheumatology International, 12,* 217–220.

Blyth, W. A., & Hill, T. J. (1984). Establishment, maintenance, and control of herpes simplex virus (HSV) latency. In B. T. Rouse & C. Lopez (Eds.), *Immunobiology of herpes simplex virus infection* (pp. 9–32). Boca Raton, FL: CRC Press.

Bonneau, R. H. (1996). Stress-induced effects on integral immune components involved in herpes simplex virus (HSV)-specific memory cytotoxic T lymphocyte activation. *Brain, Behavior, and Immunity, 10,* 139–163.

Bonneau, R. H., Brehm, M. A., & Kern, A. M. (1997). The impact of psychological stress on the efficacy of anti-viral adoptive immunotherapy in an immunocompromised host. *Journal of Neuroimmunology, 78,* 19–33.

Bonneau, R. H., Sheridan, J. F., Feng, N., & Glaser, R. (1991a). Stress-induced suppression of herpes simplex virus (HSV)-specific cytotoxic T lymphocyte and natural killer cell activity and enhancement of acute pathogenesis following local HSV infection. *Brain, Behavior, and Immunity, 5,* 170–192.

Bonneau, R. H., Sheridan, J. F., Feng, N., & Glaser, R. (1991b). Stress-induced effects on cell-mediated innate and adaptive memory components of the murine immune response to local and systemic herpes simplex virus (HSV) infection. *Brain, Behavior, and Immunity, 5,* 274–295.

Bonneau, R. H., Sheridan, J. F., Feng, N., & Glaser, R. (1993). Stress-induced modulation of the primary cellular immune response to herpes simplex virus infection is mediated by both adrenal-dependent and adrenal-independent mechanisms. *Journal of Neuroimmunology, 42,* 167–176.

Bonneau, R. H., Zimmerman, K. M., Ikeda, S. C., & Jones, B. C. (1998). Differential effects of stress-induced adrenal function on components of the herpes simplex virus-specific memory cytotoxic T lymphocyte response. *Journal of Neuroimmunology, 82,* 191–199, (1998).

Bost, K. L., Smith, E. M., Wear, L. B., & Blalock, J. E. (1987). Presence of ACTH and its receptors on a B lymphocytic cell line: a possible autocrine function for a neuroendocrine hormone. *Journal of Biological Regulators and Homeostatic Agents, 1,* 23–27.

Brenner, G. J., & Moynihan, J. A. (1997). Stressor-induced alterations in immune response and viral clearance following infection with herpes simplex virus-type 1 in BALB/c and C57BL/6 mice. *Brain, Behavior, and Immunity, 11,* 9–23.

Brooks, K. H. (1990). Adrenocorticotropin (ACTH) functions as a late-acting B cell growth factor and synergizes with interleukin 5. *Journal of Molecular and Cellular Immunology, 4,* 327–335.

Brown, D. H., Lafuse, W. P., & Zwilling, B. S. (1998). Host resistance to mycobacteria is compromised by activation of the hypothalamic-pituitary-adrenal axis. *Annals of the New York Academy of Sciences, 840,* 773–786.

Brown, D. H., Sheridan, J. F., Pearl, D., & Zwilling, B. S. (1993). Regulation of mycobacterial growth by the hypothalamus-pituitary-adrenal axis: Differential responses of *Mycobacterium bovis* BCG-resistant and -susceptible mice. *Infection and Immunity, 61,* 4793–4800.

Brown, S. L., & Van Epps, D. E. (1986). Opioid peptides modulate production of interferon γ by human mononuclear cells. *Cellular Immunology, 103,* 19–26.

Carr, D. J., DeCosta, B. R., Jacobsen, A. E., Rice, K. C., & Blalock, J. E. (1990). Corticotropin-releasing hormone augments natural killer cell activity through a naloxone-sensitive pathway. *Journal of Neuroimmunology, 28,* 53–61.

Carr, D. J., & Klimpel, G. R. (1986). Enhancement of the generation of cytotoxic T cells by endogenous opiates. *Journal of Neuroimmunology, 12,* 75–87.

Carr, D. J., Noisakran, S., Halford, W. P., Lukacs, N., Asensio, V., & Campbell, I. L. (1998). Cytokine and chemokine production in HSV-1 latently infected trigeminal ganglion cell cultures: Effects of hyperthermic stress. *Journal of Neuroimmunology, 85,*111–121.

Cohen, S., Tyrrell, D. A. J., & Smith A. P. (1991). Psychological stress and susceptibility to the common cold. *New England Journal of Medicine, 325,* 606–612.

Coker, C. M. (1956a). Some effects of cortisone in mice with acquired immunity to *Trichinella spiralis. Journal of Infectious Diseases, 98,* 39–44.

Coker, C. M. (1956b). Cellular factors in acquired immunity to *Trichinella spiralis* as indicated by cortisone treatment of mice. *Journal of Infectious Diseases, 98,* 187–197.

Collins, F. M. (1989). Mycobacterial disease: Immunosuppression and acquired immunodeficiency syndrome. *Clinical Microbiology Reviews, 2,* 360–377.

Coussons-Read, M. E., Daniels, M., & Gilmour, M. I. (1998). Morphine alters the immune response to influenza virus infection in Lewis rats. *Advances in Experimental Medicine and Biology, 437,* 73–82.

Cox, J. H., Knight, B. C., & Ivanyi, J. (1989). Mechanisms of recrudescence of *Mycobacterium bovis* BCG infection in mice. *Infection and Immunity, 57,* 1719–1724.

Daigle, J., & Carr D. J. J. (1998). Androstenediol antagonizes herpes simplex virus type 1-induced encephalitis through the augmentation of type I IFN production. *Journal of Immunology, 160,* 3060–3066.

Dannenberg, A. M. (1993). Immunopathogenesis of pulmonary tuberculosis. *Hospital Practice, 15,* 33–40.

Denis, M., Forget, A., Pelletier, M., & Skamene, E. (1988a). Pleiotropic effects of the Bcg gene. I. Antigen presentation in genetically susceptible and resistant congenic mouse strains. *Journal of Immunology, 140,* 2395–2400.

Denis, M., Forget, A., Pelletier, M., & Skamene, E. (1988b). Pleiotropic effects of the Bcg gene. III. Respiratory burst in Bcg congenic macrophages. *Clinical and Experimental Immunology, 73,* 370–375.

Dobbs, C. M., Feng, N., Beck, F. M., & Sheridan, J. F. (1996). Neuroendocrine regulation of cytokine production during experimental influenza virus infection: Effects of restraint stress-induced elevation of endogenous corticosterone. *Journal of Immunology, 157,* 1870–1877.

Dobbs, C. M., Vasquez, M., Glaser, R., & Sheridan, J. F. (1993). Mechanisms of stress-induced modulation of viral pathogenesis and immunity. *Journal of Neuroimmunology, 48,* 151–160.

Edwards, E. A., & Dean, L. M. (1977). Effects of crowding of mice on humoral antibody formation and protection to lethal antigenic challenge. *Psychosomatic Medicine, 39,* 19–24.

Eisenstein, T. K., & Hilburger, M. E. (1998). Opioid modulation of immune responses: Effects on phagocyte and lymphoid cell populations. *Journal of Neuroimmunology, 83,* 36–44.

Faith, R. E., Liang, H. J., Murgo, A. J., & Plotnikoff, N. P. (1984). Neuroimmunomodulation with enkephalins: Enhancement of human natural killer (NK) cell activity in vitro. *Clinical Immunology and Immunopathology, 31,* 412–418.

Felten, S. Y., & Felten, D. L. (1991). Innervation of lymphoid tissue, In Ader, R., Felten, D. L., & Cohen, N. (Ed.), *Psychoneuroimmunology* (2nd ed.) (pp. 27–69). San Diego, CA: Academic Press.

Felten, S. Y., & Olschowka, J. A. (1987). Noradrenergic sympathetic innervation of the spleen. II. Tyrosine hydroxylase (TH)-positive nerve terminals from synaptic-like contacts on lymphocytes in the splenic white pulp. *Journal of Neuroscience Research, 18,* 37–48.

Feng, N., Pagniano, R., Tovar, C. A., Bonneau, R. H., Glaser, R., & Sheridan, J. F. (1991). The effect of restraint stress on the kinetics, magnitude, and isotype of the humoral immune response to influenza virus infection. *Brain, Behavior, and Immunity, 5,* 370–382.

Forget, A., Skamene, E., Gros, P., Miailke, A. C., & Turcotte, R. (1981). Differences in response among inbred mouse strains to infection with small doses of *Mycobacterium bovis. Infection and Immunity, 32,* 42–47.

Freire-Garabal, M, Balboa, J. L., Fernandez-Rial, J. C., Nunez, M. J., & Belmonte, A. (1993). Effects of alprazolam on influenza virus infection in stressed mice. *Pharmacology, Biochemistry, and Behavior, 46,* 167–172.

Friedman, S. B., Ader, R., & Grota, L. J. (1973). Protective effect of noxious stimulation in mice infected with rodent malaria. *Psychosomatic Medicine, 35,* 535–537.

Fuchs, B. A., Albright, J. W., & Albright, J. F. (1988). β-Adrenergic receptors on murine lymphocytes: Density varies with cell maturity and lymphocyte subtype and is decreased after antigen administration. *Cellular Immunology, 114,* 231–245.

Galant, S. P., Durisetti, L., Underwood, S., & Insel, P. A. (1978). β-Adrenergic receptors on polymorphonuclear leukocytes: Adrenergic therapy decreases receptor number. *New England Journal of Medicine, 299,* 933–936.

Gebhardt, B. M., & Kaufman, H. E. (1995). Popranolol suppresses reactivation of herpesvirus. *Antiviral Research, 27,* 255–261.

Gilman, S. C., Schwartz, J. M., Milner, R. J., Bloom, F. E., & Feldman, J. D. (1982). β-Endorphin enhances lymphocyte proliferative responses. *Proceedings of the National Academy of Sciences, USA, 79,* 4226–4230.

Gilmore, W., & Weiner, L. P. (1988). β-Endorphin enhances interleukin-2 (il-2) production in murine lymphocytes. *Journal of Neuroimmunology, 18,* 125–138.

Gilmore, W., & Weiner, L. P. (1989). The opioid specificity of beta-endorphin enhancement of murine lymphocyte proliferation. *Immunopharmacology, 17,* 19–30.

Green, G. M., & Kass, E. H. (1965). The influence of bacterial species on pulmonary resistance to infection in mice subjected to hypoxia, cold stress and ethanol intoxication. *British Journal of Experimental Pathology, 46,* 360–366.

Gros, P., Skamene, E., & Forget, A. (1981). Genetic control of natural resistance to *Mycobacterium bovis* (BCG) in mice. *Journal of Immunology, 127,* 2417–2421.

Gross, W. B. (1984). Effect of a range of social stress severity on *Escherichia coli* challenge infection. *American Journal of Veterinary Research, 45,* 2074–2076.

Gross, W. B. (1988). Effect of environmental stress on the response of ascorbic-acid treated chickens to *Escherichia coli* challenge infections. *Avian Diseases, 32,* 432–436.

Gross, W. B., Falkinham, III, J. D., & Payeur, J. B. (1989). Effect of environmental–genetic interactions on *Mycobacterium avium* challenge infection. *Avian Diseases, 33,* 411–415.

Hahn, P. Y., Yoo, P., Ba, Z. F., Chaudry, I. H., & Wang, P. (1998). Up regulation of Kupffer cell beta-adrenoceptors and cAMP levels during the late stage of sepsis. *Biochimica et Biophysica Acta, 1404*(3), 377–384.

Hall, D. M., Suo, J. L., & Weber, R. J. (1998). Opioid mediated effects on the immune system: Sympathetic nervous system involvement. *Journal of Neuroimmunology, 83,* 29–35.

Hamilton, D. R. (1974). Immunosuppressive effects of predator induced stress in mice with acquired immunity to *Hymenolepis nana. Journal of Psychosomatic Research, 18,* 143–153.

Harbour, D. A., Hill, T. J., & Blyth, W. A. (1983). Recurrent herpes simplex in the mouse: Inflammation in the skin and activation of virus in the ganglia following peripheral stimulation. *Journal of General Virology, 64,* 1491–1498.

Hermann G., Tovar, C. A., Beck, F. M., Allen, C., & Sheridan, J. F. (1993). Restraint stress differentially affects the pathogenesis of an experimental influenza virus infection in three inbred strains of mice. *Journal of Neuroimmunology, 47,* 83–94.

Hermann G., Tovar, C. A., Beck, F. M., & Sheridan, J. F. (1994). Kinetics of glucocorticoid response to restraint stress and/or experimental influenza viral infection in two inbred strains of mice. *Journal of Neuroimmunology, 49,* 25–33.

Hermann, G., Beck, F. M., & Sheridan, J. F. (1995). Stress-induced glucocorticoid response modulates mononuclear cell trafficking during experimental influenza virus infection. *Journal of Neuroimmunology, 56,* 179–186.

Hermann G., Beck, F. M., Tovar, C. A., Malarkey, W. B., Allen, C., & Sheridan, J. F. (1994). Stress-induced changes attributable to the sympathetic nervous system during experimental influenza viral infection in DBA/2 inbred mouse strain. *Journal of Neuroimmunology, 53,* 173–180.

Hill, A. V. (1998). The immunogenetics of human infectious diseases. *Annual Reviews in Immunology, 16,* 593–617.

Hill, T. J. (1985). Herpes simplex virus latency. In B. Roizman (Ed.), *The herpesviruses* (pp. 175–240). New York: Plenum.

Hill, T. J., Blyth, W. A., & Harbour, D. A. (1978). Trauma to the skin causes recurrence of herpes simplex in the mouse. *Journal of General Virology, 39,* 21–28.

Holt, P. S., & Porter, R. E. (1992). Microbiological and histopathological effects of an induced-molt fasting procedure on a *Salmonella enteritidis* infection in chickens. *Avian Diseases, 36,* 610–618.

Hurd, J., & Robinson, T. W. (1977). Herpes virus reactivation in a mouse model. *Journal of Antimicrobial Chemotherapy, 3*(Suppl. A), 99–106.

Irwin, M. R., & Hauger, R. (1988). Adaptation to chronic stress: Temporal pattern of immune and neuroendocrine correlates. *Neuropsychopharmacology, 1,* 239–243.

Irwin, M. R., Hauger, R. L., Brown, M., & Britton, K. T. (1988). CRF activates the autonomic nervous system and reduces natural killer cytotoxicity. *American Journal of Physiology, 255,* R744–R747.

Irwin, M. R., Vale, W., & Britton, K. T. (1987). Central corticotropin-releasing factor suppresses natural killer cytotoxicity. *Brain, Behavior and Immunity, 1,* 81–87.

Ishigami, T. (1919). The influence of psychic acts on the progress of pulmonary tuberculosis. *American Reviews of Tuberculosis, 2,* 470–484.

Jackson, G. J. (1955). The effect of cortisone on *Plasmodium berghi* infections in the white rat. *Journal of Infectious Diseases, 97,* 152–159.

Jensen, M. M., & Rasmussen, A. F., Jr. (1963). Stress and susceptibility to viral infections. II. Sound stress and susceptibility to vesicular stomatitis virus. *Journal of Immunology, 90,* 21–23.

Johnson, E. W., Blalock, J. E., & Smith, E. M. (1988). ACTH receptor-mediated induction of leukocyte cyclic AMP. *Biochemical Biophysical Research Communications, 157,* 1205–1211.

Johnson, H. M., Smith, E. M., Torres, B. A., & Blalock, J. E. (1982). Regulation of the in vitro antibody response by neuroendocrine hormones. *Proceedings of the National Academy of Sciences, USA, 79,* 4171–4174.

Johnson, H. M., Torres, B. A., Smith, E. M., Dion, L. D., & Blalock, J. E. (1984). Regulation of lymphokine (interferon-γ) production by corticotropin. *Journal of Immunology, 132,* 246–250.

Johnson, R. W., Arkins, S., Dantzer, R., & Kelley K. W. (1997). Hormones, lymphohemopoietic cytokines and the neuroimmune axis. *Comparative Biochemistry and Physiology, Part A. Physiology, 116,* 183–201.

Johnson, S. C., & Zwilling, B. S. (1985). Continuous expression of I-A antigen by peritoneal macrophages from mice resistant to *Mycobacterium bovis* (BCG). *Journal of Leukocyte Biology, 38,* 635–645.

Johnsson, T., & Rasmussen Jr., A. F. (1965). Emotional stress and susceptibility to poliomyelitis virus infection in mice. *Archives. Ges. Virusforsch, 17,* 392–397.

Karp, J. D., Moynihan, J. A., & Ader, R. (1997). Psychosocial influences on immune responses to HSV-1 infection in BALB/c mice. *Brain, Behavior, and Immunity, 11,* 47–62.

Kern, J. A., Lamb, R. J., Reed, J. C., Daniele, R. P., & Nowell, P. C. (1988). Dexamethasone inhibition of interleukin 1 beta production by human monocytes. *Journal of Clinical Investigation, 81,* 237–244.

Kiecolt-Glaser, J., Glaser, R., Gravenstein, S., Malarkey, W. B., & Sheridan, J. F. (1996). Chronic stress alters the immune response to influenza virus vaccine in older adults. *Proceedings of the National Academy of Sciences, USA, 93,* 3043–3047.

Kochi, A. (1991). The global tuberculosis situation and the new control strategy of the World Health Organization. *Tubercule, 72,* 1–6.

Koff, W. C., & Dunegan, M. A. (1985). Modulation of macrophage-mediated tumoricidal activity by neuropeptides and neurohormones. *Journal of Immunology, 135,* 350–354.

Kohut, M. L., Davis, J. M., Jackson, D. A., Colbert, L. H., Strasner, A., Essig, D. A., Pate, R. R., Ghaffar, A., & Mayer, E. P. (1998). The role of stress hormones in exercise-induced suppression of alveolar macrophage antiviral function. *Journal of Neuroimmunology, 81,* 193–200.

Konstantinos, A. (1995). *The early proinflammatory cytokine response to influenza viral infection in the murine lung and its modulation by restraint stress.* Thesis, The Ohio State University.

Kriesel, J. D., Gebhardt, B. M., Hill, J. M., Maulden, S. A., Hwang, I. P., Clinch, T. E., Cao, X., Spruance, S. L., & Araneo, B. A. (1997). Anti-interleukin-6 antibodies inhibit herpes simplex virus reactivation. *Journal of Infectious Disease, 175,* 821–827.

Kusnecov, A. V., Grota, L. J., Schmidt, S. G., Bonneau, R. H., Sheridan, J. F., Glaser, R., & Moynihan, J. A. (1992). Decreased herpes simplex viral immunity and enhanced pathogenesis following stressor administration in mice. *Journal of Neuroimmunology, 38,* 129–137.

Landmann, R., Burgisser, E., West, M., & Buhler, F. R. (1985). β-Adrenergic receptors are different in subpopulations of human circulating lymphocytes. *Journal of Receptor Research, 4,* 37–50.

Laver, W. G., Bischofberger N., & Webster R. G. (1999). Disarming flu viruses. *Scientific American, January,* 78–87.

Lee, S. W., Tso, A. P., Chan, H., Thomas, J., Petrie, K., Eugui, E. M., & Allison, A. C. (1988). Glucocorticoids selectively inhibit the transcription of the interleukin 1 β gene and decrease the stability of interleukin 1 β mRNA. *Proceedings of the National Academy of Sciences, USA, 85,* 1204–1208.

Leo, N. A., Callahan, T. A., & Bonneau, R. H. (1998). Peripheral sympathetic denervation alters both the primary and memory cellular immune response to herpes simplex virus infection. *Neuroimmunomodulation, 5,* 22–35.

Lew, W., Oppenheim, J. J., & Matsushima K. (1988). Analysis of the suppression of Il-1α and Il-1β production in human peripheral blood mononuclear adherent cells by a glucocorticoid hormone. *Journal of Immunology, 140,* 1895–1902.

Loria, R. M., & Padgett, D. A. (1992). Androstenediol regulates systemic resistance against lethal infections in mice. *Archives of Virology, 127,* 103–115.

Loveland, B. E., Jarrot, B., & McKenzie, I. F. C. (1981). Beta-adrenergic receptors on murine lymphocytes. *International Journal of Immunopharmacology, 3,* 45–55.

Maestroni, G. J., & Conti, A. (1996). Melatonin and the immune–hematopoietic system therapeutic and adverse pharmacological correlates. *Neuroimmunomodulation, 3,* 325–32.

Mandler, R. N., Biddison, W. E., Mandler, R., & Serrate, S. A. (1986). β-Endorphin augments the cytolytic activity and interferon production of natural killer cells. *Journal of Immunology, 136,* 934–939.

Matthews, P. M., Froelich, C. J., Sibbitt, W. L., & Bankhurst, A. D. (1983). Enhancement of natural cytotoxicity by β-endorphin. *Journal of Immunology, 130,* 1658–1662.

McCain, H. W., Lamster, I. B., & Bilotta, J. (1986). Modulation of human T-cell suppressor activity by beta endorphin and glycyl-L-glutamine. *International Journal of Immunopharmacology, 8,* 443–446.

McCain, H. W., Lamster, I. B., Bozzone, J. M., & Grbic, J. T. (1982). β-endorphin modulates human immune activity via non-opiate receptor mechanisms. *Life Sciences, 31,* 1619–1624.

McNerney, R. (1999). TB: The return of the phage. A review of fifty years of mycobacteriophage research. *International Journal of Tuberculosis and Lung Diseases, 3,* 179–184.

Mehrishi, J. N., & Mills, I. H. (1983). Opiate receptors on lymphocytes and platelets in man. *Clinical Immunology and Immunopathology, 27,* 240–249.

Mellon, R. D., & Bayer, B. M. (1999). The effects of morphine, nicotine and epibatidine on lymphocyte activity and hypothalamic-pituitary-adrenal axis responses. *Journal of Pharmacology and Experimental Therapeutics, 288*(2), 635–642.

Miller, A. H. (1998). Neuroendocrine and immune system interactions in stress and depression. *Psychiatric Clinics of North America, 21,* 443–463.

Miller, C. S., Danaher, R. J., & Jacob, R. J. (1998). Molecular aspects of herpes simplex virus I latency, reactivation, and recurrence. *Critical Reviews in Oral Biology and Medicine, 9,* 541–562.

Miller, M. (1995). *Neuroendocrine regulation of natural killer cell activity during viral infection.* The Ohio State University, Honors Thesis.

Motulsky, H. J., & Insel, P. A. (1982). Adrenergic receptors in man. *New England Journal of Medicine, 307,* 18–29.

Noisakran, S., Halford, W. P., Veress, L., & Carr, D. J. J. (1998). Role of the hypothalamic pituitary adrenal axis and IL-6 in stress-induced reactivation of latent herpes simplex virus type 1. *Journal of Immunology, 160,* 5441–5447.

Northrop, J. P., Crabtree, G. P., & Mattila, P. S. (1992). Negative regulation of interleukin 2 transcription by the glucocorticoid receptor. *Journal of Experimental Medicine, 175,* 1235–1245.

Padgett, D. A., MacCallum, R. C., & Sheridan, J. F. (1998a). Stress exacerbates age-related decrements in the immune response to an experimental influenza viral infection. *Journal of Gerontology (Series A, Biological Sciences and Medical Sciences), 53,* B347–353.

Padgett, D. A., Sheridan, J. F., Dorne, J., Berntson, G. G., Candelora, J., & Glaser R. (1998b). Social stress and the reactivation of latent herpes simplex virus type 1. *Proceedings of the National Academy of Sciences, USA, 95,* 7231–7235.

Payne, F. E., Larson, A., Walker, D. L., Foster, L., & Meyer, K. F. (1955). Studies on immunization against plague. IX. The effects of cortisone on mouse resistance to attenuated strains of *Pasteurella pestis. Journal of Infectious Diseases, 96,* 168–173.

Pitchenik, A. E., & Fertel, D. (1992). Tuberculosis and nontuberculosis mycobacterial disease. *Medical Clinics of North America, 76,* 121–171.

Pitzalis, C., Sharrack, B., Gray, I. A., Lee, A., & Hughes, R. A. (1997). Comparison of the effects of oral versus intravenous methylprednisolone regimens on peripheral blood T lymphocyte adhesion molecule expression, T cell subsets distribution and TNF alpha concentrations in multiple sclerosis. *Journal of Neuroimmunology, 74(1–2),* 62–68.

Ramsey, J. M. (1982). *Basic pathophysiology: Modern stress and the disease process* (pp. 30–73). Menlo Park, CA: Addison-Wesley .

Rasmussen, A. F., Marsh, J. T., & Brill, N. O. (1957). Increased susceptibility to herpes simplex in mice subjected to avoidance-learning stress or restraint. *Proceedings of the Society for Experimental Biology and Medicine, 96,* 183–189.

Russo-Marie F. (1992). Macrophages and the glucocorticoids. *Journal of Neuroimmunology, 40,* 281–286.

Sacerdote, P., di San Secondo, V. E., Sirchia, G., Manfredi, B., & Panerai, A. E. (1998). Endogenous opioids modulate allograft rejection time in mice: possible relation with Th1/Th2 cytokines. *Clinical Experimental Immunology, 113,* 465–469.

Sanders, V. M. (1998). The role of norepinephrine and beta-2-adrenergic receptor stimulation in the modulation of Th1, Th2, and B lymphocyte function. *Advances in Experimental Medical Biology, 437,* 269–278.

Sawtell, N. M. (1998). The probability of in vivo reactivation of herpes simplex virus type 1 increases with the number of latently infected neurons in the ganglia. *Journal of Virology, 72,* 6888–6892.

Sawtell, N. M., & Thompson, R. L. (1992a). Herpes simplex virus type 1 latency-associated transcription unit promotes anatomical site-dependent establishment and reactivation from latency. *Journal of Virology, 66,* 2157–2169.

Sawtell, N. M., & Thompson, R. L. (1992b). Rapid in vivo reactivation of herpes simplex virus type-1 in latently infected murine ganglionic neurons after transient hyperthermia. *Journal of Virology, 66,* 2150–2156.

Selye, H. (1998). A syndrome produced by diverse nocuous agents. 1936. *Journal of Neuropsychiatry and Clinical Neuroscience, 10,* 230–231.

Sharp, B. M., Roy, S., & Bidlack, J. M. (1998). Evidence for opioid receptors on cells involved in host defense and the immune system. *Journal of Neuroimmunology, 83,* 45–56.

Sheridan, J. F., Dobbs, C., Jung, J., Chu, X., Konstantinos, A., Padgett, D., & Glaser R. (1998). Stress-induced neuroendocrine modulation of viral pathogenesis and immunity. *Annals of the New York Academy of Sciences, 840,* 803–808.

Sheridan, J. F., Feng, N., Bonneau, R. H., Allen, C., Huneycutt, B. S., & Glaser, R. (1991). Restraint-induced stress differentially effects anti-viral cellular and humoral immune responses. *Journal of Neuroimmunology, 31,* 245–255.

Singer, I. (1954). The effect of cortisone on infections with *Plasmodium berghi* in the white mouse. *Journal of Infectious Diseases, 94,* 164–172.

Smith, E. M., Bronsan, P., Meyer, W. J., & Blalock, J. E. (1987). An ACTH receptor on human mononuclear leukocytes. *New England Journal of Medicine, 317,* 1266–1269.

Snyder, D. S., & Unanue, E. R. (1992). Corticosteroids inhibit murine macrophage Ia expression and interleukin-1 production. *Journal of Immunology, 129,* 1803–1805.

Steiner, I. (1996). Human herpes viruses latent infection in the nervous system *Immunological Reviews, 152,* 157–173.

Stevens, J. G. (1975). Latent herpes simplex virus and the nervous system. *Current Topics in Microbiology and Immunology, 70,* 31–50.

Stevens-Felten, S. Y., & Bellinger, D. L. (1997). Noradrenergic and peptidergic innervation of lymphoid organs. *Chemical Immunology, 69,* 99–131.

Swiergiel, A. H., Smagin, G. H., Johnson, L. J., & Dunn, A. J. (1997). The role of cytokines in the behavioral responses to endotoxin and influenza virus infection in mice: effects of acute and chronic administration of the interleukin-1-receptor antagonist (IL-1ra). *Brain Research, 776,* 96–104.

Thompson, R. L., & Sawtell, N. M. (1997). The herpes simplex virus type 1 latency-associated transcript gene regulates the establishment of latency. *Journal of Virology, 71,* 5432–5440.

Vacca, A., Martiinitti, S., Screpanti, I., Maroder, M., Fellis, M. P., Farina, A. R., Gismondi, A., Santoni, A., Frati, L., & Gulino, A. (1990). Transcriptional regulation of the interleukin 2 gene by glucocorticoid hormones. *Journal of Biological Chemistry, 265,* 8075–8080.

van de Stolpe, A., & van der Saag, P. T. (1996). Intercellular adhesion molecule-1. *Journal of Molecular Medicine, 74(1),* 13–33.

Vollmer, E. P. (1951). The course of pneumococcal infection in mice during treatment with antibacterial substances and adrenocortical extract. *Journal of Infectious Diseases, 88,* 27–31.

Wagner, E. K., & Bloom, D. C. (1997). Experimental investigation of herpes simplex virus latency. *Clinical Microbiology Reviews, 10,* 419–443.

Webster, E. L., Battaglia, G., & De Souza, E. B. (1989). Functional corticotropin-releasing factor (CRF) receptors in mouse spleen: Evidence from adenylate cyclase studies. *Peptides, 10,* 395–401.

Webster, E. L., Torpy, D. J., Elenkov, I. J., & Chrousos, G. P. (1998). Corticotropin-releasing hormone and inflammation. *Annals of the New York Academy of Sciences, 840,* 21–32.

Webster, E. L., Tracey, D. E., Jutila, M. A., Wolfe, Jr., S. A., & De Souza, E. B. (1990). Corticotropin-releasing factor receptors in mouse spleen: Identification of receptor-bearing cells as resident macrophages. *Endocrinology, 127,* 440–452.

Wiegeshaus, E., Balasubramanian, V., & Smith, D. W. (1989). Immunity to tuberculosis from the perspective of pathogenesis. *Infection and Immunity, 57,* 3671–3676.

Wissink, S., van de Stolpe, A., Caldenhoven, E., Koenderman, L., & van der Saag, P. T. (1997). NF-kappa B/Rel family members regulating the ICAM-1 promoter in monocytic THP-1 cells. *Immunobiology, 198(1–3),* 50–64.

Zamri-Saad, M., Jasni, S., Naridi, A. B., & Sheikh-Omar, A. R. (1991). Experimental infection of dexamethasone-treated goats with *Pasteurella haemolytica* A2. *British Veterinary Journal, 147,* 565–568.

Zhang, D., Kishihara, K., Wang, B., Mizobe, K., Kubo, C., & Nomoto, K. (1998). Restraint stress-induced immunosuppression by inhibiting leukocyte migration and Th1 cytokine expression during the intraperitoneal infection of *Listeria monocytogenes. Journal of Neuroimmunology, 92*(1–2), 139–151.

Zwilling, B. S., Brown, D., & Pearl, D. (1992). Induction of major histocompatibility complex class II glycoproteins by interferon-

γ: Attenuation of the effects of restraint stress. *Journal of Neuroimmunology, 37,* 115–122.

Zwilling, B. S., Dinkins, M., Christner, R., Faris, M., Griffin, A., Hilburger, M., McPeek, M., & D. Pearl. (1990). Restraint stress induced suppression of major histocompatibility complex class II expression by murine peritoneal macrophages. *Journal of Neuroimmunology, 29,* 125–130.

# 56

# Stress, Immunity, and Susceptibility to Upper Respiratory Infection

SHELDON COHEN, GREGORY E. MILLER

## I. INTRODUCTION

Studies examining whether stress confers increased susceptibility to infectious disease date back to the 1950s. Considerable evidence has accumulated since that time in support of a relationship between stress and the incidence of *self-reported* colds and influenza (reviewed by Cohen & Williamson, 1991). The most convincing work on stress and infectious disease, however, has come from studies that provide biological verification of illness. For example, prospective epidemiological studies have demonstrated that family stress is associated with a higher incidence of serologically verified upper respiratory infection (Clover, Abell, Becker, Crawford, & Ramsey, 1989; Graham, Douglas, & Ryan, 1986; Meyer & Haggerty, 1962). In contrast, early viral-challenge studies, where volunteers completed psychological stress measures and were subsequently administered an experimental pathogen, yielded inconsistent findings concerning the association between stress and infectious susceptibility (Broadbent, Broadbent, Phillpotts, & Wallace,

1984; Greene, Betts, Ochitill, Iker, & Douglas, 1978; Locke & Heisel, 1977; Totman, Kiff, Reed, & Craig, 1980). However, recent studies employing larger sample sizes and more sophisticated methodologies provide strong evidence for a relationship between increased stress and illness risk (Cohen, Tyrrell, & Smith, 1991; Cohen et al., 1998; Cohen, Doyle, & Skoner, 1999; Stone et al., 1993).

If psychological stress does heighten vulnerability to infectious illness, what are the mechanisms through which this might occur? When the demands imposed by life events exceed a person's ability to cope, a psychological stress response is elicited (Lazarus & Folkman, 1984). The stress response consists of negative cognitive states such as helplessness and negative emotional states such as sadness or fear. These states set into motion a series of biological and behavioral changes that alter immune function and as a consequence may put persons at higher risk for developing infection and illness when exposed to an infectious pathogen. For instance, stress may influence immunity via central nervous system (CNS) innervation of lymphoid organs or through neuroendocrine–immune pathways. Direct neural pathways linking the CNS to the immune system have been identified (Felten et al., 1987; Felten & Felten, 1994). In the case of hormonal pathways, catecholamines secreted by the adrenal-medulla in response to stress and stress-triggered pituitary-mediated hormones such as cortisol and prolactin have been associated with modulation of immune function (Felten & Felten, 1994; Rabin, Kusnecov, Shurin, Zhou, & Rasnick,

1995). Moreover, receptors for a number of hormonal products have been found on lymphocytes and ligation of these receptors induces changes in lymphocyte function (see Blalock, 1994).

Behavioral changes that occur as adaptations or coping responses to psychological stress may also influence immunity. For example, persons experiencing stress often engage in poor health practices, e.g., smoking, poor diets, and poor sleeping habits (Cohen & Williamson, 1988; Conway, Vickers, Ward, & Rahe, 1981), that may have immunomodulatory effects (Kiecolt-Glaser & Glaser, 1988). Aggressive or affiliative behaviors triggered by prolonged psychological stress may also influence immunity. In other words, it may be the coping behaviors themselves, and not the precipitating stressor, that trigger sympathetic or endocrine responses (Cohen, Evans, Stokols, & Krantz, 1986; Manuck, Harvey, Lechleiter, & Neal, 1978).

Accumulating evidence on the role of the social environment and health has raised questions about potentially positive psychosocial effects on host resistance. Prospective studies have documented that people who participate in multiple social domains (e.g., family, friend, work, group membership) live longer (reviewed by Berkman, 1995), are more likely to survive myocardial infarction (reviewed by Berkman, 1995; cf. Orth-Gomer, Rosengren, & Wilhelmsen, 1993), are less likely to report being depressed (reviewed by Cohen & Wills, 1985), and are less likely to suffer a recurrence of cancer (reviewed by Helgeson, Cohen, & Fritz, 1998) than their more isolated counterparts. The health risks of being isolated are comparable in magnitude to the risks associated with cigarette smoking, blood pressure, and obesity and remain even after controlling for these and other traditional risk factors.

Although there is little evidence on the role of social behaviors in host resistance to infectious agents, there are several reasons to hypothesize that individuals with more diverse social networks may be at reduced risk for the development of upper respiratory infections (see Cohen, 1988; Cohen, Gottlieb, & Underwood, in press). First, social relationships may foster behaviors that promote resistance to infection, such as regular exercise and abstinence from tobacco. Second, when stressful life events occur, social relationships may serve a buffering function that protects individuals from the emotional and physiological sequelae associated with stress. Several studies have demonstrated that the presence of a supportive other can blunt autonomic nervous system and hypothalamo-pituitary-adrenal axis responses to stress (e.g., Kamarck, Manuck, & Jennings, 1990;

Kirschbaum, Klauer, Sigrun-Heide, & Hellhammer, 1995).

In the remainder of this chapter we describe our own research on stress, social participation, and susceptibility to upper respiratory infection. In these studies, we assess the psychosocial characteristics of healthy volunteers and subsequently expose them to a virus that causes a common cold. Approximately 40% of those exposed develop a verifiable illness. Hence we can ask whether their psychosocial status preceding exposure predicts whether their bodies are able to resist infection and illness. This paradigm eliminates the possibilities that associations we find between psychosocial characteristics and susceptibility are attributable to *previous exposure* to the virus (we assess and control for pre-challenge antibody), to *differential exposure to the virus* (we expose volunteers to controlled doses of virus), to *illness causing changes in psychosocial predictors* (we assess psychosocial factors before viral exposure in healthy volunteers), or to illness *causing changes in psychological, behavioral, and biological processes we pursue as links between psychosocial factors and disease susceptibility* (we assess these factors before viral exposure as well).

## II. THE BRITISH COMMON COLD STUDY: PSYCHOLOGICAL STRESS AND COLDS

Our initial study was carried out at the Medical Research Council's Common Cold Unit between 1986 and 1989. Detailed descriptions of the methodology used in this investigation have been published elsewhere (Cohen et al., 1991; Cohen, Tyrrell, & Smith, 1993). Briefly, 154 men and 266 women between the ages of 18 and 54 volunteered for the study. All were judged to be in good health following a physical examination, defined as having no acute or chronic medical condition and no regular medication regimen. During their first 2 days on the clinical unit, volunteers were given a thorough medical examination and completed psychological stress, personality, and health practice questionnaires. Subsequently, volunteers were exposed via nasal drops to a low infectious dose of one of five respiratory viruses: rhinovirus types 2 ($n = 86$), 9 ($n = 122$), and 14 ($n = 92$), respiratory syncytial virus ($n = 40$), and coronavirus type 229E ($n = 54$). An additional 26 volunteers received saline.

For 2 days before and 7 days after viral challenge, volunteers were quarantined in large apartments (alone or with one or two others). Starting 2 days before viral challenge and continuing through 6 days postchallenge, each volunteer was examined daily by a clinician using a standard respiratory sign-symptom protocol. Examples of items on the protocol include sneezing, watering of eyes, nasal stuffiness, sore throat, hoarseness, and cough. The protocol also included an objective count of the number of tissues used daily by a volunteer and body temperature (oral) assessed twice each day. Samples of nasal secretions were also collected daily to assess whether volunteers were infected by the experimental virus. Approximately 28 days after challenge a second serum sample was collected to assess changes in viral-specific antibody as an indirect measure of infection. All investigators were blind to volunteers' psychological status and to whether they received virus or saline.

## A. Measures

### 1. Psychological Stress

Recall that when environmental demands outstrip an individual's ability to cope, a stress response is triggered, consisting of negative emotional and cognitive states. To capture the various components of this process, we had volunteers complete questionnaires assessing (a) the number of major stressful life events they judged as having a negative impact, (b) the perception that current demands exceeded their ability to cope, and (c) their current negative affect. The major stressful life events scale consisted of events that might happen in the life of the respondent (41 items) or close others (26 items). The Perceived Stress Scale (Cohen & Williamson, 1988) was used to assess the degree to which situations in life were perceived as stressful. Items in the scale were designed to tap how unpredictable, uncontrollable, and overloading respondents found their lives. The negative affect scale included 15 items from the Zevon and Tellegen (1982) list of negative emotions. We also created an index of psychological stress that was based on all three of the scales described above. This was accomplished by quartiling each scale and summing quartile ranks for each subject, resulting in a scale with scores ranging from 3 to 12.

### 2. Clinical Colds

Volunteers were considered to have a cold if they were *both* infected and meeting illness criteria. Infection status was determined directly by culturing nasal secretion samples for viral proteins or indirectly through establishing fourfold increases in viral-specific antibody from baseline to 28 days postexposure. The illness criterion was based on clinician judgement of the severity of each volunteer's cold at the end of the trial, on a scale ranging from nil (0) to

severe (4). Ratings of mild cold (2) or greater were considered positive clinical diagnoses. Thirty-eight percent (148) developed clinical colds (infection + illness). None of the 26 saline controls developed colds.

### 3. Health Practice Measures

We also examined whether health practices operated as a pathway through which stress contributed to disease susceptibility. Health practice measures included smoking status, alcohol consumption, exercise frequency, subjective sleep quality, and diet.

### 4. Personality Measures

Because psychological stress could reflect stable personality styles rather than responses to environmental stressors, self-esteem and personal control (two personality characteristics closely associated with stress) were assessed prior to viral challenge. A third personality characteristic, introversion–extraversion, was also assessed.

### 5. Standard Control Variables

The analyses presented below include statistical controls for a set of variables that could provide alternative explanations for any relationship between stress and illness. These standard control variables include age, gender, education, weight, allergic status, season of the year during which the trial was conducted, the number of others the subject was housed with during the trial, whether housemates were infected or not, type of experimental virus the subject was infected with, and prechallenge serostatus for the experimental virus.

## B. Results

### 1. Stress and Susceptibility to Clinical Illness

As Figure 1 illustrates, subjects with more stress had higher rates of colds, irrespective of whether stress was measured as life events, perceived stress, or negative affect or by using the stress index. To determine whether any of these effects might be attributable to relations between stress and health practices, we ran an additional set of conservative analyses including smoking rate, drinking rate, diet, exercise, and sleep quality in the equations along with the 10 standard control variables and the stress index. This procedure tests whether stress is associated with greater susceptibility after the possible effects of these variables are subtracted. The addition of health practices did not significantly alter the results. To determine whether these relations might be attributable

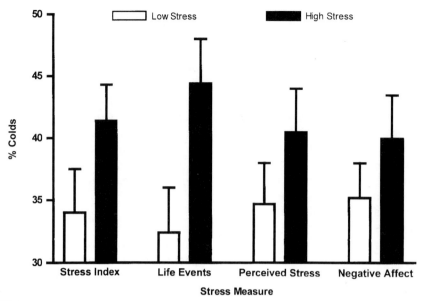

**FIGURE 1**   Observed association between each of the stress measures and rates of clinical colds. Standard errors are indicated. [Figure from Cohen, S., Tyrrell, D. A. J., & Smith, A. P. (1993). Negative life events, perceived stress, negative affect, and susceptibility to the common cold. *Journal of Personality and Social Psychology, 64*, 135. Reprinted with permission from the American Psychological Association.]

to the stress scales actually reflecting personality characteristics, we ran an additional analysis in which the three personality factors were added to the equation. Again, the relations between stress and illness were independent of these personality characteristics.

### 2. Are Stress Effects Consistent across the Five Viruses?

The analyses described thus far have collapsed across viruses. However, a test of whether the effects of stress were consistent across the viruses (stress by virus type interaction term) indicated that they were. The influence of stress on each virus is depicted in Figure 2. This suggests the possibility that the relation between psychological stress and upper respiratory illness is nonspecific, i.e., not dependent on the pathogenesis of the specific virus. Figure 2 also suggests the dose–response type relation that occurred in all cases, with each increase in stress associated with an increase in colds. (A detailed analysis of the dose–response issue is reported in Cohen et al. (1991).)

### C. Discussion

We found that higher levels of stress—whether measured as life events, perceived stress, or negative affect—were associated with increases in clinical illness. In all cases, these relations could not be explained by factors thought to be associated with stress including age, gender, education, weight, allergic status, the virus that the subject was exposed to, or environmental characteristics associated with the design of the study. The relations were also not explicable in terms of either stress-induced differences in health practices or associations between stress and the three personality characteristics we measured: self-esteem, personal control, and introversion–extraversion.

The consistency of the stress–illness relation across three very different viruses—rhinovirus, coronavirus, and respiratory syncytial virus (as well as among rhinovirus types)—was impressive. This observation suggests that stress is associated with the suppression of a general resistance process in the host, leaving persons susceptible to multiple infectious agents (or at least agents attacking the upper respiratory tract), or that stress is associated with the suppression of many different immune processes, with similar results. It is also possible that stress is associated with some general change in the host, such as the ability to produce mucus or the quality of mucus production.

### III. THE PITTSBURGH COMMON COLD STUDY: STRESS, SOCIAL NETWORKS, AND COLDS

Although the study described above yielded compelling evidence for a relationship between stress and

**% with Colds**

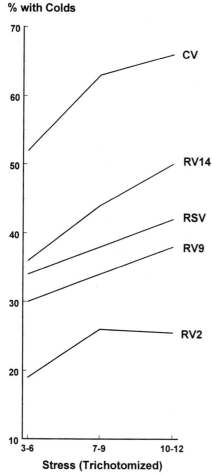

**Stress (Trichotomized)**

**FIGURE 2**  Association between the psychological stress index and the rate of clinical colds for each of the five viruses. CV, coronavirus; RSV, respiratory syncytial virus; RV, rhinovirus.

susceptibility to upper respiratory infection, it provided little information about the characteristics of stressors that place individuals at risk for illness. The objective of our second study was to gather more information about this issue. We were interested in answering questions such as: Do acutely stressful events have the same impact on susceptibility as more chronic, ongoing stressors? Do certain classes of stressors have a more potent impact than others? Does illness risk vary as a function of the duration of a stressor? The Pittsburgh study also provided us with an opportunity to examine the role of social participation in illness susceptibility. We were interested in examining both the direct effects of social participation on risk for colds and the extent to which having social ties could buffer volunteers from the increased susceptibility associated with stressful life events.

This study was carried out in Pittsburgh, Pennsylvania, between 1993 and 1996. Descriptions of the methods used have been published elsewhere

(Cohen, Doyle, Skoner, Rabin, & Gwaltney, 1997; Cohen et al., 1998). Briefly, 276 adults (125 men and 151 women) between the ages of 18 and 55 participated in the study. All volunteers initially came to the hospital for medical eligibility screenings and were judged to be in good health. Social networks, select health practices (smoking, alcohol consumption, exercise, sleep quality, diet), demographic factors, body weight, and height were also assessed at the screening and used as baseline data for those who were found to be eligible. Eligible subjects returned to the hospital both 4 and 5 weeks after screening to have blood drawn for assessment of a marker of immune function—natural killer cell activity—that was based on both blood draws, and antibody to the experimental virus based on the second blood draw. A personality questionnaire was administered twice, once at each blood draw. Volunteers returned an additional time during the period after initial screening but before being exposed to the virus to complete an intensive stressful life events interview.

Subjects were quarantined within 1 week following the second blood draw. Baseline assessment of self-reported respiratory symptoms and two objective indicators of illness (nasal mucociliary clearance, and nasal mucus production) were assessed during the first 24 h of quarantine (before viral exposure). Urine samples for the assessment of cortisol, epinephrine, and norepinephrine were also collected at this time. At the end of the first 24 h of quarantine, volunteers were given nasal drops containing a low infectious dose of one of two types of rhinovirus (RV39 [$n = 147$] or Hanks [$n = 129$]). The quarantine continued for 5 days after exposure. During this period volunteers were housed individually, but were allowed to interact with each other at a distance of 3 feet or more. Nasal secretion samples for verifying infection by virus culture were collected on each of the 5 days. On each day, volunteers completed a respiratory symptoms questionnaire and were tested for objective markers of illness. Approximately 28 days after challenge, another blood sample was collected for verifying infection by determination of changes in antibody to the challenge virus. All investigators were blinded to subjects' status on social network, personality, endocrine, health practice, immune, and pre-challenge antibody measures.

## A. Measures

### 1. Social Stress

A semistructured interview, the Bedford College Life Events and Difficulties Schedule (LEDS) was used to assess life events (Brown & Harris, 1989; Harris, 1991). The LEDS uses strict criteria for whether or not an event occurs, classifies each event on the basis of severity of threat and emotional significance, and allows dating of the onset and resolution of each event and hence a determination of event duration. Raters blind to the individual's subjective response to an event are provided with extensive information regarding each event and the context in which it occurred. They rate the threat and emotional significance of events based on the likely response of an average person to an event occurring in the specified context. A person is considered under stress if they have an event that is rated as moderately or severely threatening.

### 2. Social Participation

Social network participation was assessed by questionnaire. The Social Network Index assesses participation in 12 types of social relationships (Cohen et al., 1997). These include relationships with a spouse, parents, parents-in-law, children, other close family members, close neighbors, friends, workmates, schoolmates, fellow volunteers (e.g., charity or community work), members of groups without religious affiliations (e.g., social, recreational, professional), and members of religious groups. One point is assigned for each kind of relationship (possible score of 12) for which respondents indicate that they speak (in person or on the phone) to someone in that relationship at least once every 2 weeks. The total number of persons with whom they speak at least once every 2 weeks (number of network members) was also assessed.

### 3. Clinical Colds

Volunteers were considered to have a cold if they were *both* infected and meeting illness criteria. They were classified as infected if the challenge virus was isolated on any of the five postchallenge study days or there was a substantial rise (fourfold increase in antibody titer) in serum antibody level to the experimental virus. The illness criterion in this trial was based on selected *objective* indicators of illness—the amount of mucus produced during quarantine and mucociliary clearance function. By basing the definition of illness entirely on objective indicators, we were able to exclude interpretations of our data based on psychological influences on symptom presentation. Mucus weights were determined by collecting used tissues in sealed plastic bags. After correcting for the weight of the bag and tissue, and the mucus weight at baseline, the postchallenge weights were summed across the 5 days to create an adjusted total mucus

weight score. Nasal mucociliary clearance function refers to the effectiveness of nasal cilia in clearing mucus from the nasal passage toward the throat. Clearance function was assessed as the time required for a dye administered into the nose to reach the throat. Each daily time was adjusted for baseline and the adjusted average time in minutes was calculated across the postchallenge days of the trial. To meet clinical illness criteria, subjects had to have a total adjusted mucus weight of at least 10 g or an adjusted average mucociliary nasal clearance time of at least 7 min.

### 4. Standard Control Variables

Standard control variables were again used to examine alternative explanations for any relationship between psychosocial factors and illness. These included age, gender, ethnicity, education, body mass index (weight in kilograms divided by the square of height in meters), season during which the trial was conducted, type of experimental virus, and prechallenge antibody titers to the experimental virus.

### 5. Personality

Because either stress or social participation might merely be markers of stable personality styles, we assessed the "Big Five" personality factors (Goldberg, 1992). These factors are thought to represent the basic structure of personality (e.g., Goldberg, 1992). The factors are commonly described as: introversion–extraversion, agreeableness, conscientiousness, emotional stability, and openness.

## B. Results

### 1. Acute Stressful Life Events, Chronic Difficulties, and Susceptibility

The longer the stressful life event, the greater the risk for developing a clinical illness (Figure 3). Moreover, this association could be accounted for primarily by two types of events: enduring (1 month or longer) interpersonal problems with family and friends and enduring work (under- or unemployment; Figure 4). These effects held across two rhinoviruses and were equal for persons with and without neutralizing antibody to the virus prior to inoculation.

### 2. Social Networks and Susceptibility

As apparent from Figure 5, the rate of colds decreased as social network diversity increased. The adjusted relative risks of developing a cold were 4.2,

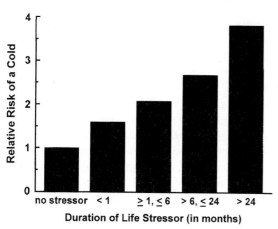

**FIGURE 3** Relative risk (odds ratio adjusted for standard controls) of developing a cold contrasting persons with stressors of varying duration with those without any stressor. Participants are grouped by their longest stressor. [Figure from Cohen, S., Frank, E., Doyle, W. J., Skoner, D. P., Rabin, B. S., & Gwaltney, J. M., Jr. (1998). Types of stressors that increase susceptibility to the common cold in healthy adults. *Health Psychology, 17,* 219. Reprinted with permission from the American Psychological Association.]

1.9, and 1 respectively. There were no interactions between the standard control variables and social network diversity in predicting colds. Hence, the relations were similar for the two virus types, for different preexposure antibody levels, age, gender, race, education, and body mass, and across the two seasons.

Total number of network members was not associated with colds. Moreover, entering number of network members into the first step of the regression

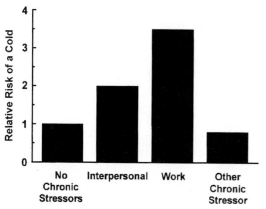

**FIGURE 4** Relative risk (odds ratio adjusted for standard controls) of developng a cold contrasting persons with interpersonal, work, and other chronic stressors with those having no chronic stressors. [Figure adapted from Cohen, S., Frank, E., Doyle, W. J., Skoner, D. P., Rabin, B. S., & Gwaltney, J. M., Jr. (1998). Types of stressors that increase susceptibility to the common cold in healthy adults. *Health Psychology, 17,* 219. Reprinted with permission from the American Psychological Association.]

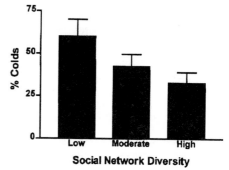

**FIGURE 5** Observed incidence of colds by social network diversity. Low diversity is described as one to three types of social relationships, moderate four to five; and high six or more. Standard errors are indicated. [Figure adapted from Cohen, S., Doyle, W. J., Skoner, D. P., Rabin, B. S., & Gwaltney, J. M., Jr. (1997). Social ties and susceptibility to the common cold. *Journal of the American Medical Association, 277,* 1943.]

equation along with standard controls did not reduce the association between diversity and colds. Hence the diversity of the network is more important than the number of network members and its association with colds is independent of the number of members.

The association of social participation and susceptibility was independent of the association between chronic stressors and susceptibility. Moreover, the interaction between chronic stress and network diversity did not achieve statistical significance, indicating that network diversity did not function as a stress buffer, but rather had a direct (irrespective of stress level) association with cold susceptibility.

### 3. Pathways Linking Social Networks and Stressful Life Events to Susceptibility

Preliminary analyses indicated that those with low levels of social participation were more likely to be smokers and less likely to exercise. Similarly, those with enduring chronic stressors were more likely to be smokers. There were also marginal associations between having a chronic stressor and less exercise and poorer sleep efficiency. All of these health practices were also associated with susceptibility to colds, with smokers, those getting less exercise, and those with poor sleep quality all at greater risk. However, these health practices could explain only a small fraction of the relation between these psychosocial characteristics and susceptibility to infectious illness. Although higher levels of epinephrine and norepinephrine were associated with greater risk for developing a cold, neither of these hormones (nor cortisol) was associated with social network or chronic stress indices. Hence, neither could operate as pathways linking these variables to illness susceptibility. Our measure of immune function, natural killer cell cytotoxicity, was not associated with either psychosocial characteristics or cold risk.

### 4. Personality as an Alternative Explanation

Of the Big five factors, we found that only introversion–extraversion was associated with susceptibility to colds. Those with scores below the median ("introverts") were at 2.7 times greater risk. Although none of the personality factors were associated with chronic stress, introversion was associated with lower levels of social network diversity. However, the relation between network diversity and colds occurred above and beyond (independent of) the association of introversion and colds.

## C. Discussion

This study provided additional evidence that psychological stress contributes to susceptibility to upper respiratory infection (see Cohen et al., 1991, 1993; Graham et al., 1986; Meyer & Haggerty, 1962; Stone et al., 1993). It also provided information about the characteristics of stressors that are likely to heighten risk for illness. Although acutely stressful life events did not confer increased susceptibility, enduring stressors lasting 1 month or longer were associated with a higher incidence of clinical colds. The relationship between chronic stress and illness was independent of volunteers' age, gender, ethnicity, education, body mass, and prechallenge virus-specific antibody levels. It also was independent of the season during which the challenge was conducted and the type of experimental virus administered.

The link between chronic stress and illness risk was primarily attributable to chronic problems in the interpersonal or work domains. Volunteers experiencing chronic interpersonal stressors such as conflicts with friends, family, or spouses were at nearly three times the risk of developing a cold as those without enduring stressors. Volunteers who were chronically underemployed or unemployed were almost five times as likely to become ill in comparison with volunteers without a chronic stressor. Because many types of chronic stressors had a low base rate in our sample, these findings should not be taken to mean that interpersonal or work stressors are the only types of enduring difficulties that heighten illness risk. Instead, our findings suggest that when these stressors occur, they can have potent influences on

susceptibility. The magnitude of this influence seems to depend in part on the duration of the stressor itself. The longer the duration of the stressor, the greater the risk for illness.

This study also demonstrated that social isolation constitutes a major risk factor for the development of illness. Volunteers who were relatively socially isolated (one to three relationships) were 4.2 times more likely to develop illness than those with very diverse networks (six or more relationships). Interestingly, it was the diversity of participants' social networks, rather than the total number of relationships that they had, that predicted susceptibility. This suggests that it is something about occupying a variety of social roles (e.g., spouse, parent, co-worker, friend) that promotes resistance to infection. How this occurs is not clear, although the present study suggests that it is *not* likely to be through a stress-buffering mechanism.

What can account for the relations between chronic stress, social participation, and susceptibility to infectious illness? Our results left us with few ideas. Neither health practices nor endocrine or immune assessments provided an explanation. Because the health practice measures were all related to susceptibility in the expected manner, we are confident that we did a good job of assessing this pathway. As a consequence, it seems unlikely that these health practices play a major role in linking social environments to resistance to infectious illness. Although we assessed the health practices that we thought would be most likely to provide a pathway, it is possible that other practices such as caffeine intake, use of mouthwash, or regular hand washing, might link stress or social participation to illness susceptibility.

Elevated epinephrine and norepinephrine were also associated with increased risk for illness. Because epinephrine and norepinephrine were assessed during the 24 h before viral exposure, it is possible they were indicating a stress type reaction to the beginning of quarantine rather than a basal level of response to volunteers' background environments.

Natural killer cell activity was not associated with either the psychosocial variables or risk for illness. We chose natural killer cell activity as our primary marker of immune function for two reasons. First, natural killer cells are surveillance cells that identify infected (and otherwise altered cells) and kill them. In theory, higher levels of natural killer cell activity should help limit infection and hence prevent illness. Second, there is evidence that chronic psychological stress is associated with suppression of NK activity (reviewed in Herbert & Cohen, 1993). However, NK activity did not operate as a pathway linking stress or social participation to illness susceptibility in our study. Measuring immunity in peripheral blood is not always the most appropriate procedure and may be the problem here (Cohen & Herbert, 1996). In theory, NK activity in the lung might be the essential issue in the case of respiratory infections. It is also possible the NK activity in the blood might make a difference, but that the ability of the immune system to compensate for deficits in single subsystems obscures any relation. At any rate, we found no evidence for immune mediation of the relations between stress and infectious illness or social participation and infectious disease. Again, we think that this may be attributable to problems in measurement.

## IV. PITTSBURGH INFLUENZA STUDY: CYTOKINES AS MEDIATORS

Up until now, the major outcome in our studies has been whether persons exposed to a virus develop a clinical illness. Clinical illness has been defined as a combination of infection by the virus (assessed by viral shedding or increased viral-specific antibody) and symptom expression (doctor diagnosed or verified by objective markers such as mucus weights). Our recent work has moved toward providing a more refined understanding of how psychosocial factors influence disease susceptibility. To do this, one needs to distinguish between the role that psychosocial factors play in susceptibility to infection and the role that they play in expression of illness among infected persons. (In our earlier trials, approximately 80% of exposed subjects develop infection, but only 40% are diagnosed as clinically ill.) We have started to address this issue by developing a challenge model that allows examination of illness expression among infected persons. To accomplish this, we used an influenza A virus that results in infection in 95% or more of subjects without previous exposure (i.e., without neutralizing antibody) to the virus. We then examine the extent to which psychosocial factors predict illness expression among infected subjects.

A major focus of this trial was to test the possibility that proinflammatory cytokines might play a role in illness expression. Recent advances in the understanding of how cytokines function in upper respiratory infection offers a promising new direction for this research. Psychological stressors have been shown to activate the production of proinflammatory cytokines such as IL-1, IL-6, IFN-$\gamma$, and TNF-$\alpha$ (Ackerman, Martino, Heyman, Moyna, & Rabin, 1998). Local increases in the concentrations of one of these cytokines, IL-6, have been linked to greater cold symptomatol-

ogy among persons with verified upper respiratory infection (Gentile, Doyle, Whiteside, Hayden, & Skoner, in press; Hayden et al., 1998). Since the secretion of cytokines in response to infection is thought to be mediated by glucocorticoids (Dobbs, Feg, Beck, & Sheridan, 1996), it is conceivable that stress could exacerbate cold symptomatology through a cortisol-triggered upregulation of proinflammatory cytokine production.

We recently conducted a relatively small trial to test the viability of studying illness expression per se and examining the role of cytokines in the link between stress and expression. This trial was designed to determine whether psychological stress was associated with the expression of symptoms and production of mucus in infected subjects (Cohen et al., 1999) and whether stress-associated elevations in cytokine production in response to a virus might explain an association between stress and illness expression. *After* completing a measure of psychological stress (the Perceived Stress Scale (PSS)), 55 subjects were experimentally infected with the A Kawasaki Influenza virus. Subjects were monitored in quarantine for 8 days (baseline and 7 days after inoculation) for upper respiratory symptoms, mucus production, and nasal lavage levels of interleukin (IL)-6.

As in previous trials we included standard controls for age, season of the year, gender, race, and body mass. The association between perceived stress and symptoms, mucus weights, and IL-6 are presented in Figures 6, 7, and 8. Higher psychological stress

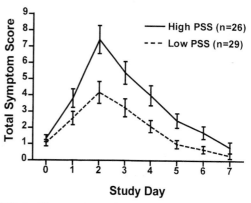

**FIGURE 6** The association between psychological stress (low, below median, high, above median) and symptoms of upper respiratory illness among subjects infected with an influenza A virus. Viral inoculation occurred at the end of day 0. Standard errors are indicated. [Figure from Cohen, S., Doyle, W. J., & Skoner, D. P. (1999). Psychological stress, cytokine production, and severity of upper respiratory illness. *Psychosomatic Medicine, 61,* 177. Reprinted with permission from the American Psychosomatic Society.]

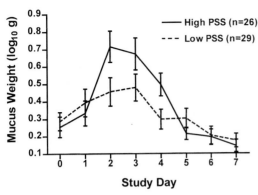

**FIGURE 7** The association between psychological stress (low, below median, high, above median) and mucus weights among subjects infected with an influenza A virus. Viral inoculation occurred at the end of day 0. Standard errors are indicated. [Figure from Cohen, S., Doyle, W. J., & Skoner, D. P. (1999). Psychological stress, cytokine production, and severity of upper respiratory illness. *Psychosomatic Medicine, 61*, 177. Reprinted with permission from the American Psychosomatic Society.]

assessed prior to the viral challenge was associated with greater symptom scores, greater mucus weights, and higher IL-6 lavage concentrations in response to infection. The IL-6 response was temporally related to both markers of illness expression, and mediation analyses indicated that these data were consistent with IL-6 acting as a major pathway through which stress was associated with increased symptoms of illness. However, this is correlational data and must be interpreted with care. This pattern of data is also consistent with rises in IL-6 occurring in response to tissue damage associated with illness symptoms or IL-6 responding in concert with other unassayed pro-

inflammatory chemicals that might play the causal role here.

## V. CONCLUSIONS

These studies that we have presented convincingly demonstrate that psychological stress is associated with increased vulnerability to the common cold. This relationship emerges whether stress is measured as life events, perceived stress, or negative emotional states. It also emerges across seven different experimental viruses, suggesting that stress dampens resistance in a way that renders the host vulnerable to a variety of infectious agents that invade the respiratory tract. The characteristics of stressors that influence illness risk also have been clarified to some extent. More enduring stressors such as underemployment and conflicts with family or friends confer increased susceptibility, while acutely stressful life events do not. The mechanisms by which this occurs are not yet clear. Our work suggests that stress-elicited changes in health behaviors such as smoking or exercise are not responsible. Moreover, thus far we have been unable to identify endocrine mediators of the relationship between stress and illness. As we noted above, this may be attributable to measurement problems. We have, however, had some initial success in our attempt to identify immune pathways with our evidence that IL-6 response to infection overlaps with stress and illness expression. We are continuing to examine the potential role of proinflammatory cytokines and hope that this work will provide a more complete understanding of the pathways which link psychological stress with vulnerability to upper respiratory infection.

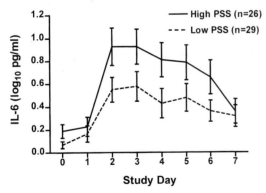

**FIGURE 8** The association between psychological stress (low, below median, high, above median) and IL-6 in nasal secretions among subjects infected with an influenza A virus. Viral inoculation occurred at the end of day 0. Standard errors are indicated. [Figure from Cohen, S., Doyle, W. J., & Skoner, D. P. (1999). Psychological stress, cytokine production, and severity of upper respiratory illness. *Psychosomatic Medicine, 61*, 178. Reprinted with permission from the American Psychosomatic Society.]

### References

Ackerman, K. D., Martino, M., Heyman, R., Moyna, N. M., & Rabin, B. S. (1998). Stressor-induced alteration of cytokine production in multiple sclerosis patients and controls. *Psychosomatic Medicine, 60*, 484–491.

Berkman, L. F. (1995). The role of social relations in health promotion. *Psychosomatic Medicine, 57*, 245–254.

Blalock, J. E. (1994). The syntax of neuroendocrine–immune communication. *Immunology Today, 15*, 504–511.

Broadbent, D. E., Broadbent, M. H. P., Phillpotts, R. J., & Wallace, J. (1984). Some further studies on the prediction of experimental colds in volunteers by psychological factors. *Journal of Psychosomatic Resesarch, 28*, 511–523.

Brown, G. W., & Harris, T. O. (1989). *Life events and illness.* New York: Guilford Press.

Clover, R. D., Abell, T., Becker, L. A., Crawford, S., & Ramsey, C. N. (1989). Family functioning and stress as predictors of influenza B infection. *The Journal of Family Practice, 28*, 536–539.

Cohen, S. (1988). Psychosocial models of the role of social support in the etiology of physical disease. *Health Psychology, 7,* 269–297.

Cohen, S., Doyle, W. J., & Skoner, D. P. (1999). Psychological stress, cytokine production, and severity of upper respiratory illness. *Psychosomatic Medicine, 61,* 175–180.

Cohen, S., Doyle, W. J., Skoner, D. P., Rabin, B. S., Gwaltney, J. M., Jr. (1997). Social ties and susceptibility to the common cold. *Journal of the American Medical Association, 277,* 1940–1944.

Cohen, S., Evans, G. W., Stokols, D., & Krantz, D. S. (1986). *Behavior, health, and environmental stress.* New York: Plenum.

Cohen, S., Frank, E., Doyle, W. J., Skoner, D. P., Rabin, B. S., & Gwaltney, J. M., Jr. (1998). Types of stressors that increase susceptibility to the common cold. *Health Psychology, 17,* 214–223.

Cohen, S., Gottlieb, B., & Underwood, L. (in press). *Social support measurement and intervention: A guide for health and social scientists.* New York: Oxford University Press.

Cohen, S., & Herbert, T. B. (1996). Health Psychology: Psychological factors and physical disease from the perspective of human psychoneuroimmunology. In J. T. Spence, J. M. Darley, & D. J. Foss (Eds.), *Annual Review of Psychology* , (Vol. 47). El Camino, CA: Annual Review.

Cohen, S., Tyrrell, D. A. J., & Smith, A. P. (1991). Psychological stress and susceptibility to the common cold. *New England Journal of Medicine, 325,* 606–612.

Cohen, S., Tyrrell, D. A. J., & Smith, A. P. (1993). Life events, perceived stress, negative affect and susceptibility to the common cold. *Journal of Personality and Social Psychology, 64,* 131–140.

Cohen, S., & Williamson, G. M. (1991). Stress and infectious disease in humans. *Psychological Bulletin, 109,* 5–24.

Cohen, S., & Williamson, G. M. (1988). Perceived stress in a probability sample of the United States. In S. Spacapan & S. Oskamp (Eds.), *The Social Psychology of Health.* Newbury Park, CA: Sage Publications.

Cohen, S., & Wills, T. A. (1985). Stress, social support and the buffering hypothesis. *Psychological Bulletin, 98,* 310–357.

Conway, T. L, Vickers, R. R., Ward, H. W., & Rahe, R. H. (1981). Occupational stress and variation in cigarette, coffee, and alcohol consumption. *Journal of Health and Social Behavior, 22,* 155–165.

Dobbs, C. M., Feg, N., Beck, F. M., & Sheridan, J. F. (1996). Neuroendocrine regulation of cytokine production during experimental influenza viral infection. *Journal of Immunology, 157,* 1870–1877.

Felten, S. Y., & Felten, D. L. (1994). Neural-immune interactions. *Progress in Brain Research, 100,* 157–162.

Felten, D. L., Felten, S. Y., Bellinger, D. Y., Carlson, S. L., Ackerman, K. D., Madden, K. S., Olschowka, J. A., & Livnat, S. (1987). Noradrenergic sympathetic interactions with the immune system structure and function. *Immunological Reviews, 100,* 225–260.

Gentile, D., Doyle, W. J., Whiteside, T., Hayden, F. G., & Skoner, D. P. (in press). Increased interleukin-6 levels in nasal lavages following experimental influenza A virus infection. *The Journal of Clinical Investigation.*

Goldberg, L. R. (1992). The development of markers for the Big-Five factor structure. *Psychological Assessment, 4,* 26–42.

Graham, N. M. H., Douglas, R. B., & Ryan, P. (1986). Stress and acute respiratory infection. *American Journal of Epidemiology, 124,* 389–401.

Greene, W. A., Betts, R. F., Ochitill, H. N., Iker, H. P., & Douglas, R. G. (1978). Psychosocial factors and immunity: Preliminary report. *Psychosomatic Medicine, 40,* 87.

Harris, T. O. (1991). Life stress and illness: The question of specificity. *Annals of Behavioral Medicine, 13,* 211–219.

Hayden, F. G., Fritz, R. S., Lobo, M. C., Alvord, W. G. Strober, W., & Straus, S. E. (1998). Local and systemic cytokine responses during experimental influenza A virus infection. *The Journal of Clinical Investigation, 101,* 643–649.

Helgeson, V. S., Fritz, H. L., & Cohen, S. (1998). Social ties and cancer. In J. C. Holland & W. Breitbart (Eds.), *Psycho-Oncology.* New York: Oxford University Press.

Herbert, T. B., & Cohen, S. (1993). Stress and immunity: A meta-analytic review. *Psychosomatic Medicine, 55,* 364–379.

House, J. S., Robbins, C., & Metzner, H. L. (1982). The association of social relationships and activities with mortality: Prospective evidence from the Tecumseh Community Health Study. *American Journal of Epidemiology, 116,* 123–140.

Kamarck T. W., Manusck, S. B., & Jennings, J. R. (1990). Social support reduces cardiovascular reactivity to a psychological challenge: A laboratory model. *Psychosomatic Medicine, 52,* 42–58.

Kiecolt-Glaser, J. K., & Glaser, R. (1988). Methodological issues in behavioral immunology research with humans. *Brain, Behavior, and Immunity, 2,* 67–78.

Kirschbaum, C., Klauer, T., Sigrun-Heide, F., & Hellhammer, D. H. (1995). Sex-specific effects of social support on cortisol and subjective responses to acute psychological stress. *Psychosomatic Medicine, 57,* 23–31.

Lazarus, R. S., & Folkman, S. (1984). *Stress, appraisal, and coping.* New York: Springer.

Locke, S. E., & Heisel, J. S. (1977). The influence of stress and emotions and the human immune response. *Biofeedback and Self-Regulation, 2,* 320.

Manuck, S. B., Harvey, A., Lechleiter, S., & Neal, K. (1978). Effects of coping on blood pressure responses to threat of aversive stimulation. *Psychophysiology, 15,* 544–549.

Meyer, R. J., & Haggerty, R. J. (1962). Streptococcal infections in families. *Pediatrics, 29,* 539–549.

Orth-Gomer, K., Rosengren, A., & Wilhelmsen, L. (1993). Lack of social support and incidence of coronary heart disease in middle-aged Swedish men. *Psychosomatic Medicine, 55,* 37–43.

Rabin B. S., Kusnecov A., Shurin M., Zhou D., & Rasnick S. (1995). Mechanistic aspects of stressor-induced immune alteration. In R. Glaser & J. K. Kiecolt-Glaser (Eds.), *Handbook of human stress and immunity.* New York: Academic Press.

Stone, A. A., Bovbjerg, D. H., Neale, J. M., Napoli, A., Valdimarsdottir, H., & Gwaltney, J. M., Jr. (1993). Development of common cold symptoms following experimental rhinovirus infection is related to prior stressful life events. *Behavioral Medicine, 8,* 115–120.

Totman, R., Kiff, J., Reed, S. E., & Craig, J. W. (1980). Predicting experimental colds in volunteers from different measures of recent life stress. *Journal of Psychosomatic Research, 24,* 155–163.

Zevon, M. A., & Tellegen, A. (1982). The structure of mood change: An idiographic/ nomothetic analysis. *Journal of Personality and Social Psychology, 43,* 111–122.

# 57

# Physical Activity and Upper Respiratory Infection

ROY J. SHEPHARD, PANG N. SHEK

## I. INTRODUCTION

Interest in the influence of physical activity on resistance to infectious disease has been stimulated by recurring reports that whereas moderate training enhances immune responses, excessive amounts of exercise—whether a single marathon run or a period of excessive training leading up to international competition—can suppress immune function for several hours to a week. The impact upon personal health of such changes in the immune response has been a source of controversy for many years (Cannon, 1993). Many exercise scientists now believe that although susceptibility to bacterial infections remains unaltered, the affected individual is at increased risk of upper respiratory infections (Brenner, Shek, & Shephard, 1994; Nieman, 1994; Gabriel & Kindermann, 1995; Peters-Futre, 1997). Others still argue that

special factors associated with high-performance competition give a false impression of an increased vulnerability to viral infections (Cannon, 1993).

This chapter summarizes normal mechanisms of defense against acute viral infections and considers briefly how protection may be modified by participation in acute and chronic physical activity. It then examines empirical epidemiological evidence suggesting an altered susceptibility to upper respiratory infections after participation in various types of exercise and training programs. Possible causes of spurious associations are explored, and the modulating influence of environmental factors, including psychological stressors, is discussed. Finally, brief comment is offered regarding the prevention and treatment of exercise-induced immunosuppression.

## II. NORMAL MECHANISMS OF DEFENSE AGAINST VIRAL INFECTIONS

The body offers both physical/mechanical and biological barriers to viral infection (Table I); both of these may be compromised if a person engages in heavy physical activity (Shephard, 1997).

### A. Physical and Mechanical Barriers

Susceptibility to any viral particles, which are suspended in the inspired air, depends on patterns of respiratory airflow and the mechanical barriers

**TABLE I   Normal Mechanisms of Defense against Invading Viral Infections**

**Physical and mechanical barriers**
  1. Nasal filtration
  2. Mucus secretion and expectoration
  3. Endothelial membrane

**Biological barriers**
  1. NK cells
       Lysis of infected cells
  2. Interferon
       Enhanced NK cell activity
       Inhibition of viral replication
  3. Specific antibodies
       Prevention of membrane penetration by virus
       Opsonization of virus
  4. Cytotoxic lymphocytes
       Lysis of infected cells
  5. Phagocytes
       Phagocytosis, presentation of viral protein to CD4+ cells
  6. Complement and acute phase protein
       Attraction of phagocytes to infected area
       Increase of viral susceptibility to lysis

imposed by mucus and endothelium. The turbinate bones create a turbulent airflow through the nasal passages, and this tends to precipitate any larger suspended particles in the nose. However, because of their small average size, virus-containing droplets tend to remain in suspension. The endothelium lining the airways functions as a physical barrier. Its effectiveness is enhanced because of mucus secretion by the goblet cells. The tracheal ciliae cause a steady flow of mucus to the throat, where it is either swallowed or expectorated. Coughing and sneezing supplement the effects of ciliate motion.

### B. Biological Barriers

The body's immediate biological response to infection is an acute inflammation of the affected tissue. Increases in local blood flow and vascular permeability facilitate the entry of leukocytes and plasma proteins into the affected region of the body. The immediate innate mechanisms available to counter viral infections include natural killer (NK) cells, phagocytes, and secretory IgA present in nasal and bronchial mucus.

NK cells have the ability to lyse infected cells and/or secrete toxic molecules onto their surface in the absence of major histocompatibility complex (MHC) proteins or cytokine messengers. Nevertheless, various cytokines, particularly interferon (IFN)-$\gamma$, a substance that also inhibits viral replication, enhance NK-cell activity. Phagocytes ingest viral particles, subse-

quently destroying them with potent enzymes and chemicals. Soluble elements such as complement and acute-phase protein play a supportive role, attracting phagocytes to the infected region and rendering the viral particles more vulnerable to lysis. Specific antibodies also contribute to early protection, either by preventing the virus from penetrating the endothelial cell membrane or by opsonization (a process that facilitates subsequent phagocytosis of the viral particle).

The main basis of biological defense against viral infections is the proliferation of specific cytotoxic lymphocytes. This process peaks some 7 days after the onset of infection. It depends on a sequence of events that includes macrocytic phagocytosis, killing of the microorganism by lysozymes and/or oxidizing agents, a processing of viral surface proteins, their presentation to T cells in association with MHC-restricted protein, and the secretion of various cytokines (particularly interleukin-1 and IFN-$\alpha$). B cells, antibodies, and complement also act against certain viruses.

## III. IMPACT OF ACUTE AND CHRONIC PHYSICAL ACTIVITY ON BARRIERS TO INFECTION

The effectiveness of both physical/mechanical and biological barriers to viral infection is modified during and immediately following a single bout of strenuous physical activity. Defenses may also be compromised by a period of heavy training such as preparation for international competition.

### A. Changes to Physical and Mechanical Barriers

The high respiratory flow rates that are developed during vigorous physical activity lead to a progressive cooling and drying of the respiratory mucosa in certain climates. The movement of the endothelial ciliae is slowed, and the viscosity of the mucus is increased. Both ciliary function and expectoration are impaired, reducing the rate of clearance of pathological microorganisms from the respiratory tract. Furthermore, drying and cooling of the endothelium may adversely affect the function of mucosal B cells, reducing the local secretion of antibodies.

Above a critical threshold intensity of exercise, the effects of a large respiratory minute volume are exacerbated by the onset of mouth breathing. The normal air warming, humidifying, and filtering mechanisms of the nose are then largely bypassed. The tracheal mucosa becomes exposed more directly not only to cold, dry air but also to respiratory pathogens, other particulate matter, and air contaminants. We might expect these various physical and mechanical factors to increase susceptibility to both viral and bacterial infections during vigorous exercise. In practice, there is little evidence of increased susceptibility to bacteria, so we must conclude that changes in barrier functions are not a major cause of the increased risk of upper respiratory infection which has been observed in heavy exercisers. This verdict is reinforced by the fact that increased susceptibility to viruses seems contingent on undertaking a volume of exercise equivalent to a marathon run; a run of 20–30 km, which might have an almost equal impact on physical barriers to infection, does not seem to modify the body's defenses.

## B. Changes in Biological Defense Mechanisms

The main basis for any change in susceptibility to upper respiratory infection seems an exercise-induced modulation of either nonspecific or specific immune defences. Regular moderate physical activity appears to enhance the efficacy of these biological mechanisms, whereas a bout of very heavy exercise or a period of intensive training weakens their effectiveness. Based on limited immunological and epidemiological evidence, several authors have proposed that the resistance to infection follows a J-shaped response curve, with excessive amounts of exercise creating a "window of opportunity" when viruses can become established in the body.

Given the normal mechanisms of biological defence outlined above, factors that might decrease the resistance to viral disease include: (1) a decrease in the number and/or function of natural killer cells; (2) a delayed or a reduced production of interferon; (3) a decreased availability of specific antibodies; (4) a decrease in the CD4+/CD8+ ratio; (5) an impaired lymphocyte proliferative response to mitogens; and (6) secondary infection due to impaired neutrophil function

### 1. Natural Killer Cells

A bout of vigorous exercise induces an acute increase in circulating NK cell count, usually with a matching rise of cytolytic activity (Shephard, 1997). The immediate rise in NK-cell numbers is correlated with the increase of heart rate, and it can be mimicked by injections of catecholamine:norepinephrine during moderate exercise, and epinephrine with more in-

tensive effort. The primary mechanism is probably a demargination of cells, secondary to an altered expression of adhesion molecules, but the exercise-induced increase in cardiac output may also play some role (Shephard, 1997).

Catecholamine secretion may lead not only to an overall increase in circulating NK-cell count, but also to the demargination and recruitment of NK cells with a high interleukin-2 response capacity. In theory, both changes might enhance cytolytic activity and thus the body's resistance to viral infection. However, in practice, the usual duration of an exercise bout and thus the period when NK count is increased is too brief to have any substantial influence on susceptibility. Moreover, if exercise is prolonged for several hours, the NK cell count and cytolytic activity gradually return toward initial resting values, even as activity continues (Shephard & Shek, 1999).

Both NK cell counts and cytolytic activity quickly fall below normal levels once exercise has ceased. In many studies, normal resting levels of NK cell function are restored within a few hours, leaving only a brief "window of opportunity" for a marauding virus. It is hard to imagine how 2–3 h of reduced NK-cell activity could account for a two- to sixfold increase in the incidence of upper respiratory infections (Nieman, 1994) that some have described following a marathon or ultramarathon run. Nevertheless, a few authors have described longer-lasting exercise-induced depressions of NK cell counts and/or cytolytic activity (Shephard & Shek, 1999). Shek, Sabiston, Buguet, and Radomski (1995) reported the most dramatic effect. In their study, both NK counts and cytolytic activity were still substantially depressed 7 days following a single 90- to 120-min bout of exercise at 65% of the individual's aerobic power. Such a prolonged change in NK cell function could limit cytolysis over the entire period when the NK cells are expected to play a dominant role in defending the body against microorganisms; in such circumstances, a substantial increase in the individual's risk of developing an acute viral illness might be anticipated, particularly if exposure to the pathogen followed closely upon the exercise bout.

Candidate hypotheses for the suppression of NK-cell activity following vigorous exercise include a lack of interleukin (IL)-2 and an accumulation of prostaglandins (Shephard, 1997). The first explanation can be discounted, since the addition of recombinant IL-2 to isolated NK cells postexercise does not restore their cytolytic activity. On the other hand, various prostaglandins ($PGE_1$, $PGE_2$, $PGA_1$, and $PGA_2$) are known to inhibit the cytotoxic activity of NK cells. In the context of heavy physical activity or excessive training, the most likely explanation seems an increased PGE$_2$ production induced by muscle trauma.

Repeated bouts of moderate exercise can increase the NK-cell count (Shephard, 1997) and this could explain why habitual exercisers sometimes have an increased resistance to infection.

### 2. Interferon

Any exercise-induced changes in the concentrations of interleukins and interferons could exert a direct effect on viral replication and also could alter the surface properties of the NK cells, changing their lytic activity (Mackinnon, 1992). However, a delayed or decreased production of interferon seems an unlikely explanation of increased viral susceptibility. Indeed, moderate physical activity may increase IFN production, and the output of IFN-$\alpha$ is unchanged by several weeks of exhausting exercise (Shephard, 1997).

### 3. Immunoglobulins

Concentrations of salivary IgA and serum IgG are essentially unchanged by a bout of moderate physical activity. In contrast, very vigorous physical activity can decrease the concentration of IgA in both saliva and nasal washings. Salivary concentrations remain depressed even after correction of data to a common salivary protein concentration and thus a constant output of saliva. One report found that concentrations remained low for 18 h following a 31-km race (Shephard, 1997).

Moderate training may increase salivary IgA concentrations, but in general, the response to an acute bout of exercise is independent of initial physical condition. IgA levels fall progressively in international competitors as they increase the intensity of their training. Partial recovery is seen during precompetitive tapering. The heavy training schedules of top competitors may also cause minor decreases in serum IgG concentrations (Mackinnon, 1996) and there have been suggestions that international athletes can profit from the administration of exogenous immunoglobulins (see below).

Decreases in mucosal IgA concentrations could have an important influence on susceptibility to upper respiratory infections in the first few hours after viral exposure, given that secretory IgA inhibits attachment of the virus to the respiratory epithelium, penetration of the epithelial cells, and subsequent intracellular replication. In support of the practical significance of changes in IgA levels, several studies have noted a temporal link between decreases in salivary IgA concentrations and an increased prevalence of upper respiratory infections (Mackinnon, 1996). In one such study, 92% of athletes who developed upper respiratory infections had low secretory IgA concentrations 2 days before developing clinical manifestations of illness.

### 4. CD4+/CD8+ Ratio

An appropriate CD4+/CD8+ ratio is important to both mitogen-induced lymphocyte proliferation and viral resistance. A decrease in the ratio leads to a downregulation of several immune responses. Decreases in CD4+ count limit the output of cytokines that activate NK and T cells and stimulate the proliferation and maturation of B cells; the immediate consequences include a decrease in cytotoxic activity and a lesser production of immunoglobulins. The CD4+/CD8+ ratio may drop below the critical value of 1.5 in response to a bout of maximal exercise, a longer period of submaximal exercise, or a spell of excessive training (Shephard, 1997). Monitoring of the CD4+/CD8+ ratio may thus help to identify athletes who have pursued training to the point where their vulnerability to infection is increased.

Nevertheless, inferences which are based on the CD4+/CD8+ ratio alone can be misleading. The CD4+/CD8+ ratio may be decreased for 1 to 2 h following vigorous exercise, but at the same time there may be increases in the absolute numbers of both CD4+ (T-helper) and CD8+ (T-cytotoxic/suppressor) cells. Further information is needed regarding the importance of the absolute CD4+ count as opposed to the CD4+/CD8+ ratio. It also remains unclear how far an increase in CD4+/CD8+ ratio and thus a greater activation of NK cells can compensate for a decrease in NK cell numbers (and vice versa).

### 5. Mitogen Responsiveness

Cell proliferation and the generation of specific cytotoxic lymphocytes offer the main basis of long-term defense against viral infections. Thus, it seems important that a bout of heavy physical activity or prolonged and rigorous military training can reduce the proliferative response of peripheral blood mononuclear cells (PBMCs) to both mitogens and antigens (Shephard, 1997). This effect of an acute bout of exercise sometimes persists for several hours, contributing to the overall window of opportunity for viral infection. On the other hand, a training program can diminish the depression of mitogen responsiveness initially associated with a given acute exercise challenge.

It has been suggested that the normal proliferative response to IL-2 is suppressed by high postexercise concentrations of prostaglandin. However, we have been unable to normalize lymphocyte proliferation by adding various quantities of IL-2 to isolated PBMCs (Shephard, 1997).

### 6. *Impaired Neutrophil Function*

Upper respiratory tract infections are often complicated and prolonged by secondary bacterial infections. A dramatic increase in the circulating numbers of neutrophils is seen during and immediately following exercise, but this does not necessarily lead to an increase in phagocytosis and thus greater resistance to bacterial infection. One study found that a 20-km race doubled the neutrophil count, but at the same time the percentage of phagocytosing cells was reduced to 49% of normal, so that there was little net change in neutrophil activity. Other investigators have described reductions in neutrophil adherence and phagocytosis following heavy exercise (Lötzerich, Wilczkowiak, Stein, & Peters, 1997; Shephard, 1997).

Evidence from training studies also suggests that activity-induced changes in neutrophil function do not have great importance in terms of upper respiratory infections. For example, an Australian investigation found that the oxidative burst of isolated neutrophils was reduced following 12 weeks of intensive training, but this did not increase susceptibility to respiratory infections.

### 7. *Other Possible Factors*

Other acute exercise-induced changes in immune function that could influence susceptibility to upper respiratory infection include increases in C-reactive protein and decreases in resting levels of serum complement and C-reactive protein (Shephard, 1997).

### 8. *Overall Responsiveness to Vaccines*

Very heavy exercise can impair the overall response to vaccines. Thus Bruunsgaard et al. (1997) noted a reduced response to tetanus and diphtheria toxoid, as well as to purified pneumococcus polysaccharide in the first few days after participation in an ironman triathlon.

## IV. PHYSICAL ACTIVITY AND THE RISK OF UPPER RESPIRATORY ILLNESS

Interactions between physical activity and susceptibility to infection are complex, depending on (among other factors) the type of viral challenge, the quality and quantity of the physical activity undertaken, its timing relative to the course of the disease process,

and the level of other environmental and psychological stressors.

Participation in a program of regular moderate physical activity seems to reduce the risk of upper respiratory infections in both animals and human subjects. On the other hand, both anecdotal reports and clinical studies suggest that a single bout of exhausting exercise or a period of very heavy physical training may have a detrimental effect on resistance, particularly if activity is undertaken during the infectious stage of the illness.

### A. Experimental Data

Limited data obtained in laboratory animals support the view that whereas moderate exercise has a beneficial effect, an excessive and/or "stressful" dose of exercise weakens host resistance to an experimental viral infection. Moreover, heavy physical activity seems to increase the virulence of certain viruses. For example, mice that have been inoculated with the influenza virus show an increased mortality if they are forced to swim during the early stages of infection (Ilbäck, Friman, Beisel, Johnson, & Berendt, 1984). Likewise, fatiguing treadmill exercise increases mortality and decreases the time to death in mice which have been inoculated with herpes simplex virus (Hertler, Davis, Kohut, Ghaffar, & Mayer, 1995).

An early human study administered filtered nasal secretions containing respiratory viruses to volunteers who were then exercised on the treadmill. Details of the exercise bout are scant, but it was concluded that the resulting fatigue caused an "insignificant" increase in the frequency with which colds were observed (Jackson et al., 1960). A more recent study instilled nasal drops containing one of five respiratory viruses or a placebo. The incidence of subsequent infection was correlated with indices of psychological stress, but was unrelated to a composite physical activity score based on walking, jogging, running, swimming, aerobic exercise, and domestic chores (Cohen, Tyrrell, & Smith, 1991). A further laboratory study assessed the severity of an experimental rhinovirus infection in terms of symptoms and the volume of mucus secreted; moderate exercise (40 min at 70% of the heart rate reserve three times per week) did not change the duration or the severity of the illness (Weidner et al., 1997).

### B. Human Epidemiological Data

Human epidemiological data support the view that whereas moderate amounts of physical activity either have no effect or reduce susceptibility to upper respiratory infection, prognosis is worsened once the volume of activity exceeds a specific threshold. Moreover, there is some indication of a dose–response relationship between the volume of physical activity that has been undertaken and the increase in susceptibility to respiratory viruses, suggesting that the observed adverse association is causal in nature (Table II).

## 1. Moderate Exercise

A single bout of moderate physical activity has little influence on immune responses. Some authors have found that participation in a program of regular, moderate physical activity has a protective effect against viral disease, although, perhaps because old people have a poorer initial immune function and a lower average initial level of physical activity, the benefit has been most obvious in seniors.

Osterback and Qvarnberg (1987) found no difference in the incidence of infections between children who participated in extracurricular activities (gymnastics, swimming, and ice hockey) and other elementary students who were physically less active, including those who were enrolled in a music program. Possibly, the intrinsic level of physical activity in young children already reaches the minimum threshold for optimal protection against viral disease.

Schouten, Verschuur, and Kemper (1988) observed a negative correlation between the incidence of respiratory tract symptoms and a moderate level of sports participation in young adult women. However, when data for young men were included in the sample, there was no longer any significant relationship between the frequency of upper respiratory complaints and either maximal oxygen intake or the dose of exercise (a moderate average of 700 MET · min per week).

Nieman et al. (1990) noted that 45 min of exercise, five times per week at 60% of the heart rate reserve, reduced the duration of symptoms but did not affect the incidence of upper respiratory infection in a group of women ages 25 to 45 years. On the other hand, among women ages 67 to 85 years, the incidence of upper respiratory tract infections was lowest in a highly conditioned subgroup, was at an intermediate level in a subgroup of regular walkers, and was greatest in calisthenic and control subgroups (Nieman et al., 1993). Likewise, Karper, and Boschen (1993) reported that 50 to 60 min of moderate exercise, performed 3 days per week, decreased the likelihood of respiratory tract infections in women ages 60 to 72 years.

## 2. Heavy Exercise and/or Overtraining

There now is a strong consensus that heavy exercise and/or overtraining increases the risk of respiratory symptomatology. However, few investigators have obtained clinical confirmation of infection or have looked for associated changes in immune function.

Douglas and Hanssen (1978) found that university rowers reported respiratory symptoms more frequently than nonathletic controls. The athletes also perceived their symptoms as being more severe. Linde (1987) noted that orienteers reported a higher incidence of respiratory infections (2.5 episodes per year) than nonorienteers (1.7 episodes per year). Symptoms also were said to persist marginally longer in orienteers than in controls (an average of 7.9 vs 6.4 days). Seyfried, Tobin, Brown, and Ness (1985) found overall morbidity rates of 7% in recreational swimmers, compared with 3% in control subjects. The swimmers had more complaints for each of the potential routes of infection (respiratory, gastrointestinal, eye, ear, and skin), although the most frequent reports were of respiratory ailments.

Peters and Bateman (1983) examined symptoms in the 2 weeks following participation in an ultramarathon event. During this time, 33% of the runners reported respiratory symptoms, compared with 15% of the nonrunners. In those who took 5.5 to 6.0 h to cover the 56-km distance, there was only a small increase in the likelihood of upper respiratory symptoms; but the prevalence of complaints increased progressively with running speed to reach three times control in those who had completed the event in less than 4 h. Nieman, Johanssen, and Lee (1989) also observed that, on average, a group of runners who participated in a 42-km marathon race had five times the likelihood of reporting an upper respiratory illness as equally trained runners who, for various reasons, had not participated in the event. On the other hand, participation in less demanding 5- to 21-km "fun runs" had no apparent impact on the incidence of respiratory infections.

Heath et al. (1991) found that the likelihood of developing a respiratory infection over a 12-month period was related to the individual's weekly running mileage in a dose-dependent manner. Risk factors included running more than 15 km per week, living alone, and a low body mass index. Likewise, Nieman, Johanssen, Lee, and Arabatzis (1990) found that marathon runners who trained over a distance of more than 97 km per week had twice the likelihood of developing upper respiratory complaints than those who ran less than 32 km per week, even after their

**TABLE II** Epidemiological Studies Examining the Influence of Acute and Chronic Physical Activity upon Susceptibility to Upper Respiratory Infections[a]

| Author | Population | Type of exercise | Upper respiratory infections |
|---|---|---|---|
| **Moderate exercise** | | | |
| Osterback and Qvamberg, 1987 | 76 M/61 F; 11–14 years | Interview: sports involvement | No difference from controls |
| Schouten et al., 1988 | 92 M/107 F; 20–23 years | Questionnaire: activity level & fitness | No effect in males, symptoms of URI less in active females |
| Nieman et al., 1990 | 36 F; 25–45 years | 45 min at 60% HR reserve 5 days/week | Reduced duration of URI symptoms |
| Karper and Boschen, 1993 | 6 M/10 F; 60–72 years | Moderate exercise 3 days/week | Reduced number of infections relative to initial state |
| Seyfried et al., 1985 | 8000 M and F; all ages to 70 years | Recreational swimming | Increased URI relative to nonswimmers |
| Nieman et al., 1993 | 44 F (elderly) | Walking 37 min 5 days/week | Reduced incidence of URI relative to controls |
| Weidner et al., 1997 | 34 M and F; 18–29 years | 40 min at 70% HR reserve 3 days/week | No change in duration or severity of experimental URI |
| **Strenuous exercise** | | | |
| Douglas and Hanssen, 1978 | 61 Rowers and 126 cadets | University rowing | Increased frequency and severity of URI in rowers |
| Strauss et al., 1988 | 87 M | University athletics | 86% report URI over 8 weeks |
| Peters and Bateman, 1983 | 145 M/5 F; 18–65 years | Ultramarathoners vs non-runners | URI symptoms increased in faster runners |
| Linde, 1987 | 55 M/28 F; 19–34 years | Orienteers vs nonorienteers | Incidence and duration of URI greater in orienteers |
| Nieman et al., 1990 | 2311 M and F; 35–37 years | Marathon runners | URI sixfold increase in faster runners after race |
| **Heavy training** | | | |
| Nieman et al., 1990 | 2311 M and F; 35–37 years | Marathon runners | URI twofold increase with training |
| Heath et al., 1991 | 447 M/83 F; 13–75 years | Distance running | URI increased if > 15 km/week |
| Lee et al., 1992 | 96 Air Force cadets | Initial training | Immune function depressed but no change in URI |
| Linenger et al., 1993 | 482 M | Special warfare training | High incidence of URI |
| Shephard et al., 1995 | 551 M/199 F; 40–81 years | Masters athletes | URI increased in 16% if > 70–80 km/week |
| Verde et al., 1992 | 10 M | Runners, 3-week 38% increase of training | Respiratory symptoms in 3/10 |

*Note.* M, male; F, female; HR, heart rate; URI, upper respiratory infections.

[a]For details of references not listed in the bibliography, see Brenner et al. (1994).

data had been adjusted for the potential confounding influences of age, stress, and illness at home.

Shephard, Kavanagh, and Mertens (1995) questioned Masters athletes (age-classified older competitors). The majority of subjects (76%) considered themselves less vulnerable to colds than their sedentary colleagues, and only 1.5% thought they were more vulnerable. Nevertheless, the vulnerable individuals were found primarily among the endurance competitors. Moreover, some 16% of the sample were conscious of a mileage at which their susceptibility was enhanced; usually, problems did not develop until they were covering a weekly distance of 70 to 80 km.

Heavy military training has also been reported to increase the incidence of respiratory infections (Linenger, Fink, Thomas, & Johnson, 1993) with a reduction of in vitro immune responsiveness (Lee, Meehan, Robinson, Mabry, & Smith, 1992). However, other investigators have maintained that in some categories of athlete (cross-country skiers, gymnasts, oarsmen, swimmers, and wrestlers) upper respiratory infections occur no more frequently than would be expected in sedentary people (Strauss, Lanese, & Leizman, 1988; Budgett & Fuller, 1989; Berglund & Hemmingson, 1990). Presumably, much depends on the type and volume of training that the individual currently is undertaking.

## V. POSSIBLE CAUSES OF SPURIOUS ASSOCIATIONS

Data suggesting that moderate physical activity protects against viral infections, but that very strenuous exercise has an adverse effect on susceptibility, are in accord with our current understanding of the responses of the immune system to various volumes of physical activity. Nevertheless, it remains important to exclude extraneous influences that could cause spurious associations between a bout of strenuous exercise and decreased resistance to infection.

Weidner (1994) has argued that for reports to be accepted, there should be a clear definition of physical activity, individual assessment of activity patterns using a reliable and valid measuring instrument, clear details of the dose of exercise (frequency, intensity, and duration), an assessment of prior activity and program adherence, and a detailed evaluation of symptoms. Few of the available reports satisfy all of these important criteria.

Critical issues that raise the specter of spurious associations include an altered exposure to pathogens, inappropriate diagnostic criteria, effects secondary to nutritional disturbances or muscle injury, and the impact of environmental and psychological stressors.

Through linkages between the hypothalamus and the immune system, a variety of environmental and psychological factors modulate the impact of acute and chronic physical activity upon the immune defenses against viral infection. Moreover, because of the pressures that surround international competition, both environmental and psychological challenges may be more severe in athletes than in laboratory subjects who perform exercise at similar relative intensities.

### A. Exposure to Pathogens

The locale of competition and any associated air travel may not only increase an individual's range of exposure to infected individuals, but also bring an athlete in contact with microorganisms which have not been encountered previously. Thus, the incidence of infection may be increased during and immediately following an international competition, even if an individual's inherent susceptibility to disease remains unchanged.

### B. Diagnostic Criteria

Infants and young children sustain four to eight upper respiratory infections per year, but in young adults, the annual incidence is often only one to two episodes per person. Thus, in order to look for exercise-induced changes in susceptibility to such infections, it is necessary to examine large populations.

In many epidemiological studies, the diagnosis of respiratory illness has been based on questionnaire responses rather than on detailed clinical examination. The symptoms associated with an upper respiratory infection (soreness of the throat and nasopharynx, nasal catarrh, and cough, with minimal fever) unfortunately are nonspecific, and they are easily confused with other consequences of vigorous exercise—particularly the respiratory irritation, coughing, and bronchospasm which may be caused by exposure to chemically polluted, cold, or dry air. For example, Schwellnus, Kiessig, Derman, and Noakes (1997) found a substantial reduction of upper respiratory symptoms following the topical administration of an anti-inflammatory agent (Fusafungine) as an oral and nasal spray.

The percentage of questionnaires that are returned is also rather low—for instance, 47 percent in the study of Nieman et al. (1990)—and it may be that the likelihood of response to a large-scale survey is biased in favour of those who develop an infection, or who fear doing so.

At the collegiate level of competition, only about one-third of upper respiratory infections are reported to a physician (Weidner, 1994). However, top-level athletes have ready access to medical services, and they perceive even a minor illness as limiting their competitive performance. Relative to the general public or even a collegiate athlete, they are thus more likely to report upper respiratory illnesses and to demand medical treatment for them. The decision to seek medical advice also depends heavily on an individual's perceived state of health. The anxiety associated with participation in an international competition or deterioration in performance subsequent to a period of overtraining tends to worsen perceived health. In consequence, the likelihood that an athlete will seek a medical consultation around the time of competition is further increased, even if the prevalence of organic disease is unchanged. This, in turn, could create a spurious association between high level competition and the prevalence of viral illnesses.

## C. Disturbances of Nutrition

Nutritional deficiencies are a well-recognized cause of impaired immune function in clinical malnutrition. An athlete shows much smaller deficiencies of essential nutrients than the person with clinical malnutrition, but may nevertheless fail to satisfy the demands imposed by either a single bout of prolonged physical activity or a repeated depletion of glycogen stores. Newsholme (1994) pointed out that glycogen depletion is followed by a 10–20% decrease in plasma glutamine levels, and he suggested that this glutamine deficiency might be sufficient to limit the rapid proliferation of immune cells. A recent report found low plasma glutamine levels ($<450\,\mu mol/L$) in all 11 of 51 top athletes who developed upper respiratory infections (Kingsbury, Kay, & Hjelm, 1998).

Other authors have suggested that deficiencies of arginine, L-carnitine, essential fatty acids, vitamin $B_6$, folic acid, vitamin E, and trace elements such as zinc, magnesium, and copper all contribute to an impairment of immune function in the athlete (Shephard & Shek, 1998b). Nehlsen-Cannarella et al. (1997) reported that a moderate (10 kg) diet-induced weight loss was sufficient to impair the function of T and B cells, monocytes, and granulocytes.

## D. Muscle Injury

The international competitor often develops cumulative subclinical tissue injuries in the working muscles during periods of intensive training. These lesions cause local and systemic acute-phase reactions. In the short term, the release of C-reactive protein stimulates the phagocytic action of monocytes. However, the chemotactic migration of leukocytes to injured tissue subsequently may increase vulnerability in other parts of the body, and the generation of reactive species during the repair process may also lead to a suppression of immune function in a manner analogous to that of clinical sepsis (Northoff, Enkel, & Weinstock, 1995).

Support for this last mechanism is provided by studies that show that the administration of vitamin C and other anti-oxidants can protect against exercise-induced infections (Hemilä, 1996; Peters, 1997; Peters-Futre, 1997).

## E. Environmental Factors

Immune function is modulated by a variety of environmental stresses such as extremes of heat and cold, high and low ambient pressures, inhalation of polluted air, sleep deprivation, time-zone shifts, and exposure to high and low gravitational forces (Shephard & Shek, 1998c). Relative to the average sedentary person, the active individual has a greater chance of exposure to most of these stresses. For example, many athletes frequently develop quite high core temperatures. Because of solar radiation, heat stress can be much more severe for an athletic competitor than for a laboratory subject, even if both ostensibly perform a comparable amount of physical activity at the same ambient temperature.

Likewise, the inhalation of air polluted by contaminants such as ozone can in itself induce an acute-phase response on the part of alveolar macrophages, and by virtue of the large respiratory minute volume that is sustained over an event, an endurance athlete is at particular risk of such an effect.

The neurohormonal responses to environmental stressors may in themselves have a marked effect on immune function—for example, the catecholamines secreted in response to severe cold, or the cortisol and cytokines (IL-1 and IL-6) associated with a rise in core temperature. Finally, if the individual is not habituated to an unusual environment, it may prove psychologically stressful, with resulting consequences for immune function.

## F. Psychological Stressors

Many types of psychological stress, from a first parachute jump to a critical university examination, impair aspects of immune function with an impact upon susceptibility to upper respiratory infections, including NK activity, lymphocyte proliferation, and salivary IgA levels (Shephard, 1997).

Vigorous physical activity—especially enforced exercise in animals and competition in humans—induces many of the neurohormonal responses associated with psychological stress, including substantial secretions of epinephrine and norepinephrine, cortisol, and growth hormone. In the competitive athlete, the inherent response to physical activity is supplemented by pressures due to the contest itself; expectations of the coach, sponsors, and general public; and the demands of international travel, including disturbance of circadian rhythms and long periods of absence from a normal home environment.

There have been reports that as much as a quarter of the variance in virus shedding from individuals inoculated with a rhinovirus can be traced to restricted social contacts and an excessive amount of time spent in goal-directed activities (Totman, Kiff, Reed, & Craig, 1980); such a lifestyle has now become almost inevitable during preparation for international athletic competition. All of these various factors increase the likelihood of upper respiratory infection in athletes, particularly around the time of major competition.

## VI.  PREVENTION OF INFECTION

Given that heavy physical activity can enhance the risk of upper respiratory infection, it is important to stress tactics of prevention, particularly for the competitive athlete. A number of practical measures reduce the likelihood of clinical infection. These include controlling exposure to pathogens, optimizing training and diet, minimizing environmental and psychological stresses, and offering preventive chemotherapy and/or immunotherapy.

### A.  Control of Exposure

Impairment of immune function sometimes leads to reactivation of a latent Epstein–Barr virus, which is widely prevalent in the young adult population. However, the development of a clinical infection generally involves exposure to an external pathogen.

Where practicable, athletes should avoid contact with young children and others who are showing symptoms of an upper respiratory infection. Hand contact is an important route for the transmission of respiratory viruses. The hands should be washed carefully before food is eaten. Some pathogens can also enter the body via the mucosa of the nose and eyes; neither should be rubbed with dirty hands.

### B.  Optimizing Training and Diet

Given reports that link impaired immune function to overtraining, any conditioning program should be matched carefully to the individual's initial physical status, and responses should be monitored closely. Declining performance, excessive fatigue, muscle soreness, a depression of mood, and adverse responses to simple psychological tests (such as the Profile of Mood States) are all indications that the intensity of training should be reduced (Shephard & Shek, 1998a).

Given the contribution of nutrition to immune function, it is important to ensure an adequate intake of overall food energy, good-quality protein, and antioxidants. In particular, vitamin C supplements can significantly reduce the incidence, duration, and severity of upper respiratory tract infections in endurance athletes (Hemilä, 1996; Peters, 1997; Peters-Futre, 1997; Shephard & Shek, 1998b). Competitors in a number of sports tend to develop a negative energy balance, particularly if the event demands prolonged physical activity or if performance is judged in part on physical appearance. It is less clear whether the negative energy balance is sufficiently severe to limit immune function. At least in animal studies, food deprivation must be quite severe before immune function deteriorates.

### C.  Minimizing Environmental and Psychological Stress

Another important preventive tactic is to minimize all forms of stress, not only psychological but also such environmental influences as excessive heat, cold, high altitude exposure, time zone shifts, and sleep deprivation.

### D.  Chemotherapy and Immunotherapy

Athletes are well advised to update their schedule of inoculations against the viruses prevalent at the venue of a major international competition. If the serum immunoglobulin levels are low, the administration of immunomodulating preparations (including intramuscular injections of human immunoglobulins) may also reduce the severity of disease if not the risk of bronchopulmonary infections (Shephard, 1997). For instance, a German study (Frohlich, Simon, Schmidt, Hitschhold, & Bierther, 1987) found that monthly injections of immunoglobulin led to a threefold reduction in the incidence of infections relative to control subjects. In contrast, world-class canoeists who were given nasal IgA showed no apparent benefit relative to controls, but this was perhaps not surprising, since the controls remained healthy and showed no evidence of subnormal levels of IgA (Lindberg & Berglund, 1996).

Intradermal kits (for example, Multitest Merieux, a cocktail of seven common antigens) allow repeated assessments of immunocompetence over the course of training. Salivary or mucosal immunoglobulins also can be monitored, although the link between low immunoglobulin levels and an increased susceptibility to infection remains tenuous.

Given the probable suppression of immune function by prostaglandins, immune function may also be helped by the administration of nonsteroidal anti-inflammatory agents such as indomethacin. Benefit is particularly likely if there is evidence of local muscular inflammation and soreness.

## VII. TREATMENT OF INFECTION

Occasional anecdotes tell of athletes achieving their best competitive times despite upper respiratory infections (Eichner, 1993), but generally such episodes cause a deterioration of physical performance. Often, the end result of a minor infection is that the competitor misses either a training session or an actual competition (Weidner, 1994).

Some deterioration of physical performance is to be anticipated as a consequence of systemic infections, given increases in resting core temperature, heart rate, and oxygen consumption and an altered activity of performance-related enzymes in both skeletal and cardiac muscle (Ilbäck, Friman, Crawford, & Neufeld, 1991). Laboratory tests show that infection reduces the time to exhaustion in experimental animals, and in humans, aerobic power and isometric and isokinetic strength all tend to be reduced. Nevertheless, it remains difficult to be certain how far these changes reflect a reduced motivation to maximal effort rather than an inherent effect of the disease process (Shephard, 1997).

In some instances, a postviral fatigue syndrome (Behan, Behan, Gow, Cavanagh, & Gillespie, 1993) may continue to limit both aerobic and anaerobic effort for a year or longer, but normal performance is usually regained quite rapidly once the acute illness has passed.

If an athlete develops an acute infection, it is important for the team physician to determine whether he or she has manifestations of a systemic viral disorder (Eichner, 1993). A simple upper respiratory infection requires no more than some moderation of training, with use of a decongestant by day and an antihistamine at night. However, if competition is approaching, care must be taken to ensure that prescribed medications do not breach antidoping rules. On the other hand, if the individual has developed a systemic viral illness, exercise must be approached with caution. Heavy training or competition can increase the severity of disease, and myocarditis can lead (albeit rarely) to death from cardiac arrest during exercise. Warning signs of systemic infection include fever, myalgia, fatigue, cough, vomiting, diarrhea, and lymphadenopathy. At least for recreational athletes, it is prudent to rest until symptoms of the infection have passed.

## VIII. CONCLUSIONS

Both a single bout of exhausting physical activity and very heavy training cause what seem a substantial array of immune disturbances. Further, these changes could reduce resistance to viral infections, in keeping with much of the available epidemiological data. However, interpretation of current findings must remain cautious. There are many possible causes of spurious associations between vigorous physical activity and upper respiratory infection. Moreover, many of the supposedly supporting immunological changes have been observed in specimens of peripheral blood, where changes in cell counts and activity may reflect no more than a demargination of previously sequestered cells, followed by their migration into recently active or injured tissues. There may thus be little true change in either cell count or antiviral activity in the body as a whole.

A further important issue in many acute experiments is that even if immune function has been suppressed, this disturbance has persisted for only a few hours. Exposure to infection would thus need to be closely coincident with the exercise bout if susceptibility to disease were to be increased. Finally, a moderate training program not only enhances resting immune function but also attenuates acute exercise-induced disturbances. Thus, although athletes may show an acute depression of an immune parameter such as NK cell count during or following a bout of intensive exercise, the absolute level of immune function may remain greater than that of sedentary individuals throughout the period of observation.

### Acknowledgment

The studies of Dr. Shephard are supported in part by the Defence and Civil Institute of Environmental Medicine.

# References

Behan, P. O., Behan, W. M., Gow, J. W., Cavanagh, H., & Gillespie, S. (1993). Enteroviruses and postviral fatigue syndrome. *CIBA Foundation Symposium, 173*, 146–159.

Berglund, B., & Hemmingson, P. (1990). Infectious disease in elite cross-country skiers: A one-year incidence study. *Clinical Sports Medicine, 2*, 19–23.

Brenner, I. K. M., Shek, P. N., & Shephard, R. J. (1994). Infection in athletes. *Sports Medicine, 17*, 86–107.

Bruunsgaard, H., Hartkopp, A., Mohr, T., Konradsen, H., Heron, I., Mordhorst, C. H., & Pedersen, B. K. (1997). In vivo cell-mediated immunity and vaccination response following prolonged, intense exercise. *Medicine and Science in Sports and Exercise, 29*, 1176–1181.

Budgett, R. G., & Fuller, G. N. (1989). Illness and injury in international oarsmen. *Clinical Sports Medicine, 1*, 57–61.

Cannon, G. (1993). Exercise and resistance to infection. *Journal of Applied Physiology, 74*, 973–981.

Cohen, S., Tyrrell, D. A. J., & Smith, A. P. (1991). Psychological stress and susceptibility to the common cold. *New England Journal of Medicine, 325*, 606–612.

Douglas, D. J., & Hanssen, P. G. (1978). Upper respiratory tract infections in the conditioned athlete. *Medicine and Science in Sports and Exercise, 10*, 55. [abstract]

Eichner, E. R. (1993). Infection, Immunity, and Exercise: What to tell patients? *Physician and Sportsmedicine, 21*(1), 125–135.

Frohlich, J., Simon, G., Schmidt, A., Hitschhold, T., & Bierther, M. (1987). Disposition to infections in athletes during treatment with immunoglobulins. *International Journal of Sports Medicine, 8*, 119. [abstract]

Gabriel, H., & Kindermann, W. (1995). Infections and sports: Frequency, causes and preventive aspects. *Deutsche Zeitschrift für Sportmedizin, 46*, 73–85.

Heath, G. W., Ford, E. S., Craven, T. E., Macera, C. A., Jackson, K. L., & Pate, R. R. (1991). Exercise and the incidence of upper respiratory tract infections. *Medicine and Science in Sports and Exercise, 23*, 152–157.

Hemilä, H. (1996). Vitamin C and common cold incidence: A review of studies with subjects under heavy physical stress. *International Journal of Sports Medicine, 17*, 379–383.

Hertler, L. M., Davis, J. M., Kohut, M. L., Ghaffar, A., & Mayer, E. P. (1995). Effect of exercise on resistance to viral infection in mice. *Medicine and Science in Sports and Exercise, 27*, S67. [abstract]

Ilbäck, N. G., Friman, D. J., Crawford, D. J., & Neufeld, H. A. (1991). Effects of training on metabolic responses and performance capacity in Streptococcus pneumonia infected rats. *Medicine and Science in Sports and Exercise, 23*, 422–427.

Ilbäck, N. G., Friman, G., Beisel, W. R., Johnson, A. J., & Berendt, R. F. (1984). Modifying effects of exercise on clinical course and biochemical response of the myocardium in influenza and tularemia in mice. *Infection and Immunity, 45*, 498–504.

Jackson, G. G., Dowling, H. F., Anderson, T. O., Riff, L., Saporta, J., & Turck, M. (1960). Susceptibility and immunity to common upper respiratory viral infections– The common cold. *Annals of Internal Medicine, 53*, 719–738.

Karper, W. B., & Boschen, M. B. (1993). Effect of exercise on acute respiratory tract infections and related symptoms. *Geriatric Nursing, 14*, 15–18.

Kingsbury, K. J., Kay, L., & Hjelm, M. (1998). Contrasting plasma free amino acid patterns in elite athletes: Association with fatigue and infection. *British Journal of Sports Medicine, 32*, 25–33.

Lee, D. J., Meehan, R. T., Robinson, C., Mabry, T. R., & Smith, M. L. (1992). Immune responsiveness and the risk of illness in U.S. Air Force Academy cadets during basic cadet training. *Aviation, Space and Environmental Medicine, 63*, 517–523.

Lindberg, K., & Berglund, B. (1996). Effect of treatment with nasal IgA on the incidence of infectious disease in world-class canoeists. *International Journal of Sports Medicine, 17*, 235–238.

Linde, F. (1987). Running and upper respiratory tract infections. *Scandinavian Journal of Sport Sciences, 9*, 21–23.

Linenger, J. M., Fink, S., Thomas, B., & Johnson, C. W. (1993). Musculoskeletal and medical morbidity associated with rigorous physical training. *Clinical Journal of Sports Medicine, 3*, 229–234.

Lötzerich, H., Wilczkowiak, I.-U., Stein, N., & Peters, C. (1997). Influence of training and competition on the phagocyte activity of athletes. *International Journal of Sports Medicine, 18*, S111. [abstract]

Mackinnon, L. T. (1992). *Exercise and immunology*. Champaign, IL: Human Kinetics Publishers.

Mackinnon, L. T. (1996). Exercise and immunoglobulins. *Exercise Immunology Review, 2*, 1–34.

Nehlsen-Cannarella, S. L., Nieman, D. C., Henson, D. A., Butterworth, D. E., Fagoaga, O. R., Warren, B. J., & Rainwater, M. K. (1997). Immune response to obesity and moderate weight loss. *International Journal of Sports Medicine, 18*, S111. [abstract]

Newsholme, E. A. (1994). Biochemical mechanisms to explain immunosuppression in well-trained and overtrained athletes. *International Journal of Sports Medicine, 15*, S142–S147.

Nieman, D. C. (1994). Exercise infection and immunity. *International Journal of Sports Medicine, 15*, S131–141.

Nieman, D. C., Henson, D. A., Gusewitch, G., Warren, B. J., Dotson, R. C., Butterworth, D. E., & Nehlsen-Cannarella, S. L. (1993). Physical activity and immune function in elderly women. *Medicine and Science in Sports and Exercise, 25*, 823–831.

Nieman, D. C., Johanssen, L. M., & Lee, J. W. (1989). Infectious episodes in runners before and after a roadrace. *Journal of Sports Medicine and Physical Fitness, 29*, 289–296.

Nieman, D. C., Johanssen, L. M., Lee, J. W., & Arabatzis, K. (1990). Infectious episodes in runners before and after the Los Angeles marathon. *Journal of Sports Medicine and Physical Fitness, 30*, 316–328.

Nieman, D. C., Nehlsen-Cannarella, S. L., Markoff, P. A., Balk-Lamberton, A. J., Yang, H., Chritton, D. B. W., & Arabatzis, K. (1990). The effects of moderate exercise training on natural killer cells and acute upper respiratory tract infections. *International Journal of Sports Medicine, 11*, 467–473.

Northoff, H., Enkel, S., & Weinstock, C. (1995). Exercise, injury and immune function. *Exercise Immunology Review, 1*, 1–25.

Osterback, L., & Qvarnberg, Y. (1987). A prospective study of respiratory infections in 12-year-old children. *Acta Paediatrica Scandinavica, 76*, 944–949.

Peters, E. M. (1997). Exercise, immunology and upper respiratory tract infections. *International Journal of Sports Medicine, 18*(Suppl. 1), S69–S77.

Peters, E. M., & Bateman, E. D. (1983). Ultramarathon running and upper respiratory tract infections. *South African Medical Journal, 64*, 582–584.

Peters-Futre, E. M. (1997). Vitamin C, ultramarathon running and URTI: The missing link? *Exercise Immunology Review, 3*, 32–52.

Schouten, W. J., Verschuur, R., & Kemper, H. C. G. (1988). Physical activity and upper respiratoryt tract infections in a population of young men and women: The Amsterdam growth and health study. *International Journal of Sports Medicine, 9*, 451–455.

Schwellnus, M., Kiessig, M., Derman, W., & Noakes, T. (1997). Fusafungine reduces symptoms of upper respiratory tract infections (URTI) in runners after a 56 km race. *Medicine and Science in Sports and Exercise, 29*, S296. [abstract]

Seyfried, P. L., Tobin, R. S., Brown, N. E., & Ness, P. F. (1985). A prospective study of swimming related illness. I. Swimming associated health risk. *American Journal of Public Health, 75*, 1068–1070.

Shek, P. N., Sabiston, B. H., Buguet, A., & Radomski, M. W. (1995). Strenuous exercise and immunological changes: A multiple-time-point analysis of leukocyte subsets, CD4/CD8 ratio, immunoglobulin production and NK cell response. *International Journal of Sports Medicine, 16*, 466–474.

Shephard, R. J. (1997). *Physical activity, training and the immune response*. Carmel, IN: Cooper.

Shephard, R. J., Kavanagh, T., & Mertens, D. J. (1995). Personal health benefits of Masters athletic competition. *British Journal of Sports Medicine, 29*, 35–40.

Shephard, R. J., & Shek, P. N. (1998a). Acute and chronic over-exertion: Do depressed immune responses provide useful markers? *International Journal of Sports Medicine, 19*, 159–171.

Shephard, R. J., & Shek, P. N. (1998b). Immunological hazards from nutritional imbalance in athletes. *Exercise Immunology Review, 4*, 22–48.

Shephard, R. J., & Shek, P. N. (1998c). Immune deficits induced by strenuous exertion under adverse environmental conditions—Manifestations and countermeasures. *Critical Reviews in Immunology, 18*, 545–568.

Shephard, R. J., & Shek, P. N. (1999). Effects of exercise and training on natural killer cell counts and cytolytic activity: A meta-analysis. *Sports Medicine, 28*, 177–191.

Strauss, R. H., Lanese, R. R., & Leizman, D. J. (1988). Illness and absence among wrestlers, swimmers and gymnasts at a large university. *American Journal of Sports Medicine, 16*, 653–655.

Totman, R., Kiff, J., Reed, S. E., & Craig, J. W. (1980). Predicting experimental colds in volunteers from different measures of recent life stress. *Journal of Psychosomatic Research, 24*, 155–163.

Weidner, T. G. (1994). Literature review: Upper respiratory illness and sport and exercise. *International Journal of Sports Medicine, 15*, 1–9.

Weidner, T. G. (1994). Reporting behaviors and activity levels of intercollegiate athletes with an URI. *Medicine and Science in Sports and Exercise, 26*, 22–26.

Weidner, T. G., Cranston, T. E., Kaminsky, L. A., Dick, E. C., Schurr, T. S., & Sevier, T. (1997). The effect of exercise training on the severity and duration of an upper respiratory illness. *International Journal of Sports Medicine, 18*, S117–S118.

# Psychological Risk Factors and Immune System Involvement in Cardiovascular Disease

WILLEM J. KOP, NICHOLAS COHEN

## I. INTRODUCTION

An increasing number of clinical and experimental studies indicate an important contribution of inflammatory processes in the progression of coronary atherosclerosis (Danesh, Collins, & Peto, 1997; Kol & Libby, 1998; Libby, Egan, & Skarlatos, 1997; Ridker, 1998; Ross, 1999). Evidence also suggests that both chronic and acute psychological factors promote the risk of coronary artery disease (CAD) (Kop, 1997; Krantz, Kop, Santiago, & Gottdiener, 1996). These psychological risk factors include chronic personality traits such as hostility and episodic factors such as depression as well as acute mental distress (Barefoot, Dahlstrom, & Williams, 1983; Carney, Freedland, Rich, & Jaffe, 1995; Frasure-Smith, Lesperance, & Talajic, 1995; Krantz et al., 1996; Williams et al., 1980). However, the mediating role of immunological processes in the relationship between these psychological risk factors and future coronary syndromes has not been explored. This review describes

potential interactions of psychological and immunological factors in the pathophysiology of CAD progression. We will distinguish between CAD and its clinical consequences such as myocardial infarction and sudden cardiac death. A brief overview of immune system involvement in CAD (section 1) will be followed by a summary of research on psychological CAD risk factors and potential psychoneuroimmunological pathways by which these psychological factors may promote CAD progression (section 2). This chapter concludes with an outline of possible clinical implications and directions for future research.

## II. IMMUNOLOGICAL FACTORS IN CORONARY DISEASE PROGRESSION

Clinical manifestations of CAD may be symptomatic (i.e., chest pain, shortness of breath, or fatigue) or take the form of acute coronary syndromes such as myocardial infarction (MI) and sudden cardiac death (Alonzo, Simon, & Feinleib, 1975; Braunwald, 1988). In most instances, acute coronary syndromes occur in the presence of underlying coronary atherosclerotic disease. In this section, we will first describe characteristics of vascular injury in stages of CAD progression and then discuss the association between the severity of atherosclerotic disease and the onset of acute coronary syndromes (section A). The atherosclerotic consequences of inflammation and infections will then be reviewed (sections B and C).

## A. Stages of Coronary Atherosclerosis and the Onset of Acute Coronary Syndromes

Given that atherosclerosis causes damage to the coronary vessel wall, the gradual progression of atherosclerotic plaques can be viewed as a "response to injury." Fuster, Falk and colleagues have formulated a pathophysiological classification of coronary vascular injury in which three types of lesions are distinguished (Falk & Fuster, 1995; Fuster, Badimon, Badimon, & Chesebro, 1992a, b). Each lesion type indicates a stage of increasing severity of CAD based on the extent of damage to the arterial wall. This three-level classification of severity of coronary disease will be used here to clarify effects of immunological and psychosocial factors on CAD progression and its clinical manifestations.

The initial stages of coronary atherosclerosis (Type I lesions, or fatty streaks) are characterized by functional alterations of the endothelium (the lining cells of the vessel wall) without substantial morphological changes in the vessel (Figure 1). Mild endothelial damage is promoted by several factors including hypercholesterolemia, circulating vasoactive amines, chemical irritants such as tobacco smoke, and inflammatory processes (Fuster et al., 1992a, b). Type I injury leads to the accumulation of lipids, macrophages, and T-lymphocytes in the vascular wall (Ross, 1999). Platelets, endothelial cells, and macrophages may secrete several growth factors that initiate

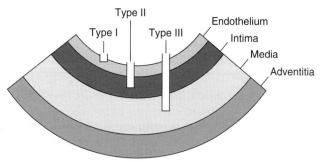

**FIGURE 1** Categorization of coronary lesion severity. Endothelial cells separate the inner layers of the vessel from the blood circulation. The type of lesion can be classified on the basis of the extent of arterial damage: Type I, endothelial damage; Type II, intimal damage; Type III, medial damage (adapted from Fuster et al., 1992a).

migration of smooth muscle cells to other layers of the vessel wall and growth (proliferation) of these cells. Endothelial dysfunction and smooth muscle cell proliferation may result in Type II lesions.

At a more advanced stage of atherosclerosis (i.e., Type II lesions), the vessel damage involves the endothelium and more inward layers (i.e., the intima). At this stage, coronary lesions are characterized by fibrin deposits in the intima, and/or the development of lesions composed of lipid-laden phagocytes, called foam cells. As a result of compensatory vessel dilatation (remodeling), the arterial luminal narrowing is generally minimal at this stage. This lipid-laden lesion is coated by a capsule-like fibrous layer of smooth muscle cells and collagen to which platelets may adhere. Because of its thin layer, Type II lesions can easily rupture, causing blood-clot formation and development of Type III lesions.

Atherosclerotic plaques at the advanced stage of CAD (Type III lesions) are characterized by severe damage to all three layers of the vessel wall, including the elastic lamina. Platelets may activate several growth factors that cause the smooth muscle cells to proliferate and migrate from the medial vascular layer to the intima. Following the formation of the initial platelet clot, an extracellular matrix may develop which includes fibrotic organization of the clot. Thus, both platelet adhesion and aggregation as well as coagulation and fibrinolytic processes are involved in the formation and stabilization of the blood clot (thrombus). The nature and speed of the processes causing progression from Type II to Type III lesions have major clinical consequences.

Acute coronary syndromes are often the first clinical sign of CAD and occur in vulnerable individuals with Type III lesions (Fuster et al., 1992a; Muller, Abela, Nesto, & Tofler, 1994). An abrupt decrease in coronary blood supply can be caused by thrombus formation and/or vasoconstriction. Myocardial infarction develops as a consequence of acute sustained cardiac ischemia which results from an imbalance between the supply of oxygenated blood to the heart muscle and cardiac demand (Krantz et al., 1996). Sudden cardiac death is often preceded by acute myocardial ischemia (Davies & Thomas, 1984) and, therefore, may be triggered by the same pathophysiological factors as those involved in myocardial ischemia and infarction. It is noteworthy that the relationship between anatomical severity of CAD and the onset of coronary syndromes is not linear, and evidence suggests that MI and sudden cardiac death tend to occur in Type III coronary lesions that do not significantly impair coronary blood flow ($< 75\%$ luminal stenosis). Furthermore, as noted previously, coronary disease progression does not progress in a constant manner and lesions undergo periodic spurts of growth (Bruschke et al., 1989).

Typical anginal symptoms such as chest pain and shortness of breath indicative of CAD may be present in obstructive coronary disease and/or gradual local increase of the atherosclerotic plaque (e.g., when the thrombus formed at the site of a Type III lesion is small). The ischemia caused by increased cardiac demand in the presence of reduced coronary supply accounts for the activity-induced symptoms of chest pain and other angina equivalents.

The onset of acute coronary syndromes may develop in the setting of these relatively stable atherosclerotic plaques as a result of plaque rupture. Recent evidence indicates that Type III coronary lesions progress to total occlusion three times as often as less severe lesions (Type I and II) ( Ambrose et al., 1988; Giroud, Li, Urban, Meier, & Rutishauer, 1992). In addition to rupture of relatively stable Type III lesions, sudden progression of a nonobstructive Type III lesion to a large and occlusive thrombus may result in acute coronary occlusion and subsequent myocardial infarction (Falk & Fuster, 1995). It is estimated that plaque rupture and thrombus formation account for approximately 50% of cases of acute coronary syndromes (Ross, 1999).

In summary, atherosclerosis progresses from minor endothelial injury (Type I lesions) via intimal damage (Type II lesions) to thrombus formation (Type III lesions). Initially, platelet adhesion and aggregation, arterial engulfment of macrophages, as well as smooth muscle cell proliferation play a crucial role. At later stages of coronary artery disease, thrombosis and impaired fibrinolysis contribute to the development of Type III lesions. Prolonged severe coronary lesions often result in gradual vessel narrowing, which may be accompanied by anginal complaints. In this situation of stable progressive CAD, acute coronary syndromes may not occur at all due to the protective effects of well-developed collateral coronary blood supply. In contrast, the disruption of relatively small atherosclerotic plaques is involved in the pathogenesis of acute myocardial infarction. Thus, it is important to differentiate between the stage of anatomical CAD progression (i.e., lesion type) and its clinical manifestation as an acute coronary syndrome. The immunological aspects of CAD progression are likely to parallel the nonlinear progression of coronary disease; the next two sections review the relationships of immunological factors and microorganisms to the severity of CAD and its clinical manifestations.

## B. Immunological Processes in Coronary Disease

Immunological factors are involved in all stages of CAD. At the initial stages of atherosclerosis (Type I and II lesions) immunological factors play a role in arterial lipid deposition as well as the proliferation and migration of smooth muscle cells. In addition, immune factors affect CAD progression indirectly by their association with known risk factors for CAD progression (e.g., hypertension, smoking, lipids). Both mechanisms may initiate a vicious circle of inflammation, lipid modification, and further inflammation that is maintained in the arterial segment due to the presence of these lipids (Ross, 1999). In general, the initial inflammatory response to arterial injury is beneficial, but if the damaging agent is not removed by the inflammatory response and inflammation persists, then this protective response becomes injurious. As in other chronic inflammatory diseases, the subsequent walling off of the damaged area may ultimately diminish the function of the artery and become part of the disease process (Ross, 1999). At more advanced stages of CAD (Type II and III lesions), immunological processes can act as precipitants of acute coronary syndromes by playing a role in plaque activation and promoting thrombus formation.

The role of immunological factors in coronary disease is supported by prospective epidemiological studies. This research has indicated that non-specific markers of systemic inflammation (most prominently C-reactive protein) are associated with an increased risk for cardiovascular events (Kuller, Tracy, Shaten, & Meilahn, 1996; Liuzzo et al., 1994; Ridker, Cushman, Stampfer, Tracy, & Hennekens, 1997; Thompson, Kienast, Pyke, Haverkate, & van de Loo, 1995; Tracy et al., 1997). In addition to these clinical studies, advances in monoclonal antibody as well as DNA technology have made it possible to gain insight into the different types and functions of endothelial cells and smooth muscle cells in the progression of coronary atherosclerosis. It is now well-established that immunological and growth-mediating factors play significant roles at various stages of CAD progression in addition to known contributions of thrombogenic and fibrinolytic factors.

As noted above, the human atherosclerotic plaque does not merely consist of a gradual accumulation of lipids into the arterial wall. Instead, coronary lesions contain living cells with a variety of specialized regulatory functions influencing the progression of atherosclerosis. Vascular cells of atherosclerotic lesions (endothelial and smooth muscle cells as well as leukocytes) can produce and respond to a wide range of cytokines. Although the immune component of atherosclerosis is not completely understood, a complex array of immunological factors including multiple feedback loops is involved. In this section, we will selectively review research supporting the cascade of inflammatory processes in CAD progression; the potential importance of immune responses to infectious microorganisms will be discussed afterward (section C). We will review aspects of the immune system relevant to CAD progression (macrophages, lymphocytes, cytokines, acute-phase proteins, adhesion molecules) including the clinical and experimental evidence supporting associations between these immune parameters and coronary disease (Figure 2).

### 1. Macrophages

Macrophages play multiple functions in the progression of CAD. The initial stages of atherosclerosis (Type I and II lesions) are characterized by formation of layers of lipid-laden foam cells, macro-

phages that have ingested circulating lipids. Macrophageous foam cells appear to originate from circulating monocytes that penetrate the vascular wall, lipid-laden smooth muscle cells, and extracellular lipids. Although the picture is far from complete, it has been convincingly documented that macrophages: (1) influence the uptake and metabolism of lipids; (2) promote the transportation and oxidation of low-density lipoprotein (LDL) cholesterol; (3) contribute to the release of several growth factors involved in the transition from Type I to Type II lesions by inducing smooth muscle cell proliferation; and (4) generate toxic products (products of lipid oxidation; free radicals) that increase atherosclerosis due to intimal damage (Type II lesions). Oxidized lipids are purported to interfere with the normal phagocytic/scavenger function of macrophages that would prevent progressive CAD under normal circumstances (Adams, 1994; Libby & Hansson, 1991).

At the advanced stages of atherosclerosis (Type II and III lesions), macrophages have been reported to

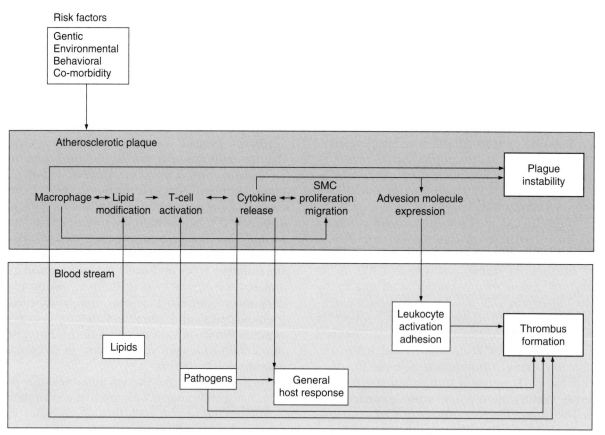

**FIGURE 2**  Immunological parameters involved in the progression of coronary artery disease and its clinical manifestations as acute coronary syndromes. Arterial lipid and leukocyte deposition characterize early stages of coronary disease and include involvement of adhesion molecules. At the advanced disease stage, several immune parameters may increase the risk of acute coronary syndromes by promoting plaque instability and thrombus formation.

produce protein- and/or peptide-dissolving enzymes (proteases) that may result in disruption of the organized extracellular matrix leading to formation of unstable Type III lesions. In addition, macrophages can promote thrombus formation by secreting tissue factor and plasminogen activator inhibitor (Libby & Hansson, 1991).

## 2. Lymphocytes

T lymphocytes can be found in early atherosclerotic lesions; in contrast, B cells and natural killer (NK) cells are not prevalent in the atherosclerotic plaque. T cells in the developing atherosclerotic plaque may be deposited passively but become important contributors to the progression of atherosclerosis when activated immunologically. T-cell activity in areas of smooth muscle cells and endothelial cells is marked by interferon-$\gamma$ (IFN-$\gamma$). Although IFN-$\gamma$ is a cytokine secreted by both NK cells as well as T helper cells, IFN-$\gamma$ in atherosclerotic plaques primarily reflects the presence of activated T cells since NK cells are virtually absent in atherosclerotic plaques. A clear demonstration of T-cell involvement in atherosclerosis has been provided by Hansson and colleagues using the arterial intimal growth response to experimentally induced vascular damage (Hansson et al., 1991). Additional evidence for T cell activity comes from the observation that T cells in atherosclerotic plaques exhibit interleukin-2 (IL-2) receptors. These indicators of activated T cells are also observed at later stages of atherosclerosis.

Several factors may result in T cell activation in atherogenesis such as oxidized lipoproteins, especially apolipoprotein-B fragments, antigens exposed to blood due to necrosis, and viral infection (herpestypes and cytomegalovirus; see section C). T cell activation results in secretion of cytokines that intensify the inflammation and stimulate metalloproteinase production by macrophages. The latter effect may result in instability of the atherosclerotic plaque, potentially leading to acute coronary syndromes. Furthermore, activation of T lymphocytes is promoted in turn by several cytokines of which the interleukins are the most extensively studied.

## 3. Cytokines

Cytokines are low-molecular-weight peptides that affect the behavior of a variety of cell types. Cytokines, released in response to microorganisms or other challenges, result in a characteristic response of the organism referred to as inflammation. In addition, cytokines increase the adhesive function of the vascular endothelium such that leukocytes and other substances adhere to the vessel wall. Originally cytokines were thought only to be produced by and affect leukocytes, hence the generic name interleukin (IL). We now know, however, that endothelial and smooth muscle cells (as well as other cell types) also synthesize proinflammatory cytokines (primarily IL-1 and IL-6). Proinflammatory cytokines, as well as cellular adhesion molecules, are involved in binding of monocytes to the vascular endothelium.

When coronary atherosclerosis is present, blood cells in the vessel wall do not only express immunoactive substances, but may also react to immunological stimulation. IL-6 contributes most to stimulation of T- and B-cell activity; IL-1 appears to be important in cell–cell contact (Libby, & Hansson, 1991). For example, IL-1 is generally not present in unstimulated vascular cells, but its production is known to increase in response to bacterial endotoxin. IL-8 may both promote and inhibit leukocyte accumulation in the atherosclerotic plaque. Further, when the cytokine tumor necrosis factor-$\alpha$ (TNF-$\alpha$) is produced by smooth muscle cells, it may contribute to atherosclerosis progression as well. Moreover, following bacterial endotoxin stimulation, higher levels of IL-1 and TNF-$\alpha$ level are found in atherosclerotic rabbit arteries than in normal arteries. Loppnow and Libby (1992) found that the low basal level of IL-1 in isolated human atherosclerotic plaques was markedly increased after exposure to endotoxin. Damage of the vessel wall activates the endothelium leading to adhesion of leukocytes. These leukocytes also migrate into the subendothelial layers, further promoting secretion of growth factors and cytokines. In addition to their important local effects, cytokines have "long-range" effects that contribute to the general host defense. No information is available as to the role of cytokines in advanced stages of atherosclerosis (Type III lesions) and the onset of acute coronary syndromes, although activation of unstable plaques may, in part, be mediated by cytokines. In summary, several cytokines are involved in the early stages of atherosclerosis, and cytokines probably play an important role in the adverse effects of low-grade inflammation and subclinical infections.

## 4. Acute-Phase Proteins

The acute phase response is part of the initial response to infection and involves secretion of several proteins from the liver, including C-reactive protein (CRP), serum amyloid A, and fibrinogen. The release of acute-phase proteins is initiated by cytokines (primarily IL-6, but also IL-1, and TNF-$\alpha$ ), shifting the production from so-called housekeeping proteins (e.g., albumin) to acute-phase reactants. Acute-phase proteins are part of the nonspecific (innate) immune system and mimic certain actions of antibodies. Levels of acute-phase proteins rise dramatically within 24–48 h after an acute inflammatory stimulus, but the regulation of these proteins in low-level diseases is not well understood.

C-reactive protein has recently been associated with elevated risk for cardiac events (Kol & Libby, 1998; Libby, et al., 1997; Ridker, 1998; Ross, 1999) and some reports indicate that the magnitude of adverse risk associated with CRP is more pronounced within 1 year of assessment and decreases with longer follow-up durations (Tracy et al., 1997). At present, it is not well established to what extent the association between acute phase reactants and adverse cardiovascular risk is mediated by a generalized systemic inflammatory condition or to what extent these proteins directly affect vascular thrombus formation. The importance of the acute phase protein fibrinogen in CAD progression is well-documented, but since its purported action is attributed primarily to coagulation, the role of fibrinogen will not be discussed in detail. The elevated risk associated with increased levels of CRP is independent of other risk factors such as lipid levels and fibrinogen (Ridker et al., 1997). Of interest is the finding that the relationship between elevated C-reactive protein and cholesterol levels was multiplicative rather than additive (Ridker, Glynn, & Hennekens, 1998).

### 5. Adhesion Molecules

Adhesion molecules, involved in binding cells to one another, include the integrins and selectins. Adhesion of leukocytes to the endothelium is stimulated by IL-1 and TNF-$\alpha$, two cytokines that also regulate the interaction between the endothelium and platelet adhesion, as well as clotting and fibrinolytic factors, thereby promoting stabilized clot formation (Bevilacqua, Schleef, Gimbrone, & Loskutoff, 1986; Stern, Nawroth, Handley, & Kisiel, 1985). The function of adhesion molecules is primarily local, but circulating levels of adhesion molecules can be used as markers of ongoing inflammatory processes because they may reflect "shedding" from the sites of inflammation. For example, the adhesion molecules L-selectin can be detached from leukocytes (e.g., by a metalloproteinase) allowing, assessment of these molecules in plasma (Ross, 1999).

During the initial stages of atherosclerosis, the binding of leukocytes to the endothelium involves mediation by adhesion molecules. In addition, white blood cells may also penetrate the endothelium in new lesions. This migration is probably activated by cytokines (IFN-$\gamma$, IL-1, IL-6, IL-8, and TNF-$\alpha$), oxidized lipoproteins, and chemotactic complement activation product. An important adhesion molecule stored in platelets and the endothelium, P-selectin, is released by thrombin. Until integrin activation occurs, neutrophil adhesion to the endothelium is very sensitive to shear stress. Shear stress is generally high ($\pm$ 12 dyn/cm$^2$) in arterial vessels, but can be substantially lower in areas immediately distal of a coronary lesion or in the microcirculation. T cells and monocytes may "stick" at the sites of low shear as a result of upregulation of the adhesion molecules on both the endothelium and leukocytes (Ross, 1999).

Adhesion molecules (i.e., intercellular adhesion molecule-1 (ICAM-1)) have a long-term prognostic value for incident myocardial infarction (Ridker, Hennekens, Roitman-Johnson, Stampfer, & Allen, 1998). Moreover, ICAM-1 levels are correlated with C-reactive protein levels. In case of sudden (stress-induced) changes in coronary diameter, activated neutrophils and monocytes may injure the coronary vessel distal to the obstruction, promote platelet activation and coagulation, and activate cytokines resulting in a net vasoconstriction distal to the obstruction (Entman & Ballantyne, 1993). Moreover, adhesion molecules affect hemostasis and thrombus formation, which may be one of the mechanisms by which these molecules contributes to the transition from chronic to acute CAD (Libby et al., 1997; Libby, & Hansson, 1991).

## C.  Bacterial and Viral Infection

The role of chronic infection in coronary disease progression is supported by seroepidemiological studies demonstrating elevated levels of antibodies to various pathogens in patients with CAD. The proposed theory is that microorganisms activate leukocytes and/or cause transformation of vascular cells including endothelial and smooth muscle cells. Beck and colleagues demonstrated that individuals with gingivitis were at increased risk of developing future cardiovascular diseases such as myocardial infarctions and cerebrovascular events (Beck et al., 1996). Some evidence suggests that *Helicobacter pylori* is a risk indicator of MI , especially the more virulent *H. pylori* strain (cytotoxin-associated gene-A) which is found in 43% patients with cardiovascular disease compared to 17% in controls (Pasceri et al., 1998). However, a recent review of the literature revealed that the association between *H. pylori* and coronary syndromes is confounded by background factors, primarily low socioeconomic status (Danesh et al., 1997). Additional research has focused on circulating antibodies to other bacteria and viruses in patients with CAD, including *Chlamydia pneumoniae* and cytomegalovirus (CMV). For example, significantly more antibody titers to *C. pneumoniae* have been reported in CAD patients than in control subjects without CAD (27/40 in myocardial infarction patients, 15/30 in patients with established CAD, compared to 7/41 controls) (Saikku et al., 1988). This finding is consistent with observations of Melnick et al. (1993) who observed that 70% of patients undergoing surgery for atherosclerotic disease had antibodies to CMV compared to 43% in non-diseased controls. An overall assessment of the literature on *C. pneumonia* and CMV reveals that these pathogenic microorganisms are associated with a two-fold risk of coronary syndromes (Danesh et al., 1997).

In concordance with these epidemiological data, recent investigations indicate that certain pathogens are frequently observed in atherosclerotic plaques. Muhlestein and colleagues observed Chlamydia antigens in 79% of the atherosclerotic plaques of 90 CAD patients, compared to 4% in arteries of healthy controls (Muhlestein et al., 1996). Further animal research by Muhlestein and colleagues indicates that infecting rabbits with Chlamydia promoted plaque formation, especially in hyperlipidemic animals, and that this effect could be neutralized by antibiotic treatment with azithromyzin.

Several theories explaining the presence of bacteria and viruses in atherosclerotic plaques have been advanced: (1) Microorganisms in atherosclerotic plaques may reflect the consequences of an inflammatory response initiated by these infectious organisms. This "low-grade" inflammation hypothesis postulates that infectious sites release toxins and activate surface molecules, initiating an inflammatory response of the vascular endothelial cells. This hypothesis is supported by the observation that increased levels of exposure to *H. pylori* is associated with increasing levels of C-reactive protein (Mendall, Patel, Ballam, Strachan, & Northfield, 1996). In addition, systemic endotoxemia or cytokinemia may evoke an "echo" effect — namely an increased local cytokine production in the atherosclerotic lesion by resident cells such as macrophages. (2) An alternative theory is that microorganisms adversely affect the local coagulation–fibrinolysis balance. In support of this notion are numerous studies demonstrating direct viral effects on the anti-coagulatory function of the vascular endothelium (for review see Libby et al. (1997)). For example, *herpes simplex* infection of the endothelium

promotes local thrombotic tendency by increasing the surface expression of tissue factor. (3) Another theory is that microorganisms play an accelerating role, rather than acting as the pathogenic stimulus, *per se*. A stronger version of this theory is that microorganisms are merely "innocent bystanders". The facts that only microbial DNA and RNA are found in atherosclerotic arteries, and efforts to culture microorganisms from atherosclerotic tissue have generally failed, may suggest that infections are not a primary cause of coronary disease progression.

Assuming that infectious diseases do play a role in CAD, research has identified potential direct as well as indirect pathophysiological mechanisms (Danesh et al., 1997; Kol & Libby, 1998; Libby et al., 1997). Figure 3 shows that at all stages of CAD **direct effects** of microorganisms include: (1) promotion of a pro-thrombotic state of the endothelium, including coagulation and fibrinolytic factors; (2) increased expression of several endothelial-leukocyte contact adhesion molecules (e.g., ICAM-1 by *C. pneumoniae*, and P-selectin by CMV); (3) cytokine production by endothelial and smooth muscle cells; and (4) lytic cytopathic changes leading to leukocyte migration and vascular inflammation. The effects of these microorganisms do not necessarily require a productive infection. Viruses have additional direct effects on smooth muscle cells such as: increased cell proliferation with apparently monoclonal expansion, decreased cell apoptosis, cholesterol esterification, and cytokine production. Such vascular effects have not been demonstrable for bacteria. **Indirect effects** of microorganisms involve injury and activation of the endothelium and smooth muscle cells. These indirect effects are mediated via lymphocytes and macrophages (see Figure 3).

In addition to the potential **chronic** atherogenic consequences of infection, other factors may play a role in the onset of **acute** coronary syndromes. Cytokines released during a systemic infection may "activate" leukocytes and smooth muscle cells of an existing atherosclerotic plaque which may trigger plaque rupture. Furthermore, infections may cause increased cardiac demand because of tachycardia and increased cardiac contractility (Libby et al., 1997). During Gram-negative bacterial sepsis, circulating endotoxins provoke substantial alterations in physiology, including hypotension and decreased systemic vascular resistance. Furthermore, endotoxin diffusely activates the endothelium, thereby promoting the development of disseminated intravascular coagulation often accompanying Gram-negative sepsis. Finally, febrile illnesses are known to increase the wall-stress challenge to the atheromatous lesion, which may lead

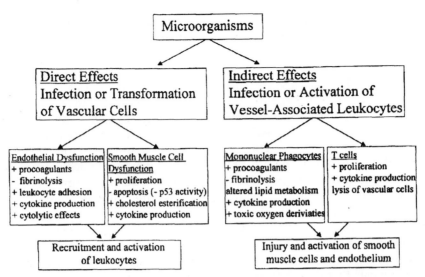

**FIGURE 3**   Direct and indirect effects of infectious agents on cells of the arterial wall. Microorganisms can infect vascular cells and viruses can also alter cell transformation. Surviving infected cells may display deleterious functions that could promote atherosclerotic lesion progression. Cytokine production in endothelial and smooth muscle cells have reciprocal influences. Indirect pathways include infection of leukocytes that are already present in the atherosclerotic plaque. These infected leukocytes may be activated to express maladaptive functions and may interact with the endothelium and smooth muscle cells to promote lesion progression (adapted from Libby et al., 1997).

to acute coronary syndromes in individuals with vulnerable plaques (Libby et al., 1997).

Although these clinical and experimental observations suggest a role of infectious processes in the progression of coronary disease, the evidence is less straightforward than for that of the aforementioned role of inflammation in atherosclerosis (section B). Several points cast doubt on a primary role of infections in CAD. First, the clinical epidemiological observations are, to a certain extent, confounded by factors such as smoking status, age, access to health care, low socioeconomic status, and possibly chronic psychological distress; because these factors by themselves may promote the onset of infectious diseases and are also involved in CAD progression and its clinical manifestations. Prospective studies that controlled for these factors have generally not supported an independent contribution of microorganisms to the progression of CAD (Danesh et al., 1997; Folsom, Nieto, Sorlie, Chambless, & Graham, 1998; Wald, Law, Morris, & Bagnall, 1997). In addition, no associations are found between the severity of CAD and *H. pylori* seropositivity, and as yet, no microorganisms have been cultured from atherosclerotic plaques. The evidence linking *C. pneumoniae* and cytomegalovirus to CAD progression is stronger and raises intriguing questions for future research. The construct of "pathogen burden" may reveal further insight in the role of infectious diseases

in CAD progression. However, it is not entirely clear what is assessed by adding the number of microorganisms an individual has been exposed to and, in addition, this approach suffers some statistical drawbacks (e.g., loss of variability and combining exposure variables with different effect sizes for CAD progression).

In summary, although several studies suggest a potential role of infection in coronary atherosclerosis, both clinical and experimental studies are far from conclusive in this regard. Several factors may explain why an existing association between infection and CAD progression is not consistently found. First, analogous to conditions in which microbial infections play a crucial role (e.g., peptic ulcers), it is conceivable that a subgroup of individuals exists whose HLA haplotypes predisposes them to susceptibility to a pathogen, thereby accounting for a lack of the cytokine-associated components of an anti-microbial immune response. Second, it is possible that viruses trigger the onset of atherosclerotic disease without persisting in the infected tissue. Third, the measurement procedures used to detect microorganisms may substantially influence the research findings and techniques such as microimmunofluorescence require expertise and often produce variable results (Libby et al., 1997). To summarize, the involvement of inflammatory processes in coronary disease is well-documented, but further research is needed to determine whether inflammation is a primary trigger or a secondary response to the ongoing atherosclerotic disease process.

## III. PSYCHOLOGICAL RISK FACTORS FOR CORONARY ARTERY DISEASE

An extensive literature addresses the role of psychological factors in the progression of CAD and its clinical manifestations. The severity of underlying CAD influences the nature and magnitude of the associations between psychological factors with the onset of acute coronary syndromes (Kop, 1997) Analogous to the traditional CAD risk factors, it has proven useful to distinguish between chronic and acute psychological factors in the progression of CAD (Kop, 1999; Krantz et al., 1996). Chronic psychological risk factors may promote the onset of initial stages of atherosclerosis (Type I and II lesions) by their sympathetic nervous system-mediated pathophysiological consequences (e.g., catecholamine-induced hypercoagulability, lipid deposition, and inflammatory processes) and/or as a result of their association with known CAD risk factors (e.g., hypertension, smoking, lipids). At more advanced stages of CAD (Type III lesions), acute psychological risk factors may trigger cardiac ischemia or malignant arrhythmias leading to acute coronary syndromes. A review of the literature on cardiovascular behavioral medicine has provided evidence supporting a three-category classification of psychological risk factors for coronary syndromes that is based on their duration and temporal proximity to the occurrence of coronary syndromes (Table I): (1) chronic psychological risk factors involved in the gradual progression of CAD (e.g., stable personality traits such as hostility); (2) episodic psychological risk factors with a duration from several months to 2 years that tend to recur over time (e.g. psychological states such as depression); and (3) acute psychological risk factors that precipitate coronary syndromes within hours (e.g., outbursts of anger or mental activities). It is also known that the exposure duration of psychological distress influences the nature of its immunological correlates (Benschop, Rodriguez-Feuerhahn, & Schedlowski, 1996; Herbert & Cohen, 1993). In the following sections, we will briefly review evidence for the adverse cardiovascular risk associated with each these three categories of psychological factors. We will also describe the potential immunological mediators involved as possible pathophysiological mechanisms (see Table I and also Figure 4).

### A. Chronic Psychological Risk Factors

#### 1. Relationship with Coronary Disease

Psychological studies in cardiovascular disease have extensively investigated hostility and, previously, the Type A behavior pattern. The influential studies by Friedman and Rosenman in the late 1950s (Friedman & Rosenman, 1959) on Type A behavior found that this antagonistic personality trait is significantly associated with incident myocardial infarction as well as with relevant cardiovascular risk factors (Friedman & Rosenman, 1959; Suarez, Williams,

**TABLE I**  Classification of Psychological Risk Factors for Myocardial Infarction and Sudden Cardiac Death

| Psychological risk factor | Chronic | Episodic | Acute |
|---|---|---|---|
| Example | Hostility<br>Low SES | Depression<br>Exhaustion | Anger<br>Mental activity |
| Temporal relation to coronary syndrome | >10 Years | <2 Years | <1 Hour |
| Associated CV Risk | Hyperlipidemia<br>Hypertension<br>Prolonged sympathetic activation | ↑Blood clotting<br>↓Fibrinolysis<br>Shift of sympatho/vagal balance<br>↑Platelet activation | ↑Catecholamines<br>↑Cardiac demand<br>↓Coronary supply<br>↓Plasma volume |
| Immune response | ↓Macrophage function<br>↑Infections (latent) | Immunosuppression<br>↑Infections (active)<br>↑Cytokines | Partial immune activation |
| Primary pathological[a] result | Atherosclerosis | Altered homeostasis | Plaque rupture<br>Ischemia<br>Arrhythmia |

[a]Only the primary pathophysiological pathways are presented; not shown are the multiple associations within and between cardiovascular (CV) risk factors and pathophysiological consequences.

Kuhn, Zimmerman, & Schanberg, 1991; Welin et al., 1985). Later studies suggested that hostility is the toxic component of Type A behavior. Hostility is assumed to be a stable personality trait characterized by cynical mistrust, aggressive responding, and an overall antagonistic attitude (Engebretson & Matthews, 1992; Barefoot et al., 1983). Most studies report an association between hostility/Type A behavior and severity of underlying coronary disease (Siegman, Dembroski, & Ringel, 1987; Williams et al., 1988) as well as first myocardial infarction (Barefoot et al., 1983; Meesters & Smulders, 1994; Shekelle, Gale, Ostfeld, & Paul, 1983). Research with primates supports a relationship between hostile behavior and severity of CAD (Manuck, Marsland, Kaplan, & Williams, 1995). In contrast, **recurrent** coronary syndromes are less consistently predicted by hostility/Type A behavior (Ragland, 1989; Shekelle, Gale, & Norusis, 1985). Moreover, the association between hostility and MI is more pronounced in younger (< 55 years of age) than older men (Meesters & Smulders, 1994; Siegman et al., 1987; Williams et al., 1988), suggesting a role of hostility at early stages of CAD progression.

## 2. Pathophysiological Mechanisms

The purported pathophysiological mechanisms involve elevated sympathetic nervous system tone and increased reactivity, resulting in accelerated CAD progression. Direct effects of elevated sympathetic tone include damage of vasculature due to arterial lipid deposition and elevated intraarterial pressure that promote early stages of CAD (Type I and II lesions). In addition to the consequences of sympathetic hyperactivity, chronic psychological risk factors affect CAD progression indirectly by their association with persistent cardiovascular risk factors such as hypertension, circulating lipids, and blood clotting factors (for reviews see: Suarez et al., 1991; Williams, Suarez, Kuhn, Zimmerman, & Schanberg, 1991).

Another potential mechanism explaining increased risk of CAD progression and its clinical manifestations involves elevated catecholamine, hemodynamic, and hemostatic responses to acute challenges among hostile individuals. This so-called ''hyperreactivity'' plays a crucial role at the advanced stage of coronary atherosclerosis (Type III lesions). Increased catecholamine reactivity to stress in hostile individuals (Friedman, Byers, Diamant, & Rosenman, 1975; Suarez et al., 1991) may specifically effect acute physiological responses leading to increased cardiac demand, as well as coronary constriction (Muller et al., 1994) and

increased clotting tendency (Markovitz, & Matthews, 1991). These acute challenge-induced (patho)physiological changes may increase the risk of ischemia and subsequent coronary syndromes.

## 3. Immunological Correlates

Relatively little is known about the relationship between psychological trait-associated changes in immune function with respect to CAD. It has been argued that atherosclerosis may initially be promoted by immunosuppressive effects of persistent psychological distress, whereas at later stages of atherosclerosis, the reduced immunocompetence may become ineffective because of the silencing effects of the atherosclerotic process itself (Fricchione, Bilfinger, Hartman, Liu, & Stefano, 1996). At present, no evidence supports this notion as it pertains to chronic psychological risk factors for CAD; this theory, however, may provide for immunological considerations in explaining episodic risk factors (section B). Since the early 1940s, it has been well documented that lipids and macrophages interact at the early stages of CAD (Leary, 1941). Some evidence supports associations between hostility and hyperlipidemia or elevated levels of oxidized lipids. One potential mechanism would be that hostility promotes early CAD progression by adversely affecting the normal phagocytic function of macrophages (Adams, 1994).

Relevant to the aforementioned reactivity hypothesis, Mills and colleagues have demonstrated that the hostility trait is related to laboratory speech task-induced immune response, particularly with elevated levels of NK cells (Mills, Dimsdale, Nelesen, & Dillon, 1996). However, the pattern of results appears rather complex because the overall task response was in the direction of suppressed immunocompetence, and furthermore, other indicators of hostility (e.g., anger expression) were related to lower NK-cell levels and higher B-cell responses. Christensen and colleagues (1996) observed that high-hostile subjects exhibited a significantly greater increase in NK-cell cytotoxicity than low-hostile subjects in response to a self-disclosure task (Christensen et al., 1996). The authors concluded that the elevated short-term increase in NK-cell activity observed in hostile persons reflects an exaggerated acute arousal response. Lee and colleagues investigated the predictive value of hostility to a stressful condition in a setting of basic cadet training in first-year Air Force Academy cadets (Lee, Meehan, Robinson, Smith, & Mabry, 1995). Hostility measures assessed prior to arrival at the academy did not predict the level of PHA-, PMA-, and anti-CD3-

stimulated lymphocyte proliferation or risk of illness. However, hostility levels reported **during** the training predicted risk of illness in the 4 weeks following psychosocial assessment (odds ratio, 7.1; 95% confidence interval, 1.4–36.1).

### 4. Summary and Interpretation

Clinical studies examining hostility and other chronic psychological factors are limited by their essentially correlational study designs. At present, no convincing evidence is available to support the notion that chronic psychological traits are associated with persistent alterations of those immunological parameters known to be associated with gradual CAD progression. However, the elevated risk factors associated with chronic psychological risk factors (e.g., hyperlipidemia) may interact with inflammatory or infectious processes, thereby indirectly promoting CAD progression. In addition to these indirect effects, some evidence suggests elevated immune responses to emotional challenges in hostile individuals. It is well documented that sympathetic nervous system tone and reactivity is elevated among hostile individuals. The direct consequences of increased sympathetic nervous system activity for the psychoimmunological component of gradual CAD progression requires further investigation.

In addition to hostility, other psychological traits such as trait anxiety as well as sociological factors—particularly low socioeconomic status—may act as additional sources of persistent exposure to psychological distress. Low socioeconomic status is associated with adverse cardiovascular health outcome (Marmot, Shipley, & Rose, 1984) as well as cardiovascular risk factors and behaviors (Kraus, Borhani, & Franti, 1980; Winkleby, Jatulis, Frank, & Fortmann, 1992) including measures of chronic low-grade inflammation (Marshall, 1993). Thus, both hostility and low socioeconomic status can be construed as chronic risk indicators that promote atherosclerosis and affect cardiovascular risk (Table I). These chronic factors may also increase the likelihood of developing proximate psychological risk factors such as episodes of exhaustion and frequent occurrences of acute psychological arousal (see section D; Figure 4).

## B. Episodic Psychological Risk Factors

### 1. Relationship with Coronary Disease

Characteristic of episodic risk factors are their limited duration (from several months to 2 years) as well as their recurring nature (Kop, 1999; Carney et al., 1995). Currently, depression is considered to be one of the core episodic risk factors in cardiovascular behavioral medicine research. Numerous studies indicate that depression is predictive of first and recurrent myocardial infarction and sudden cardiac death (for review see for example: Appels, 1997; Carney et al., 1995; Kop, 1997). At present, it is still debated whether depression reflects one single underlying pathologic process, or whether it represents a group of distinct disorders with overlapping characteristics (Gold, Goodwin, & Chrousos, 1988). Independent of the research on depression and CAD, clinical and experimental studies have shown that extreme fatigue is among the most common premonitory symptoms of acute coronary syndromes (Appels & Otten, 1992; Kuller, Cooper, & Perper, 1972). This state is referred to as "vital exhaustion" (i.e., lack of energy, increased irritability, and demoralization). Prospective studies in healthy and CAD populations have demonstrated the predictive value of exhaustion for adverse cardiovascular events (Appels & Mulder, 1988; Kop, Appels, Mendes de Leon, de Swart, & Bar, 1994). The extent to which exhaustion reflects the same construct as depression is not fully understood, but some evidence suggests that depression and exhaustion are not entirely overlapping constructs (Appels, 1997) and have different biological concomitants (Gold et al., 1988; Raikkonen, Lassila, Keltikangas-Jarvinen, & Hautanen, 1996; Kop, 1999). Episodic risk factors are associated with a two- to threefold elevated risk for incident or recurrent coronary syndromes. Despite the significant predictive value for adverse cardiovascular health outcome, episodic risk factors are not consistently associated with elevated CAD severity (Kop, Appels, Mendes de Leon, & Bar, 1996; Kop, Appels, Mendes de Leon, de Swart, & Bar, 1993).

### 2. Pathophysiological Mechanisms

A large literature has addressed the neuroendocrine correlates of depression. The most common finding is that depression, especially melancholia, is associated with increased activation of the corticotropin releasing hormone (CRH) system and hence elevated cortisol levels. Some evidence also indicates that atypical forms of depression, characterized by hyperphagia and hypersomnia, are characterized by inactivation of the CRH system. Therefore, it could be that depression and exhaustion have different neurohormonal concomitants. Both norepinephrine released from the locus ceruleus as well as hypothalamic CRH are the main effectors of the general adaptation response (Selye, 1977) and both systems show differential hyperactivation versus hypoactivation in (melancholic) depression and atypical depression, respectively (Gold et al., 1988). One neurohormonal theory of depression postulates that the inhibiting effect of glucocorticoids on CRH secretion is deteriorated in depressed individuals. In addition to these neuroendocrine correlates, episodic risk factors are related to hemostatic cardiovascular risk factors including impaired fibrinolysis (Kop, Hamulyak, Pernot, & Appels, 1998; Pietraszek, Takada, Nishimoto, Ohara, & Takada, 1991; Raikkonen et al., 1996) as well as sympathetic overactivity and decreased parasympathetic activity (Carney et al., 1995). An overall imbalance of normal homeostatic functions may be characteristic of episodic risk factors. One study showed that exhaustion was associated with increased markers of impaired fibrinolysis (elevated PAI-1 levels), whereas no consistent effects on blood coagulation factors were found (e.g., factors VII and VIII) (Kop et al., 1998). In contrast to chronic psychological risk factors, most studies have not found elevated hemodynamic responsiveness in individuals with episodic risk factors (Carney et al., 1995; Kop et al., 1997). It is not known whether this negative finding reflects a blunted hyperresponsiveness due to prolonged challenges to the cardiovascular system as a result of what has been described as increased allostatic load (Seeman, Singer, Rowe, Horwitz, & McEwen, 1997; McEwen, 1998). Thus, episodic risk factors may elevate the risk of acute coronary syndromes in the setting of advanced CAD (i.e., Type III lesions) by their association with impaired measures of hemostasis involved in thrombus formation, plaque rupture, and arrhythmias.

### 3. Immunological Correlates

The immunological correlates of depression have been reviewed in detail elsewhere (Maes, 1995; Stein, Miller, & Trestman, 1991; Weisse, 1992). In brief, depression is associated with several immune parameters, including increased numbers of peripheral leukocytes (particularly neutrophils and monocytes), decreased lymphocytes, and elevated cytokine production. In addition to numeric measures of immune function, depression is also associated with reduced "functional" measures including lower NK cell activity and a decreased proliferative response of lymphocytes to mitogenic stimulation (Weisse, 1992; Herbert, & Cohen, 1993). Patients with clinical depression also have increased antibody levels of several herpes viruses, including CMV. Psychoneuroimmunology literature generally categorizes the immunosuppressive correlates of depres-

sion along with the long-term immunological consequences of distressing behavioral or emotional states (e.g., bereavement, separation, and daily hassles). Consistent with the literature of depression, preliminary evidence suggests decreased albumin and increased leukocytes and fibrinogen levels in exhausted subjects (Kop et al., 1998). Thus, it could be argued that increased antibody titers to pathogens such as CMV among depressed individuals result from an overall immunosuppressed state of the specific adaptive immunity including suppressed T-cytotoxic cells that normally suppress pathogens; this compromised adaptive specific immunity is accompanied by a compensatory increase in components of the innate immune system (see also Goodkin & Appels, 1997). Increases in infectious activity are accompanied by elevated macrophage activity, cytokine expression, and other indicators of inflammatory processes.

### 4. Summary and Interpretation

Immunosuppression of the specific adaptive immune system is well-documented in episodic psychological factors, particularly depression. Some of the correlates of depression (e.g., elevated leukocytes and increased antibody levels to viruses) are also associated with elevated risk for acute coronary syndromes. These markers of a pro-inflammatory state in depression may promote CAD progression by enhancing macrophage and lipid deposition processes at early stages of atherosclerosis. More importantly, low-grade inflammation may alter the stability of atherosclerotic plaques (Type III lesions) and increase the risk of plaque rupture leading to acute coronary syndromes. The latter mechanism is probably more important since the duration of episodic risk factors may not be long enough to initiate and sustain an atherosclerotic process. This notion is further supported by the finding that no consistent associations have been found between episodic risk factors and CAD severity. Studies relating depression and other episodic risk factors to biological measures relevant to the pathophysiology of CAD are limited in the sense that no inferences regarding causality can be made due to the correlational nature of the study design. Some evidence indeed suggests that inflammatory processes may cause central nervous system responses as well as psychological states similar to depression and exhaustion (Dantzer & Kelley, 1989; Goodkin & Appels, 1997). Because of the recurring nature of episodic risk factors, longitudinal studies may further our understanding of the time trajectory of immunological and psychological factors in patients at risk for acute coronary syndromes. The pattern of immunological correlates of depression is quite complex and at present, it is not determined whether the main determinant is based on a neuroendocrine pathway or whether adverse health behaviors related to these episodic risk factors (e.g., smoking and poor diet) are causally involved in the observed expression of low-grade inflammation.

## C. Acute Psychological Risk Factors

### 1. Relationship with Coronary Disease

Epidemiological studies suggest that acute outbursts of anger as well as natural disasters can provoke coronary syndromes such as myocardial infarction (Dobson, Alexander, Malcolm, Steele, & Miles, 1991; Meisel et al., 1991; Mittleman et al., 1995; Trichopoulos, Katsouyanni, Zavitsanos, Tzonou, & Dalla-Vorgia, 1983). As described in section I, A, coronary syndromes often result from cardiac ischemia and/or arrhythmias. Laboratory and field studies have demonstrated that mental activities and emotions are potent triggers of myocardial ischemia (Krantz et al., 1996) and life-threatening arrhythmias (Verrier, 1987). Specifically, 30 to 60% of patients with stable CAD develop ischemic responses to laboratory tasks such as public speech, anger recall, mental arithmetic with harassment, and the Stroop color word test. Moreover, transient ambulatory ischemia is triggered by both mental and physical activities and is more prevalent among patients who demonstrate mental stress-induced ischemia in the laboratory.

### 2. Pathophysiological Mechanisms

Acute mental arousal is associated with a shift toward increased activity of the sympathetic nervous system and a decreased parasympathetic (vagal) activity, accompanied by elevated circulating catecholamines and increased cardiac demand (i.e., elevated blood pressure, heart rate, and cardiac contractility). The exact pattern of physiological and biological responses to acute emotional and mental challenges are determined by many factors, including demographic characteristics, task characteristics, presence of comorbidity, and cardiovascular risk factors. The pathophysiological consequences of acute psychological risk factors in patients with cardiac disease may result from increased cardiac demand and decreased coronary supply (Krantz et al., 1996). Markers of decreased coronary supply in response to mental challenge tasks include: impaired dilation of the coronary vessels (Kop et al., in press; Yeung et al., 1991); decreases in plasma volume (Patterson, Gottdiener, Hecht, Vargot, & Krantz, 1993); and increased platelet activity and blood clotting tendency (Jern et al., 1989; Patterson et al., 1995). The resulting imbalance between increased cardiac demand and decreased coronary blood supply may potentially lead to cardiac ischemia. The mechanisms accounting for cardiac arrhythmias induced by mental arousal have been reviewed elsewhere (Verrier, 1987) and include direct cardiac influences of the central nervous system as well as the autonomic nervous system, particularly vagal withdrawal. Furthermore, hemodynamic responses to acute stressors can lead to plaque rupture, and increased platelet aggregation may promote acute coronary thrombus formation.

### 3. Immunological Correlates

Lymphocytes have receptors for neurohormones associated with sympathetic-adreno-medullary axis and hypothalamo-pituitary-adrenal (HPA) axis activity. The effects of acute mental arousal on the immune system are complex (Ader, Cohen, & Felten, 1995) and both increased and decreased numbers of lymphocytes and NK cells have been reported. Most studies show increases in B cells and CD8+ T cells and decreases in CD4+ T cells in response to acute challenge tasks. However, both task characteristics (e.g., predictability of the stimulus, social interaction component) and subject characteristics (e.g., concomitant chronic psychological disorder, disease status, and health behaviors) affect the direction and magnitude of the acute immune response to mental challenges. Consistent with the immune system changes following arousal, modulation of autonomic nervous system activity by surgical or pharmacological procedures elicits disparate responses of the immune system. The effects of acute laboratory challenge tasks on immune parameters are mediated in part by the increased hemoconcentration following laboratory tasks (Marsland et al., 1997). Cytokines (IL-1$\alpha$ and IL-2) are reported to increase with psychological challenge (e.g., undergoing a coronary angioplasty: Schulte et al., 1994), suggesting at least a partial activation of the immune system (see also Dantzer & Kelley, 1989). Consistent with the notion of immune activation is that acute-phase proteins (CRP and fibrinogen) (Dugue, Leppanen, Teppo, Fyhrquist, & Grasbeck, 1993; Jern et al., 1989) as well as adhesion molecules (Mills & Dimsdale, 1996) increase during mental challenge tasks. Although inflammation and coagulation are related processes, the mechanism by which inflammatory factors promote atherosclerosis do not necessarily involve thrombotic processes. Some evidence suggests that the immune system changes following sympathetic activation precedes the HPA response (Landmann et al., 1984). In general, the magnitude of the immunosuppressive response is correlated with the hemodynamic increase (Benschop et al., 1995, 1998; Herbert et al., 1994; Zakowski, McAllister, Deal, & Baum, 1992), which probably reflects increased sympathetic nervous system activation as a common factor.

### 4. Summary and Interpretation

Acute psychological challenges induce a partial activation of the immune system. Although the overall acute challenge response is quite complex, increased CD8+ T cells, cytokines, acute-phase proteins (e.g., C-reactive protein and fibrinogen), and circulating adhesion molecules accompany acute mental and emotional arousal. These immune system changes may be relevant with respect to triggering acute coronary syndromes because increased immune activation may lead to activation and subsequent rupture of vulnerable atherosclerotic plaques (Libby et al., 1997). Moreover, immune activation may directly interact with several blood clotting factors and indirectly promote thrombus formation and coronary vasoconstriction by interfering with normal endothelial function. Acute immune activation may also result in reduced perfusion of coronary arteries distal to the culprit lesion and decrease perfusion of the microcirculation (Entman & Ballantyne, 1993). The immune activation component of the **acute** response to challenges therefore may be more important than the immunosuppressive component in the pathophysiology of acute coronary syndromes.

## D. Conclusions and Interpretation: Interaction between Psychological and Immunological risk Factors for Coronary Syndromes

The reviewed evidence regarding chronic, episodic, and acute psychological risk factors for coronary syndromes may have distinct consequences for the immunological component of CAD progression and its clinical manifestations. Figure 4 presents a simplified diagram that distinguishes among: (1) psychological factors, (2) physiological and immunological correlates, and (3) the atherosclerotic consequences. It is hypothesized that physiological and immunological correlates of psychological risk factors are involved in the progression of CAD (from Type I to Type III lesions) as well as the transition from Type III

lesions into acute coronary syndromes (lower part of Figure 4).

At the psychological level, chronic factors increase the likelihood of developing episodic and acute risk factors. For example, exhaustion is considered to be the end stage of prolonged uncontrollable psychological distress (Appels, 1990; Selye, 1977). Consequently, exhaustion is likely to be more prevalent among individuals who experience continued psychological distress, e.g., in hostile individuals. Several studies have found additive effects of exhaustion superimposed on these chronic sources of psychological distress (Falger & Schouten, 1992; Kop, 1999; Mendes de Leon, Kop, de Swart, Bar, & Appels, 1996). Furthermore, chronic psychological risk factors for coronary syndromes are associated with elevated responsiveness to acute challenges (Suarez et al., 1991).

1. *Chronic psychological risk factors* are involved in CAD progression and its clinical manifestations by two main pathways: elevations of adverse background factors and exaggeration of the acute challenge responses. First, the effects of chronic psychological risk factors on background factors are primarily mediated by increased sympathetic tone (Williams et al., 1991) and adverse health behaviors (Suarez et al., 1991). An important result is development of an adverse lipid profile and lipid oxidation. The immunological correlates of chronic psychological factors are primarily indirectly related to CAD progression by way of decreased phagocytic function of macrophages as well as by the higher incidence of infectious disease. Macrophages are involved in arterial lipid deposition and, in addition, infections may develop into potential latent risk factors. These immunological consequences may promote the onset of early atherosclerotic lesions (Type I) and their progression into more severe vascular damage (Type II lesions). Second, chronic psychological risk factors are associated with exaggerated physiological responses to acute challenges. This hyperreactivity may promote early atherosclerosis by increasing vessel damage, but is primarily relevant in the onset of acute coronary syndromes. Increased immunological responses may be one mechanism by which chronic psychological risk factors elevate risk of plaque rupture, thrombus formation, and, consequently, coronary syndromes. Similarly, latent infections may play a role in this two-way involvement of chronic psychological factors. As Kol and Libby (1998) state: "Given that most of the known effects on vascular cells do not require a productive infection, a latent infection might induce chronic alterations in the vascular wall, promoting atherogenesis. Distinctively

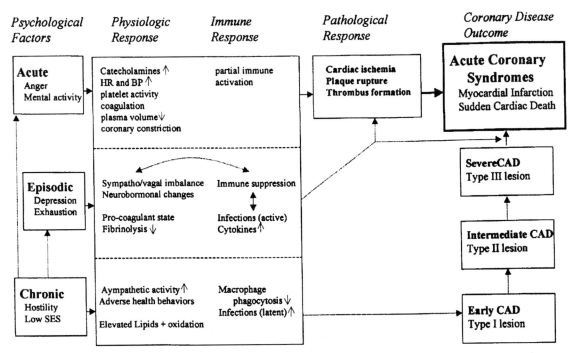

**FIGURE 4** Pathophysiologic model of the relationships between chronic, episodic, and acute psychological risk factors for coronary syndromes. Acute psychological factors result in physiological responses leading to cardiac effects (increased cardiac demand, decreased coronary supply) as well as partial immune activation that may cause plaque instability. In vulnerable patients, these cardiac effects may have pathophysiological results including myocardial ischemia, thrombus formation, and plaque rupture. Episodic psychological factors have physiological correlates that are involved in the progression of severe coronary disease to acute coronary syndromes. Chronic psychological factors promote the onset of early atherosclerosis, especially in the setting of genetic vulnerability, adverse health behaviors, and other environmental risk factors. In addition, chronic psychological factors are related to increased frequency and response magnitude of acute psychological factors and promote the risk of developing episodic factors (HR, heart rate; BP, blood pressure) (modified from Kop, 1999).

from local infection in the vessel wall, acute systemic infections might trigger acute coronary syndromes through the increase in hemodynamic stress on preexisting lesions and by induction of a prothrombotic state.''

2. *Episodic psychological risk factors* are associated with a sympathetic/parasympathetic imbalance, whereas hyperreactivity is generally not observed (Carney et al., 1995). Among the episodic risk factors, research has focused primarily on major depression and (vital) exhaustion. Although elevated cortisol levels are commonly associated with episodic risk factors, particularly in melancholic depression, some evidence suggests inactivation of the CRH system in states characterized by fatigue and hypersomnia (Gold et al., 1988). The onset of initial depressive episodes is often triggered by psychological stressful situations, but some evidence suggests that these precipitating events are less apparent at later episodes of the depressive disorder (Gold et al., 1988). Assuming an immune-suppressed state in episodic risk factors, it could be argued that activation of latent

viruses in atherosclerotic plaques is facilitated by systemic factors. An example of such a process is that glucocorticoids enhance transcription (reactivation) of latent herpes virus. Dantzer and colleagues (1989) have postulated a bidirectional relationship between immune system and psychological characteristics. The immune system (e.g., IL-1 and TNF-$\alpha$) can indeed activate the HPA axis (Dantzer & Kelley, 1989; Sapolsky, Rivier, Yamamoto, Plotsky, & Vale, 1987; White, 1997). This negative feedback loop may account for the immunosuppressive state in episodic risk factors. Moreover, infections can cause characteristics of a classical stress response including increased glucocorticoid levels and enhanced catecholamine turnover (Dantzer & Kelley, 1989). Finally, evidence of immunological influences on the central nervous system is supported by observations that cytokines mediate nonspecific responses to infection, such as malaise, fatigue, fever, slow-wave sleep, apathy, and irritability. Fatigue and malaise are common side-effects of the parenteral administration of certain cytokines. For example, systemic administration of Il-

1 increases plasma levels of glucocorticoids and ACTH; because elevated glucocorticoids inhibit the synthesis of cytokines (IL-1 and IL-2), a negative feedback loop may exist between cytokines and the neuroendocrine system which, under normal circumstances, downregulates the inflammatory response and reduces proliferation of lymphocytes (Dantzer & Kelley, 1989). Thus, episodic factors may promote cardiac disease progression by their immunosuppressive correlates which are important primarily at the early stages of CAD and by their associated elevated cytokines which are more crucial at later disease stages in the transition from Type III lesions to acute coronary syndromes.

3. *Acute psychological risk factors* trigger acute coronary syndromes primarily by the ischemic and/or arrhythmic consequences of increased autonomic nervous system activity, including cardiac demand (increased blood pressure, heart rate, and cardiac contractility) and decreased coronary supply (coronary vasoconstriction, decreased plasma volume). The immediate immune system response to acute psychological factors includes a partial immune activation. Immune activation promotes intimal cell growth and plays a direct and amplifying role in plaque disruption and thrombus formation. Indirectly, immune activation may promote cardiac ischemia by effecting endothelial function and promoting vasoconstriction. Moreover, active infectious states may be related to increased cardiac demand and promote the onset of ischemia.

Pharmacological intervention strategies aimed at the immune system component of recurrent cardiac events have focused on reducing immune activation in patients with established atherosclerosis, primarily in the setting of preventing coronary artery renarrowing after coronary angioplasty. The effects of corticosteroids (i.e., methylprednisolone) and angiopeptin have been examined because angioplasty induces vessel injury resulting in immune activation and subsequent intimal cell growth. Glucocorticoids have diminishing effects on monocyte influx and decreasing leukocyte activity, but generally, corticosteroid interventions have been ineffective in preventing restenosis (Pepine et al., 1990; Stone et al., 1989). Furthermore, corticosteroid administration shortly after myocardial infarction results in adverse clinical outcomes, including a larger infarct size (Roberts, De Mello, & Sobel, 1976). Angiopeptin is a somatostatin analogue that reduces intimal hyperplasia by inhibiting growth factors and promoting endothelial function. Although no significant beneficial effects were found in coronary renarrowing after angioplasty, angiopeptin significantly reduces secondary event rates (Eriksen et al., 1995). Simple antibiotics in addition to lipid-lowering drugs and antihypertensive medication, may be effective in reducing recurrent cardiac events (Gupta et al., 1997). Currently, azithromyzin trials are being conducted (one initiated by Pfizer, the other by the NIH) to assess this agent in a larger sample of CAD patients. Other ongoing trials have been initiated using clarithromycin (Abbott, Chicago, IL) and roxithromycin (Hoechst, Marion Roussel, Kansas City, MI) (Gura, 1998; Gurfinkel, Bozovich, Daroca, Beck, & Mautner, 1997). Some evidence suggests beneficial effects of anti-oxidant therapy (e.g., probucol and vitamin E) because these agents have antiinflammatory effects, possibly by interfering with the upregulation of adhesion molecules and reduction of smooth muscle cell proliferation (Yokoi et al., 1997). The reported beneficial effects of lipid lowering using statins may in fact be mediated in part by their anti-inflammatory effects. At present, however, the benefits of pharmacological interventions targeted at the immune system components of atherosclerosis in secondary events have at best statistically significant results but the clinical success (i.e., effect size) is relatively limited. No studies to date have addressed either the immune components at early stages of atherosclerosis, or the interaction between psychological factors and pharmacological therapy outcome.

Several behavioral intervention studies in patients with CAD indicate positive effects of relaxation (Appels, Bar, Lasker, Flamm, & Kop, 1997; van Dixhoorn, Duivenvoorden, Staal, Pool, & Verhage, 1987), stress management (Blumenthal et al., 1997), Type A behavior/hostility intervention (Friedman et al., 1986), and social support (Frasure-Smith & Prince, 1985) (for review see Linden, Stossel, & Maurice, 1996). The overall pattern of results suggests a twofold higher incidence of cardiac events among patients who did not receive psychosocial intervention, but negative studies are reported as well (e.g., Frasure-Smith et al., 1997). Intervention studies in cardiac patients generally result in improved health behaviors and reduced cardiovascular risk profiles (e.g., lipid profile and blood pressure). However, because of the multiple levels of intervention, the mechanisms underlying these positive effects are not well understood. Theoretically, it is possible that part of the beneficial effects of behavioral treatment programs in coronary disease patients is mediated by immunological consequences of such interventions. Given the role of inflammatory processes at all stages of coronary disease progression and the known relationships between psychological factors and immune function, future research in this area is likely to provide intriguing new information that may improve the development of more targeted behavioral interventions.

## Acknowledgments

Preparation of this work was supported by a grant from the NIH (HL58638) and the Dutch Heart Foundation (94098) to W.J.K and a grant from the Fetzer Institute to N.C. The opinions and assertions expressed herein are those of the authors and are not to be construed as reflecting the views of the USUHS or the US Department of Defense.

## References

Adams, D. O. (1994). Molecular biology of macrophage activation: A pathway whereby psychosocial factors can potentially affect health. *Psychosomatic Medicine, 56,* 316–327.

Ader, R., Cohen, N., & Felten, D. (1995). Psychoneuroimmunology: interactions between the nervous system and the immune system. *Lancet, 345,* 99–103.

Alonzo, A. A., Simon, A. B., & Feinleib, M. (1975). Prodromata of myocardial infarction and sudden death. *Circulation, 52,* 1056–1062.

Ambrose, J. A., Tannenbaum, M. A., Alexopoulos, D., Hjemdahl-Monsen, C. E., Leavy, J., Weiss, M., Borrico, S., Gorlin, R., & Fuster, V. (1988). Angiographic progression of coronary artery disease and the development of myocardial infarction. *Journal of the American College of Cardiology, 12,* 56–62.

Appels, A. (1990). Mental precursors of myocardial infarction. *British Journal of Psychiatry, 156,* 465–471.

Appels, A. (1997). Depression and coronary heart disease: Observations and questions. *Journal of Psychosomatic Research, 43,* 443–452.

Appels, A., Bar, F., Lasker, J., Flamm, U., & Kop, W. (1997). The effect of a psychological intervention program on the risk of a new coronary event after angioplasty: A feasibility study. *Journal of Psychosomatic Research, 43,* 209–217.

Appels, A., & Mulder, P. (1988). Excess fatigue as a precursor of myocardial infarction. *European Heart Journal, 9,* 758–764.

Appels, A., & Otten, F. (1992). Exhaustion as precursor of cardiac death. *British Journal of Clinical Psychology, 31,* 351–356.

Barefoot, J. C., Dahlstrom, W. G., & Williams, R. B. (1983). Hostility, CHD incidence, and total mortality: A 25-year follow-up study of 255 physicians. *Psychosomatic Medicine, 45,* 59–63.

Beck, J., Garcia, R., Heiss, G., Vokonas, P. S., & Offenbacher, S. (1996). Periodontal disease and cardiovascular disease. *Journal of Periodontology, 67,* 1123–1137.

Benschop, R. J., Geenen, R., Mills, P. J., Naliboff, B. D., Kiecolt-Glaser, J. K., Herbert, T. B., van der Pompe, G., Miller, G. E., Matthews, K. A., Godaert, G. L., Gilmore, S. L., Glaser, R., Heijnen, C. J., Dopp, J. M., Bijlsma, J. W., Solomon, G. F., & Cacioppo, J. T. (1998). Cardiovascular and immune responses to acute psychological stress in young and old women: A meta-analysis. *Psychosomatic Medicine, 60,* 290–296.

Benschop, R. J., Godaert, G. L., Geenen, R., Brosschot, J. F., de Smet, M. B., Olff, M., Heijnen, C. J., & Ballieux, R. E. (1995). Relationships between cardiovascular and immunological changes in an experimental stress model. *Psychological Medicine, 25,* 323–327.

Benschop, R. J., Rodriguez-Feuerhahn, M., & Schedlowski, M. (1996). Catecholamine-induced leukocytosis: Early observations, current research, and future directions. *Brain, Behavior, and Immunity, 10,* 77–91.

Bevilacqua, M. P., Schleef, R. R., Gimbrone, M. A., & Loskutoff, D. J. (1986). Regulation of the fibrinolytic system of cultured human vascular endothelium by interleukin 1. *Journal of Clinical Investigation, 78,* 587–591.

Blumenthal, J. A., Jiang, W., Babyak, M. A., Krantz, D. S., Frid, D. J., Coleman, R. E., Waugh, R., Hanson, M., Appelbaum, M., O'Connor, C., & Morris, J. J. (1997). Stress management and exercise training in cardiac patients with myocardial ischemia. Effects on prognosis and evaluation of mechanisms. *Archives of Internal Medicine, 157,* 2213–2223.

Braunwald, E. (1988). Anonymous, *Heart disease.* Philadelphia, London, Toronto, Montreal, Sydney, Tokyo: Saunders.

Bruschke, A. V., Kramer, J. R., Bal, E. T., Haque, I. U., Detrano, R. C., & Goormastic, M. (1989). The dynamics of progression of coronary atherosclerosis studied in 168 medically treated patients who underwent coronary arteriography three times. *American Heart Journal, 117,* 296–305.

Carney, R. M., Freedland, K. E., Rich, M. W., & Jaffe, A. S. (1995). Depression as a risk factor for cardiac events in established coronary heart disease: A review of possible mechanisms. *Annals of Behavioral Medicine, 17,* 142–149.

Christensen, A. J., Edwards, D. L., Wiebe, J. S., Benotsch, E. G., McKelvey, L., Andrews, M., & Lubaroff, D. M. (1996). Effect of verbal self-disclosure on natural killer cell activity: moderating influence of cynical hostility. *Psychosomatic Medicine, 58,* 150–155.

Danesh, J., Collins, R., & Peto, R. (1997). Chronic infections and coronary heart disease: is there a link? *Lancet, 350,* 430–436.

Dantzer, R., & Kelley, K. W. (1989). Stress and immunity: An integrated view of relationships between the brain and the immune system. *Life Sciences, 44,* 1995–2008.

Davies, M. J., & Thomas, A. (1984). Thrombosis and acute coronary-artery lesions in sudden cardiac ischemic death. *New England Journal of Medicine, 310,* 1137–1140.

Dobson, A. J., Alexander, H. M., Malcolm, J. A., Steele, P. L., & Miles, T. A. (1991). Heart attacks and the Newcastle earthquake. *Medical Journal of Australia, 155,* 757–761.

Dugue, B., Leppanen, E. A., Teppo, A. M., Fyhrquist, F., & Grasbeck, R. (1993). Effects of psychological stress on plasma interleukins-1 beta and 6, c-reactive protein, tumour necrosis factor alpha, anti-diuretic hormone and serum cortisol. *Scandinavian Journal of Clinical Laboratory Investigation, 53,* 555–561.

Engebretson, T. O., & Matthews, K. A. (1992). Dimensions of hostility in men, women, and boys: Relationships to personality and cardiovascular responses to stress. *Psychosomatic Medicine, 54,* 311–323.

Entman, M. L., & Ballantyne, C. M. (1993). Inflammation in acute coronary syndromes. *Circulation, 88,* 800–803.

Eriksen, U. H., Amtorp, O., Bagger, J. P., Emanuelsson, H., Foegh, M., Henningsen, P., & Saumamaki, K. (1995). Randomized double-blind Scandinavian trial of angiopeptin versus placebo for the prevention of clinical events and restenosis after coronary balloon angioplasty. *American Heart Journal, 130,* 1–8.

Falger, P. R., & Schouten, E. G. (1992). Exhaustion, psychological stressors in the work environment, and acute myocardial infarction in adult men. *Journal of Psychosomatic Research, 36,* 777–786.

Falk, E., & Fuster, V. (1995). Coronary plaque disruption. *Circulation, 92,* 657–671.

Folsom, A. R., Nieto, F. J., Sorlie, P., Chambless, L. E., & Graham, D. Y. (1998). Helicobacter pylori seropositivity and coronary heart disease incidence. Atherosclerosis risk in communities (aric) study investigators. *Circulation, 98,* 845–850.

Frasure-Smith, N., Lesperance, F., Prince, R. H., Verrier, P., Garber, R. A., Juneau, M., Wolfson, C., & Bourassa, M. G. (1997). Randomised trial of home-based psychosocial nursing intervention for patients recovering from myocardial infarction. *Lancet*, *350*, 473–479.

Frasure-Smith, N., Lesperance, F., & Talajic, M. (1995). Depression and 18-month prognosis after myocardial infarction. *Circulation*, *91*, 999–1005.

Frasure-Smith, N., & Prince, R. (1985). The ischemic heart disease life stress monitoring program: Impact on mortality. *Psychosomatic Medicine*, *47*, 431–445.

Fricchione, G. L., Bilfinger, T. V., Hartman, A., Liu, Y., & Stefano, G. B. (1996). Neuroimmunologic implications in coronary artery disease. *Advances in Neuroimmunology*, *6*, 131–142.

Friedman, M., Byers, S. O., Diamant, J., & Rosenman, R. H. (1975). Plasma catecholamine response of coronary-prone subjects (type A) to a specific challenge. *Metabolism*, *24*, 205–210.

Friedman, M., & Rosenman, R. (1959). Association of specific overt behavior pattern with blood and cardiovascular findings: Blood cholesterol level, blood clotting time, incidence of arcis senilis and clinical coronary artery disease. *Journal of the American Medical Association*, *169*, 1286–1296.

Friedman, M., Thoresen, C. E., Gill, J. J., Ulmer, D., Powell, L. H., Price, V. A., Brown, B., Thompson, L., Rabin, D. D., Breall, W. S., & et al. (1986). Alteration of type a behavior and its effect on cardiac recurrences in post myocardial infarction patients: Summary results of the recurrent coronary prevention project. *American Heart Journal*, *112*, 653–665.

Fuster, V., Badimon, L., Badimon, J. J., & Chesebro, J. H. (1992a). The pathogenesis of coronary artery disease and the acute coronary syndromes (1). *New England Journal of Medicine*, *326*, 242–250.

Fuster, V., Badimon, L., Badimon, J. J., & Chesebro, J. H. (1992b). The pathogenesis of coronary artery disease and the acute coronary syndromes (2). *New England Journal of Medicine*, *326*, 310–318.

Giroud, D., Li, J. M., Urban, P., Meier, B., & Rutishauer, W. (1992). Relation of the site of acute myocardial infarction to the most severe coronary arterial stenosis at prior angiography. *American Journal of Cardiology*, *69*, 729–732.

Gold, P. W., Goodwin, F. K., & Chrousos, G. P. (1988). Clinical and biochemical manifestations of depression. Relation to the neurobiology of stress (1). *New England Journal of Medicine*, *319*, 348–353.

Goodkin, K., & Appels, A. (1997). Behavioral–neuroendocrine–immunologic interactions in myocardial infarction. *Medical Hypotheses*, *48*, 209–214.

Gupta, S., Leatham, E. W., Carrington, D., Mendall, M. A., Kaski, J. C., & Camm, A. J. (1997). Elevated chlamydia pneumoniae antibodies, cardiovascular events, and azithromycin in male survivors of myocardial infarction. *Circulation*, *96*, 404–407.

Gura, T. (1998). Infections: a cause of artery-clogging plaques? *Science*, *281*, 35–37.

Gurfinkel, E., Bozovich, G., Daroca, A., Beck, E., & Mautner, B. (1997). Randomised trial of roxithromycin in non-q-wave coronary syndromes: roxis pilot study. Roxis study group. *Lancet*, *350*, 404–407.

Hansson, G. K., Holm, J., Holm, S., Fotev, Z., Hedrich, H. J., & Fingerle, J. (1991). T lymphocytes inhibit the vascular response to injury. *Procedings of the National Academy of Sciences, USA*, *88*, 10530–10534.

Herbert, T. B., & Cohen, S. (1993a). Depression and immunity: A meta-analytic review. *Psychological Bulletin*, *113*, 472–486.

Herbert, T. B., & Cohen, S. (1993b). Stress and immunity in humans: A meta-analytic review. *Psychosomatic Medicine*, *55*, 364–379.

Herbert, T. B., Cohen, S., Marsland, A. L., Bachen, E. A., Rabin, B. S., Muldoon, M. F., & Manuck, S. B. (1994). Cardiovascular reactivity and the course of immune response to an acute psychological stressor. *Psychosomatic Medicine*, *56*, 337–344.

Jern, C., Eriksson, E., Tengborn, L., Risberg, B., Wadenvik, H., & Jern, S. (1989). Changes of plasma coagulation and fibrinolysis in response to mental stress. *Thrombosis and Haemostasis*, *62*, 761–771.

Kol, A., & Libby, P. (1998). The mechanisms by which infectious agents may contribute to atherosclerosis and its clinical manifestations. *Trends in Cardiovascular Medicine*, *8*(5), 191–199.

Kop, W. J. (1997). Acute and chronic psychological risk factors for coronary syndromes: Moderating effects of coronary artery disease severity. *Journal of Psychosomatic Research*, *43*, 167–181.

Kop, W. J. (1999). Chronic and acute psychological risk factors for clinical manifestations of coronary artery disease. *Psychosomatic Medicine*, *61* (4), 476–487.

Kop, W. J., Appels, A., Howell, R. H., Krantz, D. S., Bairey Merz, C. N., Caravalho, J. J., Lundgren, N., & Gottdiener, J. S. for the TOMIS Investigators (1997). Relationship between vital exhaustion and stress-induced myocardial ischemia. *Annals of Behavioral Medicine.* *19*, 159. [abstract]

Kop, W. J., Appels, A., Mendes de Leon, C. F., & Bar, F. W. (1996). The relationship between severity of coronary artery disease and vital exhaustion. *Journal of Psychosomatic Research*, *40*, 397–405.

Kop, W. J., Appels, A. P., Mendes de Leon, C. F., de Swart, H., & Bar, F. W. (1993). The effect of successful coronary angioplasty on feelings of exhaustion. *International Journal of Cariology*, *42*, 269–276.

Kop, W. J., Appels, A. P., Mendes de Leon, C. F., de Swart, H. B., & Bar, F. W. (1994). Vital exhaustion predicts new cardiac events after successful coronary angioplasty. *Psychosomatic Medicine*, *56*, 281–287.

Kop, W. J., Gottdiener, J. S., Tangen, C., McBurnie, M., Fried, L. P., Walston, J., Newman, A., Hirsch, C., & Tracy, R. P. (1998). Elevated fibrinogen and albumin in exhausted elderly: Mechanisms for adverse cardiovascular outcome in the cardiovascular health study. *Circulation*, *98*, I-555. [abstract]

Kop, W. J., Hamulyak, K., Pernot, K., & Appels, A. (1998). Relationship between blood coagulation and fibrinolysis to vital exhaustion. *Psychosomatic Medicine*, *60*, 352–358.

Kop, W. J., Krantz, D. S., Howell, R. H., Ferguson, M. A., Papademetriou, V., Lu, D., Popma, J. J., Quigley, J., Vernalis, M., & Gottdiener, J. S. (in press). Effects of mental stress on coronary epicardial vasomotion and flow velocity in coronary artery disease: Relationship with hemodynamic stress responses. (Submitted for publication) *Journal of the American College of Cardiology*.

Krantz, D. S., Kop, W. J., Santiago, H. T., & Gottdiener, J. S. (1996). Mental stress as a trigger of myocardial ischemia and infarction. *Cardiology Clinics*, *14*, 271–287.

Kraus, J. F., Borhani, N. O., & Franti, C. E. (1980). Socioeconomic status, ethnicity, and risk of coronary heart disease. *American Journal of Epidemiology*, *111*, 407–414.

Kuller, L., Cooper, M., & Perper, J. (1972). Epidemiology of sudden death. *Archives of Internal Medicine*, *129*, 714–719.

Kuller, L. H., Tracy, R. P., Shaten, J., & Meilahn, E. N. (1996). Relation of c-reactive protein and coronary heart disease in the mrfit nested case-control study. Multiple risk factor intervention trial. *American Journal of Epidemiology*, *144*, 537–547.

Landmann, R. M., Muller, F. B., Perini, C., Wesp, M., Erne, P., & Buhler, F. R. (1984). Changes of immunoregulatory cells induced by psychological and physical stress: Relationship to plasma catecholamines. *Clinical and Experimental Immunology, 58,* 127–135.

Leary, T. (1941). The genesis of atherosclerosis. *Archives of Pathology, 32* (4), 507–555.

Lee, D. J., Meehan, R. T., Robinson, C., Smith, M. L., & Mabry, T. R. (1995). Psychosocial correlates of immune responsiveness and illness episodes in us air force academy cadets undergoing basic cadet training. *Journal of Psychosomatic Research, 39,* 445–457.

Libby, P., Egan, D., & Skarlatos, S. (1997). Roles of infectious agents in atherosclerosis and restenosis: An assessment of the evidence and need for future research. *Circulation, 96,* 4095–4103.

Libby, P., & Hansson, G. K. (1991). Involvement of the immune system in human atherogenesis: Current knowledge and unanswered questions. *Laboratory Investigation, 64,* 5–15.

Linden, W., Stossel, C., & Maurice, J. (1996). Psychosocial interventions for patients with coronary artery disease: A meta-analysis. *Archives of Internal Medicine, 156,* 745–752.

Liuzzo, G., Biasucci, L. M., Gallimore, J. R., Grillo, R. L., Rebuzzi, A. G., Pepys, M. B., & Maseri, A. (1994). The prognostic value of c-reactive protein and serum amyloid a protein in severe unstable angina. *New England Journal of Medicine, 331,* 417–424.

Loppnow, H., & Libby, P. (1992). Functional significance of human vascular smooth muscle cell-derived interleukin 1 in paracrine and autocrine regulation pathways. *Experimental Cell Research, 198,* 283–290.

Maes, M. (1995). Evidence for an immune response in major depression: A review and hypothesis. *Progress in Neuropsychopharmacology, Biology, and Psychiatry, 19,* 11–38.

Manuck, S. B., Marsland, A. L., Kaplan, J. R., & Williams, J. K. (1995). The pathogenicity of behavior and its neuroendocrine mediation: An example from coronary artery disease. *Psychosomatic Medicine, 57,* 275–283.

Markovitz, J. H., & Matthews, K. A. (1991). Platelets and coronary heart disease: Potential psychophysiologic mechanisms. *Psychosomatic Medicine, 53,* 643–668.

Marmot, M. G., Shipley, M. J., & Rose, G. (1984). Inequalities in death—Specific explanations of a general pattern? *Lancet,* 1003–1006.

Marshall, B. J. (1993). Helicobacter pylori: A primer for 1994. *Gastroenterologist, 1,* 241–247.

Marsland, A. L., Herbert, T. B., Muldoon, M. F., Bachen, E. A., Patterson, S., Cohen, S., Rabin, B., & Manuck, S. B. (1997). Lymphocyte subset redistribution during acute laboratory stress in young adults: Mediating effects of hemoconcentration. *Health Psychology, 16,* 341–348.

McEwen, B. S. (1998). Protective and damaging effects of stress mediators. *New England Journal of Medicine, 338,* 171–179.

Meesters, C. M., & Smulders, J. (1994). Hostility and myocardial infarction in men. *Journal of Psychosomatic Research, 38,* 727–734.

Meisel, S. R., Kutz, I., Dayan, K. I., Pauzner, H., Chetboun, I., Arbel, Y., & David, D. (1991). Effect of Iraqi missile war on incidence of acute myocardial infarction and sudden death in Israeli civilians. *Lancet, 338,* 660–661.

Melnick, J. L., Adam, E., & Debakey, M. E. (1993). Cytomegalovirus and atherosclerosis. *European Heart Journal, 14(Suppl. K),* 30–38.

Mendall, M. A., Patel, P., Ballam, L., Strachan, D., & Northfield, T. C. (1996). C reactive protein and its relation to cardiovascular risk factors: A population based cross sectional study. *British Medical Journal, 312,* 1061–1065.

Mendes de Leon, C. F., Kop, W. J., de Swart, H. B., Bar, F. W., & Appels, A. P. (1996). Psychosocial characteristics and recurrent events after percutaneous transluminal coronary angioplasty. *American Journal of Cardiology, 77,* 252–255.

Mills, P. J., & Dimsdale, J. E. (1996). The effects of acute psychologic stress on cellular adhesion molecules. *Journal of Psychosomatic Research, 41,* 49–53.

Mills, P. J., Dimsdale, J. E., Nelesen, R. A., & Dillon, E. (1996). Psychologic characteristics associated with acute stressor-induced leukocyte subset redistribution. *Journal of Psychosomatic Research, 40,* 417–423.

Mittleman, M. A., Maclure, M., Sherwood, J. B., Mulry, R. P., Tofler, G. H., Jacobs, S. C., Friedman, R., Benson, H., & Muller, J. E. (1995). Triggering of acute myocardial infarction onset by episodes of anger. Determinants of Myocardial Infarction Onset Study Investigators. *Circulation, 92,* 1720–1725.

Muhlestein, J. B., Hammond, E. H., Carlquist, J. F., Radicke, E., Thomson, M. J., Karagounis, L. A., Woods, M. L., & Anderson, J. L. (1996). Increased incidence of chlamydia species within the coronary arteries of patients with symptomatic atherosclerotic versus other forms of cardiovascular disease. *Journal of the American College of Cardiology, 27,* 1555–1561.

Muller, J. E., Abela, G. S., Nesto, R. W., & Tofler, G. H. (1994). Triggers, acute risk factors and vulnerable plaques: The lexicon of a new frontier. *Journal of the American College of Cardiology, 23,* 809–813.

Pasceri, V., Cammarota, G., Patti, G., Cuoco, L., Gasbarrini, A., Grillo, R. L., Fedeli, G., Gasbarrini, G., & Maseri, A. (1998). Association of virulent helicobacter pylori strains with ischemic heart disease. *Circulation, 97,* 1675–1679.

Patterson, S. M., Gottdiener, J. S., Hecht, G., Vargot, S., & Krantz, D. S. (1993). Effects of acute mental stress on serum lipids: Mediating effects of plasma volume. *Psychosomatic Medicine, 55,* 525–532.

Patterson, S. M., Krantz, D. S., Gottdiener, J. S., Hecht, G., Vargot, S., & Goldstein, D. S. (1995). Prothrombotic effects of environmental stress: Changes in platelet function, hematocrit, and total plasma protein. *Psychosomatic Medicine, 57,* 592–599.

Pepine, C. J., Hirshfeld, J. W., Macdonald, R. G., Henderson, M. A., Bass, T. A., Goldberg, S., Savage, M. P., Vetrovec, G., Cowley, M., Taussig, A. S., et al. (1990). A controlled trial of corticosteroids to prevent restenosis after coronary angioplasty. M-HEART Group. *Circulation, 81,* 1753–1761.

Pietraszek, M. H., Takada, Y., Nishimoto, M., Ohara, K., & Takada, A. (1991). Fibrinolytic activity in depression and neurosis. *Thrombosis Research, 63,* 661–666.

Ragland, D. R. (1989). Type A behavior and outcome of coronary disease. *New England Journal of Medicine, 319,* 1480–1481.

Raikkonen, K., Lassila, R., Keltikangas-Jarvinen, L., & Hautanen, A. (1996). Association of chronic stress with plasminogen activator inhibitor-1 in healthy middle-aged men. *Arteriosclerosis, Thrombosis and Vascular Biology, 16,* 363–367.

Ridker, P. M. (1998). Inflammation, infection, and cardiovascular risk: how good is the clinical evidence? *Circulation, 97,* 1671–1674.

Ridker, P. M., Cushman, M., Stampfer, M. J., Tracy, R. P., & Hennekens, C. H. (1997). Inflammation, aspirin, and the risk of cardiovascular disease in apparently healthy men . *New England Journal of Medicine, 336,* 973–979.

Ridker, P. M., Glynn, R. J., & Hennekens, C. H. (1998). C-reactive protein adds to the predictive value of total and hdl cholesterol in determining risk of first myocardial infarction. *Circulation, 97,* 2007–2011.

Ridker, P. M., Hennekens, C. H., Roitman-Johnson, B., Stampfer, M. J., & Allen, J. (1998). Plasma concentration of soluble intercellular adhesion molecule 1 and risks of future myocardial infarction in apparently healthy men. *Lancet, 351,* 88–92.

Roberts, R., De Mello, V., & Sobel, B. E. (1976). Deleterious effects of methylprednisolone in patients with myocardial infarction. *Circulation, 53,* I204–I206.

Ross, R. (1999). Atherosclerosis — An inflammatory disease. *New England Journal of Medicine, 340*(2), 115–126.

Saikku, P., Leinonen, M., Mattila, K., Ekman, M. R., Nieminen, M. S., Makela, P. H., Huttunen, J. K., & Valtonen, V. (1988). Serological evidence of an association of a novel chlamydia, twar, with chronic coronary heart disease and acute myocardial infarction. *Lancet, 2,* 983–986.

Sapolsky, R., Rivier, C., Yamamoto, G., Plotsky, P., & Vale, W. (1987). Interleukin-1 stimulates the secretion of hypothalamic corticotropin-releasing factor. *Science, 238,* 522–524.

Schulte, H. M., Bamberger, C. M., Elsen, H., Herrmann, G., Bamberger, A. M., & Barth, J. (1994). Systemic interleukin-1 alpha and interleukin-2 secretion in response to acute stress and to corticotropin-releasing hormone in humans. *European Journal of Clinical Investigation, 24,* 773–777.

Seeman, T. E., Singer, B. H., Rowe, J. W., Horwitz, R. I., & McEwen, B. S. (1997). Price of adaptation—allostatic load and its health consequences. Macarthur studies of successful aging. *Archives of Internal Medicine, 157,* 2259–2268.

Selye, H. (1977). *The stress of life.* New York: McGraw Hill.

Shekelle, R. B., Gale, M., & Norusis, M. (1985). Type A score (Jenkins Activity Survey) and risk of recurrent coronary heart disease in the aspirin myocardial infarction study. *American Journal of Cardiology, 56,* 221–225.

Shekelle, R. B., Gale, M., Ostfeld, A. M., & Paul, O. (1983). Hostility, risk of coronary heart disease, and mortality. *Psychosomatic Medicine, 45,* 109–114.

Siegman, A. W., Dembroski, T. M., & Ringel, N. (1987). Components of hostility and the severity of coronary artery disease. *Psychosomatic Medicine, 49,* 127–135.

Stein, M., Miller, A. H., & Trestman, R. L. (1991). Depression, the immune system, and health and illness: Findings in search of meaning. *Archives of General Psychiatry, 48,* 171–177.

Stern, D., Nawroth, P., Handley, D., & Kisiel, W. (1985). An endothelial cell-dependent pathway of coagulation. *Procedings of the National Academy of Sciences, USA, 82,* 2523–2527.

Stone, G. W., Rutherford, B. D., McConahay, D. R., Johnson, W. L., Giorgi, L. V., Ligon, R. W., & Hartzler, G. O. (1989). A randomized trial of corticosteroids for the prevention of restenosis in 102 patients undergoing repeat coronary angioplasty. *Catheterization and Cardiovascular Diagnosis, 18,* 227–231.

Suarez, E. C., Williams, R. B., Kuhn, C. M., Zimmerman, E. H., & Schanberg, S. M. (1991). Biobehavioral basis of coronary-prone behavior in middle-age men. II. Serum cholesterol, the Type A behavior pattern, and hostility as interactive modulators of physiological reactivity. *Psychosomatic Medicine, 53,* 528–537.

Thompson, S. G., Kienast, J., Pyke, S. D., Haverkate, F., & van de Loo, J. C. (1995). Hemostatic factors and the risk of myocardial infarction or sudden death in patients with angina pectoris. European concerted action on thrombosis and disabilities angina pectoris study group. *New England Journal of Medicine, 332,* 635–641.

Tracy, R. P., Lemaitre, R. N., Psaty, B. M., Ives, D. G., Evans, R. W., Cushman, M., Meilahn, E. N., & Kuller, L. H. (1997). Relationship of c-reactive protein to risk of cardiovascular disease in the

elderly. Results from the cardiovascular health study and the rural health promotion project. *Arteriosclerosis, Thrombosis and Vascular Biology, 17,* 1121–1127.

Trichopoulos, D., Katsouyanni, K., Zavitsanos, X., Tzonou, A., & Dalla-Vorgia, P. (1983). Psychological stress and fatal heart attack: The Athens (1981) earthquake natural experiment. *Lancet, 1,* 441–443.

van Dixhoorn, J., Duivenvoorden, H. J., Staal, J. A., Pool, J., & Verhage, F. (1987). Cardiac events after myocardial infarction: possible effect of relaxation therapy. *European Heart Journal, 8,* 1210–1214.

Verrier, R. L. (1987). Mechanisms of behaviorally induced arrhythmias. *Circulation, 76,* I48–I56.

Wald, N. J., Law, M. R., Morris, J. K., & Bagnall, A. M. (1997). Helicobacter pylori infection and mortality from ischaemic heart disease: Negative result from a large, prospective study. *British Medical Journal, 315,* 1199–1201.

Weisse, C. S. (1992). Depression and immunocompetence: A review of the literature. *Psychological Bulletin, 111,* 475–489.

Welin, L., Tibblin, G., Svardsudd, K., Tibblin, B., Ander-Peciva, S., Larsson, B., & Wilhelmsen, L. (1985). Prospective study of social influences on mortality. The study of men born in 1913 and 1923. *Lancet,* 915–918.

White, P. D. (1997). The relationship between infection and fatigue. *Journal of Psychosomatic Research, 43,* 345–350.

Williams, R. B., Barefoot, J. C., Haney, T. L., Harrell, F. E., Blumenthal, J. A., Pryor, D. B., & Peterson, B. (1988). Type A behavior and angiographically documented coronary atherosclerosis in a sample of 2,289 patients. *Psychosomatic Medicine, 50,* 139–152.

Williams, R. B., Haney, T. L., Lee, K. L., Kong, Y. H., Blumenthal, J. A., & Whalen, R. E. (1980). Type A behavior, hostility, and coronary atherosclerosis. *Psychosomatic Medicine,* 539–549.

Williams, R. B., Suarez, E. C., Kuhn, C. M., Zimmerman, E. A., & Schanberg, S. M. (1991). Biobehavioral basis of coronary-prone behavior in middle-aged men. I. Evidence for chronic SNS activation in Type As. *Psychosomatic Medicine, 53,* 517–527.

Winkleby, M. A., Jatulis, D. E., Frank, E., & Fortmann, S. P. (1992). Socioeconomic status and health: How education, income, and occupation contribute to risk factors for cardiovascular disease. *American Journal of Public Health, 82,* 816–820.

Yeung, A. C., Vekshtein, V. I., Krantz, D. S., Vita, J. A., Ryan, T. J., Ganz, P., & Selwyn, A. P. (1991). The effect of atherosclerosis on the vasomotor response of coronary arteries to mental stress. *New England Journal of Medicine, 325,* 1551–1556.

Yokoi, H., Daida, H., Kuwabara, Y., Nishikawa, H., Takatsu, F., Tomihara, H., Nakata, Y., Kutsumi, Y., Ohshima, S., Nishiyama, S., Seki, A., Kato, K., Nishimura, S., Kanoh, T., & Yamaguchi, H. (1997). Effectiveness of an antioxidant in preventing restenosis after percutaneous transluminal coronary angioplasty: The probucol angioplasty restenosis trial. *Journal of the American College of Cardiology, 30,* 855–862.

Zakowski, S. G., McAllister, C. G., Deal, M., & Baum, A. (1992). Stress, reactivity, and immune function in healthy men. *Health Psychology, 11,* 223–232.

# 59

# The Impact of Stress, Catecholamines, and the Menstrual Cycle on NK Activity and Tumor Development: From in Vitro Studies to Biological Significance

SHAMGAR BEN-ELIYAHU, GUY SHAKHAR

## I. INTRODUCTION

The field of psychoneuroimmunology (PNI) faces several challenges, two of which have guided the work described in this chapter. The first challenge is to elucidate mechanisms mediating the interactions among the psychological, neuroendocrinological, and immunological levels. This calls for a reductionistic approach aiming at a precise identification of the processes that constitute these interactions. The second challenge is to elucidate the biological significance, or the clinical relevance, of these interactions. That is, to identify conditions under which these interactions affect, if at all, the physical or psychological well being of humans. This requires establishing the relative weight of these interactions among the many factors that determine the health and behavior of the organism. Pursuing these two related directions in PNI research is crucial for developing measures to promote the well being of patients.

The work described in this chapter pertains to the deleterious aspects of acute stress in relation to tumor development. Whereas surgery is essential for removing the primary tumor in most cancer patients, surgical procedures have been implicated in the promotion of metastasis via numerous mechanisms, including the suppression of natural killer (NK) cell activity by stress hormones. Our studies aim at elucidating neuroendocrine mechanisms that suppress NK activity and the specific clinical circumstances in which such suppression occurs and promotes tumor metastasis. We hope that our empirical findings, as well as our hypotheses and speculations, are helpful in outlining prophylactic measures and strategies for enhancing the survival rates of cancer patients, particularly those undergoing surgery for the removal of metastasizing tumors.

## A.  Natural Killer (NK) Cells and Tumor Development

Natural killer cells are considered important in cellular resistance to viral disease (Lotzova, 1991) and malignancy (Brittenden, Heys, Ross, & Eremin, 1996; Whiteside & Herberman, 1995). Natural killer cells are predominantly large granular lymphocytes (LGL). In humans, these cells are negative for CD3, express CD16 and/or CD56 surface antigens, and comprise 10 to 15% of peripheral blood lymphocytes (Carson & Caligiuri, 1996). In the rat, NK cells can be identified using a single surface antigen as being NKR-P1$^{bright}$ (Chambers et al., 1989). The mechanism by which NK cells recognize their targets involves the detection of aberrations in, or the absence of, MHC-I molecules (Dohring & Colonna, 1997). By the time malignant cells have evolved to a metastasizing stage, they had usually suppressed the expression of functional MHC-I molecules, making them invulnerable to CTLs. This and the fact that a large proportion of NK cells reside in the blood and the tissues targeted by metastasizing cells (e.g., lung and liver) make NK cells most important at this stage (Algarra, Collado, & Garrido, 1997; Garrido et al., 1997). Lysis of target cells occurs instantly, without prior sensitization or MHC restriction. Apart from lysing single tumor cells, NK cells have been shown to infiltrate and diminish established micrometastases (Whiteside & Herberman, 1995).

Animal studies have shown that NK cells play an important role in controlling the development of leukemia and some solid tumors (Brittenden et al., 1996), and play a pivotal role in controlling metastatic development of various types of tumor (Barlozzari, Leonhardt, Wiltrout, Herberman, & Reynolds, 1985; Ben-Eliyahu & Page, 1992; Ben-Eliyahu, Yirmiya, Liebeskind, Taylor, & Gale, 1991; Gorelik, Wiltrout, Okumura, Habu, & Herberman, 1982; Hanna, 1985; Vujanovic, Basse, Herberman, & Whiteside, 1996; Wiltrout et al., 1985). Human studies have indicated an association between levels of NK cell activity (NKCA) and susceptibility to several different types of cancer. For example, patients displaying lower levels of NKCA (e.g., Chediak–Higashi syndrome, and X-linked lymphoproliferative syndrome) have

been reported to show a higher incidence of cancer (Paller, 1995). Importantly, higher levels of NKCA and tumor infiltration by NK cells at the time of tumor removal, have been associated with a better prognosis following the excision of breast, liver, colon, head, or neck tumors (Brittenden et al., 1996; Coca et al., 1997; Levy, Herberman, Maluish, Schlien, & Lippman, 1985; Schantz, Brown, Lira, Taylor, & Beddingfield, 1987; Taketomi et al., 1998).

## B.  Three Complementary Approaches for the Study of NK Activity

Three different approaches are commonly used in PNI to study the effects of stress or various hormones on NKCA or to study the role of NK cells in mediating the effects of stress on disease progression.

**Ex vivo studies** are those in which NKCA is assessed in vitro following in vivo manipulations of the organism (such as drug administration or exposure to stressful conditions). To the researcher's advantage, NK cells are exposed in vivo to the entire array of physiological changes induced by the manipulation. This aspect is crucial for studying neuroimmunomodulation, but caution should be practiced when basing conclusions as to **in vivo** levels of NKCA on the findings of ex vivo studies. Cytotoxicity is assessed after extracting the autologous serum and its soluble factors (e.g., hormones), and outside the physiological context (e.g., epithelial cells). Additionally, the common practice of excluding several types of leukocytes before assessing cytotoxicity prevents the continued interaction of NK cells with the excluded leukocytes and the cytokines they release. Such exclusion procedures (enrichment of NK cells) also introduce a delay between blood withdrawal and the actual assessment of cytotoxicity and may interfere biochemically with NKCA. For these reasons some in vivo influences on NKCA may dissipate or be distorted due to the delay and the conditions of its assessment. Some hormonal effects on NKCA have indeed been reported to be transient or dependent upon the presence of serum factors (Hellstrand, Hermodsson, & Strannegard, 1985). These effects are unlikely to be evident in ex vivo studies. In humans, we have recently been using a whole blood NK assay that can begin shortly after blood withdrawal, and in which serum and all blood cells are retained throughout the assessment of cytotoxicity. Indeed, some findings, such as higher NK cytotoxicity in schizophrenic patients, were evident when employing the whole-blood procedure, but waned when serum was removed from the same blood samples (whole-washed blood assay) (Yovel et al., in press).

Unfortunately, in rats, serum must be removed to achieve reasonable levels of cytotoxicity. Importantly, the whole-blood assay in humans and the whole washed blood assay in rats were shown to specifically reflect cytotoxicity carried out by NK cells, rather than by other cell populations or serum cytolytic factors (Ben-Eliyahu, Page, Shakhar, & Taylor, 1996a; Ree & Platts, 1983).

**In vitro studies** are those in which stress hormones or other compounds are added to the standard medium of the in vitro assay, and cytotoxicity is assessed in their presence. Good control over the variables affecting NK cytotoxicity can be achieved, but the effects are studied in the limited and artificial context of the in vitro environment. Neither the in vitro nor the ex vivo approaches can indicate the biological significance of changes in NKCA, i.e., the degree to which alteration in NKCA would affect the host's resistance to disease. Considering these limitations, we and others have also employed a third approach: in vivo assessment of NKCA using animal models of diseases.

**In vivo studies** are those in which an NK-dependent process (index) is evaluated in the living animal under different conditions. This approach allows studying NKCA in the complete and natural environment, and at the same time can reflect alterations in NKCA in the biologically relevant terms of resistance to a certain disease. This statement, however, should be tempered. First, no known NK-dependent index is likely to be affected solely by NKCA. Other factors affected by the in vivo manipulation may influence the NK-dependent index. The more NK-sensitive the index is, and the less sensitive it is to other factors, the better it reflects changes in NKCA. Second, the biological significance of the findings depends on the resemblance between the conditions in which the NK-dependent process is assessed, and the conditions in which it occurs naturally.

Many of our in vivo studies make use of the inbred Fischer 344 rat and a tumor line syngeneic to this strain, the mammary adenocarcinoma MADB106. Following intravenous inoculation, MADB106 cells concentrate in the lungs' capillary beds, extravasate within hours, and thereafter are retained in the lung tissue, where they start to establish colonies. Studies have shown these two related outcomes — lung tumor cell retention (LTR) and the number of lung tumor colonies (visible within weeks) — to be highly correlated and tightly controlled by NK-cell activity. Specifically, earlier research has shown a significant increase in LTR and a 10-fold increase in the number of lung metastases when NKCA was reduced with anti-asialo GM$_1$. These effects were prevented by adoptive transfer of relatively few purified NK cells, but not of T cells or macrophages (Barlozzari et al., 1985; Barlozzari, Reynolds, & Herberman, 1983). More recently, we have made use of anti-NKR-P1, a mAb that selectively depletes NK cells and eliminates NKCA without affecting other immune functions (Ben-Eliyahu & Page, 1992; Chambers et al., 1989; van den Brink, Hunt, & Hiserodt, 1991). Administration of anti-NKR-P1 caused a 200-fold increase in MADB106 LTR and metastatic colonization (Ben-Eliyahu & Page, 1992; Ben-Eliyahu, Page, Yirmiya, & Taylor, 1996b). No such effects were evident if the antibody was administered 24 h after tumor inoculation, by which time tumor cells have already invaded in the lung tissue (Ben-Eliyahu & Page, 1992). Finally, increased NKCA (induced by poly (I:C)) was associated with a marked decrease in LTR and metastatic colonization (Ben-Eliyahu & Page, 1992), and various conditions that suppressed NKCA (e.g., the presence of ethanol or adrenergic agonists) increased LTR and metastatic colonization of the MADB106 tumor (Ben-Eliyahu et al., 1991, 1996b; Shakhar & Ben-Eliyahu, 1998; Yirmiya, Ben-Eliyahu, Shavit, Liebeskind, & Taylor, 1991a). Together, these studies indicate that: (a) LTR is an early indicator of metastatic colonization of the MADB106 tumor, (b) both LTR and metastatic colonization sensitively reflect in vivo levels of NK activity, in the context of a naturally occurring pathology, and (c) MADB106 metastatic colonization is sensitive to NKCA predominantly during the first 24 h following tumor inoculation. Thus, the assessment of LTR at 24 h or earlier focuses on the impact of NK cells on the metastatic process and minimizes the impact of later-acting factors.

Additionally, we have used selective in vivo depletion of NK cells (using anti-NKR-P1) in order to assess the role of NK cells in mediating the impact of various manipulations on MADB106 metastasis. In some conditions, depletion did not prevent the LTR-enhancing impact of the in vivo manipulation, whereas in other conditions it did. In the latter case, such prevention would suggest exclusive mediation by NK cells (Ben-Eliyahu, Page, Yirmiya, & Shakhar, 1999). Depletion can therefore be used to assess the extent to which NK cells mediate the effects of an in vivo manipulation on the NK-dependent index.

**In sum,** these three approaches are complementary in studying NKCA. Each approach has its merits and drawbacks, but collectively they can provide a comprehensive picture of neuroendocrine modulation of NKCA, from cellular mechanisms to health implications.

## C. Redistribution of NK Cells: Implications for the Study of NKCA and Tumor Development

Catecholamines and glucocorticoids, have been shown to rapidly and markedly affect the distribution of NK cells among different immune compartments (e.g., spleen, liver, lungs, circulating blood, marginating pool of the blood, etc.) (Benschop, Nijkamp, Ballieux, & Heijnen, 1994; Dhabhar, Miller, McEwen, & Spencer, 1995). For example, infusion of catecholamines was reported to cause an up to sixfold increase in the proportion of NK cells within the circulating leukocyte population (Benschop, Rodriguez-Feuerhahn, & Schedlowski, 1996a; Schedlowski et al., 1996). These hormones are also known to affect the functional capacity of the individual NK cell (Hellstrand & Hermodsson, 1989; Masera et al., 1989). **These two factors—the number of NK cells and activity per NK cell—independently affect NKCA per milliliter of blood or per a given number of lymphocytes, splenocytes, or PBMCs, in which NKCA is commonly assessed.** Almost without exception, ex vivo studies in PNI do not purify NK cells in order to measure cytotoxicity on a per-NK-cell basis. Purification would be impractical and suffer from the drawbacks described above. However, many studies assessing NKCA per a constant number of lymphocytes (without counting NK cells) refer to their findings as alterations in NKCA, without considering possible alterations in the number of NK cells as a factor underlying their findings. Because stress markedly affects the distribution of NK cells, and because the number of NK cells remains fixed after they are harvested, such studies may predominantly reflect changes in the number of NK cells, rather then alteration in cytotoxicity on a per NK cell basis. NKCA may be **suppressed** on a per NK cells basis, but the study would report an **increase** in NKCA, which is actually the result of a large increase in the proportion of NK cells. Because the blood is the only source of NK cells available for most human studies, it is our opinion that one should assess alterations in cytotoxicity on a per-NK-cell basis. Because such alterations are likely to be mediated by systemic release of immune modulators, they could be expected to occur in all perfused immune compartments (in addition to possible modulation by organ-specific innervation) and thus be more biologically significant. In contrast, rapid alterations in the number of blood NK cells occur at the expense of other immune compartments.

Cytotoxicity on a per NK cell basis can be directly assessed following purification of NK cells, or can be inferred retrospectively based on the number of NK cells within the cell population tested for cytotoxicity. Because purification may delay the assay, disrupt NKCA, or blunt the in vivo effects, retrospective calculation seems a better alternative. However, variations in the method of retrospective calculation of cytotoxicity per NK cell, may yield divergent results. In various studies, we have assessed percentage of specific lysis of target cells per milliliter of blood (rather than per NK cell), using eight different concentrations of target cells for each subject (serial twofold dilution of target cells) (Yovel et al., in press). The exact NK-to-target ratios used for each subject were retrospectively determined, based on FACS analysis yielding NK cell counts per milliliter of blood. The eight retrospectively determined NK-to-target ratios used for each subject yield an overlapping range of more than four NK-to-target ratios common to all subjects, thus enabling a comparison between individuals on a per-NK-cell basis. In other studies, we avoided the complications of redistribution by assessing NKCA at time points in which numbers of circulating NK cells were found (and confirmed in each assay) to be at baseline levels (Ben-Eliyahu et al., 1999; Shakhar & Ben-Eliyahu, 1998).

An in vivo index of NKCA may also be affected by redistribution of NK cells. Such an index may reflect NK-dependent processes limited to a few immune compartments. Clearly the use of several different in vivo indices is desirable, as is recording organ-specific alterations in NK cell numbers.

## II. THE EFFECT OF ACUTE STRESS ON NKCA AND ITS IMPACT ON MALIGNANT PROGRESSION

A series of our studies conducted in rats examined the deleterious impact of various conditions of acute stress on NKCA and tumor development. To establish the biological significance of alterations in NKCA, we also provided evidence that they underlie, at least partially, the effects of stress on tumor development.

### A. Stress Paradigms

We employed four different stress paradigms, simulating natural as well as clinical conditions: **(1) Swim stress,** in which rats go through five cycles of 3 min swim and 3 min rest (a total of 30 min). Water is maintained at 37 °C and a weight of 45 g/kg is attached to the rat's tail. One hour later, serum corticosterone levels are markedly elevated, and rats are slightly wet and cold (1–2 °C hypothermic) (Ben-

Eliyahu, Yirmiya, Shavit, & Liebeskind, 1990). **(2) Surgical (laparotomy) stress**, in which a 4-cm midline incision is made in the abdominal muscle wall under halothane anesthesia. The small intestine is externalized, rubbed, and returned to the abdominal cavity, then the skin and muscle layer are sutured. For at least 5 h following laparotomy, increased corticosterone levels and suppressed exploratory behavior are evident (Page, McDonald, & Ben-Eliyahu, 1998). **(3) Social confrontation stress**, in which a male intruder is introduced into a cage accommodating an established male–female colony. Episodes of confrontation occur at a higher rate during the first hours, but dominant and submissive posturing, as well as occasional confrontations, continue for days (Stefanski, 1998). **(4) Hypothermic stress**, in which body temperature is lowered under anesthesia (70 mg/kg of thiopental) by an average of 5 °C for approximately 3 h, whereas in control conditions rats are either anesthetized and maintained in normothermia or not disturbed (Ben-Eliyahu, Shakhar, Rosenne, Levinson, & Beilin, in press). Hypothermia and several types of anesthesia have been suggested to contribute to several postoperative complications such as immune suppression and infections (Kurz, Sessler, & Lenhardt, 1996).

## B. The Effects of Stress on NKCA

Stress was shown to suppress NKCA in all four stress paradigms, although for different durations. Splenic NKCA against both the YAC-1 and the syngeneic MADB106 tumor lines was suppressed at 1 h following swim stress, and throughout the first day following surgical stress (Ben-Eliyahu et al., 1991; Page, Ben-Eliyahu, Yirmiya, & Liebeskind, 1991). No assessment of the proportion of NK cells within splenocytes was conducted in these early studies. In our later studies, marked alterations in the number of NK cells per milliliter of blood, and in their percentage within lymphocytes, were evident in most stress paradigms. Typically, NK cell numbers increased immediately following stress and then decreased below baseline levels, rebounded, and eventually returned to baseline within 24 to 48 h (Ben-Eliyahu et al., 1999). In these studies we assessed NKCA per milliliter of blood, and simultaneously assessed numbers of NK cells (NKR-P1$^{bright}$) using FACS analysis. We then retrospectively calculated NKCA on a per-NK-cell basis. Following swim stress, NKCA per cell was suppressed at 1 h, but not at 12 h, while following surgical stress it was suppressed throughout the first day, but not 6 days later (Ben-Eliyahu et al., 1999). Hypothermia, and to a lesser

degree thiopental anesthesia, suppressed blood NKCA, at 5 and 9 h following initiation of hypothermia, without significantly affecting numbers of NK cells (Ben-Eliyahu et al., 1999b). Twelve hours after the beginning of social confrontation, blood NKCA per milliliter and per cell was suppressed, and a decrease in circulating numbers of NK cells was evident (manuscript in preparation).

## C. The Effects of Stress on Tumor Progression

Swim stress, surgical stress, social confrontation, and hypothermia caused a two- to fivefold increase in MADB106 lung tumor retention, and/or a similar increase in the number of lung metastases detected 3 weeks later (Ben-Eliyahu et al., 1991; 1999, 1999b; Page, Ben Eliyahu, Yirmiya, & Liebeskind, 1993; Stefanski & Ben Eliyahu, 1996). Interestingly, in the social confrontation paradigm, although almost all intruder rats became subdominant, a higher frequency of submissive behavior (signaling social defeat) was associated with higher levels of lung tumor retention (Stefanski & Ben Eliyahu, 1996). Swim stress also increased the mortality rate from another NK-sensitive neoplasm, the CRNK-16 leukemia (Ben-Eliyahu et al., 1999). This syngeneic malignancy is the predominant cause of natural death among F344 rats (Ward & Reynolds, 1983). In all the above studies, tumor cells were injected concurrently with the observation of physiological or behavioral responses to the stimuli (high corticosterone levels, confrontational behavior, hypothermia, or immobility), that is, 1 h after swim stress; 4, 6, or 24 h after surgery; 3 or 6 h after initiation of hypothermia; and 1 or 12 h after the beginning of social confrontation. Notably, at later times these effects dissipated, but in no case did we find increased resistance to metastatic development.

## D. NK Mediation of Stress-Induced Metastatic Enhancement

Apart from influencing NK cells, stress affects other factors that may facilitate tumor development. To determine whether stress-induced suppression of NKCA is biologically significant, one should estimate the relative importance of NK suppression in mediating the effects of stress on tumor development. We have used several approaches to address this issue, and the following describes the evidence for NK cell mediation. First, we have demonstrated that stress-induced increase in metastatic development follows a very similar time course to that of stress-induced suppression of NKCA (ex vivo). This was shown employing two stress paradigms, swim stress and surgical stress, which differ in the duration of their effects: Swim stress suppressed NKCA and increased tumor metastasis at 1 h, but not 12 h, following stress, whereas surgery induced both effects up to 24 h after surgery, but not at 7 days (Ben-Eliyahu et al., 1999).

Second, NK cells control the metastatic process of the MADB106 during the first 24 h following tumor inoculation, but not later (Barlozzari et al., 1985; Ben-Eliyahu & Page, 1992). Thus, if NK cells mediate the effects of stress, metastatic development should not be affected if the stress is introduced 24 h or more after tumor inoculation. Indeed, our findings indicated that, when rats were subjected to swim stress or surgery 24 h after tumor inoculation, no increase in the number of lung metastases was evident (Ben-Eliyahu et al., 1991; Page et al., 1993).

Third, we have conducted selective in vivo depletion of NK cells (using the anti-NKR-P1 mAb) and compared the effects of stress on tumor metastasis in normal rats with its effects in NK-depleted rats. If the effects of stress are mediated exclusively by NK cells, stress will not affect tumor metastasis in NK-depleted rats (even though the baseline number of metastases will be higher). On the other hand, if other factors participate in mediating the effects of stress, these effects will still be evident in NK-depleted rats. Whereas surgery increased tumor retention in both normal and NK-depleted rats, swim stress, which had a larger effect than surgery in normal rats, had no effect in NK-depleted rats (Ben-Eliyahu et al., 1999) (Figure 1). These findings indicate a major role for NK cells in mediating the effects of swim stress on MADB106 metastasis and a nonexclusive role in surgical stress. It is noteworthy that in other studies (unpublished data), the effects of surgical stress were also prevented by the depletion of NK cells. Thus, certain, but as yet unknown, characteristics of the host may determine whether factors other than NK cells play a role in mediating surgically induced increased metastasis.

Last, we compared the effects of swim stress on metastasis, using two different lines of tumor cells that metastasize to the lungs: the NK-sensitive MADB106 line and the NK-insensitive C4047 colon cancer (Ben-Eliyahu et al., 1996b). Increased tumor retention was evident only in rats injected with the NK-sensitive line (Ben-Eliyahu et al., 1999).

Taken together, these four converging lines of evidence suggest that NK cells play a critical role in mediating the effects of stress on MADB106 metastasis. In the case of surgical stress other factors may also participate.

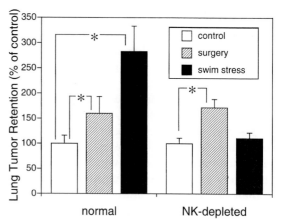

**FIGURE 1**   The effects of swim stress and surgery on lung tumor retention of the NK-sensitive MADB106 line in normal and in NK-depleted rats. Values are expressed as a percentage of the relevant control value ( ± SEM). Depletion caused a 60-fold increase in tumor retention in control rats (not shown). Swim stress increased tumor retention in normal rats, but had no effect in NK-depleted rats, suggesting that the effect of swim stress is primarily mediated by NK cells. On the other hand, surgery caused a similar effect in normal and NK-depleted rats, indicating that surgery can increase tumor retention via mechanisms other than NK cells and negating the possibility of a ceiling effect in NK-depleted rats. Asterisks indicate significant differences.

### E.  Integrating Remarks

Whereas in earlier studies we did not assess the proportion of NK cells in splenocytes, all other studies have indicated suppressed NKCA on a per NK cell basis. Still missing from our stress studies is a complete time course of the number of NK cells and their activity per cell in the major immune compartments. This would help to clarify the relationship between levels of NKCA per cell and those measured in human blood and its levels in immune compartments not accessible in humans. Additionally, it would broaden our understanding of NK cell redistribution and its impact on disease progression and in vivo indices used in rats.

The stress paradigms reported above employ specific conditions that undoubtedly activate both HPA axis and sympathetic responses. Excluding social confrontation, the stressors are acute stimuli, and their effects last for no more than a day. Using the social confrontation paradigm for a prolonged duration (7 days), Stefanski et al. reported ongoing suppression of NKCA (Stefanski & Engler, 1999). Both the acute and the chronic effects are of potential clinical relevance, which will be discussed in the last section.

The biological significance of our findings stems from the converging evidence provided by the various stress paradigms and by the two syngeneic NK-sensitive tumor models used. Nevertheless, the use of more natural and comprehensive models of malignant progression, such as spontaneously metastasizing tumors, would strengthen the clinical relevance of our findings. Our research adds to a growing body of evidence based on various tumor models and stress paradigms (Maier, Watkins, & Fleshner, 1994; Moynihan & Ader, 1996; Yirmiya et al., 1991b) and makes a unique contribution in respect to understanding the effects of stress on NKCA assessed on a per-cell basis and its role in mediating the tumor-enhancing effects of stress.

## III. ADRENERGIC INVOLVEMENT IN STRESS-INDUCED SUPPRESSION OF NKCA AND TUMOR RESISTANCE

The physiological response to stressful stimuli is complex, involving the activation of multiple neural circuits and the secretion of various hormones known to affect immunity. Hormones such as corticosteroids, opioids, growth hormones, ACTH, prolactin, and catecholamines have been shown to modulate NKCA in vitro (Bozzola et al., 1990; Callewaert, Moudgil, Radcliff, & Waite, 1991; Cesano et al., 1994; Hellstrand & Hermodsson, 1989; Mandler, Biddison, Mandler, & Serrate, 1986; McGlone, Lumpkin, & Norman, 1991; Yirmiya et al., 1991b). However, no coherent picture has yet emerged with respect to the in vivo effects of most stress hormones on NKCA, and only a few studies have assessed their role in mediating the effects of stress on NKCA and tumor resistance (e.g.,

Brenner, Felten, Felten, & Moynihan, 1992; Deguchi, Isobe, Matsukawa, Yamaguchi, & Nakagawara, 1998; Irwin, Vale, & Rivier, 1990; Kraut & Greenberg, 1986). We assessed the role of catecholamines, and, having implicated them in mediating the effects of stress on tumor development, proceeded to study their impact on the distribution, activity, and in vivo competence of NK cells.

### A. Preventing the Effects of Stress by Sympathetic Blockade

To study the extent to which the tumor-promoting effects of stress are mediated by adrenal catecholamines, we used three different stress paradigms in rats and three distinct methods of preventing adrenoceptor stimulation: (a) administration of the ganglionic blocker chlorisondamine (3 mg/kg), (b) adrenal demedullation, and (c) administration of $\beta$-blockers such as butoxamine (25 mg/kg) or nadolol (.2–.4 mg/kg). In the swim stress paradigm, these treatments prevented or reduced the stress-induced increase in LTR and the number of MADB106 metastases, without significantly affecting nonstressed rats (Figure 2A) (Ben-Eliyahu, 1998b). The tumor-enhancing effects of social confrontation and of hypothermic stress were reduced by adrenal demedullation, butoxamine, or nadolol (Ben-Eliyahu et al., 1999b; Stefanski & Ben Eliyahu, 1996). Collectively, these findings (i) demonstrate that adrenal catecholamines play a major role in mediating the effects of stress on MADB106 metastasis, (ii) indicate that peripheral activation of $\beta$-receptors is involved, and (iii) suggest that NKCA, known to restrain MADB106 metastasis, is suppressed by catecholamines.

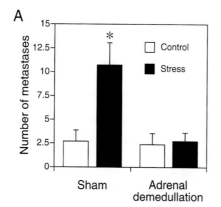
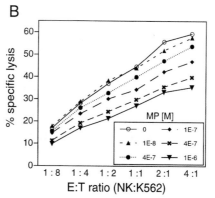

FIGURE 2  (A) Number of MADB106 lung metastases under control or swim-stress conditions in adrenal demedullated or sham operated rats. Adrenal demedullation prevented the tumor enhancing effects of stress. (B) Human NK activity at different effector to target (E:T) ratios. In vitro exposure to the $\beta$-adrenergic agonist, metaproterenol (MP), suppressed cytotoxicity in a dose-dependent manner.

## B. Mimicking the Effects of Stress by β-Adrenoceptor Activation

### 1. Tumor Enhancing Effects

To determine whether adrenergic activation is capable of affecting an NK-sensitive metastatic process, we studied the in vivo effects of adrenaline and of a nonselective β-adrenergic agonist, metaproterenol (MP) (Shakhar & Ben-Eliyahu, 1998). The latter is characterized by a relatively long half-life (about 2 h in rats) with a higher affinity to $\beta_2$ than to $\beta_1$ receptors (Dengler & Hengstmann, 1976; Muacevic, 1985). Adrenaline (.4 mg/kg, ip) caused a fivefold increase in MADB106 LTR. Similarly, MP (.6 to 9 mg/kg, sc), administered 1 h before or at the time of tumor inoculation, elevated LTR and the number of lung metastases in a dose-dependent manner, reaching a 20-fold increase (1 mg/kg, simultaneously with tumor). The β-selective antagonist nadolol (.2 mg/kg) blocked this effect. Importantly, the levels of adrenergic stimulation induced can be considered physiological, as the minimal dose of adrenaline needed to increase heart rate (Muacevic, 1985), also affected the metastatic process. To verify whether the above effects were mediated by alteration in NKCA, we compared the effect of MP (.6 mg/kg) in NK-depleted rats with its effects in untreated rats. MP had no significant effects in the NK-depleted animals, but caused a threefold increase in tumor retention in the untreated rats (Shakhar & Ben-Eliyahu, 1998). The lack of an MP effect in NK-depleted rats is unlikely to stem from a ceiling effect, since other stress paradigms mentioned earlier were shown to increase tumor retention in NK-depleted rats (Ben-Eliyahu et al., 1999). NK cells, therefore, seem to mediate the effects of MP.

### 2. Redistribution of NK Cells

Stress induces marked redistribution of NK cells (Benschop et al., 1996a), which may underlie some of the reports of increased blood NKCA and decreased splenic NKCA following stress. Thus, we tested the role of redistribution in the adrenergic effects on NKCA. FACS analysis was used to record the number of NK cells (NKR-P1[bright]) per microliter of blood and their percentage within the white blood cells (WBCs) at different intervals after the administration of MP (1 mg/kg) to rats (Shakhar & Ben-Eliyahu, 1998).

The number of NK cells per microliter of blood doubled within 10 min, declined to baseline levels within 1 h, and remained fairly constant (at approximately 300 cells/μL) thereafter. The number of PBMCs decreased to 50% of baseline levels over a period of 1 h following treatment and returned to

normal levels after 3 h. This creates an interesting situation: although the number of NK cells per microliter of blood returns to baseline levels fairly rapidly, the decrease in the number of PBMCs keeps the percentage of NK cells elevated for considerably longer. Our initial findings in humans indicate a similar but more striking picture: Administration of adrenaline (0.1 μg/kg/min) instantly induced a 10-fold increase in the number of circulating NK cells, which remained elevated throughout the 1-h infusion period, and quickly returned to baseline thereafter. This finding coincides with the observations of several groups (Benschop et al., 1996a). The cellular mechanism leading to an elevated number of circulating NK cells has been suggested to involve their detachment from endothelium and the stronger pull of an increased blood flow (Benschop et al., 1994). The spleen is believed to be a major source of this sudden outflow of NK cells, although other immune compartments have also been proposed (Benschop et al., 1996b; Iversen, Arvesen, & Benestad, 1994; Landmann, Durig, Gudat, Wesp, & Harder, 1985; Schedlowski et al., 1996; Toft, Tonnesen, Svendsen, Rasmussen, & Christensen, 1992).

### 3. Ex Vivo Suppression of NKCA

Ex vivo assessment of NKCA per milliliter of blood was conducted in rats 1 h after administration of adrenaline or MP. This timing was chosen in order to avoid complications introduced by changes in NK cell numbers, as these numbers were expected to return to baseline levels by this time. The doses of adrenaline and MP used (ip 0.1, 0.2, or 0.4 mg/kg; sc 0.02, 0.06, 0.2, or 0.6 mg/kg, respectively) were again chosen to reflect physiological levels of adrenergic activation.

Both adrenaline and MP suppressed NKCA per milliliter of blood in a dose-dependent manner, reaching 50% suppression. Significant suppression was evident for all except the lowest doses of both drugs. No significant changes in the number of NK cells per milliliter blood were evident at this time (Shakhar & Ben-Eliyahu, 1998) (adrenaline results—manuscript in preparation).

### 4. In Vitro Suppression of NKCA

In agreement with previous research (Hellstrand & Hermodsson, 1989; Takamoto, Hory, Koga, & Yokoyama, 1991; Whalen & Bankhurst, 1990), we found that in vitro exposure of human NK cells to β-adrenergic agonists suppresses NKCA in a dose-dependent manner. Suppression occurs in whole blood, as well as when separated PBMCs are used. With regard to MP, suppression starts as low as $1E^{-8}$

M, reaches $ED_{50}$ levels at $2E^{-7}$ M, and maximizes at about $1E^{-5}$ M (Fig. 2B) (David, Shakhar, Rosenne, Page, & Ben-Eliyahu, 1998). Interestingly, this robust and reproducible finding in humans is somewhat inconsistent in rats. Although several of our experiments yielded a significant in vitro suppression of NKCA, a number of our attempts failed to do so. Other investigators have also reported a lack of in vitro adrenergic effects in rodents (Madden & Livnat, 1991). On the other hand, our ex vivo and in vivo effects in rats are easily reproduced. It remains to be seen what factors determine whether catecholamines are capable of suppressing NKCA in vitro.

## C. Intracellular Mechanisms

The intracellular basis of adrenergic suppression of NKCA is fairly well understood. Human NK cells express a variety of adrenoceptors, including $\beta$-1, $\beta$-2, $\alpha$-1, and $\alpha$-2 (Jetschmann et al., 1997; Landmann, 1992), and adrenoceptors have also been identified on rat lymphocytes (Murray et al., 1993). Of these receptors, the $\beta$-2 subtype has been repeatedly implicated in the various influences of catecholamines on NK cells, be it suppression of cytotoxicity, detachment from endothelial cells, or redistribution (Benschop, Oostveen, Heijnen, & Ballieux, 1993; Hellstrand & Hermodsson, 1989; Schedlowski et al., 1996).

The intracellular mechanism mobilized by $\beta$-2 adrenoceptor stimulation involves the activation of $G_s$ proteins and adenilate cyclase, resulting in cAMP synthesis. The involvement of this pathway in the suppression of NKCA is supported by the findings that other agents that elevate intracellular cAMP, such as prostaglandins, cholera toxin, and forskolin, also suppress NKCA (Whalen & Bankhurst, 1990). The inhibitory effects of cAMP are mediated through PKA type-I activation (Torgersen et al., 1997). How these processes interfere with intracellular events leading to NK cytolytic activity is as yet unknown. There are some indications, however, that cAMP interferes with the generation of inositol trisphosphate, a $Ca^{2+}$-mobilizing second messenger that plays a part in the events leading to NK cell cytotoxicity (Windebank et al., 1988).

## D. A Role for Corticosteroids?

Corticosterone (CORT) is the major glucocorticoid released during stress in rats and, when applied in vitro at high physiological concentrations, is known to suppress NKCA (Cox, Holbrook, & Friedman, 1983). This could raise the possibility that CORT mediates the effects of stress on NKCA and tumor metastasis.

However, several of our findings suggest that elevated physiological levels of corticosteroids do not suppress NKCA in vivo, as was also indicated in humans (Bodner, Ho, & Kreek, 1998).

The stress-induced increase in MADB106 tumor metastasis was reversed by several methods of sympathetic blockade (ganglionic blocker, $\beta$-adrenergic antagonist, or adrenal demedullation), none of which prevents the release of CORT. Furthermore, we found no significant effect of CORT administration (1, 3, or 9 mg/kg, sc) on MADB106 tumor metastasis. These doses produce serum levels of CORT equal to or higher than stress levels. These studies suggest that elevated levels of CORT are not sufficient to suppress NKCA in vivo. It could be suggested, though, that elevated CORT levels are a necessary condition for other factors to affect NKCA. We tested this hypothesis with respect to MP, which suppresses NKCA and elevates CORT levels (unpublished data). Rats were pretreated with metyrapone, a CORT synthesis inhibitor, and the ex vivo levels of NKCA, as well as serum CORT levels, were assessed. Metyrapone prevented the MP-induced rise in CORT levels, but did not impede the NK-suppressive effects of MP. Therefore, it is unlikely that the effect of MP on NKCA is dependent upon the rise in corticosterone levels.

## E. Extending the Findings to Human NKCA

Our findings, and those of other groups, present a coherent picture of stress-induced changes in rodent NKCA. Following stress, the release of catecholamines, primarily from the adrenal medulla, activates $\beta$-adrenoceptors on NK cells. This activation causes a sharp, but transient, redistribution of NK cells and reduces their individual cytotoxicity. One outcome of these changes is a reduction in host ability to resist NK-sensitive metastatic processes.

Current technology does not allow in vivo studies of NKCA in humans, but the in vitro suppressive effects of catecholamines and the changes in NK cell distribution are even more pronounced in humans than in rats. In contrast, ex vivo findings in rodents and humans are incompatible. Most studies performed with human subjects have reported that catecholamine administration, acute stress, or exercise elevate NKCA rather than suppress it (Nomoto, Karasawa, & Uehara, 1994; Schedlowski et al., 1993a; Strasner et al., 1997; Tonnesen, Christensen, & Brinklov, 1987; Tonnesen, Tonnesen, & Christensen, 1984; Tvede, Kappel, Halkjaer-Kristensen, Galbo, & Pedersen, 1993). As suggested earlier, this elevation may reflect the documented increase in the proportion of

NK cells within the cell population tested for NKCA (usually PBMCs), rather than an actual increase in individual NK cell cytotoxicity. Studies that have used various methods to calculate NKCA per cell yielded inconsistent findings, including elevated, decreased, or unchanged levels of NKCA (Bachen et al., 1995; Kappel et al., 1991; Nieman et al., 1995; Schedlowski et al., 1993a, b).

We are now conducting experiments to address this unsettled issue in humans. Two major concerns in this study are: (1) distinguishing the large $\beta$-adrenergic effect on blood NK cell numbers from changes in individual cell cytotoxicity and (2) avoiding a decay of adrenergic effects while preparing NK cells for the cytotoxicity assay.

## IV. THE EFFECTS OF THE MENSTRUAL CYCLE ON NKCA AND TUMOR DEVELOPMENT: MODULATION OF THE STRESS RESPONSE

The controversial clinical observation described below provided the incentive to conduct the studies reported in this section. Our working hypotheses are derived from this clinical phenomenon, and our findings suggest ways of interpreting it, of further studying it in humans, and of developing prophylactic measures to circumvent it.

### A. Tumor Recurrence in Relation to Timing of Surgery within the Menstrual Cycle: Analysis in PNI Terms

An intriguing and controversial issue in surgical treatment of breast cancer is whether the timing of surgery in relation to the menstrual cycle affects the long-term rates of disease recurrence and survival. At least three independent groups of researchers reported an increase of up to 200% in the 10-year mortality rate in women undergoing surgery during days 2–14 of their menstrual cycle relative to those operated on during other periods of their menstrual cycle (Badwe et al., 1991; Saad et al., 1994; Senie, Rosen, Rhodes, & Lesser, 1991). However, several other groups suggested that the perimenstrual period is the one to be characterized by a higher mortality rate (Hrushesky, Bluming, Gruber, & Sothern, 1989). Other groups failed to detect any relationship between the two variables (for review see Lemon & Rodriguez-Sierra, 1996). The considerable number of independent studies observing this relationship suggests that this clinical phenomenon is real, but may depend upon yet unknown clinical circumstances or

routines used perioperatively in some, but not all hospitals. Importantly, whenever this phenomenon was observed, it was limited to patients whose lymph nodes were positive when the primary tumor was removed, and the increased rate of mortality was due to remote malignant recurrence (Lemon & Rodriguez-Sierra, 1996).

It would be reasonable to assume that this clinical phenomenon occurs because **a metastatic process** is initiated or released from control around the time of surgery. Otherwise, mortality could not be influenced by the menstrual period in which the **surgery itself** was performed. We hypothesize that the surgery facilitated or disinhibited the metastatic process and that certain aspects of the menstrual cycle (e.g., a particular sex hormone) have only modulated patient susceptibility to metastasis. The menstrual cycle alone cannot explain this clinical observation: Had the menstrual cycle affected tumor metastasis in a significant manner, then the cumulative effects of menstrual phases preceding and following surgery would have masked any effect of the specific menstrual phase during which the **surgery** was performed. **Therefore, the context of surgery is necessary for the effects of the menstrual cycle to be manifested.** This could occur in either of two ways; (i) The menstrual cycle continuously affects the metastatic process, but this effect is normally insignificant, and becomes clinically relevant only in the vulnerable condition induced by the surgery. (ii) The effects of the menstrual cycle occur only in the context of surgery.

In either case, both the effects of the menstrual cycle and the effects of surgery on tumor development could be mediated by the immune system. Surgical procedures in humans are immune suppressive, specifically in respect to NKCA (Beilin et al., 1996; Brittenden et al., 1996; Pollock, Lotzova, & Stanford, 1991, 1992; Salo, 1992; Tonnesen, Brinklov, Schou, & Christensen, 1985). Furthermore, a negative correlation was reported between levels of NKCA and rate of tumor recurrence in women undergoing surgery for the removal of breast cancer and other types of tumors (Levy et al., 1985; Schantz, Brown, Lira, Taylor, & Beddingfield, 1987). With respect to the menstrual cycle, it appears that its impact is not mediated by direct effects of sex hormones on the malignant tissue, because the clinical phenomenon occurred irrespective of whether or not the excised tumor expressed receptors for sex hormones (Lemon & Rodriguez-Sierra, 1996). Therefore, sex hormones are likely to impact tumor development indirectly via host mechanisms affecting metastatic development, such as the immune system. Indeed, suppressed

NKCA was reported during pregnancy and in animals chronically injected with sex steroids (Gabrilovac et al., 1988; Hanna & Schneider, 1983; Screpanti, Santoni, Gulino, Herberman, & Frati, 1987). Other host mechanisms may also contribute to the effects of surgery or the effects of the menstrual cycle, most notably, angiogenesis (Ludwig, Aebersold, & Rothen, 1998).

To identify mechanisms related to our hypotheses, we tested the impact of the estrous cycle and of sex hormones on the rat's resistance to metastasis of the MADB106 mammary tumor. NKCA throughout the ovarian cycle was also studied in women and rats. As our studies progressed, it became apparent that the context of surgical stress or $\beta$-adrenoceptor activation is important for the manifestation of the effects of the ovarian cycle on NKCA and tumor resistance. Direct evidence supporting this claim is presented in section C.

## B. The Effects of the Ovarian Cycle on NKCA and Metastasis

Our findings indicate that the estrous cycle modulates the resistance of the F344 rat to MADB106 metastasis. Rats inoculated with tumor during the proestrus/estrus phase (elevated estradiol levels) demonstrated significantly higher levels of LTR relative to those inoculated during the metestrus/diestrus phase. This finding was replicated several times in rats not operated upon, and tested and shown one time in the context of surgery (laparotomy) (Ben-Eliyahu et al., 1996a; Page & Ben-Eliyahu, 1997). Additionally, in ovariectomized (OVX) rats, the induction of physiological levels of estradiol for 2 days prior to tumor injection significantly increased LTR. No such effect was observed if the same total dose was administered in a single day (Ben-Eliyahu et al., 1996a). The 2-day exposure to estradiol in OVX rats correspond to natural levels of estradiol in cycling F344 rats, which increase 36 h before the day of proestrus. Later studies (unpublished) indicated that 2 days of exposure to progesterone in OVX rats can induce the same effect. Although no such condition occurs naturally in rats, it does occur in women.

We have also conducted **ex vivo** studies assessing NKCA throughout the ovarian cycles of women and rats. In rats, we were able to show, in two different experiments, decreased NKCA during the proestrus/estrus phase (Ben-Eliyahu et al., 1996a), the same phase that was characterized by increased susceptibility to MADB106 metastasis. This correspondence would suggest that fluctuations in tumor susceptibility are mediated by NK cells. However, the findings of decreased NKCA were hard to replicate. The numbers of NK cells per milliliter of blood, on the other hand, showed more consistent changes throughout the estrous cycle, increasing during the proestrus/estrus phase (Ben-Eliyahu et al., 1996a). In women, we were unable to find consistent changes in the number or activity of NK cells along the menstrual cycle (Yovel, Shakhar, Rosenne, Frenk, & Ben-Eliyahu, 1998). Although there are two reports in the literature of menstrual-related fluctuations in NKCA, the findings of these reports are inconsistent (Sulke, Jones, & Wood, 1985; White, Jones, Cooke, & Kirkham, 1982).

As our studies progressed and lab techniques became more routine, we observed that the in vivo effects of the estrous cycle in normal rats, which were previously significant, gradually decreased, occasionally becoming insignificant. This led us to hypothesize that the context of stress, be it severe as in surgical stress or mild as in unintended procedural stress (e.g., the injection of tumor cells), is critical for the ovarian cycle to manifest its effects. The expression of adrenergic receptors on lymphocytes is reported to fluctuate along the menstrual cycle (Wheeldon et al., 1994). This may provide a possible mechanism via which the ovarian cycle modulates the adrenergic suppression of both NKCA and resistance to MADB106 metastasis. We have therefore conducted the following experiments to test this hypothesis.

## C. Modulation of Adrenergic Suppression of NKCA by the Ovarian Cycle

In the following studies we made special effort to minimize the stress of experimental procedures and repeated our in vivo study under two conditions: with administration of a $\beta$-agonist (MP) and without it. This study was repeated twice, yielding the same findings. As expected, MP increased LTR of the MADB106. However this increase was significantly higher during the proestrus/estrus phase as compared to the metestrus/diestrus phase (Figure 3A). In contrast, no effects of the estrous cycle were evident in rats not injected with MP. Because our previous studies indicated that the effects of MP on LTR are mediated by NK cells, it seems that the estrous cycle modulates the suppressive effects of $\beta$-adrenergic stimulation on NKCA. To directly test this hypothesis, we conducted a study in which the effects of MP on NKCA were assessed in vitro using blood taken from rats during different phases of the estrous cycle. Significantly lower doses of MP were needed to suppress NKCA in blood drawn during the proestrus/estrus phase then during the metestrus/diestrus phase (manuscript in preparation). We then

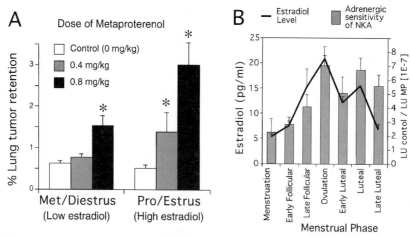

**FIGURE 3**   (A) Retention of MADB106 cells (mean ± SEM) in the lungs of rats treated with metaproterenol (MP) at different phases of the estrous cycle. MP increased lung retention of this NK-sensitive tumor, more so during phases marked by high estradiol levels. (B) Sensitivity of human NK activity to in vitro β-adrenergic stimulation—the ratio between NKCA (LU) in 0 and in 1E-7 [M] concentrations of MP—measured at different menstrual phases. Note that the levels of estradiol in these subjects (pg/mL, mean ± SEM) parallel the sensitivity of NK cytotoxicity to MP.

conducted the same study in women and found that approximately one-third of the concentration of MP was needed to achieve the same levels of NK suppression in blood drawn during the luteal phase, as compared to blood drawn during the follicular phase (David et al., 1998).

## D.  Integrating Remarks

Several studies indicate that medical conditions affected by adrenergic mechanisms, such as asthma and migraines, exacerbate during certain phases of the menstrual cycle (Cavallini et al., 1989; Wheeldon et al., 1994). Our findings in women and rats indicate that the ovarian cycle modulates β-adrenergic suppression of NKCA. In the rat, this modulation coincided with the effects of the estrous cycle on the tumor-enhancing effects of β-adrenergic stimulation and of surgery. These findings support our hypothesis that the release of catecholamines, induced by surgery or other conditions of sympathetic activation, is necessary for the menstrual cycle to significantly affect NKCA or tumor development. These findings are also consistent with our interpretation of the clinical phenomenon maintaining that surgery induces enhanced metastatic development, whereas the menstrual cycle only modulates this effect.

It is difficult to assess the relevance of our findings to the clinical phenomenon, since they are limited to one immune measure and one tumor model. The period of enhanced susceptibility to β-adrenergic suppression of NKCA and of tumor resistance coincided with the natural exposure to high levels of

estradiol in rats. In women, it occurs during the luteal phase which is characterized by high levels of both progesterone and estradiol (Fig. 3B). This period, however, does not coincide with the period associated with increased risk of cancer recurrence observed clinically. There is a backward shift of 1 week according to one set of clinical observations (Hrushesky et al., 1989), or approximately 2 weeks according to another set of studies (Badwe et al., 1991). This shift raises doubts as to the exact period following surgery in which suppression of NKCA could promote metastatic development.

Finally, if our findings are related to the clinical phenomenon, then the prevention of immune suppression will benefit all patients undergoing intrusive procedures while bearing metastasizing tumors, and will reduce the need to control the timing of surgery.

## V.  ACTIVATION OF NK CELLS AS A PROPHYLACTIC MEASURE AGAINST THE EFFECTS OF STRESS

Several approaches can be used to prevent the effects of stress on NKCA and tumor resistance. One approach would be to prevent the secretion of immunosuppressive hormones, or to use specific receptor antagonists. However, the systemic effects of such manipulations may render them impractical in clinical conditions in which these hormones are needed (e.g., adrenaline during surgery to maintain blood pressure). An alternative approach that is advantageous in this respect will be to activate the patient's immune system prior to surgery and make it resistant to the immunosuppressive effects of stress hormones. In vitro studies have suggested that activation of NK cells with several cytokines may prevent adrenergic- and prostaglandin-mediated suppression of NKCA (Leung & Koren, 1984). Our current studies in rats aim at making such an approach feasible in vivo, and our preliminary findings described below appear promising.

## A. LPS and poly I-C as Immunostimulants

Both lipopolysccharide (LPS) and polyriboinosinic:polyribocytidylic acid (poly I-C) elicit an immediate immune response, although the cytokine profile induced by these compounds is somewhat different. Poly I-C in its various forms (e.g., poly I-C-LC), is a biological response modifier (BRM) used in animals and humans. Its systemic administration is considered a model for viral infection due to its double-stranded RNA structure and because it elicits an immune response resembling the response to viral infections (Guha-Thakurta & Majde, 1997; Kimura et al., 1994). Specifically, this response involves the release of various cytokines (including IFN-$\alpha$, -$\beta$, -$\gamma$; IL-1, -2, -6, -12; TNF-$\alpha$), facilitation of cellular immune functions (such as cytotoxicity by NK, T, and macrophage cells), and altered expression of various cellular adhesion molecules (Doukas, Cutler, & Mordes, 1994; Manetti et al., 1995; Victoratos, Yiangou, Avramidis, & Hadjipetrou, 1997). The cytokine response to poly I-C is mediated by macrophages/monocytes and endothelial cells (Doukas et al., 1994; Manetti et al., 1995; Reynolds, Brunda, Holden, & Herberman, 1981). Poly I-C has been used in various regimens in animal models and in clinical trials to stimulate immunity and increase resistance to tumor development. Whereas animal models indicated a marked beneficial effect of poly I-C against tumor development (Ben-Eliyahu & Page, 1992; Black et al., 1992; Talmadge et al., 1985), clinical trials have not achieved such success (Ewel et al., 1992; Salazar et al., 1996).

LPS is a major component of the cell wall of Gram-negative bacteria and is thought to be the major activating signal for NK cells in response to bacterial infection (Lindemann, 1988). Systemic administration of LPS is considered a model for bacterial infection, and its recognition by monocytes which in turn release cytokines such as IL-6 stimulates NK cells (Miranda, Puente, Blanco, Wolf, & Mosnaim, 1998). In a macrophage cell line in which the responses to poly I-C and LPS were compared, LPS failed to induce IFN-$\alpha$, but induced IFN-$\beta$ and IL-1$\alpha$ more rapidly than poly I-C, in addition to higher levels of IL-6 mRNA (Kimura et al., 1994).

## B. Prevention of the Effects of Stress and Catecholamines on Tumor Metastasis

LPS was administered to rats intermittently for 8 days (every other day, 75, 100, 125, and 150 μg/kg), while control rats were injected with saline. Nine hours following the last injection, rats from both groups were either exposed to swim stress or injected with MP (0.8 mg/kg), adrenaline (0.4 mg/kg), or saline (no stress). An hour later, MADB106 cells were injected to all rats, and LTR was assessed 24 h later. Whereas swim stress, MP, and adrenaline significantly increased LTR in control rats, much smaller effects were evident in LPS-treated rats. LPS also decreased baseline levels of LTR in the stress-free group. In subsequent studies, we replicated the findings once, but failed to do so in three other attempts, despite the fact that LPS was as effective in reducing body weight as in successful studies. The reasons for this inconsistency are unclear to us. From here on after, we used poly I-C as an NK stimulator and found it to be very effective in all five experiments conducted.

A single injection of poly I-C (0.03, 0.1, 0.3, 1, or 4 mg/kg, ip) 1 day before tumor inoculation almost completely abolished the 20-fold tumor-enhancing effects of MP (1 mg/kg, sc, simultaneously with the tumor). Baseline levels of LTR were reduced by 50% in poly I-C-treated rats (Figure 4). Whereas the higher doses of poly I-C caused a dose dependent decrease in body weight, the lower doses (.1 and below) did not. The effects of a single poly I-C injection (.1 mg/kg) on tumor resistance became significant at 12 h, maximized at 24 to 36 h, and almost disappeared at 72 h. Chronic intermittent administration of poly I-C (four injections of .1 mg/kg every other day) was as effective as a single injection of any of the higher doses, without reducing body weight. Because the sickness-syndrome induced by immune stimulation could be stressful (Maier, Goehler, Fleshner, & Watkins, 1998; Yirmiya, 1996), we assessed whether there are short-term deleterious effects of poly I-C on tumor resistance. The higher doses of poly I-C facilitated MADB106 metastasis during the first hours following injection (at 4 but not at 12 h), an effect that was hardly noticeable using the lower doses and was reduced by a previous injection of a low dose of poly I-C (.1 mg/kg) (manuscript in preparation).

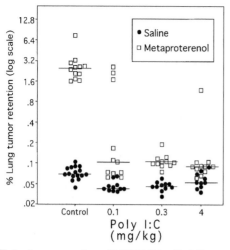

**FIGURE 4** Lung retention of MADB106 cells following administration of metaproterenol to rats pretreated with various doses of poly I-C (horizontal lines indicate medians, notice outliers). Metaproterenol significantly increased the retention of this NK-sensitive tumor, and poly I-C markedly attenuated this effect.

The current findings are insufficient to determine the mechanism mediating these in vivo effects of poly I-C, but NK cells appear to be involved. One may suggest that poly I-C recruits other immune mechanisms to resist MADB106 metastasis, thus making NKCA and its adrenergic suppression irrelevant. We refuted this hypothesis by demonstrating that the large increase in LTR induced by selective depletion of NK cells was not prevented by acute or chronic preadministration of poly I-C. Thus, poly I-C-induced alterations in cellular function of NK cells appear central in counteracting the tumor enhancing effects of adrenergic stimulation. Indeed, several in vitro studies indicated that poly I-C, interferons, and IL-2 not only increase human NKCA, but also markedly reduce the suppression of NKCA by adrenergic agonists, prostaglandins, and other drugs that elevate cAMP (Davis, Earp, & Stempel, 1984; Hellstrand & Hermodsson, 1989; Leung & Koren, 1982, 1984).

## VI. CLINICAL IMPLICATIONS: STRESS AND SURGICAL PROCEDURES IN PATIENTS WITH METASTASIZING TUMORS

Our findings in rats suggest that: (a) adrenergic suppression of NKCA facilitates perioperative metastatic development, (b) these effects are modulated by the estrous cycle, and (c) adrenergic suppression of resistance to metastasis can be prevented by activating NK cells using BRMs such as poly I-C.

**These relations may also exist in humans:** surgery is characterized by high levels of sympathetic activity (Frank et al., 1995), and has been shown to suppress NKCA (Han, 1972; Pollock et al., 1992 ). Our in vitro studies indicate that adrenergic stimulation suppresses human NKCA, and the degree of this suppression is regulated by the menstrual cycle. Finally, lower levels of NKCA have been found to indicate poorer prognosis in surgical cancer patients (Brittenden et al., 1996; Levy et al., 1985; Schantz et al., 1987).

The circumstances in which stress and adrenergic suppression of NKCA may affect health should be clarified. Although it seems unlikely that everyday stress seriously jeopardizes one's health, we do believe that our findings are relevant when high risk of infectious disease or metastatic spread is combined with elevated sympathetic activity or other conditions leading to compromised NKCA.

These conditions are met in major surgical procedures (e.g., cardiac bypass) conducted on patients that carry dormant infections, or in the surgical treatment of advance cancer. Postsurgical infection is a life-threatening complication that is facilitated by immune suppression (Holzheimer, Haupt, Thiede, & Schwarzkopf, 1997). A large proportion of cancer-related deaths are due to metastatic development, as the primary tumor can be removed in many cases. Unfortunately, surgical excision of the primary tumor has long been suspected to facilitate metastatic development (Ben-Eliyahu, 1998a; Eilber & Morton, 1970; Han, 1972), although only recently have mechanisms mediating this effect been proposed (Folkman, 1995; Page, Ben-Eliyahu, & Liebeskind, 1994; Shakhar & Ben-Eliyahu, 1998). Surgery and its associated stress involves elevated sympathetic activity: Aside from the expected emotional responses, sympathetic activation also results from perioperative hypothermia and pain. Prostaglandins (PG) are abundant following intrusive procedures due to tissue damage and are known to suppress NKCA via the same intracellular mechanisms activated by adrenergic agents (Torgersen et al., 1997). Indeed, marked suppression of NKCA is observed following surgical procedures, and often lasts for an extended period (Pollock et al., 1991). Transitory dysfunction of NK cells may create a window of opportunity for metastases to be established. This may result from loss of control over dormant micro-metastases, or from an inability to destroy tumor cells released perioperatively. As surgical intervention is usually imperative, it is important to develop prophylactic measures to reduce such unnecessary risks.

A more detailed understanding of cellular mechanisms involved in the in vivo suppression of NKCA would help to develop prophylactic measures at the cellular level. However, our current understanding is sufficient to outline the following strategies and prophylactic measures to be used perioperatively in clinical trials: (a) minimizing the release of catecholamines by the use of tranquilizers, psychological intervention, maintenance of normothermia during surgery, and adequate pain relief; (b) administrating $\beta$-adrenergic antagonists and prostaglandin synthesis inhibitors, when possible; (c) scheduling surgery according to menstrual phases characterized by reduced risk for metastasis (specifically when perioperative adrenergic stimulation cannot be prevented); and (d) stimulating innate immunity perioperatively and continuously thereafter. As indicated here and in our recent publications, we confirmed the efficiency of some of these measures in rats (Ben-Eliyahu, 1998a; Page et al., 1993, 1998). The use of such interventions is feasible clinically, as they are based upon approved drugs and procedures.

Finally, it is crucial that the proposed measures are employed perioperatively, rather then months later. Our findings suggest that poly I-C may be beneficial both by stimulating NKCA and by preventing adrenergic suppression under such stressful conditions. Most clinical trials employed poly I-C treatment or psychological intervention only months following surgery and had limited success (Ewel et al., 1992; Salazar et al., 1996). Better results may be obtained if these procedures are used in an attempt to prevent metastatic development that is induced perioperatively and promoted by surgical procedures and immune suppression.

**It is our belief that such strategies, if adopted, will increase the survival rate of cancer patients undergoing surgical procedures for the removal of metastasizing tumors.**

## Acknowledgments

We dedicate this chapter in memory of John C. Liebeskind, our friend and teacher. We thank our collaborators, Gayle G. Page, Raz Yirmiya, Volker Stefanski, Yehuda Shavit, Keren David, Galit Yovel, Ilan Yakar, and Ella Rosenne, for their enthusiasm and dedicated work. Much of this research was supported by NCI-NIH Grant CA73056-02 (S.B-E.), by a grant from the Chief Scientist of the Israeli Ministry of Health (S.B-E.), and by NIH Grant NR03915 (Gayle G. Page).

## References

Algarra, I., Collado, A., & Garrido, F. (1997). Altered MHC class I antigens in tumors. *International Journal of Clinical Laboratory Research, 27*(2), 95–102.

Bachen, E. A., Manuck, S. B., Cohen, S., Muldoon, M. F., Raible, R., Herbert, T. B., & Rabin, B. S. (1995). Adrenergic blockade ameliorates cellular immune responses to mental stress in humans. *Psychosmatic Medicine, 57*(4), 366–372.

Badwe, R. A., Gregory, W. M., Chaudary, M. A., Richards, M. A., Bentley, A. E., Rubens, R. D., & Fentiman, I. S. (1991). Timing of surgery during menstrual cycle and survival of premenopausal women with operable breast cancer. *Lancet, 337*(8752), 1261–1264.

Barlozzari, T., Leonhardt, J., Wiltrout, R. H., Herberman, R. B., & Reynolds, C. W. (1985). Direct evidence for the role of LGL in the inhibition of experimental tumor metastases. *Journal of Immunology, 134*(4), 2783–2789.

Barlozzari, T., Reynolds, C. W., & Herberman, R. B. (1983). In vivo role of natural killer cells: involvement of large granular lymphocytes in the clearance of tumor cells in anti-asialo GM1-treated rats. *Journal of Immunology, 131*(2), 1024–1027.

Beilin, B., Shavit, Y., Hart, J., Mordashov, B., Cohn, S., Notti, I., & Bessler, H. (1996). Effects of anesthesia based on large versus small doses of fentanyl on natural killer cell cytotoxicity in the perioperative period. *Anesthesia and Analgesia, 82*(3), 492–497.

Ben-Eliyahu, S. (1998a). Does surgery for the removal of cancer promotes metastasis? Mediating mechanisms and potential prophylactic measures. *Neuroimmunomodulation, 5*, 5. [conference abstract]

Ben-Eliyahu, S. (1998b). Stress, natural killer cell activity, and tumor metastasis: The role of catecholamines and corticosteroids. In A. Levi, E. Grauer, D. Ben-Nathan, & E. R. De-Kloet (Eds.), *New frontiers in stress research: Modulation in brain function* (pp. 203–215). Amsterdam: Harwood Academic.

Ben-Eliyahu, S., & Page, G. G. (1992). In vivo assessment of natural killer cell activity in rats. *Progress in NeuroEndocrineImmunology, 5*, 199–214.

Ben-Eliyahu, S., Page, G. G., Shakhar, G., & Taylor, A. N. (1996a). Increased susceptibility to metastasis during pro-oestrus/oestrus in rats: Possible role of oestradiol and natural killer cells. *British Journal of Cancer, 74*(12), 1900–1907.

Ben-Eliyahu, S., Page, G. G., Yirmiya, R., & Shakhar, G. (1999). Evidence that stress and surgical interventions promote tumor development by suppressing natural killer cell activity. *International Journal of Cancer, 80*(6), 880–888.

Ben-Eliyahu, S., Page, G. G., Yirmiya, R., & Taylor, A. N. (1996b). Acute alcohol intoxication suppresses natural killer cell activity and promotes tumor metastasis. *Nature Medicine, 2*(4), 457–460.

Ben-Eliyahu, S., Shakhar, G., Rosenne, E., Levinson, Y., & Beilin, B. (1999b). Hypothermia in anesthetized rats suppresses natural killer cell activity and compromises resistance to tumor metastasis: A role for adrenergic mechanisms. *Anesthesiology, 91*, 732–740.

Ben-Eliyahu, S., Yirmiya, R., Liebeskind, J. C., Taylor, A. N., & Gale, R. P. (1991). Stress increases metastatic spread of a mammary tumor in rats: Evidence for mediation by the immune system. *Brain, Behavior, and Immunity, 5*(2), 193–205.

Ben-Eliyahu, S., Yirmiya, R., Shavit, Y., & Liebeskind, J. C. (1990). Stress-induced suppression of natural killer cell cytotoxicity in the rat: A naltrexone-insensitive paradigm. *Behavioral Neuroscience, 104*(1), 235–238.

Benschop, R., Rodriguez-Feuerhahn, M., & Schedlowski, M. (1996a). Catecholamine-induced leukocytosis: Early observations, current research, and future directions. *Brain, Behavior, and Immunity, 10*(2), 77–91.

Benschop, R. J., Jacobs, R., Sommer, B., Schurmeyer, T. H., Raab, J. R., Schmidt, R. E., & Schedlowski, M. (1996b). Modulation of the immunologic response to acute stress in humans by beta-blockade or benzodiazepines. *Faseb Journal, 10*(4), 517–524.

Benschop, R. J., Nijkamp, F. P., Ballieux, R. E., & Heijnen, C. J. (1994). The effects of beta-adrenoceptor stimulation on adhesion of human natural killer cells to cultured endothelium. *British Journal of Pharmacology, 113*(4), 1311–1316.

Benschop, R. J., Oostveen, F. G., Heijnen, C. J., & Ballieux, R. E. (1993). Beta 2-adrenergic stimulation causes detachment of natural killer cells from cultured endothelium. *European Journal of Immunology, 23*(12), 3242–3247.

Black, P. L., Hartmann, D., Pennington, R., Phillips, H., Schneider, M., Tribble, H. R., & Talmadge, J. E. (1992). Effect of tumor burden and route of administration on the immunotherapeutic properties of polyinosinic-polycytidylic acid stabilized with poly-L-lysine in carboxymethyl cellulose [Poly(I,C)-LC]. *International Journal of Immunopharmacology, 14*(8), 1341–1353.

Bodner, G., Ho, A., & Kreek, M. J. (1998). Effect of endogenous cortisol levels on natural killer cell activity in healthy humans. *Brain, Behavior, and Immunity, 12*(4), 285–296.

Bozzola, M., Valtorta, A., Moretta, A., Cisternino, M., Biscaldi, I., & Schimpff, R. M. (1990). In vitro and in vivo effect of growth hormone on cytotoxic activity. *Journal of Pediatrics, 117*(4), 596–599.

Brenner, G. J., Felten, S. Y., Felten, D. L., & Moynihan, J. A. (1992). Sympathetic nervous system modulation of tumor metastases and host defense mechanisms. *Journal of Neuroimmunology, 37*(3), 191–201.

Brittenden, J., Heys, S. D., Ross, J., & Eremin, O. (1996). Natural killer cells and cancer. *Cancer, 77*(7), 1226–1243.

Callewaert, D. M., Moudgil, V. K., Radcliff, G., & Waite, R. (1991). Hormone specific regulation of natural killer cells by cortisol. Direct inactivation of the cytotoxic function of cloned human NK cells without an effect on cellular proliferation. *FEBS Letters, 285*(1), 108–110.

Carson, W., & Caligiuri, M. (1996). Natural Killer Cell Subsets and Development. *Methods, 9*(2), 327–43.

Cavallini, A., Micieli, G., Sances, G., Tesorio, N., Martignoni, E., & Nappi, G. (1989). Disordered sympathetic reactivity in menstrual migraine. A cardiopressor and biochemical evaluation. *Functional Neurology, 4*(1), 85–89.

Cesano, A., Oberholtzer, E., Contarini, M., Geuna, M., Bellone, G., & Matera, L. (1994). Independent and synergistic effect of interleukin-2 and prolactin on development of T- and NK-derived LAK effectors. *Immunopharmacology, 28*(1), 67–75.

Chambers, W. H., Vujanovic, N. L., DeLeo, A. B., Olszowy, M. W., Herberman, R. B., & Hiserodt, J. C. (1989). Monoclonal antibody to a triggering structure expressed on rat natural killer cells and adherent lymphokine-activated killer cells. *Journal of Experimental Medicine, 169*(4), 1373–1389.

Coca, S., Perez-Piqueras, J., Martinez, D., Colmenarejo, A., Saez, M. A., Vallejo, C., Martos, J. A., & Moreno, M. (1997). The prognostic significance of intratumoral natural killer cells in patients with colorectal carcinoma. *Cancer, 79*(12), 2320–2328.

Cox, W. I., Holbrook, N. J., & Friedman, H. (1983). Mechanism of glucocorticoid action on murine natural killer cell activity. *Journal of the National Cancer Institute, 71*(5), 973–981.

David, K., Shakhar, G., Rosenne, E., Page, G. G., & Ben-Eliyahu, S. (1998). Exposure to estradiol modulates adrenergic suppression of NK activity and tumor resistance in the female rat. *Neuroimmunomodulation, 5*, 13. [conference abstract]

Davis, V. L., Earp, H. S., & Stempel, D. A. (1984). Interferon inhibits agonist-induced cyclic AMP accumulation in human lymphocytes. *American Review of Respiratory Disease, 130*(2), 167–170.

Deguchi, M., Isobe, Y., Matsukawa, S., Yamaguchi, A., & Nakagawara, G. (1998). Usefulness of metyrapone treatment to suppress cancer metastasis facilitated by surgical stress. *Surgery, 123*(4), 440–449.

Dengler, H. G., & Hengstmann, J. H. (1976). Metabolism and pharmacokinetics of orciprenaline in various animal species and man. *Archives Internationales de Pharmacodynamie et de Therapie, 223*(1), 71–87.

Dhabhar, F. S., Miller, A. H., McEwen, B. S., & Spencer, R. L. (1995). Effects of stress on immune cell distribution. Dynamics and hormonal mechanisms. *Journal of Immunology, 154*(10), 5511–5527.

Dohring, C., & Colonna, M. (1997). Major histocompatibility complex (MHC) class I recognition by natural killer cells. *Critical Reviews in Immunology, 17*(3-4), 285–299.

Doukas, J., Cutler, A. H., & Mordes, J. P. (1994). Polyinosinic:polycytidylic acid is a potent activator of endothelial cells. *American Journal of Pathology, 145*(1), 137–147.

Eilber, F. R., & Morton, D. L. (1970). Impaired immunologic reactivity and recurrence following cancer surgery. *Cancer, 25*(2), 362–367.

Ewel, C. H., Urba, W. J., Kopp, W. C., Smith, J. W. d., Steis, R. G., Rossio, J. L., Longo, D. L., Jones, M. J., Alvord, W. G., Pinsky, C. M., et al. (1992). Polyinosinic-polycytidylic acid complexed with poly-L-lysine and carboxymethylcellulose in combination with interleukin 2 in patients with cancer: Clinical and immunological effects. *Cancer Reseach, 52*(11), 3005–3010.

Folkman, J. (1995). Tumor Angiogenesis. In P. M. H. J medelsohn, M A Israel, L A Liotta, W B Saunders (Ed.), *The molecular basis of cancer* .

Frank, S. M., Higgins, M. S., Breslow, M. J., Fleisher, L. A., Gorman, R. B., Sitzmann, J. V., Raff, H., & Beattie, C. (1995). The catecholamine, cortisol, and hemodynamic responses to mild perioperative hypothermia. A randomized clinical trial. *Anesthesiology, 82*(1), 83–93.

Gabrilovac, J., Zadjelovic, J., Osmak, M., Suchanek, E., Zupanovic, Z., & Boranic, M. (1988). NK cell activity and estrogen hormone levels during normal human pregnancy. *Gynecologic and Obstetric Investigation, 25*(3), 165–172.

Garrido, F., Ruiz-Cabello, F., Cabrera, T., Perez-Villar, J. J., Lopez-Botet, M., Duggan-Keen, M., & Stern, P. L. (1997). Implications for immunosurveillance of altered HLA class I phenotypes in human tumours. *Immunology Today, 18*(2), 89–95.

Gorelik, E., Wiltrout, R. H., Okumura, K., Habu, S., & Herberman, R. B. (1982). Role of NK cells in the control of metastatic spread and growth of tumor cells in mice. *International Journal of Cancer, 30*(1), 107–112.

Guha-Thakurta, N., & Majde, J. A. (1997). Early induction of proinflammatory cytokine and type I interferon mRNAs following Newcastle disease virus, poly [rI:rC], or low-dose LPS challenge of the mouse. *Journal of Interferon and Cytokine Research, 17*(4), 197–204.

Han, T. (1972). Postoperative immunosuppression in patients with breast cancer. *Lancet, 1*(7753), 742–743.

Hanna, N. (1985). The role of natural killer cells in the control of tumor growth and metastasis. *Biochimica et Biophysica ACTA, 780*(3), 213–226.

Hanna, N., & Schneider, M. (1983). Enhancement of tumor metastasis and suppression of natural killer cell activity by beta-estradiol treatment. *Journal of Immunology, 130*(2), 974–980.

Hellstrand, K., & Hermodsson, S. (1989). An immunopharmacological analysis of adrenaline-induced suppression of human natural killer cell cytotoxicity. *International Archives of Allergy and Applied Immunology, 89*(4), 334–341.

Hellstrand, K., Hermodsson, S., & Strannegard, O. (1985). Evidence for a beta-adrenoceptor-mediated regulation of human natural killer cells. *Journal of Immunology, 134*(6), 4095–4099.

Holzheimer, R. G., Haupt, W., Thiede, A., & Schwarzkopf, A. (1997). The challenge of postoperative infections: Does the surgeon make a difference? *Infections Control and Hospital Epidemiology, 18*(6), 449–456.

Hrushesky, W. J., Bluming, A. Z., Gruber, S. A., & Sothern, R. B. (1989). Menstrual influence on surgical cure of breast cancer. *Lancet, 2*(8669), 949–952.

Irwin, M., Vale, W., & Rivier, C. (1990). Central corticotropin-releasing factor mediates the suppressive effect of stress on natural killer cytotoxicity. *Endocrinology, 126*(6), 2837–2844.

Iversen, P. O., Arvesen, B. L., & Benestad, H. B. (1994). No mandatory role for the spleen in the exercise-induced leucocytosis in man. *Clinical Science, 86*(5), 505–510.

Jetschmann, J. U., Benschop, R. J., Jacobs, R., Kemper, A., Oberbeck, R., Schmidt, R. E., & Schedlowski, M. (1997). Expression and invivo modulation of alpha- and beta-adrenoceptors on human natural killer (CD16+) cells. *Journal of Neuroimmunology, 74*(1-2), 159–164.

Kappel, M., Tvede, N., Galbo, H., Haahr, P. M., Kjaer, M., Linstow, M., Klarlund, K., & Pedersen, B. K. (1991). Evidence that the effect of physical exercise on NK cell activity is mediated by epinephrine. *Journal of Applied Physiology, 70*(6), 2530–2534.

Kimura, M., Toth, L. A., Agostini, H., Cady, A. B., Majde, J. A., & Krueger, J. M. (1994). Comparison of acute phase responses induced in rabbits by lipopolysaccharide and double-stranded RNA. *American Journal of Physiology, 267*(6 Pt. 2), R1596–R1605.

Kraut, R. P., & Greenberg, A. H. (1986). Effects of endogenous and exogenous opioids on splenic natural killer cell activity. *Natural Immunity and Cell Growth Regulation, 5*(1), 28–40.

Kurz, A., Sessler, D. I., & Lenhardt, R. (1996). Perioperative normothermia to reduce the incidence of surgical-wound infection and shorten hospitalization. *New England Journal of Medicine, 334*(19), 1209–1215.

Landmann, R. (1992). Beta-adrenergic receptors in human leukocyte subpopulations. *European Journal of Clinical Investigation, 1*, 30–36.

Landmann, R., Durig, M., Gudat, F., Wesp, M., & Harder, F. (1985). Beta-adrenergic regulation of the blood lymphocyte phenotype distribution in normal subjects and splenectomized patients. *Advances in Experimental Medicine and Biology, 186*, 1051–1062.

Lemon, H. M., & Rodriguez-Sierra, J. F. (1996). Timing of breast cancer surgery during the luteal menstrual phase may improve prognosis. *Nebraska Medical Journal, 81*(4), 110–115.

Leung, K. H., & Koren, H. S. (1982). Regulation of human natural killing. II. Protective effect of interferon on NK cells from suppression by PGE2. *Journal of Immunology, 129*(4), 1742–1747.

Leung, K. H., & Koren, H. S. (1984). Regulation of human natural killing. III. Mechanism for interferon induction of loss of susceptibility to suppression by cyclic AMP elevating agents. *Journal of Immunology, 132*(3), 1445–1450.

Levy, S. M., Herberman, R. B., Maluish, A. M., Schlien, B., & Lippman, M. (1985). Prognostic risk assessment in primary breast cancer by behavioral and immunological parameters. *Health Psychology, 4*(2), 99–113.

Lindemann, R. A. (1988). Bacterial activation of human natural killer cells: Role of cell surface lipopolysaccharide. *Infection and Immunity, 56*(5), 1301–1308.

Lotzova, E. (1991). Natural killer cells: Immunobiology and clinical prospects. *Cancer Investigation, 9*, 173–184.

Ludwig, C. U., Aebersold, D. M., & Rothen, C. (1998). Perioperative angiogenesis and outcome in premenopausal women with breast cancer. *Lancet, 352*(9122), 147.

Madden, K. S., & Livnat, S. (1991). Catecholamine action and immunologic reactivity. In R. Ader, D. L. Felten, & N. Cohen (Eds.), *Psychoneuroimmunology* (2nd ed.). San Diego: Academic Press.

Maier, S. F., Goehler, L. E., Fleshner, M., & Watkins, L. R. (1998). The role of the vagus nerve in cytokine-to-brain communication. *Annals of the New York Academy of Sciences, 840*, 289–300.

Maier, S. F., Watkins, L. R., & Fleshner, M. (1994). Psychoneuroimmunology. The interface between behavior, brain, and immunity. *American Psychologist, 49*(12), 1004–1017.

Mandler, R. N., Biddison, W. E., Mandler, R., & Serrate, S. A. (1986). beta-Endorphin augments the cytolytic activity and interferon production of natural killer cells. *Journal of Immunology, 136*(3), 934–939.

Manetti, R., Annunziato, F., Tomasevic, L., Gianno, V., Parronchi, P., Romagnani, S., & Maggi, E. (1995). Polyinosinic acid: Polycytidylic acid promotes T helper type 1-specific immune responses by stimulating macrophage production of interferon-alpha and interleukin-12. *European Journal of Immunology, 25*(9), 2656–2660.

Masera, R., Gatti, G., Sartori, M. L., Carignola, R., Salvadori, A., Magro, E., & Angeli, A. (1989). Involvement of Ca2+-dependent pathways in the inhibition of human natural killer (NK) cell activity by cortisol. *Immunopharmacology, 18*(1), 11–22.

McGlone, J. J., Lumpkin, E. A., & Norman, R. L. (1991). Adrenocorticotropin stimulates natural killer cell activity. *Endocrinology, 129*(3), 1653–1658.

Miranda, D., Puente, J., Blanco, L., Wolf, M. E., & Mosnaim, A. D. (1998). In vitro effect of bacterial lipopolysaccharide on the cytotoxicity of human natural killer cells. *Research Communications in Molecular Pathology and Pharmacology, 100*(1), 3–14.

Moynihan, J. A., & Ader, R. (1996). Psychoneuroimmunology: Animal models of disease. *Psychosmatic Medicine, 58*(6), 546–558.

Muacevic, G. (1985). Determination of bioavailability on the basis of tachycardia after intravenous and oral administration of fenoterol, orciprenaline and salbutamol in non-anaesthetized rats. *Arzneimittelforschung, 35*(1a), 406–408.

Murray, D. R., Polizzi, S. M., Harris, T., Wilson, N., Michel, M. C., & Maisel, A. S. (1993). Prolonged isoproterenol treatment alters immunoregulatory cell traffic and function in the rat. *Brain, Behavior, and Immunity, 7*(1), 47–62.

Nieman, D. C., Henson, D. A., Sampson, C. S., Herring, J. L., Suttles, J., Conley, M., Stone, M. H., Butterworth, D. E., & Davis, J. M. (1995). The acute immune response to exhaustive resistance exercise. *International Journal of Sports Medicine, 16*(5), 322–328.

Nomoto, Y., Karasawa, S., & Uehara, K. (1994). Effects of hydrocortisone and adrenaline on natural killer cell activity. *British Journal of Anaesthesia, 73*(3), 318–321.

Page, G. G., Ben Eliyahu, S., Yirmiya, R., & Liebeskind, J. C. (1993). Morphine attenuates surgery-induced enhancement of metastatic colonization in rats. *Pain, 54*(1), 21–28.

Page, G. G., & Ben-Eliyahu, S. (1997). Increased surgery-induced metastasis and suppressed natural killer cell activity during proestrus/estrus in rats. *Breast Cancer Research and Treatment, 45*(2), 159–167.

Page, G. G., Ben-Eliyahu, S., & Liebeskind, J. C. (1994). The role of LGL/NK cells in surgery-induced promotion of metastasis and its attenuation by morphine. *Brain, Behavior, and Immunity, 8*(3), 241–250.

Page, G. G., Ben-Eliyahu, S., Yirmiya, R., & Liebeskind, J. C. (1991). Surgical stress promotes metastatic growth and suppresses natural killer cell function in rats. *Journal of Pain and Symptom Management, 6*, 180.

Page, G. G., McDonald, J. S., & Ben-Eliyahu, S. (1998). Pre-operative versus postoperative administration of morphine: Impact on the neuroendocrine, behavioural, and metastatic-enhancing effects of surgery. *British Journal of Anaesthesia, 81*(2), 216–223.

Paller, A. S. (1995). Immunodeficiency syndromes. X-linked agammaglobulinemia, common variable immunodeficiency, Chediak–Higashi syndrome, Wiskott–Aldrich syndrome, and X-linked lymphoproliferative disorder. *Dermatological Clinics, 13*(1), 65–71.

Pollock, R. E., Lotzova, E., & Stanford, S. D. (1991). Mechanism of surgical stress impairment of human perioperative natural killer cell cytotoxicity. *Archives of Surgery, 126*(3), 338–342.

Pollock, R. E., Lotzova, E., & Stanford, S. D. (1992). Surgical stress impairs natural killer cell programming of tumor for lysis in patients with sarcomas and other solid tumors. *Cancer, 70*(8), 2192–2202.

Ree, R. C., & Platts, A. A. (1983). A modified short-term cytotoxicity test: Assessment of natural cell mediated cytotoxicity in whole blood. *Journal of Immunological methods, 62*, 79–83.

Reynolds, C. W., Brunda, M. J., Holden, H. T., & Herberman, R. B. (1981). Role of macrophage in in vitro augmentation of rat, mouse, and human natural killer activities. *Journal of the National Cancer Institute, 66*(5), 837–842.

Saad, Z., Bramwell, V., Duff, J., Girotti, M., Jory, T., Heathcote, G., Turnbull, I., Garcia, B., & Stitt, L. (1994). Timing of surgery in relation to the menstrual cycle in premenopausal women with operable breast cancer. *British Journal of Neurosurgery, 81*(2), 217–220.

Salazar, A. M., Levy, H. B., Ondra, S., Kende, M., Scherokman, B., Brown, D., Mena, H., Martin, N., Schwab, K., Donovan, D., Dougherty, D., Pulliam, M., Ippolito, M., Graves, M., Brown, H., & Ommaya, A. (1996). Long-term treatment of malignant gliomas with intramuscularly administered polyinosinic-polycytidylic acid stabilized with polylysine and carboxymethylcellulose: An open pilot study. *Neurosurgery, 38*(6), 1096–1103; discussion 1103–1104.

Salo, M. (1992). Effects of anaesthesia and surgery on the immune response. *Acta Anaesthesiologica Scandinavica, 36*(3), 201–220.

Schantz, S. P., Brown, B. W., Lira, E., Taylor, D. L., & Beddingfield, N. (1987). Evidence for the role of natural immunity in the control of metastatic spread of head and neck cancer. *Cancer Immunology, Immunotherapy, 25*(2), 141–148.

Schedlowski, M., Falk, A., Rohne, A., Wagner, T. O., Jacobs, R., Tewes, U., & Schmidt, R. E. (1993a). Catecholamines induce alterations of distribution and activity of human natural killer (NK) cells. *Journal of Clinical Immunology, 13*(5), 344–351.

Schedlowski, M., Hosch, W., Oberbeck, R., Benschop, R. J., Jacobs, R., Raab, H. R., & Schmidt, R. E. (1996). Catecholamines modulate human NK cell circulation and function via spleen-independent beta 2-adrenergic mechanisms. *Journal of Immunology, 156*(1), 93–99.

Schedlowski, M., Jacobs, R., Stratmann, G., Richter, S., Hadicke, A., Tewes, U., Wagner, T. O., & Schmidt, R. E. (1993b). Changes of natural killer cells during acute psychological stress. *Journal of Clinical Immunology, 13*(2), 119–126.

Screpanti, I., Santoni, A., Gulino, A., Herberman, R., & Frati, L. (1987). Estrogen and antiestrogen modulation of the levels of mouse natural killer activity and large granular lymphocytes. *Cellular Immunology, 106*(2), 191–202.

Senie, R. T., Rosen, P. P., Rhodes, P., & Lesser, M. L. (1991). Timing of breast cancer excision during the menstrual cycle influences duration of disease-free survival. *Annales De Medecine Interne, 115*(5), 337–342.

Shakhar, G., & Ben-Eliyahu, S. (1998). In vivo beta-adrenergic stimulation suppresses natural killer activity and compromises

resistance to tumor metastasis in rats. *Journal of Immunology, 160*(7), 3251–3258.

Stefanski, V. (1998). Social stress in loser rats: Opposite immunological effects in submissive and subdominant males. *Physiology and Behavior, 63*(4), 605–613.

Stefanski, V., & Ben-Eliyahu, S. (1996). Social confrontation and tumor metastasis in rats: Defeat and beta-adrenergic mechanisms. *Physiology and Behavior, 60*(1), 277–282.

Stefanski, V., & Engler, H. (1999). Social stress, dominance and blood cellular immunity: Effects on distribution and function of immune cells. *Journal of Neuroimmunology, 94*(1-2), 144–152.

Strasner, A., Davis, J. M., Kohut, M. L., Pate, R. R., Ghaffar, A., & Mayer, E. (1997). Effects of exercise intensity on natural killer cell activity in women. *International Journal of Sports Medicine, 18*(1), 56–61.

Sulke, A., Jones, D., & Wood, P. (1985). Variation in natural killer activity in peripheral blood during the menstrual cycle. *British Medical Journal (Clinical Research Edition), 290*(6472), 884–886.

Takamoto, T. Y., Hory, Y., Koga, H., & Yokoyama, M. M. (1991). Norepinephrin inhibits human natural killer cell activity in vitro. *International Journal of Neuroscience, 58*, 127.

Taketomi, A., Shimada, M., Shirabe, K., Kajiyama, K., Gion, T., & Sugimachi, K. (1998). Natural killer cell activity in patients with hepatocellular carcinoma: A new prognostic indicator after hepatectomy. *Cancer, 83*(1), 58–63.

Talmadge, J. E., Adams, J., Phillips, H., Collins, M., Lenz, B., Schneider, M., & Chirigos, M. (1985). Immunotherapeutic potential in murine tumor models of polyinosinic- polycytidylic acid and poly-L-lysine solubilized by carboxymethylcellulose. *Cancer Reseach, 45*(3), 1066–1072.

Toft, P., Tonnesen, E., Svendsen, P., Rasmussen, J. W., & Christensen, N. J. (1992). The redistribution of lymphocytes during adrenaline infusion. An in vivo study with radiolabelled cells. *APMIS, 100*(7), 593–597.

Tonnesen, E., Brinklov, M. M., Schou, O. A., & Christensen, N. J. (1985). Natural killer cell activity in a patient undergoing open-heart surgery complicated by an acute myocardial infarction. *Acta Pathologica, Microbiologica, et Immunologica Scandandinavica. Section C, 93*(5), 229–231.

Tonnesen, E., Christensen, N. J., & Brinklov, M. M. (1987). Natural killer cell activity during cortisol and adrenaline infusion in healthy volunteers. *European Journal of Clinical Investigation, 17*(6), 497–503.

Tonnesen, E., Tonnesen, J., & Christensen, N. J. (1984). Augmentation of cytotoxicity by natural killer (NK) cells after adrenaline administration in man. *Acta Pathologica, Microbiologica, et Immunologica Scandinavica. Section C, 92*(1), 81–83.

Torgersen, K. M., Vaage, J. T., Levy, F. O., Hansson, V., Rolstad, B., & Tasken, K. (1997). Selective activation of cAMP-dependent protein kinase type I inhibits rat natural killer cell cytotoxicity. *Journal of Biological Chemistry, 272*(9), 5495–5500.

Tvede, N., Kappel, M., Halkjaer-Kristensen, J., Galbo, H., & Pedersen, B. K. (1993). The effect of light, moderate and severe bicycle exercise on lymphocyte subsets, natural and lymphokine activated killer cells, lymphocyte proliferative response and interleukin 2 production. *International Journal of Sports Medicine, 14*(5), 275–282.

van den Brink, M. R., Hunt, L. E., & Hiserodt, J. C. (1991). In vivo treatment with monoclonal antibody 3.2.3 selectively eliminates natural killer cells in rats. *Journal of Experimental Medicine, 171*(1), 197–210.

Victoratos, P., Yiangou, M., Avramidis, N., & Hadjipetrou, L. (1997). Regulation of cytokine gene expression by adjuvants in vivo. *Clinical and Experimental Immunology, 109*(3), 569–578.

Vujanovic, N. L., Basse, P., Herberman, R. B., & Whiteside, T. L. (1996). Antitumor Functions of Natural Killer Cells and Control of Metastases. *Methods*, 9(2), 394–408.

Ward, J. M., & Reynolds, C. W. (1983). Large granular lymphocyte leukemia. A heterogeneous lymphocytic leukemia in F344 rats. *American Journal of Pathology*, 111(1), 1–10.

Whalen, M. M., & Bankhurst, A. D. (1990). Effects of beta-adrenergic receptor activation, cholera toxin and forskolin on human natural killer cell function. *Biochemical Journal*, 272(2), 327–331.

Wheeldon, N. M., Newnham, D. M., Coutie, W. J., Peters, J. A., McDevitt, D. G., & Lipworth, B. J. (1994). Influence of sex-steroid hormones on the regulation of lymphocyte beta 2-adrenoceptors during the menstrual cycle. *British Journal of Clinical Pharmacology*, 37(6), 583–588.

White, D., Jones, D., Cooke, T., & Kirkham, N. (1982). Natural killer (NK) activity in peripheral blood lymphocytes of patients with benign and malignant breast disease. *British Journal of Cancer*, 46(4), 611–616.

Whiteside, T. L., & Herberman, R. B. (1995). The role of natural killer cells in immune surveillance of cancer. *Current Opinion in Immunology*, 7(5), 704–710.

Wiltrout, R. H., Herberman, R. B., Zhang, S., Chirigos, M. A., Ortaldo, J. R., Green, K. M., & Talmadge, J. E. (1985). Role of organ-associated NK cells in decreased formation of experimental metastases in lung and liver. *Journal of Immunology*, 134, 4267–4274.

Windebank, K. P., Abraham, R. T., Powis, G., Olsen, R. A., Barna, T. J., & Leibson, P. J. (1988). Signal transduction during human natural killer cell activation: Inositol phosphate generation and regulation by cyclic AMP. *Journal of Immunology*, 141(11), 3951–3957.

Yirmiya, R. (1996). Endotoxin produces a depressive-like episode in rats. *Brain Research*, 711(1-2), 163–174.

Yirmiya, R., Ben-Eliyahu, S., Shavit, Y., Liebeskind, J. C., & Taylor, A. N. (1991a). Effects of opiates and ethanol on NK activity and tumor metastases in rats. *Journal of Neuroimmunology*, 1, 75.

Yirmiya, R., Shavit, Y., Ben-Eliyahu, S., Gale, R. P., Liebeskind, J. C., Taylor, A. N., & H, W. (1991b). Modulation of immunity and neoplasia by neuropeptides released by stressors. In K. P. McCubbin & C. B. Nemepoff (Ed.), *Stress neuropeptides and systemic diseases* (pp. 261–286). San Diego: Academic Press.

Yovel, G., Mazeh, D., Sirota, P., Shakhar, G., Rosenne, E., & Ben-Eliyahu, S. (in press). Higher natural killer cell activity in schizophrenics: The impact of smoking, medication, and serum factors. *Brain, Behavior, and Immunity*.

Yovel, G., Shakhar, G., Rosenne, E., Frenk, H., & Ben-Eliyahu, S. (1998). Effects of gender, menstrual cycle, and oral contraceptives on number and activity of human NK cells: A role for serum factor? *Society for Neuroscience Abstracts*, 24(2), 1854 (736.8).

# 60

# Psychosocial Effects on Immune Function and Disease Progression in Cancer: Human Studies

JULIE M. TURNER-COBB, SANDRA E. SEPHTON, DAVID SPIEGEL

## I. INTRODUCTION

Our understanding of cancer has largely been driven by tumor biology, with the assumption that the characteristics of the tumor itself almost entirely determine disease course. While clearly a great deal of variance in outcome is determined by the source tissue and degree of dedifferentiation of the tumor, it makes sense that host resistance to tumor invasion may also play a role in the progression of the disease. These latter are to varying degrees subject to influence of the central nervous system, via behavior, peripheral innervation, endocrine, and immune function. Examination of the possibility that psychological and social factors may influence the incidence or progression of cancer involves answers to four challenging questions:

1. What is the evidence of a mind–body effect on cancer?
2. What are possible mediating physiological pathways?
3. Is there evidence for psychosocial impact on these pathways?
4. Is there evidence that these pathways can affect the course of cancer?

Evidence of relationships between psychosocial factors and the progression of cancer is accumulating, and immune and endocrine mediators providing the link between them are being identified. In this chapter, we review the possible role of immune and neuroendocrine mediators of cancer progression and survival and discuss available evidence of possible psychosocial effects on disease course. In conclusion, we discuss possible future research directions.

## II. PSYCHONEUROIMMUNE EFFECTS IN CANCER

At one time, direct effects of stress on immune function were thought of as unlikely. However, stress-induced immunosuppression is now well documented. It has also been established that psychosocial factors can modulate stress effects on immunity. For example, supportive social relationships may buffer stress and thereby reduce immunosuppression, with the possible outcome of ameliorating disease. Applying this model to cancer, however, requires several fairly controversial assumptions. These underlying assumptions or hypotheses include, first, that immune defenses are capable of regulating tumor growth, second, that psychosocial factors induce change in the types of immune mechanisms active in tumor defense, and third, that psychosocial effects on immunity are of sufficient magnitude to be clinically significant (Cohen & Rabin, 1998). What follows is a brief discussion of the evidence for each of these assumptions.

## A. Immune Defenses against Cancer

### 1. Immunosurveillance Theory

The "immunosurveillance" theory, as applied to cancer defense, asserts that the immune system is capable of protecting against newly formed tumor cells and tumor growth (Vile, Cong, & Dorudi, 1996). The clinical relevance of immunosurveillance in cancer has been called into question because immune recognition of tumor cells and cytotoxic responses against cancer are only mildly effective. It is now generally believed that anti-cancer immune defenses have only modest effects in controlling disease. Although many questions remain unanswered about the mechanisms of anti-cancer immunity, evidence does verify modest immune defenses against cancer by both nonspecific and specific killing mechanisms.

### 2. Immune Mechanisms of Tumor Defense

Clinical observations have implicated immune activity in successful cancer defense, for example, in cases of spontaneous regression of tumors (Rosenberg, 1991). Immunosuppressive medications given to patients after an organ transplant intended to prevent transplant tissue rejection have the side-effect of increasing the incidence of tumors, including leukemias, lymphomas, and skin cancers (Nossal, 1993). Tumor infiltrate that is rich in immune cells indicates a prognostic advantage with certain cancers (Oliver & Nouri, 1992). Moreover, in animal work, the injection of killed tumor cells confers the ability to subsequently resist tumor growth when live cells of the same type are administered (Beverley, 1991).

### 3. Tumor Antigens

Tumor cell membrane proteins that can be recognized by the immune system are considered tumor antigens. However, since they are transformed variants of host cells, cancer cells do not usually express unique antigens which would enable them to be recognized by the immune system as "nonself." Exceptions include animal cancers induced by viruses or high levels of carcinogen. Rather, they express unusual proportions of "self" antigen. For example, in colon cancer, proteins that are normally expressed only during fetal life may be turned on. Breast cancer cells may express altered glycoprotein antigens with modified carbohydrate side-chains, thereby displaying different epitopes. Thus, the term "tumor antigen" usually denotes these types of quantitative rather than qualitative differences in antigen expression (King, 1996).

### 4. Specific Immunity against Tumors

Cytotoxicity may be either cell-mediated or antibody-complement-mediated (King, 1996). Both mechanisms require that the tumor have an associated antigen capable of eliciting an immune response. In cases where tumor cells also carry major histocompatibility complex (MHC) antigens, immune cells are better able to recognize and kill them. The tumor antigen–MHC class I complex is recognized by a CD8 cytolytic T cell (CTL) which has been activated under the influence of cytokines released by CD4 T helper cells. This MHC-restricted CTL response to a specific tumor antigen requires two antecedents: (1) that antigen be presented to the CTL by MHC class I proteins on the tumor cells and (2) that antigen is also presented to a CD4 T helper cell which then releases cytokines (Vile et al., 1996).

CTLs may play a role in inhibiting the spread of cancer cells by recognizing tumor antigens and lysing tumor cells at the site of metastases (Shu, Plautz, Krauss, & Chang, 1997). However, the precise mechanism by which T cells mediate cytotoxicity is unknown (Kagi et al., 1994; Kagi, Ledermann, Burki, Zinkernagel, & Hengartner, 1996). CTLs may secrete cytotoxic granules resulting in cell death (Kagi et al., 1994, 1996). Alternatively, when activation of T-helper cells results in the secretion of stimulating cytokines, CTLs may kill the cell by direct contact (Geppert & Lipsky, 1989). CTLs may recognize and kill tumor cells that express the Fas ligand (a protein that can induce death of cells expressing this antigen) (Nagata, 1997). Tumor necrosis factor (TNF), a member of the same gene family as Fas, may also engender killing by CTLs using a similar mechanism (Korner & Sedgwick, 1996). The role of B lymphocytes in tumor defense should not be overlooked. Antibody responses may be important in generating antibody-dependent cellular cytotoxicity (ADCC) or antibody-dependent complement-mediated lysis of tumor cells (Lloyd, 1991).

## 5. Nonspecific Immunity against Tumors

Natural killer (NK) cells, although thought to have evolved mainly as anti-viral cells, are active in tumor surveillance and can kill tumor cells of many different types (Herberman, 1985; Trinchieri, 1989; Whiteside & Herberman, 1995). NK cells have the unique ability to recognize and kill a wide variety of both autologous (self) and allogeneic (nonself) target cells without previous sensitization (Trinchieri, 1989). NK cells are a functionally distinct population of lymphocytes with a lineage different from T and B cells (Herberman, 1986; Roder & Pross, 1982). They comprise 5–15% of lymphocytes in peripheral blood (Whiteside & Herberman, 1994) and are morphologically identified as large granular lymphocytes. Those with natural killer activity are positive for CD16 and CD56 but negative for CD3 surface antigens, while functionally distinct subsets exhibit variations of these and other markers (Bonavida, Lebow, & Jewett, 1993). Natural killer cells are also distinguished by their cytokine profile of activation (for a review see Naume & Espevik, 1994). NK cells from peripheral blood are ineffective in killing most freshly isolated tumor cells. In the presence of interleukin (IL)-2, however, NK cells can develop into lymphokine-activated killer (LAK) cells capable of lysing a broad array of fresh tumor cells (Whiteside & Herberman, 1994). A small subset develops into A-NK cells, which exhibit powerful anti-tumor activity (Vujanovic et al., 1995).

NK cells may actually recognize their targets as foreign to the body due to the failure of the target to express self MHC class I molecules (the "missing self" hypothesis) (Karre, Ljunggren, Piontek, & Kiessling, 1986; Ljunggren & Karre, 1990; Raulet, Correa, Corral, Dorfman, & Wu, 1995). MHC molecules are sometimes lost in tumor cell lines (discussed later), so this capability of NK cells makes them an important line of cancer defense. There is evidence, for example, that in vitro cytotoxicity of NK cells drawn from peripheral blood is a predictor of the rate of metastatic breast cancer progression (Levy, Herberman, Lippman, D'Angelo, & Lee, 1991). NK cells kill or "lyse" their targets by releasing factors that initiate target cell death by disintegrating the cell membrane and then fragmenting the target cell's DNA (Berke, 1995; Smyth & Trapani, 1995).

Macropohages and granulocytes may also be important in anti-tumor immune defenses because they, too, can carry out nonspecific cell lysis. Tumor-associated macrophages are a major component of the infiltrate of several human tumors (Mantovani, Bottazzi, Colotta, Sozanni, & Ruco, 1992).

## 6. Problems in Anti-cancer Immunity

Although the immune system does provide some protection against tumor development and growth, it is not as primary a defense against cancer as it is against infectious disease. Indeed, for several reasons, anti-cancer immune capabilities seem to be modest.

Clinical evidence supports this notion. Although cancer risk is increased by the medications given after organ transplantation, patients receiving these strongly immunosuppressive drugs still have a relatively low incidence of cancer; only 4 to 11% of such patients develop tumors (Penn, 1993). One explanation is that tumors take an extended time to develop. Indeed, it may take a decade for an initial dysplastic event to result in a clinically detectable tumor. Furthermore, because transplant patients often have a variety of other medical problems that may shorten their life span, they may die of other causes before tumors are detectable (Penn, 1993).

Despite these possible explanations, uncertainty remains as to the relevance of immunosurveillance in cancer for several other reasons. While organ transplant patients have a higher incidence of cancers with a viral etiology and a higher risk for unusual types of cancer, their risk for common cancers is only moderately increased. This suggests that the increase in tumor incidence after organ transplant may result primarily from the suppression of viral immune responses rather than from suppression of anti-cancer immunity (Garssen & Goodkin, 1999). These results illustrate the relative effectiveness of viral immune responses as compared with anti-tumor responses.

Tumor cells have various mechanisms by which they can evade and subvert immune mechanisms for their own survival (Somers & Guillou, 1994). Tumors may prevent T-cell immune responses from working efficiently. For example, the production of intercellular adhesion molecule-1 (ICAM-1) by the tumor may block the attachment of cytotoxic T cells. In patients with more advanced cancer, decreased numbers of CTLs may be unable to inhibit the spread of tumor cells (Liang, Wang, Chang, & Chuang, 1993). This is consistent with the finding of lower percentages of CTLs in patients with metastases compared to those without metastases (Liang et al., 1993). Another example of tumor-mediated immune suppression is the production of the antigen p43 by breast tumor cells. This molecule has been shown to bind to CTLs in patients with early-stage breast cancer but not in those with benign disease (Rosen et al., 1994). In this manner P43 may interfere with the cytotoxic function of CTLs. The immune dysregulation produced by p43 has subsequently been reported to influence the cytokine profile, with a greater type 2 response (IL-10 and IL-4) being observed in malignant breast cancer patients compared to those with benign breast disease (Rosen et al., 1994).

Specific cellular immune responses against tumor cells may fail for a number of other reasons. First, tumor cells have the capacity to mutate rapidly, and thus become invisible to the immune system. Second, if the CD4+ helper arm of the presentation pathway is not working, CTLs will not lyse the tumor. Major histocompatibility complex (MHC) class I membrane proteins, which are expressed on the surface of all normal cell types, may be lost in cancer cells. Many tumor cells downregulate or lose expression of these molecules. Indeed, about half of breast and colon cancers have lost MHC class I expression (King, 1996). Since MHC molecules are necessary for presentation of antigen to immune cells, loss of MHC may cause a tumor to be relatively undetectable to the immune system.

Not only are many tumors poorly immunogenic because they lack "nonself" antigen, there is a physical barrier to immune surveillance in that the access of cytotoxic cells and antibodies to tumor cells within a mass is hindered by poor circulation and poorly controlled tumor growth.

Last, tumor growth rates are highly variable. Some tumors grow so aggressively that they proliferate more rapidly than the immune system can mount an effective response against them (Vile et al., 1996). For these reasons, the application of immunosurveillance theory to cancer is currently seen as less viable. The immune system is better equipped to defend against infectious disease than against cancer. Nevertheless, the immune system does kill tumor cells and does provide modest protection against cancer growth. Tumors that are slow-growing, antigenic, and positive for MHC class one antigens are more susceptible to immune attack (Vile et al., 1996). Furthermore, the efficacy of immunity against viral disease may carry some benefit for cancer patients. Infectious disease has been listed as the leading cause of cancer-related death, suggesting a related immunodeficiency problem in cancer survival (White, 1993). For a review of this area see Bovbjerg and Valdimarsdottir (1998).

## B. Psychosocial Effects on Anti-tumor Immune Mechanisms

There are numerous studies that attest to psychosocial effects on immunity. Some of these studies have been conducted among cancer patients. Any psycho-logical factor that can upregulate immune mechanisms that defend against cancer may also have the potential to retard the progression of disease with some varieties of tumors. However, much research is needed to determine the combinations of psychosocial factors and types of tumors in which such mechanisms may operate.

### 1. Chronic Stress

In general, research findings suggest that "chronic stressors are associated with continued down-regulation of immune function rather than adaptation" (Kiecolt-Glaser & Glaser, 1992). A substantial literature has accumulated in support of the notion that psychosocial factors influence the relationship between a stressor, its converse, relaxation, and immunity (Snyder, Roghmann, & Sigal, 1993; for reviews see Bergsma, 1994; Kiecolt-Glaser & Glaser, 1992; Van Rood, Bogaards, Goulmy, & Houwelingen, 1993). In their meta-analysis of 23 human studies of exam or experimental stress and relaxation on immune response, Van Rood and colleagues (Van Rood et al., 1993) report that white blood cells, Epstein–Barr virus, and herpes simplex virus titers were found to increase under stress. Interleukin 2 receptor expression and T-cell proliferation in response to phytohemagglutinin were found to decrease under stress. Other immunological variables such as monocytes, B cells, T helper/inducer cells, T suppressor/cytotoxic cells, T helper/suppressor ratio, and NK cells showed inconsistency in direction of change (Van Rood et al., 1993). These authors (Van Rood et al., 1993) found consistency in direction of change with relaxation such that white blood cell concentration decreased and salivary immunolgobulin A and NK-cell activity increased during or after it. Snyder and his associates (Snyder et al., 1993) have also reported a lower lymphocyte proliferation response 3 weeks following exposure to a novel antigen in subjects who had experienced more negative stress or psychological distress. Thus this provides evidence in support of a model in which "psychosocial processes mediate the relationship between stressful events and primary immune response" (Snyder et al., 1993).

Natural killer cells are clearly reactive to stress in a number of populations (Herbert & Cohen, 1993). For example, increased NK-cell numbers and/or NK-cell activity has been noted immediately after brief psychological stress such as cognitive conflict tasks, mental arithmetic, and parachute jumping (Landmann et al., 1984; Naliboff et al., 1991; Schedlowski et al., 1993). In contrast, acute stress-induced increases in NK-cell numbers and function may be followed by decreases below baseline shortly afterward (Schedlowski et al., 1993), and decrements of NK cells have been plainly manifest after sustained stress or interpersonal difficulties such as examinations, caring for a chronically ill spouse, divorce, separation, and bereavement (Esterling, Kiecolt-Glaser, Bodnar, & Glaser, 1994; Daniels, Smith, Bloom, & Weiner, 1987; Kiecolt-Glaser, Ricker et al., 1984, 1987a, b). Lower NK cell counts have been associated with depressed mood (Kemeny, Cohen, Zegans, & Conant, 1989; Stein, Miller, & Trestman, 1991) and lower cytotoxicity has been associated with anxiety (Ironson et al., 1990). Among patients with advanced stage cancer, decrements of NK cells and higher cortisol levels have been observed in those with depression (Lechin et al., 1990).

## 2. Social Support and Emotional Expression

While some studies have not found social support to be associated with changes in immune function (e.g., Kiecolt-Glaser et al., 1985b; Schlesinger & Yodfat, 1991), in general, supportive relationships seem to modulate stress-induced immunosuppression (e.g., medical students undergoing examination stress) (Kiecolt-Glaser et al., 1984). Remarkably, psychosocial factors such as social support and interpersonal relationships seem to mitigate the effect of stress on NK cells, even among cancer patients. In a sample of stage I and II breast cancer patients, Levy and her colleagues (Levy, 1990) reported an association between NK-cell activity (NKCA) and perceived support from their spouse or intimate other. They also found a relationship between NKCA and perceived support from their physician, as well as with the active coping strategy of active social support seeking. This is particularly significant considering that, among patients who were immunologically assessed approximately 1 week postsurgically and then followed 5 years later, NKCA was a strong predictor of disease recurrence, with higher cytotoxicity being related to a longer disease-free interval (Levy et al., 1991). Levy and colleagues conclude that the quality of family support and overall mood may potentially predict disease progression in patients whose cancer does recur.

A recent study of immune function in women after surgical treatment for regional breast cancer found that higher stress levels were a significant predictor of poorer NK cytotoxicity, poorer NK-cell response to interferon-$\gamma$, and decreased T-cell responses to mitogen stimulation (Andersen et al., 1998. Lekander, Furst, Rotstein, Blomgren, and Fredrikson (1996) report social support to be related to aspects of immune status in women treated with adjuvant chemotherapy for breast cancer. Perceived attachment

was found to significantly influence white blood cell levels, and number and percentages of granulocytes in women after, but not during, chemotherapy. These authors point out that although causality is not discernible from their study, if the overall white blood cell count can be positively affected by social support then this is important to the recovery process following treatment. This obviously depends on confirmation of the immune-cancer assumption.

Other studies have found evidence for a relationship between social support and blastogenic responses of lymphocytes to mitogens (e.g., Baron, Cutrona, Hicklin, Russell, & Lubaroff, 1990; Glaser et al., 1992; Linn, Linn, & Kilmas, 1988; Snyder et al., 1993; Theorell, Orth-Gomer, & Eneroth, 1990; Thomas, Goodwin, & Goodwin, 1985). In fact, Kiecolt-Glaser and her associates (Kiecolt-Glaser, Dura, Speicher, Trask, & Glaser, 1991) found an interaction between chronic stress and helpful support in relation to blastogenic responses, such that caregivers who were low in helpful social support showed greater negative changes in functional immune response even after statistical controls for age, income, and depression.

Furthermore, in a series of studies investigating biopsychosocial aspects of cutaneous malignant melanoma (Temoshok et al., 1985), expression of negative emotions (sadness and anger) was positively related to the disease outcome and number of lymphocytes at the tumor site and negatively related to mitotic rate of the tumor. In addition, although beyond the scope of this chapter, animal studies have provided some evidence that stress-associated increases in tumor growth may occur concomitant with NK-cell activity suppression (Ben-Eliyahu, Yirmiya, Liebeskind, Taylor, & Gale, 1991; Rowse, Weinberg, Bellward, & Emerman, 1992; Shavit et al., 1985). For example, shock resulted in reduced NK activity and survival time in rats implanted with a mammary adenocarcinoma (Shavit et al., 1985). Ben-Eliyahu and his colleagues (1991) attempted to clarify the mechanism whereby NK cells mediate effects of stress upon tumor growth. Rats injected with MADB-106 lung tumor cells were subjected to an acute stressor. Stressed animals showed a significant reduction in NK-cell activity at the time most critical for NK cells to fight tumor cells. This resulted in stressed rats having a twofold increase in tumor metastases over control rats (Ben-Eliyahu et al., 1991).

Yet are we any closer to elucidating the physiological mediators of such psychosocial factors specifically in relation to survival of cancer? Some studies of cancer progression suggest that effects of stress on immunity have potential clinical relevance, although such effects are as yet controversial in regard to cancer. In studies of other diseases including upper-respiratory infections and autoimmune diseases, significant effects of stress on both the onset and the severity of disease have been noted in humans (Cohen & Herbert, 1996; Turner Cobb & Steptoe, 1996; Turner Cobb & Steptoe, 1998) and animals (Sheridan et al., 1998).

## C. Relevance of Psychoneuroimmune Effects in Cancer

Are psychosocial effects on immunity of sufficient magnitude to be clinically significant? One of the arguments frequently made against the plausibility of stress-induced immunosuppression potentiating cancer progression is that laboratory measurements of immunosuppression may not reflect clinically meaningful influences on disease. For example, an in vitro decrease in lymphocyte natural killer cell activity does not necessarily correlate with an actual increase of tumor burden in vivo, since a number of other physiological mechanisms are operating simultaneously within the body. Many of the immune measures that have commonly been used in studies of psychosocial effects on immunity, such as mitogen proliferation assays and measurement of Epstein–Barr virus antibody titers, may be affected by the same mechanisms that stimulate disease progression while having little impact on the disease process itself. This is an important concern, since the salience of in vitro changes to in vivo illness is critical.

Stress has been associated with a reduction in the performance of immune functions that are involved in tumor defense. However, evidence is suggestive rather than conclusive concerning whether or not the reductions have meaningful effects on immune resistance to tumors.

## III. NEUROENDOCRINE EFFECTS ON ANTI-CANCER IMMUNITY

Neuroendocrine interactions may be a vital link between psychosocial influences on immune functioning and cancer progression.

### A. Hypothalamo-Pituitary-Adrenal (HPA) Axis Effects on Immunity

One link between psychosocial influences and immunity appears to be via glucocorticoid hormones. Stress-induced activation of the HPA axis results in increased glucocorticoid levels, which have been implicated in tumor growth in both animal and human studies (Lointier, Wildrick, & Boman, 1992; Sapolsky & Donnelly, 1985). Two general mechanisms

have been established whereby HPA axis activity may influence immune functions important in cancer defense. First, the cytotoxicity of immune cells against tumor targets may be suppressed, and second, movement of immune cells between the blood and tissues (trafficking) may be affected in such a way that fewer immune cells locate to cancerous tissues.

Hormones of the HPA axis are generally immunosuppressive (Munck & Guyre, 1991). Receptors for glucocorticoids, ACTH and CRH, have been found on lymphocytes (Audhya, Jain, & Hollander, 1991; Berczi, 1986; Smith, Brosman, Meyer, & Blalock, 1987). Effects of elevated glucocorticoid levels include lymphocytopenia, thymus involution, and loss of tissue mass in the spleen and peripheral lymph nodes (Vogel & Bower, 1991). The effects of glucocorticoids on activity and trafficking of immune cells are well established (Kronfol, Nair, Zhang, Hill, & Brown, 1997; Gatti et al., 1993). Stress hormones are also known to influence cell adhesion molecules on lymphocytes (Felten & Olschowka, 1987) providing a possible mechanism by which stress could alter lymphocyte trafficking and therefore immune function (Lorton, Bellinger, Felten, & Felten, 1991; Madden, Felten, Felten, Sundaresan, & Livnat, 1989). There is good evidence for this hypothesis in work by Dhabhar and his colleagues, who demonstrated that stress and the circadian corticosterone rhythm induce significant changes in leukocyte distribution in animals (Dhabhar & McEwen, 1996; Dhabhar, Miller, Stein, McEwen, & Spencer, 1994). Furthermore, they found that acute stress has different effects on a cutaneous delayed type hypersensitivity (DTH) response to that of chronic stress, and the differences are mediated by glucocorticoids (Dhabhar & McEwen, 1996).

### B. Dysregulation of the Cortisol Response Is Linked with Immune Dysregulation and Tumor Progression

Cancer patients repeatedly endure physical and emotional events that may activate the HPA axis stress response. Such repeated activation has been associated with HPA axis dysregulation (McEwen, 1998). In healthy individuals, cortisol levels are usually highest prior to awakening and decrease during the day (Posener, Schildkraut, Samson, & Schatzberg, 1996), but up to 70% of patients with advanced breast cancer show flattened circadian profiles, consistently high levels, or erratic fluctuations (Touitou, Bogdan, Levi, Benavides, & Auzeby, 1996; van der Pompe, Antoni, & Heijnen, 1996). The specific causes of circadian dysregulation in cancer are undetermined.

However, cortisol dysregulation has been linked both with cancer prognosis (Mormont & Levi, 1997; Sephton, Sapolsky, Kraemer, & Spiegel, 2000) and with psychological stress. Among patients with breast and ovarian cancer, severe endocrine disruption is seen in more advanced disease (e.g., patients with poor performance status and liver metastases were found to have more markedly abnormal rhythms) (Touitou et al., 1995, 1996). For a review of alterations in circadian rhythmicity in cancer, see Mormont and Levi (1997).

Flattened profiles and erratic fluctuations of cortisol noted in cancer patients may affect anti-cancer immunity. Indeed, circadian patterns of immune activity and immune cell trafficking have been linked with circadian cortisol patterns (Kronfol et al., 1997). Disregulated patterns of immune activity and immune cell trafficking have been observed in patients with dysregulated cortisol profiles (Gatti et al., 1993; Kronfol et al., 1997). Breast and ovarian cancer patients with altered cortisol rhythms show disruptions in patterns of circulating leukocytes, neutrophils, platelets, and serum proteins (Touitou et al., 1995).

It is possible that such immune and endocrine dysregulation tends to favor tumor growth. Circadian cycles are evident in the activity and proliferation of both normal and malignant tissue (Focan, 1995; Wood & Hrushesky, 1995). Indeed, because of this the time of administration of anticancer drugs can effect their toxicity to healthy tissues and on the tumor cell death rate (Smaaland, Laerum, & Abrahamsen, 1995). Cancer patients with altered endocrine and immune rhythms may be less likely to benefit from chronomodulated chemotherapy administration. Further- more, immune mechanisms that confer cytotoxicity against tumors also follow circadian rhythms (Angeli, Gatti, Sartori, & Masera, 1992; Palm et al., 1996). Thus, tumor defense may be compromised when immune rhythms are altered, especially if periods of rapid tumor proliferation are not matched by periods of greater immune activity.

These immune and endocrine pathways suggest a means by which psychological and social factors might influence the rate of disease progression.

## IV. PSYCHOSOCIAL FACTORS AND CANCER SURVIVAL

### A. Stress and Cancer

The literature has been divided in regard to the hypothesized adverse effect of stress on cancer progression. Ramirez and colleagues (1989) compared women with breast cancer who had relapsed versus those who had not, and found a higher prevalence of major life stressors such as bereavement and loss of a job among those with advancing disease. However, Barraclough and his associates (1992), using a prospective design, found no connection between stress and disease progression. A recent meta-analysis (Petticrew, Fraser, & Regan, 1999) reports finding no good evidence of a relationship between stressful life events and breast cancer incidence. This review, which relies heavily on the European literature, reported no effect of bereavement on cancer incidence among 11 studies (OR 1.06, 95% CI 0.95–1.18, ns). However, there was a twofold effect for other stressors (OR 2.63, 95% CI 2.34–2.96). Despite this, they based their final null conclusion on six studies they deemed to be of "higher quality" because of the use of population controls, blinding of interviewers, and other methodological issues. In these studies there was no effect of stress on cancer incidence, but they did not address the issue of progression.

Some of the variation in findings may be due to differences in stress response characteristics (Spiegel, 1999). It is this coping arena that has produced particularly compelling evidence concerning psychosocial factors and disease progression in cancer, most notably by Greer, Pettingale, and Morris and their colleagues in a series of studies (Greer, Morris, & Pettingale, 1979, 1994; Greer & Watson, 1985; Morris, Pettingale, & Haybittle, 1992; Pettingale, Morris, Greer, & Haybittle, 1985). Their findings suggest that a "fighting spirit" is associated with a more positive prognosis. Conversely, repressive coping has consistently been found to be associated with more rapid cancer progression (Kneier & Temoshok, 1984; Temoshok et al., 1985). Also, avoidance or denial, fatalism or stoic acceptance, anxious preoccupation, and helplessness/hopelessness responses are associated with a poorer cancer prognosis. Not all studies however, have found evidence for such a link (for example, Cassileth, Lusk, Miller, Brown, & Miller, 1985; Dean & Surtees, 1989). In our laboratory we have found that an important element of cancer progression is the expression of negative emotion or distress associated with fear of the disease (Spiegel, 1993). Suppression of negative emotion may also reduce expression of positive emotion since expression of both types of emotion are closely linked rather than being at opposite ends of one continuum (Lane et al., 1997). Attempts to suppress negative affect not only seem to suppress positive emotion as well, but actually seem to increase rather than decrease dysphoria (Koopman, Hermanson, Diamond,

Angell, & Spiegel, 1998; Lane et al., 1997). The amount of variance accounted for by such factors and their relative contribution to disease progression particularly in relation to disease variables is still unclear (for recent review, see Fox, 1998). However, it is likely that the manner of responding to stress may either reduce or amplify its effects, both psychologically and physiologically (Spiegel, 1999).

## B. Social Support

The role of social support provides the strongest evidence of psychosocial impact on illness and hence constitutes a potential resource for resilience. The last decade has given rise to a number of large-scale studies demonstrating the impact of social relations on health in general (for reviews see Cohen, 1988; House, Landis, & Umberson, 1988; Uchino, Cacioppo, & Kiecolt-Glaser, 1996). In fact, it has been demonstrated (House et al., 1988) that the strength of the relationship between social integration and age-adjusted mortality is comparable to the effect of such standard health behavior risk factors as smoking and serum cholesterol levels. Focusing on cancer as the disease outcome, positive, supportive social relations from a number of sources, including marriage (Goodwin, Hunt, Key, Hunt, & Samet, 1987; Maunsell, Jacques, & Deschenes, 1993), daily contact with others (Arnetz, Theorell, Levi, Kallner, & Eneroth, 1983), and the presence of confidants, reduces mortality risk from cancer, as well as other diseases. Ell, Nishimoto, Mediansky, Mantell, and Hamovitchm (1992) examined associations between social support and survival for patients diagnosed with breast, colorectal, or lung cancer, revealing that psychosocial factors operate differently depending on the site and severity of the cancer. Emotional support from primary network members was found to have a protective influence in terms of survival for patients with earlier stages of disease, particularly among women with breast cancer (Ell et al., 1992). No effect was found with more advanced disease or among just lung or colorectal cancer patients. A more recent study (Penninx et al., 1998) also reports evidence for buffering effects of emotional support which were differential across diseases. Emotional support was not found to buffer depression in cancer, diabetes or lung disease but it did act as a buffer for cardiac or arthritis patients. Other studies of breast cancer patients (Hislop, Waxler, Coldman, Elwood, & Kan, 1987; Maunsell et al., 1993; Waxler-Morrison, Hislop, Mears, & Kan, 1991) have also found the marital relationship, supportive friendships, confiding in a confidant, size of social network, and employ-

ment status to be associated with longer survival. Others, however, did not find evidence for such an effect (Barraclough et al., 1992; Marshall & Funch, 1983).

An important factor not to be overlooked in this relationship between psychosocial influences on cancer survival is the impact of demographic factors including socioeconomic status (SES) and race. Lower SES has been found to be inversely associated with the overall pattern of cancer mortality (for review see Balfour & Kaplan, 1998). In a study of three specific types of cancer, breast, cervix, and uterine corpus, using large a subject pool, SES was found to predict survival from breast and uterine corpus cancer while race was associated with survival in each of the three types examined (Greenwald, Polissar, & Dayal, 1996). SES and race were found to be independent predictors of survival (Greenwald et al., 1996). A number of health behavior and health care access factors are obviously implicated in this survival relationship. However, endocrine factors may play an important role in the link between differential SES utilization of psychosocial resistance factors and health outcome. The role of social hierarchy in influencing hormonal responses has been demonstrated in an ongoing series of naturalistic baboon studies which have consistently found that endocrine responses reflect instability or demotion in social rank (Sapolsky, 1989, 1995; Sapolsky, Alberts, & Altmann, 1997; Sapolsky & Spencer, 1997). In relation to the mechanism by which social support enhances coping with life stress, it is worth pointing to studies where religion and church attendance have been associated with positive physiological health outcomes (Koenig et al., 1997; Matthews et al., 1998). It is possible that at least a part of the physiological enhancement that is experienced through religion and church attendance, is related to the increased acceptance and elevation in social hierarchy frequently sought and received through such a support system.

## C. Intervention Effects on Cancer Survival

To the extent that stress hastens cancer progression and social support as well as higher social status buffers against these stress effects, it makes sense that intensive psychosocial intervention might have positive medical as well as psychological effects. Several different types of psychosocial interventions have been developed to facilitate positive psychosocial adjustment of cancer patients and are well documented by a number of recent reviews (e.g., Bottomley, 1997; Cwikel, Behar, & Zabora, 1997; Fawzy, Fawzy, Arndt, & Pasnau, 1995; Loscalzo, 1998). Such work is based on the assumption that social support may act as a buffer between stress and illness and thereby reduce or eliminate the physiological reaction to the stress of cancer (Cohen & Wills, 1985; Levine, Coe, & Wiener, 1989; Spiegel, 1999). In fact, the evidence for improved psychosocial adjustment is so convincing that for several years there has been a call for integrating such intervention into standard medical treatment (Spiegel, 1993). A number of intervention studies have focused specifically on survival as an outcome of receiving psychotherapeutic intervention.

One of the early studies (Grossarth-Maticek, Schmidt, Vetter, & Arndt, 1984) reported evidence for such a survival effect. However, the results are less than conclusive as the methodology generated a number of serious criticisms. Some years later, findings from our laboratory (Spiegel, 1992; Spiegel, Bloom, Kraemer, & Gottheil, 1989) reported that supportive–expressive group psychotherapy was effective in increasing the length of life of women with metastatic breast carcinoma by an average of 18 months. Replication of this survival study is currently being conducted in our laboratory, and in addition a multicenter trial is underway in Canada to examine survival effects of supportive–expressive group psychotherapy (Goodwin et al., 1996). Other studies have also found evidence of a significant relationship between provision of psychosocial intervention and increased length of life, both in lymphoma and leukemia patients (Richardson, Zarnegar, Bisno, & Levine, 1990) and in newly diagnosed malignant melanoma patients (Fawzy et al., 1990a, 1993). As these authors (Fawzy et al., 1993) point out, psychosocial interventions are not proposed as alternatives to conventional medical treatment, rather their use may be most beneficial in conjunction with biomedical trials (Spiegel, 1993). Some cancer intervention studies, however, have not found a survival effect with supportive interventions (Gellert, Maxell, & Siegel, 1993; Ilnyckyj, Farber, Cheang, & Weinerman, 1994; Linn, Linn, & Harris, 1982). Most recently Cunningham et al. (1998) examined disease progression in a sample of metastatic breast cancer patients using a mixture of supportive plus cognitive behavioral therapy and failed to find a treatment survival effect. However, the study employed an inadequate "dose" of intervention and used a smaller sample than the original study. In addition, the control sample received a different intervention, further limiting power to detect a treatment effect. However, such an effect was found for a subgroup of study subjects who attended additional outside support groups.

## V. EVIDENCE OF IMMUNE AND ENDOCRINE ALTERATION VIA PSYCHOSOCIAL INTERVENTION

Thus far we have examined the psychosocial factors implicated in cancer progression, discussed psychosocial intervention studies that have investigated cancer progression and survival; and explored physiological assumptions and recent developments in immune and neuroendocrine research. Studies in the latter half of the 1990s have sought to understand the physiological mediators of psychosocial effects on disease progression or cancer survival and it is the influence of these mediators to which we now turn (Table I). includes controlled intervention trials that have examined cancer progression or "survival" as an outcome measure in addition to those which have examined immune and/or endocrine effects of psychosocial intervention (listed in chronological order).

In regard to intervention studies, as Kiecolt-Glaser and Glaser (1992) point out, enhancement of immune function is most beneficial for populations which are immunocompromised, while such an enhancement in those whose immune functioning is already optimum may be impossible or even harmful. Cancer is associated with immunosuppression both directly through metabolic, metastatic, and other mechanisms and indirectly through the effects of chemotherapy and radiotherapy. Group interventions have been found to be particularly useful in illuminating the links between changes in emotional state and immunity in cancer patients.

An early intervention study in this field gives some evidence of the potential effects of psychosocial interventions for metastatic cancer patients (Gruber, Hall, Hersh, & Dubois, 1988). Using guided imagery and relaxation, these authors report an increase in immune cell function over the treatment period as evidenced by an increase in interleukin-2 levels and T-cell mitogens (Gruber et al., 1988). However, the lack of a control group and the low number of subjects ($n = 10$) are problematic in evaluating the clinical relevance of this study. Most recently, a detailed study by van der Pompe and associates (van der Pompe, Duivenvoorden, Antoni, Visser, & Heijnen, 1997) evaluated the effectiveness of a random assignment, 13-week experiential–existential group psychotherapy program with breast cancer patients treated for primary breast cancer and diagnosed with positive axillary or supraclavicular lymph nodes. The study consisted of 11 breast cancer patients in the intervention group versus 12 breast cancer patients in the wait-list control group. In addition there was a comparison group of 15 age-matched healthy women

**TABLE I  Influence of Psychosocial Intervention on Survival and/or Immune/Endocrine Alteration**

| Authors | Psychosocial intervention | Cancer type | Immune effects | Endocrine effects | Survival effect |
|---|---|---|---|---|---|
| Cunningham et al., 1998 | Supportive plus cognitive behavioral therapy | Metastatic breast cancer ($n = 66$) | Not reported | Not reported | Not found except for subgroup of intervention subjects who attended outside support groups |
| van der Pompe, Duivenvoorden, Antoni, Visser, and Heijnen, 1997 | Group psychotherapy; experimental-existential | Metastatic breast cancer ($n = 23$) | Lower levels of NK cells, CD8 and CD4 cells, lower proliferative response to pokeweed mitogen for intervention group | Lower levels of plasma cortisol, prolactin | Not reported |
| Schedlowski, Jung, Schimanski, Tewes, and Schmoll, 1994 | Relaxation, information and education, coping skills | Breast cancer, stages I and II ($n = 24$) | Short and longer term increase in lymphocyte numbers for intervention group | Short and longer term reductions in plasma cortisol for intervention group | Not reported |
| Fawzy et al., 1993; Fawzy et al., 1990b | Health education, stress management/behavioral training, coping skills, and psychosocial group support | Malignant melanoma ($n = 61$) | Effect found for intervention group; increase in LGLs and NK cells; reduction in CD4 cells | Not reported | Increase in survival rate for intervention group at 5 to 6-year follow-up |
| Gellert, Maxell, and Siegel, 1993 | Individual support, peer counseling, and family therapy | Breast cancer ($n = 34$) | Not reported | Not reported | Not found |
| Spiegel, Bloom, Kraemer, and Gottheil, 1989 | Group psychotherapy—supportive-expressive | Metastatic breast cancer ($n = 86$) | Not reported | Not reported | Average increase in survival by 18 months for intervention group |
| Linn, Linn, and Harris, 1982 | Supportive counseling—individual | Tumors of various sites ($n = 120$ men including 65 with lung cancer) | Not reported | Not reported | Not found |

Note. NK, natural killer; LGL, large granular lymphocyte.

(van der Pompe et al., 1997). Following the 13 weeks of intervention, patients in the group who had a comparatively high baseline immune level showed lower percentages of natural killer cells, CD8 cells, and CD4 cells and a lower proliferative response to pokeweed mitogen than the cancer control group.

Our laboratory has, for some years, been conducting a replication trial of the earlier intervention study where a survival effect was found (Spiegel et al., 1989), incorporating immune and endocrine measures (Sephton et al., 2000; Turner-Cobb, Koopman, Sephton, Blake-Mortimer, & Spiegel, 2000). However, as can be seen from Table I, only one study to date has been reported which directly examines immune mediators of psychosocial intervention in conjunction with cancer progression or survival. That is a 6-week structured psychiatric group intervention study by Fawzy and his colleages (1990b). This evaluation of the effects of a 6-week group intervention for stage I or II malignant melanoma patients reported a significant increase in CD57 large granular lymphocytes (LGLs) at the end of the 6-week intervention. This increase in LGLs in the intervention group was found to take place in the CD8 T-cell subpopulation rather than in NK cells. At a 6-month follow-up, the presumed immunoenhancement among those who had been through group treatment was evident in interferon-$\alpha$-augmented CD56 NK-cell cytotoxicity rather than CD8 cell counts. Interestingly, while this higher NK-cell activity was predictive of a lower rate of recurrence, it did not predict survival time (Fawzy, 1994; Fawzy et al., 1990b). The authors suggest that the NK cell system may be especially responsive to psychological or behavioral changes. In addition, CD4 helper T cells were unexpectedly reduced at 6 months, explained by the authors as due to selective redistribution (Fawzy et al., 1990b) or possibly due to immune cell trafficking (Dhabhar et al., 1995, 1994). Changes over time in immune status were negatively associated with changes over time in mood states (Fawzy, 1994).

## VI. OTHER POSSIBLE MECHANISMS OF PSYCHOSOCIAL EFFECTS IN CANCER

The few studies that have shown increased cancer survival time after psychosocial intervention are provocative. However, it is not clear that psychosocial effects on cancer progression were mediated by immune changes. Indeed, in the only such intervention study in which immunological measures were tracked, NK cell function was improved in the psychosocial treatment group, but the immunoen-

hancement was unrelated to the change in survival time (Fawzy et al., 1993). There are a number of other mechanisms by which stress may influence cancer progression.

### A. Health Behaviors

Stress and psychosocial factors may act indirectly, via altered health-related behaviors. For example, during stressful periods, alcohol consumption may rise, sleep quality may be diminished, there may be poorer nutritional value in the diet, and exercise may be avoided. All of these factors could contribute to weakening of cancer defenses.

### B. Stress Effects on DNA Repair Mechanisms

Stress may act on a chromosomal level to influence tumor formation. For example, neurochemical correlates of depression may diminish a cell's ability to repair damaged DNA, with the result that tumors are more likely to develop (Dattore, Shantz, & Coyne, 1980). When severely depressed patients were compared with controls, the depressed group showed a significant reduction of DNA repair in X-irradiated lymphocytes (Kiecolt-Glaser, Stephens, Lipetz, Speicher, & Glaser, 1985a).

### C. Endocrine Effects on Cancer Progression

In addition to affecting cancer progression by influencing immunity, endocrine factors may also influence tumor growth directly. Glucocorticoids have been implicated in tumor growth both in animal and in vitro studies (Lointier et al., 1992; Sapolsky & Donnelly, 1985). Cortisol may accelerate tumor growth via effects on metabolic processes (Romero et al., 1992). Cortisol normally inhibits glucose uptake by healthy cells, while tumor cells may become resistant to this effect and therefore have a metabolic advantage (Romero et al., 1992; Rowse et al., 1992). Another hypothesis suggests that hormones of the HPA axis may actually promote the expression of breast cancer oncogenes (Licinio, Gold, & Wong, 1995).

Other hormones that are altered by stress and influence cortisol function include prolactin, growth hormone, and thyroid hormones, which may also influence the course of the disease. There is evidence that a majority of breast carcinomas have prolactin receptors (Bonneterre et al., 1982). Furthermore, the presence of prolactin at physiological levels stimulates the growth of such tumors in tissue culture (Malarkey, Kennedy, Allred, & Milo, 1983; Bhatavdekar et al., 1990; Shiu et al., 1987) and may therefore influence the rate of disease progression. Oxytocin is also particularly interesting as has been associated with tumor inhibition (Cassoni, Sapino, Papotti, & Bussolati, 1996) and is known as the hormone of affiliation (Carter, Lederhendler, & Kirkpatrick, 1997). Thus, there is evidence for facilitative effects on tumor growth by stress hormones via several different mechanisms.

## VII.  FUTURE DIRECTIONS

Despite the developments of the past decade within this area of psychoneuroimmunology research, many questions are still unanswered and a wealth of research opportunities remain unexplored. Necessities for future research include:

### A.  Replication of Psychosocial Intervention Trials

In order to provide conclusive evidence of the influence of psychosocial factors on disease outcome, it will be important to replicate intervention trials that have revealed survival effects. Our laboratory has been conducting a trial to replicate the study by Spiegel and his colleagues (1989), adding extensive immune and endocrine measures including in vivo responses such as delayed type hypersensitivity as well as in vitro responses. While such physiological responses would not prove the clinical significance of psychosocial effects on tumor defenses, they may provide a meaningful indication of the magnitude and clinical relevance of psychosocial influences on immune mechanisms in relation to survival.

### B.  Endocrine Dysregulation

Alterations of diurnal cortisol profiles have also been noted among healthy individuals who are under psychological stress due to work overload (Schulz, Kirschbaum, Pruessner, & Hellhammer, 1998), unemployment (Ockenfels, Porter, Smyth, Kirschbaum, & Hellhammer, 1995), depression (Nemeroff, 1991), and posttraumatic stress (Yehuda, Teicher, Levengood, Trestman, & Siever, 1994; Yehuda, Teicher, Trestman, & Levengood, 1996). The stresses of having breast cancer (e.g., anxiety about diagnosis and prognosis, taxing treatments, disruption in social, vocational, and family functioning) may also disrupt

normal circadian cortisol rhythms, an effect potentially open to mediation by social support.

Neuroendocrine dysregulation provides a possible mechanism underlying our finding a decade ago that participation by metastatic breast cancer patients in weekly group psychotherapy was associated with significantly longer survival time (Spiegel et al., 1989). A recent reanalysis of those data demonstrated that the survival advantage was not due to differences in subsequent medical treatment (Kogon, Pearl, Carlson, & Spiegel, 1997). However, this analysis showed that those patients who had undergone adrenalectomy and were therefore on nonphysiological replacement levels of cortisol had shorter survival times. Any effects of group support on disease progression may involve modulation of the HPA stress response system. It has been found that excessive glucocorticoid secretion damages the hippocampus which results in further glucocorticoid secretion. This relationship has been described as a "dysregulatory cascade" (Sapolsky, Krey, & McEwen, 1986). The association between hippocampal damage and loss of negative feedback inhibition may also be associated with cortisol slope and a reduction in cognitive ability.

### C.  Research on Hippocampal Involvement

Recent evidence from stress research (McEwen, 1998; McEwen & Stellar, 1993) indicates that HPA dysregulation in response to chronic stressors may result from hippocampal damage. The hippocampus is rich in glucocorticoid receptors, and a history of severe stress has been associated with reduced hippocampal volume (Bremner, Licinio, Darnell, & Krystal, 1997; Bremner, Randall, & Scott, 1995; Stein, Koverola, Hanna, Torchia, & McClarty, 1997). Research to examine the involvement of the hippocampus in cortisol circadian rhythmicity of patients with breast cancer might provide better understanding of neurological regulation of HPA dysfunction observed to be associated with poor cancer prognosis (Bartsch, Bartsch, Fluchter, Attanasio, & Gupta, 1985; Bartsch, Bartsch, Fluchter, Mecke, & Lippert, 1994; Mormont & Levi, 1997; Touitou et al., 1995). To the extent that abnormal levels of cortisol may be a mediator between stress response and cancer progression, impairment in HPA regulation perhaps involving the hippocampus, hypothalamus, pituitary, and/or adrenal gland, could elucidate the type of dysregulation that could affect cancer progression. In particular, high cortisol levels, alterations in diurnal variation, or abnormal cortisol stress response may have differential effects on disease progression. A better understanding of the neurological cause of neuroendocrine/neurochemical dysregulation may potentiate possible treatments designed to restore HPA function and increase survival time by slowing tumor growth. Cortisol rhythm alteration is significant in relation to immune function because of its regulatory relationship with circadian patterns of immune activity and immune cell trafficking (Dhabhar et al., 1995; Gatti, Cavallo, Sartori, Marinine, & Angeli, 1986; Nair & Schwartz, 1984; Pedersen & Beyer, 1986).

Hippocampal damage and hypercortisolemic states have been seen in people with posttraumatic stress disorder (Bremner et al., 1995, 1997; Stein et al., 1997; Yehuda, Boisoneau, Lowy, & 1995; Yehuda, Resnick, Kahana, & Giller, 1993; Yehuda et al., 1994, 1996). This process has been identified as representing "allostatic load" (McEwen, 1998), the collective somatic burden associated with repeated stress responses. Adverse health consequences can ensue from chronic overactivity of endocrine and cardiovascular stress response systems (McEwen, 1997). Exposure to frequent or severe stress over a period of time may lead to increased sensitization of the HPA axis, resulting in a pronounced stress response (Rosmond, Dallman, & Bjorntorp, 1998). Key brain areas like the hippocampus are vital to transducing context assessment cues into physiological responses that include endocrine and autonomic function (McEwen, 1997).

## D. Exploration of a Wide Range of Hormones

Exploration of other hormones that are altered by stress and which influence cortisol function need further study to understand this process and its relation to disease progression in humans. These hormones, which include ACTH (van der Pompe et al., 1996), DHEA (Dorgan et al., 1997; Massobrio et al., 1994; Secreto & Zumoff, 1994), prolactin (Bhatavdekar et al., 1990), oxytocin (Cassoni et al., 1996), and melatonin (Bartsch, Bartsch, Jain, Laumas, & Wetterberg, 1981), may enable researchers to better define the neural substrate of cortisol dysregulation (Bartsch et al., 1981; Magri et al., 1997). Studies to examine whether the dysregulation is specific to cortisol or involves more general disruption of circadian hormonal rhythms are vital, particularly in relation to psychosocial processes.

In conclusion, we have moved far from evaluating the relative contributions of psychosocial versus physiological factors, into the realms of understanding the psychophysiological interactions among immune, neuroendocrine, and psychosocial mechanisms

involved in cancer progression. Sufficient data exist to indicate an interaction among psychosocial factors, including stress and support, immune function, including natural killer, T- and B-cell activity, endocrine function, and cancer progression. At the same time, the relationships are complex, interact with standard prognostic variables and medical/surgical treatment, and vary with type of cancer. As the field develops, we may be better able to account for more of the variance in outcome by combining psychoneuroimmune and endocrine factors with other standard medical variables. It is clear that provision of psychosocial support to cancer patients provides psychological benefit, and it may positively affect immune, endocrine and other host resistance variables as well. While there are still more questions than answers, it is clear that the questions are worth asking.

## References

Andersen, B. L., Farrar, W. B., Golden-Kreutz, D., Kutz, L. A., MacCallum, R., Courtney, M. E., & Glaser, R. (1998). Stress and immune responses after surgical treatment for regional breast cancer. *Journal of the National Cancer Institute, 90,* 30–36.

Angeli, A., Gatti, G., Sartori, M. L., & Masera, R. G. (1992). Chronobiological aspects of the neuroendocrine–immune network. Regulation of human natural killer (NK) cell activity as a model. *Chronobiologia, 19,* 93–110.

Arnetz, B. B., Theorell, T., Levi, L., Kallner, A., & Eneroth, P. (1983). An experimental study of social isolation of elderly people: Psychoendocrine and metabolic effects. *Psychosomatic Medicine, 45,* 395–406.

Audhya, T., Jain, R., & Hollander, C. (1991). Receptor-mediated imunomodulation by corticotropin releasing factor. *Cellular Immunology, 134,* 77–84.

Balfour, J. L., & Kaplan, G. A. (1998). Social class/ socioecnomic factors. In J. Holland (Ed.), *Psycho-oncology.* New York: Oxford University Press.

Baron, R. B., Cutrona, C. E., Hicklin, D., Russell, D. W., & Lubaroff, D., M. (1990). Social support and immune function among spouses of cancer patients. *Journal of Personality and Social Psychology, 59,* 344–352.

Barraclough, J., Pinder, P., Cruddas, M., Osmond, C., I., T., & Perry, M. (1992). Life events and breast cancer prognosis. *British Medical Journal, 304,* 1078–1081.

Bartsch, C., Bartsch, H., Fluchter, S. H., Attanasio, A., & Gupta, D. (1985). Evidence for a moduailtn of melatonin secretion in men with benign and malignant tumors of the prostate: Relationship with the pituitary hormones. *Journal of Pineal Research, 2,* 121–132.

Bartsch, C., Bartsch, H., Fluchter, S. H., Mecke, D., & Lippert, T. H. (1994). Dimished pineal function coincides with disturbed circadian endocrine rhythmicity in untreated primary cancer patients. Consequence of premature aging or of tumor growth? *Annals of the New York Academy of Sciences, 719,* 502–525.

Bartsch, C., Bartsch, H., Jain, A. K., Laumas, K. R., & Wetterberg, L. (1981). Urinary melatonin levels in human breast cancer patients. *Journal of Neural Transmission, 52,* 281–294.

Ben-Eliyahu, S., Yirmiya, R., Liebeskind, J. C., Taylor, A. N., & Gale, R. P. (1991). Stress increases metastatic spread of a mammary tumor in rats: Evidence for mediation by the immune system. *Brain, Behavior and Immunity, 5,* 193–205.

Berczi, I. (1986). The influence of pituitary-adrenal axis on the immune system. In I. Berczi (Ed.), *Pituitary function and immunity.* Boca Raton, FL: CRC Press.

Bergsma, J. (1994). Illness, the mind, and the body: Cancer and immunology: an introduction. *Theoretical Medicine, 15,* 337–347.

Berke, G. (1995). Unlocking the secrets of CTL and NK cells. *Immunology Today, 16,* 343–346.

Beverley, P. (1991). Immunology of cancer. In L. M. Franks & N. M. Teich (Eds.), *Introduction to the cellular and molecular biology of cancer.* New York: Oxford University Press.

Bhatavdekar, J. M., Shah, N. G., Balar, D. B., Patel, D. D., Bhaduri, A., Trivedi, S. N., Karelia, N. H., Ghosh, N., Shukla, M. K., & Giri, D. D. (1990). Plasma prolactin as an indicator of disease progression in advanced breast cancer. *Cancer, 65,* 2028–2032.

Bonavida, B., Lebow, L. T., & Jewett, A. (1993). Natural killer cell subsets: maturation, differentiation and regulation. *Natural Immunity, 12,* 194–208.

Bonneterre, J., Peyrat, J. P., Vandewalle, B., Beuscart, R., Vie, M. C., & Cappelaere, P. (1982). Prolactin receptors in human breast cancer. *European Journal of Cancer and Clinical Oncology, 18,* 1157–1982.

Bottomley, A. (1997). Where are we now? Evaluating two decades of group interventions with adult cancer patients. *Journal of Psychiatric and Mental Health Nursing, 4,* 251–265.

Bovbjerg, D. H., & Valdimarsdottir, H. (1998). psychoneuroimmunology: Implications for psycho-oncology. In J. Holland (Ed.), *Psycho-oncology.* New York: Oxford University Press.

Bremner, J. D., Licinio, J., Darnell, A., & Krystal, J. H. (1997). Elevated CSF corticotropin-releasing factor concentrations in posttraumatic stress disorder. *American Journal of Psychiatry, 154,* 624–629.

Bremner, J. D., Randall, P., & Scott, T. M. (1995). MRI-based measurement of hippocampal volume in patients with combat-related posttraumatic stress disorder. *American Journal of Psychiatry, 152,* 973–981.

Carter, C. S., Lederhendler, I., & Kirkpatrick, B. (1997). The integrative neurobiology of affiliation. Introduction. *Annals of the New York Academy of Sciences, 807,* xiii–xviii.

Cassileth, B. R., Lusk, E. J., Miller, D. S., Brown, L., & Miller, C. (1985). Psychological correlates of survival in advanced malignant disease. *New England Journal of Medicine, 312,* 1551–1555.

Cassoni, P., Sapino, A., Papotti, M., & Bussolati, G. (1996). Oxytocin and oxytocin-analogue F314 inhibit cell proliferation and tumor growth of rat and mouse mammary carcinomas. *International Journal of Cancer, 66,* 817–820.

Cohen, S. (1988). Psychosocial models of the role of social support in the etiology of physical disease. *Health Psychology, 7,* 269–297.

Cohen, S., & Herbert, T. B. (1996). Health psychology: Psychological factors and physical disease from the perspective of human psychoneuroimmunology. *Annual Review of Psychology, 47,* 113–142.

Cohen, S., & Rabin, B. S. (1998). Psychologic stress, immunity, and cancer: editorial; comment. *Journal of the National Cancer Institute, 90,* 3–4.

Cohen, S., & Wills, T. A. (1985). Stress, social support, and the buffering hypothesis. *Psychological Bulletin, 98,* 310–357.

Cunningham, A. J., Edmonds, C. V., Jenkins, G. P., Pollack, H., Lockwood, G. A., & Warr, D. (1998). A randomized controlled trial of the effects of group psychological therapy on survival in women with metastatic breast cancer. *Psycho-Oncology, 7,* 508–517.

Cwikel, J. G., Behar, L. C., & Zabora, J. R. (1997). Psychosocial factors that affect the survival of adult cancer patients: A review of research. *Journal of Psychosocial Oncology, 15,* 1–34.

Dattore, P., Shantz, F., & Coyne, L. (1980). Premorbid personality differentiation of cancer and non-cancer groups. A test of the hypothesis of cancer proness. *Journal of Consulting and Clinical Psychology, 48,* 388–394.

Dean, C., & Surtees, P. G. (1989). Do psychological factors predict survival in breast cancer? *Journal of Psychosomatic Research, 33,* 561–569.

Dhabhar, F. S., & McEwen, B. S. (1996). Stress-induced enhancement of antigen-specific cell-mediated immunity. *Journal of Immunology, 156,* 2608–2615.

Dhabhar, F. S., Miller, A. H., McEwen, B. S., & Spencer, R. L. (1995). Effects of stress on immune cell distribution. Dynamics and hormonal mechanisms. *Journal of Immunology, 154,* 5511–5527.

Dhabhar, F. S., Miller, A. H., Stein, M., McEwen, B. S., & Spencer, R. L. (1994). Diurnal and acute stress-induced changes in distribution of peripheral blood leukocyte subpopulations. *Brain, Behavior, and Immunity, 8,* 66–79.

Dorgan, J. F., Stanczyk, F. Z., Longcope, C., Stephenson, H. E., Jr., Chang, L., Miller, R., Franz, C., Falk, R. T., & Kahle, L. (1997). Relationship of serum dehydroepiandrosterone (DHEA), DHEA sulfate, and 5-androstene-3 beta, 17 beta-diol to risk of breast cancer in postmenopausal women. *Cancer Epidemiology, Biomarkers and Prevention, 6,* 177–181.

Ell, K., Nishimoto, R., Mediansky, L., Mantell, J., & Hamovitchm M. (1992). Social relations, social support and survival among patients with cancer. *Journal of Psychosomatic Research, 36,* 531–541.

Esterling, B. A., Kiecolt-Glaser, J. K., Bodnar, J. C., & Glaser, R. (1994). Chronic stress, social support, and persistent alterations in the natural killer cell response to cytokines in older adults. *Health Psychology, 13,* 291–298.

Fawzy, F. I. (1994). Immune effects of a short-term intervention for cancer patients. *Advances, 10,* 32–33.

Fawzy, F. I., Cousins, N., Fawzy, N. W., Kemeny, M. E., Elashoff, R., & Morton, D. (1990a). A structured psychiatric intervention for cancer patients. I. Changes over time in methods of coping and affective disturbance. *Archives of General Psychiatry, 47,* 720–725.

Fawzy, F. I., Fawzy, N. W., Arndt, L. A., & Pasnau, R. O. (1995). Critical review of psychosocial interventions in cancer care. *Archives of General Psychiatry, 52,* 100–113.

Fawzy, F. I., Fawzy, N. W., Hyun, C. S., Elashoff, R., Guthrie, D., & Fahey, J. L. (1993). Malignant melanoma: Effects of an early structured psychiatric intervention, coping, and affective state on recurrence and survival 6 years later. *Archives of General Psychiatry, 50,* 681–689.

Fawzy, F. I., Kemeny, M. E., Fawzy, N. W., Elashoff, R., Morton, D., Cousins, N., & Fahey, J. L. (1990b). A structured psychiatric intervention for cancer patients. II. Changes over time in immunological measures. *Archives of General Psychiatry, 47,* 729–735.

Felten, S. Y., and Olschowka, J. (1987). Noradrenergic sympathetic innervation of the spleen. II. Tyrosine hydroxylase (TH)-positive nerve terminals form synaptic like contacts on lymphocytes in the splenic white pulp. *Journal of Neuroscience Research, 18,* 37–48.

Focan, C. (1995). Circadian rhythms and cancer chemotherapy. *Pharmacology and Therapeutics, 67,* 1–52.

Fox, B. H. (1998). Psychosocial factors in cancer incidence and progression. In J. C. Holland (Ed.), *Psycho-oncology.* New York: Oxford University Press.

Garssen, B., & K. Goodkin (1999). On the role of immunological factors as mediators between psychosocial factors and cancer progression. *Psychiatry Research, 85,* 51–61.

Gatti, G., Cavallo, R., Sartori, M. L., Marinine, C., & Angeli, A. (1986). Cortisol at physiological concentrations and prostaglandin E2 are additive inhibitors of human natural killer cell activity. *Immunopharmacology*, 11, 119–128.

Gatti, G., Masera, R. G., Pallavicini, L., Sartori, M. L., Staurenghi, A., Orlandi, F., & Angeli, A. (1993). Interplay in vitro between ACTH, beta-endorphin, and glucocorticoids in the modulation of spontaneous and lymphokine-inducible human natural killer (NK) cell activity. *Brain, Behavior, and Immunity*, 7, 16–28.

Gellert, G. A., Maxell, R. M., & Siegel, B. S. (1993). Survival of breast cancer patients receiving adjunctive psychosocial support therapy: A 10-year follow-up study. *Journal of Clinical Oncology*, 11, 66–69.

Geppert, T., & Lipsky, P. (1989). Antigen presentation at the inflammatory site. *Critical Reviews in Immunology*, 9, 313–362.

Glaser, R., Kiecolt-Glaser, J. K., Bonneau, R. H., Malarkey, W., Kennedy, S., & Hughes, J. (1992). Stress-induced modulation of the immune response to recombinant hepatitis B vaccine. *Psychosomatic Medicine*, 54, 22–29.

Goodwin, J. S., Hunt, W. C., Key, C. R., & Samet, J. M. (1987). The effect of marital status on stage, treatment, and survival of cancer patients. *Journal of the American Medical Association*, 258, 3125–3130.

Goodwin, P. J., Leszcz, M., Koopmans, J., Arnold, A., Doll, R., Chochinov, H., Navarro, M., Butler, K., & Pritchard, K. I. (1996). Randomized trial of group psychosocial support in metastatic breast cancer: The BEST (Breast-Expressive-Supportive Therapy) study. *Cancer Treatment Reviews*, 22, 91–96.

Greenwald, H. P., Polissar, N. L., & Dayal, H. H. (1996). Race, socioeconomic status and survival in three female cancers. *Ethnicity and Health*, 1, 65–75.

Greer, S., Morris, T., & Pettingale, K. W. (1979). Psychological response to breast cancer: Effect on outcome. *Lancet*, 2, 785–787.

Greer, S., Morris, T., & Pettingale, K. W. (1994). Psychological response to breast cancer: Effect on outcome. In A. Steptoe & J. Wardle (Eds.). *Psychosocial processes and health: A reader*. Cambridge, England UK: Cambridge University Press.

Greer, S., & Watson, M. (1985). Towards a psychobiological model of cancer: Psychological considerations. *Social Science and Medicine*, 20, 773–777.

Grossarth-Maticek, R., Schmidt, P., Vetter, H., & Arndt, S. (1984). Psychotherapy research in oncology. In A. Steptoe & A. Mathews (Eds.), *Health care and human behavior*. London: Academic Press.

Gruber, B. L., Hall, N. R., Hersh, S. P., & Dubois, P. (1988). Immune system and psychological changes in metastatic cancer patients using relaxation and guided imagery: A pilot study. *Scandinavian Journal of Behaviour Therapy*, 17, 25–46.

Herberman, R. (1985). Natural killer cells: Characteristics and possible role in resistance against tumor growth. In A. E. Reif & M. S. Mitchell (Eds.), *Immunity to cancer*. San Diego: Academic Press.

Herberman, R. (1986). Natural killer cell activity and antibody-dependent cell-mediated cytotoxicity. In N. Rose, H. Friedman, and J. Fahey (Eds.), *Manual of clinical laboratory immunology* (3rd ed.). Washington, DC: American Society for Microbiology.

Herbert, T. B., & Cohen, S. (1993). Stress and immunity in humans: A meta-analytic review. *Psychosomatic Medicine*, 55, 364–379.

Hislop, T. G., Waxler, N. E., Coldman, A. J., Elwood, J. M., & Kan, L. (1987). The prognostic significance of psychosocial factors in women with breast cancer. *Journal of Chronic Diseases*, 40, 729–735.

House, J. S., Landis, K. R., & Umberson, D. (1988). Social relationships and health. *Science*, 241, 540–545.

Ilnyckyj, A., Farber, J., Cheang, M., & Weinerman, B. (1994). A randomized controlled trial of psychotherapeutic intervention in cancer patients. *Annals of the Royal College of Physicians and Surgeons of Canada*, 27, 93–96.

Ironson, G., Lapierre, A., Antoni, M., O'Hearn, P., Schneiderman, N., Klimas, N., & Fletcher, M.A. (1990). Changes in immune and psychological measures as a function of anticipation and reaction to news of HIV-1 antibody status. *Psychosomatic Medicine*, 52, 247–270.

Irwin, M., Daniels, M., Smith, T. L., Bloom, E., & Weiner, H. (1987). Impaired natural killer cell activity during bereavement. *Brain, Behavior, and Immunity*, 1, 98–104.

Kagi, D., Ledermann, B., Burki, K., Seiler, P., Odermatt, B., Olsen, K. J., Podack, E. R., Zinkernagel, R. M., & Hengartner, H. (1994). Cytotoxicity mediated by T cells and natural killer cells is greatly impaired in perforin-deficient mice. *Nature*, 369, 31–37.

Kagi, D., Ledermann, B., Burki, K., Zinkernagel, R., & Hengartner, H. (1996). Molecular mechanisms of lymphocyte-mediated cytotoxicity and their role in immunological protection and pathogenesis in vivo. *Annual Review of Immunology*, 14, 207–232.

Karre, K., Ljunggren, H. G., Piontek, G., & Kiessling, R. (1986). Selective rejection of H-2-deficient lymphoma variants suggests alternative immune defence strategy. *Nature*, 319, 675–678.

Kemeny, M. E., Cohen, F., Zegans, L. S., & Conant, M. A. (1989). Psychological and immunological predictors of genital herpes recurrence. *Psychosomatic Medicine*, 51, 195–208.

Kiecolt-Glaser, J., Stephens, R., Lipetz, P., Speicher, C., & Glaser, R. (1985a). Distress and DNA repair in human lymphocytes. *Journal of Behavioral Medicine*, 8, 311–320.

Kiecolt-Glaser, J. K., Dura, J. R., Speicher, C. E., Trask, O. J., & Glaser, R. (1991). Spousal caregivers of dementia victims: Longitudinal changes in immunity and health. *Psychosomatic Medicine*, 53, 345–362.

Kiecolt-Glaser, J. K., Fisher, L. D., Ogrocki, P., Stout, J. C., Speicher, C. E., & Glaser, R. (1987a). Marital quality, marital disruption, and immune function. *Psychosomatic Medicine*, 49, 13–34.

Kiecolt-Glaser, J. K., Garner, W., Speicher, C.E., Penn, G., & Glaser, R. (1984). Psychosocial modifiers of immunocompetence in medical students. *Psychosomatic Medicine*, 46, 7–14.

Kiecolt-Glaser, J. K., & Glaser, R. (1992). Psychoneuroimmunology: Can psychological interventions modulate immunity? Special issue: Behavioral medicine: An update for the 1990's. *Journal of Consulting and Clinical Psychology*, 60, 569–575.

Kiecolt-Glaser, J. K., Glaser, R., Shuttleworth, E. C., Dyer, C. S., Ogrocki, P., & Speicher, C. E. (1987b). Chronic stress and immunity in family caregivers of Alzheimer's disease victims. *Psychosomatic Medicine*, 49, 523–535.

Kiecolt-Glaser, J. K., Glaser, R., Williger, D., Stout, J., Messick, G., Sheppard, S., Ricker, D., Romisher, S. C., Briner, W., Bonnell, G., & Donnerberg, R. (1985b). Psychosocial enhancement of immunocompetence in a geriatric population. *Health Psychology*, 4, 25–41.

Kiecolt-Glaser, J. K., Ricker, D., George, J., Messick, G., Speicher, C. E., Garner, W., & Glaser, R. (1984). Urinary cortisol levels, cellular immunocompetency, and loneliness in psychiatric inpatients. *Psychosomatic Medicine*, 46, 15–23.

King, R. (1996). *Cancer biology*. Edinburgh Gate, Harlow, England: Addison Wesley Longman.

Kneier, A. W., & Temoshok, L. (1984). Repressive coping reactions in patients with malignant melanoma as compared to cardiovascular disease patients. *Journal of Psychosomatic Research, 28*, 145–155.

Koenig, H. G., Cohen, H. J., George, L. K., Hays, J. C., Larson, D. B., & Blazer, D. G. (1997). Attendance at religious services, interleukin-6, and other biological parameters of immune function in older adults. *International Journal of Psychiatry in Medicine, 27,* 233–250.

Kogon, M. M., B., A., Pearl, D., Carlson, R. W., & Spiegel, D. (1997). Effects of medical and psychotherapeutic treatment on the survival of women with metastatic breast carcinoma. *Cancer, 80,* 225–230.

Koopman, C., Hermanson, K., Diamond, S., Angell, K., & Spiegel, D. (1998). Social support, life stress, pain and emotional adjustment to advanced breast cancer. *Psycho-Oncology, 7,* 101–111.

Korner, H., & Sedgwick, J. (1996). Tumor necrosis factor and lymphotoxin: Molecular aspects and role in tissue-specific autoimmunity. *Immunology and Cell Biology, 74,* 465–472.

Kronfol, Z., Nair, M., Zhang, Q., Hill, E. E., & Brown, M. B. (1997). Circadian immune measures in healthy volunteers: Relationship to hypothalamic-pituitary-adrenal axis hormones and sympathetic neurotransmitters. *Psychosomatic Medicine, 59,* 42–50.

Landmann, R. M., Muller, F. B., Perini, C., Wesp, M., Erne, P., & Buhler, F. R. (1984). Changes of immunoregulatory cells induced by psychological and physical stress: Relationship to plasma catecholamines. *Clinical and Experimental Immunology, 58,* 127–135.

Lane, R. D., Reiman, E. M., Bradley, M. M., Lang, P. J. Ahern, G.L., Davidson, R. J., & Schwartz, G.E. (1997). Neuroanatomical correlates of pleasant & unpleasant emotion. *Neuropsychologia, 35,* 1437–1444.

Lechin, F., van der Dijs, B., Vitelli-Florez, G., Lechin-Baez, S., Azocar, J., Cabrera, A., Lechin, A., Jara, H., Lechin, M., & Gomez, F., et al. (1990). Psychoneuroendocrinological and immunological parameters in cancer patients: Involvement of stress and depression. *Psychoneuroendocrinology, 15,* 435–451.

Lekander, M., Furst, C. J., Rotstein, S., Blomgren, H., & Fredrikson, M. (1996). Social support and immune status during and after chemotherapy for breast cancer. *Acta Oncologica, 35,* 31–37.

Levine, S., Coe, C., & Wiener, S. G. (1989). Psychoendocrinology. In F. R. Brush & S. Levine (Eds.), *Psychoneuroendocrinology of stress: A psychobiological perspective.* New York: Academic Press.

Levy, S., M. (1990). Perceived social support and tumor estrogen/progesterone receptor status as predictors of natural killer cell activity in breast cancer patients. *Psychosomatic Medicine, 52,* 73–85.

Levy, S. M., Herberman, R. B., Lippman, M., D'Angelo, T., & Lee, J. (1991). Immunological and psychosocial predictors of disease recurrence in patients with early-stage breast cancer. *Behavioral Medicine,* 67–75.

Liang, J., Wang, C., Chang, K., & Chuang, C. (1993). Circulating intercellular adhesion molecule-1 and lymphocyte subsets involved in immune response of breast cancer. *Chung Hua Min Kuo Wei Sheng Wu Chi Mien / Hsuen Tsa Chih, 26,* 1–5.

Licinio, J., Gold, P. W., & Wong, M. L. (1995). A molecular mechanism for stress-induced alterations in susceptibility to disease. *Lancet, 346,* 104–106.

Linn, B. S., Linn, M. W., & Kilmas, N. G. (1988). Effects of psychosocial stress on surgical outcomes. *Psychosomatic Medicine, 50,* 230–244.

Linn, M. W., Linn, B. S., & Harris, R. (1982). Effects of counseling for late stage cancer patients. *Cancer, 49,* 1048–1055.

Ljunggren, H. G., & Karre, K. (1990). In search of the "missing self": MHC molecules and NK cell recognition. *Immunology Today, 11,* 237–244.

Lloyd, K. (1991). Humoral immune responses to tumor-associated carbohydrate antigens. *Seminars in Cancer Biology, 2,* 421–425.

Lointier, P., Wildrick, D. M., & Boman, B. M. (1992). The effects of steroid hormones on a human colon cancer cell line in vitro. *Anticancer Research, 12,* 1327–1330.

Lorton, D., Bellinger, D. L., Felten, S. Y., & Felten, D. L. (1991). Substance P innervation of spleen in rats: Nerve fibers associate with lymphocytes and macrophages in specific compartments of the spleen. *Brain, Behavior and Immunity, 5,* 29–40.

Loscalzo, M. (1998). Interventions. In J. C. Holland (Ed.), *Psycho-oncology.* New York: Oxford University Press.

Madden, K. S., Felten, S. Y., Felten, D. L., Sundaresan, P. R., & Livnat, S. (1989). Sympathetic nerual modulation of the immune system. I. Depression of T cell immunito in vivo and vitro following chemical sympathectomy. *Brain, Behavior and Immunity, 3,* 72–89.

Magri, F., Locatelli, M., Balza, G., Molla, G., Cuzzoni, G., Fioravanti, M., Solerte, S. B., & Ferrari, E. (1997). Changes in endocrine circadian rhythms as markers of physiological and pathological brain aging. *Chronobiology International, 14,* 385–396.

Malarkey, W. B., Kennedy, M., Allred, L. E., & Milo, G. (1983). Physiological concentrations of prolactin can promote the growth of human breast tumor cells in culture. *Journal of Clinical Endocrinology and Metabolism, 56,* 673–677.

Mantovani, A., Bottazzi, B., Colotta, F., Sozanni, S., & Ruco, L. (1992). The origin and function of tumor-associated macrophages. *Immunology Today, 13,* 265–270.

Marshall, J. R., & Funch, D. P. (1983). Social environment and breast cancer: a cohort analysisi of patient survival. *Cancer, 52,* 1546–1550.

Massobrio, M., Migliardi, M., Cassoni, P., Menzaghi, C., Revelli, A., & Cenderelli, G. (1994). Steroid gradients across the cancerous breast: An index of altered steroid metabolism in breast cancer? *Journal of Steroid Biochemistry and Molecular Biology, 51,* 175–181.

Matthews, D. A., McCullough, M. E., Larson, D. B., Koenig, H. G., Swyers, J. P., & Milano, M. G. (1998). Religious commitment and health status: a review of the research and implications for family medicine. *Archives of Family Medicine, 7,* 118–124.

Maunsell, E. B., Jacques, B., & Deschenes, L. (1993). Social support and survival among women with breast cancer. *Cancer, 76,* 631–637.

McEwen, B. S. (1997). Hormones as regulators of brain development: Life-long effects related to health and disease. *Acta Paediatrica, 422* (Supplement), 41–44.

McEwen, B. S. (1998). Protective and damaging effects of stress mediators. *The New England Journal of Medicine, 338,* 171–179.

McEwen, B. S., & Stellar, E. (1993). Stress and the individual. Mechanisms leading to disease. *Archives of Internal Medicine, 153,* 2093–2101.

Mormont, M. C., & Levi, F. (1997). Circadian-system alterations during cancer processes: A review. *International Journal of Cancer, 70,* 241–247.

Morris, T., Pettingale, K. W., & Haybittle, J. (1992). Psychological response to cancer diagnosis and disease outcome in patients with breast cancer and lymphoma. *Psycho-Oncology, 1,* 105–114.

Munck, A., & Guyre, P. (1991). Glucocorticoids and immune function. In R. Ader, D. Feten, & N. Cohen (Eds.), *Psychoneuroimmunology.* San Diego: Academic Press.

Nagata, S. (1997). Apoptosis by death factor. *Cell, 88,* 355–365.

Nair, M. P., & Schwartz, S. A. (1984). Immunomodulatory effects of corticosteroids on natural killer and antibody-dependent cellular cytotoxic activities of human lymphocytes. *Journal of Immunology, 132,* 2876–2882.

Naliboff, B., Benton, D., Solomon, G., Morley, J., Fahey, J., Bloom, E., Makinodan, T., & Gilmore, S. (1991). Immunological change in young and old adults during brief laboratory stress. *Psychosomatic Medicine, 53,* 121–132.

Naume, B., & Espevik, T. (1994). Immunoregulatory effects of cytokines on natural killer cells. *Scandinavian Journal of Immunology, 40*, 128–134.

Nemeroff, C. B. (1991). Corticotropin-releasing factor. In C. B. Nemeroff (Ed.), *Neuropeptides and psychiatric disorders*. Washington, DC: American Psychiatric Press.

Nossal, G. J. (1993). Life, death, and the immune system. *Scientific American, 269*, 20–30.

Ockenfels, M. C., Porter, L., Smyth, J., Kirschbaum, C., & Hellhammer, D. H. (1995). Effect of chronic stress associated with unemployment on salivary cortisol: Overall cortisol levels, diurnal rhythm and acute stress reactivity. *Psychosomatic Medicine, 57*, 460–467.

Oliver, R., & Nouri, A. (1992). T cell immune response to cancer in humans and its relevance for immunodiagnosis and therapy. *Cancer Surveys, 13*, 173–204.

Palm, S., Postler, E., Hinrichsen, H., Maier, H., Zabel, P., & Kirch, W. (1996). Twenty-four-hour analysis of lymphocyte subpopulations and cytokines in healthy subjects. *Chronobiology International, 13*, 423–424.

Pedersen, B. K., & Beyer, J. M. (1986). Characterization of the in vitro effects of glucocorticoids on NK cell activity. *Allergy, 41*, 220–224.

Penn, I. (1993). The effect of immunosuppression on pre-existing cancers. *Transplantation, 55*, 742–747.

Penninx, B. W. J. H., van Tilburg, T., Boeke, A. J. P., Deeg, D. J. H., Kriegsman, D. M. W., & van Eijk, J. T. M. (1998). Effects of social support and personal coping resources on depressive symptoms: Different for various chronic diseases? *Health Psychology, 17*, 551–558.

Petticrew, M., Fraser, J. M., & Regan, M. F. (1999). Adverse life-events and risk of breast cancer: A meta-analysis. *British Journal of Health Psychology, 4*, 1–17.

Pettingale, K. W., Morris, T., Greer, S., & Haybittle, J. (1985). Mental attitudes to cancer: an additional prognostic factor. *Lancet, 1*, 750.

Posener, J. A., Schildkraut, J. J., Samson, J. A., & Schatzberg, A. F. (1996). Diurnal variation of plasma cortisol and homovanillic acid in healthy subjects. *Psychoneuroendocrinology, 21*, 33–38.

Ramirez, A. J., Craig, T. K. J., Watson, J. P., Fentiman, I. S., North, W. R. S., & Rubens, R. D. (1989). Stress and relapse of breast cancer. *British Medical Journal, 298*, 291–293.

Raulet, D. H., Correa, I., Corral, L., Dorfman, J., & Wu, M. F. (1995). Inhibitory effects of class I molecules on murine NK cells: Speculations on function, specificity and self-tolerance. *Seminars in Immunology, 7*, 103–107.

Richardson, J. L., Zarnegar, Z., Bisno, B., & Levine, A. (1990). Psychosocial status at initiation of cancer treatment and survival. *Journal of Psychosomatic Research, 34*, 189–201.

Roder, J., & Pross, H. (1982). The biology of the human natural killer cell. *Journal of Clinical Immunology, 2*, 249–263.

Romero, L., Raley-Susman, K., Redish, D., Brooke, S., Horner, H., & Sapolsky, R. (1992). A possible mechanism by which stress accelerates growth of virally-derived tumors. *Proceeding of the National Academy of Sciences, 89*, 11084.

Rosen, H. R., Ausch, C., Reiner, G., Reinerova, M., Svec, J., Tüchler, H., Schiessel, R., & Moroz, C. (1994). Downregulation of lymphocyte mitogenesis by breast cancer-associated. *Cancer Letters, 82*, 105–111.

Rosenberg, S. (1991). Immunotherapy and gene therapy of cancer. *Cancer Research, 51* (Supplement), 5074s–5079s.

Rosmond, R., Dallman, M. F., & Bjorntorp, P. (1998). Stress-related cortisol secretion in men: Relationships with abdominal obesity and endocrine, metabolic and hemodynamic abnormalities. *Journal of Clinical Endocrinology and Metabolism, 83*, 1853–1859.

Rowse, G. L., Weinberg, J., Bellward, G. D., & Emerman, J. T. (1992). Endocrine mediation of psychosocial stressor effects on mouse mammary tumor growth. *Cancer Letters, 65*, 85–93.

Sapolsky, R. M. (1989). Hypercortisolism among socially subordinate wild baboons originates at CNS level. *Archives of General Psychiatry, 46*, 1047–1051.

Sapolsky, R. M. (1995). Social subordinance as a marker of hypercortisolism. Some unexpected subtleties. *Annals of the New York Academy of Sciences, 771*, 626–639.

Sapolsky, R. M., Alberts, S. C., & Altmann, J. (1997). Hypercortisolism associated with social subordinance or social isolation among wild baboons. *Archives of General Psychiatry, 54*, 1137–1143.

Sapolsky, R. M., & Donnelly, T. M. (1985). Vulnerability to stress-induced tumor growth increases with age in rats: Role of glucocorticoids. *Endocrinology, 117*, 662–666.

Sapolsky, R. M., Krey, L. C., & McEwen, B. S. (1986). The neuroendocrinology of stress and aging: The glucocorticoid cascade hypothesis. *Endocrine Reviews, 7*, 284–301.

Sapolsky, R. M., & Spencer, E. M. (1997). Insulin-like growth factor I is suppressed in socially subordinate male baboons. *American Journal of Physiology, 273*, R1346–R1351.

Schedlowski, M., Jacobs, R., Stratmann, G., Richter, S., Hadicke, A., Tewes, U., Wagner, T. O., & Schmidt, R. E. (1993). Changes of natural killer cells during acute psychological stress. *Journal of Clinical Immunology, 13*, 119–126.

Schedlowski, M., Jung, C., Schimanski, G., Tewes, U., & Schmoll, H.-J. (1994). Effects of behavioral intervention on plasma cortisol and lymphocytes in breast cancer patients: An exploratory study. *Psycho-Oncology, 3*, 181–187.

Schlesinger, M., & Yodfat, Y. (1991). The impact of stressful life events on natural killer cells. 2nd International Society for the Investigation of Stress Conference: Stress, immunity and AIDS (1989, Athens, Greece). *Stress Medicine, 7*, 53–60.

Schulz, P., Kirschbaum, C., Pruessner, J. C., Hellhammer, D. H. (1998). Increased free cortisol secretion after awakening in chronically stressed individuals due to work overload. *Stress Medicine, 14*, 91–97.

Secreto, G., & Zumoff, B. (1994). Abnormal production of androgens in women with breast cancer. *Anticancer Research, 14*, 2113–2117.

Sephton, S. E., Sapolsky, R. M., Kraemer, H., & Spiegel, D. (2000). Early mortality in metastatic breast cancer patients with absent or abnormal diurnal cortisol rhythms. *Journal of the National Cancer Institute, 92*, 994–1000.

Shavit, Y., Terman, G. W., Martin, F., C., Lewis, J. W., Liebeskind, J. C., & Gale, R. P. (1985). Stress, opioid peptides, the immune system, and cancer. *The Journal of Immunology, 135*, 834s–837s.

Sheridan, J. F., Dobbs, C., Jung, J., Chu, X., Konstantinos, A., Padgett, D., & Glaser, R. (1998). Stress-induced neuroendocrine modulation of viral pathogenesis and immunity. *Annals of the New York Academy of Sciences, 840*, 803–808.

Shiu, R. P., Murphy, L. C., Tsuyuki, D., Myal, Y., Lee-Wing, M., & Iwasiow, B. (1987). Biological actions of prolactin in human breast cancer. *Recent Progress in Hormone Research, 43*, 277–303.

Shu, S., Plautz, G., Krauss, J., & Chang, A. (1997). Tumor immunology. *Journal of the American Medical Association, 278*, 1972–1981.

Smaaland, R., Laerum, O. D., & Abrahamsen, J. F. (1995). Circadian cell kinetics in humans. Aspects related to cancer chemotherapy. *In Vivo, 9*, 529–537.

Smith, E., Brosman, P., Meyer, W., & Blalock, J. (1987). A corticotropin receptor on human mononuclear lymphocytes: Corelation with adrenal ACTH receptor activity. *New England Journal of Medicine, 312*, 1266–1269.

Smyth, M. J., & Trapani, J. A. (1995). Granzymes: Exogenous proteinases that induce target cell apoptosis. *Immunology Today, 16,* 202–206.

Snyder, B., K., Roghmann, K. J., & Sigal, L. H. (1993). Stress and psychosocial factors: Effects on primary cellular immune response. *Journal of Behavioral Medicine, 16,* 143–161.

Somers, S., & Guillou, P. J. (1994). Tumour cell strategies for escaping immune control: Implications for psychoimmunotherapy. In C. E. Lewis, C. O'Sullivan, and J. Barraclough (Eds.), *The psychoimmunology of cancer: Mind and body in the fight for survival?* New York: Oxford University Press.

Spiegel, D. (1992). Effects of psychosocial support on patients with metastatic breast cancer. *Journal of Psychosocial Oncology, 10,* 113–120.

Spiegel, D. (1993). Psychosocial intervention in cancer. *Journal of the National Cancer Institute, 85,* 1198–1205.

Spiegel, D. (1999). Healing words. Emotional expression and disease outcome. *Journal of the American Medical Association, 281,* 1328–1329.

Spiegel, D., Bloom, J. R., Kraemer, H. C., & Gottheil, E. (1989). Effect of Psychosocial treatment on survival of patients with metastatic breast cancer. *Lancet, 2,* 888–891.

Stein, M., Miller, A. H., & Trestman, R. L. (1991). Depression, the immune system, and health and illness. Findings in search of meaning. *Archives of General Psychiatry, 48,* 171–177.

Stein, M. B., Koverola, C., Hanna, C., Torchia, M. G., & McClarty, B. (1997). Hippocampal volume in women victimized by childhood sexual abuse. *Psychological Medicine, 27,* 951–959.

Temoshok, L., Heller, B. W., Sagebiel, R. W., Blois, M. S., Sweet, D. M., DiClemente, R. J., & Gold, M. L. (1985). The relationship of psychosocial factors to prognostic indicators in cutaneous malignant melanoma. *Journal of Psychosomatic Research, 29,* 139–153.

Theorell, T., Orth-Gomer, K., & Eneroth, P. (1990). Slow-reacting immunoglobulin in relation to social support and changes in job strain: A preliminary note. *Psychosomatic Medicine, 52,* 511–516.

Thomas, P. D., Goodwin, J. M., & Goodwin, J. S. (1985). Effect of social support on stress-related changes in cholesterol level, uric acid level, and immune function in an elderly sample. *American Journal of Psychiatry, 142,* 735–737.

Touitou, Y., Bogdan, A., Levi, F., Benavides, M., & Auzeby, A. (1996). Disruption of the circadian patterns of serum cortisol in breast and ovarian cancer patients: Relationships with tumour marker antigens. *British Journal of Cancer, 74,* 1248–1252.

Touitou, Y., Levi, F., Bogdan, A., Benavides, M., Bailleul, F., & Misset, J. L. (1995). Rhythm alteration in patients with metastatic breast cancer and poor prognostic factors. *Journal of Cancer Research and Clinical Oncology, 121,* 181–188.

Trinchieri, G. (1989). Biology of natural killer cells. *Advances in Immunology, 47,* 187–376.

Turner-Cobb, J. M., Sephton, S., Koopman, C., Blake-Mortimer, J., & Spiegel, D. (2000). Social support and salivary cortisol in women with metastatic breast cancer. *Psychosomatic Medicine, 62,* 337–345.

Turner Cobb, J. M., & Steptoe, A. (1996). Psychosocial stress and susceptibility to upper respiratory tract illness in an adult population sample. *Psychosomatic Medicine, 58,* 404–412.

Turner Cobb, J. M., & Steptoe, A. (1998). Psychosocial influences on upper respiratory infectious illness in children. *Journal of Psychosomatic Research, 45,* 319–330.

Uchino, B. N., Cacioppo, J. T., & Kiecolt-Glaser, J. K. (1996). The relationship between social support and physiological processes: A review with emphasis on underlying mechanisms and implications for health. *Psychological Bulletin, 119,* 488–531.

van der Pompe, G., Antoni, M. H., & Heijnen, C. J. (1996). Elevated basal cortisol levels and attenuated ACTH and cortisol responses to a behavioral challenge in women with metastatic breast cancer. *Psychoneuroendocrinology, 21,* 361–374.

van der Pompe, G., Duivenvoorden, H. J., Antoni, M. H., Visser, A., & Heijnen, C. J. (1997). Effectiveness of a short-term group psychotherapy program on endocrine and immune function in breast cancer patients: An exploratory study. *Journal of Psychosomatic Research, 42,* 453–466.

Van Rood, Y. R., Bogaards, M., Goulmy, E., & Houwelingen, H. C. (1993). The effects of stress and relaxation on the in vitro immune response in man: A meta-analytic study. *Journal of Behavioral Medicine, 16,* 163–181.

Vile, R., Cong, H., & Dorudi, S. (1996). The immunosurveillance of cancer: Specific and nonpecific mechanisms. In A. Dalgleish & M. Browning (Eds.), *Tumor immunology.* Cambridge: Cambridge University Press.

Vogel, W., & Bower, D. (1991). Stress, Immunity and Cancer. In N. Plotnikoff, A. Murgo, R. Faith, & J. Wybran (Eds.), *Stress and immunity.* Boca Raton: CRC Press.

Vujanovic, N. L., Yasumura, S., Hirabayashi, H., Lin, W. C., Watkins, S., Herberman, R. B., & Whiteside, T. L. (1995). Antitumor activities of subsets of human IL-2-activated natural killer cells in solid tissues. *Journal of Immunology, 154,* 281–289.

Waxler-Morrison, N., Hislop, T. G., Mears, B., & Kan, L. (1991). Effects of social relationships on survival for women with breast cancer: A prospective study. *Social Science and Medicine, 33,* 177–183.

White, M. H. (1993). Prevention of infection in patients with neoplastic disease: Use of a historical model for developmental strategies. *Clinical Infectious Diseases, 17,* S355–S358.

Whiteside, T. L., & Herberman, R. B. (1994). Role of human natural killer cells in health and disease. *Clinical and Diagnostic Laboratory Immunology, 1,* 125–133.

Whiteside, T. L., & Herberman, R. B. (1995). The role of natural killer cells in immune surveillance of cancer. *Current Opinions in Immunology, 7,* 704–710.

Wood, P. A., & Hrushesky, W. J. (1995). Biological perspectives on circadian cancer therapy. *Journal of Infusional Chemotherapy, 5,* 182–190.

Yehuda, R., Boisoneau, D., Lowy, M. T., & Giller, E. L., Jr. (1995). Dose-response changes in plasma cortisol and lymphocyte glucocorticoid receptors following dexamethasone administration in combat veterans with and without posttraumatic stress disorder. *Archives of General Psychiatry, 52,* 583–593.

Yehuda, R., Resnick, H., Kahana, B., & Giller, E. L. (1993). Long-lasting hormonal alterations to extreme stress in humans: Normative or maladaptive? *Psychosomatic Medicine, 55,* 287–297.

Yehuda, R., Teicher, M. H., Levengood, R. A., Trestman, R. L., & Siever, L. J. (1994). Circadian regulation of basal cortisol levels in posttraumatic stress disorder. *Annals of the New York Academy of Sciences, 746,* 378–380.

Yehuda, R., Teicher, M. H., Trestman, R. L., & Levengood, R. A. (1996). Cortisol regulation in posttraumatic stress disorder and major depression: A chronobiological analysis. *Biological Psychiatry, 40,* 79–88.

# 61

# Psychosocial Influences on the Progression of HIV Infection

STEVE W. COLE, MARGARET E. KEMENY

## I. INTRODUCTION

Infection with human immunodeficiency virus type 1 (HIV-1) has a highly variable course, with some infected individuals remaining asymptomatic for many years and others quickly progressing to full-blown AIDS (Munoz et al., 1989; Phair et al., 1992; Sheppard et al., 1993). Some of the variables believed to underlie differential HIV progression rates include the specific viral strains contracted (Koot et al., 1993; Levy, 1993), genetic characteristics of the host immune system (e.g., the host's HLA genotype and mutations in the chemokine receptor system mediating viral infection) (Roger, 1998; Winkler et al., 1998), demographic characteristics such as age and gender (Melnick et al., 1994; Phillips et al., 1991; Saah et al., 1994), drug abuse (Munoz et al., 1988), malnutrition (Abrams, Duncan, & Hertz-Picciotto, 1993; Baum et al., 1995; Guenter et al., 1993), and coinfections with other pathogens (Bentwich, Kalinkovich, & Weisman, 1995; Lusso & Gallo, 1995; Webster et al.,

1989). However, these factors cannot fully explain the variability in HIV disease progression and a great deal of research has focused on identifying other potential cofactors. As reviewed in other chapters of this volume, a substantial body of research has shown that the nervous and endocrine systems can modulate various aspects of immune system function including leukocyte traffic and localization, antigen processing and presentation, cellular activation, and effector functions such as antibody production and cellular cytotoxicity. Such relationships raise the possibility that psychosocial characteristics of the host could conceivably influence the rate of HIV progression by modulating immunologic processes that support HIV pathogenesis, by modulating anti-HIV immune responses, or by modulating immunologic resistance to the opportunistic infections and neoplasms that result in clinical AIDS. In this Chapter, we survey evidence on the possibility that psychobiologic factors might influence the progress of HIV infection. We begin by summarizing the basic biological processes underlying HIV disease progression and then review evidence that neurophysiologic processes can influence some of these parameters. To evaluate the relevance of such findings for HIV infection *in vivo*, we survey existing studies linking psychosocial factors to HIV progression. We conclude by highlighting some of the methodological obstacles that make it difficult to evaluate the role of psychobiologic factors in HIV infection, and we highlight some promising areas for future inquiry.

## II. HIV PATHOGENESIS

### A. Acute Infection

HIV infection typically spreads via transfer of free virions or infected lymphocytes in blood or genital fluids. Upon entry into a new host, HIV virions bind to cells expressing the CD4 surface protein (mainly monocytes/macrophages and CD4+ T lymphocytes; Dalgleish et al., 1984; Ho, Rota, & Hirsch, 1986) via gp120, a glycoprotein expressed on the HIV viral envelope. The presence of additional coreceptors (e.g., the chemokine receptors CCR5 or CXCR4) permits the HIV viral envelope to fuse with the host cell membrane (Choe et al., 1996; Deng et al., 1996; Dragic et al., 1996; Feng, Broder, Kennedy, & Berger, 1996). Following fusion, viral RNA is released into the host cell cytoplasm where it begins reverse transcription into proviral DNA. Upon activation of the host cell (e.g., in CD4+ T lymphocytes, via engagement of the T-cell receptor and costimulatory molecules), reverse transcription proceeds to completion and the HIV provirus migrates to the nucleus and integrates into the host cell chromosome. Once integrated, transcription of viral genes is activated by some of the same DNA-binding proteins that regulate normal cellular function (e.g., the Sp1 and NF-$\kappa$B transcription factors) (Garcia & Gaynor, 1994; Nabel & Baltimore, 1987). Following transcription and translation, viral RNA and core proteins associate with viral envelope proteins at the plasma membrane, and a mature virion forms by budding from the cell surface.

HIV infection spreads quickly among CD4+ cells in part because HIV replicates rapidly (Ho et al., 1995; Perelson, Neumann, Markowitz, Leonard, & Ho, 1996; Wei et al., 1995). As a result, circulating levels of virus and the infected fraction of CD4+ T lymphocytes climb markedly within 3 to 6 weeks of initial infection while the total number of circulating CD4+ T lymphocytes shows a limited decline (Pantaleo, Graziosi & Fauci, 1993). The host immune system typically mounts a significant antiviral response marked by generalized immunologic activation, an increase in CD8+ T lymphocyte numbers and activation (Cossarizza et al., 1995; Pantaleo et al., 1994), production of HIV-specific antibodies, and HIV-specific cellular cytotoxicity (Borrow, Lewicki, Hahn, Shaw, & Oldstone, 1994). The immune system also generates soluble factors that downregulate HIV replication without destroying HIV-infected cells (Levy, Mackewicz, & Barker, 1996). This acute antiviral response is often accompanied by a mononucleosis-like syndrome of clinical symptoms (including fever, malaise, head and muscle aches, sore throat, skin rash, swollen lymph nodes, nausea, and diarrhea (Cooper et al., 1985; Kaslow et al., 1987)) that often resolves within 2–4 weeks. Presumably as a result of the acute antiviral response, circulating levels of free virus and virally infected cells often drop dramatically between 6 and 12 weeks after infection (Borrow et al., 1994; Graziosi, 1993; Pitak et al., 1993). Mildly elevated CD8+ T-lymphocyte levels and anti-HIV effector functions typically persist, and circulating CD4+ T-lymphocyte levels may remain stable, plunge dramatically, or decline slowly over time (Detels et al., 1988; Lang, 1989; Margolick et al., 1993).

### B. Clinical Latency

Following the "acute seroconversion reaction" associated with primary infection, an HIV-infected individual may remain healthy for many years (median time to AIDS is approximately 10 years) (Munoz et al., 1989). In some cases, this "clinical latency period" (also known as CDC Category A HIV infection) (Centers for Disease Control, 1992) is accompanied by minor symptomatology (e.g., fatigue, fever, diffuse aches, night sweats, diarrhea, and thrush, which define CDC Category B HIV infection) that often resolves spontaneously or following symptomatic treatment (Kaslow et al., 1987). Despite the absence of serious clinical symptoms and the low levels of HIV in circulating blood, HIV continues to replicate rapidly in lymph nodes and other lymphoid organs (Embertson et al., 1993; Pantaleo et al., 1993). However, follicular dendritic cells (FDCs) appear to trap many free HIV virions before they leave lymphoid tissues and newly infected cells often remain sequestered in lymphatic organs following infection, producing marked lymphadenopathy (Embertson et al., 1993; Pantaleo, Graziosi, & Fauci, 1993). Because lymphoid tissues represent the primary site of HIV replication, biological parameters in circulating blood (e.g., plasma viral load, CD4+ T lymphocyte levels) may provide less accurate information about disease pathogenesis and progression than would more direct measures of virologic and immunologic activity in lymphoid tissues (e.g., *in situ* measures based on tissue biopsy). The lymphoid microenvironment sustains significant damage during clinical latency and its progressive deterioration eventually results in heightened plasma viremia and greater circulation of HIV-infected cells. Disruption of the lymphoid microenvironment may also contribute to the progressive immunodysregulation that begins during the earliest states of infection (Frost & McLean, 1994; Heeney, 1995; Helbert, L'age-Stehr, & Mitchison, 1993).

Even during its clinically latent period, HIV infection can alter the function of a variety of physiologic systems. Migration of HIV-infected cells (particularly monocytes/macrophages) to the brain and other organs may blunt and slow autonomic nervous system (ANS) responses (Cohen & Laudenslager, 1989; Kumar, Morgan, Szapocznik, & Eisdorfer, 1991), alter activity in the hypothalamo-pituitary-adrenal axis (HPA) and other neuroendocrine circuits (Grinspoon & Bilezikian, 1992; Membrino et al., 1987; Merinich, McDermott, Asp, Harrison, & Kidd, 1993; Villette et al., 1990), and induce mild cognitive impairments (Heaton et al., Atkinson, & Wallace, 1994) or, in the later stages of infection, frank dementia (Price et al., 1988). Sleep, nutrition, appetite, and metabolism are often altered as well (Darko, Mitler, & Henriksen, 1995; De Simone, Famularo, Cifone, & Mitsuya, 1996; Moldawer & Sattler, 1998; Mulligan & Bloch, 1998; Norman et al., 1992; Strawford & Hellerstein, 1998). In the immune system, alterations in cytokine production and cellular immune response appear early in HIV infection and increase significantly over time (Clerici et al., 1993; Fan, Bass, & Fahey, 1993; Graziosi et al., 1994; Israel-Biet et al., 1991; Mossman, 1994; Nakajima et al., 1989; Schroff, Gottlieb, Prince, Chai, & Fahey, 1983; Scott-Algara, Vuillier, Marasescu, De Saint Martin, & Dighiero, 1991; Von Sydow, Sonnerborg, Gaines, & Strannegard, 1991). Several aspects of hematopoiesis and humoral immune response are also affected, and HIV-infected individuals often contract fungal and bacterial infections that are normally well resisted (Levy, 1993; Pantaleo, Graziosi & Fauci, 1993). Leukocyte mobility and compartmentalization may also be altered (Pantaleo et al., 1993; Phillips et al., 1997; Ullum et al., 1994).

However, the most prominent immunologic alteration during Category A/B infection is a progressive decline in the level of circulating CD4+ T lymphocytes. The course of decline is quite variable (Detels et al., 1988; Lang et al., 1989; Margolick et al., 1993) and its basis is not fully understood. Possible mechanisms include death of infected cells, collateral damage to bystander cells during anti-HIV immune responses, dysregulation of hematopoietic homeostasis, and inflammation-induced redistribution of CD4+ T cells out of circulation and into lymphoid tissues. Even late in the course of infection, CD4+ T-cell levels rebound rapidly when viral replication is halted, suggesting that the immune system retains a substantial ability to replenish lost cells (Ho et al., 1995; Wei et al., 1995). Moreover, some of the most lethal strains of HIV are only weakly cytopathic to CD4+ T lymphocytes (Mosier, Gulizia, MacIsaac,

Torbett, & Levy, 1993). These observations suggest that CD4+ T-cell declines may stem from alterations in lymphoid homeostatic mechanisms rather than CD4+ T-cell death per se (Heeney, 1995; Rosenberg, Anderson, & Pabst, 1998; Wolthers, Schuitemaker, & Midema, 1998). Although the mechanisms responsible for declining CD4+ T-cell levels remain poorly understood, there is strong consensus that viral replication and de novo infection of CD4-bearing cells constitute the basic engine of HIV pathogenesis (Ho, 1996). Viral replication rates and plasma viral load represent the strongest biological predictors of clinical disease onset, although immunologic markers such as CD4+ T-cell levels and cellular activation markers can provide additional prognostic information (Fahey et al., 1990; Ho, 1996; Mellors et al., 1996). Exhaustion of anti-HIV cytotoxic lymphocyte responses may also play a role in precipitating AIDS onset (Effros & Pawelec, 1997). Biological markers of HIV progression are summarized in Table I.

## C. AIDS

As immune system function deteriorates, the body becomes vulnerable to a host of opportunistic infections and neoplastic diseases that constitute full-blown AIDS (also known as CDC Category C HIV infection) (Centers for Disease Control, 1992). Other factors that may influence AIDS onset include the

---

**TABLE I  Biological Parameters Associated with HIV Progression**

Indicators of disease progression[a]
  Increasing viral load (e.g., peripheral blood HIV RNA)
  Declining circulating CD4+ T lymphocyte level
  Increasing expression of cellular activation markers
    (e.g., HLA-DR, CD38)
  Increasing levels of serum activation markers
    (e.g., neopterin, $\beta_2$ microglobulin)
  Appearance of syncytium-inducing (T-cell-tropic) viral strains

Correlates of disease progression[b]
  Reduced cellular proliferation to recall antigens/mitogens
  Altered cytokine production (e.g., reduced IL-2 and IL-12,
    increased IL-6, IL-10, IFN-$\gamma$, and TNF-$\alpha$)
  Increased serum IgA and IgG levels
  Increased lymphocyte apoptosis
  Decreased telomere length in CD8+ T cells
  Reduced natural killer cell cytotoxicity
  Declining serum dehydroepiandosterone concentration

---

[a]Defined by increasing risk of AIDS onset or HIV-related mortality.

[b]Not conclusively validated as independent predictors of AIDS onset or HIV-related mortality, but associated with other biological indicators of disease progression.

host's age and gender (Melnick et al., 1994; Phillips et al., 1991; Saah et al., 1994), the presence of coinfections with other pathogens (e.g., helminths, HHV-6, and a recently identified herpes virus associated with Kapossi's Sarcoma) (Bentwich, Kalinkovich, & Weisman, 1995; Chang et al., 1994; Lusso & Gallo, 1995; Webster et al., 1989), and the particular AIDS-defining condition contracted. In the absence of effective antiretroviral therapy, AIDS is generally fatal (10th and 90th percentile survival times are 6 months and 3 years) (Saah et al., 1994). With the advent of powerful antiretroviral medications, AIDS onset can often be significantly delayed and partial immune reconstitution typically occurs following suppression of plasma virus titers (Autran et al., 1997; Li et al., 1998; Powderly, Landay, & Lederman, 1998). However, current antiretroviral therapies cannot fully eradicate HIV from latently infected cells (e.g., quiescent T lymphocytes) (Finzi et al., 1997). Because current antiretroviral molecules do not readily penetrate the blood-brain barrier, central nervous system (CNS) tissue may also represent an ongoing site of pathogenesis even when peripheral viral load is suppressed.

## III.  NEURO–IMMUNE INTERACTIONS AND HIV PATHOGENESIS

Psychological events can influence physiologic function through CNS control of the ANS and its innervation of a wide variety of peripheral tissue systems and through CNS control of circulating hormone and neuropeptide levels (e.g., cortisol, $\beta$-endorphin, growth hormone, and prolactin) (Chrousos & Gold, 1992; Cryer, 1980; Frankenhauser, 1975; Loewy & Spyer, 1990; Mason, 1975; Rose, 1980; Sapolsky, 1993; Weiner, 1992). The presence of sympathetic nervous system (SNS) neurons in the parenchyma of all primary and secondary lymphoid organs provides a microanatomic nexus for neural regulation of immune system function (Felten et al., 1987; Straub, Westermann, Scholmerich, & Falk, 1998). Because lymphoid organs represent the primary site of HIV pathogenesis, neuroimmune interactions in these sites could conceivably influence some of the most fundamental processes involved in HIV disease progression, including viral replication, anti-HIV immune responses, generalized immunologic responsiveness, and lymphoid tissue homeostasis and destruction. Stress-induced release of HPA and SNS neuromediators is known to influence viral disease pathogenesis in several in vivo animal models (Chang & Rasmussen, 1964, 1965; Friedman, Glasgow, &

Ader, 1969; Jensen & Rasmussen, 1963; Johnson, Lavender, Hultin, & Rasmussen, 1965; Padgett et al., 1998; Rasmussen, Marsh, & Brill, 1957; Sheridan et al., 1998; Yamada, Jensen, & Rasmussen, 1964). Whether similar effects occur in HIV infection remains unclear, in part because no good small animal model for HIV infection currently exists. However, in vitro studies have shown that neuroeffector molecules of both the HPA axis (e.g., glucocorticoids) and the SNS (e.g., norepinephrine) can influence HIV replication—the driving force behind clinical disease progression in vivo.

### A.  Hypothalamo-Pituitary-Adrenal Axis and HIV Pathogenesis

Markham, Salahuddin, Veren, Orndorff, and Gallo (1986) found a two- to fivefold increase in HIV replication when they added 5 μg/mL hydrocortisone to cultures of HIV-infected peripheral blood mononuclear cells (PBMC). These results occurred regardless of whether cells were isolated from HIV-infected patients or infected in vitro following isolation from normal donors. Because similar effects were not observed in purified T cells, Markham and colleagues proposed that glucocorticoids influence viral replication indirectly—perhaps by altering monocyte cytokine production which might subsequently regulate HIV expression by T cells. Consistent with this hypothesis, they showed that antibody neutralization of interferon (IFN)-$\alpha$ activity exerted a similar effect and subsequent addition of hydrocortisone had no further influence. Addition of human chorionic gonadotropin (10 μg/mL) and insulin (10 μg/mL) also increased viral replication, although less dramatically than did hydrocortisone. Soudeyns, Geleziunas, Shyamala, Hiscott, and Wainberg (1993) also found that dexamethasone and physiologic concentrations of cortisol could increase HIV replication in an acutely infected T-cell line. While these data suggest that glucocorticoids can regulate HIV replication in vitro, the mechanism of these effects remains poorly defined.

Some studies suggest that glucocorticoids can increase transcription of genes under control of the HIV-1 promoter (the viral long terminal repeat, or LTR) (Furth, Westphal, & Hennighausen, 1990; Spandidos, Zoumpourlis, Kotsinas, Tsiriyotis, & Sekeris, 1990), implying that glucocorticoids might increase HIV replication by upregulating viral gene expression. However, those studies were conducted using cell lines of a different lineage than those normally infected in vivo, and other studies using myeloid and lymphoid cell lines have documented significant suppressive effects of glucocorticoids on HIV-1 long terminal repeat (LTR)-driven transcription (Laurence, Sellers, & Sikder, 1989; Mitra, Sikder, & Laurence, 1993). These suppressive effects are consistent with a large body of data showing that pharmacologic concentrations of glucocorticoids can suppress activity of the NF-$\kappa$B transcription factor (Auphan, Didonato, Rosette, Helmberg, & Karin, 1995; Scheinman, Cogswell, Lofquist, & Baldwin, 1995), which plays a critical role in regulating cytokine production and enhancing HIV-1 replication (Nabel & Baltimore, 1987). It is unclear whether glucocorticoid suppression of HIV-1 gene expression occurs at physiologic concentrations and whether it is mediated by NF-$\kappa$B suppression or by other mechanisms (e.g., by blocking access of other DNA-binding proteins to the viral LTR) (Mitra, Sikder, & Laurence, 1995). Because all existing studies of glucocorticoid regulation of HIV gene expression utilize only an LTR-reporter gene construct, it is also unclear whether glucocorticoid influences on other aspects of the viral life cycle (e.g., infectivity, nuclear localization, reverse transcription, RNA stability/translation, virion assembly, etc.) might offset suppression of HIV gene expression.

Glucocorticoid effects on HIV replication could be mediated in part by alterations in host cell viability following HIV infection. HIV-infected T lymphocytes are particularly vulnerable to activation-induced cell death (apoptosis resulting from activation of the T-cell receptor in the absence of a costimulatory signal via, e.g., CD28). Lu et al. (1995) have shown that pharmacologic doses of prednisone or hydrocortisone can increase the resistance of HIV-infected T lymphocytes to activation-induced cell death in vitro. As a result, the survival of HIV-infected T cells was prolonged despite accompanying suppression of T-cell proliferation. These data were obtained from isolated T-cell cultures, and it is unclear whether similar effects might occur in the presence of costimulatory signals such as those delivered by antigen presenting cells in vivo. In contrast to Markham and colleagues, Lu and colleagues found no increase in HIV replication during glucocorticoid treatment. This difference may stem from greater suppression of cellular activation (which is required for HIV gene expression) in the later study's use of higher glucocorticoid doses (10–100 µg/mL) and apoptosis-inducing culture conditions (anti-CD3 stimulation in the absence of CD28 costimulation).

Another mechanism that may mediate effects of glucocorticoids on HIV replication involves regulation of the cell cycle and its effect on virus production. Virion production is enhanced in the $G_2$ phase of the cell cycle, and the HIV-encoded protein Vpr may enhance viral replication by arresting the cell cycle at this stage (Goh et al., 1998). Vpr appears to induce this effect by binding to the cytoplasmic glucocorticoid receptor and thereby suppressing the activity of NF-$\kappa$B (Ayyavoo, 1997). Ayyavoo and colleagues (1997) showed that both glucocorticoids and Vpr can suppress mitosis and activation-induced cell death in a manner that could be blocked by the glucocorticoid receptor antagonist RU486. No data on HIV production or cell cycle staging were reported, but this group's observation that HIV gene products activate the glucocorticoid signaling pathway suggests that exogenous glucocorticoids could conceivably foster viral replication (e.g., via cell cycle arrest) and exacerbate HIV-induced cytopathology. However, such speculation should be tempered by data showing that HIV-infected cells respond differently to exogenous glucocorticoids than do uninfected cells (e.g., in showing resistance to glucocorticoid-induced apoptosis and IFN-$\alpha$ suppression).

Clerici and colleagues have proposed that heightened cortisol production during HIV infection might alter cytokine production profiles in ways that enhance viral replication and suppress cell-mediated immune responses (Clerici et al., 1997; Vago, Clerici, & Norbiato, 1994). Significant alterations in cortisol levels are not consistently found during the asymptomatic phase of infection, but dysregulation of the HPA axis becomes more prominent following AIDS onset and several studies have documented reduced responsiveness to glucocorticoids in monocytes from AIDS patients (Kawa & Thompson, 1996; Norbiato, Bevilacqua, Vago, & Clerici, 1998; Norbiato, Galli, Righini, & Moroni, 1994). In such individuals, the affinity of the monocyte glucocorticoid receptor for its ligand is significantly diminished and exogenous glucocorticoids fail to suppress the production of IFN-$\alpha$ as they normally would. Thus regulatory interactions between the HPA axis and the immune system may be altered during HIV infection in ways that preserve anti-viral responses (IFN-$\alpha$ suppresses HIV replication). Other studies have linked glucocorticoid resistance in monocytes from HIV-infected donors to diverse alterations in cytokine production (Norbiato, Bevilacqua, Vago, Taddei, & Clerici, 1997), but none of these studies has correlated glucocorticoid resistance with viral replication rates or subsequent disease progression. Glucocorticoid resistance has only been observed in patients with advanced disease, and there is little direct evidence that glucocorticoid regulation of cytokine production can influence HIV pathogenesis during the protracted clinical latency period.

Glucocorticoids may regulate HIV pathogenesis through a variety of more speculative mechanisms. For example, glucocorticoids can synergize with HIV protein constructs to suppress natural killer (NK)-mediated cytotoxicity (Nair, Saravolatz, & Schwartz, 1995; Nair & Schwartz, 1995), suggesting that HPA activation could indirectly speed disease progression by hampering immune responses to other pathogens. Pharmacologic glucocorticoid concentrations can significantly alter lymphocyte localization (Cupps & Fauci, 1982), raising the possibility that HPA activation might accelerate traffic through lymphoid organs and thus accelerate de novo infection. Glucocorticoids also influence thymopoiesis (Jondal, Xue, McConkey, & Okret, 1995; Vacchio, Ashwell, & King, 1998), raising the possibility that HPA activation might contribute to the dysregulation of T-cell homeostasis and replenishment. However, no data indicate whether such dynamics actually occur during HIV infection.

A small number of studies have examined the effects of pharmacologic glucocorticoids on HIV disease progression. In three of four such studies reviewed by Laurence, Sellers, and Sikder (1989), progression to AIDS was accelerated during prednisone therapy for idiopathic thrombocytopenia. Similar observations have been reported by other groups (Pedersen, Nielsen, Dickmeis, & Jordal, 1989; Shafer et al., 1985). Andrieu, Lu, and Levy (1995) reported no significant changes in serum HIV RNA levels during a 1-year trial of prednisolone in 44 asymptomatic HIV+ individuals. However, it is difficult to draw clear conclusions from any of these studies because they are all plagued by the presence of confounding variables (e.g., concurrent splenectomy), limited sample sizes, insufficient follow-up duration, and a focus on selected patient subpopulations (e.g., those suffering from thrombocytopenia). Thus little is known about the effects of pharmacologic glucocorticoids on HIV disease progression in general, and even less is known about their influence at the physiologic concentrations relevant to psychosocial processes. Although several studies have examined cross-sectional correlations between endogenous glucocorticoid levels and immunologic indices of HIV progression, we are not aware of any that report a prospective prediction of HIV progression from individual differences in HPA axis activity during the asymptomatic period of infection.

## B. Sympathetic Nervous System and HIV Pathogenesis

Cole, Korin, Fahey, and Zack (1998) found that the SNS neuroeffector molecule norepinephrine could increase HIV replication by 5- to 10-fold in PBMC infected in vitro with a T-cell-tropic strain of HIV-1. Norepinephrine's effects were dose dependent between $10^{-8}$ and $10^{-5}$ M and were mediated by $\beta_2$-adrenoreceptor activation of the adenylyl cyclase-cAMP–protein kinase A (PKA) signaling cascade. PKA-induced suppression of interleukin (IL)-10 and IFN-$\gamma$ appeared to mediate the effects of norepinephrine since addition of either exogenous IL-10 or IFN-$\gamma$ blocked norepinephrine's enhancement of HIV replication.

In subsequent work (Cole, Jamieson, & Zack, 1999), this group also showed that norepinephrine and other cAMP-inducing ligands can significantly upregulate lymphocyte cell surface expression of CXCR4—the chemokine receptor mediating infection by T-cell-tropic strains of HIV-1. Norepinephrine-induced increases in CXCR4 expression rendered T lymphocytes significantly more vulnerable to infection by T-cell-tropic HIV-1. Norepinephrine-induced upregulation also enhanced CXCR4's physiologic function as a mediator of chemotaxis in response to SDF-1, suggesting one molecular mechanism by which the nervous system may regulate lymphocyte traffic and localization. In contrast to cAMP-inducing ligands' enhancement of CXCR4 expression on lymphocytes, cAMP signaling significantly suppressed CXCR4 expression on CD14+ cells (monocyte/macrophages). Thivierge, Le Gouill, Tremblay, Stankova, and Rola-Pleszczynski (1998) reported a similar suppressive effect of cAMP signaling on macrophage expression of CCR5—the chemokine receptor mediating infection by macrophage-tropic strains of HIV-1. This group showed that cAMP signaling could significantly suppress vulnerability to infection by CCR5-tropic strains of HIV-1. Thus differential regulation of chemokine receptors on lymphoid vs. myeloid cells by norepinephrine and other cAMP-inducing agents may simultaneously reduce vulnerability to infection by macrophage-tropic HIV while promoting vulnerability to T-cell-tropic viral strains. Differential effects cAMP on lymphoid vs. myeloid chemokine receptor expression may also have implications for nervous system regulation of immune responses via altered localization of distinct leukocyte subsets.

Without focusing on SNS neurotransmitters per se, several other groups have shown that activation of the cAMP–PKA system can accelerate HIV replication in lymphoid and myeloid cell lines (Chowdhury et al., 1993; Nokta & Pollard, 1992). Although these studies did not identify the mechanism of cAMP's effects, others have shown that cAMP can increase the expression of genes under control of the HIV-1 LTR (Krebs, Mehrens, Pomeroy, Goodenow, & Wigdahl, 1998; Rabbi, Al-Harthi, & Roebuck, 1997; Rabbi, Al-Harthi, Saifuddin, & Roebuck, 1998; Rabbi, Saifuddin,

Gu, Kagnoff, & Roebuck, 1997; Schwartz, Canonne-Hergaux, Aunis, & Schaeffer, 1997). Basal cAMP activity appears to be required for HIV replication (Gibellini et al., 1998; Lapointe, Lemieux, Olivier, & Darveau, 1996) and HIV infection itself increases cellular cAMP–PKA activity above basal levels (Haraguchi, Good, & Day, 1995; Hofmann, Nishanian, Nguyen, Insixiengmay, & Fahey, 1993b; Hofmann, Nishanian, Nguyen, Liu, & Fahey, 1993a; Nokta & Pollard, 1991; Rabbi et al., 1997). HIV-induced cAMP activity appears to contribute to some of the functional deficits observed in infected lymphocytes, including impaired proliferation and IL-2 suppression (Aanadahl et al., 1998; Hofmann et al., 1993a, b). As a result, activation of cellular signaling pathways that inhibit cAMP activity (e.g., the type 1A serotonin receptor) can significantly improve the function of HIV-infected lymphocytes in vitro (Eugen-Olsen et al., 1997). Suppression of HIV-induced cAMP activity can also repair functional deficits in infected monocytes (Thomas et al., 1997). However, no studies have determined whether exogenous cAMP inducers such as SNS catecholamines might exacerbate the functional deficits induced by HIV activation of the cAMP–PKA system.

To determine the in vivo relevance of HIV-induced cAMP activation, Hoffman et al. (1996) administered a single dose of the cAMP-suppressing serotonin receptor agonist buspirone to 10 asymptomatic HIV+ individuals and documented a small transient increase in circulating CD4+ T cells and a decrease in serum HIV RNA levels. Over the course of a subsequent 6-week trial of buspirone in 9 asymptomatic HIV+ individuals, this group found a similar transient increase in CD4+ T-cell levels accompanied by an unexpected increase in plasma HIV-1 RNA levels that reversed upon drug discontinuation. This paradoxical increase in circulating viral load may have resulted from buspirone's unanticipated enhancement of cAMP levels in circulating lymphocytes. Although buspirone clearly does not represent an effective antiviral intervention, the association between paradoxical increases in cAMP and increased viral load is consistent with the hypothesis that cAMP upregulates HIV replication. However, no studies have directly explored the possibility that cAMP signaling induced by SNS catecholamines might influence clinical HIV disease progression.

## C. Other Neurally Regulated Messengers and HIV Pathogenesis

The HPA and ANS represent the most commonly studied pathways for transmitting the effects of psychological events to peripheral physiologic systems, but a wide variety of other hormones and neuroeffector molecules can also be influenced by psychosocial stimuli (Sapolsky, 1993; Weiner, 1992) and some of these factors could conceivably influence HIV pathogenesis as well. For example, Ho et al. (1996) found that the neuropeptide substance P could accelerate HIV replication by two- to eightfold in monocyte-derived macrophages isolated from some (but not all) healthy donors. Covas, Pinto, and Victorine (1994) found that in contrast to its normal effect of enhancing lymphocyte proliferation, substance P suppressed lymphocyte proliferation in HIV-infected PBMC. Laurence et al. (1992) found that pharmacologic levels of human growth hormone could significantly accelerate HIV replication in acutely infected PBMC—an effect that was correlated with increased DNA synthesis and TNF-$\alpha$ secretion. However, short-term clinical studies of recombinant human growth hormone as a treatment for HIV-induced wasting have failed to identify any significant effect on disease progression (e.g., Schambelan et al., 1996).

Reproductive endocrines are sensitive to psychosocial influences (Sapolsky, 1993; Weiner, 1992) and several groups have examined the effects of estrogen and progesterone on HIV replication. Bourinbaiar, Nagorny, and Tan (1992) found that physiologic concentrations of these steroids inhibited HIV-1 expression in a chronically infected monocytic cell line but not in a chronically infected lymphoid cell line. In a different system, Laurence et al. (1990) showed that preincubation of a chronically infected promonocytic cell line with the anti-estrogen tamoxifen prevented subsequent upregulation of HIV-1 expression by protein kinase C (PKC)-inducing stimuli. This group also showed that tamoxifen could block PKC induction of HIV-1 LTR transcriptional activity. Lee et al. (1997) found a small enhancing effect of estrogen on HIV expression in a chronically infected myeloid cell line. These inconsistent results may stem from the use of different cell lines and activation conditions, or from proliferation suppressing vs. nonsuppressing steroid concentrations. Lee et al. (1997) also found no effect of progesterone on HIV-1 expression in myeloid cells, but they did show that progesterone potentiated the HIV-suppressive effects of AZT. These effects were correlated with downregulation of HIV-1 LTR-driven gene expression. Thus reproductive hormones may influence HIV replication in cells of the monocyte/macrophage lineage, although there is little evidence that these effects occur in primary PBMC. No published studies have documented the relevance of such effects for clinical disease progression in vivo.

Adrenal androgens have also been examined as a potential influence on HIV pathogenesis, particularly following the discovery that levels of dehydroepiandosterone (DHEA) and its sulfate derivative (DHEA-S) decline profoundly over the course of clinical HIV disease progression (Centurelli and Abate, 1997). Henderson, Yang and Schwartz (1992) showed that DHEA could modestly suppress HIV replication in PBMC infected in vitro with a macrophage-tropic strain of HIV-1. The same group subsequently demonstrated suppressive effects of DHEA on HIV-1 expression in a latently infected T-cell line (Yang, Schwartz, & Henderson, 1993) and suppressive effects on the replication of clinical HIV isolates in vitro (Yang, Schwartz, & Henderson, 1994). The only published study of DHEA treatment in vivo failed to demonstrate any significant effect on HIV disease progression (Dyner et al., 1993), although the limited sample size and follow-up duration in this trial would hamper identification of any effect that actually existed.

## D. Mechanisms of Neuroimmune Influences on HIV Pathogenesis

As outlined above, a variety of neuromediators could conceivably influence HIV pathogenesis if released in physiologically significant quantities at appropriate tissue sites (e.g., in lymphoid organs). Potential mechanisms of such effects include alterations in (1) vulnerability to de novo infection (e.g., via altered cell surface receptor expression and altered leukocyte traffic and localization), (2) cellular activation and cell cycle progression (e.g., via modulation of activation processes necessary for HIV expression or arrest of the cell cycle in phases favoring HIV production), (3) cytokine production (e.g., modulation of HIV-suppressing cytokines such as IFN-$\alpha$, IFN-$\gamma$, and IL-10, or HIV-enhancing cytokines such as TNF-$\alpha$), (4) HIV gene transcription (e.g., interactions between cellular DNA-binding proteins and the HIV-1 LTR), (5) HIV protein expression, virion production, and virion content (e.g., regulation of active kinase molecules incorporated into virions), (6) host cell survival (e.g., regulation of activation-induced cell death), (7) immunologic responses to HIV-1 infected cells (e.g., via alterations in cellular cytotoxicity or production of soluble suppressor factors), (8) immunologic responses to other pathogens, the activity of which may accelerate HIV pathogenesis (Rosenberg & Fauci, 1989), and (9) immunologic responses to opportunistic pathogens underlying AIDS onset. Although several of these interactions are supported by in vitro data, it remains unclear whether such interactions actually influence HIV progression in vivo. One way of gauging the potential relevance of neuroimmune interactions in HIV infection involves examining the relationship between indicators of disease progression and psychosocial characteristics that may affect the function of the nervous and endocrine systems in vivo.

## IV. PSYCHOSOCIAL CHARACTERISTICS AND HIV PROGRESSION

Over 50 published studies have examined relationships between psychosocial characteristics and HIV progression. These studies vary widely in the psychosocial factors considered, in design and methodological rigor, and in the indicators of HIV progression examined. The present review organizes findings by the type of psychosocial characteristic examined (e.g., life stress, social support, depression, behavioral inhibition). The majority of these studies are prospective natural history analyses in which potential psychosocial cofactors are identified on the basis of their ability to prospectively predict changes in disease status over time. A number of methodological issues qualify the extent to which either negative or positive results from natural history studies can be interpreted as evidence that a given characteristic influences HIV progression. Following this general review, we examine some of these methodologic issues and resummarize current evidence on the basis of studies meeting a core set of methodologic criteria.

## A. Stress and Coping

### 1. Stressful Life Experiences

Events that dramatically alter an individual's life circumstances (e.g., natural disasters, bereavement, divorce, disemployment, disability) are often associated with alterations in neuroendocrine and SNS function, increased risk of morbidity, and in some cases, increased risk of mortality. However, physiologic responses are heavily dependent upon the individual's subjective psychological response to the event (Mason, 1975; Sapolsky, 1993; Weiner, 1992). Few studies measuring only the objective incidence of negative life events have found any association with HIV progression. Kessler et al. (1991) found no correlation between the frequency of negative life events and symptom onset among several hundred initially asymptomatic HIV+ gay men followed over 2 years. In a 12-month study of a heterogeneous sample of initially asymptomatic HIV+ men and women,

Perry, Fishman, Jacobsberg, and Frances (1992) found no relationship between the frequency of negative life events and CD4+ T-cell declines. Rabkin et al. (1991) also found no relationship between the number of negative life events and 6-month changes in CD4+ T-cell levels among 124 HIV+ gay men. In a small sample ($n = 11$) of asymptomatic gay men, Goodkin, Fuchs, Feaster, Leeka, and Rishel (1992) did find a relationship between negative life event frequency and concurrent CD4+ and total lymphocyte levels. In a larger sample of asymptomatic HIV+ gay men, Evans, Leserman, Perkins, Stern, Murphy, and Tamul (1995) employed a sophisticated interview methodology (the Life Events and Difficulty Survey (LEDS); Brown & Harris, 1978) and found that a 6-month history of negative life events was associated with concurrent reductions in CD8+ CD57+ cytotoxic T-cell levels. Using the same measure, Leserman et al. (1997) studied 66 HIV+ gay men and found that the presence of severe stress over a 1- to 2-year period was associated with lower CD8+ T-lymphocyte and NK-cell levels at the end of the study period. However, in none of the later three studies did measures of stressful life events predict *changes* in immunologic measures over time. In a study of 63 HIV+ men with a known date of seroconversion, Patterson et al. (1995) did find that the simultaneous absence of both severe stress (measured by LEDS) and depression was associated with more favorable changes in CD4+ T lymphocyte and $\beta_2$ microglobulin levels over a 6-month period. In all LEDS-based studies, stressors were eliminated if they might have been caused by disease progression itself. In a study of 24 HIV+ children, Moss, Bose, Wolters, and Brouwers (1998) found that death during a 1-year follow-up period was associated with parental reports of more negative life events during the 6 months preceding baseline assessment. However, some of the life events measured may have been a product of differential disease progression, leaving the causal relationship between stress and HIV progression unclear.

One particular form of stress often experienced by HIV-seropositive individuals is the AIDS-related death of a close friend or intimate partner (Martin & Dean, 1993). Bereavement has long been known to be associated with significant alterations in immune function (Bartrop et al., 1977; Irwin, Daniels, Smith, Bloom, & Weiner, 1987; Schleifer, Keller, Camerino, Thronton, & Stein, 1983) and a heightened risk of morbidity and mortality (particularly within the 6–12 months following a loss) (Stroebe & Stroebe, 1983). Studies by both Kessler and colleagues (1991) (with 2 years of follow-up) and Perry and colleagues (1992)

(12 months of follow-up) found no relationship between the occurrence of AIDS diagnosis or death in one's social network and subsequent risk of symptom onset or CD4+ T-cell declines. On a variety of immunologic measures, Kemeny et al. (1994) also found no cross-sectional difference between 45 gay men who experienced repeated bereavement of close friends and a matched group suffering no such losses. However, this group did find that bereavement of an intimate partner was associated with pre to postbereavement increases in serum neopterin levels and reductions in mitogen-induced lymphoproliferation in 39 HIV seropositive gay men compared to a matched group of nonbereaved individuals (Kemeny 1995). No differential changes in CD4+ T-cell levels were observed. Results from another study of 85 HIV-seropositive gay men did indicate that death of a close friend or partner early in the AIDS epidemic was associated with a greater decline in CD4+ T-cell levels over a 3- to 4-year follow-up (Kemeny & Dean, 1995). This study found no differences in AIDS onset or HIV-related mortality as a function of bereavement.

Among currently available studies, no research indicates that increased exposure to generalized stressful life events is associated with differential changes in HIV-relevant immunologic parameters, but several studies have documented detrimental changes in HIV-relevant immunologic parameters among bereaved individuals. It remains unclear whether bereavement-related changes in immunologic status would increase vulnerability to clinical outcomes such as AIDS onset or mortality.

### 2. Coping Responses to Stressful Events

Although little evidence supports an association between generic negative life events and HIV progression, analyses focusing on *psychological reactions* to *specific, highly significant* negative events have identified relationships with immunologic and clinical indices of HIV progression. Several studies suggest that specific types of psychological reaction to bereavement may be associated with differential HIV progression. In two studies by Kemeny et al. (1994, 1995), immunologic measures correlated significantly with levels of depressed mood in the nonbereaved group, but not in the bereaved group. These researchers suggested that the immunologic correlates of bereavement-induced dysphoria may differ from those associated with depression. Consistent with this hypothesis, Kemeny et al. (1994) found that measures of grief, uncomplicated by depression, predicted positive immunologic changes (e.g., reductions in immune activation) over a 2- to 3-year period in a group of bereaved seropositive gay men. In another study of bereaved HIV-seropositive gay men, Kemeny and Dean (1995) distinguished loss-related grief (e.g., intrusive thoughts of the deceased) from depression (sleep disturbance, confusion, hopelessness, and self-reproach) and found that only the self-reproach aspect of depression predicted declining CD4+ T-cell levels over the course of a 2- to 3-year follow-up. Additional evidence linking self-reproach to CD4+ T cell declines comes from a study in which Segerstrom, Kemeny, Taylor, and Reed (1996) coded stress and coping interviews with 86 HIV-seropositive gay men for attributional style. Once depressed mood was controlled, attributions that involved blaming ones' own characteristics for negative events predicted CD4+ T cell declines over an 18-month follow-up.

A growing literature indicates that confronting significant traumas such as bereavement or the threat of mortality can produce psychological benefits. In a study examining psychological responses to bereavement among asymptomatic HIV+ gay men, cognitive processing of the experience was associated with "finding meaning" or a shift in values and priorities as a result of the experience. Those who engaged in cognitive processing and "found meaning" experienced a slower decline in CD4+ T cell levels over 2–3 years and a higher survival rate over 4–9 years (Bower, Kemeny, Taylor, & Fahey, 1998).

In a controlled clinical trial, Goodkin et al. (1998) randomly assigned 74 HIV+, recently bereaved gay men to either a 10-week bereavement support group focusing on grief resolution and stress management or a standard of care control condition. Over a 6-month follow-up, control participants showed declining CD4+ T lymphocyte levels, increasing serum cortisol levels, and increasing health care utilization, while support group-treated individuals showed stable CD4+ T cell levels, serum cortisol declines, and unchanged health care utilization. Increasing cortisol levels were correlated with CD4+ T cell declines, suggesting that altered HPA axis function might mediate the immunologic effects of the intervention.

### 3. Coping, Expectations, and Responses to HIV Infection

HIV infection itself represents a powerful psychological stressor, and several studies have identified relationships between psychological responses to HIV infection and clinical and immunologic indicators of disease progression. In two separate studies of asymptomatic gay men, Goodkin and colleagues

found that an active coping response to HIV infection was associated with higher concurrent CD4+ T-lymphocyte levels (in a sample of 11) (Goodkin et al., 1992) and concurrent NK cytotoxicity (in a sample of 62) (Goodkin et al., 1990). Solano et al. (1993) found that "fighting spirit" was associated with reduced progression to AIDS over a 12-month follow-up among a heterogeneous group of 101 seropositive individuals. Mulder, Antoni, Duivenvoorden, Kauffmann, and Goodkin (1995) found similar results in a study of 51 HIV+ gay men, with those reporting more a more active coping response to HIV infection showing less progression in CDC disease stage over a 1-year follow-up (although CD4+ T-cell changes were not associated with active coping). Ironson et al. (1994) measured psychological reactions to notification of HIV serostatus in 23 HIV-seropositive gay men and found increasing denial to be associated with declining CD4+ T cell levels and a heightened risk of progression to AIDS over a 2-year follow-up.

In a series of studies exploring the health correlates of HIV-specific appraisal processes, Reed and colleagues have examined negative expectancies about HIV disease progression. In one study of 74 gay men with AIDS, Reed, Kemeny, Taylor, Wang, and Visscher (1994) documented reduced survival times among individuals with the most negative expectancies about future health. The shortest survival times occurred among those who had negative expectancies and had been bereaved during the previous year. In a second study following 75 initially asymptomatic HIV-seropositive gay men for 2.5–3.5 years, Reed, Kemeny, Taylor, and Visscher (1998) also found a heightened rate of symptom onset among bereaved individuals with negative expectancies. In a third study, Kemeny et al. (1998) documented a similar bereavement-related association between negative expectancies about future health and accelerated declines in CD4+ T lymphocyte levels, reductions in lymphoproliferation, and elevated serum activation markers during a 2- to 3-year follow-up of 127 AIDS-free seropositive gay men.

Appraisals of one's own role in HIV infection have also been examined as potential correlates of disease progression. Segerstrom and colleagues (1996) found that blaming one's self for the occurrence of HIV-related negative events (e.g., infection, disease progression, or bereavement) was associated with greater 18-month CD4+ T cell declines in 86 gay men in various stages of infection (although no differences in AIDS onset were observed). Self-blame was also associated with accelerated CD4+ T-lymphocyte declines in a separate sample of bereaved HIV+ gay men (Kemeny & Dean, 1995). Differences in generalized mood or coping processes did not account for the effects of self-blame in either study. A subsequent examination of 137 HIV+ gay men demonstrated that persistent feelings of HIV-specific shame and guilt over a 1-year period were associated with declining CD4+ T-lymphocyte levels, AIDS onset, and HIV mortality over a 7-year follow-up (Weitzman, Kemeny, Taylor, & Fahey, 1998). Thus, the self-related emotions of shame and guilt may explain the relationship between self-blame and HIV progression. Overall, the data from several prospective natural history studies indicate that passive forms of coping, negative expectancies about disease progression, and self-blame in the context of HIV infection are associated with both immunologic and clinical indicators of HIV disease progression.

Several experimental studies have examined the immunologic impact of psychological interventions designed to help participants cope with the stress of HIV infection. Three studies have evaluated interventions focusing primarily on relaxation. Coates, McKusick, Kuno, and Stites (1989) found no effects of 8 weeks of relaxation training on a variety of immunologic parameters measured in 64 gay men (including CD4+ T-cell levels, NK cytotoxicity, proliferative responses to mitogens and recall antigens, and serum IgA levels). However, using a very similar approach, Eller (1995) found that 6 weeks of progressive muscle relaxation (relative to control and guided imagery conditions) reduced depression and increased CD4+ T-cell levels in 69 gay men at all stages of disease. Audiotape-guided relaxation exercises were conducted daily in participants' homes, and there was no contact between participants. Taylor (1995) randomly assigned 10 asymptomatic seropositive men to either a no-treatment control group or 10 weeks of biofeedback, relaxation training, meditation, and hypnosis. At a 1-month follow-up, the 5 treated individuals showed significant increases in CD4+ T-cell levels and significant reductions in negative affect relative to controls.

Two sets of investigators have examined the effects of more comprehensive intervention strategies. In a study of 47 asymptomatic gay men, Antoni et al. (1991) found that 10 weeks of cognitive–behavioral stress-management training (vs. aerobic exercise and nontreated controls) buffered depressive responses and increased CD4+ T-lymphocyte and NK-cell levels following the notification of HIV-seropositive serostatus. Further analyses of this experiment by Esterling et al. (1992) also demonstrated reductions in antibody titers to Epstein–Barr Virus (EBV) and HHV-6 (indicating more effective cellular control of viral replication). A follow-up to this study also showed that participants who completed the stress management intervention experienced less pronounced declines in CD4+ T-lymphocyte levels and a reduced risk of progression to AIDS over a 2-year period (Ironson et al., 1994). In a subsequent study of 26 symptomatic HIV+ gay men, the same group found that a cognitive behavioral stress management intervention produced significant decreases in HSV-2 antibody titers over the 10-week intervention period (Lutgendorf et al., 1997). Changes in depression were correlated with changes in HSV-2 antibody titer, suggesting that the intervention's biological effects might be mediated by altering depressive states. No differential changes in CD4+ or CD8+ T-cell levels occurred, nor did HSV-1 antibody titers differ. In contrast to the effects described above, Mulder and colleagues (1995) found no effect of either 15 weeks of cognitive–behavioral group therapy or 15 weeks of experiential supportive group therapy on 26 asymptomatic gay men's CD4+ T-cell levels over a 2-year follow-up. Thus psychological interventions addressing the stress associated with HIV infection can impact HIV-relevant immunologic parameters under some circumstances, although it remains unclear whether such effects translate into meaningful differences in clinical outcomes or why beneficial effects are not consistently observed.

### 4. Generalized Coping Styles

In contrast to studies examining psychological responses to specific, highly stressful personal events such as HIV infection or bereavement, studies that examine more diffuse attitudes toward negative events in general have not consistently predicted HIV progression. Perry et al. (1992) did find that a generalized sense of hopelessness was associated with CD4+ T-cell declines over 1 year, but a similar study by Rabkin and colleagues (1991) found no such association. Solomon and Temoshok (1987) found that low scores on one dimension of Kobasa's measure of generalized hardiness (the control subscale) were associated with heightened mortality risk among 21 gay men diagnosed with *Pneumocystis carinii* pneumonia. In contrast, Solano and colleagues (1993) and Perry et al. (1992) found no associations between the same measure of hardiness and AIDS onset or CD4+ T-cell decline during earlier stages of infection. Keet and colleagues (1994) compared the generic coping responses of 61 seropositive gay men who remained AIDS-free for 7 years with those of 142 who progressed to AIDS over the same duration and found lower levels of active problem solving among the nonprogressors and no differences on six other dimensions of generic coping style. Patterson et al. (1996) found no relationship between either active or avoidant coping styles and symptom onset, CD4+ T-cell declines, AIDS onset, or mortality in a heterogeneous sample of 414 seropositive males followed for at least 1 year.

### 5. Summary of Stress and Coping Effects

Associations between stressful events and HIV progression appear most often in studies measuring (1) subjective psychological responses to, (2) specific events, with (3) highly personal consequences (e.g., notification of HIV serostatus, response to life-threatening illness, bereavement). Studies focusing on the objective incidence of a diffuse variety of negative events that vary in personal relevance have generally failed to predict disease progression. Studies of bereavement in particular suggest that associations with HIV progression may be strongest when analyses consider the specific positive and negative psychological response to the loss (e.g., distinguishing grief from depression; finding meaning). Studies of psychological response to HIV infection find most pronounced effects when measuring coping and appraisal processes specific to HIV/AIDS, rather than more generalized states of mind (e.g., global hopelessness or hardiness). Several randomized clinical trials suggest that psychological interventions addressing the substantial stress associated with bereavement and HIV infection may influence immunologic indices of disease progression.

## B. Depression

Depression can refer either to a specific affective state or a formally defined clinical syndrome including affective, behavioral, and physiologic components ("clinical depression"). Clinical depression often involves disturbances in sleep, eating, physical health, and neuroendocrine function, in addition to dysphoric affect. Moreover, the origin and physiologic correlates of chronic or recurrent depression may differ from those of transient depressive states.

Several studies have assessed relationships between depressive symptoms measured at one point in time and subsequent HIV progression. In a carefully controlled study of 277 initially asymptomatic gay and bisexual men, Burack et al. (1993) found a small but statistically significant acceleration in 5-year CD4+ T-cell decline among individuals manifesting depressive symptomatology. This study found no acceleration in times to symptom onset, AIDS

diagnosis, or death. However, a subsequent study of 395 HIV+ men from the same cohort did identify depression as a significant predictor of accelerated AIDS onset over a 9-year period (Page-Shafer, Delorenze, Satariano, & Winkelstein, 1996). The differing conclusions of these two analyses of the same cohort may stem from the longer follow-up of the later study or from potential contamination of the former study's depression measure by dysphoria associated with recently gained serostatus information (depression measures used in the study of Page-Shafer and colleagues were collected before HIV serostatus information became available, whereas those utilized by Burack and colleagues were collected during the 6 months following the availability of serostatus information). Gruzelier et al. (1996) found that depressed mood was associated with declining CD4+ T-lymphocyte levels over 30 months in a sample of 27 asymptomatic HIV+ gay men. Patterson and colleagues (1995) failed to find any direct association between depressed mood and CD4+ T-cell declines in 63 HIV+ men, but they did find that individuals who reported both low levels of depressive symptoms and low levels of life stress showed more favorable changes in CD4+ T-lymphocyte and $\beta_2$ microglobulin levels over a 6-month period. The same group reported an association between depression and mortality risk among a heterogeneous group of 393 seropositive males (Patterson et al., 1996). However, the later study failed to identify any relationship between depression and symptom onset, CD4+ T-cell decline, or AIDS-free survival. It is not clear whether all mortality in this sample stemmed from HIV-related pathology, or whether other sources of death (e.g., suicide) may also have played a role. Vedhara et al. (1997) reported that emotional distress (anxiety, depression, perceived stress, and subjectively stressful life events) was associated with the magnitude of CD4+ T-cell decline over a 1-year follow-up. However, the statistical analysis eliminated individuals with no loss of CD4+ T cells over the follow-up, thus truncating the range of immunologic change values and inappropriately restricting the sample to those who showed significant disease progression. Although several natural history studies have identified relationships between depression and various clinical and immunologic indicators of HIV progression, several other natural history studies have failed to identify such effects. In a carefully controlled 8-year follow-up of 1809 initially asymptomatic gay and bisexual men, Lyketsos et al. (1996) found no relationship between depressive symptomatology and HIV progression (including symptom onset, AIDS diagnosis, and

CD4+ T-cell declines). This group also subsequently reported no association between depression measured 6 months prior to AIDS diagnosis and subsequent mortality times in a study of 911 HIV+ gay men (Lyketsos et al., 1996). Two other large studies also failed to identify any correlation between degree of depressive affect and CD4+ T-cell declines over 6–12 months (Perry et al., 1992; Rabkin et al., 1991). Thus some evidence supports a relationship between one-time measures of depression and HIV disease progression, but such results are not universally found. A similar conclusion emerges from two studies of depression's relationship to immuologic variables that do not directly mark HIV disease progression. In an essentially cross-sectional analysis, Leserman et al. (1997) found that depressive symptoms measured within 6 months of immunologic assessment were associated with reduced NK-and CD8+ T-cell levels in 66 HIV+ men. However, the same study failed to identify any relationship between immunologic outcomes and depressive symptoms measured more prospectively (i.e., 1 year or more prior to immunologic assessment). Sahs et al. (1994) also failed to find any association between depression and concurrent NK-cell levels among 74 HIV+ gay men.

Only one study has examined the effects of chronic depression on HIV disease progression. In a study of 402 HIV+ gay men, Mayne, Vittinghoff, Chesney, Barrett, and Coates (1996) found that increasing frequency of depression over time was associated with increased mortality risk over an 8-year period. Depression was measured every 6 months, and those showing elevated depression scores during each period experienced a 67% increase in HIV mortality risk relative to those without an elevated score at any point. The proportion of periods with elevated depression scores was associated with increased mortality regardless of whether the time-dependent covariate of depression was lagged (by 1, 2, or 3 years) or not. Although more studies of chronic depression would be desirable, these data clearly suggest that chronic depression may be associated with accelerated HIV disease progression.

Rabkin and colleagues have conducted several studies exploring the impact of antidepressant medications on CD4+ T-lymphocyte levels. In an 8-week open-label trial of sertraline in 28 depressed individuals at various stages of infection, this group found significant reductions in depressive symptoms but no changes in CD4+ T-lymphocyte levels (Rabkin, Wagner, & Rabkin, 1994). In a larger placebo-controlled study of 97 depressed individuals at various stages of infection, 26 weeks of imipramine treatment also improved depressive symptoms without affecting

postintervention CD4+ T cell levels (Rabkin, Rabkin, Harrison, & Wagner, 1994). Thirty individuals who failed to respond to imipramine or suffered relapses in depression following treatment subsequently undertook a 12-week course of fluoxetine (supplemented by dextroamphetamine in 7 patients). Again, treatment significantly improved depressive symptomatology without differentially affecting postintervention CD4+ T-lymphocyte levels (Rabkin, Rabkin, & Wagner, 1994).

As reviewed above (in the section on bereavement), Kemeny et al. (1994, 1995) found positive associations between several immunologic parameters and one-time measures of depression for gay men who had not been recently bereaved, but no such association for those who had experienced a recent loss. These results suggest that excluding bereavement-related dysphoria from measures of depressive affect might result in more consistent relationships between depression and HIV progression. Many measures of clinical depression may also be contaminated by HIV-induced neuropsychiatric disturbances or physical symptomatology (Drebing et al., 1994). As a result, measurement difficulties may preclude any firm conclusions about the relationship between depression and HIV progression until confounded variables are isolated. However, as reviewed above, relationships between depression and HIV disease progression do emerge in studies that utilize extended follow-up periods and isolate depression from other sources of negative affect (e.g., bereavement-related dysphoria or reactions to serostatus notification) by measuring and controlling for confounders or by aggregating depression measurements over long periods of time.

## C. Social Support

The presence of positive social relationships can support physical health both by providing instrumental resources (e.g., financial support, physical assistance) and by buffering physiologic responses to stress (Berkman, 1995). Theorell et al. (1995) found that low levels of subjective social and emotional support predicted more rapid declines in CD4+ T-cell level (but not symptom onset) in a 5-year study of 37 initially asymptomatic hemophiliacs. In a heterogeneous group of initially asymptomatic HIV-infected individuals, Solano and colleagues (1993) also found that measures of low subjective social support predicted symptom onset 6 months later, but not 12 months later. In contrast, Persson, Gullberg, Hanson, Moestrup, and Ostergreen (1994a) found that among 75 HIV-seropositive gay men followed for 5–6 years, those who reported the highest levels of attachment to others experienced a *faster* decline in CD4+ T-cell level than did those who indicated having weaker attachments to others. This group also reported a cross-sectional association between high levels of social support and *faster* CD4+ T-cell declines in 47-seropositve gay men (1994b). Miller, Kemeny, Taylor, Cole, and Visscher (1997) also found this unexpected relationship in a 3-year study of 205 gay and bisexual men. In their study, high levels of subjective loneliness were associated with *slower* CD4+ T-cell declines (but no differences in AIDS onset or mortality), while objective measures of social integration (e.g., frequency of contact with friends, family members, and supportive groups or organizations) showed no relationship to any immunologic or clinical measure of disease progression. In a study of 335 initially asymptomatic men, Patterson and colleagues (1996) also found a *higher* risk of symptom onset among those with a large social networks. However, this study also found that large social networks were associated with a reduced risk of mortality and no differential risk of CD4+ T-cell decline or AIDS onset. Blomkvist et al. (1994) reported that anticipating high levels of social activity (vs. solitary activity) prospectively predicted *increased* mortality among 31 male hemophiliacs followed for 7 years. Perry et al. (1992) found no relationship between perceived social support and 12-month CD4+ T-cell declines. Part of the variability in results from natural history studies of social support and HIV progression may stem from heterogeneity in the populations studied (Miller & Cole, 1998). For example, potentially negative effects of an extensive social network could be more pronounced for gay men, who may face greater exposure to AIDS-related bereavement, caregiving burdens, and sexual HIV transmission than might the most socially integrated members of other populations.

Perhaps the strongest evidence for effects of social relationships on immunodeficiency virus infection comes from an intriguing line of research on rhesus macaques inoculated with simian immunodeficiency virus (SIV). Capitanio and Lerche (1991) found that several parameters of a young primate's social history (e.g., maternal separation, peer separation, and frequency of cage changes) predicted times from SIV inoculation to leukopenia, lymphopenia, significant weight loss, and death. In a subsequent review of data on SIV progression in 298 primates from four study sites, Capitanio and Lerche (1998) found significantly accelerated disease onset among primates subject to housing relocations and social separations during the period of time surrounding SIV inoculation.

Underscoring the possibility that social conditions may have negative effects as well, Capitanio and Lerche (1998) also found that animals housed together after SIV inoculation experienced shorter survival times than did those housed individually. In a subsequent study examining potential biological and behavioral mediators of social factors' effects on SIV progression, Capitanio, Mendoza, Lerche, and Mason (1998) found that primates randomly assigned to live in an unstable social hierarchy displayed more antagonistic social behavior, less affiliative social behavior, and (surprisingly) lower plasma cortisol levels than did animals assigned to stable social hierarchies. Animals receiving high levels of social threats had increased plasma SIV RNA levels and decreased anti-SIV IgG levels, and those displaying the highest levels of affiliative behavior showed the lowest viral loads. Consistent with these biological indicators, animals in unstable social hierarchies showed significantly shorter survival times than did those housed in stable hierarchies. The diverse results from this line of research indicate that the nature of social conditions (e.g., stable vs. unstable, antagonistic vs. affiliative) may be a critical modifier of the effects of social relationships on disease progression. These data also suggest that SIV models might potentially be employed to examine the effects of other psychosocial influences such as depression or long-term stress on immunodeficiency virus disease progression.

## D. Psychological Inhibition

Inhibiting the expression of subjectively significant thoughts, feelings, or social behaviors can heighten SNS activity (Gross & Levenson, 1993; Pennebaker & Chew, 1985), alter immunologic responses (Petrie, Booth, Pennebaker, Davison, & Thomas, 1995), and increase the risk of physical illness (Cole, 1998; Pennebaker, Kiecolt-Glaser, & Glaser, 1988). Studies have also documented a heightened incidence of immunologically mediated disorders (Bell, Jasnoskie, Kagan, & King, 1990; Broadbent, Broadbent, Phillpotts, & Wallace, 1984; Cohen et al., 1997; Gauci, King, Saxarra, Tulloch, & Husband, 1993; Kagan, Snidman, Julia-Sellers, & Johnson, 1991; Totman, Kiff, Reed, & Craig, 1980), altered immunologic responses (Cole, Kemeny, Weitzman, Schoen, & Anton, 1998), differential patterns of CNS activity (Sutton & Davidson, 1997), and heightened SNS reactivity (Block, 1957; Kagan, Reznick, & Snidman, 1991) among individuals who manifest socially inhibited personality characteristics. Similar alterations in immunologic and neuroendocrine function have been observed in animal models of inhibited social behavior (Petito, Lysle,

Gariepy, & Lewis, 1994; Suomi, 1991). To determine whether psychological inhibition might influence the course of HIV infection, Cole, Kemeny, Taylor, Visscher, and Fahey (1996) took gay men's concealment of their homosexual identity as a model of psychological inhibition and found accelerated times to a critically low CD4+ T-cell level, accelerated times to AIDS onset, and accelerated times to HIV-related mortality among "closeted" members of a sample of 80 initially healthy gay men followed for 9 years. In a subsequent analysis of the same sample, this group also found that "closeted" individuals were particularly sensitive to social rejection and rejection-sensitivity emerged as an even stronger predictor of HIV disease progression (Cole, Kemeny, & Taylor, 1997). It remains unclear whether concealment-related accelerations in HIV progression reflect a state stressor (which might be altered by "coming out of the closet") or a more general, trait-like pattern of inhibited personality characteristics rooted in individual differences in neurophysiologic function (Kagan, Reznick, & Snidman, 1991). Consistent with the later hypothesis, Gruzelier et al. (1996) studied 27 asymptomatic HIV+ gay men and found that higher levels of right hemisphere activity during resting EEG (a pattern associated with psychological inhibition in previous studies; Sutton & Davidson, 1997) were associated with lower CD8+ T-cell levels at a 30-month follow-up. Results from a battery of neuropsychological tests tapping lateralized cognitive functions also indicated that right hemisphere dominance was associated with lower CD4+ and CD8+ T-cell levels at follow-up. Eisenberger, Kemeny, and Wyatt (1998) also found that psychological inhibition (as measured by use of inhibition-related words during an interview on coping with HIV) was associated with concurrent reductions in CD4+ T lymphocyte level in a multiethnic sample of 67 HIV+ women. Thus several studies converge in suggesting that psychological inhibition may relate to clinical and immunologic indices of HIV progression.

## E. General Summary of Studies Linking Psychosocial Factors to HIV Progression

Table II summarizes all studies the authors were able to find that relate psychosocial characteristics to HIV progression or HIV-relevant immunologic parameters. (Studies were identified on the basis of previous reviews and a Medline© search using keywords "HIV" or "AIDS" in conjunction with "psychological," "social," "psychosocial," "stress," "anxiety," "depression," and "personality.") The diversity of factors studied and the varying methodologies employed lead to mixed results overall, but reasonably clear conclusions emerge when results are considered on the basis of specific genera of psychological variables. Some evidence indicates that psychological reactions to specific stressors of great relevance to an HIV-infected individual (e.g., responses to seroconversion, responses to the threat of AIDS-related illness and mortality, responses to bereavement of significant others) may relate to symptom onset, progression to AIDS, AIDS survival times, and alterations in HIV-relevant immunologic parameters (e.g., CD4+ T-cell levels, soluble markers of immunologic activation, and in vitro lymphoproliferation). Passive coping, negative HIV-specific expectancies, and self-blame have each predicted accelerated HIV progression in more than one study. Some interventions aimed at ameliorating stress in HIV+ individuals have produced immunologic benefits, although similar interventions have also failed to produce any benefit. Evidence on the effects of social relationships is mixed, with natural history studies indicating both positive and negative associations with immunologic markers of disease progression. Experimental manipulation of social conditions in primate colonies clearly indicates that social disruption can accelerate SIV disease progression. Several lines of research have also linked socially inhibited behavior to clinical and immunologic indices of HIV progression. Chronic depression has been linked to increased HIV mortality risk, while one-time measures of depression have not consistently predicted either immunologic or clinical indices of disease progression. Other psychosocial variables receiving inconsistent support as correlates of disease progression include highly generalized attitudes or expectations (e.g., global hopelessness, hardiness) and the objective frequency of negative life events (as opposed to subjective responses to those events).

Controlled experiments provide the strongest basis for causal conclusions about psychosocial factors' influence on HIV progression. Experimental studies clearly indicate that social factors (e.g., social hierarchy disruption, antagonistic behavior) can influence SIV disease progression in primate models. In humans, psychological interventions addressing stress associated with bereavement and HIV infection have produced small beneficial effects on immunologic measures of HIV disease progression (e.g., CD4+ T-cell levels), although limited follow-up durations have not permitted accurate assessment of their clinical significance (e.g., for AIDS onset or mortality risk). Moreover, similar psychological interventions have failed to produce any immunologic effects, and

**TABLE II  Studies Examining Psychosocial Factors and HIV Progression**

| Study[a] | Design[b] | Population (disease status at study entry) | Follow-up duration | Control initial CD4 | Control other influences[c] | Outcomes measured[d] | Results[e] | Meets methodological criteria[f] (P/C/CO) |
|---|---|---|---|---|---|---|---|---|
| **Generalized stressful life events** | | | | | | | | |
| Kessler et al., 1991 | PNH | Approx. 1011gay men (Cat. A/B) | 2 Years | No | No | Symptom onset / 25% CD4 drop | ns / ns | (P) |
| Rabkin et al., 1991 | PNH | 124 Gay men (Cat. A/B) | 6 Months | Yes | No | Symptom onset / CD4 level | ns / ns | |
| Goodkin et al., 1992 | CS | 11 Gay men (Cat. A/B) | None | No | No | CD4 level / Total T-cell level | sig. negative assoc. / sig. negative assoc. | |
| Perry et al., 1992 | PNH | 1221 men and women (Cat. A/B) | 1 Year | Yes | No | Symptom onset / CD4 level | ns / ns | |
| Evans et al., 1995 | CS | 96 Gay men (Cat. A/B) | None | No | Yes | CD4 level / NK level / CD8/CD57 level | ns / sig. negative assoc. / sig. negative assoc. | |
| Patterson et al., 1995 (interacting with depression) | PNH | 63 Men (all stages) | 6 Months | Yes | Yes | CD4 level / CD8 level / $\beta_2$-Microglobulin | sig. negative assoc. / ns / sig. positive assoc. | |
| Leserman et al., 1997 | CS | 66 Gay men (Cat. A/B) | 2 Years | Yes | No | CD4 level / CD8 level / CD56 level / CD57 level / CD16 level | sig. negative assoc. / ns / ns / ns / sig. negative assoc. | |
| Moss et al., 1998 | PNH | 24 Children | 1 Year | No | No | HIV mortality | sig. positive assoc. | |
| **Bereavement** | | | | | | | | |
| Kessler et al., 1991 | PNH | Approx. 1011gay men (Cat. A/B) | 2 Years | No | No | Symptom onset / 25% CD4 drop | ns / ns | (P) |
| Perry et al., 1992 | PNH | 1221 Men and women (Cat. A/B) | 1 Year | Yes | No | Symptom onset / CD4 level | ns / ns | |
| Kemeny et al., 1994 | CS | 90 Gay men (Cat. A/B) | None | Yes | Yes | CD4 level / Lymphoprolif. / Neopterin / CD8+/CD38+ | ns / ns / ns / ns | |
| Kemeny et al., 1995 | PNH | 78 Gay men (Cat. A/B) | .5–1 Year | Yes | Yes | CD4 level / Lymphoprolif. / Neopterin | sig. decrease / sig. increase / sig. decrease | |
| Kemeny and Dean, 1995 | PNH | 85 Gay men (Cat. A/B) | 3–4 Years | Yes | Yes | Symptom onset / AIDS onset / HIV mortality | ns / ns / ns | (P C CO) |
| **Responses to HIV infection** | | | | | | | | |
| Goodkin et al., 1992 (active coping) | CS | 11 Gay men (Cat. A/B) | None | No | No | CD4 level | sig. positive assoc. | |
| Goodkin et al., 1992 (active coping) | CS | 62 Gay men (Cat. A/B) | None | No | No | Total T-cell level / NK cytotoxicity | sig. positive assoc. / sig. positive assoc. | |
| Solano et al., 1993 (denial / low fighting spirit) | PNH | 100 Men and women (Cat. A/B) | 1 Year | Yes | No | Symptom onset / CD4 level | sig. Increase / ns | |

| Study | Design | Sample | Duration | | | Outcome | Result | |
|---|---|---|---|---|---|---|---|---|
| Ironson et al., 1994 (denial and intervention nonadherence) | PNH | 23 Gay men (Cat. A/B) | 2 Years | Yes | No | Symptom onset<br>AIDS onset<br>HIV mortality | sig. increase<br>sig. increase<br>sig. increase | (C CO) |
| Reed et al., 1994 (with AIDS) | PNH | 74 Gay men (with AIDS) | 4 Years | Yes | Yes | HIV mortality | sig. increase | (C CO) |
| Reed et al., 1996 (negative expectancies about future health) | PNH | 75 Gay men (Cat. A/B) | 3 Years | Yes | Yes | Symptom onset | sig. increase | (C) |
| Kemeny et al., 1996 (negative expectancies about future health) | PNH | 127 Gay men (Cat. A/B) | 2–3 Years | Yes | Yes | CD4 level<br>Lymphoprolif.<br>Neopterin level | sig. decrease<br>sig. decrease<br>sig. increase | |
| Coates et al., 1989 (stress management) | EXP | 64 Gay men (Cat. n/a) | 8 Weeks | Yes | | CD4 level<br>NK cytotoxicity<br>Lymphoprolif. | ns<br>ns<br>ns | |
| Antoni et al., 1992 (cog.–behavioral stress mgmt.) | EXP | 47 Gay men (Cat. A/B) | 10 Weeks | Yes | Yes | CD4 level | sig. less decline than control grop | (C) |
| Esterling et al., 1992 (extended analysis of Antoni et al., 1992) | | | | | | EBV Ag. level<br>HHV-6 Ag. level | sig. greater decline than control group<br>sig. greater decline than control group | |
| Eller, 1995 (relaxation) | EXP | 69 Gay men (All stages) | 6 Weeks | Yes | | CD4 level | sig. less decline than control group | (C) |
| Mulder et al., 1995 (stress management) | EXP | 26 Gay men (Cat. A/B) | 2 Years | Yes | | CD4 level | ns | (C) |
| Taylor, 1995 (stress management) | EXP | 10 Males (Cat. A/B) | 1 Month | Yes | | CD4 level | sig. less decline than control group | (C) |
| Lutgendorf et al., 1997 (cog.–behavioral stress mgmt.) | EXP | 33 Gay men (Cat. A/B) | 11 Weeks | No | | CD4 level<br>CD8 level<br>Anti-HSV-1 Ab<br>Anti-HSV-2 Ab | ns<br>ns<br>ns<br>sig. greater decline than control group | (C) |
| **Responses to generalized stressful events** | | | | | | | | |
| Solomon & Temoshok, 1987 (hardiness) | PNH | 21 Gay men (with PCP/AIDS) | 1–2 Years | No | No | HIV mortality | sig. decrease | |
| Rabkin et al., 1991 (hopelessness) | PNH | 124 Gay men (Cat. A/B) | 6 Months | Yes | No | Symptom onset<br>CD4 level | ns<br>ns | |
| Perry et al., 1992 (hopelessness) | PNH | 1221 Men and women (Cat. A/B) | 1 Year | Yes | No | Symptom onset<br>CD4 level<br>Symptom onset<br>CD4 level | sig. decrease<br>ns<br>ns<br>ns | |
| Solano et al., 1993 (hardiness) | PNH | 100 Men and women (Cat. A/B) | 1 Year | Yes | No | Symptom onset<br>CD4 decline | ns<br>ns | |
| Keet et al., 1994. (active coping) | PNH | 203 Gay men (Cat. A/B) | 7 Years | Yes | Yes | Symptom onset | sig. increase | (C CO) |
| Mulder et al., 1995 (active coping) | PNH | 51 Gay men (Cat. A/B) | 1 Year | No | Yes | CD4 level<br>CDC stage progression | ns<br>sig. decrease | |

*(Continues)*

**TABLE II** (*Continued*)

| Study[a] | Design[b] | Population (disease status at study entry) | Follow-up duration | Control initial CD4 | Control other influences[c] | Outcomes measured[d] | Results[e] | Meets methodological criteria[f] (P/C/CO) |
|---|---|---|---|---|---|---|---|---|
| Patterson et al., 1996 (active/avoidant coping) | PNH | 302–393 Males (all stages) | >1 Year | Yes | No | Symptom onset<br>CD4 decline<br>AIDS onset<br>Mortality | ns<br>ns<br>ns<br>ns | |
| Segerstrom et al., 1996 (self-blaming attribution) | PNH | 86 Gay men (all stages) | 1.5 Years | Yes | Yes | CD4 level<br>AIDS onset | sig. decrease<br>ns | (C CO) |
| Weitzman et al., 1998 (shame/guilt) | PNH | 137 Gay men (Cat. A/B) | 7 Years | Yes | Yes | CD4 level<br>AIDS onset<br>HIV mortality | sig. decrease<br>sig. increase<br>sig. increase | (C CO) |
| Vedhara et al., 1997 (emotional distress) | PNH | 47 Gay men (all stages) | 1 Year | Yes | Yes | CD4 level | sig. decrease | |
| Responses to bereavement<br>Kemeny and Dean, 1995 (grief) | PNH | 85 Gay men (Cat. A/B) | 3–4 Years | Yes | Yes | CD4 level<br>Symptom onset<br>AIDS onset<br>HIV mortality | ns<br>ns<br>ns<br>ns | (P C CO) |
| (self-reproach) | | | | | | CD4 level<br>Symptom onset<br>AIDS onset<br>HIV mortality | sig. decrease<br>ns<br>ns<br>ns | |
| Bower et al., 1998 (finding meaning) | PNH | 40 Gay men (Cat. A/B) | 4–8 Years | Yes | Yes | CD4 level<br>HIV mortality | sig. decrease<br>sig. increase | |
| Goodkin et al., 1998 (bereavement support group) | EXP | 74 Gay men (Cat. A/B) | 6 Months | Yes | | CD3 level<br>CD4 level<br><br>CD8 level<br>Cortisol level<br><br>Health care visits | ns<br>sig. less decrease than control group<br>ns<br>sig. less increase than control group<br>sig. less increase than control group | (C) |
| Depression<br>Rabkin et al., 1991 | PNH | 124 Gay men (Cat. A/B) | 6 Months | Yes | No | Symptom onset<br>CD4 level | ns<br>ns | |
| Perry et al., 1992 | PNH | 1221 Men and women (Cat. A/B) | 1 Year | Yes | No | Symptom onset<br>CD4 level | ns<br>ns | |
| Lyketsos et al., 1993 | PNH | 1809 Gay men (Cat. A/B) | 8 Years | Yes | Yes | CD4 level<br>AIDS onset<br>HIV mortality | ns<br>ns<br>ns | (P CO) |
| Burack et al., 1993 | PNH | 330 Gay men (Cat. A/B) | 5 Years | Yes | Yes | CD4 level<br>AIDS onset<br>HIV mortality | sig. decrease<br>ns<br>ns | (P C CO) |
| Sahs et al., 1994 | CS | 74 Gay men (Cat. A/B) | None | No | No | CD56 level | ns | |

| Study | Design | Sample | Duration | | | Measure | Result |
|---|---|---|---|---|---|---|---|
| Kemeny et al., 1994 (nonbereaved only) | CS | 90 Gay men (Cat. A/B) | None | | Yes | CD4 level<br>Lymphoprolif.<br>Neopterin | sig. negative association<br>sig. negative association<br>ns |
| Kemeny et al., 1995 (nonbereaved only) | PNH | 78 Gay men (Cat. A/B) | .5–1 Year | Yes | Yes | CD8+/CD38+<br>CD4 level<br>Lymphoprolif.<br>Neopterin<br>CD8–/HLA-DR+ | sig. positive association (P CO)<br>sig. decrease<br>ns<br>ns<br>sig. increase |
| Patterson et al., 1995 (interacting with stress) | PNH | 63 Men (all stages) | 6 Months | Yes | Yes | CD4 level<br>CD8 level | sig. negative assoc.<br>ns |
| Page-Shafer et al., 1996 | PNH | 395 Gay men (Cat. A/B) | 9 Years | Yes | No | $\beta_2$ microglobulin<br>AIDS onset | sig. positive assoc.<br>sig. increase. |
| Gruzelier et al., 1996 | PNH | 27 Gay men (Cat. A/B) | 30 Months | No | No | HIV mortality<br>CD4 level<br>CD8 level | ns<br>sig. negative assoc.<br>ns |
| Lyketsos et al., 1996 | PNH | 911 Gay men (Cat. A/B) | 6 Months+ | Yes | No | HIV mortality | ns |
| Mayne et al., 1996 | PNH | 402 Gay men (Cat. A/B) | 8 Years | Yes | No | HIV mortality | sig. increase |
| Leserman et al., 1997 | CS | 66 Gay men (Cat. A/B) | 2 Years | Yes | Yes | CD4 level<br>CD8 level<br>CD56 level<br>CD57 level<br>CD16 level | ns<br>sig. negative assoc.<br>sig. negative assoc.<br>ns<br>sig. negative assoc. |
| Rabkin et al., 1994 (sertraline treatment) | EXP | 28 Depressed gay men (Cat. A/B) | 8 Week | Yes | | CD4 level | ns |
| Rabkin et al., 1994 (imipramine treatment) | EXP | 97 Depressed men and women (All stages) | 26 Week | Yes | | CD4 level | ns |
| Rabkin et al., 1994 (fluoxetine treatment) | EXP | 30 Depressed men and women (All stages) | 12 Weeks | Yes | | CD4 level | ns |
| Patterson et al., 1996 | PNH | 302–393 males (All stages) | >1 Year | Yes | No | Symptom onset<br>CD4 decline<br>AIDS onset<br>Mortality | ns<br>ns<br>ns<br>sig. increase |
| **Social support (high vs. low)** | | | | | | | |
| Solano et al., 1993 | PNH | 100 Men and women (Cat. A/B) | 1 Year | Yes | No | Symptom onset<br>CD4 decline<br>HIV mortality | sig. decrease at 6 Months<br>ns<br>sig. increase |
| Blomkvist et al., 1994 | PNH | 31 Male hemophiliacs (Cat. A/B) | 7 Years | Yes | No | CD4 level | sig. greater decrease |
| Persson et al., 1994 | PNH | 75 Gay men (Cat. A/B) | 5–6 Years | Yes | No | CD4 level | sig. smaller decrease |
| Theorell et al., 1995 | PNH | 37 Male hemophiliacs (all stages) | 5 Years | Yes | No | CD4 level<br>AIDS onset | sig. increase<br>ns |
| Patterson et al., 1996 | PNH | 297–371 Males (all stages) | >1 Year | Yes | No | Symptom onset<br>CD4 decline<br>AIDS onset<br>Mortality | sig. increase<br>ns<br>ns<br>sig. increase |

(Continues)

**TABLE II** (*Continued*)

| Study[a] | Design[b] | Population (disease status at study entry) | Follow-up duration | Control initial CD4 | Control other influences[c] | Outcomes measured[d] | Results[e] | Meets methodological criteria[f] (P/C/CO) |
|---|---|---|---|---|---|---|---|---|
| Miller et al., 1998 | PNH | 205 gay men (Cat. A/B) | 3 Years | Yes | Yes | CD4 level | sig. greater decrease | (P C CO) |
| | | | | | | AIDS onset | ns | |
| | | | | | | HIV mortality | ns | |
| Perry et al., 1992 | PNH | 1221 men and women (Cat. A/B) | 1 Year | Yes | No | Symptom onset | ns | |
| | | | | | | CD4 level | ns | |
| Capitanio and Lerche, 1991 | PNH | 22 SIV-infected rhesus macaques | 2.5 Years | | | Leukopenia | sig. decrease | (C CO) |
| | | | | | | Lymphopenia | ns | |
| | | | | | | Weight loss | sig. decrease | |
| | | | | | | SIV mortality | sig. decrease | |
| Capitanio and Lerche, 1998 (low social disruption) | PNH | 298 SIV-infected rhesus macaques | 7 Years | | | SIV mortality | sig. decrease | (C CO) |
| Capitanio et al., 1998 (low social disruption) | EXP | 36 Male rhesus macaques (18 SIV+) | 2 Years+ | | | SIV mortality | sig. decrease | (C CO) |
| | | | | | | SIV viral RNA | ns decrease | |
| | | | | | | Anti-SIV IgG | ns | |
| | | | | | | Anti-tetanus Ig | sig. decrease | |
| | | | | | | Lymphoprolif. | ns | |
| (affiliative behavior) | CS | | | | | SIV viral RNA | sig. decrease | |
| | | | | | | Anti-SIV IgG | sig. increase | |
| Psychological inhibition Cole et al., 1996/1997 | PNH | 80 Gay men (Cat. A) | 9 Years | Yes | Yes | CD4 level | sig. decrease | (C CO) |
| | | | | | | AIDS onset | sig. increase | |
| | | | | | | HIV mortality | sig. increase | |
| Gruzelier et al., 1996 (right hemispheric dominance) | PNH | 27 Gay men (Cat. A) | 30 Months | No | No | CD4 level | sig. decrease | |
| | | | | | | CD8 level | sig. decrease | |
| Eisenberger et al., 1998 | CS | 67 Women (Cat. A/B) | None | No | Yes | CD4 level | sig. decrease | |

[a]For studies investigating multiple psychosocial characteristics, results for a given characteristic are included here only when other studies examined the same characteristic.
[b]PNH, prospective natural history study; CS, cross-sectional study; EXP, controlled experiment.
[c]Potential influences on HIV progression: age, gender, risk group, antiretroviral use, recreational drug use, high-risk sexual behavior.
[d]When multiple outcomes are assessed, this table includes only major indicators of HIV progression and selected immunologic variables when they were a major focus of study.
[e]Results: ns, nonsignificant at .05 level; sig., significant at .05 level.
[f]Among prospective studies: (P) negative result from well-powered study (sample size, >50; follow-up, >50; >20% median progression time, e.g., 2 years for progression from CDC Category A/B HIV infection to AIDS, 6 months for progression from AIDS to death); (C) positive result from well-controlled study (randomized experiment or statistical control for initial CD4 level and all potential confounders listed in note[c]);
(CO) examined clinical outcomes (symptom onset, AIDS onset, HIV mortality).

the reasons for inconsistent results remain unclear (possibilities include differences in population, intervention type and timing, and sample size and follow-up). Psychopharmacologic interventions aimed at ameliorating depression have consistently failed to alter immunologic indices of disease progression, although again, many of these studies are underpowered in sample size and follow-up. Although experimental manipulation of psychosocial characteristics has not always produced significant biological effects, the fact that changes are observed in some experimental settings clearly indicates that psychosocial factors are capable of influencing immunodeficiency virus disease progression.

## F. Methodological Issues and Resummarization

Poor design and analysis can prevent studies from identifying significant influences on disease progression (Cole & Kemeny, 1997; Kraemer & Thiemann, 1987). Many null findings on psychosocial correlates of HIV progression emerge from studies suffering from limited statistical power (due to insufficient sample size, poor measures of disease progression, and insufficient follow-up duration) and failure to control for confounding influences (e.g., disease progression at study entry, demographic characteristics, health-relevant behaviors such as drug-use, and antiviral treatment and adherence). Thus null findings may stem from poor study design rather than from lack of relationship between psychosocial factors and disease progression. By the same token, positive findings from cross-sectional studies (measuring psychosocial characteristics and disease status simultaneously and only once) cannot support psychosocial influences on disease progression unless it can be shown that such associations do not stem from causal effects of disease progression on psychosocial characteristics. Similar issues complicate the interpretation of psychosocial or neuroendocrine data obtained during late-stage infection (e.g., following AIDS diagnosis), when psychobiologic characteristics may reflect underlying differences in generalized physiologic dysregulation rather than causal determinants of disease progression. In addition, several "third" variables can influence both psychosocial factors and HIV progression (e.g., age, gender, risk group, biomedical prophylaxis, recreational drug use), raising the possibility of spurious associations. Studies of psychosocial influences on HIV progression should control for (or hold constant) a core set of variables known to influence disease progression, including ethnicity, age, gender, mode of transmission, antiretroviral therapy (including treatment adherence), and high-risk sexual behavior. Other potential confounders include recreational drug use (including smoking, alcohol consumption, and "street" drugs such as nitrite inhalants, amphetamines, and tranquilizers), sleep disruption, exercise, nutrition, and socioeconomic status (Adler et al., 1994; Kiecolt-Glaser & Glaser, 1988).

Because methodological problems can undermine the validity of study conclusions, it may be useful to consider evidence on psychosocial predictors of HIV progression as probative only when a study meets a core set of methodological criteria. Existing studies of psychobiologic characteristics in HIV progression are summarized in Table II. Among those, null findings from prospective studies that are at least moderately powered (sample size $\geq 50$, follow-up $\geq 20\%$ of median progression time) are denoted with a "P" in Column 9. (Because lack of power cannot explain significant results, this criterion applies only to null findings; cf. Kraemer & Thiemann, 1987). Significant results from prospective studies that control for a core set of potential confounders (age, gender, risk-group, high-risk sexual practices, antiretroviral use, and recreational drug use) are denoted by a "C" in Column 9. (Because random assignment reduces the likelihood that other influences will confound the effects of a treatment intervention, randomized experiments can be assumed to control for potential confounders.) Analysis of clinical endpoints (e.g., AIDS-defining conditions or HIV-specific mortality) provides the most valid indication of differential HIV progression, and studies that meet the core methodological criteria and report clinical outcome data are indicated by a "CO" in Column 9. Studies reporting both significant results and null results (e.g., significant effects on CD4 T cell levels but not AIDS onset) may receive all three indications.

Among the 20 prospective studies meeting core methodologic criteria, 16 have identified significant relationships between psychosocial variables and biological markers of immunodeficiency virus disease progression. Well-controlled prospective natural history studies have documented accelerated HIV disease progression as a function of depression, bereavement, psychological inhibition, self-referential emotional reactions to bereavement or HIV infection (shame, self-reproach, guilt), negative expectancies about future health, active coping, and extensive social network size. Experimental studies using primate SIV models have also shown that social disruption and aggressive interactions can significantly accelerate immunodeficiency virus disease progression. Several experimental interventions aimed at reducing stress among HIV+ individuals have documented positive effects on immunologic markers of disease progression. Among the 16 well-controlled studies reporting significant results, 8 are based on clinical outcomes (e.g., symptom onset, AIDS diagnosis, HIV/SIV mortality) and the remainder are based on changes in CD4+ T-lymphocyte levels alone. Well-controlled natural history studies have identified relationships between clinical indices of HIV progression and negative expectancies about future health, persistent shame and guilt related to HIV infection, and psychological inhibition. Experimental studies have also shown that social conditions can influence clinical outcomes in primate SIV models. Potential psychosocial influences supported by immunologic markers alone include depression, psychological reactions to bereavement, self-blame in reaction to HIV infection, extensive social network size, and cognitive-behavioral, relaxation, and stress-management interventions. Thus well-conducted studies using both experimental and prospective natural history designs have identified significant relationships between psychosocial characteristics and immunodeficiency virus disease progression.

Despite having at least moderate statistical power, four well-conducted studies have failed to identify relationships between depression, bereavement, or stressful life events and HIV disease progression. In another three cases, well-controlled studies with at least moderate statistical power have documented significant associations between psychosocial characteristics and CD4+ T cell declines but not symptom onset, AIDS diagnosis, or HIV-specific mortality (effects of social network size, psychological reactions to bereavement, and depression). The availability of nonsignificant and mixed results in published sources indicates that publication biases do not preclude access to negative findings on psychosocial predictors of HIV progression. Despite this fact, a majority of well-conducted natural history and experimental studies contain data supporting the hypothesis that psychosocial factors can influence HIV disease progression.

## V. GENERAL CONCLUSION

### A. Current Evidence

There now exists a significant body of research linking psychosocial characteristics to differential HIV disease progression (Table II). The majority of these data come from cross-sectional and prospective natural history studies, but several experimental interventions have also demonstrated causal effects of psychosocial variables on biological indicators of HIV progression in humans and SIV progression in primates. The physiologic mechanisms mediating these relationships remain unknown, but in vitro studies show that neuroeffector molecules can influence HIV replication and pharmacologic activation of hormone signal transduction pathways can influence virologic parameters and AIDS onset in vivo. Whether HIV progression can be affected by psychosocially induced neuroendocrine changes remains unclear. Simultaneous analysis of psychosocial characteristics, biological mediators, and HIV disease progression represents an important focus for further research.

### B. Directions for Future Inquiry

The dynamics of the AIDS epidemic are changing in ways that may alter the relationship between psychosocial factors and HIV progression. With the advent of clinically effective antiretroviral medications, access and adherence to treatment regimens are likely to play increasingly significant roles in disease progression. Psychosocial influences on treatment utilization thus represent an important topic for future research. Although antiretroviral medications can rapidly reduce circulating HIV titers, immunologic reconstitution proceeds more slowly (Autran et al., 1997; Li et al., 1998; Powderly et al., 1998) and the role of psychosocial factors in modulating the function of a recovering immune system remains largely unexplored. Because antiretroviral treatment often forestalls AIDS onset and may alter CD4+ T-lymphocyte trafficking (Pakker et al., 1998), future studies will also require new indices of HIV disease progression (e.g., functional measures of immunologic reconstitution, time to emergence of drug-resistant viral strains, and biopsy-based virologic measures in lymphoid tissue). Finally, the demography of the AIDS epidemic has shifted significantly during the past decade with an increasing prevalence of HIV infection in developing nations and among women and ethnic minority groups in developed countries. Psychosocial influences on HIV disease progression may differ across cultural and demographic groups, and research documenting the generality and specificity of such effects represents an important topic for future research. Economic barriers to antiretroviral use in developing nations imply that vaccination may constitute the most effective means of containing HIV worldwide. Psychosocial factors can influence both vaccine utilization and immunologic response to vaccination (Glaser, Kiecolt-Glaser, Malarkey, &

Sheridan, 1998; Petrie et al., 1995; Stone et al., 1994), suggesting another important focus for future research.

Striking demographic differences in HIV prevalence underscore the role of psychosocial factors in shaping the course of viral epidemics. The data reviewed above also indicate that psychosocial factors can potentially influence the course of HIV infection once contracted. As the nature of the AIDS epidemic changes and biomedical responses continue to evolve, psychosocial factors are likely to assume even greater significance in the health of HIV-infected individuals. Understanding the biological mechanism of such relationships remains an important topic for future research—one that would be greatly aided by more comprehensive analyses of the network of reciprocal relationships among psychosocial characteristics, central and peripheral nervous system function, and immunologic and virologic bases of HIV pathogenesis.

## References

Aanadahl, E. M., Aukrust, P., Skalhegg, B. S., Muller, F., Forland, S. S., Hansson, V., & Tasken, K. (1998). Protein kinase A type 1 antagonist restores immune responses of T cells from HIV-infected patients. *FASEB Journal, 12*, 855–862.

Abrams, B., Duncan, D., & Hertz-Picciotto, I. (1993). A prospective study of dietary intake and acquired immune deficiency syndrome in HIV-seropositive homosexual men. Journal of *Acquired Immune Deficiency Syndromes, 6*, 949.

Adler, N. E., Boyce, T., Chesney, M. A., Cohen, S., Folkman, S., Kahn, R. L., & Syme, S. L. (1994). Socioeconomic status and health: The challenge of the gradient. *American Psychology, 49*, 15.

Antoni, M. H. Baggett, L., Ironson, G., LaPerriere, A., August, S., Klimas, N., et al. (1991). Cognitive-behavioral stress management intervention buffers distress responses and immunologic changes following notification of HIV-1 seropositivity. *Journal of Consulting and Clinical Psychology, 59*, 906.

Auphan, N., Didonato, J. A., Rosette, C., Helmberg, A., & Karin, M. (1995). Immunosuppression by glucocorticoids: Inhibition of NF-κB activity through induction of IκB synthesis. *Science, 270*, 286.

Autran, B., Carcelain, G., Li, T. S., Blanc, C., Mathez, D., Tubiana, R., Katlama, C., Debre, P., & Leibowitch, J. (1997). Positive effects of combined antiretroviral therapy on CD4+ T cell homeostasis and function in advanced HIV disease. *Science, 277*, 112–116.

Ayyavoo, V., Mahboubi, A., Mahalingam, S., Ramalingam, R., Kudchodkar, S., Williams, W. V., Green, D. R., & Weiner, D. B. (1997). HIV-1 Vpr suppresses immune activation and apoptosis through regulation of nuclear factor kappaB. *Nature Medicine, 3*, 1117–1123.

Bartrop, R. W., Luckhurst, E., Lazarul, L., Kiloh, L. G., & Penny, R. (1977). Depressed lymphocyte function after bereavement. *Lancet, 1*, 834.

Baum, M. K., Shor-Posner, G., Lu, Y., Rosner, B., Sauberlich, S. E., Fletcher, M. A., et al. (1995). Micronutrients and HIV-1 disease progression. *AIDS, 9*, 1051.

Bell, J. R., Jasnoski, M. L., Kagan J., & King, D. S. (1990). Is allergic rhinitis more frequent in adults with extreme shyness? A preliminary study. *Psychosomatic Medicine, 52*, 517–525.

Berkman, L. (1995). The role of social relations in health promotion. *Psychosomatic Medicine, 57*, 245.

Block, J. (1957). A study of affective responsiveness in a lie-detection situation. *Journal of Personality and Social Psychology, 55*, 11.

Blomkvist, V., Theorell, T., Jonsson, H., Schulman, S., Berntorp, E., & Stiegendal, L. (1994). Psychosocial self-prognosis in relation to mortality and morbidity in hemophiliacs with HIV infection. *Psychotherapy and Psychosomatics, 62*, 185.

Borrow, P., Lewicki, H., Hahn, B. H., Shaw, G. M., & Oldstone, M. B. A. (1994). Virus-specific CD8+ cytotoxic T lymphocyte activity associated with control of viremia in primary human immunodeficiency virus type 1 infection. *Journal of Virology, 68*, 6103.

Bourinbaiar, A. S., Nagorny, R., & Tan, X. (1992). Pregnancy hormones, estrogen and progesterone, prevent HIV-1 synthesis in monocytes but not in lymphocytes. *FEBS Letters, 302*, 206–208.

Bower, J. E., Kemeny, M. E., Taylor, S. E., & Fahey, J. L. (1998). Cognitive processing, discovery of meaning, CD4 decline, and AIDS-related mortality among bereaved HIV seropositive gay men. *Journal of Consulting and Clinical Psychology, 66*, 979–986.

Broadbent, D. E., Broadbent, M. H. P., Phillpotts, R. J., & Wallace, J. (1984). Some further studies on the prediction of experimental colds in volunteers by psychological factors. *Journal of Psychosomatic Research, 28*, 511.

Brown, G. W., & Harris, T. (1978). *Social origins of depression: A study of psychiatric disorders in women.* New York: Free Press.

Burack, J. H., Barrett, D. C., Stall, R. D., Chesney, M. A., Ekstrand, M. L., & Coates, T. J. (1993). Depressive symptoms and CD4 lymphocyte decline among HIV-infected men. *JAMA, 270*, 2568.

Capitanio, J. P., & Lerche, N. W. (1998). Social separation, housing relocation, and survival in simian AIDS: A retrospective analysis. *Psychosomatic Medicine, 60*, 235–244.

Capitanio, J. P., & Lerche, N. W. (1991). Psychosocial factors and disease progression in simian AIDS: A preliminary report. *AIDS, 5*, 1103.

Centers for Disease Control (1992). 1993 revised classification system for HIV infection and expanded surveillance case definition for AIDS among adolescents and adults. *Morbidity and Mortality Weekly Report, 41*(RR–17), 1.

Centurelli, M. A., & Abate, M. A. (1997). The role of dehydroepiandrosterone in AIDS. *Annals of Pharmacotherapy, 31*, 639–642.

Chang, S. S., & Rasmussen, A. F., Jr. (1964). Effects of stress on susceptibility of mice to polyoma virus infection. *Bacteriology Proceedings, 64*, 134.

Chang, S. S., & Rasmussen, A. F., Jr. (1965). Stress-induced suppression of interferon production in virus-infected mice. *Nature, 205*, 623.

Chang, Y., Cesarman, E., Pessin, M. S., Lee, F., Culpepper J, Knowles, D. M., & Moore, P. S. (1994). Identification of herpesvirus-like DNA sequences in AIDS associated Kapossi's Sarcoma. *Science, 266*, 1865.

Choe, H., M. Farzan, Y. Sun, N. Sullivan, B. Rollins, P. D. Ponath, L. Wu, C. R. Mackay, G. LaRosa, W. Newman, N. Gerard, C. Gerard, & J. Sodroski.. (1996). The β-chemokine receptors CCR3 and CCR5 facilitate infection by primary HIV-1 isolates. *Cell, 85*, 1135–1148.

Chowdhury, I. H., Koyanagi, Y., Horiuchi, S., Hazeki, O., Ui, M., Kitano, K., Golde, D. W., Takada, K., & Yamamoto, N. (1993) cAMP stimulates Human Immunodeficiency Virus (HIV-1) from latently infected cells of monocyte-macrophage lineage: Synergism with TNF-α. *Virology, 194*, 345–349.

Chrousos, G. P., & Gold, P. W. (1992). The concepts of stress and stress system disorders: Overview of physical and behavioral homeostasis. *JAMA, 267*, 1244.

Clerici, M., Hakim, F. T., Venzon, D. J., Blatt, S., Hendrix, C., Wynn, T. A., & Shearer, G. M. (1993). Changes in interleukin-2 and interleukin-4 production in asymptomatic, human immunodeficiency virus-seropositive individuals. *Journal of Clinical Investigation, 91,* 759.

Clerici, M., Trabattoni, D., Piconi, S., Fusi, M. L., Ruzzante, S., Clerici, C., & Villa, M. L. (1997). A possible role for the cortisol/anticortisols imbalance in the progression of human immunodeficiency virus. *Psychoneuroendocrinology, 22* (Supplement 1), S27–S31.

Coates, T. J., McKusick, L., Knuo, R., & Stites, D. P. (1989). Stress reduction training changed number of sexual partners but not immune function in men with HIV. *American Journal of Public Health, 79,* 885.

Cohen, J. A., & Laudenslager, M. (1989). Autonomic nervous system involvement in patients with human immunodeficiency virus infection. *Neurology, 39,* 1111.

Cohen, S., Doyle, W. J., Skoner, D. P., Rabin, B. S., & Gwaltney, J. M. (1997). Social ties and susceptibility to the common cold. *JAMA, 277,* 1940–1944.

Cole, S. W. (1998). *Negative physical health effects of psychological inhibition in disclosure study control groups.* Under review.

Cole, S. W., Jamieson, B. D., & Zack, J. A. (1999) cAMP up-regulates cell surface expression of lymphocyte CXCR4: Implications for chemotaxis and HIV-1 infection. *Journal of Immunology, 162*(3), 1392–400.

Cole, S. W., & Kemeny, M. E. (1997). Psychobiology of HIV infection. *Critical Reviews in Neurobiology, 11,* 289–321.

Cole, S. W., Kemeny, M. E., & Taylor, S. E. (1997). Social identity and physical health: Accelerated HIV progression in rejection sensitive gay men. *Journal of Personality and Social Psychology, 72,* 320.

Cole, S. W., Kemeny, M. E., Weitzman, O. B., Schoen, M., & Anton, P. A. (1999). Socially inhibited individuals show heightened DTH responses during intense social engagement. *Brain, Behavior, and Immunity, 13,* 187–200.

Cole, S. W., Kemeny, M. E., Taylor, S. E., & Visscher, B. R. (1996). Elevated physical health risk in gay men who conceal their homosexual identity. *Health Psychology, 15,* 243.

Cole, S. W., Kemeny, M. E., Taylor, S. E., Visscher, B. R., & Fahey, J. L. (1996). Accelerated course of human immunodeficiency virus infection in gay men who conceal their homosexual identity. *Psychosomatic Medicine, 58,* 219.

Cole, S. W., Korin, Y. D., Fahey, J. L., & Zack, J. A. (1998). Norepinephrine accelerates HIV replication via protein kinase A-dependent effects on cytokine production. *Journal of Immunology, 161*(2), 610–616.

Cooper, D. A., Gold, J., Maclean, P., Donovan, B., Finlayson, R., Barnes, T. G., et al. (1985). Acute AIDS retrovirus infection. Definition of a clinical illness associated with seroconversion. *Lancet, i,* 537.

Cossarizza, A., Ortolani, C., Mussini, C., Borghi, V., Guaraldi, G., Mongiardo, N., et al. (1995). Massive activation of immune cells with an intact T cell repertoire in acute human immunodeficiency virus syndrome. *Journal of Infectious Disease, 172,* 105.

Covas, M. J., Pinto, L. A., & Victorino, R. M. (1994). Disturbed immunoregulatory properties of the neuropeptide substance P on lymphocyte proliferation in HIV infection. *Clinical and Experimental Immunology, 96,* 384–388.

Croxson, T. S., Chapman, W. E., Miller, L. K., Levit, C. D., Senie, R., & Zumoff, B. (1989). Changes in the hypothalamic-pituitary-gonadal axis in human immunodeficiency virus-infected homosexual men. *Journal of Clinical Endocrinology and Metabolism, 68,* 317.

Cryer, P. E. (1980). Physiology and pathophysiology of the human sympathodrenal neuroendocrine system. *New England Journal of Medicine, 303,* 436.

Cupps, T. R., & Fauci, A. S. (1982). Corticosteroid-mediated immunoregulation in man. *Immunology Review, 65,* 133.

Dalgleish, A. G., Beverley, P. C. L., Clapham, P. R., Crawford, D. H., Greaves, M. F., & Weiss, R. A. (1984). The CD4 (T4) antigen is an essential component of the receptor for the AIDS retrovirus. *Nature, 312,* 763.

Darko, D. F., Mitler, M. M., & Henriksen, S. J. (1995). Lentiviral infection, immune response peptides and sleep. *Advances in Neuroimmunology, 5,* 57–77.

De Simone, C., Famularo, G., Cifone, G., & Mitsuya, H. (1996). HIV-1 infection and cellular metabolism. *Immunology Today, 17,* 256–258.

Deng, H., R. Liu, W. Elmeier, S. Choe, D. Unutmaz, M. Burkhart, P. DiMarzio, S. Marmon, R. E. Sutton, C. M. Hill, C. B. Davis, S. C. Peiper, T. J. Schall, D. R. Littman, & N. R. Landau. (1996). Identification of a major co-receptor for primary isolates of HIV-1. *Nature, 381,* 661–666.

Detels, R., English, P. A., Giorgi, J. V., Visscher, B. R., Fahey, J. L., Taylor, J. M. G., et al. (1988). Patterns of CD4+ cell changes after HIV-1 infection indicate the existence of a codeterminant of AIDS. *Journal of Acquired Immune Deficiency Syndromes, 1,* 390.

Dragic, T., V. Litwin, G. P. Allaway, S. R. Martin, Y. Huang, K. A. Nagashima, C. Cayanan, P. J. Maddon, R. A. Koup, J. P. Moore, & W. A. Paxton (1996). HIV-1 entry into CD4+ cells is mediated by the chemokine receptor CC-CKR-5. *Nature, 381,* 667–673.

Drebing, C. E., Van Gorp, W., Hinkin, C., Miller, E. N., Satz, P., Kim, D. S., et al. (1994). Confounding factors in the measurement of depression in HIV. *Journal of Personality Assessment, 62,* 68.

Dyner, T. S., Lang, W., Geaga, J., Golub, A., Stites, D., Winger, E., Galmarini, M., Masterson, J., & Jacobson, M. A. (1993). An open-label dose-escalation trial of oral dehydroepiandrosterone tolerance and pharmacokinetics in patients with HIV disease. *Journal of Acquired Immune Deficiency Syndromes, 6,* 459–465.

Effros, R. B., & Paselec, G. (1997). Replicative senescence of T cells: Does the Hayflick Limit lead to immune exhaustion? *Immunology Today, 18,* 450–454.

Eisenberger, N., Kemeny, M. E., & Wyatt, G. (1998). *Psychological inhibition is associated with lower CD4 T cell levels in HIV positive women.* Under review.

Eller, L. S. (1995). Effects of two cognitive-behavioral interventions on immunity and symptoms in persons with HIV. *Annals of Behavioral Medicine, 17,* 339.

Embertson, J., Zupancic, M., Ribas, J. L., Burke, A., Racz, P., Tenner-Racz, K., & Haase, A. T. (1993). Massive covert infection of helper T lymphocytes and macrophages by HIV during the incubation period of AIDS. *Nature, 362,* 359.

Esterling, B. A., Antoni, M. H., Schneiderman, N., Carver, C. S., LaPerriere, A., Ironson, G., Klimas, N. G., & Fletcher, M. A. (1992). Psychosocial modulation of antibody to Epstein-Barr viral capsid antigen and human herpesvirus type-6 in HIV-1-infected and at-risk gay men. *Psychosomatic Medicine, 54,* 354–371.

Eugen-Olsen, J., Afzelius, P., Andresen, L., Iversen, J., Kronborg, G., Aabech, P., Nielsen, J. O., & Hofmann, B. (1997). Serotonin modulates immune function in T cells from HIV-seropositive subjects. *Clinical Immunology and Immunopathology, 84,* 115–121.

Evans, D., L., Leserman, J., Perkins, D. O., Stern, R. A., Murphy, C., Tamul, K., et al. (1995). Stress-associated reductions of cytotoxic T lymphocytes and natural killer cells in asymptomatic HIV infection. *American Journal of Psychiatry, 152,* 543.

Fahey, J. L., Taylor, J. M. G., Detels, R., Hofmann, B., Melmed, R., Nishanian, P., & Giorgi, J. V. (1990). The prognostic value of cellular and serologic markers in infection with human immunodeficiency virus type 1. *New England Journal of Medicine, 322,* 166.

Fan, J., Bass, H. Z., & Fahey, J. L. (1993). Elevated IFN-gamma and decreased IL-2 gene expression are associated with HIV infection. *Journal of Immunology, 151,* 5031.

Felten, D. L., Felten, S. Y., Bellinger, D. L., Carlson, S. L., Ackerman, K. D., Madden, K. S., Olschowka, J. A., & Livnat, S. (1987). Noradrenergic sympathetic neural interactions with the immune system: Structure and function. *Immunological Reviews, 100,* 225.

Feng, Y., Broder, C. C., Kennedy, P. E., & Berger, E. A. (1996). HIV-1 entry cofactor: Functional cDNA cloning of a seven-transmembrane, G protein-coupled receptor. *Science, 272,* 872.

Finzi, D., Hermankova, M., Pierson, T., Carruth, L. M., Buck, C., Chaisson, R. E., Quinn, T. C., Chadwick, K., Margolick, J., Brookmeyer, R., et al. (1997). Identification of a reservoir for HIV-1 in patients on highly active antiretroviral therapy. *Science, 278,* 1295–1300.

Fox, C. H., & Cottler-Fox, M. (1992). The pathobiology of HIV infection. *Immunology Today, 13,* 353.

Frankenhauser, M. (1975). Experimental approaches to the study of catecholamines and emotion. In L. Levi (Ed.), *Emotions—Their parameters and measurement.* New York: Raven Press.

Friedman, S. B., Glasgow, L. A., & Ader, R. (1969). Psychosocial factors modifying host resistance to experimental infections. *Annals of the New York Academy of Sciences, 164,* 381.

Frost, S. D. W., & McLean, A. R. (1994). Germinal centre destruction as a major pathway in HIV pathogenesis. *Journal of Acquired Immune Deficiency Syndromes, 7,* 236.

Furth, P. A., Westphal, H., & Hennighausen, L. (1990). Expression from the HIV-LTR is stimulated by glucocorticoids and pregnancy. *AIDS Research and Human Retroviruses, 6,* 553–560.

Garcia, J. A., & Gaynor, R. B. (1994). Regulatory mechanisms involved in the control of HIV-1 gene expression. *AIDS, 8,* S3–S17.

Gauci, M., King, M. G., Saxarra, H., Tulloch, B. J., & Husband, A. J. (1993). A Minnesota Multiphasic Personality Inventory profile of women with allergic rhinitis. *Psychosomatic Medicine, 55,* 533–540.

Gibellini, D., Bassini, A., Pierpaoli, S., Bertolaso, L., Milani, D., Capitani, S., La Placa, M., & Zauli, G. (1998). Extracellular HIV-1 Tat protein induces the rapid Ser133 phosphorylation and activation of CREB transcription factor in both Jurkat lymphoblastoid T cells and primary peripheral blood mononuclear cells. *Journal of Immunology, 160,* 3981–3898.

Glaser, R., Kiecolt-Glaser, J. K., Malarkey, W. B., & Sheridan, J. F. (1998). The influence of psychological stress on the immune response to vaccines. *Annals of the New York Academy of Sciences, 840,* 649–655.

Goh, W. C., Rogel, M. E., Kinsey, C. M., Michael, S. F., Fultz, P. N., Nowak, M. A., Hahn, B. H., & Emerman, M. (1998). HIV-1 Vpr increases viral expression by manipulation of the cell cycle: A mechanism for selection of Vpr in vivo. *Nature Medicine, 4,* 65–71.

Goodkin, K., Blaney, N. T., Feaster, D., Fletcher, M. A., Baum, M. K., Mantero-Atienza, E., et al. (1990). Active coping style is associated with natural killer cell cytotoxicity in asymptomatic HIV-1 seropositive homosexual men. *Journal of Psychosomatic Research, 36,* 635.

Goodkin, K., Feaster, D. J., Asthana, D., Blaney, N. T., Kumar, M., Baldewicz, T., Tuttle, R. S., Maher, K. J., Baum, M. K., Shapshak, P., & Fletcher, M. A. (1998). A bereavement support group intervention is longitudinally associated with salutary effects on the CD4 cell count and number of physician visits. *Clinical and Diagnostic Laboratory Immunology, 5,* 382–391.

Goodkin, K., Fuchs, I., Feaster, D., Leeka, J., & Rishel, D. (1992). Life stressors and coping style are associated with immune measures in HIV-1 infection—A preliminary report. *International Journal of Psychiatric Medicine, 22,* 155.

Gorman, J. M., Kertzner, R., Cooper, T., Goetz, R. R., Lagomasino, I., Novacenko, H., et al. (1991). Glucocorticoid level and neuropsychiatric symptoms in homosexual men with HIV infection. *American Journal of Psychiatry, 41,* 148.

Graziosi, C., Pantaleo, G., Butini, L., Demarest, J. F., Saag, M. S., Shaw, G. M., and Fauci, A. S. (1993). Kinetics of human immunodeficiency virus type 1 (HIV-1) DNA and RNA synthesis during primary HIV-1 infection. *Proceedings of the National Academy of Science, USA, 90,* 6405.

Graziosi, C., Pantaleo, G., Gantt, K. R., Fortin J.-P., Demarest, J. F., Cohen, O. J., et al.(1994). Lack of evidence for the dichotomy of TH1 and TH2 predominance in HIV-infected individuals. *Science, 265,* 248.

Grinspoon, S. K., & Bilezikian, J. P. (1992). HIV disease and the endocrine system. *New England Journal of Medicine, 327,* 1360.

Gross, J. J., & Levenson, R. W. (1993). Emotional suppression: Physiology, self-report, and expressive behavior. *Journal of Personality and Social Psychology, 64,* 970.

Gruzelier, J., Burgess, A., Baldeweg, T., Riccio, M., Hawkins, D., Stygall, J., Catt, S., Irving, G., & Catalan, J. (1996). Prospective associations between lateralised brain function and immune status in HIV infection: Analysis of EEG, cognition, and mood over 30 months. *International Journal of Psychophysiology, 23,* 215–224.

Guenter, P., Muurahainen, N., Simons, G., Kosok, A., Cohan, G. R., Rudenstein, R., & Turner, J. L. (1993). Relationships among nutritional status, disease progression, and survival in HIV infection. *Journal of Acquired Immune Deficiency Syndromes, 6,* 1130.

Haraguchi, S., Good, R. A., & Day, N. K. (1995). Immunosuppressive retroviral peptides: cAMP and cytokine patterns. *Immunology Today, 16,* 595–603.

Haynes, B. F., Pantaleo, G., & Fauci, A. S. (1996). Toward an understanding of the correlates of protective immunity to HIV infection. *Science, 271,* 324.

Heaton, R. K., Velin, R. A., McCutchan, J. A., Gulevich, S. J., Atkinson, J. H., Wallace, M. R., et al. (1994). Neuropsychological impairment in human immunodeficiency virus infection: Implications for employment. *Psychosomatic Medicine, 56,* 8.

Heeney, J. L. (1995). AIDS: A disease of impaired Th cell renewal? *Immunology Today, 16,* 515.

Helbert, M. R., L'age-Stehr, J., & Mitchison, N. A. (1993). Antigen presentation, loss of immunologic memory, and AIDS. *Immunology Today, 14,* 340.

Helbert, M. R., L'age-Stehr, J., & Mitchison, N. A. (1993). Antigen presentation, loss of immunological memory and AIDS. *Immunology Today, 13,* 340.

Henderson, E., Yang, J.-Y., & Schwartz, A. (1992). Dehydroepiandosterone (DHEA) and synthetic DHEA analogs are modest inhibitors of HIV-1 IIIB replication. *AIDS Research and Human Retroviruses, 8,* 625–631.

Ho, D. D. (1996). Viral counts count in HIV infection. *Science, 272,* 1124.

Ho, D. D., Neumann, A. U., Perelson, A. S., Chen, W., Leonard, J. M., & Markowitz, M. (1995). Rapid turnover of plasma virions and CD4 lymphocytes in HIV-1 infection. *Nature, 373,* 123.

Ho, D. D., Rota, T. R., & Hirsch, M. S. (1986). Infection of monocyte/macrophages by human lymphotropic virus type III. *Journal of Clinical Investigation, 77*, 1712.

Ho, W. Z., Cnaan, A., Li, Y. H., Zhao, H., Lee, H. R., Song, L., & Douglas, S. D. (1996). Substance P modulates human immunodeficiency virus replication in human peripheral blood monocyte-derived macrophages. *AIDS Research and Human Retroviruses, 12*, 195–198.

Hoffman, B., Afzelius, P., Iverson, J., Kronborg, G., Aabech, P., Benfield, T., Dybkjaer, E., & Nielsen, J. O. (1996). Buspirone, a serotonin receptor agonist, increases CD4 T-cell counts and modulates the immune system in HIV-seropositive subjects. *AIDS, 10*, 1339–1347.

Hoffman, B., Nishanian, P., Nguyen, T., Liu, M., & Fahey, J. (1993a). Restoration of T-cell function in HIV infection by reduction of intracellular cAMP levels with adenosine analogues. *AIDS, 7*, 659.

Hofmann, B., Nishanian, P., Nguyen, T., Insixiengmay, P., & Fahey, J. L. (1993b). Human immunodeficiency virus proteins induce the inhibitory cAMP/protein kinase A pathway in normal lymphocytes. *Proceedings of the National Academy of Sciences, USA, 90*, 6676–6680.

Ironson, G., Friedman, A., Klimas, N., Antoni, M., Fletcher, M. A., LaPerriere, A., Simoneau, J., & Schneiderman, N. (1994). Distress, denial, and low adherence to behavioral interventions predict faster disease progression in gay men infected with human immunodeficiency virus, *International Journal of Behavioral Medicine, 1*, 90.

Irwin, M., Daniels, M., Smith, T., Bloom, E., & Weiner, H. (1987). Impaired natural killer cell activity during bereavement. *Brain, Behavior, and Immunity, 1*, 98

Israel-Biet, D., Cadranel, J., Beldjord, K., Andrieu, J. M., Jeffrey, A., & Even, P. (1991). Tumor necrosis factor production in HIV-seropositive subjects. *Journal of Immunology, 147*, 490.

Jensen, M. M., & Rasmussen, A. F., Jr. (1963). Stress and susceptibility to viral infection. I. Response of adrenals, liver, thymus, slpeen and peripheral leukocyte counts to sound stress. *Journal of Immunology, 90*, 17.

Johnson, T., Lavender, J. F., Hultin, F., & Rasmussen, A. F., Jr. (1965). The influence of avoidance-learning stress on resistance to Coxsackie B virus in mice. *Journal of Immunology, 91*, 569.

Jondal, M., Xue, Y., McConkey, D. J., & Okret, S. (1995). Thymocyte apoptosis by glucocorticoids and cAMP. *Current Topics in Microbiology and Immunology, 200*, 67–79.

Kagan, J., Reznick, J. S., & Snidman, N. (1988). Biological bases of childhood shyness. *Science, 240*, 67.

Kagan, J., Snidman, N., Julia-Sellers, M., & Johnson, M. O. (1991). Temperament and allergic symptoms. *Psychosomatic Medicine, 53*, 32.

Kaslow, P. A., Phair, J. P., Friedman, H. B., Lyter, D., Solomon, R. E., Dudley, J., et al. (1987). Infection with the human immunodeficiency virus: Clinical manifestations and their relationship to immune deficiency. A report from the Multicenter AIDS Cohort Study. *Annals of Internal Medicine, 107*, 474.

Kaslow, R. A., Duquesnoy, R., VanRaden, M., Kingsley, L. Marrari, M., Friedman, H., et al. (1990). A1, Cw7, B8, DR3 HLA antigen combination associated with rapid decline of T-helper lymphocytes in HIV-1 infection. A report from the Multicenter AIDS Cohort Study. *Lancet, 335*, 927.

Kawa, S. K., & Thompson, E. B. (1996). Lymphoid cell resistance to glucocorticoids in HIV infection. *Journal of Steroid Biochemistry and Molecular Biology, 57*, 259–263.

Keet, I. P. M., Krol, A., Klein, M. R., Veugelers, P., de Wit, J., Roos, M., et al. (1994). Characteristics of long-term asymptomatic infection with Human Immunodeficiency Virus Type 1 in men with normal and low CD4+ cell counts. *Journal of Infectious Disease, 169*, 1236.

Kemeny, M. E., & Dean, L. (1995). Effects of AIDS-related bereavement on HIV progression among New York City gay men. *AIDS Education and Preview, 7*, 36s.

Kemeny, M. E., Reed, G. M., Taylor, S. E., & Visscher, B. R. (1999). Negative HIV-specific expectancies and AIDS-related bereavement as predictors of symptom onset in asymptomatic HIV-positive gay men. *Health Psychology, 18*, 354.

Kemeny, M. E., Weiner, H., Duran, R., Taylor, S. E., Visscher, B., & Fahey, J. L. (1995). Immune system changes following the death of a partner in HIV positive gay men. *Psychosomatic Medicine, 57*, 547.

Kemeny, M. E., Weiner, H., Taylor, S. E., Schneider, S., Visscher, B., & Fahey, J. L. (1994). Repeated bereavement, depressed mood, and immune parameters in HIV seropositive and seronegative gay men. *Health Psychology, 13*, 14.

Kertzner, R. M., Goetz, R., Todak, G., Cooper, T., Lin, S. H., Reddy, M. K., et al. (1993). Cortisol levels, immune status, and mood in homosexual men with and without HIV infection. *American Journal of Psychiatry, 150*, 1674.

Kessler, R. C., Foster, C., Joseph, J., Ostrow, D., Wortman, C., Phair, J., et al. (1991). Stressful life events and symptom onset in HIV infection. *American Journal of Psychiatry, 148*, 733.

Kiecolt-Glaser, J. K., & Glaser, R. (1988). Methodological issues in behavioral immunology research with humans. *Brain, Behavior, and Immunity, 2*, 67,

Koot, M., Keet, I. P., Vos, A. H., de Goede, R. E., Roos, M. T., Coutinho, R. A., et al. (1993). Prognostic value of HIV-1 syncytium-inducing phenotype for rate of CD4+ cell depletion and progression to AIDS. *Annals of Internal Medicine, 118*, 681.

Kraemer, H. C., & Thiemann, S. (1987). *How many subjects? Statistical power analysis in research.* Newbury Park, CA: Sage.

Krebs, F. C., Mehrens, D., Pomeroy, S., Goodenow, M. M., & Wigdahl, B. (1998). Human immunodeficiency virus type 1 long terminal repeate quasispecies differ in basal transcription and nuclear factor recruitment in human glial cells and lymphocytes. *Journal of Biomedical Science, 5*, 31–44.

Kumar, M., Morgan, R., Szapocznik, J., & Eisdorfer, C. (1991). Norepinephrine response in early HIV infection. *Journal of Acquired Immune Deficiency Syndromes, 4*, 782.

Lang, W., Perkins, H., Anderson, R. E., Royce, R., Jewell, N., & Winkelstein, W. (1989). Patterns of T lymphocyte changes with human immunodeficiency virus infection: From seroconversion to the development of AIDS. *Journal of Acquired Immune Deficiency Syndromes, 2*, 63.

Lapointe, R., Lemieux, R. Olivier, M., & Darveau, A. (1996). Tyrosine kinase and cAMP-dependent protein kinase activities in CD40-activated human B lymphocytes. *European Journal of Immunology, 26*, 2376–2382.

Laurence, J., Cooke, H., & Sikder, S. K. (1990). Effect of tamixifen on regulation of viral replication and human immunodeficiency virus (HIV) long terminal repeat-directed transcription in cells chronically infected with HIV-1. *Blood, 75*, 696–703.

Laurence, J., Grimison, B., & Gonenne, A. (1992). Effect of recombinant human growth hormone on acute and chronic human immunodeficiency virus infection in vitro. *Blood, 79*, 467–472.

Laurence, J., Sellers, M. B., & Sikder, S. K. (1989). Effect of glucocorticoids on chronic human immunodeficiency virus (HIV) infection and HIV promoter-mediated transcription. *Blood, 74*, 291–297.

Lee, A. W., Mitra, D., & Laurence, J. (1997). Interaction of pregnancy steroid hormones and zidovudine in inhibition of HIV type 1 replication in monocytoid and placental Hofbauer cells: Implications for the prevention of maternal-fetal transmission of HIV. *AIDS Research and Human Retroviruses, 13,* 1235–1242.

Leserman, J., Petitto, J. M., Perkins, D. O, Folds, J. D., Golden, R. N., & Evans, D. L. (1997). Severe stress, depressive symptom, and changes in lymphocyte subsets in human immunodeficiency virus-infected men. *Archives of General Psychiatry, 54,* 279–85.

Levy, J. A. (1993). Pathogenesis of human immunodeficiency virus infection. *Microbiology Review, 57,* 183.

Levy, J. A., Mackewicz, C. E., & Barker, E. (1996). Controlling HIV pathogenesis: The role of the noncytotoxic anti-HIV response of CD8+ T cells. *Immunology Today, 17,* 217.

Li, T. S., Tubiana, R., Katlama, C, Calvez, V., Ait Mohand, H., & Autran, B. (1998). Long-lasting recovery in CD4 T-cell function and viral-load reduction after highly active antiretroviral therapy in advanced HIV-1 disease. *Lancet, 351,* 1682–1686.

Loewy, A. D., & Spyer, K. M. (1990). *Central regulation of autonomic functions.* New York: Oxford University Press.

Lu, W., Salerno-Goncalves, R., Yuan, J., Sylvie, D., Han, D.-S., and Andrieu, J.-M. (1995). Glucocorticoids rescue CD4+ T lymphocytes from activation-induced apoptosis triggered by HIV-1: Implications for pathogenesis and therapy. *AIDS, 9,* 35–42.

Lundberg, U., & Frankenhauser, M. (1980). Pituitary-adrenal and sympathetic-adrenal correlates of distress and effort. *Journal of Psychosomatic Research, 24,* 125.

Lusso, P., & Gallo, R. C. (1995). Human herpesvirus 6 in AIDS. *Immunology Today, 16,* 67.

Lutgendorf, S. K., Antoni, M. H., Ironson, G., Klimas, N., Kumar, M., Starr, K., McCabe, P. (1997). Cognitive-behavioral stress management decreases dysphoric mood and herpes simplex virus-type 2 antibody titers in sympomatic HIV-seropositive gay men. *Journal of Consulting and Clinical psychology, 65,* 31–43.

Lyketsos, C. G., Hoover, D. R., Guccione, M., Senterfitt, W., Dew, M. A., Wesch, J., et al. (1996). Depressive symptoms as predictors of medical outcomes in HIV infection. *JAMA, 270,* 2563.

Margolick, J. B., Donnenberg, A. D., Munoz, A., Park, L. P., Bauer, K. D., Giorgi, J. V., et al. (1993). Changes in T and non-T lymphocyte subsets following seroconversion to HIV-1: Stable CD3+ and declining CD3– populations suggest regulatory responses linked to loss of CD4 lymphocytes. *Journal of Acquired Immune Deficiency Syndromes, 6,* 153.

Markham, P. D., Salahuddin, S. Z., Veren, K., Orndorff, S., & Gallo, R. C. (1986). Hydrocortisone and some other hormones enhance the expression of HTLV-III. *International Journal of Cancer, 37,* 67.

Martin, J. L., & Dean, L. (1993). Effects of AIDS-related bereavement and HIV-related illness on psychological distress among gay men: A seven-year longitudinal study (1985–1992). *Journal of Consulting and Clinical Psychology, 61,* 94.

Mason, J. W. (1975). Emotion as reflected in patterns of endocrine integration. In L. Levi. (Ed.), *Emotions—Their parameters and measurement.* New York: Raven Press.

Mayne, T. J., Vittinghoff, E., Chesney, M. A., Barrett, D. C., & Coates, T. J. (1996). Depressive affefct and survival among gay and bisexual men infected with HIV. *Archives of Internal Medicine, 156,* 2233–2238.

Mellors, J. W., Rinaldo, C. R., Gupta, P., White, R. M., Todd, J. A., & Kingsley, L. A. (1996). Prognosis in HIV-1 infection predicted by the quantity of virus in plasma. *Science, 272,* 1167.

Melnick, S. L., Sherer, R., Louis, T. A., Hillman, D., Rodriguez, E. M., Lackman, C., et al. (1994). Survival and disease progression according to the gender of patients with HIV infection. The Terry Beirn Community Programs for Clinical Research on AIDS. *JAMA, 272,* 1915.

Membrino, L., Irony, I., Dere, W., Klein, R., Biglieri, E. G., & Cobb, E. (1987). Adrenocortical function in acquired immunodeficiency syndrome. *Journal of Clinical Endocrinology and Metabolism, 65,* 482.

Merinich, J. A., McDermott, M. T., Asp, A. A., Harrison, S. M., & Kidd, G. S. (1993). Evidence of endocrine involvement early in the course of Human Immunodeficiency Virus infection. *Journal of Clinical Endocrinology and Metabolism, 70,* 566.

Miller, G. E., & Cole, S. W. (1998). Social relationships and the progress of human immunodeficiency virus infection: A review of evidence and possible underlying mechanisms. *Annals of Behavioral Medicine, 20,* 181–89.

Miller, G. E., Kemeny, M. E., Taylor, S. E., Cole, S. W., & Visscher, B. R. (1997). Social relationships and immune processes in HIV seropositive gay men. *Annals of Behavioral Medicine, 119,* 139–151.

Mitra, D., Sikder, S., & Laurence, J. (1993). Inhibition of tat-activated HIV-1 LTR-mediated gene expression by glucocorticoids. *AIDS Research and Human Retroviruses, 9,* 1055.

Mitra, D., Sikder, S. K., & Laurence, J. (1995). Role of glucocorticoid receptor binding sites in the human immunodeficiency virus type 1 long terminal repeat in steroid-mediated suppression of HIV gene expression. *Virology, 214,* 512–521.

Moldawer, L. L., & Sattler, F. R. (1998). Human immunodeficiency virus-associated wasting and the mechanisms of cachexia associated with inflammation. *Seminars in Oncology, 25* (1 Suppl. 1), 73–81.

Mosier, D. E., Gulizia, R. J., MacIsaac, P. D., Torbett, B. E., & Levy, J. A. (1993). Rapid loss of CD4+ T cells in Human-PBL-SCID mice by noncytopathic HIV isolates. *Science, 260,* 689.

Mosmann, T. R. (1994). Cytokine patterns during the progression to AIDS. *Science, 265,* 193.

Moss, H., Bose, S., Wolters, P., & Brouwers, P. (1998). A preliminary study of factors associated with psychological adjustment and disease course in school-age children infected with the human immunodeficiency virus. *Journal of Developmental and Behavioral Pediatrics, 19,* 18–25.

Mulder, C. L., Antoni, M. H., Duivenvoorden, H. J., Kauffmann, R. H., Goodkin, K. (1995). Active confrontational coping predicts decreased clinical progression over a one-year period in HIV-infected homosexual men. *Journal of Psychosomatic Research, 39,* 957–65.

Mulder, C. L., Antoni, M. H., Emmelkamp, P. M., Veugelers, P. J., Sandfort, T. G., van de Vijver, F. A., & de Vries, M. J. (1995). Psychosocial group intervention and decline of immunologic parameters in asymptomatic HIV-infected homosexual men. *Psychotherapy and Psychosomatics, 63,* 185.

Mulligan, K., & Bloch, A. S. (1998). Energy expenditure and protein metabolism in human immunodeficiency virus infection and cancer cachexia. *Seminars in Oncology, 25* (2 Suppl. 6), 82–91.

Munoz, A., Carey, V., Saah, A. J., Phair, J. P., Kingsley, L. A., Fahey, J. L., et al. (1988). Predictors of decline in CD4 lymphocytes in a cohort of homosexual men infected with human immunodeficiency virus. *Journal of Acquired Immune Deficiency Syndromes, 1,* 396.

Munoz, A., Wang, M. C., Bass, S., Taylor, J. M., Kingsley, L. A., Chimel, J. S., et al. (1989). Acquired immunodeficiency syndrome (AIDS)-free time after human immunodeficiency virus type 1 (HIV-1) seroconversion in homosexual men. Multicenter AIDS Cohort Study Group. *American Journal of Epidemiology, 130,* 530.

Nabel, G., & Baltimore, D. (1987). An inducible transcription factor activates expression of human immunodeficiency virus in T cells. *Nature, 326,* 711–713.

Nair, M. P., & Schwartz, S. A. (1995). Synergistic effect of cortisol and HIV-1 envelope peptide on the NK activities of normal lymphocytes. *Brain, Behavior, and Immunity, 9,* 20–30.

Nair, M. P., Saravolatz, L. D., & Schwartz, S. A. (1995). Selective inhibitory effects of stress hormones on natural killer (NK) cell activity of lymphocytes from AIDS patients. *Immunological Investigations, 24,* 689–699.

Nakajima, K., Martinez-Maza, O., Hirano, T., Breen, E. C., Nishanian, P. G., Salazar-Gonzalez, F., Fahey, J. L., & Kishimoto, T. (1989). Induction of IL-6 (B cell stimulatory factor-2/IFN-beta 2) production by HIV. *Journal of Immunology, 142,* 531.

Neugebaur, R., Rabkin, J. G., Williams, J. B., Reimen, R. H., Goetz, R., & Gorman, J. M. (1992). Bereavement reactions among homosexual men experiencing multiple losses in the AIDS epidemic. *American Journal of Psychiatry, 149,* 137.

Nokta, M., & Pollard, R. (1991). Human immunodeficiency virus infection: Association with altered intracellular levels of cAMP and cGMP in MT-4 cells. *Virology, 181,* 211–217.

Nokta, M., & Pollard, R. B. (1992). Human immunodeficiency virus replication: Modulation by cellular levels of cAMP. *AIDS Research and Human Retroviruses, 8,* 1255.

Norbiato, G., Bevilacqua, M., Vago, T., & Clerici, M. (1998). Glucocorticoid resistance and the immune function in the immunodeficiency syndrome. *Annals of the New York Academy of Sciences, 840,* 835–847.

Norbiato, G., Bevilacqua, M., Vago, T., Taddei, A., & Clerici, M. (1997). Glucocorticoids and the immune function in the human immunodeficiency virus infection: A study in hypercortisolemic and cortisol-resistant patients. *Journal of Clinical Endocrinology and Metabolism, 82,* 3260–3263.

Norbiato, G., Galli, M., Righini, V., & Moroni, M. (1994). The syndrome of acquired glucocorticoid resistance in HIV infection. *Baillieres Clinical Endocrinology and Metabolism, 8,* 777–787.

Norman, S. E., Chediak, A. D., Freeman, C., Kiel, M., Mendez, A., Duncan, R., et al. (1992). Sleep disturbance in men with asymptomatic human immunodeficiency virus (HIV) infection. *Sleep, 15,* 150.

Padgett, D. A., Sheridan, J. F., Dorne, J., Berntson, G. G., Candelora, J., & Glaser, R. (1998). Social stress and the reactivation of latent herpes simplex virus type 1. *Proceedings of the National Academy of Sciences, USA, 95,* 7231–7235.

Page-Shafer, K., Delorenze, G. N., Satariano, W. A., & Winkelstein, W. (1996). Comorbidity and survival in HIV-1 infected men in the San Francisco Men's Health Survey. *Annals of Epidemiology, 6,* 420–430.

Pakker, N. G., Notermans, D. W., de Boer, R. J., Roos, M. T., de Wolf, F., Hill, A., Leondard, J. M., Danner, S. A., Miedema, F., & Schellekens, P. T. (1998). Biphasic kinetics of peripheral blood T cells after triple combination therapy in HIV-1 infection: A composite of redistribution and proliferation. *Nature Medicine, 4,* 208–214.

Pantaleo, G., Craziosi, C., Demarest, J. F., Butini, L., Montroni, M., Fox, C. H., et al. (1993). HIV infection is active and progressive in lymphoid tissue during the clinically latent stage of disease. *Nature, 362,* 355.

Pantaleo, G., Demarest, J. F., Soudeyns, H., Graziosi, C., Francois, D., Adelsberger, J. W., et al. (1994). Major expansion of CD8+ T cells with a predominant V-beta usage during the primary immune response to HIV. *Nature, 370,* 463.

Pantaleo, G., Graziosi, C., & Fauci, A. S. (1993). The immunopathogenesis of human immunodeficiency virus infection. *New England Journal of Medicine, 328,* 327.

Patterson, T. L., Shaw, W. S., Semple, S. J., Cherner, M., McCutchan, A., Atkinson, J. H., et al. (1996). Relationship of psychosocial factors to HIV disease progression. *Annals of Behavioral Medicine, 18,* 30.

Patterson, T. L., Semple, S. J., Temoshok, L. R., Atkinson, J. H., McCutchan, J. A., Straits-Troster, K., Chandler, J. L., Grant, I., & HIV Neurobehavioral Research Center Group (1995). *Psychiatry, 58,* 299–312.

Pedersen, C., Nielsen, J. O., Dickmeis, E., & Jordal, R. (1989). Early progression to AIDS following primary HIV infection. *AIDS, 3,* 45–47.

Pennebaker, J. W., & Chew, C. H. (1985). Behavioral inhibition and electrodermal activity during deception. *Journal of Personality and Social Psychology, 49,* 1427.

Pennebaker, J. W., Kiecolt-Glaser, J. K., & Glaser, R. (1988). Disclosure of traumas and immune function: Health implications for psychotherapy. *Journal of Consulting and Clinical Psychology, 56,* 239

Perelson, A. S., Neumann, A. U., Markowitz, M., Leonard, J. M., & Ho, D. D. (1996). HIV-1 dynamics in vivo: Virion clearance rate, infected cell life-span, and viral generation time. *Science, 271,* 1582–1586.

Perry, S., Fishman, B., Jacobsberg, L., & Frances, A. (1992). Relationships over 1 year between lymphocyte subsets and psychosocial variables among adults with infection by human immunodeficiency virus. *Archives of General Psychiatry, 49,* 396.

Persson, L., Gullberg, B., Hanson, B. S., Moestrup, T., & Ostergreen, P. O. (1994a). *Influences of social network and social support on the development of the CD4-lymphocyte level—A prospective population study of HIV-infected homo- and bi-sexual men in Malmo, Sweden.* Paper presented at the Second International Conference on Psychosocial Aspects of AIDS, Brighton, UK.

Persson, L., Gullberg, B., Hanson, B. S., Moestrup, T., & Ostergren, P. O. (1994b). HIV infection: Social network, social support, and CD4 lymphocyte values in infected homosexual men in Malmo, Sweden. *Journal of Epidemiology and Community Health, 48,* 580.

Petito, J. M., Lysle, D. T., Gariepy, J.-L., & Lewis, M. H. (1994). Association of genetic differences in social behavior and cellular immune responsiveness: Effects of social experience. *Brain, Behavior, and Immunity, 8,* 111.

Petrie, K. J., Booth, R. J., Pennebaker, J. W., Davison, K. P., & Thomas, M. G. (1995). Disclosure of trauma and immune response to a hepatitis B vaccination program. *Journal of Consulting and Clinical Psychology, 63,* 787.

Phair, J., Jacobson, L., Detels, R., Rinaldo, C., Saah, A., Schrager, L., et al. (1992). Acquired immune deficiency syndrome occurring within 5 years of infection with human immunodeficiency virus type 1: The Multicenter AIDS Cohort Study. *Journal of Acquired Immune Deficiency Syndromes, 5,* 490.

Phillips, A. N., Lee, C. A., Webster, A., Janossy, G., Timms, A., Bofill, M., & Kernoff, P. B. (1991). More rapid progression to AIDS in older HIV-infected people: The role of CD4+ T-cell counts. *Journal of AIDS, 4,* 970.

Phillips, E. J., Ottaway, C. A., Freedman, J., Kardish, M., Li, J., Singer, W., & Fong, I. W. (1997). The effect of exercise on lymphocyte redistribution and leucocyte function in asymptomatic HIV-infected subjects. *Brain, Behavior, and Immunity, 11,* 217–227.

Pitak, M., Saag, M. S., Yang, L. C., Clark, S. J., Kappes, J. C., Luk, K.-C., et al. (1993). High levels of HIV-1 in plasma during all stages of infection determined by competitive PCR. *Science, 249,* 1749.

Powderly, W. G., Landay, A., & Lederman, M. M. (1998). Recovery of the immune system with antiretroviral therapy: The end of opportunism? *JAMA, 280,* 72–77.

Price, R. W., Brew, B., Sidtis, J., Rosenblum, M., Scheck, A. C., & Cleary, P. (1988). The brain and AIDS: Central nervous system HIV-1 infection and AIDS dementia complex. *Science, 239*, 586.

Rabbi, M. F., Al-Harthi, L., & Roebuck, K. A. (1997). TNF-$\alpha$ cooperates with the protein kinase A pathway to synergistically increase HIV-1 LTR transcription via downstream TRE-like cAMP response elements. *Virology, 237*, 422–429.

Rabbi, M. F., Al-Harthi, L., Saifuddin, M., & Roebuck, K. A. (1998). The cAMP-dependent protein kinase A and protein kinase C-beta pathways synergistically interact to activate HIV-1 transcription in latently infected cells of monocyte/macrophage lineage. *Virology, 245*, 257–269.

Rabbi, M. F., Saifuddin, M., Gu, D. S., Kagnoff, M. F., & Roebuck, K. A. (1997). U5 region of the human immunodeficiency virus type 1 long terminal repeat contains TRE-like cAMP-responsive elements that bind both AP-1 and CREB/ATF proteins. *Virology, 233*, 235–245.

Rabkin, J., Williams, J. B. W., Remien, R. H., Goetz, R., Kertzner, R., & Gorman, J. M. (1991). Depression, distress, lymphocyte subsets, and human immunodeficiency virus symptoms on two occasions in HIV-positive homosexual men. *Archives of General Psychiatry, 48*, 111.

Rabkin, J. G., Rabkin, R., Harrison, W., & Wagner, G. (1994). Effect of imipramine on mood and enumerative measures of immune status in depressed patients with HIV illness. *American Journal of Psychiatry, 151*, 516.

Rabkin, J. G., Rabkin, R., & Wagner, G. (1994). Effects of fluoxetine on mood and immune status in depressed patients with HIV disease. *Journal of Clinical Psychiatry, 55*, 92.

Rabkin, J. G., Wagner, G., & Rabkin, R. (1994). Effects of sertraline on mood and immune status in patients with major depression and HIV illness: An open trial. *Journal of Clinical Psychiatry, 55*, 433.

Rasmussen, A. F., Jr., Marsh, J. T., & Brill, N. Q. (1957). Increased susceptibility to herpes simplex in mice subjected to avoidance-learning stress or restraint. *Proceedings of the Society for Experimental Biology and Medicine, 96*, 183.

Reed, G. M., Kemeny, M. E., Taylor, S. E., & Visscher, B. R. (1998). *Negative HIV-specific expectancies and AIDS-related bereavement as predictors of symptom onset in asymptomatic HIV seropositive gay men.* Under review.

Reed, G. M., Kemeny, M. E., Taylor, S. E., Wang, H.-Y. J., & Visscher, B. R. (1994). Realistic acceptance as a predictor of decreased survival time in gay men with AIDS. *Health Psychology, 13*, 299.

Roger, M. (1998). Influence of host genes on HIV-1 disease progression. *FASEB Journal, 12*, 625–632.

Rose, R. M. (1980). Endocrine responses to stressful psychological events. *Psychiatric Clinics of North America, 3*, 251.

Rosenberg, Y. J., Anderson, A. O., & Pabst, R. (1998). HIV-induced decline in blood CD4/CD8 ratios: Viral killing or altered lymphocyte trafficking? *Immunology Today, 19*, 10–17.

Rosenberg, Z., & Fauci, A. S. (1989). Mini-review: Induction of expression of HIV in latently or chronically infected cells. *AIDS Research and Human Retroviruses, 5*, 1.

Saah, A. J., Hoover, D. R., He, Y., Kingsley, L. A., Phair, J. P., & the Multicenter AIDS Cohort Study (1994). Factors influencing survival after AIDS: Report from the Multicenter AIDS Cohort Study (MACS). *Journal of Acquired Immune Deficiency Syndromes, 7*, 287.

Sahs, J. A., Goetz, R., Reddy, M., Rabkin, J. G., Williams, J. B. W., Kertzner, R., & Gorman, J. M. (1994). Psychological distress and natural killer cells in gay men with and without HIV infection. *American Journal of Psychiatry, 151*, 1479–1484.

Sapolsky, R. M. (1993). *Why zebras don't get ulcers: A guide to stress, stress-related disease, and coping.* New York: Freeman.

Schambelan, M., Mulligan, K., Grunfeld, C., Daar, E. S., LaMarca, A., Kotler, D. P., Wang, J., Bozzette, S. A., & Breitmeyer, J. B. (1996). Recombinant human growth hormone in patients with HIV-associated wasting. A randomized, placebo-controlled trial. *Serostim Study Group. Annals of Internal Medicine, 125*, 873–882.

Scheinman, R. I., Cogswell, P. C., Lofquist, A. K., & Baldwin, A. S. (1995). Role of transcriptional activation of I$\kappa$B in mediation of immunosuppression by glucocorticoids. *Science, 270*, 283.

Schleifer, S. J., Keller, S. E., Camerino, M., Thronton, J. C., & Stein, M. (1983). Suppression of lymphocyte stimulation following bereavement. *JAMA, 240*, 374.

Schroff, R. W., Gottlieb, M. S., Prince, H. E., Chai, L. L., & Fahey, J. L. (1983). Immunological studies of homosexual men with immunodeficiency and Kaposi's sarcoma. *Clinical Immunology and Immunopathology, 27*, 300–314.

Schwartz, C., Canonne-Hergaux, F., Aunis, D., & Schaeffer, E. (1997). Characterization of nuclear proteins that bind to the regulatory TGATTGGC motif in the human immunodeficiency virus type 1 long terminal repeat. *Nucleic Acids Research, 25*, 1177–1184.

Scott-Algara, D., Vuillier, F., Marasescu, M., De Saint Martin, J., & Dighiero, G. (1991). Serum levels of IL-2, IL-1$\alpha$, TNF-$\alpha$, and soluble receptor of IL-2 in HIV-1 infected patients. *AIDS Research and Human Retroviruses, 7*, 381.

Segerstrom, S., Kemeny, M. E., Taylor, S. E., & Reed, G. (1996). Causal attributions predict rate of immune decline in HIV-seropositive gay men. *Health Psychology, 15*, 485–493.

Shafer, R. W., Offit, K., Macris, N. T., Hobar, G. M., Ancona, L., & Hoffman, I. R. (1985). Possible risk of steroid administration in patients at risk for AIDS. *Lancet, 2*, 934.

Sheppard, H. W., Lang, W., Ascher, M. S., Vittinghoff, E., & Winkelstein, W. (1993). The characteristics of non-progressors: Long term HIV-1 infection with stable CD4+ T-cell levels. *AIDS, 7*, 1159.

Sheridan, J. F., Dobbs, C., Jung, J., Chu, X., Konstantinos, A., Padgett, D., & Glaser, R. (1998). Stress-induced neuroendocrine modulation of viral pathogenesis and immunity. *Annals of the New York Academy of Sciences, 840*, 803–808.

Solano, L., Costa, M., Salvati, S., Coda, R., Aiuti, F., Mezzaroma, I., & Bertini, M. (1993). Psychosocial factors and clinical evolution in HIV-1 infection: A longitudinal study. *Journal of Psychosomatic Research, 37*, 39.

Solomon, G. F., & Temoshok, L. (1987). A psychoneuroimmunologic perspective on AIDS research: Questions, preliminary findings, and suggestions. *Journal of Applied Social Psychology, 17*, 286.

Soudeyns, H., Geleziunas, R., Shyamala, G., Hiscott, J., & Wainberg, M. A. (1993). Identification of a novel glucocorticoid response element within the genome of the human immunodeficiency virus type 1. *Virology, 194*, 758–768.

Spandidos, D. A., Zoumpourlis, V., Kotsinas, A., Tsiriyotis, C., & Sekeris, C. E. (1990). Response of human immunodeficiency virus long terminal repeat to growth factors and hormones. *Anticancer Research, 10*, 1241–1245.

Straub, R. H., Westermann, J., Scholmerich, J., & Falk, W. (1998). Dialogue between the CNS and the immune system in lymphoid organs. *Immunology Today, 19*, 409–413.

Strawford, A., & Hellerstein, M. (1998). The etiology of wasting in the human immunodeficiency virus and acquired immunodeficiency syndrome. *Seminars in Oncology, 25* (2 Suppl. 6), 76–81.

Stroebe, M. S., & Stroebe, W. (1983). Who suffers more? Sex differences in health risks of the widowed. *Psychological Bulletin, 93*, 297.

Stone, A. A., Neale, J. M., Cox, D. S., Napoli, A., Valdimarsdottir, H., & Kennedy-Moore, E. (1994). Daily events are associated with a secondary immune response to an oral antigen in men. *Health Psychology, 13,* 440–446.

Suomi, S. J. (1991). Uptight and laid-back monkeys: Individual differences in the response to social challenges. In S., Branch, W., Hall, and E., Dooling, (Eds.), *Plasticity of development.* Cambridge, MA: MIT Press.

Sutton, S. K., & Davidson, R. J. (1997). Prefrontal brain asymmetry: A biological substrate of the behavioral approach and inhibition systems. *Psychological Science, 8,* 204–210.

Taylor, D. N. (1995). Effects of a behavioral stress-management program on anxiety, mood, self-esteem, and T-cell count in HIV-positive men. *Psychology Reports, 76,* 451.

Taylor, J. M. G., Fahey, J. L., Detels, R., & Giorgi, J. V. (1989). CD4 percentage, CD4 number, and CD4:CD8 ratio in HIV infection: Which to choose and how to use. *Journal of Acquired Immune Deficiency Syndromes, 2,* 114–124.

Theorell, T., Blomkvist, V., Jonsson, H., Schulman, S., Berntrop, E., & Stigendal, L. (1995). Social support and the development of immune function in human immunodeficiency virus infection. *Psychosomatic Medicine, 57,* 32.

Thivierge, M., Le Gouill, C., Tremblay, M. J., Stankova, J., & Rola-Pleszczynski (1998). Prostaglandin E2 induces resistance to human immunodeficiency virus-1 infection in monocyte-derived macrophages: Downregulation of CCR5 expression by cyclic adenosine monophosphate. *Blood, 92,* 40–45.

Thomas, C. A., Weinberger, O. K., Ziegler, B. L., Greenberg, S., Schieren, I., Silverstein, S. C., & El Khoury, J. (1997). Human immunodeficiency virus-1 env impairs Fc receptor-mediated phagocytosis via a cyclic adenosine monophosphate-dependent mechanism. *Blood, 90,* 3760–3765.

Totman, R., Kiff, J. Reed, S. A., & Craig, J. W. (1980). Predicting experimental colds in volunteers from different measures of recent life stress. *Journal of Psychosomatic Research, 24,* 155.

Ullum, H., Palmo, J., Halkjer, Kristenson, J., Diamant, M., Klokker, M., Kruuse, A., et al. (1994). The effect of acute exercise on lymphocyte subsets, natural killer cells, proliferative responses, and cytokines in HIV-seropositive persons. *Journal of Acquired Immune Deficiency Syndromes, 7,* 1122.

Vacchio, M. S., Ashwell, J. D., & King, L. B. (1998). A positive role for thymus-derived steroids in formation of the T-cell repertoire. *Annals of the New York Academy of Sciences, 840,* 317–327.

Vago, T., Clerici, M., & Norbiato, G. (1994). Glucocorticoids and the immune system in AIDS. *Baillieres Clinical Endocrinology and Metabolism, 8,* 789–802.

Vedhara, K., Nott, K. H., Bradbeer, C. S., Davidson, E. A., Ong, E. L., Snow, M. H., Palmer, D., Nayagam, A. T. (1997). Greater emotional distress is associated with accelerated CD4+ cell decline in HIV infection. *Journal of Psychosomatic Research, 42,* 379–90.

Villette, J. M., Bourin, P., Doinel, C., Mansour, I., Fiet, J., Boudou, P., et al. (1990). Circadian variation in plasma levels of hypophyseal, adrenocortical and testicular hormones in men infected with the human immunodeficiency virus. *Journal of Clinical Endocrinology and Metabolism, 70,* 572.

Von Sydow, M., Sonnerborg, A., Gaines, H., & Strannegard, O. (1991). Interferon-alpha and tumor necrosis factor alpha in serum of patients in various stages of HIV-1 infection. *AIDS Research and Human Retroviruses, 7,* 375.

Webster, A., Lee, C. A., Cook, D. G., Grundy, J. E., Emery, V. C., Kernoff, P. B., et al. (1989). Cytomegalovirus infection and progression towards AIDS in haemophiliacs with human immunodeficiency virus infection. *Lancet, 2,* 63.

Wei, X., Ghosh, S. K., Taylor, M. E., Johnson, V. A., Emini, E., Deutsch, P., et al. (1995). Viral dynamics in human immunodeficiency virus type 1 infection. *Nature, 373,* 117.

Weiner, H. (1992). *Perturbing the organism: The biology of stressful experience.* Chicago: University of Chicago Press.

Weitzman, O., Kemeny, M. E., & Fahey, J. L. (1998). *Persistent shame and guilt predicts CD4 decline, AIDS onset, and mortality.* Under review.

Wilson, I. B., & Cleary, P. D. (1997). Clinical predictors of declines in physical functioning in persons with AIDS: Results of a longitudinal study. *Journal of Acquired Immune Deficiency Syndromes and Human Retrovirology, 16,* 343–349.

Winkler, C., Modi, W., Smith, M. W., Nelson, G., Wu, X., Carrington, M., et al. (1998). Genetic restriction of AIDS pathogenesis by an SDF-1 chemokine gene variant. *Science, 279,* 389–393.

Wolthers, K. C., Schuitemaker, H., & Midema, F. (1998). Rapid CD4+ T-cell turnover in HIV-1 infection: A paradigm revisited. *Immunology Today, 19,* 44–48.

Yamada, A., Jensen, M. M., & Rasmussen, A. F., Jr. (1964). Stress and susceptibility to viral infections. III. Antibody response and viral retention during avoidance learning stress. *Proceedings of the Society for Experimental Biology and Medicine, '116,* 667.

Yang, J.-Y., Schwartz, & Henderson, E. E. (1993). Inhibition of HIV-1 latency reactivation by dehydroepiandrosterone (DHEA) and an analog of DHEA. *AIDS Research and Human Retroviruses, 9,* 747–754.

Yang, J.-Y., Schwartz, A., & Henderson, E. E. (1994). Inhibition of 3'azido-3'deocythymidine-resistant HIV-1 infection by dehydroepiandrosterone in vitro. *Biochemical and Biophysical Research Communications, 201,* 1424–1432.

# 62

# Stress and Wound Healing

PHILLIP T. MARUCHA, JOHN F. SHERIDAN, DAVID PADGETT

## I. INTRODUCTION

Wound healing is a highly conserved physiological response designed to reestablish the normal structure and function of a tissue after injury. Tissue damage may be the result of physical injury, e.g., trauma/surgery, or tissue destruction caused by infections, autoimmune reactions, or neoplasms. Wound healing represents a cascade of discrete events which includes the localized release of biologically active molecules, induction of gene expression, trafficking of cellular elements, contraction of the damaged tissue, production of a temporary or provisional matrix, reepithelialization of the wound surface, and reconstruction of the underlying connective tissue. The rate of healing is dependent upon a number of factors including the location of the wound, the size and depth of the injured area, the presence of bacteria, and the age and overall health of the host. The optimal expression of inflammation through the course of wound healing protects the host from infection and regulates the activities of tissue cells that will repair the injured tissue.

Inflammation is strongly integrated with other physiological responses, particularly those of the nervous and endocrine systems. For example, stress causes physiologic changes, such as the rise in plasma glucocorticoids (GC), which can suppress inflammation and result in a decrease in wound healing kinetics (Kiecolt-Glaser, Marucha, Malarky, Mercado, & Glaser, 1995; Marucha, Kiecolt-Glaser, & Favagehi, 1998; Padgett, Marucha, & Sheridan, 1998). Stress is generally defined as a state of altered homeostasis resulting from either an external or internal stimulus, with the response to stress involving a variety of adaptive neuroendocrine mechanisms designed to restore homeostasis. Stressors induce a bodywide set of physiologic adaptations mediated primarily through the activation of the hypothalamo-pituitary-adrenal axis (HPA) and sympathetic nervous system (SNS). These pathways intersect and modulate inflammatory and immune responses. The highly integrated nature of these systems is due in large part to the sharing of common receptors and ligands, and suggests that physiologic changes in one system may affect the state of activation of the others. For example, cytokines produced during an inflammatory response activate immune function and also stimulate the central nervous system (CNS), leading to the release of neurotransmitters and adrenal hormones. Proinflammatory cytokines, like IL-1, signal hypothalamic neurons to release corticotropin-releasing hormone (CRH), which in turn activates pituitary-adrenal counterregulation of inflammation through the potent anti-inflammatory effects of GC. Thus, the response to stress would be expected to have an impact on the outcome of wound healing since wound healing is regulated by inflammatory mediators. In addition, when delayed healing is associated with reduced recruitment/function of phagocytic cells caused by stress, there is a greater risk of infection. When the wound is part of a therapeutic treatment, (e.g., periodontal or cosmetic surgery), the beneficial effect of that treatment may not be obtained if healing is impaired.

## II. STRESS AND HEALING

The effects of stress on wound healing have been documented in several recent studies in humans and animals. Using a standardized, full thickness, skin biopsy, Kiecolt-Glaser et al. (1995) demonstrated that it took chronically stressed Alzhiemer's caregivers 24% longer than age matched controls to heal a 3.5-mm cutaneous punch biopsy. This represented a 9-day delay in wound closure compared to that seen in the unstressed individuals. Stress was measured on the day of wounding using the perceived stress scale (Cohen & Hoberman, 1983). Caregivers scored significantly higher on the scale than the controls (20.5 vs. 13.7). In another study, Marucha et al. (1998) used a standardized oral wound to investigate the role of short-term stress in dental students. Second-year dental students had full thickness wounds placed on the roofs of their mouths during summer vacation and 3 days before a set of challenging examinations. Healing was delayed 40% during the examination period as compared to the wounds placed in the same individuals during the vacation period. As expected, the perceived stress scale scores on the day of wounding for the examination period was significantly greater than during the vacation period (16.0 vs. 7.4). Thus, in both older adults subjected to chronic stress and in younger adults subjected to short term stress, wound healing was delayed.

In order to investigate the mechanisms that contributed to the stress-induced delay in wound repair, a mouse model of cutaneous wound healing was developed by Padgett et al. (1998). Female, hairless SKH-1 mice, 6–8 weeks of age were subjected to restraint stress 3 days before and for 5 days following dorsal application of a 3.5-mm punch wound. The data showed that wounds on stressed mice took more than 3 additional days to heal as compared to those of control mice. Similar to the human studies, this represented a 27% delay in healing. In addition, cross-sectional histological analysis of the wound revealed reduced inflammation in restrained mice during the initial stages after wounding. The reduced inflammatory response in the stressed animals correlated with activation of the HPA axis and elevated serum corticosterone levels. When the action of

glucocorticoids was blocked by using the receptor antagonist, RU 40555, normal healing and cellularity of the wound was restored. Thus, the reduction in inflammation and delayed healing correlated with serum corticosterone levels and suggest that disruption of neuroendocrine homeostasis modulates wound healing.

Despite the differences in tissue sites (mucosa versus skin) and the differences in the morphology of mouse and human skin, the findings were consistent among each of these studies—healing was delayed by stress. Furthermore, measurement of healing revealed that differences in wounds between stressed and nonstressed conditions were apparent very early during the repair process regardless of the model.

## III. WOUND HEALING MODELS

The nature of the wound influences the nature of healing. Surgical wounds heal most rapidly when the edges of the wound are placed in close approximation using sutures or staples. This is termed "healing by first or primary intention." By definition, no granulation tissue occurs between the healing margins of such wounds. The rate of healing is influenced more by the skill of the surgeon suturing the edges of the wound together and less by the actual size of the wound.

In contrast, healing by "second intention" is when the wound margins are not approximated as in unsutured wounds (e.g., biopsies or abrasions). For healing of such wounds, granulation tissue is required for epithelial migration and connective tissue repair. Since the epithelium migrates from the wound margin, the rate of healing is determined by the geometry of the wound. Therefore, long narrow wounds heal faster than circular wounds of the same overall area.

The measurement of wound healing depends upon the model used (i.e., the type of wound) and the component of healing that is under study. Tracing the outline of the wound, or photoplanimetry, is one of the most common ways to measure wounds healing by second intention. By measuring changes in wound size over time, the kinetics of closure may be established and the effects of an intervention may be assessed. Therefore, measuring wounds by photoplanimetery and using standardized wounds overcomes many of the difficulties presented by wound geometry. Since wound size changes are a consequence of both wound contraction and reepithelialization, it may be important to measure the relative contributions of each. Wound contraction can be measured by marking the border of the wound and measuring the change in size of the original border over time (Cross, Naylor, Coleman, & Teo, 1995). Later assessments of healing include the re-establishment of barrier function of the epithelium and the quality of connective tissue repair. The epithelial barrier has been measured by assessing permeability to mannitol, and fluorescein (Brevetti, Napierkowski, & Maher, 1997; Mishima, 1982; Moore, Carlson, & Madara, 1989). The quality of connective tissue repair has been measured by the quantity and the types of collagen found in the healing wounds and by the measurement of wound strength (Hastings, Van Winkle, Barker, Hines, & Nichols, 1975; Paul et al., 1997). Wound strength measurements are accomplished by increasing tension on wounds until they fail. This has been used most extensively in measuring the outcomes of sutured wounds (Cohen & Mast, 1990). Histological and molecular analysis of healing have become our most powerful tools for understanding the events controlling wound healing (Martin, 1997; Riches, 1996; Schaffer & Nanney, 1996). Thus, using a combination of polymerase chain reaction, (PCR), immunohistochemistry and in situ hybridization, the pattern of gene expression in the healing tissue can be elucidated. As this is achieved, it will be possible to determine the influence of stress on each component of the wound healing cascade.

## IV. THE BIOLOGY OF WOUND HEALING

Wound repair is a relatively seamless series of events that is initiated whenever tissue is damaged (Figure 1). Although extreme diversity exists in the various types of wounds and in their severity, wound repair consists of a rather predictable set of responses (for reviews of wound healing, (see Clark, 1991, 1997; Martin, Hopkinson-Woolley, & McCluskey, 1992; Thomas, O'Neil, Harding, & Shepherd, 1995). After injury, signals are released that initiate and regulate all aspects of tissue repair. Histological analysis has revealed that there is a regular sequence of differing cell populations that appear in a cutaneous wound as it heals. However, wound repair is not a simple step-by-step linear process, but rather it is an integrative and dynamic process involving inflammation, fibroblast proliferation, secretion of ground substances, production of collagen, angiogenesis, contraction, and epithelialization. Unencumbered, these wound repair processes follow a relatively specific time sequence and can be temporally categorized into three major phases: (a) an inflammatory phase which consists of

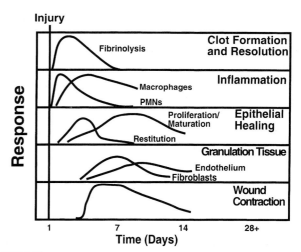

**FIGURE 1** A model for the kinetics of components of the wound healing response. Each line represents the intensity of the response. Each component is connected to other components in the process. Thus, alteration in one response will effect other responses during healing. (Reprinted with permission from J. M. Davidson. Davidson, Buckley-Sturrock, Woodward (1992). Wound repair. In Gallin, Goldstein, and Snyderman (Eds.), *Inflammation: Basic principles and clinical correlates* (pp. 809–820). New York: Raven Press.)

the extravasation of blood constituents with resultant platelet aggregation, blood coagulation and migration of inflammatory cells to the wound site; (b) a granulation/proliferative phase of healing which involves the migration and proliferation of keratinocytes, fibroblasts and endothelial cells, leading to reepithelialization, neovascularization, and granulation tissue formation; and (c) a long remodeling phase where wound strength and architecture are determined. Although these stages overlap, the latter stages of healing are strongly dependent upon the initial events of the healing process (DiPietro, 1995; Hubner et al., 1996; Martin, 1997).

### A. Hemostasis and Early Inflammatory Responses

As severe tissue injury can destroy blood vessels, there is the potential for significant blood loss. Therefore, hemorrhage from injured blood vessels is rapidly stopped and further damage to the site is minimized. Vasoconstriction, in concert with the clotting systems, aids in halting blood flow from damaged blood vessels. The immediate response is the activation of Hageman factor and the complement, kinin, clotting, and plasmin cascades (Kaplan & Silverberg, 1987; Kaplan et al., 1997; Walsh, 1987). Blood coagulation and platelet aggregation generate a fibrin-rich clot that plugs severed vessels and fills any discontinuity in the wounded tissue. Since intact barriers provide an important defense against infection, the clot plays an important role in protection from infection. Successful hemostasis is dependent on platelet adhesion and aggregation. The circulating platelet is an anucleate discoid cell containing numerous types of granules including alpha granules, lysozomes, and dense granules (Blockmans, Deckmyn, & Vermylen, 1995; Mannaioni, DiBello, & Masini, 1997). Alpha granules are the most numerous organelles within the platelet's cytoplasmic milieu. They serve as storage sites for soluble proteins that contribute to both hemostasis and wound repair.

Although hemostasis is a major function of blood coagulation, the clot also provides a scaffold, called the provisional matrix, that aids in the recruitment of reparative cells to the wound site. Specifically, fibrin in conjunction with fibronectin acts as a highway for the subsequent influx of neutrophils and monocytes and for the migration of fibroblasts (Clark, 1997; Thomas et al., 1995). In principal, blood clotting is the first step in the inflammatory phase of wound repair as platelets, in concert with the injured parenchyma, produce factors that increase blood flow and increases blood vessel permeability (Clark, 1991; Mannaioni et al., 1997). Likewise, bradykinin from the kinin system, fibrinopeptides released during fibrinogen cleavage, and histamine released from mast cells all increase blood flow to the site. Furthermore, anaphylotoxins, fibrinopeptides, and another product released from mast cells, neutrophil chemotactic factor, are chemotactic. The increased transudation of plasma, i.e., the development of edema, and the activation of these pathways produces an environment rich in recruitment factors. In addition, platelets also release chemotactic and growth factors such as platelet-derived growth factor (PDGF), and transforming growth factor-$\alpha$ (TGF-$\alpha$) and TGF-$\beta$ (Hosgood, 1993; Pierce et al., 1989). Therefore, shortly after clot formation and mere hours after the initial injury, inflammatory cells responding to platelet-released growth and chemotactic factors arrive and predominate in the wound bed.

## B. The Inflammatory Phase: The Role of the Neutrophil

The hallmark of the inflammatory phase of wound healing is the recruitment of phagocytic leukocytes. Neutrophils and monocytes/macrophages are attracted into injured tissues concurrently, but neutrophils predominate during the first 24–48 h due to their abundance in the circulation (Martin et al., 1992) and

their responsiveness to the earliest signals released at the site of injury (Carlos & Harlan, 1994; Springer, 1994). Neutrophil recruitment into peripheral tissues in response to an inflammatory or infectious stimulus is a multistep process that requires the sequential adherence of circulating neutrophils to vascular endothelium, diapedesis across the endothelial barrier, and migration directed to the inflammatory focus (Carlos & Harlan, 1994; Springer, 1994).

Leukocyte–endothelial interactions involve a cascade of molecular events that are highly dependent upon the inflammatory signals produced by the injured tissue. Locally produced chemoattractants (e.g., C5a, fMLP), inflammatory cytokines (IL-1, TNF-$\alpha$) and the $\alpha$-chemokines (IL-8, KC, IP-10, etc.) will create an adhesive endothelial surface that will capture circulating neutrophils undergoing random contact with the endothelium, resulting in low affinity, adhesion-dependent leukocyte rolling (Carlos & Harlan, 1994; Springer, 1994). This first step in leukocyte adhesion is mediated by the selectin family of adhesion molecules, L-selectin on the neutrophil surface, and E- and P-selectin on the endothelial cell, and their ligands Sialyl Lewis X (SLe$^x$) and sialomucins (CD34) (Akahori et al., 1997; Carlos & Harlan, 1994). Local activation of the loosely adherent leukocytes then leads to high-affinity adhesion ("sticking") to the endothelium. This process is mediated by the surface expression of Mac-1 (CD11b/CD18) by the neutrophil and the upregulation of ICAM-1 expression on the endothelial cell (Borregaard et al., 1994; Carlos & Harlan, 1994). In addition to their roles as chemoattractant molecules, IL-8 and PDGF also stimulate the production of elastase and collagenase molecules which facilitate cell extravasation through blood vessel basement membranes and into the tissue parenchyma (Briggaman, Schechter, Fraki, & Lazarus, 1984; Schechter, 1989).

Once in the wound area, neutrophils protect from infection, clear debris from the injured site, and produce and release factors important in the recruitment of additional phagocytic cells. If substantial wound contamination does not occur, neutrophil infiltration usually ceases rather quickly, and many effete neutrophils become entrapped within the wound clot which sloughs during tissue regeneration. Neutrophils within viable tissue undergo programmed cell death within a few days and are phagocytosed by tissue macrophages (Riches, 1996; Thomas et al., 1995). These processes mark the end of neutrophil-rich inflammation. However, while they predominate, neutrophils are the major producers of proinflammatory cytokines including IL-1$\beta$, that aid in the recruitment of monocytes (Martin et al., 1992;

McDonald, Bald, & Cassatella, 1997; Thomas et al., 1995).

Contamination of the wound, however, provokes a persistent neutrophil-rich inflammatory response. Currently neutrophils are thought to be primarily involved in the first line of defense against invading organisms and the elimination of foreign material. The oxygen free-radicals and proteases released by the neutrophils are effective for performing the defensive tasks, but they also destroy viable tissues if not limited (Martin, 1997; Ravage, Gomez, Czermak, Watkins, & Till, 1998). It is thought that, in the absence of wound contamination or infection, the neutrophils are not necessary for normal healing. For example, Bucky et al. (1994) showed that elimination of neutrophils resulted in increased wound infection but did not result in healing abnormalities.

## C. The Inflammatory Phase: The Role of the Macrophage

Whether the neutrophil infiltrate resolves or persists due to infection, monocyte accumulation begins to escalate within 48 to 96 h after wounding (Clark, 1997; DiPietro, 1995; Martin et al., 1992; Thomas et al., 1995). It is stimulated by selective monocyte chemoattractants including the proinflammatory cytokines (e.g., IL-1$\beta$ and TNF-$\alpha$) produced by the preceding influx of neutrophils and also by locally produced beta-chemokines (MIP-1$\alpha$ and MCP-1) (DiPietro, Burdick, Low, Kunkel, & Strieter, 1998; Gibran, Ferguson, Heimbach, & Isik, 1997; Lawrence & Diegelmann, 1994; Lowry, 1993; Vogt et al., 1998). Similar to neutrophil recruitment, chemoattractants stimulate circulating monocytes to attach to the endothelium of blood vessels at the site of injury and to migrate through the blood vessel wall into the tissue stroma. Once out of the circulation, monocytes mature into tissue macrophages, and they remain in the tissue until healing is complete.

Macrophages are armed to debride, or remove, damaged tissues through phagocytosis and digestion of pathogenic organisms and effete neutrophils (Riches, 1996; DiPietro, 1995). Besides promoting phagocytosis and debridement, adherence to extracellular matrix also stimulates monocytes to undergo metamorphosis into an inflammatory or reparative macrophages. These macrophages begin to produce cytokines and growth factors that are necessary for initiation and propagation of new tissue formation. As the macrophage remains in the tissue until healing is essentially complete, it will regulate many of the subsequent repair processes. Through its secretion of IL-1, the macrophage induces fibroblast-derived

collagenase that aids in the debridement of the initial wound and helps with the degradation of the provisional matrix as the scar matures (Lawrence & Diegelmann, 1994; Phan, McGarry, Loeffler, & Kunkel, 1987). The macrophage participates more directly in the remodeling phase of wound repair through the secretion of chemotactic factors, growth factors, angiogenic factors, and matrix metalloproteinases (MMP). The MMPs participate throughout the duration of wound repair in extracellular protein turnover—in other words in tissue remodeling. The pivotal role that macrophages play in wound healing is illustrated by the experiments of Leibovich and Ross (1975) who showed that macrophage-depleted animals have defective wound repair.

## D. The Proliferative/Granulation Phase: The Role of the Fibroblast

Fibroblasts play a critical role in the repair and production of connective tissue. The cytokines and growth factors that the macrophage produces recruits and stimulates fibroblasts to proliferate (Knighton & Fiegel, 1989; Schaffer & Nanney,1996). In fact, almost as soon as the macrophage arrives, fibroblasts begin to migrate to and proliferate within the wound. The recruitment of the fibroblast represents the initial step in the second major phase of wound repair. In this proliferative phase, granulation tissue forms, consisting of fibroblasts, inflammatory cells, and capillaries within a loose network of extracellular matrix. Much like macrophages, fibroblasts have several, varied functions in wound repair. Their main roles are the synthesis of matrix components (collagens, fibronectin, and glycosaminoglycans (GAGs), and the production of cytokines and growth factors required during the later stages of healing (Simeon et al., 1999).

The first fibroblasts on the scene produce large quantities of type III collagen (Woodley, O'Keefe, & Prunieras, 1985). Collagen gives a tissue its ability to resist tearing or tensile forces. As such, the network of type III collagen serves as a temporary framework holding the entire provisional matrix together. Providing the tissue with its ability to sustain compressive forces are the GAGs. Hyaluronic acid is initially the predominant GAG deposited in the extracellular matrix and is soon followed by dermatan sulfate and chondroitin sulfate (Chen & Abatangelo, 1999). The secreted collagens and GAGs provide structural support to the newly forming tissue and provide highways for the migration of the many cell types involved in the wound repair process. Therefore, the fibroblasts are responsible for producing the raw materials that help in repairing the damaged tissue. As the early inflammatory stage of wound repair changes to this granulation stage, macrophages still remain very important for the continued production of cytokines and growth factors that stimulate the proliferation of fibroblasts and also stimulate the fibroblast to deposit the new stroma (Riches, 1996; Woodley et al., 1985).

As the granulation tissue/provisional matrix begins to take shape, endothelial cells migrate in response to angiogenic stimuli and form new replacement capillaries (Goligorsky, Budzikowski, Tsukahara, & Noiri, 1999; Montrucchio et al., 1997). In addition, reepithelialization begins in earnest. Epithelial cells from the margin of the wound and also from residual epithelial structures such as hair follicles, migrate quickly to divide the damaged stroma from the wound space, and recover the surface of viable tissue. Although the stimuli for epithelial and endothelial migration and repopulation during the re-epithelialization phase have not been fully delineated, among the possibilities is the production of growth factors by the inflammatory infiltrate. These growth factors, including keratinocyte growth factor (KGF) and vascular-endothelial-growth factor (VEGF), are produced in abundance by the reparative tissue macrophages and fibroblasts (Clark, 1997; Lawrence & Diegelmann, 1994; Lowry, 1993; Martin et al., 1992; Schaffer & Nanney 1996). Although wound closure is partially accomplished by reepithelialization which begins almost immediately after wounding, wound contraction also plays an important role (Cross et al., 1995; Welch, Odland, & Clark, 1990).

### E.  The Remodeling Phase

In the final phase of wound healing, remodeling, the extracellular matrix and collagen networks are reorganized with a resultant increase in wound strength (Hastings, Van Winkle, Barker, Hines, & Nichols, 1975; Oxlund, Christensen, Seyer-Hansen, & Andreassen, 1996). During remodeling, there is a rapid synthesis and degradation of extracellular matrix proteins. The nature of the matrix components in wounds changes with time. During the transition of granulation tissue into a mature scar, collagen remodeling depends on a balance between catabolism and continued synthesis and deposition. Matrix metalloproteinases are derived from numerous sources in addition to fibroblasts. During the process of remodeling, type III collagen, the major collagen type synthesized by wound fibroblasts, is transformed into a more stable preinjury dermal phenotype that contains predominantly type I collagen (Schaffer & Nanney 1996; Simeon et al., 1999;

Woodley et al., 1985). This remodeling phase can last for years.

At the site of collagen and extracellular matrix protein production, the fibroblast is necessary for normal scar tissue formation in wounds involving dermal injury. In addition, fibroblasts not only produce the extracellular matrix components, but they are also important precursors to specialized cells that participate in other aspects of wound repair. In the normal wound repair process, some fibroblasts will progress through a transformation to myofibroblasts that initiate wound contraction. Myofibroblasts are characterized by large bundles of actin-containing microfilaments along the cytoplasmic membranes of opposing cells that are connected to one another (Moulin et al., 1999; Welch et al., 1990). These cell–cell and cell–matrix links provide a network across the wound whereby the traction of myofibroblasts on their pericellular matrix can be transmitted across the wound (Gabbianni, 1999; Grinnel, 1999). In other words, the wound is pulled together by the contraction of the myofibroblast.

Wound closure, including both reepithelialization and contraction, represents a complex and masterfully orchestrated interaction of cells, extracellular matrix, and cytokines. The final remodeling stage of wound repair, which is very important for wound closure, is dependent on deposition of new stroma and proliferation of fibroblasts during the granulation stage. In turn, granulation tissue formation is dependent upon the earlier inflammatory stages where neutrophils and macrophages have cleansed, debrided, and initiated the reparative process. Thus, the proinflammatory infiltrate appears highly critical to the overall healing process.

### F.  Growth Factors Involved in Wound Repair

Coordination among the cells involved in the cascade of wound repair is regulated by cytokines and growth factors produced primarily by the macrophage. Platelet-derived growth factor (PDGF), as the name would suggest, is produced by platelets early during initial clot formation (Blockmans et al., 1995; Hosgood, 1993; Martin et al., 1992; Pierce et al., 1989; Simeon et al., 1999). However, macrophages are also a significant source of this potent growth factor as they are involved in each of the phases of wound repair. PDGF is a potent mitogen and is chemoattractant for fibroblasts and smooth muscle cells. PDGF is also chemotactic toward neutrophils and monocytes and stimulates the activation of the reparative macrophages. It upregulates fibronectin gene expression and procollagen synthesis and increases collagenase activity, processes essential for connective tissue re-modeling (Cass, Meuli, & Adzick, 1997; Hosgood, 1993; Pierce et al., 1989).

Acidic and basic fibroblast growth factors (FGFs) are strongly mitogenic for endothelial cells and are probably the major growth factor family involved in angiogenesis, directing endothelial cell migration, proliferation, and plasminogen activator synthesis (Klein, Bond, Gupta, Yacoub, & Anderson, 1999; Uhl et al., 1993; Venkataraman, Raman, Sasisekharan, & Sasisekharan, 1999). Both FGF and keratinocyte growth factor stimulate the proliferation of keratinocytes.

Transforming growth factor-$\beta$ (TGF-$\beta$) promotes angiogenesis, plays a major role in the deposition of extracellular matrix, and also induces the differentiation of fibroblasts into myofibroblasts (Hosgood, 1993; Pierce et al., 1989). TGF-$\beta$ causes significant increases in the breaking strength of healing wounds. The enhanced tensile strength of healing wounds is accompanied by a marked increase in collagen deposition at the wound site (Pilcher, Sudbeck, Dumin, Welgus, & Parks, 1998; Sefton & Woodhouse, 1998). TGF-$\beta$ is a potential stimulator of extracellular matrix production, by promoting synthesis of both fibronectin and collagen in fibroblasts. Thus, TGF-$\beta$ plays an important role in ''scar'' formation because of its role in matrix macromolecule synthesis. Furthermore, TGF-$\beta$ is anti-inflammatory. It reduces the effects of residual proinflammatory cytokines on recruitment and activation of inflammatory cells while maintaining the ability to stimulate matrix production and remodeling (Shull et al., 1992).

Many other growth factors play essential roles in wound healing. Epidermal growth factor derived from platelets and macrophages stimulates migration and proliferation of epithelial cells and increases wound tensile strength (Hudson & McCawley, 1998; Lawrence & Diegelmann, 1994; Tomic-Canic, Komine, Freedberg, & Blumenberg, 1998). Insulin-like growth factor acts with other cytokines to stimulate fibroblast proliferation (Lawrence & Diegelmann, 1994; Leibovich & Ross, 1975; Lowry, 1993). Nerve growth factor, produced by fibroblasts and keratinocytes, stimulates the growth of sensory neurons and is an activating factor for melanocytes (Bothwell, 1997; Tron, Coughlin, Jang, & Sauder, 1990). Vascular endothelial growth factor not only stimulates endothelial cell growth, but also increases vascular permeability (Larcher, Murillas, Bolontrade, Conti, & Jorcano, 1998). Thus, there are many growth factors that play overlapping and sometimes opposing roles during wound healing. This intricate network of regulatory factors finely controls the process of wound healing.

## G. Expression of Proinflammatory Cytokines and Chemokines

The early processes of wound repair, including the recruitment and activation of inflammatory cells, are regulated by proinflammatory cytokines, e.g., IL-1 and TNF-$\alpha$. Proinflammatory cytokines also induce the expression of growth factors required for the proliferative phase of wound healing. Furthermore, in the caregiver and examination stress studies described above, stress was associated with a substantial decrease in the ability of leukocytes to produce IL-1$\beta$. For example, examination stress was associated with a reduction of IL-1$\beta$ gene expression by greater than two-thirds then the vacation period. Thus, the proinflammatory cytokines may play an important role in mediating stress effects.

IL-1 (IL-1$\alpha$ and IL-1$\beta$) and TNF-$\alpha$ are proinflammatory cytokines that are synthesized in the earliest stages of wound healing. In the mouse model IL-1 and TNF-$\alpha$ are induced at the mRNA level within 15 h of wounding (Hubner et al., 1996). All three cytokines are very strongly expressed throughout the first 3 days of wound healing and their expression parallels the influx of inflammatory cells. In situ hybridization studies revealed that the principal producers of all three cytokines in the wound tissue are PMNs and monocytes (Hubner et al., 1996). They are induced to express these cytokines in response to a number of signals at the wound site including complement activation, bacterial products, tissue injury and cytokines released by resident cells.

Keratinocytes can also produce IL-1. Cultured normal human keratinocytes express both IL-1$\alpha$ and IL-1$\beta$ mRNA, but IL-1$\alpha$ mRNA is the predominant form (Kupper et al., 1986; Lee, Morhenn, Ilnicka, Eugui, & Allison, 1991). Interestingly, the only biologically active cytokine detected in normal epidermis in the absence of disease is IL-1$\alpha$ (Blanton, Kupper, McDougall, & Dower, 1989; Kupper, 1989). Langerhans cells are dendritic cells derived from the monocytic lineage which intercalate between keratinocytes in the epidermis (Salmon, Armstrong, & Ansel, 1994). In contrast to keratinocytes, unstimulated Langerhans cells predominantly express IL-1$\beta$ mRNA over IL-1$\alpha$ mRNA in vitro (Matsue, Cruz, Bergstresser, & Takashima, 1992). Thus, a constitutive pool of proinflammatory cytokines forms part of the immunoprotective barrier of the skin. Upon tissue injury, resident cells become alerted. For example, after repeated tape stripping of human skin, there is increased TNF-$\alpha$ and IL-1$\beta$ mRNA in the epidermis accompanied by keratinocyte expression of intercellular adhesion molecule-1 (ICAM-1) and the appearance of endothelial cell adhesion molecules (ELAM-1).

The effects of increased levels of IL-1 and TNF-$\alpha$ at the wound site are multiple. Both cytokines modulate the expression of chemotactic cytokines by resident and infiltrating cells, e.g., IL-8 and macrophage chemotactic protein-1 (MCP-1) (Engelhardt et al., 1998; Goebeler et al., 1997; Zoja et al., 1991). This ensures continued activation and recruitment of neutrophils and monocytes into the wound. Both IL-1 and TNF-$\alpha$ also induce ICAM-1 expression by endothelial cells (Dustin, Rothlein, & Bhan, 1986), which is important for migration of leukocytes into the wound. Later in the inflammatory response, IL-1 and TNF-$\alpha$ orchestrate the proliferative phase of wound healing. They increase fibroblast proliferation and migration, and induce collagen synthesis (Canalis, 1986; Schmidt et al., 1984; Tracey, & Vlassara, & Cerami, 1989). In addition, IL-1 and TNF-$\alpha$ induce the production of matrix metalloproteinases (MMPs), such as collagenase and stromelysin (Madlener et al., 1996). MMPs cleave proteins of the extracellular matrix, thereby releasing the migrating keratinocytes at the wound edge from their attachment to the basal lamina and dermal substratum. Therefore, IL-1 and TNF-$\alpha$ are the initial inflammatory mediators at the wound site which will mobilize effector cells from the peripheral circulation into the tissues and will also recruit resident epidermal cells from the vicinity.

## V. NEUROENDOCRINE REGULATION OF WOUND HEALING

### A. Influence of Glucocorticoids on Wound Repair

Clinically, glucocortcoids were introduced into therapy in the middle of the 20th century and continue to be the mainstay in the treatment of many different inflammatory diseases ranging from allergy to autoimmunity. However, the desirable anti-inflammatory effects can be costly to other physiologic systems. One of the adverse consequences of glucocorticoid use is inhibition of wound repair (Anstead, 1998; Diethelm, 1977; Goldman, 1987). Clinically, the treatment of surgical patients with glucocorticoids is associated with an increased risk of wound infection, and overall, the use of glucocorticoids increases the risk of wound complications twofold to fivefold (Diethelm, 1977).

It is the potent anti-inflammatory effect of cortisol which accounts for its profound inhibitory effect on wound healing. After administration of exogenous glucocorticoids, neutrophil (Clark, Gallin, & Fauci, 1979, Perretti & Flower, 1994) and monocyte (Norris, Capin, & Weston, 1982) recruitment is decreased, and macrophage phagocytosis and bacterial killing are suppressed (Fauci, Dale, & Balow, 1976). This results in delayed wound debridement and impaired foreign body and bacterial elimination. Reepithelialization and wound closure are also delayed by glucocorticoids. In addition, keratinocyte proliferation is inhibited (Edwards & Dunphy, 1958; Lenco, McKnight, & Macdonald, 1975) producing a thinned and abnormal epidermal layer. As a consequence to these deficits, the tensile strength of the final scar is reduced (Bitar, 1998).

### B. Mechanism of Glucocorticoid Regulation of Wound Repair

Glucocorticoids have been used to reduce expression of proinflammatory cytokines such as IL-1, TNF-$\alpha$, GM-CSF, and G-CSF, expression of chemoattractant molecules such as MIP-1$\alpha$, MCP-1, and KC (Bendrups, Hilton, Meager, & Hamilton, 1993; Russo-Marie, 1992; Snyder & Unanue, 1982), and endothelial cell expression of E-selectin (Brostjan, Anrather, Csizmadia, Natarajan, & Winkler, 1997). Each of these is important, if not necessary, for efficient wound repair. Therefore, it should not be surprising that their suppression by glucocorticoids would alter the outcome of the healing process.

Snyder and Unanue (1982) demonstrated that hydrocortisone reduced production of IL-1 by PMA-stimulated murine peritoneal macrophages. Similarly, LPS-stimulated human monocytes treated with dexamethasone had decreased expression of both IL-1$\alpha$ and IL-1$\beta$ mRNA, decreased cell-associated levels of IL-1$\alpha$ and IL-1$\beta$, and decreased secretion of IL-1$\beta$ in culture supernatants. Dexamethasone also significantly inhibited IL-1-induced IL-6 mRNA expression in synoviocytes of patients with rheumatoid arthritis (Amano, Lee, & Allison, 1993). This suggests that downregulated IL-1 gene expression caused by GC will result in reduced expression of other cytokine genes known to be induced by IL-1, thereby suppressing the cascade of mediators elicited by IL-1 during inflammation.

Dexamethasone has also been shown to diminish the rate of TNF gene transcription in murine macrophages and to exert an even more marked effect on hormone biosynthesis at a posttranscriptional level (Beutler, Krochin, Milsark, Luedke, & Cerami, 1986).

Furthermore, Hubner et al. (1996) demonstrated that GC-treatment of mice reduced induction of IL-1α, IL-1β, and TNF-α after injury. This was associated with a reduced infiltration of inflammatory cells, delayed wound reepithelialization, and impaired granulation tissue formation. Resident epithelial cells can also be a target for GC cytokine regulation. Lee et al. (1991) found that hydrocortisone decreases the expression of IL-1α mRNA in human KC. Therefore, GC can downregulate gene expression of proinflammatory cytokines IL-1 and TNF-α in peripheral and local cellular compartments, both of which participate and interact decisively in wound healing.

In addition to the influences of GC on proinflammatory cytokine production, Chedid, Hoyle, Csaky, and Rubin (1996) showed that dexamethasone significantly reduces the level of constitutively produced KGF from human dermal fibroblasts. These results suggest that downregulation of KGF expression by GC may be due to a direct effect on mesenchymal cells. However, it may also be explained by an inhibition of KGF-inducing factors in the wound, such as IL-1 and TNF-α. Indeed, it was found that the addition of TNF-α or IL-1β to dexamethasone -treated fibroblasts reversed the inhibitory effect of GC on KGF expression. Therefore, elevated levels of exogenous GC can dysregulate the profile of proinflammatory cytokines and growth factors that interact locally for a rapid and effective restoration of skin integrity.

Although the precise mechanism of action by which GCs act is not completely understood, many recent studies have begun to shed light on their influences on cytokine, chemokine, and growth factor gene transcription (Almawi, Beyhum, Rahme, & Rieder, 1996). GCs bind to cytoplasmic glucocorticoid receptors (GR), which function through a variety of mechanisms, some of which are posttranscriptional but most of which are at the level of transcriptional control. Activation of gene expression by glucocorticoids generally requires translocation of the activated glucocorticoid receptor to the nucleus (Hollenberg, Giguere, Sequi, & Evans, 1987) and subsequent binding of GC receptor dimers to a specific site on the DNA, called the glucocorticoid response element (GRE). However, transcriptional repression by the GR is not clearly defined; GC repressive GREs have not been found in cytokine promoters. Alternatively, it is thought that inhibition of cytokine gene transcription by GC may be based on protein–protein interactions between the transcription factors and glucocorticoid-induced inhibitors (Auphan, DiDonato, Rosett, Helm-berg, & Karin, 1995; Gottlicher, Heck, & Herrlich, 1998; Scheinman, Cogswell, Lofquist, & Baldwin, 1995).

NF-κB-responsive elements are required for the function of many cytokine promoters (Mercurio, DiDonato, Rosett, & Karin, 1993; Scheinman, Beg, & Baldwin, 1993). The transcription factor NF-κB, initially characterized as a heterodimer of p50 (NF-κB1) and p65 (RelA) subunits, is constitutively present in the cytosol of endothelial cells and kept inactive by association with inhibitor proteins that contain ankyrin repeat motifs (for reviews of NF-κ B structure and functions see Baeuerle and Henkel (1994), Baldwin (1996), Huxford, Huang, Malek, & Ghosh (1998). These inhibitory molecules include the IκB family (IκBα, -β, and -γ) as well as the NF-κB precursor molecules p105 and p100 (NF-κB1 and NF-κB2). Upon activation by LPS, antigen, or proinflammatory cytokines, cells rapidly degrade IκBα. NF-κB then enters the nucleus and interacts with promoter elements of defined DNA sequences, enhancing transcription initiation of the respective genes. However, GCs induce the transcription of IκBα, which increases IκBα,mRNA. This results in increased IκBα protein synthesis, which effectively inhibits NF-κB activation (Auphan et al., 1995; Scheinman et al., 1995).

Inhibition of NF-κB activation can account for many of the immunosuppressive and anti-inflammatory activities of GCs. NF-κB plays a central role in induction of a large number of important immunoregulatory genes including those encoding proinflammatory cytokines (IL-1α, IL-1β, TNF-α), α-chemokines (IL-8, KC, IP10), β-chemokines (MCP-1, MIP-1α), and growth factors (TGF-β and KGF) (Bond, Fabunmi, Baker, & Newby, 1998; Collart, Baeuerle, & Bassalli, 1990; Eckert & Welter, 1996; Haas et al., 1998; McDonald & Cassatella, 1997; Rogler et al., 1998; Tomic-Canic et al., 1998). Because of the pervasiveness of NF-κB transcriptional regulation throughout the proinflammatory, chemotactic, and cellular responses, it is a possible candidate modulating stress-associated decrements in wound healing.

## C. Nonglucorticoid Neuroendocrine Modulation of Wound Healing

Although glucocorticoids have a dramatic influence on the course of wound healing, other neuroendocrine pathways have the potential to modulate healing. Activation of the sympathetic nervous system (SNS) results in the production of plasma and tissue catecholamines. Since catecholamines are known to alter blood flow and the trafficking of inflammatory cells, stress-induced activation of the SNS may also play a regulatory role in healing. Furthermore, catecholamines are known for their contribution to local tissue edema, increasing endothelial cell adhesion (Koopman, 1995). Catecholamines have also been shown to have an inhibitory effect on epidermal cell migration (Donaldson & Mahan, 1984). This suggests that increased levels of catecholamines at the wound site, either arising from the peripheral circulation or released from local sympathetic nerve endings, may impact upon wound healing processes by altering blood flow, altering cell recruitment, increasing edema, and delaying reepithelialization.

Sensory neurons are also important in wound healing. These neurons are known to be involved in neurogenic inflammation (Baluk, 1997; Green et al., 1998). They release neuropeptides, e.g., substance P and calcitonin gene-related peptide (CGRP) which can induce inflammatory responses. For example, substance P causes the release of IL-1 from keratinocytes and fibroblasts and IL-8 from endothelial cells (Scholzen et al., 1998). It can also induce endothelial cells to express vascular cellular adhesion molecule 1 and have effects on vascular permeability. If substance P fibers are cut or ablated with capsaicin, then wound healing is delayed (Khalil & Helme, 1996; Kim, Whelpdale, Zurowski, & Pomeranz, 1998; Westerman, Carr, Delaney, Morris, & Roberts, 1993). These neurons grow during wound healing and are under the influence of nerve growth factor which is produced by keratinocytes and fibroblasts (Bothwell, 1997). Thus, there is a bidirectional relationship between tissue cells and neurons at the local site during wound healing. Since glucocrticoids are known to suppress sensory fibers in the periphery, there is a potential role for chronic stress to reduce the inflammatory response mediated by these neurons and therefore, influence wound healing.

## VI.  CONCLUSIONS

Wound healing is a process that plays an important role whenever tissue is damaged. Thus, every injury, infection, or neoplasm interfaces with the wound healing response. The available data demonstrate that the neuroendocrine system regulates many components of the wound healing cascade. Studies have shown that wound healing can be delayed by stress, by treatment with glucocorticoids, and by ablating neurons. The focus, thus far, has been on the impact of the neuroendocrine system on early inflammatory processes because these are important in the recruitment and activation of inflammatory cells and tissue cells required for healing. The timing of each event during healing is important since each component is dependent on the one that came before. Therefore, if IL-1 is not adequately expressed during early healing, then subsequent factors, e.g., MIP-1$\alpha$, will not be adequately induced. Monocytes will not be recruited to the site in sufficient numbers. They will not be able to clear apoptotic cells or produce cytokines that induce growth factors for the later phases of healing. Thus, healing will not proceed normally.

The clinical implications are many. In a hospital setting, healing that is delayed provides an increased opportunity for infection. This is especially problematic with the accompanied potential immunosuppression caused by stress and compounded by aging and systemic diseases, e.g., diabetes (Bitar, 1998; Goodson & Hunt, 1979). Biomedical science is now attempting to regenerate tissues and organs for therapeutic benefit. The success of these complex therapies will require a predictable course of wound healing within an individual. Because an individual's wound healing response can be modulated by the interactions between the immune and neuroendocrine systems, understanding the physiology of healing in the context of psychoneuroimmunology will provide significant insight of these processes. Thus, the goals of future studies should be to determine the critical pathways that are regulated by neuroendocrine inputs and identify those at risk for a poor healing outcome. In order to develop an appropriate intervention that is individualized for the type of wound, the genetic makeup of the individual, and psychological factors, the molecular mechanisms involved in neuroendocrine modulation of wound healing will have to be discovered.

## Acknowledgments

This work was supported by research grants from the National Institutes of Health. R01-DE11014 (P.T.M.), P01-AG11585 (P.T.M., J.F.S.), R01-MH46801 (J.F.S.), R29-MH56899 (D.A.P.), and the John D. and Catherine T. MacArthur Foundation Mind–Body Network (J.F.S.).

## References

Akahori, T., Yuzawa, Y., Nishikawa, K., Tamatani, T., Kannagi, R., Miyasaka, M., Okada, H., Hota, N., & Matsuo, S. (1997). Role of Sialyl Lewis$^x$-like epitope selectively expressed on vascular endothelial cells in local skin inflammation of the rat. *The Journal of Immunology, 158,* 5384–5392.

Almawi, W. Y., Beyhum, H. N., Rahme, A. A., & Rieder, M. J. (1996). Regulation of cytokine and cytokine receptor expression by glucocorticoids. *Journal of Leukocyte Biology, 60,* 563–572.

Amano, Y., Lee, S. W., & Allison, A. C. (1993). Inhibition by glucocortiocids of the formation of interleukin-1$\alpha$, interleukin-1$\beta$, and interleukin 6: Mediation by decreased mRNA stability. *Molecular Pharmacology, 43,* 176–182.

Anstead, G. M. (1998). Steroids, retinoids, and wound healing. *Advances in Wound Care, Oct. 11*(6), 277–85.

Auphan, N., DiDonato, J. A., Rosett, C., Helmberg, A., & Karin, M. (1995). Immunosuppression by glucocorticoids: Inhibition of NF-$\kappa$B activity through induction of I$\kappa$B synthesis. *Science, 270,* 286–289.

Baeuerle, P., & Henkel, T. (1994). Function and activation of NF-$\kappa$B in the immune system. *Annual Review of Immunology, 12,* 141–179.

Baldwin, A. S., Jr. (1996). The NF-$\kappa$B and I$\kappa$B proteins: New discoveries and insights. *Annual Review of Immunology, 14,* 649–681.

Baluk, P. (1997). Neurogenic inflammation in skin and airways. *Journal of Investigative Dermatology, Symposium Proceedings, 2,* 76–81.

Bendrups, A., Hilton, A., Meager, A., & Hamilton, J. A. (1993). Reduction of tumor necrosis factor alpha and interleukin-1 beta levels in human synovial tissue by interleukin-4 and glucocorticoids. *Rheumatology International, 12*(6), 217-220.

Beutler, B. N., Krochin, I. W., Milsark, C., Luedke, A., & Cerami, A. (1986). Control of cachectin (tumor necrosis factor) synthesis: Mechanisms of endotoxin resistance. *Science, 232*(4753), 977–980.

Bitar, M. S. (1998). Glucocorticoid dynamics and impaired wound healing in diabetes mellitus. *America Journal of Pathology, 152,* 547–554.

Blanton B., Kupper, T. S., McDougall, J., & Dower, S. (1989). Regulation of interleukin 1 and its receptor on human keratinocytes. *Proceedings of the National Academy of Science, USA, 86,* 1273–1277.

Blockmans, D., Deckmyn, H., & Vermylen, J. (1995). Platelet activation. *Blood Reviews, Sep.* 9(3), 143–156.

Bond, M., Fabunmi, R. P., Baker, A. H., & Newby, A. C. (1998). Synergistic upregulation of metalloproteinase-9 by growth factors and inflammatory cytokines: An absolute requirement for transcription factor NF-kappa B. *FEBS Letters, 435,* 29–34.

Borregaard, N., Kjeldsen, L., Sengelov, H., Diamond, M. S., Springer, T. A., Anderson, H. C., Kishimoto, T. K., & Bainton, D. F. (1994). Changes in subcellular localization and surface expression of L-selectin, alkaline phosphatase, and Mac-1 in human neutrophils during stimulation with inflammatory mediators. *Journal of Leukocyte Biology, 56,* 80–87.

Bothwell, M. (1997). Neurotrophin function in skin. *Journal of Investigative Dermatology, Symposium Proceedings, 2,* 27–30.

Brevetti, G. R., Napierkowski, M. T., & Maher, J. W. (1997). Assessment of esophageal leak with oral fluorescein. *America Journal of Gastroenterology, 92,* 165–166.

Briggaman, R. A., Schechter, N. M., Fraki, J., & Lazarus, G. S. (1984). Degradation of the epidermal-dermal junction by proteolytic enzymes from human skin and human polymorphonuclear leukocytes. *Journal of Experimental Medicine, Oct. 1 160*(4), 1027–1042.

Brostjan, C., Anrather, J., Csizmadia, V., Natarajan, G., & Winkler, H. (1997). Glucocorticoids inhibit E-selectin expression by targeting NF-$\kappa$B and not ATF/c-Jun. *The Journal of Immunology, 158,* 3836–3844.

Bucky, L. P., Vedder, N. B., Hong, H. Z., Ehrlich, H. P., Winn, R. K., Harlan, J. M., & May, J. W., Jr. (1994). Reduction of burn injury by inhibiting CD18-mediated leukocyte adherence in rabbits. *Plastic and Reconstructive Surgery, 93,* 1473–1480.

Canalis, E. (1986). Interleukin 1 has independent effects on deoxyribonucleic acid and collagen synthesis in cultures of rat calvariae. *Endocrinology, 118,* 74–81.

Carlos, T. M., & Harlan, J. M. (1994). Leukocyte-endothelial adhesion markers. *Blood, 84,* 2068–2101.

Cass, D. L., Meuli, M., & Adzick, N. S. (1997). Scar wars: Implications of fetal wound healing for the pediatric burn patient. *Pediatric Surgery International, 12,* 484–489.

Chedid, M., Hoyle, J. R., Csaky, K. G., & Rubin, J. S. (1996). Glucocorticoids inhibit keratinocyte growth factor production in primary dermal fibroblasts. *Endocrinology, 137,* 2232–2237.

Chen, W. Y., & Abatangelo, G. (1999). Functions of hyaluronan in wound repair. *Wound Repair, Regeneration, and Artificial Tissues, 7,* 79–89.

Clark, R. A. F. (1991). Cutaneous wound repair. In L. A. Goldsmith (Ed.), *Physiology, biochemistry, and molecular biology of the skin* (pp. 576–601). Oxford: Oxford Press.

Clark, R. A. F. (1997). Wound repair: Lessons for tissue engineering. In R. Lanza, R. Langer, and W. Chick (Eds.), *Principles of tissue engineering* (pp. 737–767). Landes.

Clark, R. A. F., Gallin, J. I., & Fauci, A. S. (1979). Effect of in vivo prednisone on in vitro eosinophil and neutrophil adherence and chemotaxis. *Blood, 53,* 633–641.

Cohen, I. K., & Mast, B. A. (1990). Models of wound healing. *Journal of Trauma, 30,* S149–S155.

Cohen, S., & Hoberman, H. M. (1983). Positive events and social supports as buffers of life change stress. *Journal of Applied Social Psychology, 13,* 99–125.

Collart, M. A., Baeuerle, P., & Bassalli, P. (1990). Regulation of tumor necrosis factor-$\alpha$ transcription in macrophages: Involvement of four $\kappa$B-like motifs and of constituitive and inducible forms of NF-$\kappa$B. *Molecular and Cellular Biology, 10,* 1498.

Cross, S. E., Naylor, I. L., Coleman, R. A., & Teo, T. C. (1995). An experimental model to investigate the dynamics of wound contraction. *British Journal of Plastic Surgery, 48,* 189–197.

Davidson, J. M., Buckley-Sturrock, A., & Woodward, S. C. (1992). Wound repair. In J. Gallin, I. Goldstein, and R. Snyderman, (Eds.), *Inflammation: Basic principles and clinical correlates* (pp. 809–820). New York: Raven Press.

Diethelm, A. G. (1977). Surgical management of complications of steroid therapy. *Annals of Surgery, Mar. 185*(3), 251–263.

DiPietro, L. A. (1995). Wound healing: The role of the macrophage and other immune cells. *Shock, 4,* 233–240.

DiPietro, L. A., Burdick, M., Low, Q. E., Kunkel, S. L., & Strieter, R. M. (1998). MIP-1alpha as a critical macrophage chemoattractant in murine wound repair. *Journal of Clinical Investigation, 101,* 1693–1698.

Donaldson, D. J., & Mahan, J. T. (1984). Influence of catecholamines on epidermal cell migration during wound closure in adult newts. *Comparative Biochemistry and Physiology, 78C,* 267–270.

Dustin, M. L., Rothlein, R., & Bhan, A. K. (1986). Induction by IL-1 and IFN-$\gamma$: Tissue distribution, biochemistry and function of a natural adherence molecule (ICAM-1). *Journal of Immunology, 137,* 245–247.

Eckert, R. L., & Welter, J. F. (1996). Transcription factor regulation of epidermal keratinocyte gene expression. *Molecular Biology Reports, 23,* 59–70.

Edwards, J. C., & Dunphy, J. E. (1958). Wound healing. II. Injury and abnormal repair. *New England Journal of Medicine, 259,* 275–285.

Engelhardt, E., Toksoy, A., Goebeler, M., Debus, S., Brocker, E. B., & Gillitzer, R. (1998). Chemokines IL-8, GRO-alpha, MCP-1, IP-10, and Mig are sequentially and differentially expressed during phase-specific infiltration of leukocyte subsets in human wound healing. *American Journal of Pathology, 153,* 1849–1860.

Fauci, A. S., Dale, D. C., & Balow, J. E. (1976). Glucocorticoid therapy: Mechanisms of action and clinical considerations. *Annals of Internal Medicine, 84,* 304–315.

Gabbiani, G. (1999). Some historical and philosophical reflections on the myofibroblast concept. *Current Topics in Pathology, 93,* 1–5.

Gibran, N. S., Ferguson, M., Heimbach, D. M., & Isik, F. F. (1997). Monocyte chemoattractant protein-1 mRNA expression in the human burn wound. *Journal of Surgical Research, 70,* 1–6.

Goebeler, M., Yoshimura, T., Toksoy, A., Ritter, U., Brocker, E. B., & Gillitzer, R. (1997). The chemokine repertoire of human dermal microvascular endothelial cells and its regulation by inflammatory cytokines. *Journal of Investigative Dermatology, 108,* 445–451.

Goldmann, D. R. (1987). Surgery in patients with endocrine dysfunction. *Medical Clinics of North America, 1*(3), 499–509.

Goligorsky, M. S., Budzikowski, A. S., Tsukahara, H., & Noiri, E. (1999). Co-operation between endothelin and nitric oxide in promoting endothelial cell migration and angiogenesis. *Clinical and Experimental Pharmacology and Physiology, 26*(3), 269–271.

Goodson, W. H., & Hunt, T. K. (1979). Wound healing and aging. *Journal of Investigative Dermatology, 73,* 88–91.

Gottlicher, M., Heck, S., & Herrlich, P. (1998). Transcriptional cross-talk, the second mode of steroid hormone receptor action. *Journal of Molecular Medicine, 76,* 480–489.

Green, P. G., Miao, F. J., Strausbaugh, H., Heller, P., Janig, W., & Levine, J. D. (1998). Endocrine and vagal controls of sympathetically dependent neurogenic inflammation. *Annals of the New York Academy of Sciences, 840,* 282–288.

Grinnell, F. (1999). Signal transduction pathways activated during fibroblast contraction of collagen matrices. *Current Topics in Pathology, 93,* 61–73.

Haas, A. F., Wong, J. W., Iwahashi, C. K., Halliwell, B., Cross, C. E., & Davis, P. A. (1998). Redox regulation of wound healing? NF-kappaB activation in cultured human keratinocytes upon wounding and the effect of low energy HeNe irradiation. *Free Radical Biology And Medicine, 25,* 998–1005.

Hastings, J. C., Van Winkle, W., Barker, E., Hines, D., & Nichols, W. (1975). The effect of suture materials on healing wounds of the bladder. *Surgical Gynecological Obstetrics, 140,* 933-937.

Hollenberg, S. M., Giguere, V., Sequi, P., & Evans, R. M. (1987). Colocalization of DNA-binding and transcriptional activation functions in the human glucocorticoid receptor. *Cell, 49,* 39–46.

Hosgood, G. (1993). Wound healing. The role of platelet-derived growth factor and transforming growth factor beta. *Veterinary Surgery, 22*(6), 490–495.

Hubner, G., Brauchle, M., Smola, H., Madlener, M., Fassler, R., & Werner, S. (1996). Differential regulation of pro-inflammatory cytokines during wound healing in normal and glucocorticoid-treated mice. *Cytokine, 8,* 548–556.

Hudson, L. G., & McCawley, L. J. (1998). Contributions of the epidermal growth factor receptor to keratinocyte motility. *Microscopy Research and Technique, 43*(5), 444–455.

Huxford, T., Huang, D. B., Malek, S., & Ghosh, G. (1998). The crystal structure of the IkappaBalpha/NF-kappaB complex reveals mechanisms of NF-kappaB inactivation. *Cell, 95,* 759–770.

Kaplan, A. P., Joseph, K., Shibayama, Y., Reddigari, S., Ghebrehiwet, B., & Silverberg, M. (1997). The intrinsic coagulation/kinin-forming cascade: Assembly in plasma and cell surfaces in inflammation. *Advances in Immunology, 66,* 225–72.

Kaplan, A. P., & Silverberg, M. (1987). The coagulation-kinin pathway of human plasma. *Blood, 70*(1), 1–15.

Khalil, Z., & Helme, R. (1996). Sensory peptides as neuromodulators of wound healing in aged rats. *Journals of Gerontology. Series A, Biological and Medical Sciences, 51,* B354–B361.

Kiecolt-Glaser, J. K., Marucha, P. T., Malarky, W. B.,. Mercado, A. M., & Glaser, R. (1995). Slowing of wound healing by psychological stress. *The Lancet, 346,* 1194–1196.

Kim, L. R., Whelpdale, K., Zurowski, M., & Pomeranz, B. (1998). Sympathetic denervation impairs epidermal healing in cutaneous wounds. *Wound Repair and Regeneration, 6,* 194–201.

Klein, S. A., Bond, S. J., Gupta, S. C., Yacoub, O. A., & Anderson, G. L. (1999). Angiogenesis inhibitor TNP-470 inhibits murine cutaneous wound healing. *Journal of Surgical Research, 82*(2), 268–274.

Knighton, D. R., & Fiegel, V. D. (1989). The macrophages: Effector cell wound repair. *Progress in Clinical and Biological Research, 299,* 217–226.

Koopman, C. F. (1995). Cutaneous wound healing, an overview. *The Otolaryngologic Clinics of North America, 28*(5), 835–845.

Kupper, T. S. (1989). Mechanisms of cutaneous inflammation. *Archives of Dermatology, 125,* 1406–1411.

Kupper, T. S., Ballard, D. W., Chua, A. O., McGuire, J. S., Flood, P. M., Horowitz, M. C., Langdon, R., Lightfoot, L., & Gubler, U. (1986). Human keratinocytes contain mRNA indistinguishable from monocyte interleukin-1 a and β mRNA. *Journal of Experimental Medicine, 164,* 2095–2100.

Larcher, F., Murillas, R., Bolontrade, M., Conti, C. J., & Jorcano, J. L. (1998). VEGF/VPF overexpression in skin of transgenic mice induces angiogenesis, vascular hyperpermeability and accelerated tumor development. *Oncogene, 17,* 303–311.

Lawrence, W. T., & Diegelmann, R. F. (1994). Growth factors in wound healing. *Clinics in Dermatology, 12,* 157–169.

Lee, S. W., Morhenn, V. B., Ilnicka, M., Eugui, E. M., & Allison, A. C. (1991). Autocrine stimulation of interleukin-1α and transforming growth factorα production in human keratinocytes and its antagonism by glucocorticoids. *Journal of Investigative Dermatology, 97,* 106–110.

Leibovich, S. J., & Ross, R. (1975). The role of the macrophage in wound repair: A study with hydrocortisone and anti-macrophage serum. *American Journal of Pathology, 78,* 71–91.

Lenco, W., Mcknight, M., & Macdonald, A. S. (1975). Effects of cortisone acetate, methylprednisolone and medroxyprogesterone on wound contracture and epithelization in rabbits. *Annals of Surgery, 181*(1), 67–73.

Lowry, S. F. (1993). Cytokine mediators of immunity and inflammation. *Archives of Surgery, 28,* 1235–1241.

Madlener, M., Mauch, C., Conca, W., Brauchle, M., Parks, W. C., & Werner, S. (1996). Regulation of the expression of stromelysin-2 by growth factors in keratinocytes: Implications for normal and impaired wound healing. *Biochemistry Journal 320*(Pt. 2), 659–664.

Mannaioni, P. F., Di Bello, M. G., & Masini, E. (1997). Platelets and inflammation: Role of platelet-derived growth factor, adhesion molecules and histamine. *Inflammation Research, 46*(1), 4–18.

Martin, P. (1997). Wound healing—Aiming for perfect skin regeneration. *Science, 276*(5309), 75–81.

Martin, P. J., Hopkinson-Woolley, & McCluskey, J. (1992). Growth factors and cutaneous wound repair. *Progress in Growth Factor Research, 4,* 25–44.

Marucha, P. T., Kiecolt-Glaser, J. K., & Favagehi, M. (1998). Mucosal wound healing is impaired by examination stress. *Psychosomatic Medicine, 60,* 362–365.

Matsue, H., Cruz, P. D., Bergstresser, P. R., & Takashima, A. (1992). Langerhans cells are the major source of mRNA for IL-1β and MIP-1α among unstimulated mouse epidermal cells. *Journal of Investigative Dermatology, 99,* 537–541.

McDonald, P. P., Bald, A., & Cassatella, M. A. (1997). Activation of NF-κB pathway by inflammatory stimuli in human neutrophils. *Blood, 89,* 3421–3433.

McDonald, P. P., & Cassatella, M. A. (1997). Activation of transcription factor NF-kappa B by phagocytic stimuli in human neutrophils. *FEBS Letters, 412,* 583–586.

Mercurio, F., DiDonato, J. A., Rosett, C., & Karin, M. (1993). p105 and p98 precursor proteins play an active role in NF-kappa B-mediated signal transduction. *Genes and Development, 7,* 705–718.

Mishima, S. (1982). Clinical investigations on the corneal endothelium-XXXVIII Edward Jackson Memorial Lecture. *American Journal of Ophthalmology, 93,* 1–29.

Montrucchio, G., Lupia, E., de Martino, A., Battaglia, E., Arese, M., Tizzani, A., Bussolino, F., & Camussi, G. (1997). Nitric oxide mediates angiogenesis induced in vivo by platelet-activating factor and tumor necrosis factor-alpha. *American Journal of Pathology, 151*(2), 557–563.

Moore, R., Carlson, S., & Madara, J. L. (1989). Rapid barrier restitution in an in vitro model of intestinal epithelial injury. *Laboratory Investigations, 60,* 237–244.

Moulin, V., Garrel, D., Auger, F. A., O'Connor-McCourt, M., Castilloux, G., & Germain, L. (1999). What's new in human wound-healing myofibroblasts? *Current Topics in Pathology, 93,* 123–133.

Norris, D. A., Capin, L., & Weston, W. L. (1982). The effect of epicutaneous glucocorticosteroids on human monocyte and neutrophil migration in vivo. *Journal of Investigative Dermatology, 78,* 386–390.

Oxlund, H., Christensen, H., Seyer-Hansen, M., & Andreassen, T. T. (1996). Collagen deposition and mechanical strength of colon anastomoses and skin incisional wounds of rats. *Journal of Surgical Research, 66,* 25–30.

Padgett, D. A., Marucha, P. T., & Sheridan, J. F. (1998). Neuroendocrine effects on wound healing in SKH-1 female mice. *Brain, Behavior, and Immunity, 12,* 64–73.

Paul, R. G., Tarlton, J. F., Purslow, P. P., Sims, T. J., Watkins, P., Marshall, F., Ferguson, M. J., & Bailey, A. J. (1997). Biomechanical and biochemical study of a standardized wound healing model. *International Journal of Biochemistry and Cell Biology, 29,* 211–220.

Perretti, M., & Flower, R. J. (1994). Cytokines, glucocorticoids and lipocortins in the control of neutrophil migration. *Pharmacology Research, 30,* 53–59.

Phan, S. H., McGarry, B. M., Loeffler, K. M., & Kunkel, S. L. (1987). Regulation of macrophage-derived fibroblast growth factor release by arachidonate metabolites. *Journal of Leukocyte Biology, 42*(2), 106-113.

Pierce, G. F., Mustoe, T. A., Lingelbach, J., Masakowski, V. R., Griffin, G. L., Senior, R. M., & Deuel, T. F. (1989). Platelet-derived growth factor and transforming growth factor-beta enhance tissue repair activities by unique mechanisms. *Journal of Cell Biology, 109*(1), 429–440.

Pilcher, B. K., Sudbeck, B. D., Dumin, J. A., Welgus, H. G., & Parks, W. C. (1998). Collagenase-1 and collagen in epidermal repair. *Archives of Dermatology Research, 290* (Suppl), S37-S46.

Ravage, Z. B., Gomez, H. F., Czermak, B. J., Watkins, S. A., & Till, G. O. (1998). Mediators of microvascular injury in dermal burn wounds. *Inflammation, 22*(6), 619–629.

Riches, D. W. H. (1996). Macrophage involvement in wound repair, remodeling and fibrosis. In R. A. F. Clark (Ed.), *The molecular and cellular biology of wound repair* (2nd ed.) (pp. 95–142). New York: Plenum.

Rogler, G., Brand, K., Vogl, D, Page, S., Hofmeister, R., Andus, T., Knuechel, R., Baeuerle, P. A., Scholmerich, J.,& Gross, V. (1998). Nuclear factor kappaB is activated in macrophages and epithelial cells of inflamed intestinal mucosa. *Gastroenterology, 115,* 357–369.

Russo-Marie, F. (1992). Macrophages and the glucocorticoids. *Journal of Neuroimmunology, 40,* 281–286.

Salmon, J. K., Armstrong, C. A., & Ansel, J. C. (1994). The skin as an immune organ. *Western Journal of Medicine, 160,* 146–152.

Schaffer, C. J., & Nanney, L. B. (1996). Cell biology of wound healing. *International Review of Cytology, 169,* 151–181.

Schechter, N. M. (1989). Structure of the dermal-epidermal junction and potential mechanisms for its degradation: The possible role of inflammatory cells. *Immunology Series, 46,* 477–507.

Scheinman, R. I., Beg, A. A., & Baldwin, A. S., Jr. (1993). NF-kappa B p100 (Lyt-10) is a component of H2TF1 and can function as an I-kappa B-like molecule. *Molecular and Cellular Biology, 13,* 6089–6101.

Scheinman, R. I., Cogswell, P. C., Lofquist, A. K., & Baldwin, A. S., Jr. (1995). Role of transcriptional activation of IκB in mediation of immunosuppression by glucocorticoids. *Science, 270,* 283–286.

Schmidt J. A., Oliver, C. N., Lepe-Zuniga, J. L., et al. (1984). Silica-stimulated monocytes release fibroblast proliferation factors identical to interleukin 1. *Journal of Clinical Investigation, 73,* 1462–1472.

Scholzen, T., Armstrong, C. A., Bunnett, N. W., Luger, T. A., Olerud, J. E., & Ansel, J. C. (1998). Neuropeptides in the skin: Interactions between the neuroendocrine and the skin immune systems. *Experimental Dermatology, 7,* 81–96.

Sefton, M. V., & Woodhouse, K. A. (1998). Tissue engineering. *Journal of Cutaneous Medical Surgery, 3*(Suppl. 1), S1–18–23.

Shull, M. M., Ormsby, I., Kier, A. B., Pawlowski, S., Diebold, R. J., Yin, M., Allen, R., Sidman, C., Proetzel, G., Calvin, D., et al. (1992). Targeted disruption of the mouse transforming growth factor-beta 1 gene results in multifocal inflammatory disease. *Nature, 359,* 693–699.

Simeon, A., Monier, F., Emonard, H., Wegrowski, Y., Bellon, G., Monboisse, J. C., Gillery, P., Hornebeck, W., & Maquart, F. X. (1999). Fibroblast–cytokine–extracellular matrix interactions in wound repair. *Current Topics in Pathology, 93,* 95–101.

Snyder, D. S., & Unanue, E. R. (1982). Corticosteroids inhibit murine macrophage Ia expression and interleukin 1 production. *Journal of Immunology, 129*(5), 1803–1085.

Springer, T. A. (1994). Traffic signals for lymphocyte recirculation and leukocyte emigration: The multistep paradigm. *Cell, 76,* 301–314.

Thomas, D. W., O'Neil, I. D., Harding, K. G., & Shepherd, J. R. (1995). Cutaneous wound healing: A current perspective. *Journal of Oral Maxillofacial Surgery, 53,* 442–447.

Tomic-Canic, M., Komine, M., Freedberg, I. M., & Blumenberg, M. (1998). Epidermal signal transduction and transcription factor activation in activated keratinocytes. *Journal of Dermatological Science, 17,* 167–181.

Tracey, K. J., Vlassara, H., & Cerami, A. (1989). Cachectin/tumor necrosis factor. *Lancet, 8647,* 1122–1126.

Tron, VA, Coughlin, M. D., Jang, D. E., & Sauder, D. N. (1990). The expression and modulation of nerve growth factor (NGF) in murine keratinocytes (PAM212). *Journal of Clinical Investigations, 85,* 1085–1089.

Uhl, E., Barker, J. H., Bondar, I., Galla, T. J., Leiderer, R., Lehr, H. A., & Messmer, K. (1993). Basic fibroblast growth factor accelerates wound healing in chronically ischaemic tissue. *British Journal of Surgery, 80*(8), 977–980.

Venkataraman, G., Raman, R., Sasisekharan, V., & Sasisekharan, R. (1999). Molecular characteristics of fibroblast growth factor-fibroblast growth factor receptor-heparin-like glycosaminogly-can complex. *Proceedings of the National Academy of Sciences, USA, 96*(7), 3658–3663.

Vogt, P. M., Lehnhardt, M., Wagner, D., Jansen, V., Krieg, M., & Steinau, H. U. (1998). Determination of endogenous growth factors in human wound fluid: Temporal presence and profiles of secretion. *Plastic and Reconstructive Surgery, 102,* 117–123.

Walsh, P. N. (1987). Platelet-mediated trigger mechanisms in the contact phase of blood coagulation. *Seminars in Thrombosis and Hemostasis, 13*(1), 86–94.

Welch, M. P., Odland, R. F., & Clark, R. A. F. (1990). Temporal relationships of F-actin bundle formation, collagen and fibronectin matrix assembly, and fibronectin receptor expression to wound contracture. *Journal of Cell Biology, 110*, 133–145.

Westerman, R. A., Carr, R. W., Delaney, C. A., Morris, M. J., & Roberts, R. G. (1993). The role of skin nociceptive afferent nerves in blister healing. *Clinical Experimental Neurology, 30*, 39–60.

Woodley, D. T., O'Keefe, E. J., & Prunieras, M. (1985). Cutaneous wound healing: A model for cell-matrix interactions. *Journal of the American Academy of Dermatology, 12*(2Pt.2), 420–433.

Zoja, C., Wang, J. M., Bettoni, S., Sironi, M., Renzi, D., Chiaffarino, F.,. Abboud, H. E., Van Damme, J., Mantovani, A., Remuzzi, G., (1991). Interleukin-1 beta and tumor necrosis factor-alpha induce gene expression and production of leukocyte chemotactic factors, colony- stimulating factors, and interleukin-6 in human mesangial cells. *American Journal of Pathology, 138*, 991–1003.

# 63

# Psychoneuroimmune Interactions in Periodontal Disease

TORBJØRN BREIVIK, PER STANLEY THRANE

## I. INTRODUCTION

The now well-established concept of a bidirectional communication between the central nervous system (CNS) and the immune system is an underresearched area in dentistry. However, increased interest in epidemiological studies investigating disease probability factors has revealed an association between destructive inflammatory conditions in the gums (periodontal disease) and negative life experiences, especially those manifested as depression (Genco et al., 1998; Monteiro da Silva, Oakly, Newman, Nohl, & Lloyd, 1996; Moss et al., 1996). Further-more, associations have been found between periodontal disease and the genetic background of an individual (Michalowicz, 1991), increasing age (Burt, 1994; Hugoson & Jordan, 1982), some Gram-negative lipopolysaccharide (LPS)-containing bacterial species (Beck, Koch, Zambon, Genco, & Tudor, 1992; Burt 1994), heavy smoking (Gonzalez et al., 1996; Martinez-Canut, Lorca, & Magan, 1996), poorly controlled and long-duration

diabetes mellitus (Dennison, Gottsegen, & Rose, 1996; Thorstensson & Hugoson, 1993), as well as HIV infection (Murray, 1994). Recent studies also suggest relationships between periodontal disease and increased risk of atherosclerosis/coronary heart disease (Beck, Offenbacher, Williams, Gibbs, & Garcia, 1998; Mattila et al., 1989). Currently, it is poorly understood how and why these risk factors are associated with increased periodontal disease susceptibility. The field of brain–neuroendocrine–immune interactions, therefore, is ripe for exploitation.

Observations from dental practice indicate that patients with severe and/or rapidly progressive forms of periodontal disease often seem to have experienced traumatic life events, such as the loss of a loved one by death or divorce. We therefore initiated experimental studies in a rat model to further explore the mechanisms underlying these observations. We induce experimental periodontal disease in rats by applying a silk ligature around the necks of some of their teeth. The resulting accumulation of oral microorganisms and a subsequent shift in the microflora from a largely aerobic to a more anaerobic flora creates a chronic inflammatory response that persists and results in tissue destruction. In this model system, we can time the onset and termination of the inflammatory response by applying or removing the plaque retainer (i.e., silk ligature). Furthermore, we can change the number of inflammatory as well as control sites and thereby regulate the overall magnitude of the inflammatory response. The resulting tissue destruction, including loss of attachment fibers and bone around the affected teeth, can be quantified radiographically and histologically. This provides us with an objective measure of disease activity (e.g., tissue breakdown) that is lacking in many of the current inflammatory model systems.

In this chapter, we will focus on the significance of the hypothalamo-pituitary-adrenal (HPA) axis on the chronic inflammatory response. Based on a series of experiments in rats, we discuss the influence of various factors on these highly complex interactions. In addition to describing our own research, we will review relevant literature and discuss the needs and directions for continuous work in this new interdisciplinary area of "brain–neuroendocrine–immune–periodontology."

## II. PERIODONTAL DISEASE

Oral microorganisms which normally colonize tooth surfaces (dental plaque) in close contact with the gingival margin, are constantly triggering immune responses of the gums. These responses may be clinical silent or may appear as inflammatory conditions, which may be nondestructive (gingivitis) or destructive (periodontitis or periodontal disease). Periodontal disease is a term comprising a group of diseases ranging from moderate to more severe and aggressive forms, resulting in various degrees of breakdown of the tooth-supporting tissues (the periodontium), including periodontal attachment fiber destruction and resorption of the alveolar bone, which lead to periodontal pocket formation and to increased tooth mobility and tooth loss in the most severe cases (Lindhe, 1995; Page, Offenbacher, Schroeder, Seymour, & Kornman, 1997).

Periodontal disease seems to have harmed mankind all through its existence. The bone lesions typical of periodontal disease have been observed in fossils from the Neanderthal man, and the disease appears to have been one of the most common diseases among Egyptians more than 4000 years ago (Page, 1995). Recent epidemiological studies also indicate that periodontal disease is one of our most common maladies, affecting hundreds of millions of people worldwide (Page, 1998). Thus, enormous efforts and resources are used in treating this disease and its consequences. Although tooth loss is not a life-threatening condition, a functional dentition and a healthy mouth undoubtedly improve the overall health and quality of life. Therefore, retention of teeth is important, and disease prevention is the ultimate goal.

Since the recognition in the 1960s that removal of dental plaque from the gingival margin area of the teeth reduces inflammation of the gums, periodontal disease has been looked upon as a bacterial infection (Löe, Theilade, & and Jensen, 1965). Periodontal disease was thought to begin during the teenage years, and to increase in prevalence almost linearly until early middle age, at which time it was considered to have affected virtually 100% of the adult population (Greene, 1963). Everyone was thought to be at risk, and the treatment strategies since then have been aimed at dental plaque control.

However, it has been observed that in some individuals the disease does not develop despite large amounts of bacterial plaque and gingival inflammation (gingivitis) during a lifetime. On the other hand, severe and rapid progressive forms of periodontal disease develop even in patients with good oral hygiene and in spite of professional periodontal plaque reducing treatment procedures. These observations have recently been confirmed by epidemiological studies showing that approximately 5–15% of most populations develop severe forms of periodontal disease, whereas a similar proportion seems to be highly resistant (Baelum, Chen, Manji, Luan, & Fejerskov, 1996; Hugoson & Jordan, 1982). Furthermore, epidemiological studies indicate that the incidence of severe destructive forms of periodontal disease has remained largely unaffected despite a general improvement of oral hygiene and treatment procedures to reduce dental plaque (Bartold, Seymour, Cullinan, & Westerman, 1998). This suggests that factors other than the total amount of microorganisms are important for the development of the disease.

Severe and/or treatment-resistant forms of periodontal disease are strongly associated with certain Gram-negative anaerobic bacteria dominating the subgingival flora (Dzink, Tanner, Haffajee, & Socransky, 1985; Socransky & Haffajee, 1992). Recent studies indicate that these microorganisms and their toxic products may be capable of damaging superficial tissue cells, but also that it is the host response mechanisms activated by these microorganisms that are responsible for most of the tissue damage (Birkedal-Hansen, 1993; Lee, Aitken, Sodek, & McCulloch, 1995; Page, 1991). Thus, although Gramnegative microorganisms may be necessary for the development of the disease, they are not sufficient for its clinical manifestation and progression. This is supported by studies showing that putative periodontal pathogens can be found in patients without periodontal disease (Dahlén, Manji, Baelum, & Fejerskov, 1989).

A number of studies have focused on putative "weaknesses" or "failures" in the immune system, leading to insufficient immune responses. However, there is now considerable evidence that the failure to control inflammatory tissue destruction often results from inappropriate rather than insufficient immune responses (Powie & Coffman, 1993).

Recent studies have focused on the balance between the two arms of the immune system, e.g., cellular and humoral immunity (Seymour et al., 1996). This balance has been shown to be highly dependent on the type of CD4+ T helper cells involved. T helper cells have recently been functionally divided into T helper 1 (Th1) and T helper 2 (Th2) cells, respectively, based on their cytokine profile. They have furthermore been shown to control each other's activity reciprocally (Heinzel, 1995; Liblau, Singer, & McDewitt, 1995; Scott & Kaufmann, 1991). A Th1-dominated pattern of cytokine release supports cellular immunity. It activates macrophages, favors a delayed type hypersensitivity reaction and immunoglobulin (Ig) isotype switching to IgG2a, stimulates CD8+ T cells, and inhibits humoral immunity. A Th2-dominated response supports humoral immunity and inhibits cellular immunity. It provides efficient help for B cell activation, for switching to IgG1, IgA, and IgE isotypes, and for antibody production. There are indications that Th1-dominated responses tend to protect against periodontal breakdown, whereas Th2-dominated responses tend to increase the breakdown (Seymour et al., 1996; Tokoro, Matsuki, Yamamoto, Suzuki, & Hara, 1997). Activation of macrophages and the high ability of IgG2a antibodies to bind to the Fc receptor on macrophages may explain, in part, the protective effect of Th1 responses. In addition, intraepithelial homing of $\gamma\delta$ CD8+ T cells seem to have an important role in the front lines of the body's defense against pathogens (Lundquist, Baranov, Teglund, Hammarstrøm, & Hammarstrøm, 1994; Williams, 1998).

The mechanisms by which the tooth-supporting tissue is destroyed are reasonably well understood (Birkedal-Hansen, 1993; Chapple, 1997; Lee et al., 1995). A dynamic balance exists between tissue breakdown and tissue rebuilding processes that involves both innate (PMNs, macrophages, and fibroblasts) and specific (lymphocytes) immune mechanisms interacting in a complex network. In periodontal disease, reactive oxygen metabolites (ROMs) and proteolytic enzymes, so-called matrix metalloproteinases (MMPs) released from polymorphnuclear phagocytic cells (PMNs) (which, together with plasma cells, are the dominating cells during active period-

ontal disease), are thought to be responsible for most of the soft tissue breakdown (Lee et al., 1995; Shapira, Borinski, Sela, & Soskolne, 1991). There is an indication that ROMs induce tissue destruction by activating latent MMPs (Shah, Baricos, & Basci, 1987). Bone resorption by osteoclasts is closely regulated by hormones and cytokines (Heymann, Guicheux, Gouin, Passuti, & Daculsi, 1998). Increased release of so-called proinflammatory cytokines such as interleukin-1$\beta$ (IL-1$\beta$), tumor necrosis factor-$\alpha$ (TNF-$\alpha$), and IL-6 can act as a powerful local stimulating signal for bone resorption (Bertolini, Nedwin, Bringman, Smith, & Mundy, 1986; Gowen, Wood, Ihrie, McGuire, & Russell, 1983; Jilka et al., 1992). These cytokines stimulate receptors on osteoblasts, which again modulate osteoclast function by release of other signals such as nitric oxide (Hukkanen et al., 1995). This suggests that the majority of tissue destruction is, in fact, derived from immune cells, and not from microorganisms present in the periodontal pocket. This has led to a change in view from periodontal disease being an infectious disease to that of an infection-induced inflammatory disease (Page, 1995).

Based on this current understanding and our rat experiments, we have put forward a hypothesis which may explain some of the variations in periodontal disease susceptibility (Breivik, Thrane, Murison, & Gjermo, 1996). We suggest that one of the factors involved may be individual differences in the reactivity of neural and neuroendocrine responses. Glucocorticoids released from the adrenal cortex via activation of the HPA axis seem to be important due to their ability to regulate the recruitment of immune cells into inflamed tissues, as well as to skew the Th1/Th2 balance toward a Th2-dominant immune response (Cronstein, Kimmel, Levin, Martiniuk, & Weissmann, 1992; Mason, 1991; Rook & Hernandez-Pando, 1997). Furthermore, we have focused on the HPA axis because most of the known periodontal disease risk factors, including increasing age, certain Gram-negative microorganisms, smoking, emotional stress, and insulin deficiency have been shown to stimulate this axis (Dallman et al., 1994; Lupien et al., 1994; Matta, Foster, & Sharp, 1993; Schwartz, Strack, & Dallman, 1997; Tilders et al., 1994). A recent epidemiological study on the association of stress, distress and coping behavior with periodontal disease supports this concept (Genco et al., 1998). This study showed a direct correlation of salivary cortisol levels and alveolar bone loss in patients with established periodontal disease who have high levels of financial strain and poor coping strategies.

## III. PSYCHOLOGICAL FACTORS AND PERIODONTAL DISEASE

The best documented correlation between emotional stress and disease in the gums has been shown in an acute necrotic ulcerative form of gingivitis and periodontitis (Horning & Cohen, 1995; Murayama, Kurihara, Nagai, Dompkowski, & Van Dyke, 1994). This is a painful rapidly destructive inflammatory disease in the gums. The disease was earlier referred to as Vincent's infection or infectious oral necrosis. In this condition, significant predisposing factors include extreme and/or unusual life stress, inadequate sleep, and recent illness (Dean & Singleton, 1945; Horning & Cohen, 1995; Pindborg, Bhat, & Roed-Petersen, 1967). During World War I, this was a common disease called "trench-mouth," and during World War II, up to 14% of the personnel in military units was found to suffer from the disease. Recent studies in industrialized countries have reported prevalence between 0.5 and 0.19%, or even less than 0.001% in Denmark (Barnes, Bowles, & Carter, 1973; Horning, Hatch, & Lutskus, 1990; Pindborg & Holmstrup, 1987). Increased incidence of this condition has been found in military personnel during stressful activities, students during examination periods, people not coping with their life situation over time, as well as in patients in periods with severe depression and/or other emotional disorders (Cohen-Cole et al., 1983; Giddon, Goldhaber, & Dunning, 1963; Giddon, Zackin, & Goldhaber, 1964; Kur, 1945; Moulton, Ewen, & Theiman, 1952; Pindborg, 1951).

In a recent study in United States, of 1426 subjects ages 25 to 74, financial strain and inadequate coping strategies were significantly associated with increased periodontal tissue breakdown after adjusting for age, gender, and smoking (Genco et al., 1998). In another study with 50 patients with adult rapidly progressive periodontal disease and 50 controls without significant periodontal destruction, depression and loneliness were found to be significantly increased in the diseased group (Monteiro da Silva et al., 1996). High depression scores were also found in patients with periodontal disease in another recent study (Moss et al., 1996). In this study, a strong association was found between serum antibody (IgG) levels to a periodontal pathogen (*Bacterioides forsythus*) and periodontal disease among individuals with a high depression scores but not among individuals with low depression score, suggesting a psychoneuroimmune link between the production of antibodies to this pathogen and periodontitis.

In addition to these emotional stress studies, there are a few studies indicating a positive correlation between adult periodontal disease and negative life events. In a case–control study of 100 dental patients matched for age and sex, periodontal disease was associated with the impact and number of negative life events and being unemployed (Croucher, Marcenes, Torres, Hughes, & Sheiham, 1997). In another study, measurements of life event stress among 50 patients in a dental clinic were significantly correlated with the measures of periodontal disease, and the disease severity increased with increasing stressors (Green, Tryon, Marks, & Huryn, 1986). The results of a small sample study of 10 women and 8 men (mean age of 39 years), from the head office of a large company, suggested that the susceptibility to periodontal disease was related to psychological factors. Moreover, reactions to stressful life events were dependent on the personality of the individual (Freeman & Gross, 1993). In a study of 50 periodontal disease patients chosen at random from a dental clinic, a positive correlation was found between anxiety state and periodontal disease (Miller, Thaller, & Soberman, 1956).

The relationship between periodontal disease and personality factors has also been studied. In a recent study, two groups of patients classified as well-responders and non-responders to periodontal treatment were compered in relation to somatic and psychosocial factors. The results indicated that the nonresponding group displayed more psychological strain and more passive-dependent personality, whereas the well-responding patients displayed more rigid personality and possibly a less stressful psychosocial situation in the past (Axtelius, Soderfeldt, Nilsson, Edwardsson, & Attstrom, 1998). In another study, 62 psychiatric patients and 40 healthy individuals were compared. It was found that certain personality factors tended to be associated with periodontal disease. There was also a positive correlation with marital adjustment, broken home, and the person's tendency for somatization (Baker, Crook, & Schwabacher, 1967) and poor coping strategies (Freeman & Gross, 1993). The severity of periodontal disease was also significantly greater among 104 psychiatric patients than in a control group of 122 nonpsychiatric subjects (Belting & Gupta, 1961). In this study, the degree of anxiety was also shown to be important. Anxiety and levels of circulating glucocorticoids, moreover, was found to correlate with periodontal disease in another study in psychiatric patients (Davis & Jenkins, 1962). In a study of 11 22- to 32-year-old veterans from the Vietnam War, diagnosed with severe alveolar bone loss, it was concluded that the only common denominator in all cases was severe emotional stress (De Marco, 1976).

Radiographs taken immediately prior to entering the military service and taken after finishing clearly illustrated a change in alveolar bone height during this short, but extremely stressful, period of life. This is supported by some early experimental stress studies in animals, indicating a positive correlation between bone loss and restraint stress, as well as cold stress (Gupta, Blechman, & Stahl, 1960; Shklar, 1966). The degree of gingival inflammation during stressful situations has also been studied (Deinzer, Ruttermann, Mobes, & Herforth, 1998), and it was found that the clinical signs of gingival inflammation increased in medical students participating in a major exam.

All in all, human studies on psychological factors and periodontal disease are few and limited. It can also be argued that behavioral changes, occurring as adaptations or coping responses to stressors, may influence disease risk. For example, persons under emotional stress tend to engage in less favorable health behaviors. They may smoke more, drink more alcohol, eat poorly, and practice poor oral hygiene, all factors, which may influence gingival and periodontal health.

On the other hand, numerous interdisciplinary psychoimmunological studies during the past 20 years have provided evidence that the immune system is not only triggered by bacterial antigens (or other antigens); external stimuli generating emotional stress responses may likewise influence and modulate the immune system via nervous and neuroendocrine systems (Ader, Cohen, & Felten, 1995; Blalock, 1994). Therefore, an experimental animal model is needed to be able to study the relative importance of various factors in a more controlled and restricted way. We have found that the rat ligature model looks most promising in this respect.

## IV. AN EXPERIMENTAL PERIODONTAL DISEASE MODEL IN RATS

Investigation of the bidirectional communication between CNS and the immune system has been greatly advanced by the use of animal models (Moynihan & Ader, 1996). Animal studies allow careful control of environmental stimuli, the genetic background of an individual (both in terms of the immune system response and the stress response system), the nature of the stressor, the nature of the antigenic challenge, and the type of immune responses generated.

We have used an experimental periodontal disease model, where a silk ligature is tied around the neck of

rat molar teeth in the gingival sulcus. The ligature, which serves as a retention device for oral microorganisms, also induces a periodontal pocket and a shift from an aerobic to a subgingival anaerobic microflora typical for periodontal disease. The contralateral molar teeth serve as control teeth for naturally occurring periodontal disease. Ligature-induced periodontal disease has for many years been used in primates, dogs, ferrets, and rats to study different treatment strategies and effects of various factors believed to influence the severity of periodontal disease (Fischer & Klinge, 1994; Kornman, Holt, & Robertson, 1981; Sallay et al., 1982; Svanberg, Lindhe, Hugoson, & Grøndahl, 1973). When antibacterial therapy was instituted during the presence of silk ligatures, no loss of periodontal attachment fibers or alveolar bone occurred (Polson, Zappa, Espeland, & Eisenberg, 1986; Zappa & Polson, 1988). This indicated that loss of the attachment and bone were due to the altered subgingival bacterial plaque and not to the mechanical trauma from the ligature itself. An advantage of this disease model is that we do not introduce exogenous antigen/pathogens, but rather change the environment, allowing growth of a pathogenic microflora much in the same way as in human periodontal disease.

The severity of the disease is measured on radiographs and on histologically properly oriented serial sections by measuring the distance from the enamel–cementum junction to the coronal margin of periodontal attachment fibers and the bone surrounding the tooth. Under healthy conditions, periodontal attachment fibers start at this junction, providing us with a fixed "landmark" on the teeth from which we can measure degree of tissue breakdown (Figure 1).

### A. Effects of Genetic Variations in the Stress Response System

To cope with environmental challenges, the organism elicits an adaptive response involving neural and neuroendocrine adjustments that is aimed at restoring homeostatic balance and to the return to status quo ante (Cannon, 1929; Selye, 1955). Strong evidence has been obtained that these stress response regulatory mechanisms are of relevance for the homeostasis of immune responses as well (Schauenstein et al., 1997). Cytokines and peptide hormones secreted from activated immune cells inform the brain about contact with antigens, and CNS-derived signals subsequently modulate the immune response. Furthermore, other external signals such as emotional stress activate this brain–neuroendocrine–immune regulatory system and modulate immune activities. The sympathetic

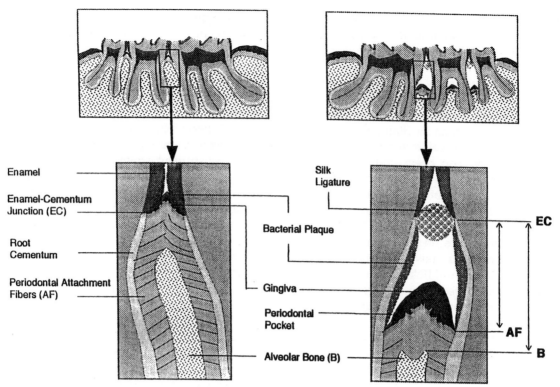

**FIGURE 1**  Schematic drawing illustrating tooth-supporting tissue breakdown on mesio-distal oriented cross sections of maxillary rat molar teeth (right) and control side without experimental periodontal disease (left). The arrowhead lines mark distances measured histometrically. Periodontal attachment fiber loss is measured as the distance between the enamel–cementum junction (EC) to the most coronal attachment fibers (AF) and alveolar bone loss as the distance between EC to the most coronal alveolar bone (B).

(adrenergic), the parasympathetic (cholinergic), and the sensory nervous system, as well as the hormonal system, including the hypothalamo-pituitary-adrenal (HPA) axis, all take part in this brain–neuroendocrine–immune network (Ader et al., 1995; Blalock, 1994; Schauenstein et al., 1997). There is evidence that genetically determined variation in the magnitude of these stress response-regulating mechanisms can determine susceptibility or resistance to diseases (Derjik & Sternberg, 1994; Mason, 1991; Sternberg, Chrousos, Wilder, & Gold, 1992).

Activation of the HPA axis is one of the major responses to stressful stimuli, including emotional stress, infection and inflammation. Furthermore, this axis is an important brain–immunoregulatory pathway. In short, the HPA axis consists of parvocellular neurons in the paraventricular nucleus of the hypothalamus producing corticotrophin-releasing hormone (CRH) and arginine vasopressin (AVP), as well as other hormones. Terminals of these neurons are located in the median eminence, where CRH and AVP are secreted into the portal blood by activation. CRH and AVP are important regulators of adrenocorticotrophic hormone (ACTH) secretion in the pituitary

gland. This peptide hormone, in turn, stimulates the secretion of glucocorticoids from the adrenal cortex (Antoni, 1986; Whitnall, 1993). Glucocorticoids (cortisol in man and corticosterone in rodents) are powerful immunosuppressive hormones, inhibiting Th1-mediated immune responses in particular (Mason, 1991; Rook & Hernandez-Pando, 1997). The response to various stimuli are dependent on neural inputs, mediated by central neurotransmitters, mainly noradrenaline and serotonin (Feldman, Conforti, & Weidenfeld, 1995; Plotsky, Cunningham, & Widmaier, 1989).

In addition, the activity of the HPA axis is regulated by negative feedback exerted by the glucocorticoids themselves. Two distinct subtypes of corticoid receptors, namely the high-affinity mineralocorticoid receptor (MR) and the lower-affinity glucocorticoid receptors (GR), mediate the effects of glucocorticoids on the brain (De Kloet, 1991). This feedback action of glucocorticoids is highly complex, as they are exerted at multiple sites within the brain and the pituitary gland. Genetically determined as well as stress-induced differences in receptor density, distribution and their binding affinity to glucocorticoids play a major role for the outcome of the feedback control (Buckingham, Loxley, Christian, & Philip, 1996). The effects of such variations will be discussed in the following subsections.

To study the effects of genetic variations in HPA activities on experimental periodontal disease, we have used the inbred Lewis and Fischer 344 strains of rats. These rats show extreme differences in their HPA axis responsivity to stressful stimuli (Sternberg et al., 1992). However, they share the same major histocompatible complex (MHC) class II molecule (RT1B) and consequently respond to the same antigenic epitopes (Caspi et al., 1996). While the HPA axis in Lewis rats responds poorly to inflammatory stimuli as well as other stressors, Fischer rats show a significantly higher HPA axis responsiveness to stressful stimuli. The low HPA axis responding Lewis rats are susceptible to a host of experimentally Th1-mediated inflammatory diseases, whereas the high responding Fischer rats are resistant to such diseases. Conversely, the Fischer rats show increased susceptibility to pathogenic microorganisms, whereas Lewis rats are resistant. In the experimental rat model, we have found that Fischer rats developed significantly more severe periodontal disease than Lewis rats (Breivik, Opstad, Gjermo, & Thrane, 1999).

Susceptibility versus resistance is thought to be dependent on the immunosuppressive effects of glucocorticoids on cell-mediated (Th1) immunity in particular. Glucocorticoid administration to cultures of murine T cells selectively inhibits the response of Th1 cells and the differentiation and/or activation of Th2 cells is favored in the presence of glucocorticoids (Daynes & Araneo, 1989; Daynes, Areano, Dowell, Huang, & Dudley, 1990). In addition to their role as potent inhibitors of inflammation via the direct suppression of cytokine production by Th-cells, glucocorticoids may further inhibit Th-cell-mediated inflammation indirectly by suppressing IL-12 and enhancing IL-10 production by antigen-resenting cells (Vieira, Kalinski, Wierenga, Kapsenberg, & de Jong, 1998; Visser et al., 1998). The ratio of cortisol/corticosterone to another immunoregulatory adrenal cortex hormone, dehydroepiandrosterone (DHEA), seems to be crucial for the Th1/Th2 balance and the control of pathogens (Rook & Hernandez-Pando, 1997). Furthermore, glucocorticoids have been found to inhibit binding of T cell to endothelial cells by modulating the expression of their adhesion molecules (Eguchi et al., 1992). This effect influences T-cell recruitment into inflamed tissues.

CNS-induced immunosuppression, however, is not uniquely linked to the activation of the HPA axis. In rats immunosuppression (decrease of mitogen-induced lymphocyte proliferation and natural killer (NK)-cell activity) has recently been found to be present only after administration of a stressor that increases $\beta$-endorphin, whereas immunosuppression was absent when the concentrations of $\beta$-endorphin were not modified (Panerai, Sacerdote, Bianchi, & Manfredi, 1997). Interestingly, this study showed that plasma corticosterone levels could be similarly elevated after stresses whether or not they suppressed immune responses, thus suggesting a pivotal role of $\beta$-endorphin.

Periodontal disease is induced by an overgrowth of Gram-negative anaerobic microorganisms in the periodontal pocket. Immunity to anaerobic pathogens appears to correlate with a delayed-type hypersensitive response in vivo accompanied by a Th1 cytokine secretion profile. We have previously suggested that the overgrowth of these microorganisms may, in part, be explained by a genetically determined and/or stress-induced neuroendocrine response (Breivik et al., 1996). This response inhibits T-cell-mediated immunity and drives the balance between cell-mediated (Th1) responses and humoral immunity (Th2 responses) toward an inappropriate Th2 cytokine profile, which may lead to immunopathology. This view is supported by a recent immunohistochemical study showing a significantly higher number of CD4+ cells in gingival and periodontal tissues of the periodontal disease-resistant Lewis rats compared to the susceptible Fischer rats (Breivik, Nerland, Murison, & Jonsson, 1998).

The immunopathology of periodontal disease appears to correlate with increased secretion of reactive oxygen metabolites and proteolytic enzymes (MMPs) from phagocytic PMNs, which are recruited in large numbers in the inflamed tissue (Lee et al., 1995) during a Th2-dominated response. We have suggested that this increased recruitment of PMNs in the inflamed tissues may be a compensation for the lack of the more effective Th1-type cell activation resulting in macrophage phagocytic immunity. In addition, intraepithelial $\gamma\delta$ T-cell activation, which is thought to play an important role in the defense against pathogenic microorganisms, may be downregulated during a Th2 response. Without such compensatory phagocytic hyperactivity by PMNs during a weak Th1 immune response, the tissue could have been invaded by microorganisms, which again could be life threatening for the host. Although life saving, the increased accumulation of PMNs and their release of tissue destructive components during phagocytosis, may be responsible for most of the local tissue destruction in periodontal disease.

In addition to the increased recruitment of PMNs to inflammatory sites during a weak Th1 response, we have found that activated peripheral leukocytes from Fischer rats, which are typical Th1 low responders (Caspi et al., 1996), release significantly more ROMs than peripheral leukocytes taken from Lewis rats, when activated by phorbol 12-myristate 13-acetaten (PMA) in vitro (Breivik et al., unpublished data). Furthermore, PMNs from Fischer rats show increased release of ROMs when they were mixed with mast cells, whereas PMNs from Lewis rats did not. This indicates that there may be a higher release of ROMs from PMNs in the inflamed tissue during phagocytosis in Fischer rats compared to Lewis rats. This is in accordance with studies showing that the release of ROMs is coupled to HPA axis reactivity (Skrede, Røshol, Ærø & Wiik, 1996; Wiik et al., 1995). The significantly increased severity of experimental periodontal disease in HPA axis high responding animals may, thus, be explained by the high recruitment of PMNs, as well as the higher release of ROMs from PMNs in periodontal disease susceptible individuals.

In addition to the studies in the inbred Lewis and Fisher rats we are now, in collaboration with the Department of Psychoneuropharmacology of the University of Nijmegen, The Netherlands, investigating the effect on experimental periodontal disease in two different lines of outbred Wistar rats. These rat lines are bidirectionally selected for the susceptibility to the dopaminergic agonist apomorphine and are termed APO-SUS (animals with a high susceptibility to apomorphine) and APO-UNSUS (animals with a low susceptibility to apomorphine). They have also been found to be high and low HPA responders to stressful stimuli, respectively (Cools & Gingras, 1998). Moreover, their individual differences in HPA axis structure and reactivity have been found to co-occur with group-specific differences in susceptibility to Th1-mediated experimental autoimmune encephalomyelitis and *Trichinella spiralis* infection (Kavelaars, Heijnen, Ellenbroek, van Loveren, & Cools, 1997).

Our data so far from these studies (Breivik, Sluyter, Hof, & Cools, 2000), as well as in Lewis and Fischer rats, suggest that differential genetic susceptibility plays a major role in the development of periodontal disease.

## B. Effects of Hippocampal Lesioning

Hippocampal neurons expressing glucocorticoid receptors play a major role in the control of the HPA axis, particularly in relation to behavioral adaptation (Jacobson & Sapolsky, 1991). Individual differences in HPA function seem to be related to the degree of hippocampal pathology later in life, by which stress-induced high glucocorticoid levels seem to play an important role for hippocampal neuron degeneration (Magariños & Mc Ewen, 1995).

As described above, the feedback control of glucocorticoids in the brain is regulated by the high-affinity MR, and the lower-affinity GR (De Kloet, 1991). In the brain, MRs are predominantly located in the hippocampus, and are important for the regulation of low circulating glucocorticoid levels in non-stressed conditions. GRs (as well as the MR) sites, on the other hand, are occupied by high glucocorticoid levels following stressful stimuli, including emotional stress, infections/inflammations, or by administration of exogenous glucocorticoids. In most brain tissues both the MRs and the GRs exert negative feedback on HPA activity. Hippocampal GRs, however, do not appear to mediate negative feedback of glucocorticoids on stress-induced HPA activity, but rather exert positive feedback through disinhibition (Joëls & De Kloet, 1994).

Differences in the distribution of these hippocampal receptors, as well as their binding capacity, are important for the outcome of the HPA activity. For example, Lewis rats, which are low HPA axis responders, show high hippocampal MR expression (Oitzl, van Haarst, & de Kloet, 1995), whereas high HPA axis responders, as for example old individuals showing hippocampal neuron degeneration and cell loss, exert a low MR expression (Hauger, Thrivikraman, & Plotsky, 1994; Raadsheer et al., 1995). Moreover, hippocampal GR number is reduced in 2-month-old male adult Wistar rats that are separated from their mother for 24 h 3 days after birth (Sutanto, Rosenfeld, de Kloet, & Levine, 1996).

Based on these data, as well as hippocampal lesion experiments showing increased HPA activity (Fendler, Karmos, & Telegdy, 1961; Herman et al., 1989), we investigated whether bilateral lesions of the hippocampal region (hippocampus proper, fascia dentata, and subiculum) had any effects on experimental periodontal disease in Wistar rats. Preliminary results of this experiment suggested that hippocampal lesioned rats developed significantly more severe periodontal tissue destruction compared to sham-operated controls (Breivik, Gjermo, Thrane, & Myhrer, 2000). This study supports our finding that HPA dysfunction may play a role in periodontal disease susceptibility.

## C. Effects of Adrenalectomy

Surgical removal of the adrenal glands leads to decreased levels of corticosterone. Since high corticosterone levels are found to increase the severity of periodontal disease in our other experiments, we hypothezed that adrenalectomy would lead to a reduction in experimental periodontal disease compared to sham-operated animals. In our first experiment, adrenalectomized rats were delivered from an animal house. We found to our surprise that the severity of periodontal disease was significantly increased, but so also was the corticosterone level. When the adrenal glands were examined, it was revealed that they were not totally removed. This, in addition to data showing that adrenalectomy increases CRH neuron activity and induces an increase of CRH mRNA and CRH levels (Sawchenko, 1987), as well as increases the amount of colocalized AVP in CRH neurons (Whitnall, 1988), may explain the higher corticosterone levels as well as the increased severity of periodontal disease in these animals. In a follow-up study, adrenalectomy was properly done and the corticosterone levels were kept low. This reduced the severity of experimental periodontal disease compared to that seen in sham-operated animals (Breivik et al., 2000). These experiments demonstrate that the corticosterone blood level may be an important modulator of periodontal disease susceptibility. This confirms our previous findings showing that animals with low corticosterone levels are resistant to developing experimental periodontal disease, whereas high corticosterone levels increase disease susceptibility.

## D. Effects of Exogenous Glucocorticoids

Sustained elevation in circulating glucocorticoids is typical in chronic stressful situations associated with fear, uncertainty, lack of control, poor predictability of upcoming events, either real or imagined (Levine, Weinberg, & Ursin, 1978). Furthermore, sustained high levels of glucocorticoids are found in depression and other neuropathologic disorders, including chronic alcoholism and Alzheimer's disease (Holsboer, Spengler, & Heuser, 1992; Raadsheer et al., 1995). Administration of exogenous glucocorticoids such as corticosterone or the synthetic glucocorticoid analogue dexamethasone, have been shown to mimic these effects. In addition, chronic administration of LPS from Gram-negative bacteria and proinflammatory cytokines, such as IL-1$\beta$, lead to sustained elevation of corticosterone (Harbuz & Lightman, 1992; Sapolsky, Rivier, Yamamoto, Plotsky, & Vale, 1987).

We have investigated the effects of these steroids in the experimental periodontal disease model in the low HPA axis-responding Lewis rats. Corticosterone was delivered by subcutaneously implanting slow releasing corticosterone pellets (200 mg of corticosterone delivered over 60 days). The intervention increased the severity of experimental periodontal disease significantly compared to matched controls (Breivik et al., 2000). Other studies have shown that elevation of glucocorticoids by exogenous administration, or by chronic stress, may increase susceptibility to viral and mycobacterium infections (Brown, Sheridan, Pearl, & Zwillig, 1993; Dobbs, Vasquez, Glaser, & Sheridan, 1993). Since both these diseases have been shown to be most effectively protected by T-cell-mediated immunity, our experiment supports recent suggestions that a Th1-dominated immune response is protective in periodontal disease. This further indicates that the positive correlation found in epidemiological studies between psychological stress and the prevalence and severity of periodontal disease may be associated with stress-induced increased gluococorticoid levels. In fact, such a correlation was found in a recent study focusing on stress and periodontal disease (Genco et al., 1998).

## E. Effects of Infection/Inflammation-Induced HPA Axis Hyperfunction

Bacterial LPS and proinflammatory cytokines, such as interleukin-1 (IL-1), IL-6, and IL-8 released by activated immune cells have been shown to stimulate the HPA axis at multiple levels, including the hypothalamic CRH and AVP producing neurons (Buckingham et al., 1996; Navarra, Schettini, & Grossman, 1997). Activation of the HPA axis by these peripheral immune messengers may be mediated to the brain by sensory afferent nerves as well additional neuronal and humoral pathways (Danzter, 1994; Tilders et al., 1994). Furthermore, prostaglandins generated in the periphery may play an important role in the immune–brain dialogue by stimulating sensory nerve endings (Navarra et al., 1997). Stimulation of the HPA axis by these immune messengers subsequently modulate the inflammatory process through the release of immunoregulating neurotransmitters and neuropeptides from nerve endings, and hormones from endocrine glands, including glucocorticoids with potent anti-inflammatory and immunosuppressive effects (Ader et al., 1995; Blalock, 1994).

Since we have found that experimental periodontal disease is more severe in rats with high blood levels of corticosterone compared to those with low corticosterone levels, it should be expected that LPS and/or proinflammatory cytokines known to activate the HPA axis would increase the severity of the periodontal disease during an infectious and/or inflammatory process. In fact, this seems to be the case. For example, in the experimental ligature-induced periodontal disease model, in vivo administration of recombinant human IL-1$\beta$ accelerates the severity of the disease over a 2-week period (Koide et al., 1995). Furthermore, we have found that the development of naturally occurring periodontal disease during an 11-week period was more severe in left maxillary molar teeth in rats where experimental periodontal disease was induced in right maxillary molar teeth, compared to naturally occurring periodontal disease in the same teeth of control rats without induction of experimental periodontal disease (Breivik et al., 2000). This indicates that infections and/or inflammations, such as periodontal disease, may increase disease development and progression through increased activation of the HPA axis. Infectious and/or inflammatory processes have, in fact, been found to induce permanent hyperactivation of the HPA axis when induced in early childhood. For example, postnatal administration of IL-1$\beta$ in mice stimulates corticosterone output and induces permanent HPA axis hyperreactivity to stressful stimuli in adulthood (Furukawa, del Rey, Monge Arditi, & Besedovsky, 1998). Moreover, prenatal immune challenges by immunization in rats have been found to permanently alter the HPA axis reactivity (Reul et al., 1994).

These and a number of other studies have shown that the development of the HPA axis depends on environmental signals, including signals derived from the immune system, in addition to genetically determined mechanisms (Besedovsky et al., 1991). Furthermore, emotional signals, particular those experienced in early life, seem to play an important role in the development of the HPA axis (Plotsky & Meany, 1993). Since the HPA axis is also activated by nicotine (Matta et al., 1993), chronic pain (Vaccarino & Couret, 1995), high-fat intake (Tannenbaum et al., 1997), and insulin deficiency (Schwartz et al., 1997), it could be expected that these factors would increase periodontal disease susceptibility via a hyperreactive HPA axis as well.

Taken together, these data suggest that activation of the HPA axis may contribute to the tissue breakdown during certain infectious and/or inflammatory processes. A growing body of evidence now suggests that many of the risk factors involved in periodontal disease, such as Gram-negative bacterial LPS and increasing age, may increase glucocorticiod secretion by impaired regulation of the glucocorticoid negative feedback. This may include downregulation of brain glucocorticoid receptors and/or degeneration and death of brain cells containing these receptors, such

as hippocampal pyramidal neurons (Liu et al., 1997; Magariños & McEwen, 1995; Weidenfeld & Yirmiya, 1996).

## F. Effects of Age-Related HPA Axis Hyperfunction

It has been known for a long time that increasing age is strongly associated with periodontal tissue destruction (reviewed in Burt 1994). In most populations, very few subjects under the age of 30 (less than 1%) show signs of severe periodontal disease, whereas about 10% are seriously affected by the disease in the age group above 50 (Baelum et al., 1996; Hugoson & Jordan, 1982). It has also been shown that the rate of progression of periodontal breakdown increases with age (Albandar, Buischi, & Barbosa, 1991). Thus, the association between increasing age and periodontal disease may be explained either as a biologic consequence of aging, or as a consequence of long-time exposure to dental plaque, or both.

Our studies indicate that the severity of experimental periodontal disease in rats correlates with increasing plasma levels of corticosterone. Since plasma glucocorticoid levels have generally been found to increase with increasing age in both rats and humans under basal and poststress conditions (Landfield & Pitler 1984; Lupien et al., 1994), we suggest that increased periodontal disease susceptibility associated with aging may be a consequence of higher glucocorticoid levels in aged individuals.

However, increased HPA activity is not an inevitable consequence of aging, either in rats or in humans (Issa, Rowe, Gauthier, & Meany, 1990; Sharma, Palacios-Bois, Schwartz, Quirion, & Nair, 1989), but seems to be associated with age-related neuropathology. For example, aged cognitive-impaired rats and humans show HPA hyperactivity that correlates with hippocampal neuron degeneration (Bodnoff et al., 1995). Furthermore, age-related neuropathology, including hippocampal neuron cell death, is associated with stress-induced high corticosterone secretion (Friedman, Green, & Sharland, 1969; Lupien et al., 1994; Magariños & McEwen, 1995). Increase in age-related high corticosterone levels has also been found in pathological conditions associated with hippocampal neuron degeneration, such as major depression and Alzheimer's disease (Raadsheer et al., 1995).

In addition to the loss of hippocampal neurons induced by cumulative exposure of high glucocorticoid levels during aging, age-related abnormalities in the neurotransmitter input into the hippocampus may alter the HPA activity directly (Yau, Dow, Fink, & Seckl, 1992). Furthermore, HPA hyperactivity may also result from hypothalamic dysfunction in aged rats. Cholinergic, noradrenergic, and serotonergic afferents all stimulate the secretion of CRH into the hypothalamic circulation (Plotsky, Otto, & Sutton, 1987; Plotsky, 1988). This stimulatory neurotransmitter input to hypothalamic CRH neurons may increase during aging (Hauger et al., 1994). Thus, age-related neuropathology of brain neurons regulating HPA activity, and the subsequent increased release of the immunoregulating hormone may play an important role for the outcome of immune responses to antigenic challenges, such as to dental plaque microorganisms in the gingival sulcus. Moreover, genetically determined as well as stress-induced high glucocorticoid levels may be responsible for some of the neuropathology seen during age-related HPA axis dysfunction (Wang, Lo, & Kau, 1997). This may also explain our finding that aged male Fischer 344 rats showed significantly more severe experimental periodontal breakdown than young adult male Fischer 344 rats. In this rat strain, age-related cognitive deficits appear to be the rule (Hauger et al., 1994).

Taken together, recent brain and neuroendocrine research, as well as our experimental periodontal disease studies in rats, provide some initial support for the idea that age-related hyperactivity of the HPA axis may contribute to the increased susceptibility to periodontal disease found in aged individuals.

## G. Effects of Experimental Stress

Increased corticosterone blood levels resulting from activation of the HPA axis by restraint increases the susceptibility of mice to *Mycobacterium ovium*, as well as influenza virus and herpes virus infections (Bonneau, Sheridan, Feng, & Glaser, 1993; Brown et al., 1993; Dobbs et al., 1993). Since these infections and periodontal disease are best protected by Th1-mediated immune responses, it should be expected that restraint stress might increase the severity of experimental periodontal disease in rats.

In a recent experimental study in Wistar rats, restraint stress accelerated ligature-induced periodontal disease (Skaleric & Gaspersic 1998). This supports the hypothesis that stress may influence periodontal disease severity. Moreover, we have found that the number of CD4+ cells (T helper cells and some macrophages) in gingival and periodontal tissues in Lewis rats (which we found are relatively higher than in Fischer rats), decreased after exposure to inescapable footshock stress (Breivik et al., 1998). This further supports the suggestion that Th1-dominated immune responses is protective in periodontal disease, and that stressful stimuli known to activate the HPA axis, such as inescapable footshock stress, influence immune cell recruitment into inflamed tissues.

## H. Effects of Early Stressful Life Events in Adult Rats

To study the putative relationship between negative life events and periodontal disease more directly, in particular, those experienced during childhood, we have used a maternal separation model in rats to examine how such early events might effect the severity of experimental periodontal disease in adulthood.

In rats, early postnatal separation of the pups from their mother leads to permanent changes in the responsivity of the HPA axis (Plotsky & Meany, 1993). Daily short-term separation (15 min) from lifeday 2 to lifeday 14 (termed handling) decreases HPA reactivity, whereas long-term (180 min) maternal separation leads to the opposite response, e.g., increased basal and stress-induced HPA activity (Plotsky & Meany, 1993). Moreover, rats separated for 24 h at postnatal day 3 show strong basal corticosterone levels in adult age (Rots, de Jong, Levine, Cools, & de Kloet, 1996). Interestingly, variation in maternal care also affects the development of individual differences in HPA axis responses to stress in rats. For example, the offspring of rat mothers that exhibit more licking and grooming of their pups during the first 10 days of life show reduced plasma corticosterone responses to stress (Liu et al., 1997). This suggests that maternal behavior may serve to "program" HPA axis responses to stressful stimuli in the offspring.

The maternal separation model in rats is also viewed as a good model for investigating depression (Nemeroff, 1998). People who have both a genetic predisposition for depression and a traumatic childhood seem to be unusually prone to the condition. In fact, most depressed patients, particularly those who are most severely affected, display HPA axis hyperactivity. Indeed, this finding is looked upon as the most reproducible one in all of biological psychiatry (Nemeroff, 1998). Thus, maternal separation in rats may represent a good model for investigating the effect of how traumatic life experiences during childhood may produce permanent changes in the HPA axis responsivity. These changes may chronically boost the output of immunomodulatory neurotransmitters, neuropeptides, and hormones, including glucocorticoids, and influence immune activities, such as in gingival connective tissues to dental bacterial plaque.

These data suggest that loss of the mother for a period of time during infancy produces permanent changes in the developing brain. Such changes, including those leading to HPA hyperactivity, may thus increase the individual's susceptibility to periodontal disease. We are now investigating the effect of experimental periodontal disease in rats separated postnatally from their mother for 24 h from lifeday 9. Preliminary data from our rat model suggest that maternal separation may influence the progression of experimentally induced periodontal disease. In addition, postnatal exposure to bacterial LPS (andotoxin, ip) or cytokines (IL-1) was shown to permanently alter the HPA axis reactivity (Furukawa et al., 1998; Shanks et al., 1995) and, thus, may also influence periodontal disease susceptibility later in life. We have recently found that postnatally endotoxin-treated Lewis rats developed significantly more periodontal breakdown at both experimental and control teeth compared to postnatally saline-treated control animals (Breivik et al., 2000).

Taken together, these data suggest that emotional as well as Gram-negative bacterial load during early postnatal life may alter the development of neural systems, which govern endocrine responses to stressful stimuli, and may thereby predispose individuals to pathology.

## V.  GENERAL DISCUSSION

In this chapter, we have focused on the relationship between negative life events and periodontal disease. Taken together, studies so far suggest that emotional stress, especially when manifested as depression, may increase the risk of microorganism-induced inflammatory diseases, such as periodontal disease. To investigate mechanisms by which emotional stress may influence periodontal disease development and progression, we have used an experimental periodontal disease model in rats.

We have shown that rats with extreme genetic differences in their HPA axis structure and reactivity to stressful stimuli, show significant differences in their susceptibility to periodontal disease. For example, the inbred HPA axis high responding Fischer rats develop significantly more severe periodontal tissue destruction than do the MHC identical HPA axis low responding Lewis rats. The same tendency is observed in two fundamental distinct lines of outbred Wistar rats, which have been selected for their high and low susceptibility to the dopaminergic agonist apomorphine and respond with a low and high HPA activity to stressful stimuli, respectively. Interestingly,

genetically determined susceptibility to periodontal disease is found in a human twin study (Michalowicz, 1994). Could variations in the HPA axis responsiveness account for a part of the genetic correlation in that study? In humans, salivary free cortisol measurement responses to a standardized psychological stressor could reveal such differences. This has been shown to be a reliable measurement for the HPA axis reactivity (Buske-Kirchbaum et al., 1997). Indeed, significantly higher salivary cortisol values are found in patients exhibiting severe periodontal disease compared to a control group with little or no periodontal disease (Genco et al., 1998).

The behavioral and neuroendocrine genetic differences between HPA axis high and low responding individuals can, however, be modulated by environmental factors. Maternal behavior and care during infancy are critical for HPA axis development (Plotsky & Meany, 1993). This is supported by studies in the rat model suggesting that maternal separation during the early postnatal period may increase the severity of experimental periodontal disease induced when they reach adulthood compared to that seen in nonseparated controls. Furthermore, we have found increased periodontal disease susceptibility in postnatally endotoxin-treated rats. This suggests that early life experiences that induce HPA hyperactivity, may increase susceptibility to periodontal disease.

Furthermore, our rat studies have suggested that aged HPA axis high responding Fischer rats develop significantly more severe experimental periodontal breakdown compared to young adult HPA axis lower responding Fischer rats. HPA axis reactivity normally increases during aging, particularly in individuals showing neuropathology (Dodt et al., 1991, Friedman et al., 1969). Since increasing age is associated with increased risk of periodontal disease (Burt, 1994), we suggest that age-induced HPA axis hyperactivity may play a role in the pathogenesis of periodontal disease.

LPS, smoking, and poorly controlled and long-duration diabetes mellitus are factors known to increase the risk of periodontal disease initiation and progression. Since the HPA axis is also activated by LPS, nicotine, and insulin deficiency, we suggest that these risk factors may increase the risk of periodontal disease via the same brain–neuroendocrine–immune regulating system. The HPA axis has been shown to be hyperactivated in more than half of the patients with major depression (Charlton & Ferrier, 1989), and periodontal disease is associated with depressive mood states, as shown above. Moreover, HPA hyperactivity has been found in Alzheimer's disease, anorexia nervosa, chronic active alcoholism, chronic pain, and high-fat intake (Holsboer et al.,

1992; Licinio, Wong, & Gold, 1996; Raadsheer et al., 1995; Tannenbaum et al., 1997; Vaccarino & Couret, 1995). Could these patients be at risk of developing periodontal disease as well?

Studies suggesting that periodontal disease may be associated with increased risk of coronary heart disease and stroke (Mattila et al., 1989; Beck et al., 1998), may also be explained by HPA hyperactivation. Elevated levels of cortisol are associated with atherosclerosis (Troxler, Sprague, Albanese, Fuchs, & Thompson, 1977), and increased HPA activity with elevation in glucocorticoids is, in addition to immunosuppression, associated with increased serum glucose and lipids as well as increased cardiovascular tone. Furthermore, long-term HPA activation also has been linked to increased risk for cardiovascular disease, diabetes, and hypertension (Brindley & Rolland, 1989). Therefore, this association may be due to shared risk factors. This suggestion is further supported by studies in patients with prolonged systemic glucocorticoid therapy, such as in patients with rheumatoid arthritis or lupus erythematosus. These patients exhibit higher prevalence of atherosclerosis and infections, as well as shorter life expectancies (Reilly, Chosh, Maddison, Rasker, & Silman, 1990; Bulkley & Roberts, 1975). A more direct causal relationship has also been suggested where blood-borne proinflammatory cytokines (TNF-$\alpha$, IL-1$\beta$) released from inflamed periodontal tissues may directly affect atherosclerotic processes (Beck et al., 1998).

The mechanisms by which sustained HPA axis hyperactivity may increase periodontal disease susceptibility seem, in part, to be mediated by glucocorticoid inhibition of T-cell-mediated immune responses. This leads to a shift toward antibody-mediated immunity, which may subsequently lead to the overgrowth of pathogenic microorganisms. The antibody-mediated immunity results in a high recruitment of phagocytic PMNs to fight the invading microorganisms. The price to be paid for sustained activation of this innate immune response, is local tissue destruction as seen during active periodontal disease.

## VI. SUMMARY AND FUTURE PERSPECTIVES

To summarize, our research suggests that an inappropriate HPA axis hyperactivity and a subsequent inappropriate Th2 immune response play a role in the etiopathogenesis of periodontal disease. Mood states such as depression, as well as other factors including proinflammatory cytokines, nicotine, or insulin deficiency, may induce biochemical changes in the brain, thereby increasing periodontal disease susceptibility.

Based on these data, the question arises whether drugs with inhibitory effects on the HPA axis may have favorable effects on periodontal disease. In rats, antidepressives increase corticosteroid receptor expression in brain regions known to regulate the HPA axis (Holsboer & Barden, 1996). Chronic treatment with antidepressives markedly increased both the mineralocorticoid receptor and the glucocorticoid receptor transcription and binding sites in the hippocampus (Przegalinski & Budziszewska, 1993; Seckl & Fink, 1992; Vedder, Weiss, Holsboer, & Reul, 1993). This has been shown to lead to increased negative feedback control, decreased HPA activity, and subsequent reduced plasma glucocorticoid levels (Rowe et al., 1997).

Based on the effect of antidepressives on the HPA axis, we have just initiated experimental studies in our rat model in which antidepressants are given over a prolonged period of time, starting 4 weeks before application of the silk ligatures. A next logical step would be to examine if antidepressants can be used in the treatment of patients with severe forms of periodontal disease. Moreover, this could give us an indication of the importance of emotional stress for the development of periodontal disease and the importance of psychological treatment strategies aimed at reducing HPA axis hyperactivities.

Psychological treatment of negative sustained mood states, such as depression, may be important in preventing age-related neuropathology and subsequent HPA hyperactivity, leading to emotional as well as somatic pathology, such as periodontal disease. Psychotherapeutic intervention in children subjected to severe stress may be expected to prevent neurodevelopemental changes and thereby reduce the risk of developing psychopathology, and perhaps also other pathological conditions, including periodontal disease, later in life. As described elsewhere in this edition of *Psychoneuroimmunology*, the HPA system represents only one of several mechanisms by which the brain regulates immune activities, and thus modulates the outcome of chronic inflammatory conditions. Further research in this interdisciplinary field of "brain–neuroendocrine–immune–periodontology" may provide new insights in periodontal disease initiation and progression.

## References

Ader, R., Cohen, N., & Felten, D. (1995). Psychoneuroimmunology: Interactions between the nervous system and the immune system. *Lancet, 345*, 99–103.

Albandar, J. M., Buischi, Y. A., & Barbosa, M. F. (1991). Destructive forms of periodontal disease in adolescents. A 3-year longitudinal study. *Journal of Periodontology, 62,* 370–376.

Antoni, F. A. (1986). Hypothalamic control of adrenocorticotropin secretion: Advances since the discovery of 41-residue corticotropin-releasing factor. *Endocrine Reviews, 7,* 351–378.

Axtelius, B., Soderfeldt, B., Nilsson, A., Edwardsson, S., & Attstrom, R. (1998). Therapy-resistant periodontitis. Psychosocial characteristics. *Journal of Clinical Periodontology, 6,* 482–491.

Baelum, V., Chen, X., Manji, F., Luan, W. M., & Fejerskov, O. (1996). Profiles of destructive periodontal disease in different populations. *Journal of Periodontal Research, 31,* 17–26.

Baker, E. G., Crook, G. H., & Schwabacher, E. D. (1967). Personality correlates of periodontal disease. *Journal of Dental Research, 40,* 396–403.

Barnes, G. P., Bowles, W. F., & Carter, H. G. (1973). Acute necrotizing ulcerative gingivitis: a survey of 218 cases. *Journal of Periodontology, 44,* 35–42.

Bartold, P. M., Seymour, G. J., Cullinan, M. P., & Westerman, B. (1998). Effect of increased community and professional awareness of plaque control on the management of inflammatory periodontal diseases. *International Dental Journal, 48,* 282–289.

Beck, J. D., Koch, G. G., Zambon, J. J., Genco, R. J., & Tudor, G. E. (1992). Evaluation of oral bacteria as risk indicators for periodontitis in older adults. *Journal of Periodontology, 63,* 93–99.

Beck, J. D., Offenbacher, S., Williams, R., Gibbs, P., & Garcia, R. (1998). Periodontitis: A Risk Factor for Coronary Heart Disease? *Annals of Periodontology, 3,* 127–141.

Belting, C. M., & Gupta, O. P. (1961). The influence of psychiatric disturbances on the severity of periodontal disease. *Journal of Periodontology, 32,* 219–226.

Bertolini, D. R., Nedwin, G., Bringman, D., Smith, D., & Mundy, G. R. (1986). Stimulation of bone resorption and inhibition of bone formation in vitro by human tumour necrosis factors. *Nature, 319,* 516–519.

Besedovsky, H. O., del Rey, A., Klusman, I., Furukawa, H., Monge Arditi, G., & Kabiersch, A. (1991). Cytokines as modulators of the hypothalamus-pituitary-adrenal axis. *Journal of Steroid Biochemistry and Molecular Biology, 40,* 613–618.

Birkedal-Hansen, H. (1993). Role of matrix metalloproteinases in human periodontal diseases. *Journal of Periodontology, 64,* 474–484.

Blalock, J. E. (1994). The syntax of immune-neuroendocrine communication. *Immunology Today, 15,* 504–511.

Bodnoff, S. R., Humphreys, A., Lehman, J., Diamond, D. M., Rose, G. M., & Meany, M. J. (1995). Elevated glucocorticoid levels produce spatial memory deficits, dampened long-term potentiation, and enhanced hippocampal neuron loss in mid-aged rats. *Journal of Neuroscience, 15,* 61–69.

Bonneau, R. H., Sheridan, J. F., Feng, N., & Glaser, R. (1993). Stress-induced modulation of the primary cellular immune response to herpes simplex virus is mediated by both adrenal-dependent and adrenal-independent mechanisms. *Journal of Neuroimmunology, 42,* 167–176.

Breivik, T., Gjermo, P., Thrane, P. S., & Myhrer, T. (2000). *Hippocampal lesioning aggreyates experimental periodontitis in Wistar rats.* Submitted for publication.

Breivik, T., Nerland, A., Murison, R., & Jonsson, R. (1998). Influence of stress on immune cell recruitment in rat gingival tissues. *Journal of Dental Research, 77,* 859. [abstract]

Breivik, T., Opstad, P. K., Gjermo, P., & Thrane, P. S. (2000). Effects of hypothalamic-pituitary-adrenal axis reactivity on periodontal tissue destruction in rats. *European Journal of Oral Sciences, 108,* 115–122.

Breivik, T., Sluyter, F., Hof, M., & Cools, A. (2000). Differential susceptibility to periodontitis in genetically selected Wistar rats lines that differ in their behavioural and endocrinological responses to stress. *Behavior Genetics,* in press.

Breivik, T., Thrane, P. S., Gjermo, P., Stephan, M., Pabst, R., & von Hoersten, S. (1999). *Postnatal endotoxin exposure permanently alters emotional behaviour and periodontal disease susceptibility in Lewis rats.* Submitted for publication.

Breivik, T., Thrane, P. S., Murison, R., & Gjermo, P. (1996). Emotional stress effects on immunity, gingivitis and periodontitis. *European Journal of Oral Sciences, 104,* 327–334.

Brindley, D. N. & Rolland, Y. (1989). Possible connections between stress, diabetes, obesity, hypertension and altered lipoprotein metabolism that may result in atherosclorosis. *Clinical Science, 77,* 453–461.

Brown, D. H., Sheridan J. F., Pearl, D., & Zwillig, B. S. (1993). Regulation of mycobacterial growth by hypothalamo-pituitary-adrenal axis: Differential responses of mycobacterium bovis BCG-resistant and susceptible mice. *Infection and Immunity, 61,* 4793.

Buckingham, J. C., Loxley, H. D., Christian, H. C., & Philip, J. G. (1996). Activation of the HPA axis by immune insults: Roles and interactions of cytokines, eicosanoids and glucocorticoids. *Physiol, 54,* 285–298.

Bulkley, B. H., & Roberts, W. C. (1975). The heart in systemic lupus erythematosus and the changes induced in it by corticsteroid therapy. A study of 36 necropsy patients. *American Journal of Medicine, 58,* 243–264.

Burt, B. A. (1994). Periodontitis and aging: Reviewing recent evidence. *Jornal of American Dental Association, 125,* 273–279.

Buske-Kirschbaum, A., Jobst, S., Wustmans, A., Kirschbaum, C., Rauh, W., & Hellhammer, D. (1997). Attenuated free cortisol response to psychological stress in children with atopic dermatitis. *Psychosomatic Medicine, 59,* 419–426.

Cannon, W. B. (1929). The wisdom of the body. *Physiological Reviews, 9,* 399–431.

Caspi, R. R., Silver, P. B., Chan, C.-C., Sun, B., Agarwal, R. K., Wells, J., Oddo, S., Fujino, Y., Najafian, F., & Wilder, R. L. (1996). Genetic susceptibility to experimental autoimmune uveoretinitis in the rat is associated with an elevated Th1 response. *Journal of Immunology, 157,* 2668–2675.

Chapple, I. L. C. (1997). Reactive oxygen species and antioxidants in inflammatory diseases. *Journal of Clinical Periodontology, 24,* 287–296.

Charlton, B. G., & Ferrier, I. N. (1989). Hypothalamo-pituitary-adrenal axis abnormalities in depression: A review & a model. *Psychological Medicine, 19,* 331–336.

Cohen-Cole, S. A., Cogen, R. B., Stevens, A. Jr.. Kirk, K., Gaitan, E., Bird, J., Cooksey, R., & Freeman, A. (1983). Psychiatric, psychosocial and endocrine correlates of acute necrotizing ulcerative gingivitis (trench mouth): A preliminary report. *Psychiatric Medicine, 1,* 215–225.

Cools, A. R., & Gingras, M. A. (1998). Nijmegen high and low responders to novelty: A new tool in the search after the neurobiology of drug abuse liability. *Pharmacology Biochemistry and Behavior, 60,* 151–159.

Cronstein, B. N., Kimmel, S. C., Levin, R. L., Martiniuk, F., & Weissmann, G. A. (1992). Mechanism for the antiinflammatory effects of corticosteroids: The glucocorticoid receptor regulates leukocyte adhesion to endothelial cells and expression of endothelial-leukocyte adhesion molecule 1 and intercellular adhesion molecule 1. *Proceedings of the National Academy of Sciences, USA, 89,* 9991–9995.

Croucher, R., Marcenes, W. S., Torres, M. C. M. B., Hughes, F., & Sheiham, A. (1997). The relationship between life events and periodontitis. A case control study. *Journal of Clinical Periodontology, 24,* 39–43.

Dahlén, G., Manji, F., Baelum, V., & Fejerskov, O. (1989). Black-pigmented *Bacteroides* species and *Actinobacillus actinomycetemcomitans* in subgingival plaque of adult Kenyans. *Journal of Clinical Periodontology, 16,* 305–310.

Dallman, M. F., Akana, S. F., Bradbury, M. J., Strack, A. M, Simon-Hanson, E., & Scribner, K. A. (1994). Regulation of the hypothalamo-pituitary-adrenal axis during stress: Feedback, facilitation and feeding. *Seminars in Neurosciences, 6,* 205–213.

Dantzer, R. (1994). How do cytokines say hello to the brain? Neural versus humoral mediation. *European Cytokine Network, 5*(3), 271–273.

Davis, C. H., & Jenkins, D. (1962). Mental stress and oral disease. *Journal of Dental Research, 41,* 1045–1049.

Daynes, R. A., & Araneo, B. A. (1989). Contrasting effects of glucocorticoids on the capasity of T cells to produce the growth factors interleukin-2 & interleukin-4. *European Journal of Immunology, 19,* 2319–2325.

Daynes, R. A., Araneo, T. A., Dowell, T. A., Huang, K., & Dudley, D. (1990). Regulation of murine lymphokine production in vivo. III. The lymphoid tissue microenvironment exerts regulatory influences over T helper cell function. *Journal of Experimental Medicine, 171,* 979–996.

Dean, H. T., & Singleton, D. E. (1945). Vincent's infection: A wartime disease. *American Journal of Public Health, 35,* 433–439.

Deinzer, R., Ruttermann, S., Mobes, O., & Herforth, A. (1998). Increase in gingival inflammation under academic stress. *Journal of Clinical Periodontology, 5,* 431–433.

De Kloet, E. R. (1991). Brain corticosteriod receptor and homeostatic control. *Frontiers in Neuroendocrinology, 62,* 543–644.

De Marco, T. J. (1976). Periodontal emotional stress syndrome. *Journal of Periodontology, 47,* 67–68.

Dennison, D. K., Gottsegen, R., & Rose L. F. (1996). Diabetes and periodontal diseases. *Journal of Periodontology, 67,* 166–176.

Derjik, R., & Sternberg, E. M. (1994). Corticosteroid action and neuroendocrine–immune interactions. *Annals of New York Academic Sciences, 746,* 33.

Dobbs, C. M., Vasquez, R., Glaser, R., & Sheridan, J. F. (1993). Mechanisms of stress-induced modulation of viral pathogenesis and immunity. *Journal of Neuroimmunology, 48,* 151.

Dodt, C., Dittman, J., Hruby, J., Spth-Schwalbe, E., Born, J., Schüttler, R., & Fehm, H.L. (1991). Different regulation of adrenocorticotropin and cortisol secretion in young, mentally healthy elderly and patients with senile dementia of Alzheimer's type. *Journal of Clinical and Endocrinological Metabolisms, 72,* 272–276.

Dzink, J. L., Tanner, A. C. R., Haffajee, A. D., & Socransky, S. S. (1985). Gramnegative species associated with active destructive periodontal lesions. *Journal of Clinical Periodontolgy, 12,* 648–659.

Eguchi, K., Kawakami, A., Nakashima, M., Ida, H., Sakito, S., Matsuoka, N., Terada, K., Sakai, M., Kawabe, Y., Fukuda, T., Ishimaru, T., Kurouji, K., Fujita, N., Aoyagi, T., Maeda, K., & Nagataki, S. (1992). Interferon-alpha and dexamethasone inhibit adhesion of T cells to endothelial cells and synovial cells. *Clinical and Experimental Immunology, 88,* 448–454.

Feldman, S., Conforti, N., & Weidenfeld, J. (1995). Limbic pathways and hypothalamic neurotransmitters mediating adrenocortical responses to neural stimuli. *Neuroscience and Biobehavioral Reviews, 19,* 235–240.

Fendler, K., Karmos, G., & Telegdy, G. (1961). The effect of hippocampal lesion on pituitary-adrenal function. *Acta Physiologica (Budapest), 20,* 283–297.

Fischer, R. G., & Klinge, B. (1994). Clinical and histological evaluation of ligature-induced periodontal breakdown in domestic ferrets immunosuppressed by Cyclosporin A. *Journal of Clinical Periodontolgy, 21,* 240–249.

Freeman, R., & Gross, S. (1993). Stress measures as predictors of periodontal disease—A preliminary communication. *Community Dentristry and Oral Epidemiolgy, 21,* 176–177.

Friedman, M., Green, M. F., & Sharland, D. E. (1969). Assessment of hypothalamic-pituitary-adrenal function in the geriatric age group. *Journal of Gerontology, 24,* 292–297.

Furukawa, H., del Rey, A., Monge Arditi, G., & Besedovsky, H. O. (1998). Interleukin-1, but not stress, stimulates glucocorticoid output during early postnatal life in mice. *New York Academy of Science Annals Forts AV LYC, 840,* 117–122.

Genco, R. J., Ho, A. W., Kopman, J., Grossi, S. G., Dunford, R. G., & Tedesco, L. A. (1998). Models to evaluate the role of stress in periodontal disease. *Annals of Periodontology, 3,* 288–302.

Giddon, D. B., Goldhaber, P., & Dunning, J. M. (1963). Prevalence of reported cases of acute necrotizing ulcerative gingivitis in university population. *Journal of Periodontology, 34,* 66–70.

Giddon, D. B., Zackin, S. J., & Goldhaber, P. (1964). Acute necrotizing ulcerative gingivitis in college students. *Journal of American Dental Association, 68,* 381–386.

Gonzalez, Y. M., De Nardin, A., Grossi., S., Machtei, E. E., Genco, R. J., & De Nardin, E. (1996). Serum cotinine levels, smoking, and periodontal attachment loss. *Journal of Dental Research, 75,* 796–802.

Goodson, J. M. (1994). Antimicrobal strategies for treatment of periodontal disease. *Periodontology 2000, 5,* 142–168.

Gowen, M., Wood, D. D., Ihrie, E. J., McGuire M. K. B., & Russell, R. G. G. (1983). An interleukin-1 like factor stimulates bone resorption in vitro. *Nature, 306,* 378–380.

Green, L. W., Tryon, W. W., Marks, B., & Huryn J. (1986). Periodontal disease as a function of life events stress. *Journal of Human Stress, 12,* 32–36.

Greene, J. C. (1963). Oral hygiene and periodontal disease. *American Journal of Public Health, 53,* 913–922.

Gupta, O. P., Blechman, H., & Stahl, S. S. (1960). Effects of stress on the periodontal tissues of young adult male rats and hamsters. *Journal of Periodontology, 31,* 413–417.

Harbuz, M. S., & Lightman, S. L. (1992). Stress and the hypothalamic-pituitary-adrenal axis: acute, chronic and immunological activation. *Journal of Endocrinology , 134,* 327.

Hauger, R. L., Thrivikraman, K. V., & Plotsky, P. M. (1994). Age-related alterations of hypothalamic-pituitary-adrenal axis function in male Fischer 344 rats. *Endocrinology, 134,* 1528–1536.

Heinzel, F. P. (1995). Th1 and Th2 cells in the cure and pathogenesis of infectious diseases. *Current Opinion in Infectious Diseases, 8,* 151–155.

Herman, J. P., Schäfer, M. K. H., Young, E. A., Thompson, R., Douglass, J., Akil, H., & Watson, S. J. (1989). Evidence for hippocampal regulation of neuroendocrine neurons of the hypothalamo-pituitary-adrenocortical axis. *The Journal of Neuroscience, 9,* 3072–3082.

Heymann, D., Guicheux, J., Gouin, F., Passuti, N., & Daculsi, G. (1998). Cytokines, growth factors and osteoclasts. *Cytokine, 10,* 155–168.

Holsboer, F., & Barden, N. (1996). Antidepressants and hypthalamo-pituitary-adrenal regulation. *Endocrine Reviews, 17,* 187–205.

Holsboer, F., Spengler, D., & Heuser, I. (1992). The role of corticotropin-releasing hormone in the pathogenesis of Cushing's disease, anorexia nervosa, alcoholism, affective disorders and dementia. *Progress in Brain Research, 93,* 385–417.

Horning, G. M., & Cohen, M. E. (1995). Necrotizing ulcerative gingivitis, periodontitis, and stomatitis: Clinical staging and predisposing factors. *Journal of Periodontology, 66,* 990–998.

Horning, G. M., Hatch, C. L., & Lutskus, J. (1990). The prevalence of periodontitis in a military treatment population. *Journal of American Dental Association, 121,* 616–622.

Hugoson, A., & Jordan, T. (1982). Frequency distribution of individuals aged 20–70 years according to severity of periodontal disease. *Community Dentistry and Oral Epidemiology, 10,* 187–192.

Hukkanen, M., Hughes, F. J., Buttery, L. D. K., Gross, S. S., Evans, T. J., Seddon, S., Riveros-Moreno, V., Macintyre, I., & Polak, J. M. (1995). Cytokine-stimulated expression of inducible nitric oxide synthase by mouse, rat, and human osteoblast-like cells and its functional role in osteoblast metabolic activity. *Endocrinology, 136,* 5445–5453.

Issa, A. M., Rowe, W., Gauthier, S., & Meany, M. J. (1990). Hypothalamic-pituitary-adrenal activity in aged, cognitively impaired and cognitively-unimpaired rats. *Journal of Neuroscience, 10,* 3247–3254.

Jacobson, L., & Sapolsky, R. M. (1991). The role of the hippocampus in feedback regulation of the hypothalamo-pituitary adrenal axis. *Endocrine Reviews, 12,* 118–134.

Jilka, R. L., Hangoc, G., Girasole, G, Passeri, G, Williams, D. C., Abrams, J. S., Boyce, B., Broxmeyer, H., & Magolagas, S. C. (1992). Increased osteoclast developement after estrogen loss: mediation by interlukin-6. *Science 3,* 88–91.

Joëls, M., & De Kloet, E. R. (1994). Mineralocorticoid and glucocorticoid receptors in the brain. Implications for ion permeability and transmitters system. *Progress in Neurobiology, 43,* 1–36.

Kavelaars, A., Heijnen, C. J., Ellenbroek, B., van Loveren, H., & Cools, A. (1997). Apomorphine-susceptible and apomorphine-unsusceptible Wistar rats differ in their susceptibility to inflammatory and infectious diseases: A study on rats with group-specific differences in structure and reactivity of hypothalamic-pituitary-adrenal axis. *Journal of Neuroscience, 17 (7),* 2580–2584.

Koide, M., Suda, S., Saitoh, S., Ofuji, Y., Suzuki, T., Yoshie, H., Takai, M., Ono, Y., Taniguchi, Y., & Hara, K. (1995). In vivo administration of IL-1$\beta$ accelerates silk ligature-induced alveolar bone resorption in rats. *Journal of Oral Pathology and Medicine, 24,* 420–434.

Kornman, K. S., Holt, S. C., & Robertson, P. B. (1981). The microbiology of ligature-induced periodontitis in the cynomolgus monkey. *Journal of Periodontal Research, 16,* 363–371.

Kur, D. A. (1945). Gingival and periodontal disease. *Journal of American Dental Association, 32,* 31–33.

Landfield, P. W., & Pitler, T. A. (1984). Prolonged Ca2$^+$-dependent after-hyperpolarization in hippocampal neurons of the aged rat. *Science, 226,* 1089–1092.

Lee, W., Aitken, S., Sodek, J., & McCulloch C. (1995). Evidence of a direct relationship between neutrophil collagenase activity and periodontal tissue destruction in vivo: role of active enzyme in human periodontitis. *Journal of Periodontal Research, 30,* 23–33.

Levine, S., Weinberg, J., & Ursin, H. (1978). Definition of the coping process and statement of the problem. In S. Levine & H. Ursin (Eds.), *Psychobiology of stress* (pp. 3–21). Academic Press, New York.

Liblau, R. S., Singer S. M., & McDewitt, H. O. (1995). Th1 and Th2 CD4$^+$ T cells in the pathogenesis of organ-specific autoimmune diseases. *Immunology Today, 16,* 34–38.

Licinio, J., Wong, M. L., & Gold, P. W. (1996). The hypothalamic-pituitary-adrenal axis in anorexia nervosa. *Psychiatry Research, 62,* 75–83.

Lindhe, J. (1995). *Textbook of clinical periodontology* (2nd ed., 5th printing). Copenhagen: Munksgaard.

Liu, D., Diorio, J., Tannenbaum, B., Caldji, C., Francis, D., Freedman, A., Sharma, S., Pearson, D., Plotsky, P. M., & Meany, M. J. (1997). Maternal care, hippocampal glucocorticoid receptors, and hypothalamic-pituitary-adrenal responses to stress. *Science, 277,* 1659–1662.

Lundqvist, C., Baranov, V., Teglund, S., Hammarstrøm, S., & Hammarstrøm, M.-L. (1994). Cytokine profile and ultrastructure of intraepithelial T cells in chronically inflamed human gingiva suggest a cytotoxic effector function. *Journal of Immunology, 153,* 2302–2312.

Lupien, S., Lecours, A. R., Lussier, I., Scwartz, G., Nair, N. P. V., & Meany, M. J. (1994). Basal cortisol levels and cognitive deficits in human aging. *Journal of Neuroscience, 14,* 2893–2903.

Löe, H., Theilade, E., & Jensen S. B. (1965). Experimental gingivitis in man. *Journal of Periodontology, 36,* 177–187.

Magariños, A. M., & McEwen, B. S. (1995). Stress-induced atrophy of apical dendrites of hippocampal CA3c neurons: Involvement of glucocorticoid secretion and excitatory amino acid receptors. *Neuroscience, 69,* 89–98.

Martinez-Canut, P., Lorca, A., & Magan, R. (1996). Smoking and periodontal disease severity. *Journal of Clinical Periodontolgy, 22,* 743–749.

Mason, D. (1991). Genetic variation in the stress response: Susceptibility to experimental allergic encephalomyelitis and implications for human inflammatory diseases. *Immunology Today, 12,* 57–60.

Matta, S. G., Foster, C. A., & Sharp, B. M. (1993). Nicotine stimulates the expression of cFos protein in the parvocellular paraventricular nucleus and brainstem catecholaminergic regions. *Endocrinology, 132,* 2149–2156.

Mattila, K. J., Nieminen, M. S., Valtonen, V. V., Rasi, V. P., Kesaniemi, Y. A., Syrjala, S. L., Jungell, P. S., Isoluoma, M., Hietaniemi, K., & Jokinen, M. J. (1989). Association between dental health and acute myocardial infarction. *British Medical Journal, 298,* 779–781.

Michalowicz, B. (1994). Genetic and heritable risk factors in periodontal disease. *Journal of Periodontology, 65,* 479–488.

Miller, S. C., Thaller, J. L., & Soberman, A. (1956). The use of the Minnesota muliphasic personality inventory as a diagnostic aid in periodontal disease—A preliminary report. *Journal of Periodontology, 27,* 44–46.

Monteiro da Silva, A. M., Oakly, D. A., Newman, H. N., Nohl, F. S., & Lloyd, H. M. (1996). Psychosocial factors and adult onset rapidly progressive periodontitis. *Journal of Clinical Periodontology, 23,* 789–794.

Moss, M. E., Beck, J. D., Kaplan, B. H., Offenbacher, S., Weintraub, J. A., Koch, G. G., Genco, R. J., Machtei, E. E., & Tedesco, L. A. (1996). Exploratory case-control analysis of psychosocial factors and adult periodontitis. *Journal of Periodontology, 67,* 1060–1069.

Moulton, R., Ewen, S., & Theiman, W. (1952). Emotional factors in periodontal disease. *Oral Surgery, Oral Medicine, Oral Pathology, 5,* 833–860.

Moynihan, J. A., & Ader, R. (1996). Psychomeuroimmunology: animal models of disease. *Psychosomatic Medicine, 58,* 546–558.

Murayama, Y., Kurihara, H., Nagai, A., Dompkowski, D., & Van Dyke, T. E. (1994). Acute necrotizing ulcerative gingivitis: Risk factors involving host defense mechanisms. *Periodontology 2000, 6,* 116–124.

Murray, P. A. (1994). HIV disease as a risk factor for periodontal disease. *Compendium of Continuing Education in Dentistry, 15,* 1052–1064.

Navarra, P., Schettini, G., & Grossman, A. B. (1997). Responses of the stress axis to immunological challenge: The role of eicosanoids and cytokines. In J. C. Buckingham, G. E. Gillies,

& A.-M. Cowell (Eds.), *Stress, stress hormones and the immune system* New York: Wiley.

Nemeroff, C. B. (1998). The neurobiology of depression. *Scientific American*, 28–35.

Oitzl, M. S., van Haarst, A. D., & De Kloet E. R. (1995). Corticosterone, brain mineralocorticoid receptors (MRs) and the activity of the hypothalamus-pituitary-adrenal axis: The Lewis rat as an example of increased central MR capacity and a hyporesponsive HPA-axis. *Psychoneuroendocinology, 20*, 655–675.

Page, R. C. (1991). The role of inflammatory mediators in the pathogenesis of periodontal disease. *Journal of Periodontal Research, 26*, 230–242.

Page, R. C. (1995). Critical issues in periodontal research. *Journal of Dental Research, 74*, 1118–1128.

Page, R. C. (1998). The pathology of periodontal diseases may affect systemic diseases: Inversion of a paradigm. *Annals of Periodontology, 3*, 108–120.

Page, R. C., Offenbacher, S., Schroeder H. E., Seymour, G. J., & Kornman, K. S. (1997). Advances in the pathogenesis of periodontitis: Summary of developments, clinical implications and future directions. *Periodontology 2000, 14*, 216–248.

Panerai, A. E., Sacerdote, P., Bianchi, M., & Manfredi, B. (1997). Intermittent but not continuos inescapable footshock stress and intracerebroventricular interleukin-1 similarly affect immune responses and immunocyte beta-endorphin concentrations in the rat. *International Journal of Clinical Pharmacology Research, 17*, 115–116.

Pindborg, J. J. (1951). Gingivitis in military personnel with special referance to ulceromembranous gingivitis. *Odontologisk Tidsskrift, 59*, 407–493.

Pindborg, J. J., Bhat, M., & Roed-Petersen, B. (1967). Oral changes in South Indian children with severe protein deficiency. *Journal of Periodontology, 38*, 218–221.

Pindborg, J. J., & Holmstrup, P. (1987). Necrotizing gingivitis related to human immunodeficiency virus (HIV) infection. *African Dental Journal, 1*, 5–8.

Plotsky, P. M. (1988). Hypophysiotropic regulation of stress-induced ACTH secretion. In G. P. Chrousos, D. L. Loriaux, & P. W. Gold, (Eds.), *Mechanisms of physical and emotional stress* (pp. 65–81). New York: Plenum.

Plotsky, P. M., Cunningham, E. T., & Widmaier, E. P. (1989). Catecholaminergic modulation of corticotropin-releasing factor and adrenocorticotropin secretion. *Endocrine Reviews, 10*, 437–458.

Plotsky, P. M., & Meany, M. J. (1993). Early, postnatal experiences alters hypothalamic corticotropin-releasing factor (CRF) mRNA, median eminence CRF content and stress-induced release in adult rats. *Molecular Brain Research, 18*, 195–200.

Plotsky, P. M., Otto, S., & Sutton, S. (1987). Neurotransmitter modulation of corticotropin releasing factor secretion into the hypophysial-portal circulation. *Life Sciences, 41*, 1311–1317.

Polson, A. M., Zappa, U. E., Espeland, M. A., & Eisenberg, A. D. (1986). Effect of metronidazole on development of subgingival plaque and experimental periodontitis. *Journal of Periodontology, 57*, 218–224.

Powie, F., & Coffman, R. L. (1993). Cytokine regulation of T cell function: potential for therapeutic intervention. *Immunology Today, 14*, 270–274.

Przegalinski, E., & Budziszewska, B. (1993). The effect of long-term treatment with antidepressant drugs on the hippocampal mineralocorticoid and glucocorticoid receptors in rats. *Neuroscience Letters, 161*, 215–218.

Raadsheer, F. C., van Heerikhuize, J. J., Lucassen, P. J., Hoogendijk, W. J. G., Tilders, F. J. H., & Swaab, D. F. (1995). Corticotropin-releasing hormone mRNA levels in the paraventricular nucleus of patients with Alzheimer's disease and depression. *American Journal of Psychiatry, 152* (9), 1372–1376.

Reilly, P. A., Chosh, J. A., Maddison, P.J., Rasker, J.J., & Silman, A. J. (1990). Mortality and survival in rheumatoid arthritis: A 25 year prospective study of 100 patients. *Annals of Rheumatic Diseases, 49*, 363–369.

Reul, J. M., Stec, I., Wiegers, G. J., Labeur, M. S., Linthorst, A. C., Arzt, E., & Holsboer, F. (1994). Prenatal immune challenge alters the hypothalamic-pituitary-adrenocortical axis in adult rats. *Journal of Clinical Investigation, 93*, 2600–2607.

Rook, G. A. W., & Hernandez-Pando, R. (1997). Pathogenetic role, in human and murine tuberculosis, of changes in the peripheral metabolism of glucocorticoids and antiglucocorticoids. *Psychoendocrinology, 22*, 109–113.

Rots, N. Y., de Jong, J., Levine, S., Cools, A. R., & de Kloet, E. R. (1996). Neonatal mother-deprived rats have as adult elevated basal pituitary-adrenal activity and apomorphine susceptibility. *Journal of Neuroendocrinology, 8*, 501–506.

Rowe, W., Steverman, A., Walker, M., Sharma, S., Barden, N., Seckl, J. R., & Meany, M. J. (1997). Antidepressants restore hypothalamic-pituitary-adrenal feedback function in aged, cognitively-impaired rats. *Neurobiology of Aging, 18*, 5, 527–533.

Sallay, K., Sanavi, F., Ring, I., Pham, P., Behling, U. H., & Nowotny, A. (1982). Alveolar bone destruction in the immunosuppressed rat. *Journal of Periodontal Research, 17*, 263–274.

Sapolsky, R, Rivier, C, Yamamoto, G., Plotsky, P., & Vale, W. (1987). Interleukin-1 stimulates the secretion of hypothalamic corticotropin-releasing factor. *Science, 238*, 522–524.

Sawchenko, P. E. (1987). Adrenalectomy-induced enhancement of CRF and vasopressin immunoreactivity in parvocellular neurosecretory neurons: Anatomic, peptide, and steroid specificity. *Journal of Neuroscience, 7*, 1093–1106

Schauenstein, K., Rinner, I., Felsner, P., Liebmann, P., Haas, H. S., Hofer, D., Wölfler, A., & Korsatko, W. (1997). The role of the autonomous nervous system in the dialogue between the brain and the immune system. In *Current update in psychoimmunology* (pp. 13–21). Springer Verlag/Wien.

Schwartz, M. W., Strack, A. M., & Dallman, M. F. (1997). Evidence that elevated plasma coricosterone levels are caused of reduced hypothalamic corticotrophin-releasing hormone gene expression in diabetes. *Regulatory Peptides, 72*, 105–112.

Scott, P., & Kaufmann, H. E. (1991). The role of T-cell subsets and cytokines in the regulation of infection. *Immunology Today, 12*, 346–348.

Seckl, J. R., & Fink, G. (1992). Antidepressants increase glucocorticoid and mineralocorticoid receptor mRNA expression in rat hippocampus in vivo. *Neuroendocrinology, 55*, 621–626.

Selye, H. (1955). Stress and disease. *Science, 122*, 626–631.

Seymour, G. J., Gemmell, E., Kjeldsen, M., Yamazaki, K., Nakajima, T., & Hara, K. (1996). Cellular immunity and hypersensivity as components of periodontal destruction. *Oral Diseases, 2*, 96–101.

Shah, S. V., Baricos, W. H., & Basci, A. (1987). Degradation of human glomerular basement membrane by stimulated neutrophils. Activation of a metalloproteinase(s) by reactive oxygen metabolites. *Journal of Clinical Investigation, 79*, 25–31.

Shanks, N., Larocque, S., & Meany, M. (1995). Neonatal endotoxin exposure alters the development of the hypothalamic-pituitary-adrenal axis: Early illness and later responsivity to stress. *The Journal of Neuroscience, 15*, 376–384.

Shapira, L., Borinski, R., Sela, M. N., & Soskolne, A. (1991). Superoxide formation and chemiluminescence of peripheral polymorphonuclear leukocytes in rapidly progressive periodontitis patients. *Journal of Clinical Periodontology, 18*, 44–48.

Sharma, M., Palacios-Bois, J., Schwartz, G., Quirion, R., & Nair, N. P. V. (1989). Circadian rhythms of malatonin and cortisol in aging. *Biological Psychiatry, 25,* 305–319.

Shklar, G. (1966). Periodontal disease in experimental animals subjected to chronic cold stress. *Journal of Periodontology, 37,* 377–383.

Shklar, G., & Glickman, I. (1953). The periodontium and salivary gland in the alarm reaction. *Journal of Dental Research, 32,* 773.

Skaleric, U., & Gaspersic, R. (1998). Restraint stress modulates the experimental periodontitis in rats. *Journal of Dental Research, 77,* 1031. [abstract].

Skrede, K. K., Røshol, H., Ærø, C. E., & Wiik, P. (1996). Peritoneal leukocytes from spontaneously hypertensive rats have reduced chemiluminescence response and lowered sensivity to dexamethasone in vivo. *Acta Physiologica Scand, 158,* 169–179.

Socransky, S. S., & Haffajee, A. D. (1992). The bacterial etiology of destructive periodontal disease. *Journal of Periodontology, 63,* 322–331.

Sternberg, E. M., Chrousos, G. P., Wilder, R. L., & Gold, P. W. (1992). The stress response and the regulation of inflammatory disease. *Annals of International Medicine, 117,* 854–866.

Strack, A. M., Sebastian, R. J., Schwartz, M. W., & Dallman, M. F. (1995). Glucocorticoids and insulin: Reciprocal signals for energy balance. *American Journal of Physiology, 268,* 142–149.

Sutanto, W., Rosenfeld, P., De Kloet, E. R., & Levine, S. (1996). Long-term effects of neonatal maternal deprivation and ACTH on hippocampal mineralocorticoid and glucocorticoid receptors. *Developmental Brain Research, 92,* 156–163.

Svanberg, G., Lindhe, J., Hugoson, A., & Gröndahl, H. G. (1973). Effect of nutritional hyperparathyroidism on experimental periodontitis in the dog. *Scandinavian Journal of Dental Research, 81,* 155.

Tannenbaum, B. M., Brindley, D. N., Tannenbaum, G. S., Dallman, M. F., McArthur, M. D., & Meany, M. J. (1997). High-fat feeding alters both basal and stress-induced hypothalamic-pituitary-adrenal activity in the rat. *American Journal of Physiology, 273,* E1168–E1177.

Thorstensson, H., & Hugoson, A. (1993). Periodontal disease experience in adult long-duration insulin-dependent diabetics. *Journal of Clinical Periodontology, 20,* 352–358.

Tilders, F. J. H., De Rijk, R. H., Van Dam, A. M., Vincent, V. A. M., Schotanus, K., & Persoons, J. H. A. (1994). Activation of the hypothalamus-pituitary-adrenal axis by bacterial endotoxins: Routes and intermediate signals. *Psychoneuroendocrinology, 19,* 209–232.

Tokoro, Y., Matsuki, Y., Yamamoto, T., Suzuki, T., & Hara, K. (1997). Relevance of local Th2-type cytokine mRNA expression in immunocompetent infiltrates in inflamed gingival tissue to periodontal diseases. *Clinical and Experimental Immunology, 107,* 166–174.

Troxler, R. G., Sprague, R. A., Albanese, R. A., Fuchs, R., & Thompson, A, J. (1977). The association of elevated plasma cortisol and early atherosclerosis as demonstrated by coronary angiography. *Atherosclerosis, 26,* 151–162.

Vaccarino, A. L., & Couret, L. C., Jr. (1995). Relationship between hypothalamic-pituitary-adrenal activity and blockade of tolerance to morphine analgesia by pain: a strain comparison. *Pain, 63,* 385–389.

Vedder, H., Weiss, I., Holsboer, F., & Reul, J. M. H. M. (1993). Glucocorticoid and mineralocorticoid receptors in rat neocortical and hippocampal brain cells in culture: Characterization and regulatory studies. *Brain Research, 605,* 18–24.

Vieira, P. L., Kalinski, P., Wierenga, E. A., Kapsenberg, M. L., & de Jong, E. (1998). Glucocorticoids inhibit bioactive IL-12p70 production by in vitro-generated human dendritic cells without Affecting their T cell stimulatory potential. *Journal of Immunology, 161,* 5245–5251.

Visser, J., van Boxel-Dezaire, A., Methorst, D., Brunt, T., de Kloet, E., & Nagelkerken, L. (1998). Differential regulation of interleukin-10 (IL-10) and IL-12 by glucocorticoids in vitro. *Blood, 91,* 4255–4264.

Wang, P. S., Lo, M.-J., & Kau, M.-M. (1997). Glucocorticoids and aging. *Journal of the Formosan Medical Association, 96,* (10).

Weidenfeld, J., & Yirmiya, R. (1996). Effects of bacterial endotoxin on the glucocorticoid feedback regulation of adrenocortical response to stress. *Neuroimmunomodulation, 3,* 352–357.

Whitnall, M. H. (1993). Regulation of the hypothalamic corticotropin-releasing hormone neurosecretory system. *Progress in Neurobiology,* 573–629.

Wiik, P., Skrede, K. K., Knardahl, S., Haugen, A.-H., Ærø, C. E., Opstad, P. K., & Bøyum, A. (1995). Effect of in vivo corticosterone and acute food deprivation on rat resident peritoneal cell chemiluminescence after activation ex vivo. *Acta Physiologica Scandinavia, 154,* 407–416.

Williams, N. (1998). T cells on the mucosal frontline. *Science, 280,* 198–200.

Yau, J. L., Dow, R. C., Fink, G., & Seckl, J. R. (1992). Medial septal cholinergic lesions increase hippocampal and glucocorticoid receptor messenger RNA expression. *Brain Research, 577,* 155–160.

Zappa, U. E., & Polson, A. M. (1988). Factors associated with occurence and reversibility of connective tissue attachment loss. *Journal of Periodontology, 59,* 100–106.

# 64

# Clinical, Experimental, and Translational Psychoneuroimmunology Research Models in Oral Biology and Medicine

FRANCESCO CHIAPPELLI, ABDUL ABANOMY, DEBORAH HODGSON,
KENNETH A. MAZEY, DIANA V. MESSADI, RONALD S. MITO,
ICHIRO NISHIMURA, IGOR SPIGELMAN

## I. INTRODUCTION

Certain structures within the oral cavity may play a critical role in the neuroendocrine–immune network (Sabbadini & Berczi, 1995). The extent to which psychoneuroimmunology may be significant within the context of oral biology and medicine remains to be established. This chapter addresses this question.

Research in oral biology and medicine aims at improving the dental patients' well-being. As such, it covers a wide spectrum of endeavors, from the behavioral to the molecular sciences. Pathologies of the soft and hard tissues within the oral cavity, events associated with the healing process, dysfunctions of stomatological structures such as the temporomandibular joint, and associated perceptions of anxiety, stress, discomfort, and pain, as observed in patients with fibromyalgia, can be associated with psychological and biological complications detrimental to the patient's overall health and quality of life. Consequential impact upon family and societal structures result. Dentists are increasingly aware of the need and importance of socio-psycho-biological assessment and intervention programs in oral biology and medicine. Three domains of health, the physical, the psychological, and the social, play an important role in tailoring restorative and preventive dental plans to the needs of individual patients (Freeman, 1997). The psychoneuroimmune perspective on oral biology and medicine is timely and important.

Psychoneuroimmunology investigates the relationship between the psychophysiological and the immunophysiological dimensions of the patient. From a philosophical standpoint, psychoneuroimmunology represents the reunification of Descartes' *res extensa* (bodily functions) and *res cogitans* (the measurable functions of the "soul"—in today's terminology, the psyche). The delicate balance between health and disease systemically, as well as locally in the oral cavity, is threatened extrinsically by environmental factors that include external pathogens and toxic substances. Ongoing processes of development and aging modulate this balance. Immune surveillance is brought about by events that are intimately intertwined and communicate via cytokines, growth factors, complement factors and complement receptors, and cell populations. Structures of the lymphatic system receive direct sympathetic and parasympathetic innervation, and cells of the immune system carry specific and functional membrane receptors for substance P, $\beta$-endorphin, and other neuropeptides commonly found at sites of inflammation and pain. Most, if not all neuropeptides identified to date are endowed with immunomodulatory properties. Immune cells are also endowed with hormone receptors, which direct the immune cells' response to steroid and nonsteroid hormones. In that fashion, immune cells respond to neurobiological stimuli elicited by the brain via direct innervation and indirectly by means of the neuroendocrine system (Chiappelli & Liu, 1999).

The brain, as it processes cognitions, memories, and emotions, generates neurobiological signals that are recognized as significant modulatory commands of immune responses peripherally as well as centrally. Invasion of pathogens and inflammatory reactions peripherally or centrally trigger the production of cytokines, which communicate to the brain either directly or indirectly via the production of cytokines by astrocytes and other cell populations within the central nervous system. Neurobiological responses ensue that modulate the immune response to the pathogens or the inflammation process. Neurobiological responses also modulate cognitions, emotions and memories, as well as other centrally mediated responses, such as feeding behavior, temperature regulation, and the like. These interactions impact upon the maintenance of health and healing processes of soft stomatological structures, as we discuss in this chapter.

## II. DENTAL PATIENTS SUFFER FROM PSYCHONEUROIMMUNOLOGICALLY RELEVANT ANXIETY

### A. Anxiety in the Dental Patient

Prehistoric archeological specimens show evidence of surgical tooth extraction, which may have been practiced as a result of trauma, abscesses, advanced caries, periodontal disease, and as a means to relieve pain. Contemporary phobic patients often elect tooth extraction to relieve chronic pain, but also to avoid anxiety caused by restorative dental procedures. Pain associated with the oral cavity provokes considerable fear and anxiety today, even with the effective anesthetic pretreatments available.

Dental patients often suffer pervasive and prolonged anxiety that may contribute to the onset and the exacerbation of systemic and oral pathologies. Ten percent of a sample of 1548 men and women from Iceland (ages 25–74) stated that their dental anxiety was "considerable," whereas 5% indicated "extensive" fear. Data showed that age and gender are significant predictors of dental anxiety, as women and younger subjects are more likely to express dental anxiety. Also, the finding that male and female patients are more prone to express anxiety if they have fewer fillings suggested an inverse relationship between the frequency of dental visits and dental anxiety. Dental anxiety was significantly more common in rural rather than urban populations and in subjects with less education (Ragnarsson, 1998).

A similar study conducted in Detroit confirmed the prevalence of dental anxiety to be about 10% of dental patients. In addition to negative attitudes toward dentists, predictors of dental anxiety included infrequent checkups and small numbers of filled surfaces. Female gender and lower income were confirmed as strong predictors of dental anxiety (Doerr, Lang, Nyquist, & Ronis, 1998).

Populations with special health care needs, such as the handicapped, display increased dental anxiety. One study of physically and mentally challenged patients revealed they are at increased risk for oral and systemic pathologies. Their condition may be a perceived and/or a real barrier to obtaining oral health care. Almost 28% reported significant anxiety about the prospect of a dental visit. Approximately half of that subgroup reported excessive fear and anxiety, extreme nervousness, or terror. This study further confirmed the inverse relationship between frequency of dental visits and excessive dental anxiety (Gordon, Dionne, & Snyder, 1998).

High anxiety dental populations may share a sense of vulnerability and helplessness, based on perceived inabilities to predict, control, or obtain desired results in upcoming dental situations. Individuals who do not rank high in the hierarchy of social dominance (Chiappelli, Franceschi, Ottaviani, Farné, & Faisal, 1993) may succumb to the submissive role once they enter the dental operatory. It is possible and even probable that these individuals may develop anxiety that would make them particularly vulnerable to perceptions of unpredictability and uncontrollability and that would trigger anxious behavior during the dental visit.

A key question is whether or not dental anxiety in these populationsis is maintained significantly over the life span. In that case, dental phobia may be consistent with epidemiological research, indicating that phobias tend to run a prolonged course (Agras, Chapin, & Oliveau, 1972). It remains to be determined if dental phobic patients continue to drain energies obsessing about dental visists, or if dental anxiety eventually dissipates away from the dental office. It is not clear whether or not the dental phobic patient is oblivious to the dental anxiety syndrome when it is not activated by the threat of dental treatment. The proportion of dental phobic patients who chronically maintain hypervigilance in anticipation of dental treatment also remains to be studied. If dental phobias are similar to other types of anxiety disorders, which tend to be chronic, then issues of self-esteem, periods of marked disability, and other factors of personality dysfunction affecting well-being are implicated and merit closer study.

## B. Dental Stressors and Clinical Training

Stressors in dentistry are characterized by unique factors not routinely encountered in other medical specialties. The oral cavity is imbued with symbolic meaning. Dental patients often experience dental procedures as intrusive and threatening of their personal space and psychosocial boundaries. Claus-trophobic dental patients are understandable when one considers the number of dental instruments that go into the small cavity of the mouth: high volume evacuator, saliva ejector, mirror, drill, rubber dam, cotton rolls, gauze, and fingers. That more people are not phobic of dentistry and do not complain of difficulty breathing or fear of suffocating is testimony to the resilience of patients in general and to the competence of dentists. Yet, more dental patients probably experience distress, repress their feelings, and endure the procedures than is commonly recognized. In the United States, estimates suggest that millions of people suffer dental anxiety and that most remain untreated.

Accurate assessment of the specificity of fears and degree of anxiety is pivotal in providing optimal dental care and treatment. Tailoring treatment to the particular psychological profile of the dental patient requires understanding of the psychodynamic and behavioral symptomatology of anxiety disorders in general and dental phobias in particular. In most instances, this knowledge is not imparted to dentists in training. Whereas dental schools generally neglect to teach the psychosocial aspects of patient care, school administrators, faculty, and practitioners alike acknowledge the importance of the dentist–patient relationship. Yet, success of dental treatment more often depends upon how well the practitioner and his staff respond to the nonverbal emotions of the dental patient, including facial and behavioral expressions, and less often upon the technical competence of the dentist.

Not only the well-being of patients, but that of dental practitioners, who are not immune to stressors, is at stake. Among health care professionals, dentists display prominent symptoms of stress (Hilliard-Lysen & Riemer, 1988; Litchfield, 1989; Mazey, 1994). Stress-related medical problems, including coronary heart disease, respiratory diseases, and substance abuse are reported to be unusually high among dentists. Research shows that dentists perceive the fearful patient as a major barrier to successful treatment and that they become more anxious while working with fearful patients (O'Shea & Corah, 1984). Enhancing the psychological training of dentists and encouraging multidisciplinary collaboration with psychologists will be important steps in ameliorating the stressful environment of dental practice (Mazey & Mito, 1993).

## C. Dental Anxiety and Specific Dental Fears

Dental stress and anxiety function as multireferential theoretical constructs bridging the gap of psyche and soma. The well-trained practitioner must be prepared to cope with systemic disturbances and identify signs and symptoms across their various modalities—namely, the physical (sweaty palms, tachycardia, nausea), the cognitive ("I can't handle this; I have to flee."), affective ("I'm afraid it's going to hurt."), and the behavioral (squirming, white-knuckling, crying).

The ability of the practitioner to diagnose high anxiety and to identify triggering factors prior to initiating dental procedures is fundamental. In clinical practice, this means that the dentist should not worry about hiding the syringe from a patient who is afraid of the sound of the drill. Similarly, a patient reclining in the dental chair who says that he is doing fine, but who displays beads of sweat on his forehead, is either denying his fear out of embarrassment or is unaware of his distress. Because excessive fear is often irrational, it is not necessarily correlated with the invasiveness or extent of the dental procedure. In the life span of a dental phobic, prolonged anticipatory anxiety is the physiological and emotional basis of phobic avoidance. The power of the phobic patient's imagination is unequaled in producing real physiological responses (tension, tachycardia, sweaty palms, blurry vision, foggy mind). Clinical training in the management of dental medical emergencies should routinely include psychological and behavioral interventions for ameliorating excessive anxiety and panic in dental patients.

### D. Idiosyncratic Dental Stressors and Anticipatory Anxiety and Fear of Pain

Dental stressors are idiosyncratic and personal to each dental patient. While one patient may fear taking X-rays because of a hyperactive gag reflex or because of anxiety about vomiting, another patient may resist reclining in the dental chair because of feelings of helplessness associated with a prior history of childhood abuse. The majority of highly anxious patients fear the pain of an injection or the pain of drilling because of previous negative experiences with those particular procedures. Patients may project their fears and anxieties onto needles and onto the sounds of drilling since they are easily identifiable as potentially harmful. For the phobic patient, the needle and drill may function as symbols for an array of fears about dentistry, which generally remain undifferentiated without further psychological probing. Detailed psychological assessment may be necessay to bring into focus the fine features of the dental fear schema of which the patient himself is unconscious. This is a critical assessment prior to initiating any psychotherapeutic intervention to assure consideration of the specific problems that make up the phobic syndrome (Table I).

**TABLE I**  Fear Differential[a]

| | |
|---|---|
| Calling for an appointment | Arriving for an appointment |
| Waiting in reception room | Sitting in dental chair |
| Seeing the dentist | Having teeth X-rayed |
| Seeing dental instruments | Smell of dental office |
| Having cleaning done | Anticipating and feeling pain |
| Seeing the needle | Anticipating injection |
| Sound of the drill | Having teeth drilled |
| Having a root canal | |
| Having an extraction | |

[a] Adapted from K. A. Mazey, and R. S. Mito (1993). Multidisciplinary treatment of dental phobia. *CDA Journal, 21,* 17–25.

With proper training in dental schools and with multidisciplinary collaboration with psychologists, dentists should develop appropriate predental treatment anxiety reduction protocols that differentiate fears. New and improved models of interventions should be directed to ameliorate dysfunctional behavior based on exaggerated gag reflex, needle phobia, inability to tolerate X-rays, or a host.

Fear of pain often stems from prior patient experience of failed anesthetics and of inability to attain numbness prior to dental treatment. This complication is sometimes caused by combinations of overwhelming patient anxiety and of acute infections in which the low pH of bacterial infection neutralizes the high pH of local anesthetics, rendering them relatively ineffective. In these instances, the patient may report pain even after the dentist has properly administered several injections of anesthesia. When dentists fail to grasp how anesthesia can be compromised by acute infections, they exacerbate the stress that the patient already is experiencing due to anticipatory anxiety and fear of pain. The well-trained clinician, on the other hand, will expect behavioral disruptions (facial tension, squirming, disturbed physiological arousal) and will look for cognitive–affective changes as well (hypervigilance, narrowing and shifting of attention, labile emotions).

Phobic patients over the years have criticized dentists for their lack of empathy. In particular, dentists have been assailed for making disparaging comments about fearful patients, accusing them of immaturity and childish behavior when they were frightened and uncooperative with simple dental procedures. The emotional core of the phobic experience is regressive and parallels the cognitive–affective schema of a child. Helplessness, exaggerated emotional response, loss of volitional control, and loss of cognitive coping skills are characteristics of an earlier developmental stage. Rather than judge these regressive features of the phobic's behavior, the dentist should anticipate that a frightened patient may present in a child-like manner and should use appropriate cognitive–behavioral interventions, including techniques used in pediatric dentistry (show-tell-do), to restore calm to the anxious patient. Hand-over-mouth techniques for managing crying or out-of-control children in pediatric dentistry should be abandoned because they worsen the young dental patient's experience of vulnerability, stress, and anxiety. Iatrogenic factors that cause or exacerbate the dental patient's stress have been largely neglected in the stress research. Given more attention, research into the complex interactions of the fearful patient and the dental practitioner will serve to improve the quality of services and enhance the therapeutic goals of oral medicine.

## E. The Psychobiology of Stress and Anxiety: Fish as an Animal Model

Psychological strain and anxiety, as in dental anxiety, often arises as the real or perceived lack of fit of the person within the extrinsic ( = outer world of the individual) or intrinsic environment ( = inner world of the individual) (Chiappelli, 1985; Chiappelli, Kung, Stefanini, & Foschi, 1998; Conway, Vickers, & French, 1992). The perception of lack of fit derives from the set of perceived and actual social roles that individuals carry in every day life, which represent an intertwined set of perceived or actual rights and responsibilities that signify the individuals' personality, social involvement, cultural background, legal status, and hierarchical position.

Individuals with different resilience to psychological stress, strain, and anxiety have different inner motivational strengths to overcome the lack of fit they may perceive or they may actually experience. Motivations rest on certain fundamental attributions that the individuals make in relation to the person–environment fit, and which include such questions as where does the cause of the lack of fit originate ("locus"), how stable or unstable is the situation that brings about the lack of fit ("stability"), is the lack of fit particular to the situation or generalizable to all situations ("globality"), and how much control is there over the situation ("controllability") (Weiner, 1985).

Attributions and perceived responsibility come to form the essential elements of an array of models of psychological helping and coping (Brickman, 1982), whose relevance to overly anxious dental patients remains to be tested. Knowledge and appraisal of given situations, either consciously or subconsciously, cognitively or instinctively, are additional critical elements of perceptions of fit, and of consequential emotions (Lazarus, 1991), psychological well-being, and the behavioral manifestations thereof.

Appraisal of fit can be subconscious and instinctive and may represent an ancestral *modus adaptandi* in the animal kingdom. Lack of fit of animals within their environment, and experimental manipulations that tend to induce the animals' lack of fit within their environment, engender the physiological "stress response" described by Cannon (1929) and by Selye (1976). Stress hormones (e.g., glucocorticoids) and peptides (e.g., opioids) have a wide range of immunomodulatory effects. From invertebrates to fish to humans, the neuroendocrine system responds to perceived or actual threats, stress, or pain with hormones and peptides of considerable immunomodulatory potency. Factors produced by activated immune cells, in turn, significantly modulate psychoneuroendocrine responses (for review, Ader, Felten, & Cohen, 1991; Besedovsky & del Rey, 1996; Blalock, 1994; Chiappelli et al., 1993; Chiappelli, Franceschi, Ottaviani, Solomon, & Taylor, 1996a; Chiappelli & Trignani, 1993; Heijnen, Kavelaars, & Ballieux, 1991; Solomon & Amkraut, 1981).

Anxiety and stress are associated with a variety of medical interventions, which can be taken as models for orosurgical and oromedical interventions. Surgical stress leads to a significant activation of the endocrine system (e.g., increased serum and saliva cortisol), which appears to be proportional to the severity of surgical stress. This observation applies to the differential degrees of stress and anxiety that patients experience from minor oral surgical procedures, to implantological procedures that are often protracted for months at the time, to mandibular reconstruction following serious trauma. The psychobiological repercussion upon the healing process is outlined below.

Whereas the assessment of cortisol in saliva was criticized in the past, it is now widely accepted. Salivary cortisol was rejected because of concerns that it may fail to reflect endogenous circadian patterns, that it may not provide an adequate index of 24-h cortisol, and that it may not manifest appropriate responses to hypothalamo-pituitary-adrenal tests. Further, it was argued that salivary collections may be contaminated with plasma from ulcers in the oral mucosa and gingival inflammation. Significant methodological developments have contributed to establish salivary levels of cortisol as a valid and reliable reflection of the unbound serum levels (Aardal-Eriksson, Karlberg, & Holm, 1998).

Taking together the context of the person–environment fit model of stress and anxiety and the psychosocial observations noted in the preceding section, it is evident that the dentist-patient dyad can induce a conscious or subconscious perception of submissiveness in many if not most dental patients. Research models can better characterize psychoneuroendocrine–immune effects of the perception of submissiveness in dental patients.

Significant immunophysiological alterations, that involve hypothalamus, pituitary, and interrenal hormones as well as the sympathetic nervous system, accompany the establishment of social hierarchy and social dominance/submissiveness in aggressive fish as in all vertebrates. The mechanism by which stressful situations affect the immune system of fish may serve as a good model for human studies since fish possess leukocytes that are akin in their function and to lesser degree in morphology to their mammalian counterparts, and since the molecular basis of the fish immune response specificity resembles that of mammals (Chiappelli et al., 1993).

During interaction between two aggressive fish (e.g., rainbow trout, European Eels, tilapia) for a period of up to 5 h, a characteristic investigative behavior ensues that leads to vigorous combat (including tail beating, ramming, chasing, mouth fighting, and biting). The frequency of mouth bites can be up to 12.33/min. The combat leads to the establishment of a dominant ($\alpha$) fish and a subordinate (submissive) ($\beta$) fish. $\beta$ Fish typically surrender and manifest a variety of physiological changes, among which profound neuroendocrine alteration (e.g., significant rise in circulating ACTH, cortisol), overall collapse of cellular immune functions (i.e., blunted natural cytotoxicity, proliferative response to T-cell mitogens), and premature death. The immunophysiological collapse observed in $\beta$ fish can be prevented in large part by naltrexone (1 mg/kg, im) 1 h prior to encounter, thus establishing the immunosuppressive role of the endogenous opioid system. $\beta$ Rainbow trout become infected with a moderately virulent strain of the Gram-negative bacterium *Aeromonas hydrophila*, the cause of motile Aeromonas septicemia in fish, via water or intramuscular injection significantly more readily than the dominant cohort (Chiappelli et al., 1993; Chiappelli & Liu, 1999) (Figure 1).

In conclusion, aquatic animals, which exhibit physiological responses similar to those of other vertebrates, may provide reliable and simple animal models of psychoneuroimmunology in the domain of oral biology and dentistry (Chiappelli & Liu, 1999).

## III. DENTAL MATERIALS MAY EXHIBIT PSYCHONEUROIMMUNOTOXIC PROPERTIES

### A. Amalgam Toxicity: Clinical Reports

The use of amalgam as a restorative material in dentistry, while very common over the past 150 years, remains controversial. What has been termed "amalgam disease" may simply be a placebo effect (Grandjean, Guldager, Larsen, Jørgensen, & Holmstrup, 1997).

Despite this optimistic outlook, a growing body of animal and human research supports the notion that heavy metals contained in amalgam, and in particular mercury (Hg), can lead to significant toxic manifesta-

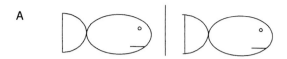

A: Fish are acclimated for 7 days in a common aquarium, but separated by a translucent partition

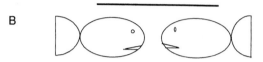

B: Fish are allowed to interact for a period of up to 5 hours. During this time, characteristic behaviors develop from investigative encounter to aggression and combat

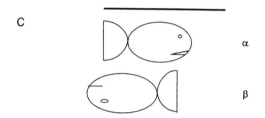

C: Interactions result in the establishment of a dominant ($\alpha$) fish and of a submisive or subordinate ($\beta$) fish

**FIGURE 1** Schematic diagram of the social confrontation paradigm in aggressive fish. (A) The preconfrontational situation where two fish are kept acclimated for 7 days in a common aquarium, but separated by a translucent partition. (B) The period of active interaction between the two fish, which usually lasts up to 5 h and which is characterized by aggressive behavior, including combat. (C) The outcome of the interaction, characterized by the establishment of a dominant ($\alpha$) and submissive ($\beta$) fish.

tions via vapor, corrosion products in swallowed saliva, and direct absorption into the blood from the oral cavity. Adverse physiological effects to dental amalgam may be local in the oral cavity or systemic, depending on the ability of released components to enter the body and, if they do enter the body, depending on their rate of absorption. Patients who bear amalgam dental fillings are chronically exposed to these heavy metals. Amalgam fillings are the most important source of mercury exposure in the general population. The average daily absorption of mercury from dental amalgam is 3–17 µg/day, a dose equivalent to 1.25- to 6.5-fold the average mercury load from other dietary sources (Ziff, 1992; Skare & Engqvist, 1994).

Certain psychopathological manifestations appear to be associated with amalgam fillings. Patients with multiple sclerosis and dental amalgam fillings have significantly poorer mental health status (more symptoms of depression, hostility, psychotism, and more obsessive–compulsive behavior) compared to cohorts whose amalgams had been replaced. Ratings of depression (Beck Depression Inventory) are significantly higher in healthy women with amalgam fillings compared to control women without amalgams. Women with amalgams show higher symptoms of fatigue and insomnia, as well as anger (State-Trait Anger Expression Inventory) than control women. Women with amalgams have lower score on items that evaluate their state of being pleasantly, satisfied, happy, secure, and indicate that they have a more difficult time making decisions. These patterns correlate positively with oral mercury content, whether the saliva is obtained before or after chewing gum (Siblerud, Motl, & Kienholz, 1994).

On the one hand, emotional suppression, the conscious suppression of emotions when emotionally aroused, has been associated with decreased overall somatic activity and increased sympathetic activity (Gross & Levenson, 1993). On the other hand, positive and negative moods, including emotional provocation and threat can have a significant impact upon a range of physiological responses, including the body's immune system (Futterman, Kemeny, Shapiro, & Fahey, 1994). These reports, taken together with the psychoneuroimmunological literature about anxiety and depressed moods (Irwin et al., 1990; Stein, Miller, & Trestman, 1991; Chiappelli et al., 1996a) suggest direct implications and applications to this particular area of research in oral biology and dental medicine and open new avenues for future investigation in the field, with specific focus to amalgam research.

Clinical findings indicate that mercury released from dental amalgams can cause, in susceptible individuals, hypersensitivity and toxic reactions, which often mimic or result in an oral pathological condition known as oral lichen planus (OLP) (vide infra). Replacement of amalgam with other restorative compounds can have strong palliative effects (Pang & Freeman, 1995; Ibbotson, Speight, Macleod, Smart, & Lawrence, 1996). Oral hypersensitivity reactions to dental amalgam mercury may be an important cofactor in the etiology and the pathogenesis of gingivitis, periodontitis, and periodontal disease (Swartzendruber, 1993), possibly through its systemic and local immunotoxic effects (vide infra).

## B. Amalgam Toxicity: Experimental Studies

Absorbed mercury can have significant systemic toxicity evident in cells of the neurological as well as the immunological systems. ADP-ribosylation of tubulin and actin is markedly inhibited by inorganic mercury implants in rat brains, thus indicating the potential of this heavy metal to alter neuron membrane structure. In monkeys, mercury from dental amalgam enriches the intestinal flora with mercury-resistant bacterial species, which in turn become resistant to eradication, thus potentially contributing to mucosal ulceration. Brown–Norway rats injected with mercury chloride ($HgCl_2$) develop an autoimmune disease characterized by T-dependent polyclonal B-cell activation, which is autoregulated and strain-specific (Dubey, Kuhn, Vial, Druet, & Bellon, 1993). The symptomatology involves an overactivation of the Th2 branch of the cytokine network (Dubey et al., 1993), interleukins responsible for the maturation of B cells into antibody secreting lymphocytes, such as IL-4, and a relative decrement in Th1 cytokine production. Taken together, these data indicate that, in susceptible organisms, mercury hypersensitivity may be manifested as a form of autoimmune disorder characterized by a shift in the ratio of Th1 and Th2 cytokines in favor of the latter, thus resulting in decreased cellular immune surveillance and hyperglobulinemia (Dubey et al., 1993).

The relevance of Th1 and Th2 patterns of cytokine responses is increasingly evident in the context of dental medicine. Periodontal and gingival disease (cf., this volume), which may result from or be exacerbated by amalgam hypersensitivity and tissue toxicity (Swartzendruber, 1993), is characterized by apical migration of the epithelial attachment, inflammatory infiltrate subjacent to the junctional epithelium, breakdown of the connective tissue fibers anchored to the cementum, and resorption of the marginal portions of the alveolar bone. Gingivitis is limited to marginal gingival tissue. The pathogenesis of periodontal/gingival disease is attributed in part to the destruction of periodontal/gingival tissue by histo- and cytotoxic factors produced and released by invading and colonizing microflora. Altered immune surveillance to these microorganisms is implicated in the onset and progression of periodontal/gingival disease and is related to systemic diseases. From the viewpoint of immunopathogenesis, periodontal/gingival disease is now recognized to be a spectrum of disorders which can be traced to shifts in T cell distributions and Th1/Th2 patterns of cytokines, which may account for the aggressiveness of periodontal/gingival disease in different clinical situations (Cole, Seymour, & Powell, 1987).

Immunotoxicologic studies of amalgam concur in implicating preferentially the T-cell compartment. For instance, a flow cytometric study indicated that occupational exposure to mercury, which was associated with plasma levels of $4.7 + 7.2 \, \mu g/L$ Hg, induced significant changes in T-cell subpopulations, but had less effect on B or NK cells (Moszczynski & Slowinski, 1994). The cytotoxic effect of mercury upon lymphocytes is irreversible after about 13 h of metal exposure. Scanning electron microscopy data indicate that mercury destroys the cell membranes by either binding to cell surfaces or by forming precipitates within the bilayer that could inhibit cellular metabolic pathways (Steffensen et al., 1994). Mercury impairs cellular immune responses by altering early responses of transmembrane signaling. Treatment of murine thymocytes or spleen cells with mercury leads to deregulated membrane-associated tyrosine phosphorylation of several cellular proteins. Mercury causes cross-linkage of the transmembrane CD4, CD3, CD45, and glycosylphosphatidylinositol-anchored Thy-1 moieties on thymocytes or T lymphocytes. Along with the aggregation of Thy-1 and CD4, the nonreceptor protein tyrosine kinase p56$^{lck}$ also aggregates with resulting activation, leading to deregulated T-cell proliferation and IL-2 production (Nakashima et al., 1994). Mercury further alters the regulation of calcium flux during rat splenic T-cell stimulation (Tan, Tang, Castoldi, Manzo, & Costa, 1993).

Mercury exposure modulates human T-cell function. Following treatment of T cells with nano- to microgram mercury (HgCl$_2$, proliferative response to mitogens in vitro was significantly impaired. Flow cytometric analysis of the expression of membrane activation markers showed a markedly blunted CD25 and CD71 expression (Shenker et al., 1992a; Shenker, Rooney, Vitale, & Shapiro, 1992b). We have confirmed these observations, and have found that $10^{-6}$–$10^{-9}$ M HgCl$_2$ abrogates the activation and cell cycle traversal of T cells following stimulation with PHA (Chiappelli, manuscript under review).

Heavy metals are also immunotoxic to B-cells. Mercury inhibits B-cell RNA and DNA synthesis. The IC$_{50}$ (the concentration required to inhibit a specific B-cell function by 50%) for HgCl$_2$ was 50 and 120 nM for RNA and DNA synthesis, respectively, within 2 h. Mercury arrests B-cell cycle traversal, B-cell maturation in vitro, and immunoglobulin secretion. Selective effects were noted on specific immunoglobulin classes, as IgG$_3$ production was most sensitive to inhibition by mercury, followed by IgG$_1$ and IgG$_{2b}$, IgM and IgG$_{2a}$ (Daum, Shepherd, & Noelle, 1993). Electron microscopy shows significant early nuclear alterations, nuclear fragmentation, and condensation of nucleoplasm. Rapid and sustained elevation in intracellular calcium levels was noted, suggesting that mercury may lead immune cells to apoptotic cell death (Shenker, Mayro, Rooney,

Vitale, & Shapiro, 1993b; Shenker, Guo, & Shapiro, 1998).

## IV. DISEASES OF THE ORAL MUCOSA AS MODELS FOR CLINICAL PSYCHONEUROIMMUNOLOGY RESEARCH

The concept that the psyche and personality styles influence disease processes of the oral mucosa is over one century old (Jacobi, 1894; Sibley, 1899; Giddon, 1966). Indeed, "...*the oral mucosa is highly reactive to psychological influences, and in some cases oral diseases may be a direct expression of emotions or conflicts, while in other instances lesions of the oral mucosa may be the indirect result of an emotional problem...an oral response to emotional stress or tension...may not only represent a conversion but may be the result of constant trauma and irritation produced by neurotic habits related to the mouth...*" For instance, aphthous stomatitis is "...*a disease of the oral mucosa comparable to ulcerative lesions of the gastrointestinal tract and...considered to represent an oral response to some underlying emotional disturbance...*" Oral lichen planus (OLP) is "...*considered a form of psychosomatic response, comparable to various dermatological conditions*" (McCarthy & Shklar, 1980). A plethora of other oral conditions exist for which "*psychological factors may play some etiologic role*" (e.g., erythema multiforme, membrane pemphigoid, inflammation of the periodontium, and gingiva), "*emotional stress serves as a predisposing factor*" (recurrent herpes labialis, necrotizing gingivitis), "*induced by neurotic habits*" (e.g., leukoplakia, dental and periodontal pathology secondary to bruxism), and "*neurotic oral symptoms*" (e.g., glossodynia, dysgeusia) (McCarthy & Shklar, 1980), as well as recurrent herpetic outbreaks (Logan, Lutgendorf, Hartwig, Lilly, & Berberich, 1998). T-cell-mediated hypersensitivity is involved in recurrent aphthous stomatitis and oral lichen planus; humoral-mediated immunity to cadherin intercellular adhesion molecules is important in the process of acantholysis in pemphigus vulgaris, and genetic defects and antibody-mediated processes give rise to junctional separation in epidermolysis bullosa and mucous membrane pemphigoid, respectively, whereas an immune complex mechanism appears to underlie the pathogenesis of erythema multiforme (Eversole, 1994).

### A. Oral Lichen Planus

Oral lichen planus (OLP), first described by Erasmus Wilson in 1859, is a complex pathology of the soft oral mucosa (82% cheek, 50% tongue, 22% lips, 17% palate, 11% gums; McCarthy, Shklar, 1980), a chronic inflammatory disorder that afflicts up to 2% of the population. The etiology of OLP may be dependent in part upon gonadal hormones since women are 1.5–2.0 times at greater risk than men. Aging plays a role in the onset of OLP since over 95% of OLP cases occur middle age (>30 years of age), with men reportedly afflicted at an earlier age (40–49 years), than women (50–59 years). The incidence of OLP does not vary significantly across ethnic groups, although whites appear to be afflicted in greater numbers than other ethnic groups. OLP and its cutaneous equivalent, LP, are associated with systemic diseases, such as primary biliary cirrhosis, coeliac disease, chronic liver disease as determined by elevated serum transaminase levels (serum glutamic–oxaloacetic transaminase or serum glutamic–pyruvic transaminase), diabetes mellitus, hypertension, graft-versus-host disease, lupus erythematous, myasthenia gravis, thymoma, and oral manifestations often observed in HIV-seropositive and AIDS patients. Antirheumatics, nonsteroidal antiinflammatory agents, antihypertensives, and antibiotics often lead to the development of lichenoid lesions and their exacerbation. OLP persists for 20 years or longer and manifests as reticular (lace-like keratotic patterns), atrophic (reticular keratosis and erythema), erosive (atrophic mucosa with ulcers), and bullous lesions (large thin-walled bullae) (Dreyer, 1983; Eversole, 1994; Bricker, 1994).

The erosive and bullous stages of the disease may predispose to oral carcinomas, although the predictive value of OLP lesions is less than that of other recognized oral carcinogenic factors (Lozada-Nur & Miranda, 1997). Up to 1 in 25 patients with the more severe OLP lesions develop squamous oral cancers, an alarming 1000-fold increase over the general population (Pogrel & Weldon, 1983; Barnard, Scully, Eveson, Cunningham, & Porter, 1993). Malignant transformation occurs in a mean time of 3.4 years after the onset of lichen planus (Silverman, Gorsky, & Lozada-Nur, 1985).

Several factors contribute to the etiology of OLP, including a complex succession of immunological events (Porter, Kirby, Olsen, & Barrett, 1997). The stimulation of Langerhans cells and of keratinocytes by a foreign antigen may lead to the production of inflammatory cytokines. The expression of these cytokines is modulated by psychoneuroendocrine factors (cf., this volume). These cytokines modulate the activation and homing of T cells and preferentially of CD4+ T lymphocytes, the expression of intercellular adhesion molecule-1 (ICAM-1) and HLA-Dr

antigens on the membranes of lymphocytes and keratinocytes, and the adhesion of T lymphocytes to the keratinocytes leading eventually to the destruction of the latter (André, Laporte, Delavault, 1990). HLA-Bw57 may predispose the onset of OLP, while HLA-Dq1 may be associated with resistance to it (Porter, Klouda, Scully, Bidwell, & Porter, 1993). Contact reactions to mercury and other dental materials can also, as noted, lead to the onset of OLP (Lind, Hurlen, Lyberg, & Aas, 1986; Bolewska & Reibel, 1989; Ostman, Anneroth, & Skoglund, 1994).

The progression from the reticular to the atrophic, erosive and bullous forms of the disorder is believed to be driven by anxiety, psychological trauma and psychosocial turmoil (Gauro, Hernández Vicente, Unamuno Pérez, & Martin-Pascual, 1977; McCarthy & Shklar, 1980). We reported significant differences in psychoimmune interactions between patients afflicted with nonerosive OLP lesions compared to those with erosive OLP lesions (Chiappelli et al., 1997), confirming earlier studies that showed that over half of patients with OLP lesions verified by histochemical diagnosis reported significant levels of life stress prior to the onset of the exacerbation of the lesions (Hampf, Malmström, Aalberg, Hannula, & Vikkula, 1987; Burkhart, Burker, Burkes, & Wolfe, 1996). Patients with OLP score high on the Hamilton anxiety scale and the Hamilton depressive scale (Colella, Gritti, De Luca, & de Vito, 1993), as well as the Profile of Moods scale (Chiappelli et al., 1997), but not on the Hospital Anxiety and Depression scale (McCartan, 1995). The research to date suggests a psychosomatic component to the etiology and prognosis of OLP, but this still remains controversial (Allen, Beck, Rossie, & Kaul, 1986; Hampf et al., 1987).

Histologically, OLP lesions show parakeratosis, epithelial hyperkeratosis, occasionally slight acanthosis, basal epithelial cell destruction, and copious infiltration of leukocytes in the submucosa. There is substantial increase in number of mast cells within OLP lesions and increased direct mast cell–nerve interaction in the lesions compared to normal tissue (Zhao, Savage, Pujic, & Walsh, 1997). T cells, Langerhans cells, and macrophages that express the adhesion molecules CD54 and CD106 are the predominant infiltrating populations, while B lymphocytes are typically scarce. CD4 lymphocytes outnumber CD8 cells by two- to threefold, and the latter line primarily the epithelial-mesenchymal interface. Infiltrating CD4 and CD8 lymphocytes express the memory T-cell phenotype (CD45RO+CD29+) (Simon, Reimer, Schardt, & Hornstein, 1983; Konttinen et al., 1989; Walsh, Tseng, Savage, & Seymour, 1989; Sugerman, Voltz, Savage, Basford, & Seymour, 1992; Sugerman,

Savage, & Seymour, 1993a; Sugerman, Savage, Walsh, & Seymour, 1993b; Karagouni, Dotsika, & Sklavounou, 1994; Walton, Thornhill, & Farthing, 1994). The percentage of peripheral blood CD4+CD45R0+ cells is 65.7% in patients with OLP, compared to 49.1% in controls, and the percentage of CD4+CD45RA+ in OLP lesion epithelium is 24% in patient biopsies, but *nil* in biopsies of healthy mucosa obtained from control subjects. Fewer Langerhans cell express CD45RO in OLP patient compared to control biopsies. OLP biopsy T lymphocytes and Langerhans cells express significantly higher levels of ICAM-1 than control tissue, suggestive of selective recruitment of immune cells in OLP, in part mediated by ICAM-1 (Walton, Macey, Thornhill, & Farthing, 1998).

Patients with OLP show impaired T-cell immunity systemically. The percentage and number of peripheral blood CD4+CD45RA+ T lymphocytes is typically less in patients with OLP than in control subjects, whereas the proportion of CD4+CD29+ T lymphocytes is increased significantly (Konttinen et al., 1989; Sugerman et al., 1992). Indicative of a state of inflammation are the elevated serum levels of TNF-$\alpha$ and IL-6 in the patients with OLP (Karagouni et al., 1994). Keratinocytes appear to be the target for T-cell-mediated destruction in OLP lesions, but the fundamental mechanism remains unknown (Sugerman et al., 1993b). To begin to gain some understanding of the nature of infiltrating T cells, OLP lesion infiltrating lymphocytes were extracted, and cell lines were obtained and expanded. The majority of clones expressed CD8+ and the $\alpha/\beta$ T-cell receptor (TcR), although three clones were CD4+ and $\alpha/\beta$ TcR. Of all the isolated clones, only one was CD4+CD8- and $\gamma/\delta$ TcR (Sugerman et al, 1993a).

We obtained physiologically and clinically significant interactions between the psychological status of patients with OLP and the maturation process of CD4+CD45RA+ cells. Peripheral blood T cells obtained from OLP patients revealed blunted responses to T-cell-specific mitogenic stimulation, and significantly decreased proliferation, production of IL-2 and IFN, two representative products of the Th1 pattern of cytokines. The expression of the $\alpha$ chain of the IL-2 receptor, CD25, an important marker of the T cells' ability to engage in the initial phases of activation, was also blunted in T cells from patients with OLP (Chiappelli et al., 1997).

To obtain a rough endocrine assessment in these patients, we measured plasma cortisol levels. There are important limitations of this measurement from the perspective of data interpretation since a one-time point determination of cortisol during a 24-h period may not be fully informative (Chiappelli & Trignani,

1993). Nevertheless, such data can suggest important neuroendocrine–immune deregulations. We drew blood from patients with oral lesions, whose pathologies were diagnosed clinically and verified histologically, between 10:00 AM and 12:00 PM, which is during the peak of the cortisol circadian cycle. Close to half the patients had cortisol levels within the normal range below 25.0 µg/dL (range, 13.2–22.0 µg/dL). The remaining patients showed relatively elevated late morning plasma cortisol levels ranging from 34.4 µg/dL and above. Cortisol levels are inversely related to circulating CD3+ cells (percentage of lymphocytes and absolute numbers) in normal individuals (Chiappelli & Trignani, 1993). This relationship was observed in the subgroup of patients with relatively mild OLP lesions and with relative hypercortisolemia ($r=-.8$), and in their cohorts with late-morning cortisol levels within the normal range ($r=-.34, p>.05$). Cortisol levels and the percentage or absolute number of circulating CD3+ cells were not significantly correlated in patients with mucous membrane pemphigoid, in patients with pemphigoid vulgaris, or in patients with the more aggressive erosive OLP lesions, despite the rather elevated late morning plasma cortisol level in these three groups of patients (39.9–45.4 µg/dL). Taken as a group, patients with OLP lesions characterized by plasma cortisol levels below 25.0 µg/dL at this time of the day, typically showed CD4/CD8 ratios about 1.0 ($1.0 \pm 0.4$). Their cohorts with late morning plasma cortisol levels that ranged above 25.0 µg/dL typically showed a CD4/CD8 ratio below 1.0 ($0.7 \pm 0.3$), with the exception of the patients who manifested the erosive lesions. The ratio in the latter subgroup fell within the normal 1.0–2.0 range ($1.3 \pm 0.5$) (Chiappelli et al., 1997). Taken together, these outcomes strongly indicate the need to study in greater detail the psycho–neuroendocrine–immune interrelationship in the pathogenesis of OLP.

## B. Aphthous Canker Sores

Recurrent aphthous stomatitis (RAS, commonly referred as canker sores) is another common, most painful and distressing condition of the oral mucosa. The etiology of RAS rests in part on the perception of stress by the patient. Its manifestation includes significant alterations in T-cell distribution and function. RAS is the most common inflammatory ulcerative condition of the oral mucosa in North American patients (McCarthy & Shklar, 1980; Rogers, 1997).

RAS typically manifests as recurrent oral ulcers, recurrent aphthous ulcers, or simple or complex aphthosis. Clinical evaluation requires classification of the ulcers on the basis of morphology (e.g., minor vs. major aphthous ulcers) and severity (simple versus complex) (Rogers, 1997). Canker sores appear as recurring self-limited ulcers of the nonkeratinized oral mucosa and oropharynx. Sores can be minor, shallow and painful ulcers less than 5 mm in diameter that have the potential to heal in 10–14 days or even months without scarring (minor recurrent aphthous stomatitis). Sores can also manifest as major ulcers that spread over substantial distances on the oral mucosa, heal in a period of weeks and often leave significant scarring. A prodromal phase is recognized by most patients as a burning sensation a few days prior to the onset of ulceration. The histopathology of RAS involves the invasion of inflammatory cells and early intraepithelial degeneration of individual cells in *stratum spinosum* (Stenman & Heyden, 1980). Differential diagnosis must exclude associated systemic disorders, such as Behçet's disease and complex aphthosis variants, such as ulcus vulvae acutum, mouth and genital ulcers with inflamed cartilage syndrome, fever, aphthosis, pharyngitis, and adenitis syndrome, and cyclic neutropenia (Rogers, 1997).

Histologically, the mucosa in canker sores appears nonspecifically lesioned. The surface epithelium has a central area of destruction, and the connective tissue is densely infiltrated with lymphocytes and neutrophils. Active fibrosis is evident at the base and sides of the ulcerated areas. Cell-to-cell and cell-to extracellular matrix contacts are directed, as in the instance of OLP, by adhesion proteins, which maintain the integrity of the mucosal lining of the oral cavity. Disease processes that destroy keratinocytes or adversely affect their adhesion to one another or to the subjacent basement membrane will result in erosions, ulcerations, and desquamations in RAS as it occurs in OLP (Eversole, 1994).

The etiology of RAS is multifactorial. These factors include trauma, smoking, stress, hormonal state, family history, food hypersensitivity, bacterial antigens, and immunologic factors (Graykowski, Barile, Lee, & Stanley, 1966; MacPhail, 1997; Rogers, 1997). Semiquantitative reverse transcriptase polymerase chain reaction shows elevated messenger expression of IL-2, IFN, and TNF-$\alpha$, but not IL-10, in biopsies obtained from patients with acute RAS lesions, compared to that seen in normal oral mucosa. Failure to suppress the inflammatory reaction initiated by trauma or other external stimuli seems to be critical in the pathogenesis of RAS (Buño, Huff, Weston, Cook, & Brice, 1998). RAS seems more common among patients with the HLA-Cw7 (23% vs. 9% in controls) and HLA-B51 (23% vs. 5% in

controls) phenotypes, the latter being common in Behçet's syndrome. RAS can have profound effects upon the quality of life of the patient, including recurrent prolonged burning pain, which hampers chewing, talking, and other oral functions (McCarthy & Shklar, 1980). Pain may be so debilitating that pain control may be used with pain medications or with adherent agents that coat the ulcers (MacPhail, 1997). Patients with persistent RAS show significant levels of anxiety, as measured by the Self-Rating Anxiety Scale (Buajeeb, Laohapand, Vongsavan, & Kraivaphan, 1990) or the Hospital Anxiety and Depression scale (McCartan, Lamey, & Wallace, 1996). In the latter study, patients manifested significantly elevated salivary cortisol levels ($p < .01$) compared to control subjects (McCartan et al., 1996). Relaxation/imagery treatment techniques can reduce recurrence of ulcers (Andrews & Hall, 1990).

RAS is an immunological disease primarily involving the T-cell compartment (Lehner, 1978; Pedersen & Pedersen, 1993). Patients with HIV infection typically have very aggressive RAS (McPhail & Greenspan, 1997). The percentage of circulating CD4+ lymphocytes is significantly lower in patients with RAS than in control subjects ($p < .0001$), whereas the percentage of CD8+ cells does not differ between the groups. Patients with RAS show significantly ($p < .01$) more CD45RA+ T lymphocytes, than control healthy subjects (Pedersen, Klausen, Hougen, & Ryder, 1991). The condition waxes and wanes, and reduced numbers of mononuclear cells, including T-lymphocytopoenia in the oral mucosa, are more pronounced during the active phase of the disease (Pedersen, Hougen, Kenrad, 1992). RAS could signify autoimmune reactions since a significantly greater number of patients with RAS than controls have elevated levels of circulating anti-DNA antibodies (Rodríguez-Archilla, Urquía, Gómez-Moreno, & Ceballos, 1994). The proportion of circulating T cells bearing the $\gamma/\delta$ TcR is significantly increased in patients with active RAS (median, 8.5%) compared with that seen in control subjects (median, 2.8%; $p < .001$) as well as patients with inactive RAS (median, 5.0%; $p < .01$). ICAM-I and ELAM are strongly expressed on systemic lymphocytes, and TNF-$\alpha$ production is increased in peripheral blood lymphocytes of healthy patients with RAS. Thalidomide, which inhibits TNF-$\alpha$ production, is often an effective treatment for RAS (MacPhail & Greenspan, 1997).

A significant role for the neuroendocrine system in the etiology of RAS is suggested by the observation of its onset with episodes with the menstrual cycle (Eversole, Shopper, & Chambers, 1982). Lesions reach maximum incidence in the postovulatory phase of the menstrual cycle, when estrogen levels drop and progesterone levels rise (McCarthy & Shklar, 1980).

Reactivation of certain latent viruses (e.g., varicella-zoster virus, cytomegalovirus) are also listed among the critical etiological factors of RAS (Pedersen & Pedersen, 1993). Herpes simplex virus (HSV) is the causative factors for various orofacial lesions, including primary herpetic stomatitis, recurrent herpes labialis, and recurrent intraoral infections. The sores associated with HSV are reminiscent of RAS. Of the two subtypes HSV-1 and HSV-2, the former is commonly associated with herpetic stomatitis and the latter with genital infections. Many primary infections with HSV are subclinical with stomatitis and pharyngitis being the most common clinical manifestations of primary infection. Intact epithelium constitutes the main defense against HSV infection, and humoral and cellular responses directed against cell surface viral glycoproteins are involved. Antibodies also mediate viral neutralization and antibody-dependent cellular cytotoxicity (ADCC).

Reactivation of the latent virus is triggered by various factors that operate via depression of the latent viral genes or deregulation of the immune surveillance mechanisms, including stress (Glaser et al., 1987). There appears to be a significant decrease in serum epinephrine levels as well as CD56+ cell number, the latter being correlated with moods of discontentment ($r = .64$, $p = .05$), from the week prior to herpes outbreak recurrence to the week of recrudescence (Logan et al., 1998). These observations are relevant in a psychoneuroendocrine–immune context because, as noted above, HSV can contribute to the onset of oral cancer.

## C. Oral Cancer

The incidence of cancer of the oral cavity has dramatically increased in the past decade, mainly due to an increase in tobacco and alcohol abuse. Males are affected twice as often as females, and most frequently after 40 years with a peak at 60 years. A total of 31,000 new cases of oral cancer are recognized every year in the United States alone, mostly occurring in the lips, tongue, floor of the mouth, palate, gingiva, alveolar and buccal mucosa, and oropharynx. Squamous cell carcinoma accounts for 96% of all oral cancers; sarcomas and salivary gland tumors account for the remainder. Although most of primary lesions are curable, oral cancer patients have a poor long-term prognosis due to increased susceptibility to secondary tumors in the pharyngeal and laryngeal cavities. The 5-year survival rates for malignancies of

the oral cavity and pharynx remains lower than 50%. Alarmingly, the head and neck is the only anatomical region in which 5-year survival rates have not improved significantly in the past decade, and over 10,000 deaths from oral cancer, about 2.4% of all cancers, will occur in the United States this year (Parker, Tong, Bolden, & Wingo, 1997).

The suspicion that the etiology of cancer can be traced to psychological distress and emotion goes back almost 2000 years, as ''melancholic'' women were observed by Galen to be more prone than women with other psychological makeups to manifest the development of breast tumors. Cancer, as we understand it today, refers to the uncontrolled growth and spread of abnormal cells, and is unquestionably linked to psychological factors, such as moods and bereavement (Fife, Beasley, & Fertig, 1996). Patients with oral cancer are often psychologically traumatized by the threat and the sequelae of the disfiguring surgical intervention. A second round of reconstructive surgery is almost always required. Relevant to the field of psychoneuroimmunology, critical role that psychoemotional stress plays in the pathogenesis of oral cancer is therefore evident.

Cellular immunity (e.g., cytotoxic T lymphocytes [CTLs], tumor-infiltrating lymphocytes [TILs], natural killer [NK] cells, lymphokine-activated killer [LAK] cells), plays a critical role in tumor recognition and rejection, but the role of the psychoneuroendocrine system in modulating immune surveillance of oral cancer, such as the endogenous opioid system (Panerai, Sacerdote, 1997, Figure 2), remains to be fully characterized. Regulatory T lymphocytes interact with oral tumor cells through the recognition of putative tumor-associated antigens, and become activated leading to modulation of the activity of cytotoxic effector cells, and the putative role of endogenous opioids and other neuropeptides in modulating these responses remains to be tested experimentally.

Cancer is a multistep process that involves initiation, promotion, and tumor progression. Initiation is induced by random genomic mutation due to limited exposure to chemical carcinogens, tumor viruses, or ionizing radiation or through genetic predisposition and results in irriversible DNA damage. Mutations in tumor suppressor genes (e.g., p53), which help regulate cell growth, have been linked to tobacco smoking in squamous cell carcinoma of the head and neck, as have human papillomavirus (HPV) 16 and 18, which can be detected in leukoplakia and in squamous cell carcinoma. Alterations in the p53 gene leads to no expression of p53 or overexpression of mutant p53 protein that acts as an oncogene product. Mutations of the p53 gene lead to growth deregula-

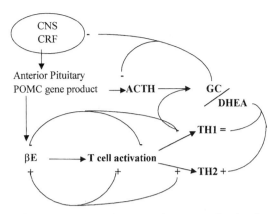

**FIGURE 2** Schematic diagram of neuro–endocrine–immune interactions, and specifically of the connection between the hypothalamo-pituitary-adrenal (HPA) axis and cell-mediated immunity (CMI). The central nervous system (CNS) produces corticotropin releasing factor (CRF) from hypothalamic neurons. CRF induces the anterior pituitary to express the proopiomelanocortin (POMC) gene, which is clipped into peptides, including β-endorphin (βE) and adrenocortico-tropic hormone (ACTH). These peptides are also produced by stimulated lymphocytes. The former modulates T-cell activation, favoring the maturation of T cells capable of producing Th2-type cytokines (e.g., IL-4 and IL-5), whereas hindering the maturation of T cells responsible for a Th1 pattern of cytokines (e.g., IL-2, interferon-γ). ACTH also down-regulates T-cell maturation leading to Th1 cytokines, whereas it induces adrenocortical cells to produce glucocorticoids (GC). The ratio of GC to dehydroepiandrosterone (DHEA) level, a steroid also produced by adrenal cortex cells, has important physiological correlates, including the modulation of T-cell maturation toward a Th1 or a Th2 pattern of cytokine production.

tion and malignant progression: mutant p53 expression vectors enhance the tumorigenicity of weak tumorigenic cell lines and increase the metastatic potential of tumor cells. The level of overexpression of the p53 protein is predictive of disease outcome in oral cancer induced by tobacco (Kaur, Srivastava, & Ralhan, 1998). Up to 30–40% of oral cancer biopsy specimens contain the viral DNA for HPV (Syrjanen, 1992). The role of HPV in carcinogenesis derives from its transforming capacity. Transformation and subsequent immortalization of normal oral epithelial cells can be demonstrated with cloned HPV-16 and -18 DNA (Park, Min, Li, Cherrick, & Doniger, 1991). Mutations of the p53 gene can be induced by HPV since high levels of p53 protein resulting from point mutation of the p53.2 gene are evident in human oral squamous cell carcinoma and these changes are associated with HPV infection. HPV-immortalized primary oral epithelial cells require exposure to nicotine and other tobacco metabolites for progression to a fully malignant tumor (Shin, Moo, Cherrick, & Park, 1994). Additional oral cancer tumor-specific genes remain to be identified.

In Western societies, close to 75% of all oral and pharyngeal cancers are attributable to joint abuse of tobacco and alcohol alone (Blot et al., 1988). Among the individuals that do use tobacco very few actually develop oral cancer; but the risk for the development of oral cancer increases with the quantity of alcoholic beverage consumed. Combined risk factors, particularly the interaction between alcohol and tobacco, are thus more strongly predictive of the development of oral cancer than each single factor individually (Chiappelli, Kung, Savage, Villanueva, & Fiala, 1996b). Chronic alcohol induces serious alterations to the histological structures of the oral mucosa, and the basal cell nuclei and the size of the basal cell layer of the oral mucosa become enlarged, thus altering the stratification of the cells as well as oral mucosal cell proliferation. Hyperregenerative mucosa has increased susceptibility to chemical carcinogens. Alcohol also inhibits detoxification of carcinogenic compounds, and may actually favor metabolic activation of compounds into carcinogenic state. Alcohol impairs cell-mediated immunity and suppresses immune surveillance of malignancies. Chronic exposure of rodents to ethanol reduces the number and activity of NKs, which participate in the defense against tumor development and metastasis. In human and animal models, toxic concentrations of alcohol have been shown to alter lymphocytic migration behavior by impairing the ability of lymphocytes to adhere to the endothelium (for review Chiappelli & Kung, 1995; Chiappelli & Liu, 1999).

Oral cancer is also associated with generalized nutritional deficits, particularly deficiencies in vitamins A, B, and C and iron, whereas vitamins A and E and β-carotene may confer protection against cancer. β-Carotene is metabolized to vitamin A and may have similar effect as vitamin A. Vitamins A and E and β-carotene act as antioxidants and free radical scavengers. Free radicals and reactive oxygen molecules are normal metabolic byproducts of tobacco and alcohol metabolism. Free radicals damage lipid membranes, denature proteins, and attack nucleic acids. Antioxidants and free radical scavengers trap these molecules, thus preventing damage to the oral mucosa. Clinical trials using β-carotene and retinoids have shown significant reductions in leukoplakia (precancerous oral lesions). Vitamin A may also retard tumor development by impairing protein kinase C signal transduction (Berger, Berger, & Schmahl, 1991; Lippman et al., 1993). Consumption of N-nitroso compounds commonly found in salt cured, pickled, and moldy foods increases the chances of oral cancer (Li, Ji, & Cheng, 1986; Lijinsky, 1987). Changes in caloric intake can influence tumor progression.

Chronic dietary restriction (60% of ad libitum diet) is associated with a significant reduction in the incidence of spontaneous, chemically induced, and transplanted tumors in rats (Albanes, 1987).

Immunosuppressive drugs, such as the corticosteroids, often utilized in the course of treatment for mucosal pathologies can increase the susceptibility of the oral mucosa to infection and neoplasia. Deregulation in the HPA axis, which brings about hypercortisolemia and an alteration in the ratio between circulating corticosteroids and the weak adrenocortical androgen, dehydroepiandrosterone (DHEA), as well as its physiologically more effective sulfated form, DHEA-S, occurs in several disease states (Chiappelli et al., 1994) and may contribute to tumorogenesis by hampering cellular immune surveillance.

An additional risk factor for oral cancer is aging. By the year 2050 it is estimated that 23% of the population will be at least 65 years old. Given that 50% of all cancers occur in the older age group (60+ years), the incidence of malignancies of all types of cancers, including oral cancers, should increase during the coming decades. During aging, as the oral mucous becomes thinner and less resilient to the impact of trauma and bacterial, fungal, and viral infection, certain aspects of immunity decline, including T-cell blastogenesis, LAK-cell activity, and the numbers of lymphocytes and polymorphonuclear leukocytes. The probability that patients will be infected with HSV or HPV increases with age, and the elderly are less resilient in terms of dealing with stress and more susceptible to stress-related disorders as well as malnutrition. With aging, the initiation of the adrenocortical response to stress remains unimpaired, but the ability to terminate the response is altered, such that in contrast to younger subjects (animal or human), high levels of corticosteroids persist for up to 24 h after exposure to a stressor (Sapolsky, Krey, & McEwen, 1986).

We are currently testing the interrelatedness of some of these factors in three experimental animal models.

i. MADB106 tumor cells, a selected variant cell line obtained from a pulmonary metastasis of a mammary adenocarcinoma chemically induced in the F344 rat, administered intravenously, reliably colonizes primarily to the lungs. Well-defined surface metastases can be counted 3–4 weeks after inoculation. Colonization of the lungs is primarily surveyed by NK-cell activity, and NK-cell activity in splenocytes and in peripheral blood lymphocytes predicts the number of metastases observed at 3 weeks as well as

the clearance of tumor cells from the lungs measured as early as 24 h postinoculation (Ben-Eliyahu, Page, Yirmiya, & Taylor, 1996). Alcohol intake (2.3–3.5 g ethanol/kg) 1 h prior to inoculation, suppresses NK-cell activity, decreases lung clearance, and increases metastasis of MADB106 tumor cells in F344 rats (Hodgson et al., 1996). Chronic ethanol (35% ethanol-derived calories) for 2 weeks prior to, and 3 weeks after, further significantly increases the number of metastases and decreases NK-cell activity. Chronic dietary restriction modulates immune surveillance to the MADB106 tumor. We find that chronic dietary restriction enhances or inhibits MADB106 tumor cell coloni-zation in lungs depending on the specific parameters of the feeding regimen: severe dietary restriction inhibits tumor spread, but moderate dietary restriction enhances MADB106 tumor cell lung metastasis (Hodgson et al., 1997). Stress results in the production of inflammatory cytokines, whose central action upon hypothalamic neurons initiates the modulatory processes observed in the periphery. Therefore, IL-1$\beta$ levels are increased centrally following exposure to stress, and intraventricular administration of IL-1$\beta$ inhibits lung clearance of MADB106 tumor cells, and increases lung colonization. This effect, mediated by the central and not peripheral actions of IL-1$\beta$, is blocked by coadministration of the IL-1 receptor antagonist. Intraventricular IL-1$\beta$ impairs lung clearance of tumor cells by suppressing NK-cell activity. This tenet of psycho-neuroimmunology applies to immune surveillance of MADB106 tumors, and most likely all tumors including cancers of the oral cavity. It is probable that this effect is obtained via the actions of adrenal catecholamines, most likely epinephrine, acting at $\beta$-adrenergic receptors in the periphery (Hodgson, Yirmiya, Chiappelli, & Taylor, 1998), in a manner not dissimilar to that reported in humans (Heijnen et al., 1991). Studies show increased resistance to the mammary tumor, MADB106, in dietary restricted rats consequential to altered NK-cell activity (Hodgson et al., 1997). Whether or not the same trend will be shown in either of two models of oral cancer remains to be tested.

ii. Increase in the risk of developing oral cancer may be linked to the consumption of N-nitroso compounds, including N-nitrosomethyl benzlamine (NMBA) (Lijinsky, 1987). The proposed mechanism of NMBA carcinogenicity is through microsomal activation to form benzaldehyde and an electrophilic metabolite which methylates DNA, and may induce DNA mutations (Singer, 1979). A high frequency of both H-ras and p53 mutations in NMBA-induced papillomas occurs in rats (Lozano, Nakazawa, Cross,

Cabral, & Yamasaki, 1994). Esophageal cancers result in adult Fischer 344 rats injected subcutaneously with 0.5 mg/kg of NMBA 3 times/week. The tongue and esophagus are assessed for the number of tumors. Cold stress (total immersion, 2C, three times, 3 min, separated by a rest period of 3 min) administered 5 days/week for 3 weeks, a stress paradigm which impairs NK-cell-mediated removal of MADB106 tumor cells, leads 100% of the animals to develop esophageal tumors within 9 weeks of the NMDA administration. The stress protocol significantly increases plasma corticosterone levels (stress, $388.6 \pm 38.9$ ng/mL control, $153.8 \pm 25.5$ ng/mL) and favors survival by 60%, perhaps because the lowered body temperature and vasoconstriction may keep the NMBA localized in the subcutaneous skin layer, reduce its spread, and minimize its carcinogenic effects.

iii. The chemical carcinogen 7,12-dimethylbenz[a]-anthracene (DMBA) produces epidermoid oral carcinomas in a relatively short period of time (Perrin, Astre, Broquerie, Saint Aubert, Joyeux, 1990). Topical application 3 times/week induces hyperplastic changes at 4 weeks, dysplasia at 4–6 weeks, carcinoma in situ at 6–8 weeks, and invasive carcinoma by the 10th to the 14th week. Carcinomas of the tongue are obtained with a single application. The tumors are typically squamous cell carcinoma and there are typically no metastases of tumor cells to other organs of the body The histopathological alterations of the oral epithelium are almost identical to those in biopsies of human oral malignant and premalignant lesions. The mechanisms underlying the development of DMBA oral tumors are as yet not fully known, although they most likely relate to overexpression of mRNA for the oncogene c-erb-B1, for TGF-$\alpha$ and epidermal growth factor, and for eosinophilia. Tissue eosinophils express TGF-$\alpha$, which mediates certain aspects of the malignant transformation process (i.e., mitogenesis and angiogenesis), as well as healing (vide infra). Adult Fisher 344 rats, treated with a single injection of DMBA (5 mg/kg) into the left lateral border of the middle third of the tongue and subjected to the cold stress outlined above, manifest significant increase (14%) in morbidity and mortality at 18 weeks.

## D. Wound Healing and Associated Growth Factors

Tooth extraction results in a sizable wound in the maxillary or the mandibular bone, as well as in periodontal soft tissues and oral mucosa. Tooth extraction is therefore an accessible experimental model for studying the process of wound healing. The tooth extraction wound healing model serves to test the hypothesis that the differences in biological structure and physiological behavior are due in part to the expression of specific genes during oral soft tissue wound healing or as a long-term consequence to the wounding (Abanomy & Nishimura, 1997). Total RNAs from wound healing sites and control oral mucosa were subjected to differential display polymerase chain reaction (DD-PCR) analysis, the products isolated, and the initial candidates further screened by RNA transfer blot analysis. Two DD-PCR clones, AA1 and AA2a, were identified as the wound site specific cDNAs, which hybridized with 3.8 and 4.2 kb mRNA species, respectively, but that could not be matched to existing sequences in the GenBank, indicating that these cDNAs may encode unique genes. Further characterization should demonstrate that psychoneuroimmunologic factors modulate the healing of oral mucosa wound through the expression of these genes.

Oral wounds heal more rapidly than skin wounds, and they heal in a manner mechanistically dissimilar to that seen in skin. Skin wounds revascularize with an abundance of capillaries that later regress; oral wounds revascularize more slowly and without ever achieving a capillary density greater than uninjured tissue. The oral mucosa fibroblasts demonstrate a significantly increased ability to reorganize extracellular matrix (ECM) in vitro compared to skin fibroblasts.

During the healing of skin wounds, resident fibroblasts and some perivascular mesenchymal cells differentiate into phenotypically distinct cells, the myofibroblasts rich in actin filaments that permit contractile and migratory capabilities. Fibronectin acts as an adhesive scaffolding on which myofibroblasts and fibroblasts migrate and later synthesize collagen. Endothelial cells permit neoangiogenesis, which parallels the migration and proliferation of fibroblasts and is important in delivering nutrients and oxygen as well as carrying away toxic waste and metabolic by-products. Endothelial cell proliferation is stimulated by cytokines, and vessel growth is promoted by the wound's low oxygen tension. As healing slows and wound remodeling occurs, capillaries slowly regress and the highly vascular-cell-rich granulation tissue transforms into a white, relatively avascular cell-poor scar.

The process of healing in the stroma occurs as follows: (1) Following removal of a tooth, the blood coagulate forms in the socket, and red blood cells are entrapped in the fibrin meshwork within 24–48 h. (2) Alterations in the vascular bed (vasodilatation and the formation of small spaces between endothelium) permit leukocytes to migrate into interstitial tissues and to initiate the innate host response to foreign microorganisms and debris accumulation. (3) Factors are produced, whose expression is modulated by neuroendocrine products, secreted as a psychoneuroendocrine response to stress, pain, and anxiety (cf., this volume), among which are platelet-derived growth factor (PDGF) and transforming growth factor-$\beta$ (TGF-$\beta$). (4) There is an influx of inflammatory cells, fibroblasts, and endothelial cells at the surface of the healing area for the formation of new epithelium by the process of epithelialization. (5) Formation of granulation tissue occurs immediately thereafter (3 to 4 days after injury) and consists of a dense population of macrophages, fibroblasts, and neovasculature within an edematous matrix of residual fibrin, fibronectin, glycoproteins, collagen, and glycosaminoglycans (GAGs). Granulation tissue is sustained in instances of open wounds until reepithelialization occurs.

The GAGs, an important component of the granulation tissue response, consist in a group of polysaccharides that contain repeating disaccharide units usually composed of glucoronic or iduronic acid and hexosamine. All GAGs, except hyaluronic acid, are coupled to core proteins through an oligosaccharide linkage. During the early phases of granulation tissue formation, hyaluronic acid is prominent in the wound matrix and aids in maintaining wound hydration and in the process of cellular migration, proliferation, and differentiation. In the later stages of granulation tissue formation, hyaluronic acid is replaced in these functions by sulfated GAGs, such as chrondroitin-4,6-sulfates, dermatan sulfate, and heparan sulfate, which contribute to tissue resilience and may have a role in collagen synthesis.

Early granulation tissue is composed largely of type III collagen synthesized by resident fibroblasts 2 to 3 days after the cells enter the wound site. The preexistence of fibronectin at the site is essential for collagen fibrin deposition. Fibronectin is one of the main matrix constituents during early wound repair; it is a glycoprotein produced mainly by fibroblasts and endothelial cells and is found in serum. It comprises the primary provisional matrix for tissue repair and is integral component of all connective tissues. Fibronectin appears, in early granulation tissue, preceding the appearance of collagenous proteins. Fibronectin also has a role in blood coagulation by binding to fibrin in the presence of factor XIII to form cross-links, which strengthen the fibrin clot, and fibroblast invasion. Matrix formation thus begins with the process of fibroplasia. Fibroblasts appear within 2 days after injury; growth factor, from platelets and macrophages stimulate the fibroblasts to proliferate and to synthesize collagen. Because the fibroblasts are metabolically active and depend on the adequacy of local oxygen supply, the rate of production of collagen is dependent on the level of the tissue oxygen tension. The rate of collagen synthesis is minimal in the first 2 weeks, and collagen deposition is minimal at 3 to 4 weeks; thus, the tensile strength of the wound is approximately 10% at 2 weeks and 25% at 3 to 4 weeks. The extracellular matrix is constantly altered by the rapid elimination of fibronectin. There is a slow accumulation of large fibrous bundles of types I collagen, which is composed mainly of three $\alpha$-polypeptide chains intertwined to form a helical structure. The collagen fibrils are composed of molecules arranged in an overlapping configuration; fibril strength is augmented through formation of intermolecular cross-links. Collagen macromolecules provide the healing tissue with stiffness and tensile strength.

Remodeling, the final phase of wound healing, begins simultaneously with granulation and tissue formation, and continues progressively for months after reepithelialization has occurred. Collagen remodeling during scar formation depends on collagen synthesis and degradation, which is initiated by various collagenase enzymes and other proteases secreted by granulocytes, macrophages, epidermal cells, and fibroblasts. Inflammatory cytokines stimulate fibroblasts to increase the synthesis and secretion of collagenase enzymes. In addition to providing structural support and strength to the new tissue, collagen also alters cell function by acting as a chemoattractant for fibroblasts in vivo and in vitro.

In the early stages of scar formation, collagen production exceeds collagen breakdown, which leads to a temporarily hypertrophied scar. As the healing process continues and the overlying epithelium thickens and matures, collagenase production increases and collagen breakdown may exceed collagen formation, causing the scar to regress to a thin, dense white tissue. Derangement in the balance between synthesis and degradation results in a net accumulation of extracellular matrix that can lead to the formation of hypertrophic scars and keloids. These conditions are more frequent in skin than the oral cavity (Clark, 1997).

The extent to which psychoneuroendocrine processes and responses modulate these events remains to be tested experimentally. It is possible that such interactions exist, considering that many of the events of wound healing are mediated by growth factors and cytokines, whose production is finely modulated by neuropeptides and hormones (cf., this volume).

In brief, the principal growth factor involved in wound healing include:

• Platelet derived growth factors (PDGF) are secreted by fibroblasts, vascular endothelial cells, smooth muscle cells, macrophages, platelets, and inflammatory cells. PDGF plays an important role in the inflammatory response, the granulation tissue formation, the scar formation, and the remodeling phases of healing. Binding of PDGF to its receptor results in autophosphorylation of tyrosine, transduction of intracellular signals, and the induction of various early response genes such as c-*fos* and c-*myc*. PDGF functions as a chemoattractant to neutrophils and macrophages and stimulates both chemotaxis and mitogenesis of fibroblasts and smooth muscle cells. PDGF stimulates synthesis of collagen, fibronectin, and hyaluronan and stimulates collagenase activity.

• Transforming growth factor $\beta$ (TGF-$\beta$) is produced by platelets, macrophages, lymphocytes, and tissues such as bone and kidney. TGF-$\beta$ stimulates anchorage-dependent cells to lose contact inhibition and to undergo anchorage independent growth in cell culture and thus plays an important role in embryonic development and in regulating repair and regeneration after tissue injury. TGF-$\beta$ is present at high concentrations in the $\alpha$ granules of platelets and is released during degranulation at the site of injury. TGF-$\beta$ regulates its own production by macrophages in an autocrine manner and can either stimulate (mesenchymal cells such as fibroblasts) or inhibit the proliferation and differentiation of many cell lines (lymphocytes and most epithelial cells) depending on concentration and the presence of other growth factors. TGF-$\beta$ is chemotactic for fibroblasts and macrophages and is one of the most potent stimulants of collagen synthesis and of the synthesis of other extracellular matrix constituents such as fibronectin, hyaluronan, and proteoglycan. TGF-$\beta$ is secreted in a latent (inactive) form, with activation occurring through proteolytic processing of the molecule by plasmin or by exposure to the low pH of the wound environment. Numerous nonneoplastic and neoplastic cells have receptors for TGF-$\beta$. Three major receptor proteins bind to TGF-$\beta$ are type I, type II, and type III, although the type I receptor mediates most of the effects of TGF-$\beta$.

• Epidermal growth factor (EGF) consists of a family of four proteins: EGF, transforming growth factor $\alpha$ (TGF-$\alpha$), amphiregulin, and heparin-binding EGF. They are similar in structure and have the same receptors, which are widely distributed in skin and mucosa. They also have more or less the same biological functions. EGF, first discovered in 1962 in extracts of murine submaxillary glands, is a small (6-kDa) polypeptide of 53 amino acids. Found in a wide variety of tissues such as kidney, lacrimal gland, submandibular gland and Brunner's gland, EGF is present in many secretions including, saliva, tears, and urine. EGF receptors are abundant on epithelial cells, and to a lesser extent on endothelial cells, fibroblasts, and smooth muscle cells. EGF is chemotactic and a potent mitogenic stimulator for epithelial cells, endothelial cells and fibroblasts. EGF stimulates angiogenesis and collagenase activity.

• Fibroblast growth factor (FGF) presents in both an acidic and a basic form ($\alpha$-FGF and $\beta$-FGF), with a 50% homology sequence. $\beta$-FGF (a single chain of 146 amino acids, with a molecular weight of 17 kDa, and the gene located on chromosome 4) is 10 times more potent as an angiogenic stimulant than $\alpha$-FGF. FGF's are produced by fibroblasts, vascular smooth muscle cells, adrenocortical cells, astrocytes, and some tumor cells, chondrocytes, and osteoblasts. $\beta$-FGF stimulates the proliferation of most major cells involved in the process of healing, including, capillary endothelial cells, vascular endothelial cells, fibroblasts and keratinocytes. $\beta$-FGF binds to heparin and heparan sulfate, as well as the extracellular matrix and in basement membranes. $\beta$-FGF favors wound neovascularization by stimulating collagen synthesis, epithelialization, fibronectin, and proteoglycan synthesis.

• Insulin-like growth factors (IGF) I and II—also called somatomedin-C—are structurally related to proinsulin and synthesized as large precursor molecules that are proteolytically cleaved to produce the biological active proteins. IGF-II is more prominent in fetal development, and IGF-I is synthesized mostly by adult tissue such as liver, heart, lung, kidney, pancreas, cartilage, brain, and muscle. IGF-I stimulates mitosis of many cells in vitro such as fibroblasts, osteocytes, and chondrocytes. IGF-I may stimulate wound healing, in synergy with PDGF, by potentiating the regeneration of dermal connective tissue and on epithelial healing, and may act as an autocrine growth factor on fibroblasts and stimulates the formation of collagen by these cells.

• Tumor necrosis factor (TNF)-$\alpha$, a cytostatic and cytolytic agent for many human and murine tumor cells, is a cytokine released by macrophages, which is mitogenic to fibroblasts and which stimulates collagen and collagenase synthesis.

- Vascular endothelial growth factor (VEGF) was recently described to enhance the permeability of local venules and small veins with a potency of 50,000 times that of histamine. Since increased vascular permeability and angiogenesis are characteristic features of wound healing, the role of this factor is imperative in the complex integrated events of wound healing formation and maturation.

## E. Lymphatic Drainage of the Oral Tissues

Immune surveillance of oral tissues is the outcome of concerted events, mediated by cells and factors of the immune system and modulated by neuroendocrine products, that occur primarily locally in structures of the lymphatic system. The stoma is rich in lymphoid tissues, which reveals the intricate nature of the lymphatic drainage of the oral cavity and related structures. The neuroendocrine system regulates lymphokinesis through the lymphatic system systemically (Chiappelli et al., 1993, 1996b) and in the oral cavity specifically (Chiappelli & Kung, 1995).

In brief, the lymphatic system is an intricate circulatory system, which is connected to the venous and the arterial circulatory systems in that the lymph is collected through the thoracic duct and the right lymphatic duct and flows into the left and right internal jugular (or the right and left subclavian) veins. The lymph, an exudate from blood rich in lymphoid cells, flows from the extremities to these ducts by traversing chains of lymph nodes. Naive lymphoid cells generally enter the lymph node by means of the arterial supply, penetrate the parenchyma of the node by crossing the high activated endothelium, engage in activation, proliferation, and maturation following their encounter with antigen-carrying antigen-presenting cells (e.g., dendritic cells, myeloid cells), and exit the medulla of the node via the efferent lymphatic as memory cells. Efferent lymphatics are afferent to the next node in the chain and carry memory cells into the cortical area of this second string of nodes (Chiappelli et al., 1993, 1996b; Chiappelli & Kung, 1995).

In the oral cavity, the vessels of the incisor and canine teeth drain into lymphatics that pass forward to join the anterior facial lymphatics, which drain into the submental and the submandibular nodes and eventually the deep ring of cervical lymph nodes. The vessels from the premolar and the molar teeth run posteriorly to pierce the buccinator and the superior constrictor muscles to drain deep into the upper cervical nodes, which then drain into the deep cervical nodes as well. The vessels from the anterior aspect of the hard palate run anterolaterally to drain into the submandibular nodes; by contrast, the vessels from the posterior aspect of the hard palate drain directly deep through the superior constrictor muscle into the cervical nodes. The extensive drainage from the soft palate drains posterolaterally to join efferent lymphatics from the tonsils into the retropharyngeal and upper deep cervical ring of lymph nodes. The vessels from the cheeks and the mucosa over the buccal aspect of the alveolar processes run deep laterally to pierce the buccinator and to flow into the submandibular nodes. The lips are drained either in the submental or the submandibular nodes; whereas the floor of the mouth is drained anteriorly directly into the deep cervical nodes and posterolaterally into the submandibular and then the deep cervical nodes. The tip of the tongue drains into the submental nodes, whereas the lateral portions and the posterior aspect of the tongue drains into the submandibular and later the deep cervical nodes.

In addition to lymphoid tissue the oral cavity is guarded by tonsillar tissue. Tonsillar tissue is distinct from intraoral lymphoid tissue in that it consists of three paired lymphoid aggregates that share features with the mucosal and the systemic lymphoid tissue. Tonsils form a lymphoid cluster between the oro- and the nasopharynx that signifies the Waldeyer rings, an important immune gate-keeper structure of the oral cavity. The palatine tonsils are situated superiorly between the glosso- and pharingopalatine arches. The lingual tonsils border the tongue posteriorly. The pharyngeal tonsils lie inferiorly to the nasopharyngeal mucosa in the nasopharynx (Chiappelli & Kung, 1995; Chiappelli et al., 1996b).

That systemic lymphoid organs are richly innervated with peptidergic and nonpeptidergic neurons that secrete neurotransmitters locally and may carry information about the activated immune state of the organ to the brain by retrograde transport is known (for review, Brown & Blalock, 1990; Chiappelli et al., 1996b). What is not known is the extent to which this interaction occurs locally in structures of the oral cavity, and the extent to which these interactions, if they occur, mediate pathological and healing processes of the stoma. Studies designed to define and to characterize the neuroendocrine regulation of lymphological processes and structures specific to the oral cavity should gain considerable momentum in the next decade.

# V. PAIN AND TEMPOROMANDIBULAR JOINT DISORDERS

Most, if not all chronic orofacial pain conditions have an immune component, which may participate in the maintenance of chronic pain states. The normal response to tissue injury includes an inflammatory component mediated by the release of neuropeptides (e.g., substance P) from activated nociceptive primary afferent fibers. Stimulation and recruitment of immune cells by substance P results in their proliferation, chemotaxis, and production of cytokines, prostaglandins, opioids, etc. (Helme, Eglezos, & Hosking, 1987b). Cytokines, prostaglandins, and various products of mast cell degranulation contribute to the sensitization of primary afferent fibers in the area surrounding the injury site. Sensitization can also be mediated by CNS mechanisms, such that both peripheral and central mechanisms contribute to the development of hyperalgesia (heightened response). As a result of hyperalgesia in the area around the damaged tissue, the organism tends to protect the area of injury. This facilitates the process of tissue repair and healing.

Selectively damaging the neuropeptide-releasing neurons with capsaicin leads to decreased immune responses to the antigen challenge, which may be restored by introducing exogenous neuropeptides (Helme, Eglezos, Dandie, Andrews, & Boyd, 1987a; Eglezos, Andrews, Boyd, & Helme, 1991). Exogenous neuropeptide application also profoundly enhances repair of damaged skin (Kjartansson & Dalsgaard, 1987). When the inflammation hyperalgesia and pain increase beyond a tolerable threshold or outlast the tissue repair process, then a pathological process obtains. Characterization of the threshold is critical to the understanding of the disease process, and in developing efficacious therapeutics for the treatment of chronic orofacial pain conditions.

That the immune system plays an active role in the development of peripheral inflammation suggests a role of the immune system in the development of persistent hyperalgesic states of the oral cavity. Activation of the immune system in response to systemic infection clearly leads to the development of "illness responses," mediated by the production and action of various cytokines within the CNS. These responses comprise a set of homeostatic physiological and behavioral changes (e.g., fever, decreased water and food intake, decreased digestion, increased sleep) that together enhance the ability of the organism to devote resources to the destruction of the invading antigen (Hart, 1988; Watkins, Maier, & Goehler, 1995a).

Preinflammatory cytokines (IL-1$\beta$, TNF-$\alpha$, and IL-6) play a critical role in producing the illness responses (Watkins, Maier, & Goehler, 1995b). The illness responses are produced not by the direct action of cytokines in the periphery but rather indirectly via the CNS. Hyperalgesia is readily induced by intracerebroventricular (icv) injections of IL-1$\beta$, in the absence of prior peripheral injury or inflammation (Oka, Aou, & Hori, 1993; Watkins et al., 1994). Increased IL-1$\beta$ production in the CNS can initiate a cascade that may culminate in a full-blown acute-phase response (Morimoto, Murakami, Nakamori, Sakata, & Watanabe, 1989). Intramuscular (im) or intraperitoneal (ip) injection of lipopolysaccharide (LPS), a membrane extract of *Escherichia coli*, induces peripheral inflammation and elevations in these cytokines at specific loci within the CNS (Taylor, Chiappelli, & Yirmiya, this volume).

## A. Temporomandibular Joint Disorders and Neuropathic Pain

The immune system plays an important role in the induction and possibly the maintenance of chronic oral inflammatory pain states. While it would seem timely to consider chronic orofacial inflammatory disorders from a psychoneuroimmune perspective, there remains a relative paucity of animal models of orofacial pain and inflammation.

Studies of temporomandibular joint (TMJ) inflammation reveal features distinct from those of other joints. The TMJ is not similar to a typical weight-bearing joint, and its pattern of use is clearly quite different from that of, for instance, the knee. The TMJ differs from most synovial joints in several important respects, including the facts that the articular surfaces consist of fibrous connective tissue rather than hyaline cartilage, the enchondral growth apparatus of the condyle differs structurally from the epiphyseal plates of the long bones and responds differently to experimental stimuli, and a complete articular disc divides the articular space into a superior and inferior compartment. The TMJ is the only articulation with both hinge and sliding movements. The choice of species and sex is important when deciding on an animal model of TMJ dysfunction. For example, the human and guinea-pig TMJ is a closed capsule, whereas the TMJ in rabbits or rats has an open capsule. Use of female animals is also more appropriate, since 70–90% of human patients presenting active TMJ disorders are female (Robinson, 1995).

Even though several laboratories have developed models of acute inflammation of the TMJ (Haas, Nakanishi, MacMillan, Jordan, & Hu, 1992; Okuda-

Akabane, 1994) or craniofacial muscles (Hu, Sessle, Raboisson, Dallel, & Woda, 1992; Yu, Sessle, & Hu, 1993), there is no current literature on the models of chronic TMJ arthritis or chronic orofacial muscle pain. Given that the TMJ arthritis and myofacial pain are considerable clinical problems, this particular area of stomatological psychoneuroimmunology should become a rich field of future research in the next decades.

A similar situation exists with regards to orofacial models of neuropathic pain. Major advances have been made using injury models of the sciatic nerve or spinal roots, and these models of partial afferent nerve injury bear considerable similarity to the human conditions in that they present with hyperalgesia, mechanical allodynia and spontaneous pain (Bennett & Xie, 1988; Seltzer, Dubner, & Shir, 1990; Mosconi & Kruger, 1996). A wealth of information has been gathered on the molecular, anatomic, and functional changes in these neuropathic pain models. The development of norepinephrine sensitivity of injured axons in these models resembles human neuropathic conditions such as reflex sympathetic dystrophy (Korenman & Devor, 1981; Burchiel, 1984; Xie, Zhang, Petersen, & LaMotte, 1995; Perl, 1994), but the immune involvement in the neuropathology of spinal peripheral nerve injury (Frisen, Risling, & Fried, 1993) remains to be fully elucidated.

Few studies have addressed the development of neuropathic pain in the trigeminal region using animal models (Vos, Strassman, & Maciewicz, 1994; Bongenhielm & Robinson, 1998), despite the high incidence of injuries to the inferior alveolar and lingual nerves following surgical procedures such as removal of impacted molar teeth (LaBlanc & Gregg, 1992). These procedures can lead to the development of neuropathic pain (Sandstedt & Sorensen, 1995). *Tic douloureux* (trigeminal neuralgia) is classically described as a neuropathic disorder unique to the trigeminal system for which animal models also need to be developed (King, Meagher, & Barnett, 1956).

Future studies should consider the involvement of cytokines in the development and the maintenance of the chronic orofacial pain states, and determine whether peripheral nerve injury necessarily results in the production of central cytokines and the development of the illness response. Although widespread hyperalgesia is readily induced by intracerebroventricular injections of IL-1$\beta$, or by systemic antigen challenges, the activation of CNS immune components after partial deafferentation is an issue that is far from being resolved.

## B. Fibromyalgia

Fibromyalgia is a noninflammatory rheumatic disorder with chronic widespread musculoskeletal pain in which the musculoskeletal system, the neuroendocrine–immune system, and the CNS appear to play a critical role (Weigent, Bradley, Blalock, & Alarcón, 1998). It is characterized by decreased pain threshold, fatigue, sleep disturbance, and, more often than not, psychological stress (Wolfe, 1995). Patients with fibromyalgia typically have high levels of hyaluronate, low levels of serotonin, and high levels of antibodies to serotonin, gangliosides, and phospholipids. A large proportion of fibromyalgia patients also have a concurrent TMJ dysfunction (McCain & Scudds, 1988; Blasberg & Chalmers, 1989).

Primary fibromyalgia is one of the "stress-associated syndromes" by virtue of onset and exacerbation following acute or chronic physical or emotional stress. Fibromyalgia may be associated with the risk of victimization, particularly adult physical abuse (Amir et al., 1997), and sexual, physical, and emotional trauma appear to be important factors in the development and maintenance of this condition and its associated disability (Walker et al., 1997). Patients with fibromyalgia have significant elevations on anxiety and depression scales (Wolfe et al., 1984). Trait anxiety may also be causally related to symptoms in fibromyalgia (Celiker, Borman, Oktem, Gökçe-Kutsal, & Basgöze, 1997).

Patients with fibromyalgia are usually females (female:male, 50:1), ages 25–40 years. Patients complain of diffuse musculoskeletal aches, pains, or stiffness associated with tiredness (particularly morning stiffness), poor and nonrefreshing sleep, multiple tender points, irritable bowel syndrome, headache, irritable bladder syndrome, dysmenorrhea, subjective swelling in the articular and periarticular areas, and numbness. Laboratory tests and roentgenologic findings in fibromyalgia are normal or negative, but significant biochemical, hormonal, and neurotransmitter abnormalities are evident (Yunus, Masi, Calabro, Miller, & Feigenbaum, 1981; Clauw, 1995).

The symptoms of fibromyalgia may correspond to the illness response, which could result in part from activation of central cytokines and neuropeptides. The cerebrospinal fluid levels in these patients have up to threefold elevated levels of substance P compared to that seen in control subjects (Russell et al., 1994). Higher values of IgG deposits and higher numbers of mast cells are observed in fibromyalgia patients than in controls (Eneström, Bengtsson, & Frodin, 1997). Fibromyalgia patients also present with low serum levels of insulin-like growth factor I (Bennett, Cook,

Clark, Burckhardt, & Campbell, 1997), low peripheral serotonin levels, and low plasma levels of neuropeptide Y, a peptide colocalized with norepinephrine (Neeck & Riedel, 1994).

Patients with fibromyalgia show significant alterations in the regulation of the hypothalamo-pituitary-adrenal and hypothalamo-pituitary-thyroid axes (Neeck & Riedel, 1994). For instance, patients show elevated pituitary ACTH release in response to CRH, concomitantly with low cortisol release. Patients characteristically present with a relative loss of diurnal variation in plasma cortisol and low 24-h urine-free cortisol levels (McCain & Tilbe, 1989). Patients with fibromyalgia have normal plasma DHEA-S levels, but low cortisol/DHEAS ratio (Nilsson, de la Torre, Hedman, Goobar, & Thörner, 1994), as well as an abnormally high prolactin response to thyrotropin-release hormone (TRH).

Prolactin is an anterior pituitary hormone whose secretion is finely regulated by several neuropeptides, by hypothalamic hormones, and by catecholamines. While dopamine, the precursor of norepinephrine, is the major physiologic prolactin inhibiting factor, TRH induces prolactin secretion. Prolactin contributes to the regulation of the menstrual cycle, fertility in women, ovarian function, osmoregulation, as well as immunoregulation (Matsuzaki, Irahara, & Aono, 1997). Taken together, these findings signify the relevance of this condition as an ideal research model for the next generation of psychoneuroimmunologists of the stoma.

## VI. CONCLUSION

Taken together, the pieces of evidence presented in this chapter lead to the realization that a significant number of dental patients (10%, up to 30% for certain populations) suffer from undue anxiety and stress, which is relevant from the viewpoint of psychoneuroimmunology. The principal elements of the psychological and the biological framework of stress research, which are developed at greater length in this volume, are outlined in reference to dental anxiety and stress, as well as in context of other anxiety-laden situations. The characteristics of the dentist/patient dyad in the context of real or perceived dominance/submissiveness and perceived fit of the patient within the environment of the dental visit and the dental procedure clearly relate to psychoneuroendocrine phenomena that enter at play in the processes of immune surveillance and healing of soft and hard structures within the oral cavity.

Heavy metals contained in amalgam may exert a significant degree of psychological and immunological toxicity in a large proportion of dental patients. While the literature remains controversial, it is unquestionable that it must be considered of high importance when addressing research and treatment in oral biology and medicine from a psychoneuroimmunological viewpoint.

The clinical and experimental fields of oral biology and medicine, particularly in terms of the diseases of the soft mucosa, temporomandibular joint disorders, and chronic pain are further rich terrains of psychoneuroimmune endeavors. There exists a wide spectrum of domains from pathologies of the soft mucosa, including oral cancer, to the processes of wound healing and lymphatic drainage, inflammatory processes resulting in chronic and acute pain syndromes that illustrate the breadth of bench research, and clinical research now open as a new frontier in psychoneuroimmunology.

## Acknowledgments

The authors thank Dr. A. N. Taylor, Dr. L. R. Eversole, Dr. E. Manfrini, Dr. E. L. Cooper, Dr. M. Faisal, Dr. Trilla Cajulis-Sekimoto, as well as the many students who took part in the studies presented here. The authors also acknowledge support from Federal and non-Federal sources for these studies: NIAID AI07126, NIDA DA07683, and UCLA Program on Psychoneuroimmunology to F.C.; NIAAA AA09850, UCLA Program on Psychoneuroimmunology to D.H.; NIDR DE10033 and DE 01598 to D.M.; DE 07212 and the Whitehall Foundation to I.S. Additional support for the flow cytometry studies was provided by NIAID AI28697 and NCI CA16042.

## References

Aardal-Eriksson, E., Karlberg, B. E., & Holm, A. C. (1998). Salivary cortisol—An alternative to serum cortisol determinations in dynamic function tests. *Clinical Chemistry and Laboratory Medicine, 36*, 215–222.

Abanomy, A. A., & Nishimura, I. (1997). Molecular cloning of cDNAs expressed in residual ridge soft tissue. *Journal of Dental Research, 76*, 584. [abstract]

Ader, R., Felten, D., & Cohen, N. (Eds.) (1991). *Psychoneuroimmunology*. San Diego, CA: Academic Press.

Agras, W. S., Chapin, N. H., & Oliveau, D. C. (1972). The natural history of phobia. *Archives of General Psychiatry, 26*, 315–317.

Albanes, D. (1987). Caloric intake, body weight, and cancer: A review. *Nutrition and Cancer, 9*, 199–217.

Allen, C. M., Beck, F. M., Rossie, K. M., & Kaul, T. J. (1986). Relation of stress and anxiety to oral lichen planus. *Oral Surgery, Oral Medicine, and Oral Pathology, 61*, 44–46.

Amir, M., Kaplan, Z., Neumann, L., Sharabani, R., Shani, N., & Buskila, D. (1997). Posttraumatic stress disorder, tenderness and fibromyalgia. *Journal of Psychosomatic Research, 42*, 607–613.

André, J., Laporte, M., & Delavault, P. (1990). Lichen planus: Etiopathogenesis. *Acta Stomatologica Belgica, 87*, 229–231.

Andrews, V. H., & Hall, H. R. (1990). The effects of relaxation/imagery training on recurrent aphthous stomatitis: A preliminary study. *Psychosomatic Medicine, 52*(5), 526–535.

Barnard, N. A., Scully, C., Eveson, J. W., Cunningham, S., & Porter, S. R. (1993). Oral cancer development in patients with oral lichen planus. *Journal of Oral Pathology and Medicine, 22,* 421–424.

Ben-Eliyahu, S., Page, G. G., Yirmiya, R., & Taylor, A. N. (1996). Acute alcohol intoxication suppresses natural killer cell activity and promotes tumor metastasis. *Nature Medicine, 2,* 457–460.

Bennett, G. J., & Xie, Y. K. (1988). A peripheral mononeuropathy in rat that produces disorders of pain sensation like those seen in man. *Pain, 33,* 87–107.

Bennett, R. M., Cook, D. M., Clark, S. R., Burckhardt, C. S., & Campbell, S. M. (1997). Hypothalamic-pituitary-insulin-like growth factor-I axis dysfunction in patients with fibromyalgia. *Journal of Rheumatology, 24,* 1384–1389.

Berger, M. R., Berger, I., & Schmahl, D. (1991). Vitamins and cancer. In I. R. Rowland (Ed.), *Nutrition, toxicity and cancer* (pp. 517–548). Ann Arbor, MI: CRC Press.

Besedovsky, H. O., & del Rey, A. (1996). Immune–neuro-endocrine interactions: Facts and hypotheses. *Endocrine Reviews, 17,* 64–102.

Blalock, J. E. (1994). The syntax of immune–neuroendocrine communication. *Immunology Today, 15,* 504–511.

Blasberg, B., & Chalmers, A. (1989). Temporomandibular pain and dysfunction syndrome associated with generalized musculoskeletal pain: A retrospective study. *Journal of Rheumatology, 19,* 87–90.

Blot, W. J., McLaughlin, J. K., Winn, D. M., Austin, D. F., Greenberg, R. S., Preston-Martin, S. Bernstein, L., Schoenberg, J. B. Stemhagen, A., & Fraumeni, J. F. Jr. (1988). Smoking and drinking in relation to oral and pharyngeal cancer. *Cancer Research, 48,* 3282–3287.

Bolewska, J., & Reibel, J., (1989). T lymphocytes, Langerhans cells and HLA-DR expression on keratinocytes in oral lesions associated with amalgam restorations. *Journal of Oral Pathology and Medicine, 18,* 525–528.

Bongenhielm, U., & Robinson, P. P. (1998). Afferent activity from myelinated inferior alveolar nerve fibres in ferrets after constriction or section and regeneration. *Pain, 74,* 123–132.

Bricker S. L. (1994). Oral lichen planus: A review. *Seminars in Dermatology, 13*(2), 87–90.

Brickman, P. (1982). Models of helping and coping. *American Psychologist, 37,* 368–384.

Brown, S. L., & Blalock, J. E. (1990). Neuroendocrine immune interactions. In J. J. Oppenheimer & E. M. Shevach (Eds.), *Immunophysiology: The role of cells and cytokines in immunity and inflammation* (chapter 17). Oxford: Oxford University Press.

Buajeeb, W., Laohapand, P., Vongsavan, N., & Kraivaphan, P. (1990). Anxiety in recurrent aphthous stomatitis patients. *Journal of the Dental Association of Thailand, 40,* 253–258.

Buño, I. J., Huff, J. C., Weston, W. L., Cook, D. T., & Brice, S. L. (1998). Elevated levels of interferon gamma, tumor necrosis factor alpha, interleukins 2, 4, and 5, but not interleukin 10, are present in recurrent aphthous stomatitis. *Archives of Dermatology, 134,* 827–831.

Burchiel, K. J. (1984). Spontaneous impulse generation in normal and denervated dorsal root ganglia: Sensitivity to alpha-adrenergic stimulation and hypoxia. *Experimental Neurology, 85,* 257–272.

Burkhart, N. W, Burker, E. J., Burkes, E. J., & Wolfe, L. (1996). Assessing the characteristics of patients with oral lichen planus. *Journal of the American Dental Association, 127,* 648, 651–652, 655–656 passim.

Cannon, W. (1929). *Bodily changes in pain, humger, fear and rage.* Boston, MA: Brandford.

Celiker, R., Borman, P., Oktem, F., Gökçe-Kutsal, Y., & Basgöze, O. (1997). Psychological disturbance in fibromyalgia: Relation to pain severity. *Clinical Rheumatology, 16,* 179–184.

Chiappelli, F. (1985). Research in stress and the relevance of counseling psychology to public health. *Health in transition: UCLA Journal of Public Health, 1,* 33–36.

Chiappelli, F., Franceschi, C., Ottaviani, E., Farné, M., & Faisal, M. (1993). Phylogeny of the neuroendocrine-immune system: Fish and shellfish as a model system for social interaction stress research in humans. *Annual Review of Fish Disease, 3,* 327–346.

Chiappelli, F., Franceschi, C., Ottaviani, E., Solomon, G. F., & Taylor, A. N. (1996a). Neuroendocrine modulation of the immune system. In R. Greger, H.-P. Koepchen, W. Mommaerts, & U. Winhorst (Eds). *Human physiology: From cellular mechanisms to integration* (Section L, chapter 90). New York, NY: Springer.

Chiappelli, F., & Kung, MA. (1995). Immune surveillance of the oral cavity and lymphocyte migration: Relevance for alcohol abusers. *Lymphology, 28,* 196–207.

Chiappelli, F., Kung, M. A., Nguyen, P., Villanueva, P., Farhadian, E. A., & Eversole, L. R. (1997). Cellular immune correlates of clinical severity in oral lichen planus: Preliminary association with mood states. *Oral Diseases, 3,* 64–70.

Chiappelli, F., Kung, M. A., Savage, M., Villanueva, P., & Fiala, M. (1996b). Nicotine and ethanol modulation of cell-mediated immune surveillance of oral squamous cell carcinoma. *International Journal of Oral Biology, 21,* 19–27.

Chiappelli, F., Kung, M. A., Stefanini, G. F., & Foschi, F. G. (1998). Alcohol and immune function. In M. E. Gershwin, B. German, & C. L. Keen (Eds.). *Nutrition and immunology: Principles and practice* (chapter 23). Totowa, NJ: Humana Press.

Chiappelli, F., & Liu N. Q. (1999). Non-mammalian models of neuroendocrine–immune modulation: Relevance for research in oral biology and medicine. *International Journal of Oral Biology* (in press).

Chiappelli, F., & Trignani, S. (1993). Neuroendocrine–immune interactions: Implications for clinical research. *Advances in the Biosciences, 90,* 185–198.

Clark, R. A. F. (1997). Wound repair: Overview and general considerations. In R. A. F. Clark, (Ed.), *The molecular and cellular biology of wound repair* (pp. 3–35). Plenum: New York, NY.

Clauw, D. J. (1995). Fibromyalgia: More than just a musculoskeletal disease. *American Family Physician, 52,* 843–851 and 853–854.

Cole, K. L., Seymour, G. J., & Powell, R. N. (1987). Phenotypic and functional analysis of T cells extracted from chronically inflamed human periodontal tissues. *Journal of Periodontology, 58,* 569–573.

Colella, G., Gritti, P., De Luca, F., & de Vito, M. (1993). The psychopathological aspects of oral lichen planus (OLP). *Minerva Stomatologica, 42,* 265–270.

Conway, T. L., Vickers, R. R., & French, J. R. (1992). An application of person-environment fit theory: Perceived versus desired control. *Journal of Social Issues, 48,* 95–107.

Daum, J. R., Shepherd, D. M., & Noelle, R. J. (1993). Immunotoxicology of cadmium and mercury on B-lymphocytes. I. Effects on lymphocyte function. *International Journal of Immunopharmacology, 15,* 383–394.

Doerr, P. A., Lang, W. P., Nyquist, L. V., & Ronis, D. L. (1998). Factors associated with dental anxiety. *Journal of the American Dental Association, 129,* 1111–1119.

Dorgan, J. F., & Schatzkin, A. (1991). Antioxidant micronutrients in cancer prevention. *Hematology/Oncology Clinics of North America, 5,* 43–68.

Dreyer, W. P. (1983). The clinical manifestations of oral lichen planus. *Journal of the Dental Association of South Africa, 38,* 619–624.

Dubey, D., Kuhn, J., Vial, M. C., Druet, P., & Bellon, B. (1993). Anti-interleukin-2 receptor monoclonal antibody therapy supports a role for Th1-like cells in HgCl$_2$-induced autoimmunity in rats. *Scandinavian Journal of Immunology, 37*, 406–412.

Eglezos, A., Andrews, P. V., Boyd, R. L., & Helme, R. D. (1991). Tachykinin-mediated modulation of the primary antibody response in rats: Evidence for mediation by an NK-2 receptor. *Journal of Neuroimmunology, 32*, 11–18.

Eneström, S., Bengtsson, A., & Frodin, T. (1997). Dermal IgG deposits and increase of mast cells in patients with fibromyalgia—Relevant findings or epiphenomena? *Scandinavian Journal of Rheumatology, 26*, 308–313.

Eversole, L. R. (1992). Diseases should not be considered entities unto themselves. *Oral Surgery, Oral Medicine, and Oral Pathology, 73*, 707.

Eversole, L. R. (1994). Immunopathology of oral mucosal ulcerative, desquamative, and bullous diseases. Selective review of the literature. *Oral Surgery, Oral Medicine, and Oral Pathology, 77*, 555–571.

Eversole, L. R., Shopper, T. P., & Chambers, D. W. (1982). Effects of suspected foodstuff challenging agents in the etiology of recurrent aphthous stomatitis. *Oral Surgery, Oral Medicine, and Oral Pathology, 54*, 338.

Fife, A., Beasley, P. J., & Fertig, D. L. (1996). Psychoneuroimmunology and cancer: Historical perspectives and current research. *Advances in Neuroimmunology, 6*, 179–190.

Freeman, R. (1997). The triangle of health. 1. The clinical arena. *Dental Update, 24*, 61–63.

Frisen, J., Risling, M., and Fried, K. (1993). Distribution and axonal relations of macrophages in a neuroma. *Neuroscience, 55*, 1003–1013.

Futterman, A. D., Kemeny, M. E., Shapiro, D., & Fahey, J. L. (1994). Immunological and physiological changes associated with induced positive and negative mood. *Psychosomatic Medicine, 56*, 499–511.

Gauro, M., Hernández Vicente, I., Unamuno Pérez, P., & Martin-Pascual, A. (1977). Psychosomatic aspects of alopecia areata and lichen. *Actas Dermo-Sifiliograficas, 68*, 563–568.

Giddon, D. B. (1966). Psychophysiology of the oral cavity. *Journal of Dental Research, 45*, 1627–1629.

Glaser, R., Rice, J., Sheridan, J., Fertel, R., Stout, J., Speicher, C., Pinsky, D., Kotur, M., Post, A., Beck, M., et al. (1987). Stress-related immune suppression: Health implications. *Brain, Behavior, and Immunity, 1*, 7–20.

Gordon, S. M., Dionne, R. A., & Snyder, J. (1998). Dental fear and anxiety as a barrier to accessing oral health care among patients with special health care needs. *Special Care in Dentistry, 18*, 88–92.

Grandjean, P., Guldager, B., Larsen, I. B., Jørgensen, P. J., & Holmstrup, P. (1997). Placebo response in environmental disease. Chelation therapy of patients with symptoms attributed to amalgam fillings. *Journal of Occupational and Environmental Medicine, 39*, 707–714.

Graykowski, E. A., Barile, M. F., Lee, W. B., & Stanley, H. R., Jr. (1966). Recurrent aphthous stomatitis. Clinical, therapeutic, histopathologic, and hypersensitivity aspects. *JAMA, 196*, 637–644.

Griep, E. N., Boersma, J. W., & de Kloet, E. R. (1993). Altered reactivity of the hypothalamic-pituitary-adrenal axis in the primary fibromyalgia syndrome. *Journal of Rheumatology, 20*, 469–474.

Gross, J. J., & Levenson, R. W. (1993). Emotional suppression: Physiology, self-report, and expressive behavior. *Journal of Personality and Social Psychology, 64*, 970–986.

Haas, D. A., Nakanishi, O., MacMillan, R. E., Jordan, R. C., & Hu, J. W. (1992). Development of an orofacial model of acute inflammation in the rat. *Archives in Oral Biology, 37*, 417–422.

Hampf, B. G., Malmström, M. J., Aalberg, V. A., Hannula, J. A., & Vikkula, J. (1987). Psychiatric disturbance in patients with oral lichen planus. *Oral Surgery, Oral Medicine, and Oral Pathology, 63*, 429–432.

Hart, B. L. (1988). Biological basis of the behavior of sick animals. *Neuroscience and Biobehavioral Review, 12*, 123–137.

Heijnen, C. J., Kavelaars, A., & Ballieux, R. E. (1991). $\beta$-Endorphin: Cytokine and neuropeptide. *Immunological Reviews, 119*, 41–63.

Helme, R. D., Eglezos, A., Dandie, G. W., Andrews, P. V., & Boyd, R. L. (1987a). The effect of substance P on the regional lymph node antibody response to antigenic stimulation in capsaicin-pretreated rats. *Journal of Immunology, 139*, 3470–3473.

Helme, R. D., Eglezos, A., and Hosking, C. S. (1987b). Substance P induces chemotaxis of neutrophils in normal and capsaicin-treated rats. *Immunology and Cell Biology, 65*, 267–269.

Hilliard-Lysen, J., & Riemer, J. W. (1988). Occupational stress and suicide among dentists. *Deviant Behavior, 9*, 333–341.

Hodgson, D. M., Chiappelli, F., Kung, M. A., Tio, D. L., Morrow, N. S., & Taylor, A. N. (1996). Effect of acute dietary restriction on the colonization of MADB106 tumor cells in the rat. *Neuroimmunomodulation, 3*, 371–380.

Hodgson, D. M., Chiappelli, F., Kung, M. A., Tio, D. L., Morrow, N. S., & Taylor, A. N. (1997). Chronic dietary restriction inhibits colonization of MADB106 tumor cells in the rat. *Nutrition and Cancer, 28*, 189–198.

Hodgson, D. M., Yirmiya, R., Chiappelli, F., & Taylor, A. N. (1998). Intracerebral HIV glycoprotein (gp120) enhances tumor metastasis via centrally released interleukin-1. *Brain Research, 781*, 244–251.

Hu, J. W., Sessle, B. J., Raboisson, P. Dallel, R., & Woda, A. (1992). Stimulation of craniofacial muscle afferents induces prolonged facilitatory effects in trigeminal nociceptive brain-stem neurones. *Pain, 48*, 53–60.

Ibbotson, S. H., Speight, E. L., Macleod, R. I., Smart, E. R., & Lawrence, C. M. (1996). The relevance and effect of amalgam replacement in subjects with oral lichenoid reactions. *British Journal of Dermatology, 134*, 420–423.

Irwin, M., Patterson, T., Smith, T. L., Caldwell, C., Brown, S. A., Gillin, J. C., & Grant, I. (1990). Reduction of immune function in life stress and depression. *Biological Psychiatry, 27*, 22–30.

Jacobi, A. (1894). Stomatitis neurotica chronica. *Transactions of the Association of American Physicians, 9*, 279–285.

Karagouni, E. E., Dotsika, E. N., & Sklavounou, A. (1994). Alteration in peripheral blood mononuclear cell function and serum cytokines in oral lichen planus. *Journal of Oral Pathology and Medicine, 23*, 28–35.

Kaur, J., Srivastava, A., & Ralhan, R. (1998). Prognostic significance of p53 protein overexpression in betel- and tobacco-related oral oncogenesis. *International Journal of Cancer, 79*, 370–375.

King, R. B., Meagher, J. N., & Barnett, J. C. (1956). Studies of trigeminal nerve potentials in normal compared to abnormal experimental preparations. *Journal of Neurosurgery, 13*, 176.

Kjartansson, J., & Dalsgaard, C. J. (1987). Calcitonin gene-related peptide increases survival of a musculocutaneous critical flap in the rat. *European Journal of Pharmacology, 142*, 355–358.

Konttinen, Y. T., Jungell, P., Bergroth, V., Hampf, G., Kemppinen, P., & Malmström, M. (1989). PHA stimulation of peripheral blood lymphocytes in oral lichen planus. Abnormality localized between interleukin-2 receptor ligand formation and gamma-interferon secretion. *Journal of Clinical and Laboratory Immunology, 28*, 33–7.

Korenman, E. M., & Devor, M. (1981). Ectopic adrenergic sensitivity in damaged peripheral nerve axons in the rat. *Experimental Neurology, 72*, 63–81.

Kotwall, C., Razack, M. S., Sako, K., & Rao, U. (1989). Multiple primary cancers in squamous cell cancer of the head and neck. *Journal of Surgical Oncology, 40*, 97–99.

LaBlanc, J. P., & Gregg, J. M. (1992). Trigeminal nerve injuries. Basic problems, historical perspectives, early successes and remaining challenges. In J. P. LaBlanc & J. M. Gregg (Eds.), *Oral and maxillofacial surgery clinics of North America: Trigeminal nerve injury: Diagnosis and management* (pp. 227-283). Philadelphia, PA: Saunders.

Lazarus, R. S. (1991). Psychological stress in the workplace. Special Issue: Handbook on job stress. *Journal of Social Behavior and Personality, 6*, 1–13.

Lehner, T. (1978). Immunological aspects of recurrent oral ulceration and Behçet's syndrome. *Journal of Oral Pathology, 7*, 424–430.

Li, M. H., Ji, C., & Cheng, S. J. (1986). Occurrence of nitroso compounds in fungi-contaminated foods: A review. *Nutrition and Cancer, 8*, 63–69.

Lijinsky, W. (1987). Carcinogenicity and mutagenicity of N-nitroso compounds. *Molecular Toxicology, 1*, 107–119.

Lind, P. O., Hurlen, B., Lyberg, T., & Aas, E. (1986). Amalgam-related oral lichenoid reaction. *Scandinavian Journal of Dental Research, 94*, 448–451.

Lippman, S. M., Batsakis, J. G., Toth, B. B., Weber, R. S., Lee, J. J., Martin, J. W., Hays, G. L., Goepfert, H., & Hong, W. K. (1993). Comparison of low-dose isotretinoin with beta-carotene to prevent oral carcinogenesis. *New England Journal of Medicine, 328*, 15–20.

Litchfield, N. B. (1989). Stress-related problems of dentists. *International Journal of Psychosomatics, 36*, 41–44.

Logan, H. L., Lutgendorf, S., Hartwig, A., Lilly, J., & Berberich, S. L. (1998). Immune, stress, and mood markers related to recurrent oral herpes outbreaks. *Oral Surgery, Oral Medicine, Oral Pathology, Oral Radiology and Endodontics, 86*, 48–54.

Lozada-Nur, F., & Miranda, C. (1987). Oral lichen planus: Epidemiology, clinical characteristics, and associated diseases. *Seminars in Cutaneous Medicine and Surgery, 16*, 273–277.

Lozano, J.-C., Nakazawa, H., Cross, M.-P., Cabral R., & Yamasaki, H. G. (1994). A mutationsin p53 and Ha ras genes in esophageal papillomas induced by N-nitrosomethylbenzylamine in two strains of rats. *Molecular Carcinogenesis, 9*, 33–39.

MacPhail, L. (1997). Topical and systemic therapy for recurrent aphthous stomatitis. *Seminars in Cutaneous Medicine and Surgery, 16*, 301–307.

MacPhail, L. A., & Greenspan, J. S. (1997). Oral ulceration in HIV infection: Investigation and pathogenesis. *Oral Diseases, 3*, S190-S103.

Matsuzaki, T., Irahara, M., & Aono, T. (1977). Physiology and action of prolactin. *Japanese Journal of Clinical Medicine, 55*, 2871–2875.

Mazey, K. A. (1994). Stress in the dental office. *CDA Journal, 22*, 13–19.

Mazey, K. A., & Mito, R. S. (1993). Multidisciplinary treatment of dental phobia. *CDA Journal, 21*, 17–25.

McCain, G. A., & Scudds, R. A. (1988). The concept of primary fibromyalgia (fibrositis): Clinical value, relation and significance to other chronic musculoskeletal pain syndromes. *Pain, 33*, 273–287.

McCain, G. A., & Tilbe, K. S. (1989). Diurnal hormone variation in fibromyalgia syndrome: A comparison with rheumatoid arthritis. *Journal of Rheumatology, 19*, 154–157.

McCarthy, P. L., & Shklar, G. (1980). *Diseases of the oral mucosa* (2nd ed.). Philadelphia: Lea & Fabiger.

McCartan, B. E. (1995). Psychological factors associated with oral lichen planus. *Journal of Oral Pathology and Medicine, 24*, 273–275.

McCartan, B. E., Lamey, P. J., & Wallace, A. M. (1996). Salivary cortisol and anxiety in recurrent aphthous stomatitis. *Journal of Oral Pathology and Medicine, 25*, 357–359.

Morimoto, A., Murakami, N., Nakamori, T., Sakata, Y., & Watanabe, T. (1989). Brain regions involved in the development of acute phase responses accompanying fever in rabbits. *Journal of Physiology (London), 416*, 645–657.

Mosconi, T., & Kruger, L. (1996). Fixed-diameter polyethylene cuffs applied to the rat sciatic nerve induce a painful neuropathy: Ultrastructural morphometric analysis of axonal alterations. *Pain, 64*, 37–57.

Moszczynski, P., & Slowinski, S. (1994). The behaviour of T-cell subpopulations in the blood of workers exposed to mercury. *Medicina del Lavoro, 85*, 239–241.

Nakashima, I., Pu, M. Y., Nishizaki, A., Rosila, I., Ma, L., Katano, Y., Ohkusu, K., Rahman, S. M., Isobe, K., & Hamaguchi, M., et al. (1994). Redox mechanism as alternative to ligand binding for receptor activation delivering disregulated cellular signals. *Journal of Immunology, 152*, 1064–1071.

Neeck, G., & Riedel, W. (1994). Neuromediator and hormonal perturbations in fibromyalgia syndrome: Results of chronic stress? *Baillieres Clinical Rheumatology, 8*, 763–775.

Nilsson, E., de la Torre, B., Hedman, M., Goobar, J., & Thörner, A. (1994). Blood dehydroepiandrosterone sulphate (DHEAS) levels in polymyalgia rheumatica/giant cell arteritis and primary fibromyalgia. *Clinical and Experimental Rheumatology, 12*, 415–417.

Oka, T., Aou, S., & Hori, T. (1993). Intracerebroventricular injection of interleukin-1 beta induces hyperalgesia in rats. *Brain Research, 624*, 61–68.

Okuda-Akabane, K. (1994). Hyperalgesic change over the craniofacial area following urate crystal injection into the rabbit's temporomandibular joint. *Journal of Oral Rehabilitation, 21*, 311–322.

O'Shea, R. M., & Corah, N. L. (1984). Sources of dentists' stress. *Journal of American Dental Association, 109*, 48–51.

Ostman, P. O., Anneroth, G., & Skoglund, A. (1994). Oral lichen planus lesions in contact with amalgam fillings: A clinical, histologic, and immunohistochemical study. *Scandinavian Journal of Dental Research, 102*, 172–179.

Panerai, A. E., & Sacerdote, P. (1997). Beta-endorphin in the immune system: A role at last? *Immunology Today, 18*, 317–319.

Pang, B. K., & Freeman, S. (1995). Oral lichenoid lesions caused by allergy to mercury in amalgam fillings. *Contact Dermatitis, 33*, 423–427.

Park, N.-H., Min, B.-M., Li, S. L., Cherrick, H. M., & Doniger, J. (1991). Immortalization of normal human oral keratinocytes with type-16 human papillomavirus. *Carcinogenesis, 12*, 1627–1631.

Parker, S. L., Tong, T., Bolden, S., & Wingo, P. A. (1997). Cancer statistics, 1997. *Ca: A Cancer Journal for Clinicians, 47*, 5–27.

Parkin, D. M., Läärä, E., & Muir, C. S. (1988). Estimates of the worldwide frequency of sixteen major cancers in 1980. *International Journal of Cancer, 41*(2), 184–197.

Pedersen, A., Hougen, H. P., & Kenrad, B. (1992). T-lymphocyte subsets in oral mucosa of patients with recurrent aphthous ulceration. *Journal of Oral Pathology and Medicine, 21*, 176–180.

Pedersen, A., Klausen, B., Hougen, H. P., & Ryder, L. P. (1991). Peripheral lymphocyte subpopulations in recurrent aphthous ulceration. *Acta Odontologica Scandinavica, 49*, 203–206.

Pedersen, A., & Pedersen, B. K. (1993). Natural killer cell function and number of peripheral blood are not altered in recurrent aphthous ulceration. *Oral Surgery, Oral Medicine, and Oral Pathology, 76*, 616–619.

Perl, E. R. (1994). Causalgia and reflex sympathetic dystrophy revisited. In J. Boivie, P. Hanson, & U. Lindblom (Eds.), *Touch, temperature, and pain in health and disease: Mechanisms and assessments.* Seattle, WA: IASP Press.

Perrin, C., Astre, C., Broquerie, E., Saint Aubert, B., & Joyeux, A. (1990). Lingual fibrosarcoma induced by 7,12-dimethylbenzanthracene in the rat. *Journal of Oral Pathology and Medicine, 19*, 13–15.

Pogrel, M. A., & Weldon, L. L. (1983). Carcinoma arising in erosive lichen planus in the midline of the dorsum of the tongue. *Oral Surgery, Oral Medicine, and Oral Pathology, 55*, 62–66.

Porter, S. R., Kirby, A., Olsen, I., & Barrett, W. (1997). Immunologic aspects of dermal and oral lichen planus: A review. *Oral Surgery, Oral Medicine, Oral Pathology, Oral Radiology and Endodontics, 83*, 358–366.

Porter, K., Klouda, P., Scully, C., Bidwell, J., & Porter, S. (1993). Class I and II HLA antigens in British patients with oral lichen planus. *Oral Surgery, Oral Medicine, and Oral Pathology, 75*, 176–180.

Ragnarsson, E. (1998). Dental fear and anxiety in an adult Icelandic population. *Acta Odontologica Scandinavica, 56*, 100–104.

Robin, O., Alaoui-Ismaïli, O., Dittmar, A., & Vernet-Maury, E. (1998). Emotional responses evoked by dental odors: An evaluation from autonomic parameters. *Journal of Dental Research, 77*, 1638–1646.

Robinson, P. D. (1995). A review of temporomandibular joint pain. *Pain Reviews, 2*, 138–151.

Rodríguez-Archilla, A., Urquía, M., Gómez-Moreno, G., & Ceballos, A. (1994). Anti-DNA antibodies and circulating immune complexes (C1q-IgG) in recurrent aphtous stomatitis. *Bulletin du Groupement International pour la Recherche Scientifique en Stomatologie et Odontologie, 37*, 31–35.

Rogers, R. S., III (1997). Recurrent aphthous stomatitis: Clinical characteristics and associated systemic disorders. *Seminars in Cutaneous Medicine and Surgery, 16*, 278–283.

Russell, I. J., Orr, M. D., Littman B., Vipraio, G. A., Alboukrek, D., Michalek, J. E., Lopez, Y., & MacKillip, F. (1994). Elevated cerebrospinal fluid levels of substance P in patients with the fibromyalgia syndrome. *Arthritis and Rheumatism, 37*, 1593–1601.

Sabbadini, E., & Berczi, I. (1995). The submandibular gland: A key organ in the neuro-immuno-regulatory network? *Neuroimmunomodulation, 2*, 184–202.

Sandstedt, P., & Sorensen, S. (1995). Neurosensory disturbances of the trigeminal nerve: A long-term follow-up of traumatic injuries. *Journal of Oral Maxillofacial Surgery, 53*, 498–505.

Sapolsky, R. M., Krey, L. C., & McEwen, B. S. (1986). The neuroendocrinology of stress and aging: The glucocorticoid cascade hypothesis. *Endocrine Review, 7*, 284–301.

Selye, H. (1976). *The stress of life.* New York, NY: McGraw-Hill.

Seltzer, Z., Dubner, R., & Shir, Y. (1990). A novel behavioral model of neuropathic pain disorders produced in rats by partial sciatic nerve injury. *Pain, 43*, 205–218.

Shenker, B. J., Berthold, P., Decker, S., Mayro, J., Rooney, C., Vitale, L., & Shapiro, I. M. (1992a). Immunotoxic effects of mercuric compounds on human lymphocytes and monocytes. II. Alterations in cell viability. *Immunopharmacology and Immunotoxicology, 14*, 555–577.

Shenker, B. J., Guo, T. L., & Shapiro, I. M. (1998). Low-level methylmercury exposure causes human T-cells to undergo apoptosis: Evidence of mitochondrial dysfunction. *Environmental Research, 77*, 149–159.

Shenker, B. J., Mayro, J. S., Rooney, C., Vitale, L., & Shapiro, I. M. (1993b). Immunotoxic effects of mercuric compounds on human lymphocytes and monocytes. IV. Alterations in cellular glu-

tathione content. *Immunopharmacology and Immunotoxicology, 15*, 273–290.

Shenker, B. J., Rooney, C., Vitale, L., & Shapiro, I. M. (1992b). Immunotoxic effects of mercuric compounds on human lymphocytes and monocytes. I. Suppression of T-cell activation. *Immunopharmacology and Immunotoxicology, 14*, 539–553.

Shin, K.-H., Moo, B.-M., Cherrick, H. M., & Park, N.-H. (1994). Combined effects of human papillomavirus-18 and N-methyl-N-nitro-N-nitrosoguanidine on the transformation of human oral keratinocytes. *Molecular Carcinogenesis, 9*, 76–86.

Siblerud, R. L., Motl, J., & Kienholz, E. (1994). Psychometric evidence that mercury from silver dental fillings may be an etiological factor in depression, excessive anger, and anxiety. *Psychological Reports, 74*, 67–80.

Sibley, W. N. (1899). Neurotic ulcers of the mouth. *British Medical Journal, 1*, 900–905.

Silverman, S., Jr., Gorsky, M., & Lozada-Nur, F. (1985). A prospective follow-up study of 570 patients with oral lichen planus: Persistence, remission, and malignant association. *Oral Surgery, Oral Medicine, and Oral Pathology, 60*, 30–34.

Simon, M., Jr., Reimer, G., Schardt, M., & Hornstein, O. P. (1983). Lymphocytotoxicity for oral mucosa in lichen planus. *Dermatologica, 167*, 11–15.

Singer, B. (1979). N-Nitroso alkylating agents: Formation and persistence of alkyl derivatives in mammalian nucleic acids as contributing factors in carcinogenesis. *Journal of the National Cancer Institute, 62*, 1329–1339.

Skare, I., & Engqvist, A. (1994). Human exposure to mercury and silver released from dental amalgam restorations. *Archives of Environmental Health, 49*, 384–394.

Solomon, G. F., & Amkraut, A. A. (1981). Psychoneuroendocrinological effects on the immune response. *Annual Review of Microbiology, 35*, 155–184.

Steffensen, I. L., Mesna, O. J., Andruchow, E., Namork, E., Hylland, K., & Andersen, R. A. (1994). Cytotoxicity and accumulation of Hg, Ag, Cd, Cu, Pb and Zn in human peripheral T and B lymphocytes and monocytes in vitro. *General Pharmacology, 25*, 1621–1633.

Stein, M., Miller, A. H., & Trestman, R. L (1991). Depression, the immune system, and health and illness. Findings in search of meaning. *Archives of General Psychiatry, 48*, 171–177.

Stenman, G., & Heyden, G. (1980). Premonitory stages of recurrent aphthous stomatitis. Histological and enzyme histochemical investigations. *Journal of Oral Pathology, 9*, 155–162

Sugerman, P. B., Savage, N. W., & Seymour, G. J. (1993a). Clonal expansion of lymphocytes from oral lichen planus lesions. *Journal of Oral Pathology and Medicine, 22*, 126–131.

Sugerman, P. B., Savage, N. W., Walsh, L. J., & Seymour, G. J. (1993b). Disease mechanisms in oral lichen planus. A possible role for autoimmunity. *Australasian Journal of Dermatology, 34*, 63–69.

Sugerman, P. B., Voltz, M. J., Savage, N. W., Basford, K. E., & Seymour, G. J. (1992). Phenotypic and functional analysis of peripheral blood lymphocytes in oral lichen planus. *Journal of Oral Pathology and Medicine, 21*, 445–450.

Swartzendruber, D. E. (1993). The possible relationship between mercury from dental amalgam and diseases. I. Effects within the oral cavity. *Medical Hypotheses, 41*, 31–34.

Syrjanen, S. M. (1992). Viral infectionsin oral mucosa. *Scandinavian Journal of Dental Research, 100*, 17–31.

Tan, X. X., Tang, C., Castoldi, A. F., Manzo, L., & Costa, L. G. (1993). Effects of inorganic and organic mercury on intracellular calcium levels in rat T lymphocytes. *Journal of Toxicology and Environmental Health, 38*, 159–170.

Vos, B. P. Strassman, A. M., & Maciewicz, R. J. (1994). Behavioral evidence of trigeminal neuropathic pain following chronic constriction injury to the rat's infraorbital nerve. *Journal of the Neurosciences, 14,* 2708–2723.

Walker, E. A., Keegan, D., Gardner, G., Sullivan, M., Bernstein, D., & Katon, W. J. (1997). Psychosocial factors in fibromyalgia compared with rheumatoid arthritis. II. Sexual, physical, and emotional abuse and neglect. *Psychosomatic Medicine, 59,* 572–577.

Walsh, L. J., Tseng, P. W., Savage, N. W., & Seymour, G. J. (1989). Expression of CDw29 and CD45R antigens on epithelial cells in oral lichen planus. *Journal of Oral Pathology and Medicine, 18,* 360–365.

Walton, L. J., Macey, M. G., Thornhill, M. H., & Farthing, P. M. (1998). Intra-epithelial subpopulations of T lymphocytes and Langerhans cells in oral lichen planus. *Journal of Oral Pathology and Medicine, 27,* 116–123.

Walton, L. J., Thornhill, M. H., & Farthing, P. M. (1994). VCAM-1 and ICAM-1 are expressed by Langerhans cells, macrophages and endothelial cells in oral lichen planus. *Journal of Oral Pathology and Medicine, 23,* 262–268.

Watkins, L. R., Maier, S. F., & Goehler, L. E. (1995a). Immune activation: The role of pro-inflammatory cytokines in inflammation, illness responses and pathological pain states. *Pain, 63,* 289–302.

Watkins, L. R., Maier, S. F., & Goehler, L. E. (1995b). Cytokine-to-brain communication: A review and analysis of alternative mechanisms. *Life Sciences, 57,* 1011–1026.

Watkins, L. R., Wiertelak, E. P., Goehler, L. E., Smith, K. P., Martin, D., & Maier, S. F. (1994). Characterization of cytokine-induced hyperalgesia. *Brain Research, 654,* 15–26.

Weigent, D. A., Bradley, L. A., Blalock, J. E., & Alarcón, G. S. (1998). Current concepts in the pathophysiology of abnormal pain perception in fibromyalgia. *American Journal of the Medical Sciences, 315,* 405–412.

Weiner, B. (1985). An attributional theory of achievement motivation and emotion. *Psychological Review, 92,* 548–573.

Wolfe, F. (1995). Fibromyalgia. In B. J. Sessle, P. S. Bryant, & R. A. Dionne (Eds.), *Temporo-mandibular disorders and related pain conditions* (pp. 31–46). Seattle, WA: IASP Press.

Wolfe, F., Cathey, M. A., Kleinheksel, S. M., Amos, S. P., Hoffman, R. G., Young, D. Y., & Hawley, D. J. (1984). Psychological status in primary fibrositis and fibrositis associated with rheumatoid arthritis. *Journal of Rheumatology, 11,* 500–506.

Wolfe, F., Russell, I. J., Vipraio, G., Ross, K., & Anderson, J. (1997). Serotonin levels, pain threshold, and fibromyalgia symptoms in the general population. *Journal of Rheumatology, 24,* 555–559.

Xie, Y., Zhang, J., Petersen, M., & LaMotte, R. H. (1995). Functional changes in dorsal root ganglion cells after chronic nerve constriction in the rat. *Journal of Neurophysiology, 73,* 1811–1820.

Yaron, I., Buskila, D., Shirazi, I., Neumann, L., Elkayam, O., Paran, D., & Yaron, M. (1997). Elevated levels of hyaluronic acid in the sera of women with fibromyalgia. *Journal of Rheumatology, 24,* 2221–2224.

Yu, X. M., Sessle, B. J., & Hu, J. W. (1993). Differential effects of cutaneous and deep application of inflammatory irritant on mechanoreceptive field properties of trigeminal brain stem nociceptive neurons. *Journal of Neurophysiology, 70,* 1704–1707.

Yunus, M., Masi, A. T., Calabro, J. J., Miller, K. A., & Feigenbaum, S. L. (1981). Primary fibromyalgia (fibrositis): Clinical study of 50 patients with matched normal controls. *Seminars in Arthritis and Rheumatism, 11,* 151–171.

Zhao, Z. Z., Savage, N. W., Pujic, Z., & Walsh, L. J. (1997). Immunohistochemical localization of mast cells and mast cell-nerve interactions in oral lichen planus. *Oral Diseases, 3,* 71–76.

Ziff, M. F. (1992). Documented clinical side-effects to dental amalgam. *Advances in Dental Research, 6,* 131–134.

# 65

# *Helicobacter pylori*, Immune Function, and Gastric Lesions

HERBERT WEINER, ALVIN P. SHAPIRO[†]

## I. INTRODUCTION

### A. Discovery of *Helicobacter pylori* and Its Presumed Role in Gastroduodenal Disease

In 1983 and 1984, Warren and Marshall (1983, 1984) reported the presence of an unidentified, corkscrew-shaped bacterium, originally called *Campylobacter pyloridis*, since renamed *Helicobacter pylori* (*H. pylori*), on the surface mucosa of the cardia, body, and antrum of the stomachs of patients with chronic gastritis and peptic ulcer (PU). Since that time, nonulcer dyspepsia (NUD) (Rokkas et al., 1987), acute and active chronic (Type B) gastritis (Marshall & Warren, 1984), atrophic

[†]Deceased.

gastritis (Kuipers, Pérez-Pérez, Meuwissen, & Blaser, 1991), gastric (GU) and duodenal ulcer (PDU) (Marshall & Warren, 1984), gastric carcinoma (Nomura et al., 1991), and lymphoma (Parsonnet et al., 1994) have been causally associated with it. *Helicobacter pylori* has been isolated from the stomachs of patients with gastrinoma (Saeed et al., 1991), bile reflux gastritis (Graham, 1995), and gastric ulcers anteceded by the ingestion of nonsteroidal anti-inflammatory drugs (NSAID) (Taha & Russell, 1993). However, it is also present much more frequently in the stomachs, both fundus and antrum, of subjects without any symptoms or any of these diseases. Furthermore, *H. pylori* was present in a variable percentage of patients with these different diseases.

In addition to isolating this organism or measuring antibodies against it, the principle line of evidence for the pathogenic role of this bacterium in these disorders is that some of them can be "cured" by antibiotic treatment, or rather, antibiotics combined with bismuth and/or antacids. The isolation and identification of *H. pylori* in diseases of the upper gastroduodenal tract, and the supposed curative role of antibiotics, has swept away all critical thought. Therefore, we shall review the evidence upon which this line of reasoning is based. This chapter makes four main points by reviewing the evidence: (1) for the causative role of *H. pylori* in a variety of apparently distinct diseases of the upper gastroduodenal tract; (2) against its unicausal role; (3) that this manner of thinking simply does not do justice to the well-established facts about PDU, for example, that it is a heterogeneous and multifactorial disease; (4) that a unified mulifactorial hypothesis about the etio-pathogenesis of gastroduodenal disease incorporating the role of *H. pylori* is needed, testable, and more likely than a unicausal one.

## II. EPIDEMIOLOGY OF
### *HELICOBACTER PYLORI*

If *H. pylori* is the sole pathogenic cause of the several diseases already mentioned, then its presence in the stomach and duodenum should be closely correlated with the incidence and prevalence of the disease. To take PU as an example, its incidence and prevalence figures are hard to come by because they continue to vary from decade to decade, country to country, social class to social class, one historical period to another (Feldman, 1948; Pflanz, 1971), and differ in the two genders (reviewed in Susser, 1967). Furthermore, most of these figures were hospital- and not population-based; even if they were, the presence of "silent" ulcer would not be detectable in a population.

Notwithstanding these quandaries, the incidence of PDU in the United States is between 1 and 3.5/1000/ year in men, and it occurred in about 25–40% of that figure in women. The frequency of GU in men was about 0.5/1000/year and in women about 0.3–0.4/ 1000/year (Sturdevant, 1976). The incidence and prevalence in these diseases is generally believed to be much lower in tropical Africa (Holcombe, 1992), where the prevalence of *H. pylori* infection was high. Regional variation in the incidence of gastric carci-noma has also been described in China (Hu, Li, & Lin, 1995).

The exact incidence figures for *H. pylori* infection based on seropositivity in the general population in different areas of the world are not precisely known. The infection is chronic, and the prevalence figures showed a consistent increase with age; they range from 20% in healthy adult volunteers to 50%, and to 90% or more in older persons above the age of 65 years (Fallingborg, Poulsen, Grove, & Teglbjaerg, 1992; Soll, 1990; Taylor & Blaser, 1991) without regard to gender. The highest prevalence rates occurred in subjects living in the underdeveloped countries and in healthy Hispanic and African-Americans living in the United States. The fact remains that many more adult people test seropositive for the bacterium than ever develop symptoms or any of the various gastroduodenal diseases (Fallingborg et al., 1992; Taylor & Blaser, 1991), suggesting that additional factors must be involved in those infected persons

that do develop these various diseases compared with that seen in those that do not.

If one ascribes causality to *H. pylori* in the pathogenesis of both PU and gastric carcinoma, why should the age-standardized prevalence patterns of infection have been the same in two geographic areas, in one in which the incidence of diseases was high, and in another in which it was low? (Hu et al., 1995). No answer has been provided for this question. Nor has the mode of transmission of *H. pylori* been identified (Taylor & Blaser, 1991).

The prevalence figures just cited indicated that *H. pylori* infection was asymptomatic in most subjects. In fact, a long-term longitudinal study showed no difference in the frequency of gastrointestinal symp-toms in subjects who tested seropositive for *H. pylori* than in those who were seronegative (Parsonnet, Blaser, Pérez-Pérez, Hargrett-Bean, & Tauxe, 1992). A similar statement can be made for chronic gastritis, which in most persons was also asymptomatic. How-ever, the diagnosis of gastritis in symptomatic patients was not always reliable; it depends on whether it was made by endoscopy or histological examination of biopsied gastric tissue, which is subject to sample bias. The correlation of these two methods is by no means strong (Dooley et al., 1989; Fallingborg et al., 1992).

### A. Prevalence of *Helicobacter pylori* in Gastroduodenal Diseases: Type B Gastritis

The most frequent association of *H. pylori* is with Type B chronic gastritis. Two forms of chronic gastritis are recognized: Type A is an autoimmune disease involving the fundus and body of the stomach, characterized by high serum gastrin and low serum pepsinogen levels, little or no pepsin activity, and achlorhydria, and in which *H. pylori* infection may or may not occur (Fong et al., 1991). Type B gastritis involves mainly the antrum of the stomach, serum gastrin levels were low and *H. pylori* infection was present in 88% of 401 patients (Fong et al., 1991; Taylor and Blaser, 1991). Autoimmunity is not the only putative cause of gastritis: NSAID, alcohol ingestion, and bile reflux may antecede it.

Type B gastritis is a very common antecedent of GU and PU, and may also precede gastric carcinoma. However, it is recognized that PU and gastric car-cinoma are usually mutually exclusive in the same patient. The prevalence of Type B gastritis was about 20% in young adults, rising to about 50% at the age of 50 years in those living in developed countries. As stated, there was a strong correlation between the presence of Type B gastritis and *H. pylori* infection (Dooley et al., 1989; Taylor & Blaser, 1991), even when gastritis was asymptomatic. The inflammation with *H. pylori* affects only gastric-type epithelial cells, and duodenal metaplastic (heterotopic) ones.

Now it has been argued that the infection causally produced the chronic gastritis, supposedly because gastric inflammation (e.g., due to bile reflux) per se is not necessary for the development of the infection. However, this argument is not conclusive. In fact, data have been published which strongly suggested that gastritis preceded colonization by *H. pylori*, and may have been a prerequisite for it (Fallingborg et al., 1992).

## B. Acute Gastritis

The association of *H. pylori* with acute gastritis was based on two self-inoculation experiments (Marshall, Armstrong, McGechie, & Glancy, 1985; Morris & Nicholson, 1987), which will be described below.

## C. Epidemic Hypochlorhydria and Acute Gastritis

The earliest phase of *H. pylori* infection has been associated with a low gastric pH, followed by a rise to a neutral pH (Morris & Nicholson, 1987). Subjects undergoing gastric secretion studies with a pH electrode have become infected with *H. pylori* and developed hypochlorhydria lasting 2–8 months and gastritis (Barthel, Westholm, Havey, Gonzalez, & Everett, 1988; Morris & Nicholson, 1989). However, hypochlorhydria, associated with *H. pylori* infection and gastritis, may be asymptomatic in healthy volunteers.

## D. Nonulcer Dyspepsia

Nonulcer dyspepsia in adults occurred with a prevalence of at least 20–30% of a population (Talley & Phillips, 1988), but was variably associated with *H. pylori* and chronic gastritis. However, the association of *H. pylori* and NUD increased with age as did the prevalence of seropositivity in asymptomatic patients (Greenberg & Bank, 1990), suggesting that in the former group the correlation was not causal. However, in other studies *H. pylori* was more commonly present (67%) in NUD patients than in normal controls (25%) when subjected to biopsy of both the gastric fundus and the antrum (Strauss et al., 1990). Yet it was not possible to discriminate the symptoms of patients with NUD who were or were not seropositive for *H. pylori* (Mearin et al., 1994).

The role of *H. pylori* in NUD was inferred from a reduction of symptoms in about 60% of patients treated with bismuth subcitrate but not with placebo (reviewed in Taylor & Blaser, 1991).

## E. Peptic Ulcer

The causal role of *H. pylori* in PU was inferred from the observations that 75 to 100% of patients with PDUs, and 35 to 86% of patients with GUs, harbored the bacterium in the gastric antrum (Taylor & Blaser, 1991). A more cautious approach might have been to state that *H. pylori* constituted a risk factor, as gastric metaplasia does too, along with many others, for PDU (Taylor & Blaser, 1991; Weiner, 1991). If so, it is a risk factor that lacks specificity for any one gastroduodenal disease for reasons that have not been made clear.

The concept that *H. pylori* infection increased the risk for the subsequent development of GU and PDU was partly based on one prospective, case–controlled study of Japanese-American, hospitalized men. (In fact, almost every study of this topic has been on male patients!) The bacterium was not isolated but rather specific immunoglobulin-G (IgG) antibodies against it were measured in the serum of patients and controls. Ninety-three percent of 150 patients with GU, and 92% of 65 patients with PDU, tested positive for antibody levels. The serum of the same number of matched controls for both groups was positive in 78%. (However, the odds ratios were, respectively, 3.2 and 4.0—both statistically significant.) Also, the higher the antibody level, the more likely it was that the two diseases were present (Nomura, Stemmerman, Chyou, Pérez-Pérez, and Blaser, 1994).

This study has much to recommend it because it avoided the pitfall of studying patients after disease onset. However, the authors of this report only briefly discussed the fact that 78% of those with positive antibody titers had no disease—a finding that must suggest that other risk factors interact with *H. pylori* to produce the two diseases.

Although *H. pylori* infection is very common in populations, while chronic gastritis with and without infection is also very prevalent, and virtually all patients with PDU are infected, why do most infected persons not develop PDU? Once again, the most likely explanation is that in order to do so, additional factors play roles. This argument is supported by the recognized fact that benign PDU does not occur in patients with atrophic and Type A gastritis with pernicious anemia—that is with achlorhydria and very low pepsin activity, yet *H. pylori* can still be recovered in gastric biopsies (Graham, 1995).

## F. Atrophic Gastritis and Gastric Carcinoma

Chronic superficial gastritis may terminate in atrophic gastritis over a period of 36 years (Siurala, Sipponen, & Kekki, 1985). It has been speculated that Type B gastritis may also evolve into atrophic gastritis after many years.

However, the association of *H. pylori* infection and gastric carcinoma has not been explained, as the bacterium has not been isolated at the gastric site of the malignancy. Yet the prevalence of the infection in the disease was as high as 89% (Parsonnet et al., 1991) and was also a risk factor (Nomura et al., 1991). Yet marked geographic variations occurred in the incidence of gastric carcinoma that may or may not be related to variations in the prevalence of the infection (Forman et al., 1990; Hu et al., 1995).

## G. Gastric Lymphoma

This rare malignancy constitutes 0.3% of all gastric neoplasms. In a case–control study of 230,593 persons followed prospectively for 14 years, 33 developed it. Those who did were significantly more likely to have a previous *H. pylori* infection (odds ratio: 6.3) than those that did not. The infection was not associated with nongastric lymphomas (Parsonnet et al., 1994).

The lymphoma under discussion derives from gastric mucosa-associated lymphoid tissue (MALT) (Isaacson, 1995). The MALT is a primary B-cell lymphoma, but the role of *H. pylori* in its induction is not known. Nonetheless, in two patients the MALT lymphoma arose from specific B-cell clones at the site of chronic gastritis, which later gave rise to the tumor, presumably by expansion and proliferation (Zucca et al., 1988).

## III. RESPONSE TO TREATMENT

One of the principal arguments that has been put forward in favor of the causative role of *H. pylori* in gastroduodenal diseases was their responses to treatment. Amoxicillin, combined with omeprazole and ranitidine, designed to eradicate *H. pylori* from the stomach and the duodenum, healed or lowered the recurrence rate of PDU in 74 and 95% of patients, respectively (Graham et al., 1992; Hentschel et al., 1993; Labenz, Rühl, Bertrams, & Börsch, 1994). However, 75% of patients with PDU in one series responded favorably to placebo without the disappearance of the infection—a statistically significant lower response rate than in those given combined treatment. However, 19% of patients in whom the

bacterium had been eradicated, later had a recurrence of a PDU (Hentschel et al., 1993).

It cannot be emphasized enough that these treatment studies on PDU and antral gastritis (Marshall, 1987) all used a combination of drugs, and that an antibiotic was no more effective than a bismuth preparation (Rauws, Langenberg, Houthoff, Zanen, & Tytgat, 1988). Single antibiotic agents, such as erythromycin (McNulty et al., 1986) or doxiciline (Unge & Gnarpe, 1988) fail to eradicate *H. pylori*; it seems necessary to combine them with either a protective coating agent and/or an inhibitor of acid secretion, as was done in the studies (Graham et al., 1992; Hentschel et al., 1993; Hosking et al., 1994; Labenz et al., 1994) reported above. As Graham (1995) has pointed out, no single study has been carried out that shows that antibiotic therapy alone can heal PUs any better than placebo does. However, bismuth subcitrate may by itself be beneficial in NUD.

Although histological improvement of chronic gastritis and the elimination of *H. pylori* has been achieved either by treatment with bismuth subcitrate or amoxicillin, the relapse rate was high (Blaser, 1987). In another study, administration with a bismuth preparation alone was much more effective than erythromycin or placebo (McNulty et al., 1986), or cimetidine (Blaser, 1987). However, still other studies have shown that amoxicillin may clear the infection in chronic antral gastritis (Glupczynski et al., 1988). Therefore, the results of treatment of antral gastritis remain inconsistent.

Antibiotic treatment has also been given to six patients with low-grade, MALT lymphomas. In five of them it produced tumor remission (Wotherspoon et al., 1993). However, there is no evidence so far that similar treatment responses occur with gastric carcinomata.

The claim that antibiotics were the key to the successful eradication of *H. pylori* and the healing of lesions is doubtful. *Helicobacter pylori* can frequently be recovered in gastric biopsies of gastrinomas. Proton-pump inhibitors, such as omeprazole, produced a remission of the PU and disappearance of *H. pylori* from antral mucosa (Koop et al., 1991; Saeed et al., 1991).

In addition, the therapeutic success of bismuth preparations alone suggests that *H. pylori* does not directly produce lesions. Bismuth in the stomach combines with mucosal glycoproteins, especially in eroded craters which become coated with the polymer to inhibit the backdiffusion of protons (Graham, 1995).

There is little doubt that improvement in symptoms, some of the histological lesions, and a fall in specific antibody titers occurred with clearing of

*H. pylori* infection. However, these events did not prove pathogenic causality any more than reversal of low cardiac output failure by digitalis tells us what its causes were.

Furthermore, chronic gastritis associated with *H. pylori* infection is asymptomatic in most patients, so that some additional (unknown) factors must determine which patients did or did not have symptoms. In fact, it has been known for 20 years that the relationship of gastroduodenal symptoms to the anatomical lesion, or physiological alteration, is complex. The symptoms of duodenal ulcer respond to placebo as frequently as to antacids, but the lesion does not (Peterson et al., 1977).

Therefore, treatment studies besides being "blind" and placebo-controlled, need to observe the effects on symptoms, on the infection, and on endoscopic, histological, bacteriological, and serological variables.

## IV. BACTERIOLOGY AND IMMUNOLOGY OF *Helicobacter pylori*

The bacteriology of the stomach and, in particular, the presence of spiral bacteria in it, has been a subject of investigation for at least 125 years (reviewed in Blaser, 1987). Seeley and Colp (1941) studied the bacteriology of PU and gastric carcinomata because they were interested in the possibility that bacteria might produce postoperative infections, rather than postulating their pathogenic role in the two diseases. The topic of unidentified spiral organisms received a major impetus following the introduction of endoscopy but it remained for Marshall (1983), Marshall & Warren (1984), and Warren & Marshall (1983) to state that they resembled *Campylobacter jejuni* and to relate their presence to gastritis and GU and PDU in biopsy specimens. The bacterium was renamed *Campylobacter pyloridis* but is now known as *Helicobacter pylori* because of its distinctive characteristics.

It is a Gram-negative, quadruple-flagellated, U-shaped organism. Its genomic sequence has been characterized: it consists of 1,667,876 base pairs (Tomb et al., 1997), with few regulatory genes.

*Helicobacter pylori* has some unusual features: it is adapted not only to live in the extremely acid environment of the stomach, but to neutralize hydrochloric acid. It does so by virtue of coding for urease, which splits urea to generate ammonia ions and carbon dioxide and hence bicarbonate ions. The ability to neutralize protons in this manner may be the basis of the epidemic hypochlorhydria already described.

*Helicobacter pylori* requires a source of iron, micro-aerobic conditions, and a temperature above 30°C to grow. Genes coding for several iron-scavenging pathways have been identified. The organism is catalase- and oxidase-positive (Taylor & Blaser, 1991).

Considerable genetic variability occurs in *H. pylori* (Majewski & Goodwin, 1988). Some strains are more virulent than others, and still other strains are capable of forming plasmids. At least 10 antigenic proteins of various sizes have been identified. Several major surface antigens are also present and show considerable diversity in their properties (Pérez-Pérez & Blaser, 1987). The genes coding for the surface antigens contain hypervariable regions allowing for the bacterium to evade and adapt to immune responses by altering their antigenic properties.

*Helicobacter pylori* produces a vigorous antibody response which forms the basis for a specific and sensitive serological test to detect its presence in the stomach (Pérez-Pérez, Dworkin, Chodos, & Blaser, 1988). The serological test is more reliable than endoscopy or gastric biopsy. It is also much more feasible than the other diagnostic tests in epidemiological research.

However, specific antibody titers may take several months to develop. They then remain stable, unless treatment was successful, after which they fall (Taylor & Blaser, 1991). However, one of the curious aspects of the untreated infection is that it is not eliminated by the (humoral) immune response. The specific antibodies are of the IgM, IgA, and IgG varieties, correlate with the infection, and are secreted into serum and gastric juice.

*Helicobacter pylori* is not the only spiral bacterium present in the stomach: *H. heilmannii* has also been isolated from it. It is only two to three times as long as *H. pylori*. Its prevalence was considerably less—occurring in about 1% of middle-aged subjects, and twice as frequently in men as in women. Compared with *H. pylori*, *H. heilmannii* was focally distributed in the gastric antrum. Its distribution in the stomach was more restricted than was *H. pylori*. The gastritis it produced was much milder, metaplasia was rare, but MALT lymphomas did appear. Occasional erosions and ulceration have been described in 4% of 202 patients; when they did occur they were associated with the ingestion of NSAID (Stolte et al., 1997).

### A. Site of Origin of the Antibodies

*Helicobacter pylori* is usually located on the luminal side of the surface of gastric, mucus-secreting cells and in the pits of the stomach, within or under the mucus layer, in close contact or partly fused with the epithelial cells, or within endocytotic vacuoles (reviewed in Blaser, 1987). Phagocytosis of the bacterium has been observed. The infected epithelial layer contains polymorphonuclear leukocytes. However, the bacterium does not seem to invade the gastric epithelium, and does not seem to affect normal duodenal mucosa. Its presence is, however, closely associated with gastritis but not with normal gastric mucosa. The mucus layer may protect the bacterium from low gastric acidity, but is depleted by the infection, exposing it to those ("aggressive") factors that are associated with ulceration.

The source of the specific antibodies has not been ascertained. However, the infected mucosa may be infiltrated with plasma cells and lymphocytes (Marshall, 1987). It is not, however, certain whether *H. pylori* reaches antibody-producing cells, most of which are usually present in the *lamina propria*. Furthermore, the presence of agglutinating antibody titers to *H. pylori* in 5–20% of noninfected subjects has raised questions about the specificity for the diseases enumerated (Hornick, 1987). However, *H. pylori* seemed to have the ability to induce the appearance of lymphoid tissue in the mucosa of the stomach (Wyatt & Rathbone, 1988). Cultured MALT lymphoma cells incubated with *H. pylori* expressed the interleukin-2 receptor, proliferated, and synthesized tumor immunoglobulin. However, this sequence of events occurred only in the presence of normal T cells in the culture medium (Hussell, Isaacson, Crabtree, & Spencer, 1993).

The topic of the roles of immunocompetent cells in the pathogenesis of gastroduodenal disease not related to infection has been neglected until lately. These cells did more than produce antibodies, or killed invading bacteria by cellular means. They also express mRNAs for histamine ($H_2$), gastrin, muscarinic ($M_{1-5}$) acetylcholine, and dopamine ($D_{1-5}$) receptors, which parietal cells did not seem to do (Mezey & Palkovitz, 1992). Therefore, immunocytes (e.g., macrophages, monocytes, CD4+ cells, and so forth), and mast cells may be under the control of efferent vagal discharge (Adelson, unpublished). However, these cellular roles have not systematically been studied in *H. pylori* infection.

## V.  HELICOBACTER PYLORI'S ROLE IN THE PATHOGENESIS OF GASTRODUODENAL DISEASES

In order to prove the role of *H. pylori* as the causative agent in several gastroduodenal diseases, a number of conditions must be met (Correa, 1991): (1) The bacterium must be present in the stomach of subjects with the disease. As already noted, prevalence studies have documented that this condition was met with few exceptions. (2) An association should occur between the rate of infection and the disease(s). As already mentioned, in patients with PDU who also have chronic antral gastritis, 93% were *H. pylori* positive; in GU the figure was 92%; and in NUD it was 50% (Marshall, 1987). The consensus to date is that *H. pylori* infection increased the risk several fold for these diseases. However, in the case of NUD the rate of infection was not greater than chance. Furthermore, in these correlational studies other risk factors—the ingestion of alcohol, salicylates, and NSAID have not usually been ruled out. (3) The infection as inferred by serological means must antecede the disease, in order to have causal validity. This condition has been met in prospective studies in PDU (Nomura et al., 1994), gastric carcinoma (Parsonnet et al., 1991), and MALT lymphoma (Parsonnet et al., 1994). However, another study, as already mentioned, showed that gastritis anteceded infection in asymptomatic subjects (Fallingborg et al., 1992)—evidence that gastritis was a prerequisite at least in some for bacterial colonization of the corpus and antrum. In gastric carcinoma, furthermore, the malignant cells were not infected; but the tumor was surrounded by an inflammatory reaction in noncancerous cells, which either were or were not infected with *H. pylori*. (4) Koch's four postulates for the pathogenic role of *H. pylori* should be met; in actuality, only two have been in the case of *H. pylori*—one of the principal arguments against *H. pylori*'s prime, causative role in gastroduodenal disease (Graham, 1995; Wormsley, 1989). Yet part of the enthusiasm for the bacterium's pathogenic role in gastroduodenal diseases—or at least acute gastritis—was generated by Marshall drinking a broth containing *H. pylori* after having had a normal gastric biopsy and having ingested cimetidine. Ten days later he underwent gastroscopy and biopsy by a colleague who reported inflammation of the gastric antral mucosa (i.e., gastritis) (Marshall et al., 1985). By the 14th day, the acute gastritis had vanished; no antibody response developed, and no peptic ulcer ever occurred. Two years later this self-experiment was repeated by Morris and Nicholson (1987). One of these investigators ingested *H. pylori* bacteria twice after baseline biopsy studies showed normal antral and fundal mucosa, and a pH of <2 of gastric juice. He first ingested $4 \times 10^7$ bacteria. Immediately after ingestion the gastric pH was 1.7. No infection developed. A second biopsy was taken which also proved normal. He subsequently ingested $3 \times 10^5$ bacteria, subcultured from a patient with chronic gastritis, 4 h after taking 800 mg of cimetidine. Three days later he experienced epigastric pain and vomiting. On the fifth day a biopsy revealed acute antral gastritis and the presence of *H. pylori* in the histological specimen. On the 8th to the 27th day, the gastric pH was above 7.4. After that time, the gastric aspirate became negative for the bacterium, but by the 61st day, reinfection occurred which was arrested by treatment with bismuth subsalicylate. A transient IgM seroconversion was documented after successful treatment, followed by an increase in specific IgG and IgA titers. A year after the initial experiment, the infection recurred, and evidence of chronic Type B gastritis was manifested, both lasting another 2 years (Morris, Ali, Nicholson, Pérez-Pérez, & Blaser, 1991).

These two reports provided strong evidence that *H. pylori* could incite acute and/or chronic gastritis symptoms and, in the second instance, a delayed serological response. Furthermore, the infection in Morris' and Nicholson's experiment was associated with evidence of an hypo- or achlorhydria (although the experimenter was premedicated with cimetidine to suppress gastric acid secretion). Although this was only a single-case report, it may help to explain the onset of ("epidemic") achlorhydria and gastritis after the stomach has been contaminated iatrogenically with *H. pylori*.

Unexplained, however, is why ingestion of the second but not the first culture only produced gastric infection in this self-experiment. Now it is true that PU is often preceded by chronic gastritis and PDU with heterotopic (gastric) tissue in the duodenum (Steer, 1984). However, the self-induced gastritis in Marshall's case was acute, and in the Morris and Nicholson case no ulcer developed. Nor have Koch's postulates ever been fulfilled for the several other diseases for which *H. pylori* has been claimed to be the pathogenetic agent.

## A. Animal Models of Pathogenesis

The fulfillment of Koch's other postulates could occur with an animal model of any of the diseases associated with *H. pylori* infection. Mice, gerbils, dogs, cats, ferrets, pigs, and monkeys have been infected with different species of *Helicobacter. Helicobacter felis* and *H. pylori* successfully infected rats and mice; *H. mustelae* did so in ferrets. In rats, the mouse-adapted *H. pylori* strain may have to be used to produce gastric colonization and inflammation, which it does several weeks after its introduction into the stomach (Li, Kalies, Mellgård, & Helander, 1998; Li, Mellgård, & Helander, 1997).

Perhaps the duration of the infection in rats in negative experiments was too short. It may take 2 months after feeding the bacterium to rats before antral inflammation and colonization occurred. Success in producing gastritis required the pretreatment of the animals with omeprazole. The gastritis histologically mimicked the human lesion. Infection delayed healing of the inflammation when compared with gastric lesions produced by acetic acid, and it enhanced apoptosis. Rats developed increased levels of specific IgM and IgG (but not IgA) antibodies (Li et al., 1998). The gastritis developed despite the absence of the two cytotoxins (Vac A and Cag A) (Li et al., 1997).

Mice develop gastritis on infection (Marchetti et al., 1995). In other experiments, rats, when fed daily suspensions of the organism for 7 days, did not develop gastritis or gastric erosions. However, when gastric erosions were first experimentally induced by stressful procedures and rats were then fed a broth suspension of *H. pylori*, inflammation in the erosion was intensified (Ross et al., 1992). In gerbils, colonization by the bacterium and mild inflammation without prior erosion formation were produced by orally administered *H. pylori* in the gastromucosal layer but only when they were pretreated with indomethacin (Yokota et al., 1991).

This second group of studies indicates that in rats and gerbils, *H. pylori* infection alone does not produce erosions but must be combined with a stressful procedure or prostaglandin inhibition. In the past such synergisms have been described—for example, between injecting aspirin and restraining rats or exposing them to cold, when neither alone would produce multiple, bleeding, gastric ulcers (Meeroff, Paulsen, & Guth, 1975).

## B. Comments about the Pathogenic Role of *Helicobacter pylori* in Human Diseases

The evidence for the direct and unicausal role of *H. pylori* in gastroduodenal diseases is contradictory and is mainly based on the two self-experiments and on correlations. The fact remains that most people by late middle-age were infected but only a small percentage developed disease—for example, only 1 in 100 or 180 persons had a PDU. In areas such as Africa where the prevalence of infection was very high, few developed PDU or gastric carcinomata. Despite the two self-experiments reviewed, direct evidence for the sole pathogenic role of *H. pylori* has been correlational. In order to make sense of the discrepancies noted, explanations have been sought in variations in virulence of the bacterium's different strains, or in reduced host resistance to it. The first of these arguments was used by Atherton (1997). These strain differences consisted specifically in the production of cytotoxins and their ability to activate neutrophils, or in other gene products. However, the author admitted that, at least, PDU was multifactorial, so that the virulence of the bacterium was but one additional variable. To make the matter even more problematic was the fact that 30–40% of patients with PDU did not harbor the virulent strains (Tee, Lambert, & Dwyer, 1995). The second argument—of reduced host resistance—has several attractive aspects, ranging from immunological ones to the effects of stressors on gastric acid production, to the role of factors such as pepsin and mucus secretion in the stomach, in other words, to the known roles of "aggressive" and protective factors.

In fact, *H. pylori* does deplete and disrupt the mucus protective layer. Thus an additional pathogenic factor is already known. In order to prove its proximate action in producing disease, other known pathogenetic variables in ulceration have already been investigated. Infected patients had excessive gastrin responses to the eating of a meal, as a result of which they had higher gastric acid secretion rates than noninfected subjects (Goldschmiedt, Redfern, Barnett, Schwarz, & Feldman, 1989). Even when no ulcer was present, infected subjects showed higher basal and serum gastrin levels to meals and to bombesin than did noninfected ones (Graham, Opekum, Lew, Klein, & Walsh, 1991: Mertz & Walsh, 1991). In addition, infection has been shown to raise pepsinogen-1 (PG-1) levels, which fell with antibiotic treatment (Mertz & Walsh, 1991). Infection was also associated with a lowering of hydrophobicity of the gastric mucus layer due probably to an endopeptidase secreted by *H. pylori*. Treatment restored the composition of the mucus (Cover, Dooley, & Blaser, 1990). The bacterium has also been found to secrete protein cytotoxins (Cover et al., 1990) and a chemotactic factor (Craig, Karnes, Territo, & Walsh, 1990) which may incite an inflammatory response and gastric mucosal metaplasia (Carrick, Lee, Hazell, Ralston, & Daskapoulos, 1989). The exact role of the cytotoxins is, however, controversial. At least two have been identified: Cag A$^+$ (cytotoxin-associated gene A) and Vac A$^+$ (vacuolating cytotoxin gene) phenotypes. Vac A$^+$ is a known bacterial virulence factor (Blaser, 1995). Fifty percent of *H. pylori* strains expressed Vac A$^+$. Four allelic variants of the protein exist. The protein incited specific antibodies against it (Cover, Cao, Murthy, Sipple, & Blaser, 1992).

At first, it was claimed that the Vac A$^+$ phenotype was associated more frequently with the occurrence of PDU than in infected patients without it (Atherton, 1997), but this assertion was not confirmed. No differences were found in the frequency of allelic variants of the protein in PDU and asymptomatic gastritis (Go, Cissel, & Graham, 1998).

However, *H. pylori* strains, which released the Vac A$^+$ protein as well as urease, adhered to and invaded, in vitro, (HEp-2) epithelial cells and produced a change in the phospholipid and glycolipid composition of their cell walls. The induction of this particular strain was achieved by mild (pH 6) acidification of the medium (Bukholm et al., 1997).

The role of the Cag A$^+$ protein in pathogenesis is also debatable; its presence was independent of whether subjects were asymptomatic or suffered from PDU (Go & Graham, 1996).

The role of other *H. pylori* proteins has also been postulated. Two flagellar genes code for four proteins which did not, however, differ in producing bacterial motility, or vacuolating cytotoxins, but they did differ in the amounts of IL-8 secretion. (Interleukin-8 is a chemotactic factor and activates neutrophils.) However, the amount of this cytokine secreted did not correlate with the type of disease (i.e., PDU, GU, carcinoma, or gastritis) (Ohta-Tada, Tagaki, Koga, Kamiya, & Miwa, 1997).

Presumably, *H. pylori* by raising gastrin secretion increased gastric acid and pepsin production, impaired mucus protection, and incited metaplasia and inflammation, leading to gastritis, duodenitis, and peptic ulceration. However, this line of reasoning was not confirmed because acid secretion was suppressed in infected patients (Furuta et al., 1998) and contradicted the data that infection lowers the gastric pH. A more likely sequence was that when the mucus layer was disrupted, backdiffusion of protons occurred. Yet *H. pylori* also produced ammonia and bicarbonate ions to neutralize them, as already mentioned.

Nonetheless, an impairment of gastrin release, gastric emptying and acid secretion remains a possibility (Hamlet & Olbe, 1996), especially as *H. pylori*-infected patients with PDU had reduced somatostatin levels in the antral mucosa (Moss, Legon, Bishop, Polak, & Calam, 1992). It has also been suggested that cytokines released by immunocompetent cells on infection may have inhibited gastric acid secretion, which IL-1$\beta$ is known to do. Or, gastrin release was stimulated in tissue culture by IL-1$\beta$, TNF-$\alpha$, IFN-$\gamma$, and IL-2 (Wallace, Cucala, Mugridge, & Parente, 1991; Weigert, Schaffer, Schuszdziarra, Classen, & Schepp, 1996).

A possible model for the role of cytokines in regulating the physiology of the human stomach is the production of gastritis with aspirin. As a consequence, inreased production of IL-1$\beta$, IL-6, and IL-8, but not of TNF-$\alpha$ or IFN-$\gamma$, was found in biopsied antral mucosa. The acid-inhibitory response on serum gastrin levels was abolished (Hamlet, Lindholm, Nilsson, & Olbe, 1998). This study, however, does not prove that the inflammatory responses to aspirin and *H. pylori* are identical: additional cytokines (e.g., IL-4, IL-12) have very recently been reported to play a putative role in some patients with *H. pylori* gastritis (Karttunen, Karttunen, Ekre, & MacDonald, 1995; Karttunen et al., 1997). (The role of IL-12 is to increase IFN-$\gamma$ secretion by T and NK cells, and its release is regulated by IL-10).

The emphasis in this line of investigation was on the factors initiated by *H. pylori* infection, which would help our understanding of inflammation, its chronicity, the recruitment of polymorphonuclear leukocytes and lymphocytes into the gastric mucosa, due presumably to a shift in balance between pro-inflammatory cytokines and those that suppress inflammation.

The healing of the infected gastric mucosa was delayed, at least, in rats (Li et al., 1998). Mucosal repair was partly promoted by epidermal growth factor (EGF) and transforming growth factor-$\alpha$ (TGF-$\alpha$), as well as gastrin and growth hormone. Additionally, the two growth factors inhibited gastric acid secretion, and increased gastric blood flow and pro-staglandin secretion (Uribe & Barrett, 1997). The immunohistochemical expression of EGF and TGF-$\alpha$ was enhanced in the mucosa of infected patients with PDU and NUD more than in noninfected controls, and it persisted for 2–4 weeks after the infection was eradicated and healing occurred by treating patients with amoxicillin, metromidazole, and omeprazole (Konturek et al., 1998).

In conclusion, the manner in which *H. pylori* incites or enhances inflammation and/or retards healing and produces the different forms of upper gastroduodenal disease is both complex and not fully understood. However, it must be clear that these processes are not linear–causal. Furthermore, this literature has so far largely overlooked additional predisposing and, especially, known host factors. They have also not mentioned that each of the diseases associated with *H. pylori* infection are heterogeneous.

## VI. THE HETEROGENEITY AND MULTIFACTORIAL NATURE OF GASTRODUODENAL DISEASES

For many years it has been known that subjects with blood group O, non-ABH secretor status, and the Lewis (a+b−) blood group phenotype were at increased risk for PU (Lam, 1993; Sipponen et al., 1989; Weiner, 1977). The Lewis blood group consists of soluble plasma antigens, which are adsorbed by, among others, gastroduodenal mucosal cells.

In a large population-based study of Danish men, the lifetime prevalence rate for PDU was significantly higher in those with the Lewis (a+b−) phenotype and who did not secrete ABH. However, those with the blood group O phenotype had the highest risk for hospitalization (Hein, Suadicani, & Gyntelborg, 1992).

This study did not, however, ask the question of a potential, differential prevalence of *H. pylori* infection in subjects carrying the various genetic markers (e.g., ABH, ABO, Lewis, and C3 complement). Nonetheless, there is some controversial evidence that the Lewis (a+) blood group antigen agglutinated potentially pathogenic bacteria, including *H. pylori* (Essery et al., 1994), and therefore acted as a receptor when attached to the gastric mucosa. However, another report assigns this role to the Lewis b antigen (Borén, Normark, & Falk, 1994).

Genetic variation in blood group and nonsecretor status accounted for 2.5–3% of the etiological variance of PDU. Another genetic variation was in serum pepsinogen (PG) levels, which in PDU fell within the upper 2.5% of the distribution in 45–50% of all patients, both before and after the development of the disease. Isoforms of PG also occurred, classified into two main groups according to their structural characteristics and localization in the stomach. Some groups of PDU patients have elevated levels of PG-I and others of PG-II. Patients with GU ulcer were more likely to have elevated PG-II levels.

Pepsinogen-I levels were inherited as an autosomal dominant trait. However, in another form of PDU, PG-I levels were normal, and the inheritance was polygenic (Rotter & Rimoin, 1977; Samloff, 1989). Inheritance of elevated PG-I levels increased the risk for disease by a factor of five to eight. Additional genetic factors accounted for 30–50% of the etiological variance of PDU (Rotter, 1981). Peptic duodenal ulcer is, therefore, multifactorial, polygenic, and genetically heterogeneous.

Some PDUs occur with rare genetic syndromes such as multiple endocrine adenomatosis, Type I, and systemic mastocytosis (Rotter, 1981). The heterogeneity of PDU has also been described in physiological terms. Variations in mucus and somatostatin secretion may occur. As mentioned, serum PG-I levels were usually greater in PDU than in GU; and basal acid secretion also was. However, only about 50% of all PDU patients were acid hypersecretors; the rest were normosecretors. Patients with GU usually had normal or low levels of acid secretion. Some but not all PDU patients had increased basal and stimulated gastrin responses and/or increased or normal rates of gastric emptying (Rotter, 1981; Wolfe & Soll, 1988). PDU and GU patients differed in the ages of onset of the diseases and in the association with the genetic markers already mentioned. Yet they may occur together, in which case they are thought to be a distinct form of ulcer diesease. In PDU disease, a positive correlation between gastric acid output and a gastrin response to a protein meal has been found, when compared with GU patients and controls who had a negative correlation (Lam & Lai, 1978).

An anatomical heterogeneity of PDU also exists: some, but not all, patients have heterotopic antral tissue in the duodenum; others have a "short bowel" syndrome; and the disease has also been associated with others, such as renal stones and chronic pulmonary diseases.

However, the exact means by which ulceration comes about remains uncertain. Some gastric acid must be present and acts as a permissive factor due to the backdiffusion of protons; its levels do not have to be elevated. Pepsin may digest mucus. Bicarbonate secretion, proton exchange, blood flow, prostaglandin secretion, the action of some cytokines, and the speed of cell regeneration act as protective factors. Any combination of factors that increase mucosal injury, such as increased pepsin secretion and/or unregulated gastrin and thus acid secretion, or factors decreasing protection such as H. pylori, aspirin, NSAID, bile salts, and/or alcohol may damage gastric epithelial cells (Richardson, 1985; Weiner, 1991).

Nonulcer dyspepsia has also been subdivided into different forms by physiological and anatomical criteria. Various changes in gastric motility have been described: in some patients, the usual three cycle per minute regular gastric rhythm sped up and/or became irregular; in others backward propagation of the rhythm was recorded; and in another group it slowed and became intermittent.

Approximately one-half of NUD patients have a normal gastric mucosa; one-third demonstrate minimal mucosal-surface erosions; and 14.5% show a chronic atrophic gastritis. However, it must also be emphasized that 65–70% of all patients with chronic gastritis are asymptomatic (reviewed in Weiner, 1992).

Gastric carcinomata are anatomically heterogeneous: they have been classified into an intestinal type and a diffuse type. Helicobacter pylori was associated almost three times more frequently with the former than the latter (Parsonnet et al., 1991). However, the process of carcinogenesis is complex and no single factor by itself accounts for it.

Two types, at least, of gastric lymphoma have also been recognized by some: non-Hodgkin's and MALT

lymphomas. However, because of their rarity (1 in 30 to 80,000 of the population in the United States) it is not certain whether H. pylori was associated in particular with one form and not the other.

## VII. OTHER RISK FACTORS FOR GASTRODUODENAL DISEASE

In order to explain the relative low probability of developing the various diseases when infected with H. pylori, additional risk factors for them have been invoked. The question is why do some infected persons develop the disease and most do not.

### A. Social, Economic, and Ethnic Factors

The prevalence of H. pylori infection was greater in underdeveloped countries and among poor people, and it increased with age. In the United States, the prevalence is two or three times greater in African-American and Hispanic populations, as estimated by endoscopy or seropositivity for H. pylori. Yet, antibodies for H. pylori were rarely found in an Australian aborigine population, which also had a low prevalence of PDU. In ethnic Chinese people living in Singapore, the rate of PDU was seven times greater than in the Malaysian population (Taylor & Blaser, 1991). Yet the prevalence of PDU was higher in Europe than in Africa despite the fact that prevalence figures for H. pylori infection run in the opposite direction in these two areas. Gastric ulcers were more frequent in Japan than in Europe (Rotter, 1981; Susser, 1976). The incidence of gastric carcinoma was also low in Africa (Holcombe, 1992).

A marked regional difference in the incidence of MALT lymphoma has been described in persons living in the Veneto region of northeastern Italy where its incidence is about 12 times greater than in the United States, and where the prevalence of H. pylori infection was also very high (Doglioni, Wotherspoon, Moschini, de Boni, & Isaacson, 1992).

What do these often contradictory figures mean? One explanation is that a number of uncontrolled or unknown variables have not been accounted for in these prevalence reports. Among the most likely of these is that when heterogeneity for the disease is present, the proportions of the various subforms differ in different populations. Also, however, these studies do not often control variations in diet, the ingestion of alcohol and drugs known to incite gastritis or PDU, or exposure and sensitivity to adverse experiences in their personal lives.

Given the known heterogeneity of the various diseases with which H. pylori has been associated and the number of risk factors, one might well ask the question whether these might account for the fact that only a minority of infected subjects—those at highest cumulative risk—develops one or other of them. So one might ask are subjects with an elevation of PG-I, as a risk factor for PDU, more or less likely to develop an infection? Or one might postulate that the excessive, postprandial gastrin response—a known characteristic of PDU patients—might be another potentiator of the consequences of infection.

We have found only one report in the literature that addressed these comprehensive questions. Seventy-five patients, who had recently developed symptomatic PDU, underwent an assessment of their exposure to stressful life events; personality profiles, mood status, age, gender, family history of PDU, smoking habits, the consumption of alcohol, coffee, and NSAID, blood type, serum PG-I levels, and *H. pylori* antibody titers. The greater the number of cumulative risk factors, the less likely were the patients to have been exposed to stressful events or to show high scores on psychopathology, or altered moods, and vice versa. An inverse correlation was especially prominent in patients with no previous history of PDU, and with higher levels of antibody titers, but not with elevated PG-I levels or blood type O (Levenstein et al., 1995).

These results not only underline the multifactorial nature of PDU, but also the complexity of the various interacting variables.

## B. Psychosocial and Precipitating Factors

The roles of certain personal habits such as alcohol and caffeine ingestion and cigarette smoking have remained controversial. The most conservative conclusion has been that smoking slowed the healing of PDU, but did not incite the disease (Richardson, 1985).

Much controversy also surrounds the issue of the personal profiles of patients at risk for PDU (Weiner, 1977, 1991). Once again it must be emphasized that PDU is a heterogeneous disease. The particular, personal profiles described may apply only to those who, for example, have elevated PG-I levels and not to those who do not (Weiner, Thaler, Reiser, & Mirsky, 1957).

The second area of psychosocial research, especially into PDU and NUD, has been designed to answer two questions: who develops symptoms and the diseases, and when; and why does one predisposed person develop them and not the other? (These questions are, however, complicated by the fact that those who seek medical care for symptoms and a

disease are often no different than those who do not. The fact remains that most people with chronic gastritis have no symptoms.)

One important personal risk factor for PDU was being unmarried while being exposed to a greater number of threatening difficulties in life (e.g., financial and housing). The conclusion of this hospital-based study applied only to women patients (Gilligan, Fung, Piper, & Tennant, 1987). They were also less educated, and were employed in lower status occupations than their healthy, matched peers.

These observations were made on women patients after the onset of disease. They may or may not apply to men. Much more convincing evidence can be obtained by prospective, population-based studies, which also control for multiple risk factors. Such a study was done on 4595 middle-aged, Alameda County (CA) men and women, initially ulcer-free, who were followed for 9 years. During this period the incidence of PDU was 8%. Those in the upper versus the lower tertile on scores for a depressed mood, social isolation, hostility, and low socioeconomic status were significantly more liable to develop PDU when all other risk factors were controlled for (Levenstein, Kaplan, & Smith, 1997). This study also confirmed the fact that men and women, especially poor ones, when confronted with concrete difficulties in life, were more likely to develop PDU. These difficulties differed in men and women. The women lacked social relationships and were concerned with problems with their children. The men were confronted with marital and financial problems and were poorly educated with blue-collar occupations. They were burdened by a sense of personal failure (Levenstein, Kaplan, & Smith, 1996). However, the study did not evaluate the subjects' *H. pylori* antibody titers or levels of serum PG-I or -II.

After many controversial findings in the past about the role of the quantity of stressful life events in PDU and NUD patients, it seems fairly certain now that the critical factor was how these events were interpreted and not their quantity (Hui, Shiu, Lok, & Lam, 1992), and how they were adapted to. Subjects who developed PDU were more dependent, had fewer supporting figures around them, and were more plaintive, anxious, and depressed (Feldman & Walker, 1984). However, these characteristics were predominantly seen in subjects with a family history of PDU and elevated PG-I levels (Feldman, Walker, Green, & Weingarden, 1986).

The conclusion that those who perceive themselves as adversely stressed were more likely to develop PDU was borne out by a long-term study lasting 13 years (Anda et al., 1992). Yet in occasional persons, a dramatic and overwhelming life event anteceded PDU development (Richardson, 1985).

What is needed in this area of research are studies of perceived life events in relationship to *H. pylori* infection and its associated diseases. Some of the questions are: do they have anything to do with who becomes infected and who does not? Do they determine who develops, for example, PDU or NUD on being infected? Do chronically unpleasant lives have anything to do with the chronicity of gastritis and other diseases such as PDU and NUD?

These may not be idle questions, because we do not know why these different diseases or their variable courses are the outcomes of the infection. When treated with ranitidine, 75 patients, followed for up to about 6 years, with documented PDU had quite different treatment results. A significantly greater percentage (29%) of the ones of low socioeconomic status, little education, in a depressed mood, exposed to stressful events, and with evident psychopathology, were symptomatic longer than those (6%) with none of these characteristics. However, the impact of stressful events was much less in those with low scores on psychopathology. These social and psychological characteristics of these patients determined the response to treatment; age, gender, the smoking of cigarettes, the ingestion of alcohol and NSAID, serum PG-I levels, *H. pylori* antibody titers, or an initial response to ranitidine did not (Levenstein et al., 1996).

Such studies need also to take into account the various subforms of these diseases, their associated risk factors, and discrete physiological disturbances. Only by clearly determining the subgroups under study is progress likely to be made.

It cannot be emphasized too strongly that no one today believes that stressful experiences by themselves are pathogenetic in PDU and NUD. Even when psychosocial factors play a role in their inception they are combined with genetic, physiological, dietary and other factors in a multifactorial manner. Multi-causality is the general rule in clinical disease development. However, the proportions of the factors in the etiological variance may differ in the different subforms of the disease (Weiner & Shapiro, 1998).

## VIII. CONCLUSION: WHAT THEN IS THE ROLE OF *HELICOBACTER PYLORI* IN GASTRODUODENAL DISEASE?

If gastroduodenal diseases are both multifactorial and heterogeneous, then one may be able to find a role for *H. pylori* in their pathogeneses. That role is not likely to be invariant, monocausal, or linear. To claim that it is flies in the face of the evidence that PU, for example, comes about by a shift in the balance of a variety of factors that damage (including *H. pylori*) and those that protect the gastric mucosa against damage (Soll, 1990; Weiner, 1991).

A review of the literature simply does not bear out the contention that *H. pylori* linearly causes a variety of gastroduodenal diseases, except possibly in the two self-experiments, in which acute gastritis was incited in one and a chronic gastritis in the other. This is the best direct evidence of its role. However, gastritis may antecede infection so that one can only agree with Fallingborg and colleagues (1992) and Graham (1995) that *H. pylori* is most likely an "opportunist" that produces its effects in some people but only when the gastric mucosa has been disrupted or damaged by inflammation, atrophy, alcohol (Uppal et al., 1991), NSAID, neoplasia, or secondary to gastrinoma, etc., or when metaplasia of the duodenal mucosa has occurred. The transient role of *H. pylori* is supported by Marshall's experiment in which he induced in himself a time-limited acute gastritis (Marshall et al., 1985). Even the association of *H. pylori* and chronic gastritis is subject to bias because most patients with it are asymptomatic. Therefore, the association only occurs in symptomatic patients and not in those without symptoms who do not come for care and study.

In conclusion, the arguments presented do not refute a multifactorial concept about (at least) peptic ulceration; in fact, they support it, and they raise the question of how *H. pylori* could possibly and by itself incite so many different diseases of the gastroduodenal tract.

## References

Adelson, D. (1998). Personal communication.

Anda, R. F., Williamson, D. F., Escobedo, L. G., Remington, P. L., Mast, E., & Madans, J. F. (1992). Self-perceived stress and the risk of peptic ulcer disease. A longitudinal study of adults. *Archives of Internal Medicine, 152,* 829–833.

Atherton, J. C. (1997). The clinical relevance of strain types of *Helicobacter pylori. Gut, 40,* 700–703.

Barthel, J. S., Westblom, T. U., Havey, A. D., Gonzalez, F., & Everett, D. (1988). Gastritis and *Campylobacter pylori* in healthy, asymptomatic volunteers. *Archives of Internal Medicine, 148,* 1149–1151.

Blaser, M. J. (1987). Gastric *Campylobacter*-like organisms, gastritis, and peptic ulcer disease. *Gastroenterology, 93,* 371–383.

Blaser, M. J. (1990). *Helicobacter pylori* and the pathogenesis of gastroduodenal inflammation. *Journal of Infectious Disease, 161,* 626–633.

Blaser, M. J. (1995). Intrastrain differences in *Helicobacter pylori. Annals of Medicine, 27*(5), 559–563.

Borén, T., Normark, S., & Falk, P. (1994). *Helicobacter pylori*: Molecular basis for host recognition and bacterial adherence. *Trends in Microbiology, 2,* 221–228.

Bukholm, G., Tannæs, P., Nedenskov, P., Esbensen, Y., Grav, H. J., Havig, T., Ariansen, S., & Guldvog, I. (1997). Colony variation of *Helicobacter pylori*: Pathogenic potential is correlated to cell wall lipid composition. *Scandinavian Journal of Gastroenterology, 32,* 445–454.

Carrick, J., Lee, A., Hazell, S., Ralston, M., & Daskalopoulos, G. (1989). *Campylobacter pylori*, duodenal ulcer, and gastric metaplasia: A possible role of functional heterotopic tissue in ulcerogenesis. *Gut, 30,* 790–797.

Correa, P. (1991). Is gastric carcinoma an infectious disease? *New England Journal of Medicine, 325,* 1127–1131.

Cover, T. L., Cao, P., Murthy, U. K., Sipple, M. S., & Blaser, M. J. (1992). Serum neutralizing antibody response to the vacuolating cytotoxin of *Helicobacter pylori*. *Journal of Clinical Investigation, 90,* 913–918.

Cover, T. L., Dooley C. P., & Blaser, M. J. (1990). Characterization of and human serologic response to proteins in *Helicobacter pylori* broth culture supernatatants with vacuolizing cytotoxin activity. *Infection and Immunity, 58,* 603–609.

Craig, P. M., Karnes, W. E., Territo, M. C., & Walsh, J. H. (1990). *Helicobacter pylori* secretes a chemotactic factor for monocytes and neutrophils. *Gastroenterology, 98,* A33. [abstract]

Doglioni, C., Wotherspoon, A. C., Moschini, A., de Boni, M., & Isaacson, P. G. (1992). High incidence of primary gastric lymphoma in northeastern Italy. *Lancet, 339,* 834–835.

Dooley, C. P., Cohen, H., Fitzgibbons, P. L., Bauer, M., Appleman, M. D., Pérez-Pérez, G. I., & Blaser, M. J. (1989). Prevalence of *Helicobacter pylori* infection and histological gastritis in asymptomatic persons. *New England Journal of Medicine, 321,* 1562–1569.

Essery, S. D., Weir, D. M., James, V. S., Blackwell, C. C., Saadi, A. T., Busuttil, A., & Tzanakak, G. (1994). Detection of microbial surface antigens that bind Lewis (a) antigen. *FEMS. Immunology and Medical Microbiology, 9,* 15–21.

Fallingborg, J., Poulsen, L. O., Grove, A., & Teglbjaerg, P. S. (1992). Frequency of *Helicobacter pylori* and gastritis in healthy subjects without gastrointestinal symptoms. *Scandinavian Journal of Gastroenterology, 27,* 338–390.

Feldman, M. (1948). Statistical study of life cycle of 1154 cases of duodenal ulcer. *Journal of the American Medical Association, 136,* 736–739.

Feldman, M., & Walker, P. (1984). A controlled study of psychosocial factors in peptic ulcer disease. *Gastroenterology, 86,* 1075.

Feldman, M., Walker, P., Green, J. L., & Weingarden, K. (1986). Life event stress and psychosocial factors in men with peptic ulcer disease: A multidimensional case–controlled study. *Gastroenterology, 91,* 1370–1379.

Feng, Y. Y., & Wang, Y. (1988). *Campylobacter pylori* in patients with gastritis, peptic ulcer, and gastric carcinoma of the stomach in Lanzhou, China. *Lancet, 1,* 1055–1056.

Fong, T. L., Dooley, C. A., Dehesa, M., Cohen, H., Carmel, R., Fitzgibbons, P. L., Pérez-Pérez, G. I., & Blaser, M. J. (1991). *Helicobacter pylori* infection and pernicious anemia: A prospective controlled study. *Gastroenterology, 100,* 328–332.

Forman, D., Sitas, F., Newell, D. G., Stacey, A. R., Boreham, J., Peto, R., Campbell, T. C., & Chen, J. (1990). Geographic association of *Helicobacter pylori* antibody prevalence and gastric cancer mortality in rural China. *International Journal of Cancer, 46,* 608–611.

Furuta, T., Baba, S., Takashima, M., Futami, H., Arai, H., Kajimura, M., Hanai, H., & Kaneko, E. (1998). Effect of *Helicobacter pylori* infection on gastric pH. *Scandinavian Journal of Gastroenterology, 33,* 357–363.

Gilligan, I., Fung, L., Piper, D. W., & Tennant, C. (1987). Life event stress and chronic difficulties. *Journal of Psychosomatic Research, 31,* 117–123.

Glupcyzynski, Y., Burette, A., Labbe, M., Deprey, C., De Reuck, M., & Delentre, M. (1988). *Campylobacter pylori*-associated gastritis: A double blind placebo-controlled trial with amoxicillin. *American Journal of Gastroenterology, 83,* 365–372.

Go, M. F., Cissell, L., & Graham, D. Y. (1998). Failure to confirm association of *vac A* gene mosaicism with duodenal ulcer disease. *Scandinavian Journal of Gastroenterology, 33,* 132–136.

Go, M. F., & Graham, D. Y. (1996). The *cag A* is in the majority of *H. pylori* strains independent of whether the individual has duodenal ulcer or asymptomatic gastritis. *Helicobacter, 1,* 107–111.

Graham, D. Y., Lew, G. M., Klein, P. D., Evans, D. G., Evans, D. J., Jr., Saeed, Z. A., & Malaty, H. M. (1992). Effect of treatment of *Helicobacter pylori* infection on the long-term recurrence of gastric or duodenal ulcer. *Annals of Internal Medicine, 116,* 705–708.

Graham, D. Y., Opekum, A., Lew, G. M., Klein, P. D., & Walsh, J. H. (1991). *Helicobacter pylori*-associated gastrin release in duodenal ulcer patients. The effects of bombesin infusion and urea ingestion. *Gastroenterology, 100,* 1571–1575.

Graham, J. R. (1995). *Helicobacter pylori*: Human pathogen or simply an opportunist? *Lancet, 345,* 1095–1097.

Goldschmiedt, M., Redfern, J. S., Barnett, C., Schwarz, B., & Feldman, M. (1989). Effect of age on gastric acid secretion and serum gastrin concentrations in healthy men and women. *Gastroenterology, 98,* A50. [abstract]

Greenberg, R. E., & Bank, S. (1990). The prevalence of *Helicobacter pylori* in non-ulcer dyspepsia: Importance of stratification according to age. *Archives of Internal Medicine, 150,* 2053–2055.

Hamlet, A., Lindholm, C., Nilsson, O., & Olbe, L. (1998). Aspirin-induced gastritis like *Helicobacter pylori*-induced gastritis disinhibits acid secretion in humans: Relation to cytokine expression. *Scandinavian Journal of Gastroenterology, 33,* 346–356.

Hamlet, A., & Olbe, L. (1996). The influence of *Helicobacter pylori* infection on postprandial duodenal acid load and duodenal bulb pH in humans. *Gastroenterology, 111,* 391–400.

Hein, H. O., Suadicani, P., & Gyntelborg, F. (1992). Genetic markers for peptic ulcer. A study of 3387 men aged 54 to 74 years. The Copenhagen male study. *Scandinavian Journal of Gastroenterology, 32,* 16–21.

Hentschel, E., Brandstätter, G., Dragosics, B., Hirsch, A. M., Nemec, H., Schütze, K., Taufer, M., & Wurzer, H. (1993). Effect of ranitidine and amoxicillin plus metroridazole on the eradication of *Helicobacter pylori* on the recurrence of duodenal ulcer. *New England Journal of Medicine, 328,* 308–312.

Holcombe, C. (1992). *Helicobacter pylori*: The African enigma. *Gut, 33,* 429–431.

Hornick, R. B. (1987). Peptic ulcer disease: A bacterial infection. *New England Journal of Medicine, 316,* 1598–1600.

Hosking, S. W., Ling, T. K. W., Chung, S. C. S., Yung, M. Y., Cheng, A. F. B., Sung, J. J. Y., & Li, A. K. C. (1994). Duodenal ulcer healing by eradication of *Helicobacter pylori* without anti-acid treatment: Randomised controlled trial. *Lancet, 343,* 508–510.

Hu, P. J., Li, Y. Y., & Lin, H. L. (1995). Gastric atrophy and regional variation in upper gastrointestinal disease. *American Journal of Gastroenterology, 90,* 1102–1106.

Hui, W. M., Shiu, L. P., Lok, A. S. F., & Lam, S. K. (1992). Life events and daily stress in duodenal ulcer disease: A prospective study of patients with active disease and in remission. *Digestion, 52,* 165–172.

Hunt, R. H. (1996). The role of *Helicobacter pylori* in pathogenesis–the spectrum of clinical outcomes. *Scandinavian Journal of Gastroenterology, 31* (Supplement 220), 3–9.

Hussell, T., Isaacson, P. G., Crabtree, J. E., & Spencer, J. (1993). The response of cells from low-grade B-cell gastric lymphomas of mucosa-associated lymphoid tissue to *Helicobacter pylori*. *Lancet*, *342*, 571–574.

Isaacson, P. G. (1995). The MALT lymphoma concept updated. *Annals of Oncology*, *6*, 319–320.

Jiang, S. J., Liu, W. Z., Zhang, D. Z., Shi, Y., Xiao, S. D., Zhang, Z. H., & Lu, D. Y. (1987). *Campylobacter*-like organisms in chronic gastritis, peptic ulcer and gastric carcinoma. *Scandinavian Journal of Gastroenterology*, *22*, 553–558.

Karttunen, R., Karttunen, T., Ekre, H.-PT., & MacDonald, T. T. (1995). Interferon gamma and interleukin 4 secreting cells in the gastric antrum in *Helicobacter pylori* positive and negative gastritis. *Gut*, *36*, 341–345.

Karttunen, R. A., Karttunen, T. J., Yousfi, M. M., El-Zimaity, H. M. T., Graham, D. Y., & El-Zaatari, F. A. K. (1997). Expression of mRNA for interferon-gamma, interleukin-10, and interleukin-12 (p40) in normal gastric mucosa and in mucosa infected with *Helicobacter pylori*. *Scandinavian Journal of Gastroenterology*, *32*, 22–27.

Konturek, P. Ch., Bobrzynski, A., Konturek, S. J., Bielanski, W., Faller, G., Kirchner, T., & Hahn, E. G. (1998). Epidermal growth factor and transforming growth factor alpha in duodenal ulcer and non-ulcer dyspepsia patients before and after *Helicobacter pylori* eradication. *Scandinavian Journal of Gastroenterology*, *33*, 143–151.

Koop, H., Stumpf, M., Eissele, R., Lamberts, R., Stockmann, F., Creutzfeldt, W., & Arno, R. (1991). Antral *Helicobacter pylori*-like organisms in different states of gastric acid secretion. *Digestion*, *48*, 230–236.

Kuipers, E. J., Pérez-Pérez, G. I., Meuwissen, S. G. M., & Blaser, M. J. (1991). *Helicobacter pylori* and atrophic gastritis. *Journal of the National Cancer Institute*, *87*, 1777–1780.

Labenz, J., & Börsch, G. (1994). Evidence for the essential role of *Helicobacter pylori* in gastric ulcer disease. *Gut*, *35*, 19–22.

Labenz, J., Rühl, G. H., Bertrams, J., & Börsch, G. (1994). Medium- or high-dose omeprazole plus amoxicillin eradicates *Helicobacter pylori* in gastric ulcer disease. *American Journal of Gastroenterology*, *89*, 726–730.

Lam, S. K. (1993). Epidemiology and genetics of peptic ulcer. *Gastroenterology Japonica*, *28*, (Supplement 5), 145–157.

Lam, S. K., & Lai, C. L. (1978). Gastric ulcers with and without associated duodenal ulcer have different pathophysiology. *Clinical Science and Molecular Medicine*, *55*, 97–102.

Levenstein, S., Kaplan, G. A., & Smith, M. W. (1996). Socio-demographic characteristics, life stressors, and peptic ulcer. A prospective study. *Journal of Clinical Gastroenterology*, *21*, 185–192.

Levenstein, S., Kaplan, G. A., & Smith, M. W. (1997). Psychological predictors of peptic ulcer incidence in the Alameda County Study. *Journal of Clinical Gastroenterology*, *24*, 140–146.

Levenstein, S., Prantera, C., Varvo, V., Arca, M., Scribano, M. L., Spinella, S., & Berto, E. (1996). Long-term symptom patterns in duodenal ulcer: Psychosocial factors. *Journal of Psychosomatic Research*, *41*, 465–472.

Levenstein, S., Prantera, C., Varvo, V., Scribano, M. L., Berto, E., Spinella, S., & Lanari, G. (1995). Patterns of biologic and psychologic risk factors in duodenal ulcer patients. *Journal of Clinical Gastroenterology*, *21*, 110–117.

Li, H., Kalies, I., Mellgård, B., & Helander, H. F. (1998). A rat model of chronic *Helicobacter pylori* infection. Studies of epithelial cell turnover and gastric ulcer healing. *Scandinavian Journal of Gastroenterology*, *33*, 370–378.

Li, H., Mellgård, B., & Helander, H. F. (1997). Innoculation of VacA- and CagA-*Helicobacter pylori* delays gastric ulcer healing in the rat. *Scandinavian Journal of Gastroenterology*, *32*, 439–444.

Majewski, S. I., & Goodwin, C. S. (1988). Restriction endonuclease analysis of the genome of *Campylobacter pylori* with a rapid extraction method: Evidence for considerable genomic variation. *Journal of Infectious Disease*, *157*, 465–471.

Marchetti, M., Arico, B., Burroni, D., Figura, N., Rappuoli, R., & Ghiara, P. (1995). Development of a mouse model of *Helicobacter pylori* that mimics human disease. *Science*, *267*, 1655–1656.

Marshall, B. J. (1983). Unidentified curved bacilli on gastric epithelium in active chronic gastritis. *Lancet*, *ii*, 1273–1275.

Marshall, B. J. (August 15, 1987). Peptic ulcer: An infectious disease. *Hospital Practice*, 87–96.

Marshall, B. J., Armstrong, J. A., McGechie, D. B., & Glancy, R. J. (1985). Attempts to fulfill Koch's postulates for pyloric *Campylobacter*. *Medical Journal of Australia*, *142*, 436–439.

Marshall, B. J., & Warren, J. R. (1984). Unidentified curved bacilli in the stomach of patients with gastritis and peptic ulceration. *Lancet*, *1*, 1311–1314.

McNulty, C. A. M., Gearty, J. C., Crump, B., Davis, M., Donovan, I. A., Melikian, V., Lister, D. M., & Wise, R. (1986). *Campylobacter pyloridis* and associated gastritis: Investigator blind placebo controlled trial of bismuth salicylate and erythromycin ethyl-succinate. *British Medical Journal*, *293*, 645–649.

Mearin, F., de Ribot, X., Balboa, A., Salas, A., Varas, M. J., Cucala, M., Bartolomé, R., Armengol, J. R., & Malagelada, J.-R. (1995). Does *Helicobacter pylori* infection increase gastric sensitivity in functional dyspepsia? *Gut*, *37*, 47–51.

Meeroff, J. C., Paulsen, G., & Guth, P. (1975). Parenteral aspirin produces and enhances gastric mucosal lesions and bleeding in rats. *Digestive Diseases and Science*, *20*, 847–852.

Mertz, H. R.,& Walsh, J. H. (1991). Peptic ulcer pathophysiology. *Medical Clinics of North America*, *75*, 799–814.

Mezey, E., & Palkovits, M. (1992). Localization of targets for anti-ulcer drugs in cells of the immune system. *Science*, *258*, 1662–1665.

Morris, A. J., Ali, M. R., Nicholson, G. I., Pérez-Pérez, G. I., & Blaser, M. J. (1991). Long-term follow up of voluntary ingestion of *Helicobacter pylori*. *Annals of Internal Medicine*, *114*, 662–663.

Morris, A. J., & Nicholson, G. (1987). Ingestion of *Campylobacter pyloridis* causes gastritis and raised fasting gastric pH. *American Journal of Gastroenterology*, *82*, 192–199.

Moss, S. F., Legon, S., Bishop, A. E., Polak, J. M., & Calam, J. (1992). Effect of *Helicobacter pylori* on gastric somatostatin in duodenal ulcer disease. *Lancet*, *340*, 930–932.

Nomura, A., Stemmerman, G. N., Chyou, P.-H., Kato, I., Pérez-Pérez, G. I., & Blaser, M. J. (1991). *Helicobacter pylori* infection and gastric carcinoma among Japanese Americans in Hawaii. *New England Journal of Medicine*, *325*, 1132–1136.

Nomura, A., Stemmerman, G. N., Chyou, P.-H., Pérez-Pérez, G. I., & Blaser, M. J. (1994). *Helicobacter pylori* infection and the risk for duodenal and gastric ulceration. *Annals of Internal Medicine*, *120*, 977–981.

Ohta-Tada, V., Tagaki, A., Koga, Y., Kamiya, S., & Miwa, T. (1997). Flagellin gene diversity among *Helicobacter pylori* strains and IL-8 secretion from gastric epithelial cells. *Scandinavian Journal of Gastroenterology*, *32*, 455–459.

Parsonnet, J., Blaser, M. J., Pérez-Pérez, G. I., Hargrett-Bean, N., & Tauxe, R. V. (1992). Symptoms and risk factors of *Helicobacter pylori* infection in a cohort of epidemiologists. *Gastroenterology*, *102*, 41–46.

Parsonnet, J., Friedman, G. D., Vandersteen, D. P., Chang, Y., Vogelman, J. H., Orentreich, N., & Sibley, R. K. (1991).

*Helicobacter pylori* and the risk of gastric carcinoma. *New England Journal of Medicine, 325,* 1127–1131.

Parsonnet, J., Hansen, S., Rodriguez, L., Gelb, A. B., Warrke, R. A., Jellum, E., Orentreich, N., Vogelman, J. H., & Friedman, G. D. (1994). *Helicobacter pylori* infection and gastric lymphoma. *New England Journal of Medicine, 330,* 1267–1271.

Pauli, G., & Yardley, J. K. (1989). Pathology of *Campylobacter pylori*-associated gastric and esophageal lesions. In M. J. Blaser (Ed.), *Campylobacter pylori in gastritis and peptic ulcer disease* (pp. 73–98). New York: Igaku Shoin Medical Publishers.

Pérez-Pérez, G. I., & Blaser, M. J. (1987). Conservation and diversity of *Campylobacter pyloridis* major antigens. *Infection and Immunity, 55,* 1256–1263.

Pérez-Pérez, G. I., Dworkin, B., Chodos, J., & Blaser, M. J. (1988). *Campylobacter pylori*-specific serum antibodies in humans. *Annals of Internal Medicine, 109,* 11–17.

Peterson, W. L., Sturdevant, R. A. L., Frankl, H. D., Richardson, C. T., Isenberg, J. L., Elashoff, R. D., Sones, J. Q., Gross, R. A., McCallum, R. W., & Fordtran (1977). Healing of duodenal ulcer with an antacid regimen. *New England Journal of Medicine, 297,* 341–345.

Pflanz, M. (1971). Epidemiological and sociocultural factors in the etiology of duodenal ulcer. *Advances in Psychosomatic Medicine, 6,* 121–151.

Rauws, E. A. J., Langenberg, W., Houthoff, H. J., Zanen, H. C., & Tytgat, G. N. (1988). *Campylobacter pyloridis*-associated chronic active antral gastritis. *Gastroenterology, 94,* 33–40.

Richardson, C. T. (1985). Pathogenetic factors in peptic ulcer disease. *American Journal of Medicine (Supplement C), 79,* 1–7.

Rokkas, T., Pursey, C., Uzoechina, E., Dorrington, L., Simmons, N. A., Felipe, M. I., & Sladen, G. E. (1987). *Campylobacter pylori* and non-ulcer dyspepsia. *American Journal of Gastroenterology, 82,* 1149–1152.

Ross, J. S., Bui, H. X., del Rosario, A., Sonbati, H., George, M., & Lee, C. Y. (1992). *Helicobacter pylori.* Its role in the pathogenesis of peptic ulcer disease in a new animal model. *American Journal of Pathology, 141,* 721–727.

Rotter, J. I. (1981). Gastric and duodenal ulcer are each many different diseases. *Digestive Diseases and Science, 26,* 154–160.

Rotter, J. I., & Rimoin, D. L. (1977). Peptic ulcer disease—A heterogeneous group of disorders. *Gastroenterology, 73,* 604–607.

Saeed, Z. A., Evans, D. G., Jr., Evans D. G., Cornelius, M. J., Maton, P. N., Jensen, R. T., & Graham, D. Y. (1991). *Helicobacter pylori* and Zollinger-Ellison syndrome. *Digestive Diseases and Science, 36,* 15–18.

Samloff, I. M. (1989). Peptic ulcer. The many proteinases of aggression. *Gastroenterology, 96,* 586–595.

Seeley, G. P., & Colp, R. (1941). The bacteriology of peptic ulcers and gastric malignancies, possibly bearing on complications following gastric surgery. *Surgery, 10,* 369–380.

Sipponen, P., Äärynen, M., Kääriäinen, I., Kettunen, P., Helske, T., & Seppälä, K. (1989). Chronic antral gastritis, Lewis (a+) phenotype, and male sex as factors in predicting coexisting duodenal ulcer. *Scandinavian Journal of Gastroenterology, 24,* 581–588.

Siurala, M., Sipponen, P., & Kekki, M. (1985). Chronic gastritis: Dynamic and clinical aspects. *Scandinavian Journal of Gastroenterology (Supplement), 20,* 69–76.

Soll, A. H. (1990). Pathogenesis of peptic ulcer and implications for therapy. *New England Journal of Medicine, 322,* 909–916.

Steer, H. W. (1984). Surface morphology of the gastroduodenal mucosa in duodenal ulceration. *Gut, 25,* 1203–1210.

Stolte, M., Kroher, G., Meining, A., Morgner, A., Bayerdörffer, E., & Bethke, B. (1997). A comparison of *Helicobacter pylori* and *H.*

*heilmannii* gastritis. *Scandinavian Journal of Gastroenterology, 32,* 28–33.

Strauss, R. M., Wang, T. C., Kelsey, P. B., Compton, C. C., Ferraro, M-J, Pérez-Pérez, G., Parsonnet, J., & Blaser, M. J. (1990). Association of *Helicobacter pylori* infection with dyspeptic symptoms in patients undergoing gastroduodenoscopy. *The American Journal of Medicine, 89,* 464–469.

Sturdevant, R. A. (1976). Epidemiology of peptic ulcer. *American Journal of Epidemiology, 104,* 9–14.

Susser, M. (1976). Causes of peptic ulcer: A selective epidemiologic review. *Journal of Chronic Disease, 20,* 435–456.

Taha, A. S., & Russell, R. I. (1993). *Helicobacter pylori* and non-steroidal anti inflammatory drugs: Uncomfortable partners in peptic ulcer disease. *Gut, 34,* 580–583.

Talley, N. J., & Phillips, S. F. (1988). Non-ulcer dyspepsia: potential causes and pathophysiology. *Annals of Internal Medicine, 108,* 865–879.

Taylor, D. N., & Blaser, M. J. (1991). The epidemiology of *Helicobacter pylori* infection. *Epidemiological Review, 13,* 42–59.

Tee, W., Lambert, J. R., & Dwyer, B. (1995). Cytotoxin production by *Helicobacter pylori* from patients with upper gastrointestinal tract disease. *Journal of Clinical Microbiology, 33,* 1203–1205.

Tomb, J. L., White, O., Kerlavage, A. R., Clayton, R. A., Sutton, G. G., Fleischman, R. D., Ketchum, K. A., Klenk, H. P., Gill S., & Dougherty, B. A. (1997). The complete genome sequence of the gastric pathogen *Helicobacter pylori. Nature, 388,* 539–547.

Unge, P., & Gnarpe, H. (1988). Pharmacokinetic, bacteriological and clinical aspects on the use of doxiciline in patients with active duodenal ulcer associated with *Campylobacter pylori. Scandinavian Journal of Infectious Diseases* (Supplement), *53,* 70–73.

Uppal, R., Lateef, S. K., Korsten, M., Paronetto, F., & Lieber, C. S. (1991). Chronic alcoholic gastritis. Roles of alcohol and *Helicobacter pylori. Archives of Internal Medicine, 151,* 760–764.

Uribe, J. M., & Barrett, K. E. (1997). Nonmitogenic actions of growth factors: An integrated view of their role in intestinal physiology and pathophysiology. *Gastroenterology, 112,* 255–268.

Wallace, H., Cucala, M., Mugridge, K., & Parente, L. (1991). Secretagogue-specific effects of interleukin-I on gastric acid secretion. *American Journal of Physiology, 261,* G559–G564.

Warren, J. R., & Marshall, B. J. (1983). Unidentified curved bacilli in gastric epithelium in active chronic gastritis. *Lancet, 1,* 1273–1285.

Weigert, N., Schaffer, K., Schusdziarra, V., Classen, M., & Schepp, W. (1996). Gastrin secretion from primary cultures of rabbit antral G cells: Stimulation by inflammatory cytokines. *Gastroenterology, 110,* 147–154.

Weiner, H. (1977). *Psychobiology and human disease* (pp. 39–41). New York, NY: Elsevier.

Weiner, H. (1991). From simplicity to complexity (1950–1990): The case of peptic ulceration I. Human studies. *Psychosomatic Medicine, 53,* 467–490.

Weiner, H. (1992). *Perturbing the organism* (pp. 102–104). Chicago, IL: University of Chicago Press.

Weiner, H. (1996). Use of animal models in peptic ulcer disease. *Psychosomatic Medicine, 58,* 524–545.

Weiner, H., & Shapiro, A. P. (1998). Is Helicobacter pylori really the cause of gastroduodenal diseases? *Quarterly Journal of Medicine, 94,* 707–711.

Weiner, H., Thaler, M., Reiser, M. F., & Mirsky, I. A. (1957). Etiology of duodenal ulcer. I. Relation of specific psychological characteristics to rate of gastric secretion. *Psychosomatic Medicine, 19,* 1–10.

Wolfe, M. M., & Soll, A. H. (1988). The physiology of gastric acid secretion. *New England Journal of Medicine, 319,* 1707–1715.

Wormsley, K. G. (1989). *Campylobacter pylori* and ulcer disease—a causal connection? *Scandinavian Journal of Gastroenterology, Supplement, 160,* 53–58.

Wotherspoon, A. C., Doglioni, G., Diss, J. C., Pan, L., Moschini, A., de Boni, M., & Isaacson, P. G. (1993). Regression of primary low grade B-cell gastric lymphoma of mucosa-associated lymphoid tissue type after eradication of *Helicobacter pylori. Lancet, 342,* 575–577.

Wyatt, J. I., & Rathbone, B. J. (1988). Immune response of the gastric mucosa to *Campylobacter pylori. Scandinavian Journal of Gastroenterology* (Supplement), *142,* 44–49.

Yokota, K., Kurebayashi, Y., Takayama, Y., Hayashi, S., Isogai, H., Isogai, E., Imai, K., Yabana, T., Yachi, A., & Oguma, K. (1991). Colonization of *Helicobacter pylori* in the gastric mucosa of mongolian gerbils. *Microbiology and Immunology, 35,* 475–480.

Zucca, E., Bertoni, F., Roggero, E., Bosshard, G., Cazzaniga, G., Pedrinis, E., Biondi, A., & Cavalli, F. (1998). Molecular analysis of the progression from *Helicobacter pylori*-associated chronic gastritis to mucosa-associated-tissue lymphoma of the stomach. *New England Journal of Medicine, 338,* 804–810.

# 66

# Alcoholism and Immune Function

SAEED HOSSEINI, TOMAS SEPULVEDA, JEONGMIN LEE,
RONALD R. WATSON

## I. INTRODUCTION

Historically, alcohol has been associated with lowered resistance to infectious disease and some cancer. We found that administration to animals of alcohol at nontoxic levels led to decreased spleen and thymus weight (Watzl & Watson, 1993; Watzl et al., 1993a). Alcohol altered cytokine secretion by lymphocytes from uninfected and retrovirus infected mice (Wang & Watson, 1994b; Watson, Wang, Huang, Lopez, & Wood, 1993). We have found that ethanol applied to cells in vitro (Rabhala & Watson, 1990), as well as consumed chronically by mice, was associated with a variety of changes in lymphoid cell number

and particularly functions (Darban, Crawford, & Watson, 1992; Shahbazian, Darban, Stazzone, & Watson, 1992; Wang, Huang, Giger, & Watson, 1993, 1994d; Watzl & Watson, 1993; Watzl et al., 1993a). Alcohol at physiological levels in animals and humans causes changes in immune regulation and function. This is supported by many researchers as we have reviewed and evaluated in various formats (Pillai & Watson, 1991, 1993; Watson, 1995; Seminara, Pawlowski, & Watson, 1990; Watson, 1993, 1989; Watson et al., 1994; Watson, Watson, Lopez, Odeleye, & Darban, 1992a; Watzl & Watson, 1992a). We found that alcohol use in humans changes production of several Th2 cell cytokines (Martinez et al., 1993). In animals alcohol use suppresses Th1 cells' cytokine production (Wang et al., 1993, 1994d; Watson et al., 1993; Watzl & Watson, 1992a), lowering levels of Interleukin-2 (IL-2) and interferon-$\gamma$ (IFN-$\gamma$). While Th2 cytokines are important for promoting B-cell functions and antibody synthesis, they also suppress Th1 cells. Alcohol-induced cytokine dysregulation reduced cellular immunity and lowered regulation of Th2 cells' secretion of cytokines IL-4, IL-6, and IL-10 (Ardestai & Watson, 1995; Beckham & Watson, 1994; Darban et al., 1993; Lopez, Colombo, Huang, & Watson, 1992; Pillai & Watson, 1991, 1993; Watson, 1995; Wang, Huang, & Watson, 1995; Wang & Watson, 1994c, 1995a, b; Watson et al., 1994; Watson & Gottesfeld, 1993; Watzl & Watson, 1992b). Chronic alcohol abuse in animals and people is a cause of immune dysfunction. Ethanol as well as retrovirus infections affect several neurological systems that regulate or modulate immune systes. Therefore, we will review

687

ethanol's actions on cells in vitro, in humans, in animals, and in animal models of AIDS.

## II. ETHANOL INDUCES IMMUNE DYSFUNCTION IN UNINFECTED MICE AND PEOPLE

We found that chronic, long-term dietary ethanol produced immune dysfunction in mice (Darban, Watson, Darban, & Shahbazian, 1992; Wang et al., 1994d; Wang, Huang, Giger, & Watson, 1994c; Wang, Huang, & Watson, 1994e; Watson et al., 1993; Watzl et al., 1993a). Ethanol has direct effects on the number and percentage of various lymphocyte subsets when applied in vitro to human lymphocytes (Rabhala & Watson, 1990) or consumed chronically (Watson et al., 1993). It modified cytokine secretion in alcoholics (Martinez et al., 1993). We found that some immune functions were suppressed due to ethanol consumption (Wang et al., 1993, 1994d,e) whereas others were partially restored by high nutrient intakes (Wang et al., 1994e; Watzl et al., 1993a; Watzl, Lopez, Shahbazian, & Watson, 1993b; Watzl & Watson, 1993) during alcohol use as nutrient deficiency was one cause of immune dysfunction. A moderate dose of alcohol given in drinking water for 11 weeks reduced IgA and CD4+ cells in the intestinal lamina propria. This did not occur when the Lieber–DeCarli diet, heavily supplemented with megadoses of vitamins, was used. Thus, some of the mechanisms of alcohol-induced immune dysfunction occur via alcohol's induction of nutrient inadequacy. This would also explain some of vitamin E's enhancement (Wang et al., 1994e) of alcohol-suppressed immune functions.

Prothymocytes leave the bone marrow and arrive at the thymus where they find the appropriate environment, which lets them complete their differentiation to become functional T cells. The generation of functional, competent T cells from precursor populations within the thymus involves several stages of cellular proliferation and differentiation (Lesley, Trotter, Schutle, & Hyman, 1990; Scollay et al., 1988), which are mediated by cytokines (Carding, Hayday, & Bottomly, 1991).

Cytokines produced by T helper cells are biologically active polypeptides, intercellular messengers and potent regulators of immune functions that regulate growth, mobility, and differentiation of leukocytes. There are two types of T helper cells that produce distinct patterns of cytokines. The Th1 cell characteristically secretes IFN-$\gamma$, tumor necrosis factor-$\alpha$ (TNF-$\alpha$), and IL-2 and orchestrates or activates cell-mediated immunity (such as macrophage and

granulocyte activation). The Th2 cells secrete IL-4, IL-5, IL-6, IL-9, and IL-10 (Mosmann & Coffman, 1989) and mediate B-cell activation to produce IgGl and IgE, eosinophil differentiation, and mast cell proliferation. In the immune system, IL-1 can regulate various aspects of T- and B-cell development and functional activation and can stimulate T cells to secrete IL-2, which is an important cytokine in the growth and differentiation of T and B cells (Mitzi, 1989). IL-4, IL-5, and IL-6 are responsible for the growth, proliferation, and differentiation of B cells into antibody-producing cells (Mitzi, 1989). In addition, cytokines produced by one subset can exert cross-regulatory or inhibitory effects on the differentiation and effector function of the other subset. For example IFN activates phagocytosis of macrophages and neutrophil cells and cytotoxicity of natural killer (NK) cells, augments Th1 cell differentiation, and inhibits the proliferation and differentiation of Th2 cells and their effector functions (Mosmann & Coffman, 1989), whereas Th2-type cytokines, particularly IL-4 and IL-10, exert strong inhibitory effects on cell-mediated inflammatory responses. Conversely IL-10 inhibits Th1 cell differentiation and production of Th1 cytokines via indirect action of IL-10 on a subpopulation of accessory cells (Scott & Kaufmann, 1991). Thus, cytokines play extremely important roles in the communication network that links inducer and effector cells during immune and inflammatory responses.

Extensive clinical and experimental studies have shown that alcohol ingestion is associated with immune modulation or suppression and can alter both specific (Saad, Domiati-Saad, & Jerrells, 1993: Steven, Kumar, Stewart, & Seelig, 1990) and nonspecific immunity (McGregor, 1986; Adams & Jordan, 1984; Meadows, Wallendai, Kosugi, Wunderich, & Singer, 1992; Watson, Prabhala, Abril, & Smith, 1988), thus leading to an increased susceptibility to a variety of infections. Alterations include changes in the cell number (Jerrells, Smith, Eckardt, Majchrowicz, & Weight, 1986) and composition of lymphoid tissues (Saad & Jerrells, 1991), impairments in T-cell proliferation (Rosselle & Mendenhall, 1982; Spinozzi et al., 1991) and B-cell antibody production (Bagasra, Howeedy, Dorio, & Kajdacsy-Balla, 1987; Jerrells, Peritt, Marietta, & Edkardt, 1989), changes in cytokine production (Na & Seelig, 1994), and changes in macrophage activation (Bagasra, Howeedy, & Kajdacsy-Balla, 1988), as well as granulocyte mobility and function (Spagnuolo & McGregor, 1975). Although the mechanisms for the effect of ethanol on the immune system are not well understood, one possibility is that alcohol intake may induce high levels of circulating glucocorticoid (Ellis, 1966; Tabakoff, Jaffe, & Ritzmann, 1978) that would be associated with alterations in the immune response. Following acute administration of ethanol, significant increases in serum levels of glucocorticoids, opioids, and catecholamines (epinephrine and norepinephrine) have been reported (Han, Lin, & Pruett, 1993; Thiagaran, Mefford, & Eskay, 1989). Previous studies have suggested that elevated levels of corticosteroids induced by ethanol may act in conjunction with other factors to downregulate the immune response, especially cell-mediated inflammatory responses (Goldstein, 1983; Hall & Goldstein, 1984). Some of these effects can be blocked by glucocorticoid antagonist, like RU 486, indicating involvement of glucocorticoids (Han et al., 1993; Han & Pruett, 1995). Therefore, it is possible that alcohol consumption may induce a suppression of Th1 cell function and an action of Th2 cells. The thymus is also very sensitive to corticosteroids, which cause apoptosis and loss of functions of thymocytes. In addition, ethanol interacts with the endogenous opioid system by: (a) production of certain ethanol metabolites including the isoquinolines that bind to opiate receptors, (b) modification of the binding properties of opiate receptors, and (c) alteration of the release, synthesis and posttranslational processing of endogenous opioid peptide (Budec, Ciric, Koko, & Asanin, 1992; Gianouakis, 1989). Thus, ethanol-induced changes in corticosteroids and opiates could be responsible for the changes in cytokine release by thymocytes, thereby altering T-cell maturation. The increased levels of corticosterone induced by ethanol are sufficient to decrease the expression of MHC class II molecules on the B-cell surface. On the other hand, it is not sufficient to decrease spleen cell number and alter subpopulation ratios (Weiss, Collier, & Pruett, 1996). Since B cells are one of the professional antigens presenting cells due to their exquisite recognition of antigen by way of surface immunoglobulins, T-cell activation will be diminished.

Ethanol consumption also reduces the number of thymocytes, thymus weight, thymocyte mitogenesis, and CD4+ and CD8+ thymocytes (Ewald & Frost, 1987, & 1988; Jerrells, Eckardt, & Weinber, 1990). Consequently, the alteration in peripheral T-cell subsets or T-cell functions by ethanol consumption could be the consequence of changes at the thymus level including thymocyte cytokine production. The inhibition of IL-2 production by ethanol use may partly contribute to the changes in T-cell subpopulations and differentiation in the thymus. IL-4 blocks T-cell development by reducing the number of double-positive thymocytes (Plum, De Smedt, & Leclercq,

1990). Ethanol ingestion decreases IL-6 production; thus ethanol should contribute to the disruption of T-cell maturation (Wang & Watson, 1994a).

Alcohol consumption suppresses IFN-$\gamma$ production by human peripheral lymphocytes (Wagner et al., 1992). The dysregulation of IFN-$\gamma$ release by thymocytes may reflect the failure of T-cell education, leading to loss of tolerance to self-antigens or reaction to nonself antigens. In addition, migration inhibiting factor activity (Rosselle, Mendenhall, & Grossman, 1989) and the levels of serum and lung TNF-$\alpha$ (Nelson, Bagby, Bainton, & Summer, 1989a) are suppressed in alcoholic animals.

IFN and TNF-$\alpha$ regulate production of other cytokines and the development of functional cellular immunity during infection with its direct cytotoxic effects against invading parasites and viruses (Ungar et al., 1991).

Ethanol impairs essential host defenses against lung infections. T cells from alcoholic patients show a decreased capacity to secrete IFN-$\gamma$, a potent activator of macrophage TNF-$\alpha$ production (Chadha et al., 1990). In addition, T cells from alcoholic patients and animals maintained on a chronic ethanol diet have a decreased proliferative response to mitogens and recall antigens (Chadha, Stadler, Albini, Nakeeb, & Thacore, 1991; Straus, Berenyi, Huang, & Straus, 1971; Thestrup-Pederseti, Ladefoged, & Anderson, 1976). Within lung tissue, the capacity of alveolar macrophage to secrete soluble mediators, recruit polymorphonuclear leukocytes, and release reactive oxygen and reactive nitrogen intermediates critical for the intracellular killing of pathogens are all adversely affected by ethanol (Antony, Godbey, Hott, & Queener, 1993; Greenberg et al., 1994; Astry, Warr, & Jakab, 1983; Dorio, Joek, Rubin, & Forman, 1988; Nelson, Bagby, & Summer 1989b; Rimland, 1983). Cytokines like TNF-$\alpha$ and granulocyte-macrophage colony-stimulating factor have bacteriostatic and bactericidal effects (Bermudez & Young, 1988; Sheflito et al., 1990). Alcohol downregulates the release of TNF-$\alpha$ and PMN recruitment in the early phase of an inflammatory response may impair the clearance of the pathogenic organisms.

## III. THE EFFECTS OF ALCOHOL ON MONOCYTES AND MACROPHAGES

Acute or chronic ethanol consumption has been shown to modulate T-cell proliferation, B-cell function, and particularly macrophage function. Monocytes or macrophages play a pivotal role in the immune system by serving as professional phagocytes in elimination of pathogens at the site of inflammation. Moreover, monocytes have tremendous capacity for immune regulation via their cytokine/mediator production and accessory cell capacity. However, the mechanisms for ethanol-induced suppression of immune functions on monocytes and macrophages are not well defined.

Acute ethanol treatment inhibits inflammatory cytokines (TNF-$\alpha$, IL-1$\beta$, and IL-6), while increasing inhibitory cytokine (TGF-$\beta$, IL-10) production in human blood monocytes that, in turn, could contribute to the overall immune abnormalities seen after alcohol use (Gallucci & Meadows, 1995; Gyongyi, Pranoti, Linda, & Donna, 1996; Szabo, Mandrekar, Verma, & Catalano, 1995). The production of TNF-$\alpha$ and IL-1$\beta$ is autoregulated via the inhibitory effects of TGF-$\beta$ and IL-10 produced by the macrophage themselves (Ahuja, Poliogianni, Yamada, Balow, & Boumpas, 1993). Ethanol has been shown to induce TGF-$\beta$ in kupffer cells, the resident hepatic macrophage population, and monocytes, and it is likely to increase IL-10 (DelPrete, DeCarli, & Almerigogna, 1992). Therefore, pathologically increased macrophage TGF-$\beta$ and/or IL-10 levels after ethanol use can potentially attenuate host defense in both inflammatory and immune responses. Decreased induction of TNF-$\alpha$, IL-1$\beta$, and IL-6 is seen at both the protein and the mRNA levels in human monocytes or macrophages after acute ethanol treatment (Mandrekar, Catalano, & Szabo, 1997). Due to the fact that NF-kB/Rel is a common regulatory element of the promoter region of the inflammatory cytokine genes, it is reasonable to hypothesize that acute ethanol treatment might affect cytokine gene expression via modulation of the nuclear regulation factors (NF-kB/Rel) in human monocytes. For example, Mandrekar and co-workers (1997) suggested that a physiologically relevant concentration of ethanol (25 mM) might affect production of inflammatory cytokines, such as TNF-$\alpha$, IL-1$\beta$, and IL-6, by disrupting NF-kB signaling in monocytes. The impairment of the ability of human macrophages and murine kupffer cells to produce these cytokines is dependent in part on a downregulation in the number of cytokine receptors on the macrophage membrane. Macrophages, in the presence of ethanol levels achievable, in serum expressed four times fewer TNF-$\alpha$ receptors than untreated macrophages (Bermudez, 1994).

Several studies have indicated a correlation between macrophage changes and disease progression, such as alcoholic liver disease and cirrhosis during chronic consumption of ethanol. The liver is the major site of ethanol metabolism; thus, its resident cell populations are exposed to higher ethanol concentrations than other organs. Normal kupffer cell function is impaired in liver disease. Studies of experimental alcoholic liver disease in rats showed that kupffer cells lysozyme content is decreased (Kelly, Heryet, & McGee, 1989). In addition, kupffer cells isolated from chronic ethanol-fed rats demonstrated markedly depressed phagocytic capacity. The kupffer cell in the damaged liver may alter its ability to produce cytokines leading to the pathological changes associated with hepatic disease. McClain, Hill, Marsano, Cohen, and Shedlofsky (1993) demonstrated that serum levels of IL-1, IL-6, IL-8, and TNF-$\alpha$ are increased in patients with alcoholic liver disease. Acute ethanol ingestion leads to stimulation of superoxide production in isolated perfused rat liver, indicating an association between an alteration in cytokine homeostasis and a variety of liver diseases (Bautista & Spitzer, 1993). Monocytes in cirrhotic patients may become activated in a process to a priming event by ethanol, and that resultant oversecretion of cytokines such as TNF-$\alpha$ and IL-6 may be involved not only in the pathogenesis of the disease but in maintenance and be linked with symptoms of cirrhosis such as weight loss and muscle wasting and low-grade fever (Deviere, Content, Denys, & Vandenbussche, 1990). Thus, the impairment of the physiological mechanism for regulation of kupffer cell immune response could be a major contributing factor leading to the development of hepatic diseases. Additionally, in the rat model, alcohol exposure can also lead to enhanced production of macrophage inflammatory proteins (MIP1 and MIP2), which are cytotoxic to alcoholic hepatocytes in vitro, and upregulate the expression of adhesion molecules, i.e., CD-18 and its counterreceptor, intracellular adhesion molecule-1 (ICAM-1), thereby causing the initiation of hepatic injury (Bautista, 1997).

Chronic consumption of alcohol has been associated with a high rate of bacterial infection as well as a state of immune suppression in humans. Although a number of functional abnormalities of the immune function have been described both in vitro and in vivo following exposure to ethanol, epidemiologic evidence only exists to associate chronic ingestion to ethanol with bacterial infections including *Streptococcus pneumonia*, *Klebsiella pneumonia*, and pulmonary and peritoneal tuberculosis (Bermudez, 1994). Infection caused by organisms belonging to the *Mycobacterium avium* complex, which is an intracellular bacterium that invades and multiplies within macrophages, is associated with both localized and disseminated disease in patients with AIDS (Bermudez, 1994; Bermudez et al., 1993). In this population, macrophages and murine kupffer cells exposed to ethanol are more permissive toward intracellular growth of *M. avium*, and histopathologic studies show massive aggregates of bacteria within macrophages of the liver, spleen, and intestinal cells.

Recently, ethanol has been shown to affect macrophage microbicidal activity by suppressing superoxide anion production of pulmonary macrophages (Nympha, Steve, Warren, & Ion, 1996). In the lung, the alveolar macrophage (AM) serves as the first line of defense against invading pathogens. Following an encounter with a pathogen, the AM releases mediators including TNF-$\alpha$, PGE2, and superoxide anion ($O_2^-$) and nitric oxide (NO), which are critical components to pulmonary host defense. Nympha and coworkers (1996) demonstrated that both acute and chronic alcohol administration to rats inhibit AM TNF-$\alpha$, $O_2^-$, and NO. Thus, an insufficient release of these AM-derived-mediators caused by alcohol consumption may increase host susceptibility to a subsequent pulmonary infection. In liver acute ethanol exposure enhanced production of superoxides and nitric oxide (Bautista & Spitzer, 1993). Removal of cells from ethanol for 4 h returned superoxides production to normal levels. The overproduction of inducible nitric oxide in kupffer cells stimulated by cytokine (IFN-$\gamma$) and endotoxin (lipopolysaccharide (LPS)) is thought to contribute to vasodilation and increased liver sinusoidal blood flow during liver disease. However, the effect of chronic ethanol exposure on superoxides and nitric oxide production by kupffer cells and other monocyte–macrophages are not well defined.

## IV. THE EFFECTS OF ALCOHOL ON HIV-INFECTED PATIENTS

What are the risk factors that make some HIV-1-infected individuals more susceptible to the development of immune dysfunction and complicating disease? Isaki and Gordis (1993) stated that, "It seems possible that assaults by ethanol on the already compromised systems of patients infected with HIV could lead to an increased incidence of recurrent opportunistic infections which are typical manifestations of AIDS." Immune regulation is substantially accomplished by cytokines from CD4+ T helper (Th1) cells. Their cytokines promote cellular immunity and suppress Th2 cells' cytokine secretion. Alcohol abuse, retrovirus infection, oxidation, and deficiencies of antioxidant vitamins promote Th2 cells' production of cytokines, thus suppressing Th1 cells' cytokine secretion for reduced cellular immunity and increased

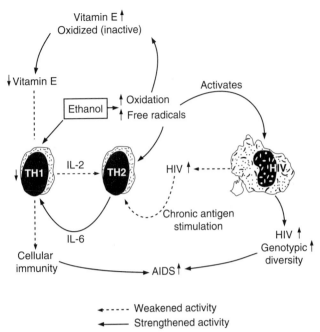

**FIGURE 1**  Schematic overview of alcohol's mechanisms for accentuation of immune dysfunction during HIV-1 infection. Alcohol use as well as murine and human retrovirus infection increases cytokine dysregulation, lowering mildly immunostimulatory antioxidant vitamins in lymphoid tissues. Supplementation with antioxidants in retrovirus-infected or alcohol-using mice slows immune dysfunction and loss of disease and cancer resistance, whereas alcohol use accentuates the immunological damage. Immune dysfunction promotes activation of HIV-1 by increased oxidation, resulting in more HIV-1 to accelerate development of AIDS.

HIV-1 production (Figure 1). Is alcohol's induced cytokine dysregulation a cause of accelerated progression to immunodeficiency and AIDS? Such knowledge would be beneficial in developing strategies for redirecting cytokine patterns. Alcohol exacerbated immune dysfunction during murine retrovirus infection by increasing cytokine dysregulation (Wang et al., 1993, 1994d), making these mice even more susceptible to oral cancer (Odeleye, Eskelson, Mufti, & Watson, 1992; Watson, 1992) and infectious agents (Darban et al., 1992; Shahbazian, Darban, Darban, Stazzone, & Watson, 1992) common to human AIDS patients. By studying cytokine production, we better understand synergism between alcohol- and retrovirus-induced immune dysfunction. Alcohol accentuated the loss of antioxidant vitamins (Wang et al., 1993, 1994d) and increased oxidative damage during murine AIDS (Wang, Liang, & Watson, 1994f). Supplementation with a moderately immunostimulatory antioxidant, vitamin E (Wang et al., 1994f), slowed the loss of Th1 cytokines and immune function in retrovirally infected mice. Therefore, the combination of low antioxidant vitamin levels, increased oxidation, immune dysfunction, and cyto-kine dysregulation due to alcohol abuse exacerbate immune and cytokine dysfunction induced by HIV-1. These changes will promote HIV-1 replication and reduce killing of HIV-1-infected cells, further exacerbating immune dysfunction. Synergism of the effects of alcohol abuse and retrovirus infection promote activation and production of HIV-1, especially genotypes and phenotypes that are particularly pathogenic. A greater HIV-1 burden would accelerate immunosuppression and progression to AIDS.

## V. ALCOHOL ACCELERATES DEVELOPMENT OF SEVERE IMMUNODEFICIENCY DURING RETROVIRUS INFECTION

What are the risk factors that make some HIV-infected individuals more susceptible to development of immune dysfunction and complicating diseases? Progressors have increased IL-4 and IL-6 production by CD8 cells, whereas HIV-1-infected nonprogressors have a Th0 pheotype and thus better immunity (Zanussi et al., 1996). Chronic immune activation in HIV-1-infected people is required for Fas/Apo-1-induced apoptosis and loss of the Th1-cell phenotype. In HIV-1-infected chimpanzees (Gougeon et al., 1997), there was no chronic immune activation. Thus cytokine dysregulation and loss of T cells did not occur and primate AIDS did not develop (Gougeon et al., 1997).

Progression from HIV infection to AIDS took a few months in people consuming large amounts of alcohol instead of the expected 7–11 years (Penkower et al., 1995). The authors hypothesized that greatly increased alcohol use stimulated HIV-1 replication and suppressed immune defenses. They concluded that the subjects eventually reduced their alcohol use due to complications of AIDS (Penkower et al., 1995). Another pilot study concluded that alcoholism promoted progression to AIDS. Heavy alcohol use is very common among intravenous drug users. The relative risk of AIDS was 3.8 times higher in heavy alcohol drinkers than moderate ones among (Lake-Bakaar & Grimson, 1996). Alcohol abuse was more common among AIDS patients than HIV-1-infected drug abusers (Lake-Bakaar & Grimson, 1996) or uninfected intravenous drug users. A study involving HIV-1-infected, heavy alcohol drinkers showed a 41% increase in CD4+ cells after cessation of alcohol use (Pol, Artu, Berthelot, & Nalpas, 1996), whereas only a 15% increase was seen in uninfected controls who quit drinking. Such changes suggest the direct (immuno-

toxic) actions of heavy alcohol use, as well as indirect ones due to undernutrition, by HIV-1-infected people, result in a 30–40% decrease in CD4 cells over 4 years (Pol et al., 1996). Retrovirus-activated lymphocytes increase their susceptibility to HIV-1 infection. In vitro ethanol modulated env-gag induced lymphocyte proliferation (Nair et al., 1994). Replication increased and syncytia formed in more HIV-1-infected cells from subjects after drinking (Bagasra, Kajdacsy-Balla, Lischner, & Pomerant, 1993), promoting their destruction. A lack of balance among immune cells and their functions may favor the retrovirus proliferation (Nair et al., 1994). Removal of CD8+ cells favored HIV replication in vitro. Alcohol use induces a relative decrease in CD8+ in some animal and human studies, which would promote HIV-1 growth (Nair et al., 1994). HIV-1 progressors had CD8 cells which produced more Th2 cell cytokines (Abehsira-Amar, Gilbert, Joliy, Thesze, & Jankovic, 1992) while nonprogressors had a Th0 cytokine phenotype. Similarly, cytokines can inhibit or promote HIV-1 production in vitro. Thus, ethanol induced modulation of cytokine production (Watzl & Watson, 1992a) or cytokine receptors should promote progression to AIDS. Human as well as murine retroviral infection (Wang et al., 1993, 1994d) also suppress Th1 cell cytokine production and cellular immunity while accentuating secretion of Th2 cell cytokines. Thus, a vicious cycle of collaboration could be induced by alcohol and retrovirus-induced dysregulation in cytokine production, suppressing disease resistance together for accelerated development of AIDS (Figure 1). Preliminary data suggest that heavy alcohol use induces cytokine dysregulation and accelerated progression to human AIDS. We found that alcohol consumption accentuated the loss of disease resistance due to murine retrovirus infection even when ethanol consumption had no effect on resistance in normal (nonretrovirus infected) mice (Alak et al., 1993; Darban et al., 1992; Shahbazian et al., 1992). Thus, alcohol was a "cofactor," causing accelerated development of murine AIDS. In our murine AIDS model alcohol consumption exacerbated cytokine dysregulation (Wang et al., 1993; Watson et al., 1993), increased immune dysfunction (Lopez, Huang, Wang, & Watson, 1994; Watson, 1992; Watson, Odeleye, Darban, & Lopez, 1992a, b), and further suppressed disease resistance to pathogens common in AIDS patients (Alak et al., 1993; Darban et al., 1992; Odeleye et al., 1992; Shahbazian et al., 1992). Alcohol exacerbated the stimulated secretion of IL-4 during murine retrovirus infection (Wang et al., 1993), suppressing disease resistance further (Alak et al., 1993). We found that treating with anti-IL-4 antisera (Wang, Ardestani, Liang, Beckham, &

Watson, 1994a) or TCR V$\beta$ peptides (Watson et al., 1995) prevented cytokine dysregulation and immune dysfunction.

# VI. ALCOHOL ABUSE EXACERBATES HIV-INDUCED DEFICIENCIES IN IMMUNOSTIMULATORY MICRONUTRIENTS FOR INCREASED IMMUNOSUPPRESSION

Single and multiple nutritional deficiencies suppress immune functions in animals and humans in the absence of alcohol or retrovirus infection (McMurray, Watson, & Reyes, 1981). Chronic alcoholism is the most common cause of undernutrition in affluent societies (Watson & Watzl, 1992), reducing dietary intake, absorption, utilization, storage, and excretion of nutrients (Watson & Watzl, 1992). Alcohol abuse increases free radicals and causes oxidative damage. Oxidation caused DNA damage, whereas supplementation with vitamin E or C or $\beta$-carotene greatly reduced the DNA damage in lymphocytes of both smokers and nonsmokers (Duthie, Ma, Ross, & Collin, 1995). As alcohol and retrovirus each separately induce losses in tissue antioxidants, together they should promote greater DNA damage and dysfunction in lymphocytes. Responses to skin testing in alcoholics without liver disease (62% undernourished) were impaired; 29% showed energy to the skin testing, emphasizing the combined immunotoxic effects of undernutrition and alcohol. We found that loss of nutrients in alcohol-fed mice played a significant role in immune dysfunction (Watzl & Watson, 1993; Watzl et al., 1993a), whereas vitamin E supplementation partially normalized antioxidant vitamin deficiencies and cytokine production in retrovirus-infected mice (Wang et al., 1994e; Wang, Huang, Eskelson, & Watson, 1994b; Wang & Watson, 1994d). Vitamin E helped overcome the additional suppression of immune systems and nutrient deficiency induced by chronic alcohol consumption (Watzl & Watson, 1993; Watzl et al., 1993a) during murine AIDS. Reduced tissue levels of nutrients were not due to a lower food intake as food consumption was unchanged (Shahbaziam, Wood, & Watson, 1994; Wang et al., 1994f; Wang, Liang, & Watson, 1994g;). HIV-1-infected people have declining amounts of vitamin E as HIV-1 progresses. HIV-1-infected men supplemented with vitamin E had a 30% lower risk of progression to AIDS (Tang, Graham, Semba, & Saah, 1997). Vitamin E deficiency compromises immunity via increased damage to immune effector cells by free radicals (Meydani, 1995). Vitamin B$_6$ supplementation

improved HIV-infected people's survival (Tang, Graham, Saah, 1996). Vitamin B$_{12}$ deficiency in HIV was associated with lower numbers of CD4 cells and accelerated progression to AIDS. In a prospective study, micronutrient supplemented HIV-infected people had slower progression to AIDS than controls (Abrams, Duncan, & Hertz-Picciotto, 1993). In summary, alcohol abuse and retrovirus infection each separately reduce immunostimulatory antioxidants. They should synergize to increase immune dysfunction for accelerated progression to AIDS. Alcohol-induced undernutrition, together with the direct immunotoxic effects of alcohol, should reduce the effectiveness of the host defense system against infections.

# VII. ALCOHOL ACCENTUATES LOSS OF DISEASE RESISTANCE TO AIDS-ASSOCIATED PATHOGENS

We found that during murine retrovirus infection alcohol consumption accelerated deaths from unknown causes. Alcohol accentuated, whereas vitamin E reduced, tumor growth in murine AIDS (Watson et al., 1992a). Alcohol use accentuates the loss of tissue vitamin E and A due to murine AIDS (Watzl & Watson, 1993), whereas vitamin A supplementation delayed premature death. Vitamin E supplementation overcame the tissue deficiencies due to the retroviral infection and slowed development of cytokine dysfunction (Wang et al., 1994b,e; Wang & Watson, 1994d). *Cryptosporidium* infection is an untreatable, AIDS-associated pathogen. We found that it persisted in adult mice when they were infected and immunosuppressed by murine retrovirus infection, while nonvirus infected controls cleared their transient *Cryptosporidium* infection rapidly. Intriguingly, dietary alcohol (Alak et al., 1993) (which ceased prior to parasite challenge) suppressed resistance to *Cryptosporidium* in retrovirus-infected mice, which had developed immune deficiency. The loss of parasite resistance was greater than that caused by murine retrovirus infection alone. The moderate, chronic alcohol intake had no effect on parasite resistance in non-retrovirus-infected controls (Alak et al., 1993), which also did not have the severe immune dysfunction of murine retrovirus infection during alcohol consumption. We found that retrovirus infection reduced secretory IgA anti-*Giardia* antibodies in the intestine (Wang et al., 1994e). They correlated with partial loss of resistance to *Giardia*, which was suppressed further by ethanol (Wang et al., 1994e). By day 21, post-parasite-challenge control mice began to clear *Giardia* from the intestinal tract (Wang et al., 1994e) whereas there were seven-fold more *Giardia* cysts in the retrovirus-infected mice (Wang et al., 1994e). Alcohol use also exacerbated *Giardia* colonization in naive mice (Wang et al., 1994e). Increased cytokine dysregulation due to alcohol use was a key underlying factor causing immune cell dysfunction and abnormal lymphoid cell distribution to the intestine, leading to severe immunodeficiency in the retrovirus-infected animals. Alcohol use also accelerated the death rate of *Streptoccocus pneumoniae*-challenged mice especially when immunologically damaged by retrovirus infection (Darban et al., 1992; Shabbazian et al., 1992). Alcohol use exacerbated AIDS-associated diseases, cytokine dysregulation, and immune function during murine retrovirus infection.

## VIII. THE EFFECTS OF ALCOHOL ON B AND T CELLS

Ethanol may predominantly target immature double positive CD4+/CD8+ lymphocytes (Jerrels et al., 1990). Effects on mature T-cell population can be induced only with long-term alcohol exposure (Jerrells, 1991). In addition, mice prenatally treated with ethanol have significant reduction in the proportion of CD4+ and CD8+ cells (Ewald & Juang, 1990). Our studies in this matter have revealed an increase in the CD4+, a decrease in the CD8+, and an increase in the CD4+/CD8+ ratio with a reduced number of both T and B cells in the spleen (Watson, 1994). Studies using total enteral nutrition as a delivery system to administer ethanol in rats have indicated that it has a direct effect on total lymphocyte population, with lower counts occurring in both the peripheral blood and spleen (Watson et al., 1995). Ethanol at high concentration (>25 mM) significantly suppresses the mitogenic response of thymocytes to phytohemagglutinin (PHA) in a dose-dependent manner. Addition of rIL-2 to the thymocyte cultures reverses the suppressive effect of ethanol over thymocyte proliferation (Yeh, Chang, & Norman, 1996).

Ethanol administration to experimental animals induces depletion of cells from thymus, spleen, and mesenteric lymph nodes (Ewald & Frost, 1987; Jerrells et al., 1990; Sibley, Fuseler, Slukvin, & Jerrells, 1995). In the thymus, immature thymocytes are the most susceptible, whereas in the spleen B cells are most affected by ethanol (Saad & Jerrells, 1991). Both T and B cells are depleted from mesenteric lymph nodes after ethanol exposure, although B-cell loss occurs earlier than T-cell loss once ethanol treatment has

started (Jerrells, Sibley, Slukvin, & Mitchellka, 1998). In vitro exposure to ethanol can induce apoptosis in mouse thymocytes (Ewald & Shao, 1993). Thymocytes and B cells are much more susceptible to ethanol-induced apoptosis than T cells. Studies have shown that thymocytes and T and B cells have different pathways that lead them to apoptosis when in contact with ethanol (Slukvin & Jerrells, 1995). Slukvin and co-workers (1995) suggests that phospholipase C could be one of the molecules activated by ethanol in thymocytes, which lead to activation of protein kinase C (PKC), and increases intracellular calcium by a nonreceptor-mediated process. Moreover, unlike thymocytes, inhibition of PKC by H7 and protein synthesis by Cycloheximide induced apoptosis of T and B cells (Illera, Peradones, Stunz, Mower, & Ashman, 1993; Paradones, Illera, Peckham, Stunz, & Ashman, 1993). It has been found that IL-4 reduces the level of spontaneous apoptosis in both T and B cells (Illera et al., 1993; Migliorati, 1992, 1994). Since IL-4 induces the production of Bcl-2 suppressor protein for apoptosis, ethanol could affect its expression and promote apoptosis of mature lymphocytes (Dancescu et al., 1992; Slukvin & Jerrells, 1995).

Finally, ethanol reduces the percentage of double-positive (CD4+CD8+) lymphocytes and causes an increase in the percentages of CD+CD8− fetal thymocytes (Taylor, Tio, & Chiappelli, 1999). The double-positive population also seems to be affected in a chronic ethanol treatment (Saad et al., 1991); however, mature populations of CD4+CD8− and CD4−CD8+ thymocytes were depleted under this condition. Therefore, ethanol treatment on intrathymic T cells maturational sequence differs significantly.

Alcoholics have higher levels of circulating immunoglobulins (Bailey et al., 1976; Drew, Clifton, LaBrooy, & Shearman, 1984; Lee, 1965; Mendenhall, Anderson, Weesner, Golberg, & Crolic, 1984; Nouri-Aria et al., 1986; Pelletier, Briantais, Buffet, Pillot, & Etienne, 1982; Thompson, Carter, Stokes, Geddes, & Goodall, 1973). Patients with acute alcoholic hepatitis express elevated levels of IgM as the disease progresses; the same happens with IgG and IgA (Mendenhall et al., 1984). In the same manner, IgE levels have also been reported to be elevated in alcoholics with liver disease (Smith et al., 1980). Antibodies against Mallory bodies, hepatocyte proteins, and antigens on the plasma membrane of liver cells have been detected in alcoholic liver disease patients (McFarlaner, 1984). These types of antibodies have been found to react with hepatocytes from ethanol-treated animals but not with the untreated ones, indicating that there is more than one cellular protein recognized in this autoimmune process induced as a result of ethanol metabolism (Crossley, Neuberger, Williams, & Eddleson, 1986). One of the main metabolites of ethanol, acetaldehyde, is known to alkylate a number of hepatic and nonhepatic proteins (Nicholls, De Jersey, Worral, & Wilce, 1992). Acetaldehyde–protein conjugates induce the production of antibodies that specifically recognize the aldehyde-modified protein, where the acetaldehyde acts as an epitope independently from the carrier protein (Israel, Hurwitz, Niemela, & Arnon, 1986). However, other studies have shown that acetaldehyde is not the only reactive intermediate produced during alcohol metabolism. During ethanol oxidation, free radical intermediates, identified as hydroxyethyl radicals, are formed by the action of cytochrome P4502E1 (CYP2E1) (Albano, Tomasi, Goria-Gatti, & Dianzani, 1988; Albano et al., 1991). Hydroxyethyl radi-cals are capable of binding to microsomal proteins with high efficiency (Albano, Parola, Comoglio, & Dianzani, 1993).

## Acknowledgment

This review supported by NHLBI Grant HL 63667.

## References

Abehsira-Amar, O., Gilbert, M., Joliy, M., Thesze, J., & Jankovic, D. L. (1992). IL-4 plays a dominant role in the differential development of Tho into Th1 and Th2 cells. *Journal of Immunology, 148*, 3820–3828.

Abrams, B., Duncan, D., & Hertz-Picciotto, I. (1993). A prospective study of dietary intake and acquired immune deficiency syndrome in HIV-seropostiive homosexual men. *Journal of AIDS, 6*, 949–958.

Adams, H. G., & Jordan, C. (1984). Infections in alcoholics. *Medical Clinics of North America, 68*, 179–200.

Ahuja, S. S., Poliogianni, F., Yamada, H., Balow, J. E., & Boumpas, D. T. (1993). Effect of TGF $\beta$ on early and late activation events in human T cells. *Journal of Immunology, 150*, 3109–3118.

Alak, J. I. B., Shahbazian, M., Huang, D., Wang, Y., Darban, H., Watson, R. R., & Jenkins, E. M. (1993). Alcohol and suppression of resistance to *Cryptosporidium parvum* infection during modulation of cytokine production murine acquired immune deficiency syndrome. *Alcoholism: Clinical and Experimental Medicine, 17*, 539–544.

Albano, E., Parola, M., Comoglio, A., & Dianzani, M.U. (1993). Evidence for the covalent binding of hydroxyethyl radicals to rat liver microsomal proteins. *Alcoholism, 28*, 453–459.

Albano, E., Tomasi, A., Goria-Gatti, L., & Dianzani, M. U. (1988). Spin trapping of free radical species produced during the microsomal metabolism of ethanol. *Chemico-Biology Interaction, 65*, 223–234.

Albano, E., Tomasi, A., Goria-Gatti, L., Persson, J. O. Terelius, Y., Ingelman-Sundberg, M., & Dianzani, M.U. (1991). Role of ethanol-inducible cytochrome P-450 (P450IIE1) in catalysing the free radical activation of aliphatic alcohols. *Biochemistry and Pharmacology, 41*, 1895–1902.

Alkhatib, G., Combadiere, C., Broder, C., Feng, Y., Kennedy, P., Murphy, P., & Berger, E. (1996). CC CKR5: A RANTES, MIP-1 alpha, MIP-1 beta receptor as a fusion cofactor for macrophage-tropic HIV-1. *Science, 272*, 1955–1958.

Allan, J. S., Coligan, J. E., & Brain, F., et al. (1988). Major glycoprotein antigens that induce antibodies in AIDS patients are encoded by HTLV-III. *Science, 228*, 1091–1094.

Antony, V. B., Godbey, S. W., Hott, J. W., & Queener, S. F. (1993). Alcohol-induced inhibition of alveolar macrophage oxidant release in vivo and in vitro. *Alcoholism: Clinical Experimental Research, 17*, 389–393.

Ardestani, S., & Watson, R. R. (1995). Immunomodulation by alcohol in mice. *Alcohol, Drugs of Abuse and Immune Functions*, 27–42.

Asjo, B., Morfeldt-Manson, L., & Alberet, J., et al. (1986). Replicative capacity of human immunodeficiency virus from patients with varying severity of HIV infection. *Lancet, 2*, 660–662.

Astry, C. L., Warr, G. A., & Jakab, G. J. (1983). Impairment of polymorphonuclear leukocyte immigration as a mechanism of alcohol-induced suppression of pulmonary antibacterial defenses. *American Review of Respiratory Disease, 128*, 113–117.

Bagasra, O., Howeedy, A., Dorio, R., & Kajdacsy-Balla, A. (1987). Functional analysis of T cell subsets in chronic experimental alcoholism. *Immunology, 61*, 63–69.

Bagasra, O., Howeedy, A., & Kajdacsy-Balla, A. (1988). Macrophage function in chronic experimental alcoholism. I. Modulation of surface receptors and phagocytosis. *Immunology, 65*, 405–409.

Bagasra, O., Kajdacsy-Balla, A., Lischner, H. W., & Pomerant, R. J. (1993). Alcohol intake increase human immunodeficiency virus type 1 replication in human peripheral blood mononuclear cells. *Journal of Infectious Disease, 167*, 789–797.

Bailey, R. J., Kresner, N., Eddleston, A. L. W. F., williams, R., Tee, E. E. H., Doniach, D., Kennedy, L. A., & Batchelor, J. R. (1976). Histocompatibility antigens, autoantibodies, and immunoglobulins in alcoholic liver disease. *British Medical Journal, 2*, 727.

Baum, M. K., Shor-Posner, G., Lu, Y., Rosner, B., Sauberlich, H. E., Fletcher, M. A., Szapoczknki, J., Eisdorer, C., Buring, J. E., & Heenekens, C., H. Micronutrients and HIV-1 disease progression. *AIDS, 9*, 1051–1056.

Bautista, A. P. (1997). Chronic alcohol intoxication induces hepatic injury through enhanced macrophage inflammatory protein-2 production and intercellular adhesion molecule-1 expression in the liver. *Hepatology, 25*, 335–342.

Bautista, A. P., & Spitzer, J. J. (1993). Superoxide formation during acute or chronic ethanol intoxication. *Advances in Biology, 86*, 211–218.

Beckham, C. J., & Watson, R. R. (1994). Ethanol-induced undernutrition and immunosuppression: Potential role in increased cancer risk in alcoholics. *Journal of Optimal Nutrition, 2*, 234–238.

Bermudez, L., & Young, L. (1988). Tumor necrosis factor (TNF or cachetin) alone or in combination with IL-2 but not interferon-gamma is associated with macrophage killing of *Mycobacterium avium* complex. *Journal of Immunology, 140*, 3006–3013.

Bermudez, L. E. (1994). Effect of ethanol on the interaction between the macrophage and Mycobacterium avium. *Alcoholism, 11*, 69–73.

Bermudez, L. E., Young, L. S., Martinelli, J., & Petrofsky, M. (1993). Exposure to ethanol upregulates the expression of *M. avium* proteins associated with bacteria virulence. *Journal of Infectious Disease, 168*, 961–968.

Budec, M., Ciric, O., Koko, V., & Asanin, R. (1992). The possible mechanism of action of ethanol on rat thymus. *Drug Alcohol Dependency, 30*, 181–185.

Carding, S. R., Hayday, A. C., & Bottomly, K.(1991). Cytokines in T-cell development. *Immunology Today, 12*, 239–245.

Cemey, A., Hugin, A. W., Hardy, R. R., et al. (1990). B-cells are required for induction of T-cell abnormalities in a murine retrovirus-induced immunodeficiency syndrome. *Journal of Experimental Medicine, 171*, 315–320.

Ceredig, R., Medveczky, J., & Skulimowski, A. (1989). Mouse fetal thymus lobes cultured in IL-2 generate CD3',TCR-,yb expressing CD4-/CD8- cells. *Journal of Immunology, 142*, 3353–3360.

Chadha, K. C., Stadler, L., Albini, B., Nakeeb, S. M., & Thacore, H. R. (1991). Effect of alcohol on spleen cells and their functions in C57BIJ6 mice. *Alcoholism, 8*, 481–485.

Chadha, K. C., Whitney, R. B., Cummings, M., Norman, M., Windle, M., & Stadler I. (1990). *Evaluation of interferon system among chronic alcoholics. Alcohol, immunomodulation, and AIDS* (pp. 123–133). New York: A. R. Liss.

Cheng-Myer, C., Seto, D., Tateno, M., & Levy, J. A. (1990). Biologic features of HIV-1 that correlate with virulence in the host. *Science, 240*, 80–82.

Choe, H., Farzan, M., Sun, Y., Sullivan, N., Rollins, B., Ponath, P. D., Wu, L., Mackay, C. R., LaRosa, G., Newman, W., Gerard, N., Gerard, C., & Sodroski, J. (1996). *Cell, 85*, 1135–1815.

Cooper, B., & Maderazo, E. G. (1989). Alcohol abuse and impaired immunity. *Infect. Surg., March 94*, 101.

Crossley, I. R., Neuberger, J., Davis, M., Williams, R., & Eddleson, A.L.W.F. (1986). Ethanol metabolism in the generation of new antigenic determinants on liver cells. *Gut, 27*, 186–189.

Dancescu, Rubio-Trujillo, M., Biron, G., Bron, G., Delespesse, G., & Sarfati, M. (1992). Interleukin 4 protects chronic lymphocytic leukemic B cells from death by apoptosis and upregulates Bcl-2 expression. *Journal of Experimental Medicine, 176*, 1319–1326.

Darban, H., Crawford, G. B., & Watson, R. R. (1993). Alcohol and the human immune system. *Advances in Biology, 86*, 5–6.

Darban, H., Watson, R. R., Darban, J., & Shahbazian, L. M. (1992). Modification of resistance to Streptococcus pneumoniae by dietary ethanol, immunization and murine retroviral infection. *Alcoholism: Clinical and Experimental Research, 16*, 844–885.

Daynes, R. A., & Araneo, B. A. (1989). Contrasting effects of glucocorticoids on the capacity of T cells to produce the growth factors interleukin-2 and interleukin-4. *European Journal of Immunology, 19*, 2319–2325.

DelPrete, G., DeCarli, M., Almerigogna, F., et al. (1992). Human IL-10 in produced by both type 1 helper and type 2 helper T cell clones and inhibits their antigen-specific proliferation and cytokine production. *Journal of Immunology, 150*, 353–360.

Deviere, J., Content, J., Denys, C., Vandenbussche, P., et al. (1990). Excessive in vitro bacterial lipopolysaccharide-induced production of monokines in cirrhosis. *Hepatology, 11*, 628–634.

Dorio, R. J. , Joek, J. B., Rubin, E., & Forman, H. J. (1988). Ethanol modulates rat alveolar macrophage superoxide production. *Biochemical Pharmacology Journal, 37*, 3528–3531.

Drew, P. A., Clifton, P. M., LaBrooy, J. T., & Shearman, D. J. C. (1984). Polyclonal B cell activation in alcoholic patients with no evidence of liver dysfunction. *Clinical and Experimental Immunology, 57*, 479.

Duthie, S. J., Ma, A., Ross, M. A., & Collin, A. R. (1995). Antioxidant supplementation decreases oxidative DNA damage in human lymphocytes. *Cancer Research, 56*, 1291–1295.

Ellis, F. W. (1966). Effect of ethanol on plasma corticosterone levels. *Journal of Pharmacology and Experimental Therapeutics. 153*, 121–127.

Ewald, S. J., & Frost, W. W. (1987). Effect of prenatal exposure to ethanol on development of the thymus. *Thymus, 9*, 211–219.

Ewald, S. J., & Frost, W. W. (1988). Flow cytometric and histological analysis of mouse thymus in fetal alcohol syndrome. *Journal of Leukocyte Biology, 44*, 434–440.

Ewald, S. J., & Juang, C. (1990, 1991). Lymphocyte populations and immune responses in mice prenatally exposed to ethanol. In

D. Seminara, R. R. Watson, & A. Pawlowski (Eds.), *Alcohol, Immunomodulation and AIDS: Proceedings of the Alcohol-Immunology AIDS Conference, Tucson Arizona, April 27–29, 1989*. New York: A. R. Liss.

Ewald, S. J., & Shao, H. (1993). Ethanol increases apoptotic cell death of thymocytes in vitro. *Alcoholism: Clinical and Experimental Research, 17*, 359–365.

Feng, Y., Broder, C., Kennedy, P., & Berger, E. (1996). HIV-1 entry cofactor: Functional cDNA cloning of a seven transmembrane, G protein-coupled receptor. *Science, 272*, 872–877.

Gallucci, R. M., & Meadows, G. G. (1995). Ethanol consumption reduces the cytolytic activity of lymphokine-activated killer cells. *Alcoholism: Clinical and Experimental Research, 19*, 402–409.

Gianouakis, C. (1989). The effect of ethanol on the biosynthesis and regulation of opioid peptides. *Experientia, 45*, 428–436.

Goldstein, D. B. (1983). Alcohol and the endocrine system. In *Pharmacology of Alcohol* (pp. 156–169). New York: Oxford Press.

Gougeon, M. L., Lecouer, H., Boudet, F., Ledru, E., Marzabal, S., Boullier, S., Roue, R., Nagata, S., & Henney, J. (1997). Lack of chronic immune activation in HIV-infected Chimpanzees correlates with the resistance of T cells to fas/Apo-1 (CD95) induced apotosis and preservation of a T helper 1 phenotype. *Journal of Immunology, 158*, 2964–2976.

Greenberg, S., Kous, J., Bagby, G., Nelson, S., Summer, W., Greenberg, J., & Xie, J. (1994). Ethanol metabolism is required for inhibition of nitric oxide gene expression by endotoxin in lung macrophages. *Alcoholism: Clinical and Experimental Research, 18*, 440. [Abstract 111]

Gyongyi, S., Pranoti, M., Linda, G., & Donna, C. (1996). Regulation of human monocyte functions by acute ethanol treatment: Decreased tumor necrosis factor-$\alpha$, IL-1$\beta$ and elevated IL-10, and TNF- production. *Alcoholism: Clinical and Experimental Research, 20*, 900–907.

Hall, N. R., & Goldstein, A. L. (1998). Endocrine regulation of host immunity. In R. L. Fenichel & M. A. Chirigos, (Eds.), *Immune modulation agents and their mechanisms, Immunology Series*, (vol. 25, pp. 533–563). New York: Dekker.

Han, Y. C., Lin, T. L., & Pruett, S. B. (1993). Ethanol-induced thymic atrophy in mouse model for binge drinking: Involvement of glucocorticoids. *Toxicology and Applied Pharmacology, 123*, 16–25.

Han, Y. C., & Pruett, S. B. (1995). Mechanisms of ethanol-induced suppression of a primary antibody response in a mouse model for binge drinking. *Journal of Pharmacology and Experimental Therapeutics, 275*, 950–957.

Helm, R. M., Wheeler, G., Burks, A. W., Hakkak, R., & Badger R. M. (1996). Flow cytometric analysis of lymphocytes from rats following chronic ethanol treatment. *Alcohol, 13*, 467–471.

Hwang, S. S., Boyle, T. J., Lyerly, H. K., & Cullen, B. R. (1991). Identification of the envelope V3 loop as the primary determinant of cell tropism. *Science, 253*, 71–74.

Illera, V. A., Perandones, C. E., Stunz, L. L., Mower, D. A., Jr., & Ashman, R. F. (1993). Apoptosis in splenic B cells. Regulation by protein kinase C and IL-4. *Journal of Immunology, 151*, 2965–2973.

Isaki, L., & Gordis, E. (1993). Alcohol and immunology—Progress and questions. *Alcoholism: Clinical and Experimental Research, 17*, 725–726.

Israel, Y., Hurwitz, E., Niemela, O., & Arnon, R. (1986). Monoclonal and polyclonal antibodies against acetaldehyde-containing epitopes in acetaldehyde-protein adducts. *Proceedings of the National Academy of Science., USA, 83*, 7923–7927.

Javaherian, K., Langlois, A. J., McDanal, D., Ross, K. L., Eckler, L. I., Jellis, C. L., Profy, A. T., Rusche, J. R., Bolognesi, D. P., Putney, S. D., & Mathews, T. J. (1986). Principal neutralizing domain of the human immunodeficeincy virus type 1 envelope protein. *Proc. National Academy of Science. USA., 86,* 6768–6772.

Jerrells, T. R. (1991). Immunodeficiency associated with ethanol abuse. In H. Friedman, (Ed.), *Drugs of abuse, and immunodeficiency.* New York: Plenum.

Jerrells, T. R., Eckardt, M. J., & Weinber, J. (1990). Mechanisms of ethanol induced immunosuppression. In R. R. Watson, & A. Pawlowski, (Eds.), *Alcohol, Immunomodulation and AIDS: Proceedings, Alcohol-Immunology AIDS Conference, Tucson, Arizona, April 27–29, 1989, Seminar, D.* New York: A. R. Loss.

Jerrells, T. R., Peritt, D., Marietta, C., & Edkardt M. (1989). Mechanisms of suppression of cellular immunity induced by ethanol. *Alcoholism: Clinical and Experimental Research, 13,* 490–493.

Jerrells, T. R., Sibley, D. A., Slukvin, I., & Mitchell, K. A. (1998). Effects of ethanol consumption on mucosal and systemic T cell dependent immune response to pathogenic microorganisms. *Alcoholism: Clinical and Experimental Research, 22* (5 Suppl.), 2125–2155.

Jerrells, T. R., Smith, W., & Eckardt, M. J. (1990). Murine Model of ethanol-induced immunosuppression. *Alcoholism: Clinical and Experimental Research, 14,* 546–550.

Jerrells, T. R., Smith, W., Eckardt, M. J., Majchrowicz, E., & Weight, F. F. (1986). Effects of ethanol administration on parameters of immunocompetency in rats. *Journal of Leukocyte Biology, 39,* 499–510.

Kelly, P. M., Heryet, A. R., & McGee, J.O.D.(1989). Kupffer cell number is normal, but their lysozyme content is reduced in alcohol liver disease. *Journal of Hepatology, 8,* 173–180.

Kenealy, W. R., Mathews, T. J., Ganfeild, M. C., Langlois, A. J., Waselefsky, D. M., & Petteway, S. R. (1989). Antibodies from human immunodeficiency virus-infected individuals bind to a short amino acid sequence that elicits neutralizing antibodies in animals. *AIDS Research and Human Retrovirus, 5,* 173–182.

Lake-Bakaar, G., & Grimson, R. (1996). Alcohol abuse and stage of HIV disease in intravenous drug abusers. *Journal of the Royal Society of Medicine, 89,* 389–392.

Lasky, L. A., Groopman, J. E., Fennie, C. W., Benz, P. M., Capon, D. J., Dowbenko, D. J., Nakamura, G. R., Nunes, W. M., Renz, M. E., & Berman, P. W. (1986). Neutralization of the AIDS retrovirus by antibodies to a recombinant envelope glycoprotein. *Science, 233,* 209–212.

Lee, F. I. (1965). Immunoglobulins in viral hepatitis and active alcoholic liver disease. *Lancet, 2,* 1043.

Lesley, J., Trotter, J., Schutle, & Hyman, R., (1990). Phenotypic analysis of the early events during repopulation of the thymus by bone marrow prothymocyte cells. *Journal of Immunology, 128,* 63–78.

Liang, B., Chung, S., Araghiniknam, M., & Lane, L. (1996). Vitamins and immunomodulation in AIDS. *Nutritional Science, 12,* 1–7.

Lopez, M. C., Colombo, L. L., Huang, D. S., & Watson, R. R. (1992). Suppressed mucosal lymphocyte populations by LP-BM5 murine leukemia virus infection producing murine AIDS. *Regional Immunology, 4,* 162–167.

Lopez, M. C., Huang, D. S., Wang, Y., & Watson, R. R. (1994). Modification of lymphocyte subsets in the intestinal immune system and thymus by ethanol consumption. *Alcoholism: Clinical and Experimental Research, 18,* 8–11.

Luciw, P. A. (1995). Human immunodeficiency viruses and their replication (pp. 1881–1952). In Fields (Eds.) *Virology* (vol. 2).

MacFarlaner, I. G. (1984). Autoimmunity in liver disease. *Clinical Science, 67,* 569–587.

Mandrekar, P., Catalano, D., & Szabo G. (1997). Alcohol-induced regulation of nuclear regulatory factor-$\kappa\beta$ in human monocytes. *Alcoholism: Clinical and Experimental Research, 21,* 988–994.

Martinez, F., Darban, H., Thomas, N. M., Cox, T. J., Woods, S., & Watson, R. R. (1993). Interleukin-6 and interleukin-8 production by mononuclear cells of chronic alcoholics during treatment. *Alcoholism: Clinical and Experimental Research, 17,* 1193–1197.

Mathews, T. J., Langlois, A. J., Robey, W. G, Chang, N. T., Gallo, R. C., Fischinger, P. J., & Bolognesi, D. P. (1986). Restricted neutralization of divergent human T-lymphotrophic virus type III isolates by antibodies to the major envelope glycoprotein. *Proceedings of the National Academy of Science, USA, 83,* 9709–9713.

Matsushita, S., Robert-Guroff, M., Rusche, J., Koifo, A., Hattori, T., Hoshino, H., Javaherian, K., Takatsuki, K., & Putney, S. (1988). Characterization of human immunodeficiency virus neutralizing monoclonal antibody and mapping of the neutralizing epitope. *Journal of Virology, 62,* 2107–2114.

McClain, C. J., Hill, D. B., Marsano, L., Cohen, D., & Shedlofsky, S. (1993). A role for cytokines in alcoholic hepatitis. *Advances Bioscience, 86,* 133–141.

McGregor, R. R. (1986). Alcohol and immune defense. *Journal of American Medical Association, 256,* 1474–1479.

McMurray, D. N., Watson, R. R., & Reyes, M. A. (1981). Effect of renutrition on humoral and cell-mediated immunity in severely malnourished children. *American Journal of Clinical Nutrition, 34,* 2117–2126.

Meadows, G. G., Wallendai, M., Kosugi, A., Wunderich, J., & Singer, D. S. (1992). Ethanol induces marked changes in lymphocyte populations and natural killer cell activity in mice. *Alcoholism: Clinical and Experimental Research, 16,* 474–479.

Mendenhall, C. L., Anderson, S., Weesner, R. E., Goldberg, S. J., & Crolic, K. A. (1984). Protein-calorie malnutrition associated with alcoholic hepatitis. *American Journal of Medicine, 76,* 211.

Meydani, M. (1995). Vitamin E. *Lancet, 345,* 170–175.

Migliorati, G., Nicoletti, I., Crocicchio, F., Pagliacci, C., D'Adamio, F., & Riccardi, C. (1992). Heat shock induces apoptosis in mouse thymocytes and protects them from glucocorticoid-induced cell death. *Cell Immunology, 143,* 348–356.

Migliorati, G., Nicoletti, I., D'Adamio, F., Spreca, A., Pagliaccci, C., & Riccardi, C. (1994). Dexamethasone induces apoptosis in mouse natural killer cells and cytotoxic T lymphocytes. *Immunology, 81,* 21–26.

Mitzi, S. (1989). Interleukin. *FASEB Journal, 3,* 2379–2388.

Mosmann, T. R., & Coffman, R. L. (1989). Thl and Th2 Cells: Different patterns of lymphokine secretion lead to different functional properties. *Annual Revision of Immunology, 7,* 145–173.

Mulder, J. W., Frissen, J., Krijenen, P. H., Endert, E., Dewolf, F., Goudsmit, J., Masterson, J. G., & Liang, J. M. (1992). DHEA as a predictor for progression to AIDS in asymptomatic human immunodeficiency virus-infected men. *Journal of Infectious Disease, 165,* 413–418.

Myers, G., Korber, B., Wain-Hobson, Jeang, K., T., et al., (1994). *Human retroviruses and AIDS. A compilation and analysis of nucleic acid and amino acid sequences.* Los Alamos, NM:Los Alamos National Laboratory.

Na, H. R., & Seelig, L. L. (1994). Effect of maternal ethanol consumption on in vitro tumor necrosis factor, interleukin-6 and interleukin-2 production by rat milk and blood leukocytes. *Alcoholism: Clinical and Experimental Research, 18,* 398–402.

Nair, M. P. N, Kumar, N. M., Kronfol, Z. A., Srarvolatz, L. A, Pottathin, R., Greden, J. H., & Schwartz, S. A. (1994). Selection effect of alcohol on cellular immune responses of lymphocytes from AIDS patients. *Alcohol, 11,* 85–90.

Nelson, S., Bagby, G. J., Bainton, B. G., & Summer, W. R. (1989a). The effects of acute and chronic alcoholism on tumor necrosis factor and the inflammatory response. *Journal of Infectious Disease, 160*, 422–429.

Nelson, S., Bagby, G., & Summer, W. R. (1989b). Alcohol suppresses lipopolysaccharide-induced tumor necrosis factor activity in serum and lung. *Life Science, 44*, 673–676.

Nicholls, R., De Jersey, J., Worral, S., & Wilce, P. (1992). Modification of proteins and other biological molecules be acetaldehyde:Adduct structure and functional significance. *International Journal of Biochemistry, 24*, 1899–1906.

Nouri-Aria, K. T., Alexander, G. J. M., Portmann, B. C., Hegarty, J. E., Eddleston, A. L. W. F., & Williams, R. (1986). T and B cell function in alcoholic liver disease. *Journal of Hepatology, 2*, 195.

Nympha, B. D., Steve, N., Warren, R. S., & Ion, V. D. (1996). Alcohol modulates alveolar macrophage tumor necrosis factor-$\alpha$, super-oxide anion, and nitric oxide secretion in the rat. *Alcoholism: Clinical and Experimental Research, 20*, 156–163.

Odeleye, O. E., Eskelson, C. D., Mufti, S. I., & Watson, R. R. (1992). Vitamin E protection against chemically-induced esophageal tumor growth in mice immunocompromised by retroviral infection. *Carcinogenesis, 13*, 1811–1816.

Odeleye, O. E., & Watson, R. R. (1991). The potential role of vitamin E in treatment of immunologic abnormalities during acquired immune deficiency syndrome. *Progress in Food and Nutrition Science, 15*, 1–19.

Palker, T. J., et al. (1988). Type-specific neutralization of the human immunodeficiency virus with antibodies to env-encoded synthetic peptides. *Proceedings of the National Academy of Science, USA, 85*, 1932–1936.

Paradones, C. E., Illera, V. A., Peckham, D., Stunz, L. L., & Ashman, R. F. (1993). Regulation of apoptosis in vitro in mature murine spleen T cells. *Journal of Immunology, 151*, 3521–3529.

Pelletier, G., Briantais, M. J., Buffet, C., Pillot, J., & Etienne, J. P. (1982). Serum and intestinal secretory IgA in alcoholic cirrhosis of the liver. *Gut, 23*, 475.

Penkower, L., Dew, M. A., Kingley, L., Zhou, S. Y., Lyketsos, C. G., Wesch, J., Senterfitt, J. W., Hoover, D. R., & Becker, J. T. (1995). Alcohol consumption as a cofactor in the progression of HIV infection and AIDS. *Alcohol, 12*, 547–552.

Pillai, R. K., & Watson, R. R. (1991). AIDS: Disease progression and immunomodulation by drugs of abuse and alcohol. *AIDS Medical Report, 4*, 25–36.

Pillai, R. K., & Watson, R. R. (1993). Immunotoxicology of drug and alcohol use: Relevance to AIDS and cancer. *Advanced Bioscience, 86*, 427–4361.

Pol, S., Artu, P., Berthelot, P., & Nalpas, B. (1996). Improvement of the CD4 cell count after alcohol withdrawal in HIV-positive patients. *AIDS, 10*, 1293–1294.

Plum, J., De Smedt, M., & Leclercq, G. (1990). Inhibitory effect of murine recombinant IL-4 on thymocyte development in fetal thymus organ cultures. *Journal of Immunology, 145*, 1066–1073.

Putney, J. R., Mathews, T. J., Robey, W. G., Lynn, D. L., Robert-Guroff, M., Meuller, W. T., Lanlois, A. J., Gharayeb, J., Petteway, S. R., Weinhold, K. J., Fischinger, P. J., Wong-Staal, F., Gallo, R. C., & Bolegnisi, D. P. HTLVII/LAV neutralizing antibodies to and *E. coli* produced fragment of the virus envelope. *Science, 234*, 1392–1395.

Rabhala, R. H., & Watson R. R. (1990). Effects of various alcohols applied in vitro on human subtypes and mitogenesis. *Progress Clinical Biology Research, 325*, 155–164.

Rimland, D. (1983). Mechanisms of ethanol induced defects of alveolar macrophage function. *Alcoholism: Clinical and Experimental Research, 8*, 73–76.

Robey, W. G., Arthur, L. O., Mathews, T. J., Lanlois, A., Copeland, T. D., Lerhe, N. W., Oroszlan, S., Bolognesi, D. P., Gilden, R. V., & Fiscinger, P. J. Prospect for prevention of human immunodeficiency virus infection: Purified 42-kDa envelope glycoprotein induces neutralizing antibody.

Rosselle, G. A., & Mendenhall, C. L. (1982). Alteration of in vitro human lymphocyte function by ethanol acetaldehyde and acetate. *Journal of Clinical and Laboratory Immunology, 9*, 33–37.

Rosselle, G. A., Mendenhall, C. L., & Grossman, C. J. (1989). Ethanol and soluble mediators of host defense. *Alcoholism: Clinical and Experimental Research, 13*, 494–498.

Rusche, J. R., Javaherian, K., McDanal, C., Petro, J., Lynn, D. L., Grimailia, R., Langlois, A., Gallo, R. C., Arthur, L. O., Fischinger, P. J., Bolognesi, D. P., Putney S. D., & Mathews, T. J. (1988). Antibodies that inhibit fusion of human immunodeficiency virus-infected cells bind a 24-amino acid sequence of the viral envelope, gp120. *Proceedings of the National Academy of Science, USA, 85*, 3198–3202.

Saad, A. J., Domiati-Saad, R., & Jerrells, T. R. (1993). Ethanol ingestion increased susceptibility of mice to Listeria monocytogenes. *Alcoholism: Clinical and Experimental Research, 17*, 75–85.

Saad, A. J., & Jerrells, T. R. (1991). Flow cytometric and immunohistochemical evaluation of ethanol-induced changes in splenic and thymic lymphoid cell populations. *Alcoholism: Clinical and Experimental Research, 15*, 796–803.

Scollay, R., Wilson, A., Damico, A., Kelly, K., Egreton, M., Pearse, M., Wu, L., & Shortamn, K. (1988). Developmental status and reconstitution potential of subpopulations of murine thymocytes. *Immunology Revision, 104*, 81–120.

Scott, P., & Kaufmann, S. H. E. (1991). The role of T-cell subsets and cytokines in the regulation of infection. *Immunology Today, 12*, 346–348.

Seminara, D., Pawlowski, A., & Watson, R. R. (1990). Alcohol, Immunomodulation and AIDS. *Progress in Clinical Biology Research, 325*, 1–457.

Shabbazian, L. M., Darban, H. R., Darban, J. R., Stazzone, A. M., & Watson, R. R. (1992). Influence of the level of dietary ethanol on resistance to Streptococcus pneumoniae in mice with murine AIDS. *Alcohol Alcoholism, 27*, 345–352.

Shahbazian, L. M., Stazzone, A., Hebert, A., & Watson, R. R. (1993). Effect of thymosin fraction 5 on immune response of C57BL/6 mice fed ethanol diet and challenged with Streptococcus pneumoniae. *Advanced Bioscience, 86*, 353–358.

Shahbaziam, L. M., Wood, S., & Watson, R. R. (1994). Ethanol consumption and early murine retrovirus infection influence liver, heart, and muscle levels of iron, zinc, and copper in C57BL/6 mice. *Alcoholism: Clinical and Experimental Research, 18*, 964–968.

Sheflito, J. E., Suzara, V. V., Blumenfeld, W., Beck, J. M., Steger, H. J., & Ermak, T. H. (1990). A new model of Pneumocystis carinii infection in mice selectively depleted of helper T lymphocytes. *Journal of Clinical Investigation, 85*, 1683–1693.

Sheppard, H. W., Lang, W., Ascher, M. S., Vittinghoff, E., & Winkelstein, W. (1993). The characterization of nonprogressors long term HIV-1 infection with stable CD4+ T-cell levels. *AIDS, 7*, 1159–1166.

Shioda, T., Levy, J. A., & Cheng-Mayer, C. (1991). Macrophage and T cell line tropism of HIV-1 are determined by specific regions of the envelope gp120 gene. *Nature, 349*, 167–169.

Sibley, D. A., Fuseler, J., Slukvin, I., & Jerrells, T. R. (1991). Ethanol-induced depletion of lymphocytes from the mesenteric lymph nodes of C57Bl/6 mice is associated with RNA but not DNA degradation. *Alcoholism: Clinical and Experimental Research, 19*, 324–331.

Skinner, M. .A., Ting, R., Langlois, A. J., Weinhold, K. J., Lyerly, H. K., Javerhian, K., & Mathews, T. J. (1988). Characteristics of a neutralizing monoclonal antibody to the HIV envelope glycoprotein. *AIDS Research and Human Retrovirus, 4*, 187–194.

Slukvin, I. I., & Jerrells, T. R. (1995). Different pathways of in vitro ethanol-induced apoptosis in thymocytes and splenic T and B lymphocytes. *Immunopharmacology, 31*, 43–57.

Smith, F. E., & Palmer D. L. (1976). Alcoholism, infection and altered host defenses: A review of clinical and experimental observations. *Journal of Chronic Diease, 29*, 35–49.

Smith, W. I., Jr., Van Thiel, D. H., Whiteside, T., Janoson, B., Magovern, J., Puet, T., & Rabin, B. S. (1980). Altered immunity in male patients with alcoholic liver disease: Evidence for defective immune regulation. *Alcoholism: Clinical and Experimental Research, 4*, 199–206.

Spagnuolo, P. J., & MacGregor, R. R. (1975). Acute ethanol effect of chemotaxis and other components of host defense. *Journal of Laboratory and Clinical Medicine, 86*, 24–31.

Spinozzi, F., Bertotto, A., Rondoni, F., Gerli, R., Scalise, F., & Grignani, F. (1991). T lymphocyte activation pathways in alcoholic liver disease. *Immunology, 73*, 140–146.

Steven, W. M., Kumar, S. N., Stewart, G. L., & Seelig, L. L. (1990). The effects of ethanol consumption on the expression of immunity of Trichinella spiralis in rats. *Alcoholism: Clinical and Experimental Research, 14*, 87–91.

Straus, B., Berenyi, M. R., Huang, J. M., & Straus, E. (1971). Delayed hypersensitivity in alcoholic cirrhosis. *Diagnosis Disease, 16*, 509–514.

Szabo, G., Mandrekar, P., Verma, B., & Catalano, D. (1995). Acute ethanol uptake prior to injury modulates monocyte TNF-$\alpha$ production and mononuclear cell apoptosis. In E. Faist (Ed.), *Immune consequences of trauma and sepsis.* Berlin: Springer-Verlag.

Tabakoff, B., Jaffe, R. C., & Ritzmann, R. F. (1978). Corticosterone concentrations in mice during ethanol drinking and withdrawal. *Journal of Pharmacy and Pharmacology., 30*, 371–374.

Takeuchi, Y., Akutsu, A., Murayama, K., Shimuzu, N., & Hoshino, H. (1991). Host range mutant of HIV-1: Modification of cell tropism by a single point mutation at the neutralization epitope in the env b gene. *Journal of Virology, 65*, 1710–1718.

Tang, A. M. Graham, N. M. H., & Saah, A. J. (1996). Effects of micronutrient intake on survival in human immunodeficiency virus type l infection. *American Journal of Epidemiology, 143*, 1244–1256.

Tang, A. M., Graham, N. M. H., Semba, R. D., & Saah, A. J. (1997). Association between serum vitamin A and E levels and HIV-1 progression. *AIDS*, in press.

Taylor, A. N., Tio, D. L., & Chlappelli, F. (1999). Thymocyte development in male fetal alcohol-exposed rats. *Alcoholism: Clinical and Experimental Research, 23*, 465–470.

Tersmette, M., Gruters, R. A., deWolf, F., et al. (1989). Evidence for a role of virulent HIV-1 variants in the pathogenesis of AIDS: Studies on sequential HIV isolates. *Journal of Virology, 63*, 2118–2125.

Tersmette, M., & Rudd, E. Y, deGoeda, B. J. M., et al. (1988). Differential syncytium-inducing capacity of HIV isolates: Frequent detection of syncytium-inducing isolates in patients with AIDS and AIDS related complex. *Journal of Virology, 62*, 2026–32.

Thestrup-Perderseti, K., Ladefoged, K., & Anderson, P. (1976). Lymphocyte transformation test with liver specific protein and phytohemagglutinin in patients with liver disease. *Journal of Clinical and Experimental Immunology, 24*, 1–8.

Thiagaran, A. B., Mefford, I. N., & Eskay, R. L. (1989). Single-dose ethanol administration activates the hypothalamic-pituitary-adrenal axis:Exploration of the mechanism of action. *Neuroendocrinology, 50*, 427–432.

Thompson, R. A., Carter, R., Stokes, R. P., Geddes, A. M., & Goodall, J. A. D. (1973). Serum immunoglobulins, complement component levels and autoantibodies in liver disease. *Clinical Experimental Immunology, 14*, 335–346.

Veronese, F. D., DeVico, A. L., Copeland, T. D., et al. (1985). Characterization of gp41 as transmembrane protein encoded by the HTLV-III/LAV envelope gene. *Science, 229*, 1402–1405.

Wagner, F., Fink, R., Hart, R., Lersch, C., Dancygier, H., & Classen, M. (1992). Ethanol inhibits interferon-gamma secretion by human peripheral lymphocytes. *Journal of Study of Alcohol, 53*, 277–280.

Wang, Y., Ardestani, S. K., Liang, B., Beckham, C., & Watson R. R. (1994a). Anti-interleukin-4 monoclonal antibody and interferon-gamma administration retards development of immune dysfunction and cytokine dysregulation during murine AIDS. *Immunology, 83*, 384–389.

Wang, Y., Huang, D. S., Eskelson, C. D., & Watson, R. R. (1994b). Long-term dietary vitamin E retards development of retrovirus-induced dysregulation in cytokine production. *Clinical and Immunology Immunopathology, 72*, 70–75.

Wang, Y., Huang, D. S., Giger, P. T., & Watson, R. R. (1993). Ethanol-induced modulation of cytokine production by splenocytes during murine retrovirus infection causing murine AIDS. *Alcoholism: Clinical and Experimental Research, l7*, 1035–1039.

Wang, Y., Huang, D. S., Giger, P. T., & Watson, R. R. (1994c). Influence of chronic dietary ethanol on cytokine production by murine splenocytes and thymocytes. *Alcoholism: Clinical and Experimental Research, 18*, 64–70.

Wang, Y., Huang, D. S., Giger, P. T., & Watson, R. R. (1994d). Suppression of in vitro cytokine production by chronic dietary ethanol fed to C57BL/6 mice. *Alcoholism: Clinical and Experimental Research.*

Wang, Y., Huang, D. S., & Watson, R. R. (1995). Alcohol and immunomodulation during murine acquired immunodeficiency syndrome. *Alcohol, Drugs of Abuse and Immune Functions*, 185–200.

Wang, Y., Huang, D. S., & Watson, R. R. (1994e). Dietary vitamin E modulation of cytokine production by splenocytes and thymocytes from alcohol-fed mice. *Alcoholism: Clinical and Experimental Research, 18*, 355–362.

Wang, Y., Liang, B., & Watson R. R. (1994f). Normalization of nutritional status by various levels of vitamin E supplementation during murine AIDS. *Nutrition Research, 14*, 1375–1386.

Wang, Y., Liang, B. & Watson, R. R. (1994g). Suppression of tissue levels of vitamin A, E, zinc and copper in murine AIDS. *Nutritional Research, 14*, 1031–1041.

Wang, Y., & Watson, R. R. (1994a). Chronic ethanol consumption prior to retrovirus infection alters cytokine production by thymocytes during murine AIDS. *Alcohol, 11*(5), 361–365.

Wang, Y., & Watson, R. R. (1994b). Chronic ethanol consumption prior to retrovirus infection is a cofactor in the development of immune dysfunction during murine AIDS. *Alcoholism: Clinical and Experimental Research, 18*, 976–981.

Wang, Y., & Watson, R. R. (1994c). Ethanol, immune responses and murine AIDS; The role of vitamin E as an immunostimulant and antioxidant. *Alcohol, 11*, 75–84.

Wang, Y., & Watson R. R. (1994d). Is vitamin E supplementation a useful agent in AIDS therapy? *Progress in Food and Nutrition Science.*

Wang, Y., & Watson, R. R. (1994e). Vitamin E supplementation at various levels alters cytokine production by thymocytes during retrovirus infection causing murine AIDS. *Thymus, 22*, 153–165.

Wang, Y., & Watson, R. R. (1995a). Is alcohol consumption a cofactor in the development of acquired immunodeficiency syndrome? *Alcohol, 12,* 105–109.

Wang, Y., & Watson, R. R. (1995b). The role of alcohol on endocrine–immune interactions. *Alcohol, Drugs of Abuse and Immune Functions,* 229–244.

Watson, R. R. (1989). Immunomodulation by alcohol: A cofactor in development of AIDS after retrovirus infection. In *Cofactors in HIV-I Infection and AIDS* (pp. 47–54). Boca Raton, FL: CRC Press.

Watson, R. R. (1992). LP-BM5, a murine model of AIDS: Role of cocaine, morphine, alcohol and carotenoids in nutritional immunomodulation. *Journal of Nutrition, 122,* 744–748.

Watson, R. R. (Ed.) (1993). *Alcohol, drugs of abuse and immunomodulation* (pp. 1–690). Elmsford, NY: Pergamon.

Watson, R. R. (1994). Alcohol, immunomodulation, and AIDS. *Alcohol, 11,* 67.

Watson, R. R. (1995). Alcohol, drugs of abuse and immune functions (pp. 1–264). Boca Raton, FL: CRC Press.

Watson, R. R., Borgs, P., Witte, M., McCuskey, R. S., Lantz, C., Johnson, M. I., Mufti, S. I., & Earnest, D. L. (1994). Alcohol, immunomodulation, and disease. *Alcohol Alcoholism, 29,* 131–139.

Watson, R. R., & Gottesfeld, Z. (1993). Neuroimmune effects of alcohol and its role in AIDS. *Advance Neuroimmunology, 3,* 151–162.

Watson, R. R., Lopez, M. C., Odeleye, O. & Darban, H. (1992a). Modulation of differentiation antigen expression and function of immune cells following short and prolonged alcohol intake during murine retrovirus infection. *Nutrient Modulation of the Immune Response,* 255–262.

Watson, R. R., Odeleye, O. E., Darban, H. R., & Lopez, M.C. (1992b). Modification of lymphoid subsets by chronic consumption of alcohol in C57BL/6 mice infected with LP-BM5 murine leukemia virus. *Alcohol Alcoholism, 7,* 417–424.

Watson, R. R., Odeleye, O. E., Eskelson, C. D., & Mufti, S. I. (1992c). Alcohol stimulation of lipid peroxidation and esophageal tumor growth in mice immunocompromised by retrovirus infection. *Alcohol, 9,* 495–500.

Watson, R. R., Prabhala, R. N., Abril, E., & Smith, T.L. (1988). Changes in lymphocyte subsets and macrophage function from high, short-term dietary ethanol in C57/BL6 mice. *Life Science, 43,* 865–870.

Watson, R. R., Wang, J. Y., Dehghanpisheh, K., Huang, D. S., Wood, S., Ardestani, S. K., Liang, B., & Marchalonis, J. J. (1995). T cell receptor V-beta complementarity determining region 1 peptide administration moderates immune dysfunction and cytokine dysregulation induced by murine retrovirus infection. *Journal of Immunology, 155,* 2282–2291.

Watson R. R., Wang, Y., Huang, D. S., Lopez, M. C., & Wood, S. (1993). Ethanol and murine retrovirus modulation of cytokine production by thymocytes. *Advanced Bioscience, 86,* 153–161.

Watson, R. R., & Watzl, B. (Eds.), (1992). *Nutrition and alcohol* (pp. 1–470). Boca Raton, FL: CRC Press.

Watzl, B., Lopez, M. C., Shabazian, M., Chen, G., Colombo, L. L., Huang, D. S., Witte, M., & Watson, R. R. (1993a). Diet and ethanol modulate immune responses in young C57BL/6 mice. *Alcoholism: Clinical and Experimental Research, 17,* 623–630.

Watzl, B., Lopez, M., Shahbazian, M., & Watson, R. R. (1993b). Splenocyte populations in alcoholic, mature C57BL/6 mice fed diets with different nutritional adequacy. *Advanced Bioscience, 86,* 13–18.

Watzl, B., & Watson, R. R. (1992a). Alcohol and cytokine secretion. *Alcohol, Immunology and Cancer,* 87–102.

Watzl, B., & Watson, R. R. (1992b). Nutrition and alcohol-induced immunomodulation. *Nutrition and Alcohol,* 429–446.

Watzl, B., & Watson, R. R. (1993). Role of nutrients in alcohol-induced immunomodulation. *Alcohol Alcoholism, 28,* 89–95.

Weiss, P. A. (1993). Cellular receptors and viral glycoproteins involved in retrovirus entry. In J. A. Levy, (Ed.), *The retroviridae* (pp. 1–108). New York: Plenum.

Weiss, P. A., Collier, S. D., & Pruett, S. B. (1996). Role of glucocorticoids in ethanol-induced decreases in expression of MHC class II molecules on B cells and selective decreases in spleen cell number. *Toxicology and Applied pharmacology, 139,* 153–162.

Westervelt, P., Trowbridge, D, B., Epstein, L. G., Blumberg, B. M., Li, Y., Hahn, B. H., Shaw, G. M., Price, R. W., & Ratner, L. (1992). Macrophage tropism determinants of HIV-1 in vivo. *Journal of Virology, 66,* 2577–2582.

Wiley, R. L., Ross, E. K., Buckler-White, A. J., Theodore, T. S., Earl, P. L., & Martin, M. A. (1989). Functional interactions of constant and variable domains of HIV that is critical for infectivity. *Journal of Virology, 62,* 139–147.

Wiley, R. L., Smith, D. H., Lasky, L. A., Theodor, T. S., Earl, P. L., Mars, B., Capon, D. J., & Martin, T. J. (1988). In vitro mutagenesis identifies a region with the envelope gene of the human immunodeficiency virus that is critical for infectivity. *Journal of Virology, 62,* 139–147.

Yeh, M., Chang, M. P., & Norman, D. C. (1996). Effects of exogenous cytokines on the ethanol-mediated suppression of murine thymocyte proliferation. *International Journal of Immunopharmacology, 18*(3), 219–226.

Zanussi, S., Simonelli, C., D'andrea, M., Caffau, C., Clerici, M., Tirelli, U., & De Paoli, P. (1996). CD8 lymphocyte phenotype and cytokine production in long-term non-progressor and in progressor patients with HIV-1 infection. *Clinical and Experimental Immunology, 105,* 220–224.

# 67

# Psychoneuroimmunology and Aging

GEORGE FREEMAN SOLOMON, JOHN E. MORLEY

## I. INTRODUCTION

Significant changes in immunological functions that have major clinical implications occur with aging. There are close bidirectional interactions between the immune system and the central and autonomic nervous systems. These interactions also have important clinical relevance. The field concerned with these interactions is psychoneuroimmunology. Psychoneuroimmunology (PNI) deals with the transduction of experiential/psychosocial factors into alteration of resistance to and course of infectious and neoplastic diseases and also the influence of such factors on diseases/processes of immunological aberration. It can be hypothesized that an immune system already compromised by aging might be more susceptible to further, more clinically significant compromise by aging. Psychoneuroimmunology is also concerned with the effects of cells and products of the immune system on the function, and even the structure, of the brain. One type of brain cell is immunological in nature. Microglia are the fixed macrophages of the central nervous system, and they produce cytokines that can affect neurons. There are a number of other modes of immune system effects on the brain. Immunological mechanisms may be important in a variety of neurogenerative disorders, particularly Alzheimer's disease, that are more prevalent in the elderly. Cytokines, particularly those proinflammatory in nature, can affect cognition (usually reversibly). Cognition may be impaired in the elderly, not only as a result of Alzheimer's disease, and immunological processes may have relevance to cognitive deficits of aging. In view of the close interrelatedness of central nervous and immune systems, factors that limit immunosenescence may also ameliorate senescent changes in brain function and structure. Because of growing evidence that immunity may play a role in pathophysiological processes important to aging that are not limited to the central nervous system, particularly atherosclerosis, psychoneuroimmunology may, thereby, have truly broad implications for processes of aging that lead to morbidity and mortality.

This chapter first will summarize those changes in immunity usually associated with aging. Since psychosocial influences on immunity are generally neuroendocrinologically mediated, we shall next discuss endocrine changes that occur with aging. Psychological processes particularly relevant to aging (e.g., bereavement, depression) that also are known to have immunological sequelae will be covered. Included will be the effects of stressors, both naturalistic and experimental, as they may affect immunity in the aging. Since a significant number of very old people remain physically healthy with low utilization of medical services, we address the question of whether such physical well-being is correlated with psychological well-being and cognitive intactness as well as with relative lack of immunosenescence. If that seems to be the case, what sorts of interventions might promote healthy aging? We shall review evidence for the influence of products of the immune system on neural function and cognition and review evidence for the role of cytokines in the pathogenesis of Alzheimer's disease. These approaches, hopefully, will be convincing in demonstrating the relevance of psychoneuroimmunology to gerontology.

## II. THE IMMUNE SYSTEM AND AGING

Numerous changes occur in the immune system with aging (Morley, 1999). The rate of change varies tremendously from individual to individual. All aging-related immune system changes tend to be in a negative direction. The predominant changes involve T lymphocytes, but aging also is associated with B-cell dysregulation, leading to an overproduction of autoantibodies and a decreased production of antibodies in response to environmental challenges (Table I).

With aging there is a decrease in in vitro cellular growth response to mitogens. Aging is associated with an increase in memory T-cells (i.e., those with previous antigen exposure) and a decrease in naive T cells (Miller, 1996). In addition, these memory T cells demonstrate a decrease in their intracellular signaling systems in response to antigenic stimulation (Wick & Grubeck-Laebenstein, 1997). The decline in T-cell population doublings with age results in replicative

### TABLE I  Effects of Aging on the Immune System

1. Reduced T-cell proliferation to mitogens
2. Increased T-cell apoptosis
3. Increased memory cells
4. Decreased naive cells
5. Thymic involution
6. Decreased immunoglobulin production to stimuli
7. Increased autoantibody production
8. Decreased IL-2, transforming growth factor-$\beta$, and granulocyte-macrophage colony-stimulating factor
9. Increased IL-3, IL-4, and IL-6

senescence and, therefore, a smaller T-cell population. Natural killer (NK) cytotoxic cells either increase in number or show no change in older compared to younger humans.

Aging has a number of effects on cytokine production. Interleukin-1 (IL-1) and tumor necrosis factor show no age-related changes. IL-3, IL-4, and IL-6 increase with aging. Interferon-$\alpha$, IL-2, and transforming growth factor-$\beta$ decrease with aging. There is an increase in soluble IL-2 receptors with aging, suggesting an increase in activation of the cytokine system in older persons.

## III. HORMONES, AGING, AND IMMUNITY

In general, the levels of circulating hormones tend to decline with aging (Table II). When circulating hormone levels are elevated in older persons, it often is secondary to a decrease in the receptor or post-receptor mechanism (Mooradian, Morley, & Korenman, 1988). The decline in hormones with aging is even more marked when the system has to respond to stress (Wittert & Morley, 1997). As many of the immune system responses to central nervous system stimulation are mediated by hormonal release, this alteration of stress response suggests that with aging there will be an attenuation in the ability of the brain/ psyche to modulate the immune system adaptively.

Diseases due to hormonal deficiency present with a series of signs and symptoms similar to some of the physiological, functional, and structural changes that occur with aging (Table III). This observation has led to the hypothesis that one or more of the hormones that decline with aging are responsible for the development of the aging process. Thus, in the past decade there has been a constant search for the "hormonal fountain of youth." In most cases this has proven to be futile. Growth hormone produced a panopoly of side-effects and minimal positive effects (Papadakis et al., 1996). Dehydroepiandrosterone (DHEA) in high doses improved strength in men but not women (Yen, Morales, & Khorram, 1995). In older men DHEA (50 mg daily for 20 weeks) resulted in an increase in monocytes and B cells (Khorram, Vu, & Yen, 1997). There was also an increase in soluble IL-2 receptors and in vitro mitogen-stimulated release of IL-2 and IL-6. Both cell number and activity of natural killer cells was increased. However, administration of DHEA to older volunteers (61 to 89 years) failed to enhance the immunization response to influenza vaccination (Danenberg, Ben-Yehuda, Zakay-Rones, Gross, & Friedman, 1997; Evans et al., 1996). The claims for the rejuvenating effects of melatonin far

**TABLE II  Changes in Circulating Hormones with Aging**

| | Decrease | No change | Increase |
|---|---|---|---|
| Pituitary | Growth hormone | Luteinizing hormone (Males)<br>Thyrotrophin | Luteinizing hormone (females)<br>Follicle-stimulating hormone<br>ACTH<br>Prolactin |
| Thyroid | Triiodothyronine (old–old) | Thyroxine | |
| Adrenal | DHEA<br>DHEA-S<br>Pregnenolone | Epinephrine | Cortisol<br>Norepinephrine |
| Pancreas | | | Insulin |
| Gastrointestinal<br>Tract | | Glucagon-like peptide I | Cholecystokinin<br>Vasoactive intestinal peptide |
| Heart | | | Atrial naturetic factor |
| Liver | Insulin-like growth factor-I | | |
| Gonads | Testosterone (males)<br>Estradiol (females) | | |

outweigh their scientific bases (Waterhouse, Reilly, & Atkinson, 1998). Melatonin decreases IL-6 levels (Neri et al., 1998). Melatonin has also been reported to improve outcomes in melanoma and small cell cancer of the lung (Lissoni et al., 1996, 1997, 1996). The memory enhancing effects of the true "mother hormone" pregnenolone appear to be limited to mice (Flood, Morley, & Roberts, 1995). Vitamin D decreased hip fracture in old women in nursing homes and increased longevity (Chapuy, Arlot, Delmas, & Meunier, 1994). The possibility that some of this effect was due to its immune enhancing effects is intriguing but not proven (Muller & Bendtzen, 1996).

Most endocrine disease in old age is due to glandular failure, e.g., hypothyroidism, diabetes

**TABLE III  Signs and Symptoms of Aging and Hypoendocrine Disorders**

| | Aging | Growth hormone | Thyroid | Testosterone |
|---|---|---|---|---|
| Decreased muscle strength | Yes | Yes | Yes | Yes |
| Osteopenia | Yes | Yes | — | Yes |
| Decreased skin thickness | Yes | Yes | — | Yes |
| Decreased cognition | Yes | Maybe | Yes | Yes |
| Immune dysfunction | Yes | Yes | Yes | Maybe |
| Fatigue | Yes | Yes | Yes | Yes |

mellitus, or due to ectopic hormone production from cancers. When hormone overproduction does occur, it often presents unusually, as with apathetic thyrotoxicosis. Thyroid disease has a long history, suggesting that it may be a psychoneuroimmune disease since the first case reported by Graves—a young woman whose onset of the disease was purportedly due to the traumatic psychic event of falling out of a wheelchair! Immune dysfunction plays a major role in the development of thyroid disease. Thyroid autoantibodies increase over the life span up to the age of 85 years (Mariotti et al., 1993). However, highly healthy centenarians have lower autoantibodies to thyroid tissue than do younger old persons (Mariotti et al., 1992). This finding suggests that failure to develop thyroid autoantibodies may confer a survival advantage on older persons.

Type II diabetes mellitus occurs in approximately 16% of older persons (Morley & Perry, 1991). Depression has been shown to play a major role in the pathogenesis of poor outcomes in older persons with diabetes (Rosenthal, Fajardo, Gilmore, Morley, & Naliboff, 1998). While this is, in part, due to the effects of depression on compliance issues, it is also related to the increased levels of hormones (e.g. cortisol, growth hormone) that antagonize insulin effects and the effects of depression on immune function.

Both androgens and estrogen, which decrease with aging, enhance NK activity. However, as pointed out above, most studies find NK activity relatively intact with aging. Both testosterone and estradiol have been demonstrated to modulate cytokine release in vitro (Li, Davis, & Brooks, 1993). Neuroendocrine–immune feedback circuits are altered by aging. For example, the stimulation of the hypothalamo-pituitary-adrenal (HPA) axis is blunted by aging. Interleukin-1 (IL-1) does not induce as great a rise in CRH-ACTH-cortisol in aging rats (Bernadini et al., 1992). This failure of feedback may be related to the higher incidence of autoantibodies in the aged (Cammarata, Rodnan, & Fennel, 1967). Strains of rats with blunted HPA axis response to stress are more susceptible to adjuvant-induced arthritis as well as experimental allergic encephalitis, which are animal models of the human autoimmune diseases rheumatoid arthritis and multiple sclerosis, respectively (Sternberg, Wilder, Chrousos, & Gold, 1991).

High insulin growth factor-1 (IGF-1) levels have been correlated with poor subsequent survival in middle-aged men (Maisson et al., 1998). Insulin-like growth factor-1, the mediator of growth hormone effects, inhibits apoptosis of hematopoetic precursor cells—including immune (Kelley et al., 1998). High circulating IGF-1 levels have been associated with an increase in the risk for breast cancer (Hankinson et al., 1998). In cell cultures, a negative IGF-1 receptor mutant inhibited adhesion of the breast cell tumor line (Dunn et al., 1998). These findings strongly suggest that the decline in IGF-1 with aging may be protective against cancer.

Levels of vitamin D often decline with aging. 1,25-Dihydroxyvitamin D3 inhibits the proliferation of T cells and the release of IL-2 and interferon-$\gamma$ (Muller & Bendtzen, 1996). The CD45RA− subset of T-helper cells is more sensitive than the CD45RA+ group to the effects of vitamin D. Thus, vitamin D deficiency may be responsible, in part, for the increase of autoantibodies with aging.

## IV. THYMIC FUNCTION, HORMONES, AND AGING

The thymus starts to involute soon after birth, and this process continues throughout life. The thymus plays a central role in T-cell differentiation and also produces immunoactive hormones. Thymulin levels decline with aging secondary to the fall in growth hormone levels (Hadden, 1998; Kelley et al., 1988). B-cell maturation is delayed with aging, resulting in altered proportions of primary and memory B cells in the periphery (Klinman & Kline, 1997). The number of circulating B cells is maintained by an increase in the half-life of B cells. These B cells tend to produce lower affinity antibodies, which are less protective against infection (Song, Price, & Cerney, 1997).

Thymopentin and thymopoetin, subject to age-related decline in thymic functions, enhance production of ACTH, $\beta$-endorphin (BE), and $\beta$-lipotropin (Malaise et al., 1987). Thymic stromal elements contain prolactin- and growth hormone-releasing properties (Spangelo & MacLeod, 1988). Their atrophy, thus, may have a relationship to growth hormone deficiency of aging. Augmentation of proliferative responses of T cells by BE is weaker in old compared to young mice, probably reflective of decrease in opioid receptor binding with aging (Norman, Morley, & Chang, 1988). In contrast, there was no difference found between the ability of BE to stimulate natural killer cell activity pre- and postexercise between young and old subjects (Fiatarone et al., 1989). Somatostatin, which has a number of immunomodulatory roles including inhibition of T-cell proliferation and stimulation of release of histamine from most cells while inhibiting its release from basophils, has been found to be decreased in brains of patients with Alzheimer's disease (Arai, Moroji, & Kosaka, 1984).

## V. AGING AND PSYCHOSOCIAL INFLUENCES ON IMMUNITY

### A. Bereavement

Obviously, the older one gets the greater the number of significant relationships that are lost and the more a person is subject to bereavements and grief. Grieving is an active process and involves psychological "work" or "working through." Grief and depression are related but not synonymous psychological constructs (Freud, 1917). Failure of the grieving process can result in depression. It has been noted in a condition other than aging also associated with immunodeficiency, HIV/AIDS, that repeated bereavements are associated with a more rapid decline in measures of immune competence (Kemeny et al., 1989). Research suggests that both lymphocyte response to mitogenic stimulation and NK cytotoxic activity are lower following bereavement as compared to prebereavement levels or those of control subjects (Bartrop, Luckhurst, Lazarus, Kiloh, & Penny, 1997; Irwin, Daniels, Risch, Bloom, & Weiner, 1988; Schleifer, Keller, Camerino, Thornton, & Stein, 1987). Studies have included both men and women. The study by Irwin and his colleagues (1987) included older women (mean age of subjects = 57), but age effects have not been analyzed in studies of bereavement and immunity. An intriguing contrary finding comparing depressed patients and women anticipating bereavement found a positive correlation between mitogen (phytohemagglutinin (PHA)) response and depression scores in the prebereavemed compared to the negative correlation in depressed patients (Spurrell & Creed, 1993). The authors suggest that the positive immune findings may be a reflection of an adaptive coping response.

## B. Depression/Sleep

Depressive illness and dysphoric symptoms, unrelated to bereavement, affect over 15% of the geriatric population (Kennedy, 1991). Depressive symptoms predict physical decline in community-dwelling older persons (Pennix et al., 1998). Studies of depression and immunity have been somewhat contradictory. Differences often are due to methodological problems such as sample size, immunological assays utilized, and lack of control for sex, age, hospitalization status, and diagnosis. A meta-analytic review accounting for the methodological problems mentioned concluded that there remains a reliable association between decreased cellular immune function and depression (Herbert & Cohen, 1993). In addition, this relationship is significantly impacted by age and by severity and duration of depression. A study with age- and sex-matched controls found that only older patients showed decreased lymphocyte response to mitogens (PHA, concanavalin A (Con A), pokeweed mitogen (PWM)), with degree of decrease proportional to age (Schleifer, Keller, Bond, Cohen, & Stein, 1989). Other studies suggest that depression reduces NK-cell cytotoxicity in an age-independent way and that return to normal follows recovery (Irwin, Lecher, & Caldwell, 1992). Both degree of depression-associated reductions in stimulation of T lymphocytes by PHA and of NK cells by IL-2 were found to be age related (Guidi et al., 1991).

Depressed patients show evidence of immune activation as well as suppression. (Activation might be related to the aforementioned increase in autoantibodies in the aged.) Depressed patients show increased IL-1 receptor antagonist concentrations, IL-1$\beta$ production, IL-1, IL-2, and IL-6 receptor plasma concentrations, and levels of C-reactive protein, HLA-DR, neopterin, and complement (Berk, Wadee, Kushke, & O'Neil-Kerr, 1997; Katila, Appelberg, Hurme, & Rimon, 1994; Maes et al., 1993, 1995; Sluzewska et al., 1996). Some have gone so far as to call depression an "inflammatory disease." Most unfortunately, in contrast to studies of immunosupression in depression, studies of immune activation have not controlled for age. It is likely that the reversible cognitive deficits associated with depres-

sion-induced pseudodementia of the elderly are induced by proinflammatory cytokines. This topic will be discussed further.

That depression-related immunodeficiency is clinically significant in the older population is suggested by findings that older persons with depressive symptoms have increased medical morbidity, costs of health services, and mortality (Alexopoulis & Chester, 1992; Unützer et al., 1997; Kouzis, Eaton, & Leaf, 1995; Whooly & Browner, 1998).

Sleep is disturbed in depression, but sleep is also often disturbed in the nondepressed aged as well (Coleman, Miles, Guilleminault, Zarcone, & Dement, 1981). Interleukin-1 increases with onset of slow-wave sleep, suggesting deep sleep's immunological as well as mental "restorative" function (Moldofsky, Lue, Eisen, Keystone, & Gorcynski, 1989). Partial sleep deprivation reduces NK cell activity (Irwin et al., 1994). However, sleep deprivation increases production of cytokines interferon-$\alpha$ and IL-1$\beta$ (Uthgennant, Schoolmann, Pietrowsky, Fehm, & Born, 1995). Clearly, attention to sleep problems of the elderly is likely important to their health.

## C. Caregiving Stress

Caregiving of demented spouses is associated with high risk of negative immune changes as well as increased risk of illness in the elderly population. With increasing longevity, caregiving of demented parents may be given by already aging offspring. Such caregiving is a chronic, ever-worsening stressor. As amply illustrated elsewhere in this text, both intensity and duration of a stressor are correlated with the magnitude of its immunological sequelae. There is an ample literature, more fully cited elsewhere in this volume, regarding health-relevant immune changes in caregivers including lowered stimulability of lymphocytes, decreased NK-cell activity, high levels of antibody to latent herpes-group viruses (reflecting lowered cellular immunological control and viral activation), and lower percentage of total T and helper T lymphocytes (Kiecolt-Glaser et al., 1987). Distress-related immunosuppression is more likely to have health consequences in older caregivers because of existing age-related compromises in immune functioning (Kiecolt-Glaser, Dura, Speicher, Trask, & Glaser, 1991). Moreover, female caregivers of patients with Alzheimer's disease are also at high risk for depression, which can further contribute to immunosuppression (Crook & Miller, 1985). Depression in caregivers of demented patients is associated with altered immunity including impaired lymphocyte proliferation capacity and declines in lymphocytes with surface signal transduction molecules (CD38+) and the cytotoxicity marker CD56+CD8+ (Castle, Wilkins, Heck, Tanzy, & Fahey, 1995). The chronic stress of caregiving but not the acute stress of housing relocation is associated in older women with significant elevations of serum levels of IL-6 over and above the elevations associated with normal aging (Lutgendorf et al., 1999). There are gender differences in at least some immunological sequelae of the stress of caregiving to demented spouses. Caregiving husbands over 60 had lower CD4 helper T-cell counts than married noncaregiving controls, but caregiving wives did not (Scanlon, Vitaliano, Ochs, Savage, & Borson, 1998). Hassles affected CD4/CD8 ratio in the men but not the women. Perhaps, a greater immunological vulnerability to stress in older men contributes to the significantly greater statistical longevity of women then that seen in men.

## D.  Stress "Buffers"

### 1.  Social Support

Networks of social support tend to diminish for aging people as friends die, work friendships disappear with retirement, and offspring move to distant places in our mobile society. Social support has been referred to as a "stress buffer." There are studies of amelioration of stress effects on immunity by social support. Older women (mean age 73) were classified as having experienced marked adversity in the past year or no stress (McNaughton, Smith, Patterson, & Grant, 1990). High-stress women had significantly lower ratios of CD4+ to CD8+ T cells, and a considerable proportion of this variance was accounted for by satisfaction with social support. Literature on the relevance of social support factors in stress of the nonelderly to immunity might be expected to have even greater relevance to the elderly. Medical students reporting being lonely have greater activation of latent herpes virus infection under the stress of examinations than do medical students with supportive relationships (Glaser, Kiecolt-Glaser, Speicher, & Holiday, 1985). It would seem likely that the incidence of loneliness is higher in the old than in the young. There is evidence that strong social networks reduce mortality (Berkman & Syme, 1979). Such epidemiological evidence is supported by experimental evidence (albeit in young people) that fixed doses of rhinovirus administered intranasally were less likely to result in colds or to lead to milder colds if subjects had strong diversified social networks of family, friends, colleagues, neighbors, etc. (Cohen, Doyle, Skoner, Rabin, & Gwaltney, 1997).

### 2.  Perceived Control

In older adults, low perceived control over significant life stressors predicts T-cell responses to mitogenic (PHA) and antigenic challenge as well as NK-cell activity after exposure to stress (Rodin, 1986; Sieber, Rodin, Larson, Ortega, & Cummings, 1992). Sense of control is not the same psychological construct as need for control. In unpublished data, the first author and Gregory Hallert found that need for control positively correlated significantly with per cell NK-cell cytotoxicity in the elderly (mean age 73), while that immunological function was negatively correlated with need for control in the young (mean age 29). Additionally, in this population, a pessimistic explanatory style was associated with a lower CD4/CD8 ratio and lower response to lymphocyte stimulation by PHA, but this association was not age-related. In another immunocompromised population, gay men with HIV/AIDS, pessimism (not well termed as "realistic acceptance"), similarly, was associated with decreased survival time (Reed, Kemeny, Taylor, Wang, & Fisher, 1994). Interventions that increase the control older monkeys have over changes in the social environment reduce the deleterious immune alterations of such changes (Coe, Erschler, Champoux, & Olson 1992). A strong sense of coherence (Antonovsky, 1987), a component of which is a belief in the controllability of the environment, is associated with lesser decrements in NK-cell activity associated with the stress of housing relocation from homes to independent living-facilities in older adults (Lutgendorf, Vitaliano, Tripp-Reimer, Harvey, & Lubarott, 1999).

## E.  Alcoholism

Alcoholism is known, by virtue of a considerable number of human and animal studies on the effects of ethanol on immunity, to have adverse immunological consequences (Watson, 1995; Yirmiya & Taylor, 1993). These include loss of lymphocytes from the thymus, spleen, and peripheral blood, reduced mitogen- and recall antigen-induced lymphocyte proliferation, reduced ability of B cells to respond to T-dependent antigens, inhibition of production of proinflammatory cytokines, induction of inhibitory immune mediator production, and reduction of the growth factors GM-CSF and G-CSF (Jerrels, Marietta, Eckhardt, Majchrowicz, & Wright, 1986). Alcoholism in the elderly is a relatively common and underrecognized problem (Adams, Yuan, Barboriak, & Rimm, 1993). Clearly, the long-held contention that alcoholism diminishes as a problem with aging because most heavy drinkers have died of complications of alcoholism before the age of 60 is not valid. A decade ago (1989) nearly 90,000 Medicare recipients (> age 65) were hospitalized for alcohol-related causes in a single year. The rate of such hospitalizations was 55 elderly men and 15 women per 10,000 compared to rates of heart attacks (myocardial infarction) of between 17 and 44/10,000 in people over 65. Depression is common among alcoholics and, as already stated, is also relatively common in the aged, in whom it is likely to be associated with immunological deficits. Alcoholism is associated with increased risk of infection and premature mortality, which may be, in part, related to alcohol-induced immunosuppression (Friedman, Klein, & Specter, 1996). It seems quite likely that alcohol is a synergistic cofactor not only in the cognitive and affective problems often associated with aging but also in immunosenescence.

### F. Experimental Stress

Several studies have shown that brief experimental stresses given to volunteer subjects in a laboratory, such as mental arithmetic, result in some transient immunological changes, particularly increases in number of circulating NK cells and increases in NK cytotoxic activity. Such increases generally correlate with at least some measures of psychophysiological arousal (Benschop et al., 1998). Acute upregulation of nonspecific "first line of defense" immunity, occurring under circumstances analogous to fight/flight situations in nature, generally has been interpreted as biologically adaptive. Only one study compared the affects of an acute laboratory stressor (time-pressured mental arithmetic) between groups of healthy young (21–41 years) and healthy old (65–85 years) subjects (Naliboff et al., 1991). In contrast to to-be-mentioned findings with acute exercise, old, unlike young, subjects did not show stress-induced increases in NK-cell cytotoxicity, while they did show increases in numbers of circulating NK cells (CD16+, CD56+). This finding indicates an actual decrease in per cell NK cytotoxicity with mental stress in the aged.

## VI. INTERVENTIONS AND IMMUNITY IN THE ELDERLY

### A. Psychological Interventions

There are few studies of psychosocial interventions aimed at enhancing immune functions in the elderly. Relaxation training has been shown significantly to increase NK cell activity in old people (Kiecolt-Glaser et al., 1985). Relaxation therapy improves NK cell

activity in caregivers of patients with Alzheimer's disease (Lewis, Kroening, Bonner, & Cooper, 1999). Control enhancing intervention studies, particularly of patients in nursing homes, suggest that increased sense of control positively affects psychological and physical health and decreases mortality (Rodin, 1986). Similarly, studies of interventions in patients with age-related diseases, particularly cancer, report health outcomes, usually not measures of possible mediating physiological variables, particularly immune. An exception, fortunately being emulated in current research (see chapter by David Spiegel), is that of a psychological intervention consisting of enhancement of problem solving skills, stress management, and psychological support in patients (ages 19–70) with malignant melanoma by Fawzy and colleagues. Psychological and immunological results appeared independent of age. The short-term (6-week) intervention reduced psychological distress and enhanced longer-term effective coping (Fawzy et al., 1990a). There were no immunological differences six weeks following intervention, but at the six-month assessment there were significant increases in NK cell numbers and activity in the intervention group (1990b). By the 18-month, 2-year, and 6-year follow-ups, immunological differences had disappeared, but increasingly significant differences in survival had emerged (Fawzy et al., 1993). Fawzy's intervention patients had significantly lower mortality than both within institution and national norms. If psychological interventions can help patients with immunologically resisted neoplasms, perhaps interventions might have a prophylactic effect in still healthy but at-risk elder persons. Such epidemiological studies, however, would require many subjects and long follow-up. Effective treatment of depression (psychopharmacological, electroconvulsive) reverses depression-associated immunological deficits—albeit probably to an already lower baseline in the elderly (Weizman et al., 1994; Avissar, Mechamkin, Roitman, & Schreiber, 1998).

### B. Exercise

Physical inactivity in capable older adults appears to increase morbidity and mortality; conversely, recreational physical activity offers benefits in reducing risk of functional decline and mortality (Simonsick et al., 1993). Studies of the effects of exercise on immunity in younger adults, which are covered extensively in another chapter of this text, suggest that acute exercise is associated with transient increases in various measures of immunity including: total leukocyte count, cytotoxic (CD8+) lymphocytes, plasma interferon and interleukin-1 levels, and natural killer cell number and activity. Exercise programs for the elderly can improve endurance (Cunningham, Rechnitzer, Howard, & Donner, 1987; Sidney & Sheppard, 1987). As has been widely documented, physical conditioning may ameliorate disease states common in old people, including osteoporosis, cardiovascular disease, and even diabetes (Hollenbech, Haskell, Rosenthal, & Reaven, 1985). Home-based moderate-intensity physical activity regimens have been shown to improve physical health (blood pressure) and psychological health, particularly anger expression (King & Brassington, 1997). The latter result may have immunological implications since emotional expressiveness has been found to be related to better cellular immunological control of latent viruses (Esterling, Antoni, Kumar, & Schneiderman, 1990).

An acute bout of maximal cycling exercise results in equivalent increases in NK-cell numbers and activity and decreases in NK-cell stimulability by IL-2 following exercise in both young (21–39 years) and healthy old (over 65) women (Fiatarone et al., 1989). Another study had similar findings, but physically trained elderly women achieved significantly greater increases in NK activity (Crist, MacKinnon, Thompson, Atterborn, & Egan, 1989). There have been few studies of endurance training in the elderly to determine whether repeated bouts of aerobic exercise resulted in upregulation of any immune measures compared to preexercise baseline. Elderly women who participated in 16 weeks of aerobic training three times a week demonstrated a 33% increase in basal NK-cell cytotoxicity (Crist et al., 1989). However, another study found that moderate aerobic training five times a week had no effect on either basal NK-cell activity or T-cell function (PHA responsiveness) in previously sedentary women (Nieman et al., 1993). A 1996 review concluded that the [relatively meager] evidence of cross-sectional comparisons of immune status of elderly subjects implies that habitual physical activity may enhance NK-cell activity and check certain aspects of age-related decline in T-cell function (Shinkai, Konishi, & Sheppard, 1996).

It is now well-known that overtraining, even in conditioned athletes, can lead to immunosuppression and illness (Keast, 1996). It must be kept in mind that in already immune compromised elderly, particularly the frail, "overtraining" may result from only moderate exercise. Frail men over the age of 70 not suffering from any known life-threatening disease were given an exercise intervention of increasing strenuousness for 60 min three times a week for 3 months (Rincón, Solomon, Benton, & Rubenstein,

1996). After 6 and 12 weeks of physical conditioning, cytotoxic activity of NKcells showed progressive decrease in spite of transient exercise-induced increases. At the end of the study, the exercise-induced increase of NK-cell activity was less than preexercise baseline at the beginning. Clearly, exercise programs must be very cautiously given and closely monitored immunologically in frail elderly persons, while healthy elderly persons probably derive comparable benefits from exercise as younger people.

## C. Medications

It is beyond the scope of this chapter to review the many claims and reports of "immunorestorative" effects of various biological substances in the elderly, particularly those that decline with aging, including thymic extracts and products, pineal extracts, sex hormones, antioxidants, and growth hormone. DHEA and melatonin already were mentioned. As will be discussed further, a correlation among intact immunological functions, health, and longevity makes further investigation of interventions that foster immunocompetence in the elderly of considerable medical importance.

## VII. HEALTHY AGING

### A. Mental Health and Course of Disease

Medicine and, to a lesser extent, behavioral and psychosomatic medicine primarily have been concerned with disease, its etiology (nowadays, thankfully, multifactorily considered), pathophysiology, psychophysiology, and treatment. Psychoneuroimmunology, with the notable exception of conditioning and intervention studies, has been concerned mainly with adverse experiential effects on immunity and adverse central nervous system sequelae of immunological processes. It seems at least as important to understand health, especially in old age, and relative health (prompt recovery or slow progression) in the face of disease. We shall, therefore, refer to some findings concerning doing relatively well with two immunologically related diseases, rheumatoid arthritis and HIV/AIDS. Although psychosocial factors in progression of autoimmune disease and AIDS are the topics of other chapters of this text, some findings that seem possibly of particular relevance to aging will be mentioned herein. Both aging and AIDS have been compared (Solomon, 1991). Slow progression of or relatively little incapacitation by and good response to medical treatment of rheumatoid arthritis were related to relative absence of psychological distress ("dysphoric affects") and effective coping (Moos & Solomon, 1964, 1965; Solomon & Moos, 1965a). Patients who did less well were less able to continue former modes of adaptation and coping and were, thereby, experiencing increases in anxiety and depression. A comparison was made between two groups of healthy relatives of patients with rheumatoid arthritis, one whose sera showed the anti-IgG autoantibody associated with that disease, "rheumatoid factor" (known to have predictive significance for later development of the disease), and one whose sera were negative for rheumatoid factor (Solomon & Moos, 1965b). Rheumatoid factor seronegative family members ranged from mentally disturbed to psychologically healthy, similar to a distribution curve of psychological/psychiatric disturbance in a random population. On the other hand, the rheumatoid factor positive relatives were psychiatrically asymptomatic and reported satisfaction with relationships and occupations. Thus, it appeared as if mental well-being might serve as a protective factor in the face of a probably genetically determined predisposition to disease. With a similar strategy, a group of unusually long-survivors of AIDS were studied before the advent of anti-retroviral therapies (Solomon, Temoshok, O'Leary, & Zich, 1987). These people turned out to be quite remarkable psychologically, tending to use 15 highly adaptive modes of coping. Rather similar findings of themes of adaptive coping have been found in studies of persons who are long survivors with HIV/AIDS (Ironson, Solomon, Cruess, Barroso, & Stivers, 1995). These themes comprise: following healthy self-care, maintaining interpersonal connectedness, maintaining a sense of meaning and purpose, and maintaining perspective (a failure of which is manifested by depression, negative affect, and hopelessness). Indeed, these findings of positive psychological factors in those doing relatively well in the face of an autoimmune disease and of acquired immunodeficiency syndrome may be relevant to healthy aging.

## B. Psychology and Immunology in the Healthy Elderly

Psychological and immunological measures were carried out in samples of young control ($N = 38$, mean age 29) and old ($N = 58$, mean age 73) physically healthy, community dwelling women (Solomon et al., 1988). In the first year of the study, immunological assays (NK-cell cytotoxicity, numbers of lymphocytes bearing NK-associated markers CD16+ and CD56+, and T-cell function assessed by PHA-induced mito-

genesis) were done every 3 months. These healthy older adults had higher NK-cell activity than the younger adults, and T-cell function did not differ between the two groups. After the first year, measures were taken annually for 30 of the healthy older subjects. For all time points measured (1986–1992), there were no significant changes in NK-cell activity or T-cell mitogenesis compared to baseline (1986, average of three measures). This immunological stability of functional measures over time in healthy elderly people is of interest in view of the generally high variability of measures of immunity in the elderly. In the older subjects, number of CD16+ and CD56+ lymphocytes significantly *increased* over time compared to baseline. Psychological measures of anxiety, depression, anger, and hopelessness were also assessed over time. All were within normal limits. Except for anxiety, which *decreased* from baseline, measures of psychological distress, like immunological measures, did not significantly change. This psychological and immunological normality (as standardized in a younger population) and stability strongly suggests a linkage between mental and physical health in older persons. Importantly, during the follow-up period, there was only one major health change (herpes zoster) and were only three deaths (two myocardial infarctions, one cancer). Looking at psychological–immune relationships, in older people there was a significant relationship between feelings of anger and NK-cell activity during the first year of study. However, no such relationship emerged in the subsequent years. Interestingly, those healthy old people who subjectively perceived themselves (nonverbally by placement of a mark along a "life-line") as nearer the end of life than would be "realistic" (by age-corrected actuarial tables) showed lower NK-cell activity (Grohr, Solomon, & Benton, 1994). The anticipation of a major future life event as farther into the future predicted lower NK-cell activity 2 years later than was the case in those persons who looked forward to a more immediate significant event. The aim of this study to determine prospectively whether life stress, relative failure of coping, and consequent psychological distress anteceded immunological changes, which, in turn, anteceded illness and death was not achieved because of the maintenance of health and life in these elderly women. At the conclusion of the study, the oldest subject was 101 years of age. Clearly, the sample was highly selected for excellent health, little medication use, and independent living, and the findings, thus, represent an atypical cohort effect.

Sense of coherence comprises senses of comprehensibility, manageability, and meaningfulness in relation to one's environment and its challenges and has been found to be a predictor of health and life satisfaction in older adults (Antonovsky, 1987). Sense of coherence ameliorates negative effects on NK-cell activity related to the stress of residential relocation in the elderly (Lutgendorf, Vitaliano, Tripp-Reimer, Harvey, & Lubaroff, 1999). Related to comprehensibility and meaningfulness may be religiosity. Attendance at religious services was found to be inversely correlated with levels of IL-6 in a large cohort of persons over age 65 (Koenig et al., 1997).

Centenarians are the best example of successful aging, since they have avoided or survived the major age-associated diseases, and most are in good mental and physical health. Their numbers are increasing. A review of prior studies and further study of centenarians concluded that several immune parameters are well conserved in those successfully achieving very advanced age (Franceschi, Monti, Sansoni, & Cossaria, 1995). In regard to cellular immunity, there is well-preserved capability of T cells to proliferate after polyclonal stimuli or contact with superantigens as well as a consistent number of "virgin" or "naive" CD4+ and CD8+ T cells (CD45RA+) capable of responding to novel antigens. Healthy centenarians lacked the autoantibodies relatively common to old age, implying successful "selection" by the thymus or some other organ. The finding that most centenarians have all V$\beta$ families of the T cell repertoire is evidence that huge numbers of T cells can be produced and selected until toward the limit of human life. However, centenarians do not escape the age-related tendency to develop CD8+ T-cell clonal expansions. Nonspecific "innate" or natural immunity is maintained not only by NK cells but also by normal cell locomotion of macrophages in response to chemotactic stimuli. Centenarians' lymphocytes have increased resistance to oxidative stress and high genomic stability (i.e., low spontaneous chromatin breaks and micronuclei frequency). As pointed out, healthy centenarians are less likely to produce thyroid autoantibodies than younger old persons (Mariotti et al., 1992). Perceptively, the immunologists reporting these findings in centenarians informally made some psychological observations (personal communication). They observed healthy centenarians to be future-oriented, tolerant of losses, and a bit narcissistic!

## VIII. COGNITION, CYTOKINES, ALZHEIMER'S DISEASE, AND AGING

Cytokines, such as interferon-$\alpha$, when given to humans to treat cancer can produce a decrease in cognition and dysphoria (Licinio, Kling, & Hauser, 1998). Cytokines produce these effects both by peripheral and central mechanisms. In rodents, cytokines have been demonstrated to stimulate ascending fibers of the vagus (Hansen, Taishi, Chen, & Krueger, 1998). These activated afferent fibers then carry messages to the midbrain and from there to the amygdala and the hippocampus. In the hippocampus, this cascade leads to interleukin-1 release from glial cells. IL-1 then inhibits acetylcholine release in the hippocampus producing a decline in learning and memory potential of the animal (Rada et al., 1991). In addition, cytokines may produce direct effects on the central nervous system since cytokines have been demonstrated to cross the blood-brain barrier (Banks, Kastin, & Ehrensing, 1994). Both of these mechanisms appear to be involved in the pathogenesis of delirium produced by infection (Figure 1).

Alzheimer's disease is the most common cause of dementia in older persons. Anatomically, the disease is defined by the presence of amyloid plaques and neurofibrillary tangles. There is evidence that the pathogenesis of Alzheimer's disease involves the overproduction of $\beta$-amyloid. $\beta$-Amyloid decreases memory retention by inhibiting acetylcholine release in the hippocampus, either directly or indirectly (Flood, Morley, & Roberts, 1994; Flood & Morley, 1998). Amyloid-$\beta$-peptide can also cause tissue destruction through generation of inflammatory cytokines and neurotoxic free radicals such as nitric oxide (Hu, Akama, Kraft, Chromy, & Van Eldik, 1998). Amyloid-$\beta$-peptide appears to produce these effects by activation of the intracellular signal transduction pathway through NF KappaB (Kitamura, 1997) and activation of the complement system (Aisen, 1996). $\beta$-Amyloid has been demonstrated to increase the production of both interleukin-6 and tumor necrosis factor from astrocytes (Forloni, Mangiarotti, Angeretti, Lucca, & DeSimoni, 1997). Circulating serum levels of IL-6 have been correlated with the severity of the dementia in Alzheimer's disease (Kalman et al., 1997).

Young persons dying 4 or more weeks following severe head injury have been found to have large numbers of amyloid plaques in the brain (Roberts, Gentleman, Lynch, & Graham, 1991). This deposition appears to be secondary to activation of glia, leading to IL-1 release. IL-1 release then promotes processing of the amyloid-$\beta$ protein precursor protein (Griffin et al., 1998). Thus, cytokines appear to play a role not only in producing cellular destruction following amyloid-$\beta$ protein activation but also in activating the amyloid-$\beta$ protein. These effects have been termed

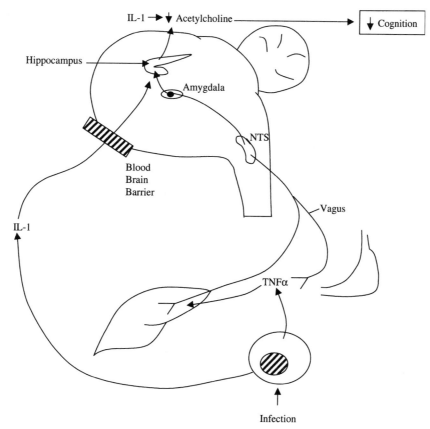

IL-1 → ↓ Acetylcholine ——————————→ ↓ Cognition

Hippocampus

Amygdala

NTS

Blood
Brain
Barrier

Vagus

IL-1

TNFα

Infection

**FIGURE 1**   Role of cytokines in the pathogenesis of delirium.

the "cytokine cycle" and are considered a key element in the pathogenesis of Alzheimer's disease (Figure 2).

Recently, as in the case of atherosclerosis (to be discussed), infectious processes have been implicated in the pathogenesis and/or exacerbation of Alzheimer's disease. *Chlamydia pneumoniae* is commonly found in brains of persons who died from Alzheimer's disease (Balin et al., 1998). *C. pneumoniae* may aggravate the disease by promoting inflammation and consequent production of proinflammatory cytokines. If an immunologically resisted microorganism is related to the pathogenesis of Alzheimer's disease, depression and stress-induced immunosuppression may be important and, by implication, psychological well-being may contribute to prevention of cognitive decline in the elderly.

## IX.  ATHEROSCLEROSIS AND IMMUNITY

Since atherosclerosis with its consequences of heart attack, stroke, and peripheral vascular disease is one of the two (along with cancer) main causes of morbidity and mortality in the elderly, it would seem worthwhile briefly to review current evidence

that immunity [neuroendocrinololgically regulated, of course] is of relevance to the pathogenesis of atherosclerosis and cardiovascular disease, which has been postulated to be an immunologically-mediated disease (Wick, Schett, & Amberger, 1995). A large literature supports important roles for stress, behavior, and personality factors in the development of atherosclerosis/cardiovascular disease, particularly coronary artery stenosis and obstruction (e.g., Chesney & Rosenman, 1985). Macrophages are the [immunologically competent cells] that take up cholesterol into the endothelium of blood vessels. A bacterium (*C. pneumoniae*) may be involved in atherogenesis. High anti-Chlamydia IgA antibody titers have been found 3–6 months before myocardial infarction (Saikku et al., 1992). A study of atherosclerotic plaques, both early stages and advanced, in Alaska natives who died from accidents found *C. pneumoniae* in over one-third (Davidson et al., 1998). Analysis of the sera of the same individuals from months to years earlier showed that those with antibody evidence of prior infection were more likely to have bacteria in plaques. Antibodies to low-density lipoproteins appear to have a protective effect against athersclerotic plaques (Travis, 1993). High cholesterol

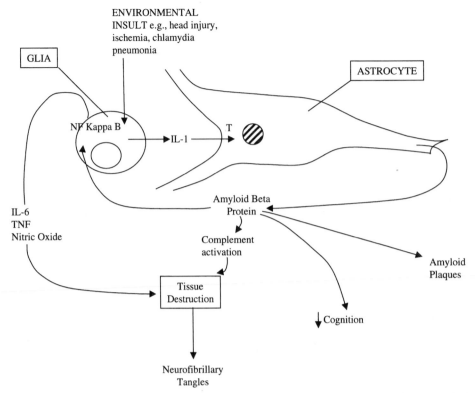

**FIGURE 2**    Role of cytokines in the pathogenesis of Alzheimer disease—"the cytokine cascade."

containing liposomes can stimulate production of anti-cholesterol antibodies.

Within atherosclerotic lesions there is evidence of immunoglobulins, complement, activated T cells, and macrophages and production of proinflammatory cytokines IL-1 and IL-6 (Aretz & Colvin, 1997). Atherosclerosis may result from cellular and humoral autoimmune responses that are triggered by the expression of heat shock proteins by endothelial cells in response to stressful stimuli that stimulate [immunoregulatory] sympathetic nervous system activity (Kaplan, Pettersson, & Manuck, 1991). Reduction of C-reactive protein, a serum marker of inflammation predictive of future myocardial infarction and stroke, by use of aspirin suggests that its prophylactic effect may be anti-inflammatory rather than anti-coagulatory (Ridker, Cushman, Stampfer, Tracy, & Henekens, 1997). Interaction of the CD40 receptor on T cells and its ligand may be important in atherosclerosis (Laman, de Smet, Schoneveld, & van Meurs, 1997). Endothelial cells respond (immunity, inflammation, thrombosis, atherogenesis) to cytokines, INF-γ, IL-1, IL-3, IL-4, IL-6, IL-10, IL-13, GM-CSF, G-CSF (Mantovani, Bussolini, & Introna, 1997).

Clinically, as demonstrated by other chapters in this volume, psychoneuroimmunology has been considered relevant to mental illness, inflammatory,

infectious, and autoimmune diseases, and to at least some cancers. Growing evidence of immunological processes (infectious, resistive, inflammatory) in atherosclerosis and cardiovascular disease has made psychoneuroimmunology also relevant to these pathophysiological processes that contribute so significantly to the morbidity and mortality of the aged.

## X.  SUMMARY AND CONCLUSIONS

Psychoneuroimmunology is relevant to the psychological and biological processes and conditions that tend to be associated with aging and, thus, is a field that is of relevance to gerontology and geriatric medicine. Immunosenescence involves various aspects of immune functions, including: decline in the naive T-cell population; decrements in T-cell functioning; increases in autoantibodies; and increases, decreases, or no change in levels of particular cytokines. However, there is high interindividual variability in age-associated immunological changes, and physically healthy old people, including centenarians, show remarkable little difference in immunity from younger persons. Moreover, such healthy old people are likely to be cognitively intact and to demonstrate psychological well-being, suggesting that aging reflects parallel processes in immune and central nervous systems. Age-related declines in hormone levels likely have relevance to changes in immunity. The less "vigorous" immune system of the old person appears to be more vulnerable to some experientially and psychologically related alterations in immune functions, particularly T-cell function in depression, a psychiatric disorder more common in the elderly. Immune activation, associated both with aging (e.g., increased IL-2 receptors) and with depression (e.g., increased IL-1 production) may contribute to cognitive problems in elderly persons. In Alzheimer's disease, $\beta$-amyloid induces production of proinflammatory cytokines by astrocytes. Immunologically resisted diseases, infectious and neoplastic, are more common in old people. Psychological factors have been found to influence the course of immunologically related diseases in young persons and, therefore, likely also do so in the elderly. Moreover, atherosclerosis involves immunological pathophysiology (inflammatory and, possibly, infectious) and, thereby, makes psychoneuroimmunology of even further relevance to aging. Interventions, both biological and psychological, that may slow age-related decrements in immunological functions deserve further investigation as ways to improve immunity and health, which appear to be closely linked in the elderly population.

# References

Adams, L. S., Yuan, Z., Barboriak, J. J., & Rimm, A. A. (1993). Alcohol-related hospitalizations of elderly people: Prevalence and geographic variation in the United States. *Journal of the American Medical Association, 270,* 1222–1225.

Aisen, P. S. (1996). Inflammation and Alzheimer's disease. *Molecular Chemistry, and Neuropathology,* 83–88.

Alexopoulis, G. S., & Chester, J. G. (1992). Outcomes of geriatric depression. *Clinical Geriatric Medicine, 8,* 363–376.

Antonovski, A. (1987). *Unraveling the mysteries of health: How people manage stress and stay well.* San Francisco: Jossey-Bass.

Arai, H., Moroji, T., & Kosaka, K. (1984). Somatostatin and VIP in post-mortem hair from patients with senile dementia of the Alzheimer's type. *Neuroscience Letters, 52,* 73–78.

Aretz, H. T., & Colvin, R. B. (1997). Endothelial biopsies. *Journal of the American Medical Association, 278,* 1197–1198.

Avissar, S., Mechamkin, Y., Roitman, G., & Schreiber, G. (1998). Dynamics of ECT normalization of low G protein function and immunoreactivity in mononuclear leukocytes of patient with major depression. *American Journal of Psychiatry, 155,* 666–671.

Balin, B. J., Gérard, H. C., Arking, E. J., Appely, D. M., Branigan, P. J., Abrams, J. T., Whittum-Dudson, J. A., & Hudson, A. P. (1998). Identification and localization of *Chlamydia pneumoniae* in Alzheimer's brains. *Medical Microbiology and Immunology, 187,* 23–42.

Banks, W. A., Kastin, A. J., & Ehrensing, C. A. (1994). Blood-borne interleukin-1 alpha is transported across the endothelial blood-spinal cord barrier of mice. *Journal of Physiology, 479* (Pt. 2), 257–264.

Benschop, R. J., Geenen, R., Mills, P. J., Naliboff, B. D., Kiecolt-Glaser, J. K., Herert, T. B., van der Pompe, G., Miller, G. E., Matthews, K. A., Godaert, G. L. R., Gilmore S. L., Glaser, R., Heijnen, C. J., Dopp, J. M., Solomon, G. F., Cacciopio, J. T., & Bijlsma, J. W. J. (1998). Cardiovascular and immune responses to acute psychological stress in young and old women: Demented patients is associated with impaired proliferative capacity, increased CD8+, and a decline in lymphocytes with surface signal transduction molecules (CD38+) and a cytotoxicity marker (CD56+CD8+): A meta-analysis. *Psychosomatic Medicine, 60,* 290–296.

Berk, M., Wadee, A. A., Kuschke, R. H., & O'Neill-Kerr, A. O. (1997). Acute phase proteins in major depression. *Journal of Psychosomatic Research, 43,* 529–534.

Berkman, L. F., & Syme, S. L. (1979). Social networks, host resistance, and mortality. *American Journal of Epidemiology, 109,* 186–204.

Bernardini, R. G., Mauceri, M. P., Iurato, A., Chiarenza, L., Lempereur, L., & Scapagnini, U. (1992). Response of the hypothalamic-pituitary-adrenal axis to interleukin 1 in the aging rat. *Progress in NeuroEndocrinImmunology, 5,* 166–171.

Castle, S., Wilkins, S., Heck, E., Tanzy, K., & Fahey, J. (1995). Depression in caregivers of demented patients is associated with impaired proliferative capacity, increased CD8+, and a decline in lymphocytes with surface signal transduction molecules (CD38+) and a cytoxicity marker (CD56+CD8+). *Clinical and Experimental Immunology, 101,* 487–493.

Chesney, M. A., & Rosenman, R. H. (1985). *Anger and hostility in cardiovascular and behavioral disorders.* Washington, DC: Hemisphere.

Coe, C. L., Erschler, W. B., Champoux, M., & Olson, J. (1992). Psychosocial factors and immune senescence in the aged primate. *Annals of the New York Academy of Sciences, 650,* 276–282.

Cohen, S., Doyle, W. J., Skoner, D. P., Rabin, B. S., & Gwaltney, J. M. (1997). Social ties and susceptibility to the common cold. *Journal of the American Medical Association, 227,* 1940–1944.

Coleman, R. M., Miles, L. E., Guilleminault, C. C., Zarcone, V. P., & Dement, W. C. (1981). Sleep–wake disorders in the elderly: A polysomnographic analysis. *Journal of the American Geriatric Society, 29,* 289–296.

Crist, D. M., MacKinnon, L. T., Thompson, R. F., Attenborn, H. A., & Egan, P. H. (1989). Physical exercise increases natural cellular-mediated immunity in elderly women. *Gerontology, 35,* 66–70.

Crook, T. H., & Miller, N. E. (1985). The challenges of Alzheimer's disease. *American Psychologist, 40,* 1245–1250.

Cunningham, D. A., Rechnitzer, P. A., Howard, J. H., & Donner, A. P. (1987). Exercise training of men at retirement: A clinical trial. *Journal of Gerontology, 42,* 17–23.

Danenberg, H. D., Ben-Yehuda, A., Zakay-Rones, Z., Gross, D. J., Friedman, G. (1997). Dehydroepiandrosterone treatment is not beneficial to the immune response to influenza in elderly subjects. *Journal of Clinical Endocrinology and Metabolism, 82,* 2911–2914.

Davidson, M., Kuo, C-C., Middough, J. C., Campbell, L. A., Wang, S-P., Newman, III, W. P., Finley, J. C., & Grayson, J. T. (1998). Confirmed infection with Chlamydia pneumoniae and its presence in early atherosclerosis. *Circulation, 98,* 628–633.

Dunn, S. E., Ehrlich, M., Sharp, N. J., Reiss, K., Solomon, G., Hawkins, R., Baserga, R., Barrett, J. C. (1998). A dominant negative mutant of the insulin-like growth factor-I receptor inhibits the adhesion, invasion, and metastasis of breast cancer. *Cancer Research, 58,* 3353–3361.

Esterling, B. A., Antoni, M. H., Kumar, M., & Schneiderman, N. (1990). Emotional repression, stress disclosure responses, and Epstein–Barr viral capsid antigen titers. *Psychosomatic Medicine, 52,* 397–410.

Evans, T. G., Judd, M. E., Dowell, T., Poe, S., Daynes, R. A., & Araneo, B. A. (1996). The use of oral dehydroepiandrosterone sulfate as an adjuvant in tetanus and influenza vaccination of the elderly. *Vaccine, 14,* 1531–1537.

Fawzy, F. I., Cousins, N., Fawsy, N. W., Kemeny, M. E., Elashoff, R., & Morton, D. (1990a). A structures psychiatric intervention for cancer patients. I. Changes over time in methods of coping and effective disturbance. *Archives of General Psychiatry, 47,* 720–726.

Fawzy, F. I., Fawzy, N. W., Hyun, C. S., Elashoff, R., Guthrie, D., Fahey, J., & Morton, D. L. (1993). Malignant melanoma: Effects of an early structured psychiatric intervention, coping, and affective state on recurrence and survival six years later. *Archives of General Psychiatry.*

Fawzy, F. I., Kemeny, M. E., Fawzy, H. W., Elashoff, R., Morton, D., Cousins, N., & Fahey, J. L. (1990b). A structured psychiatric intervention for cancer patients. II. Changes over time in immunological measures, *Archives of General Psychiatry, 47,* 729–735.

Fiatarone, M. A., Morley, J. E., Bloom, E. T., Benton, D., Solomon, G. F., & Makinodan, T. (1989). The effect of exercise on natural killer cell activity in young and old subjects. *Journal of Gerontology, 44,* M37–M45.

Flood, J. F., & Morley, J. E. (1998). Learning and memory in the SAMP8 mouse. *Neuroscience and Biobehavior Review, 22,* 1–20.

Flood, J. F., Morley, J. E., & Roberts, E. (1994). An amyloid beta-protein fragment, A beta[12–28], equipotently impairs post-training memory processing when injected into different limbic system structures. *Brain Research, 663,* 271–276.

Flood, J. F., Morley, J. E., & Roberts, E. (1995). Pregnenolone sulfate enhances post-training memory processes when injected in very low doses into limbic system structures: The amygdala is by far the most sensitive. *Proceedings of the National Academy of Sciences, USA, 92,* 10806–10810.

Forloni, G., Mangiarotti, F., Angeretti, N., Lucca, E., & De Simoni, M. G. (1997). Beta-amyloid fragment potentiates IL-6 and TNF-alpha secretion by LPS in astrocytes but not in microglia. *Cytokine, 9,* 759–762.

Fox, R. A. (1984). *Immunology and infection in the elderly.* Edinburgh: Churchill Livingstone.

Franceschi, C., Monti, D., Sansoni, P., & Cossaria, A. (1995). The immunology of exceptional individuals: The lesson of centenarians. *Immunology Today, 16,* 12–16.

Freud, S. (1917). Mourning and melancholia. In *Complete Works of Sigmund Freud* (vol. 14, pp. 237–258). London: Hogarth.

Friedman, H., Klein, T. W., & Specter, S. (Eds.) (1996). *Drugs of abuse, immunity, and infections.* Boca Raaton, FL: CRC Press.

Glaser, R., Kiecolt-Glaser, J. K., Speicher, C. E., & Holiday, J. E. (1985). Stress, loneliness, and changes in herpes virus latency. *Journal of Behavioral Medicine, 8,* 249–260.

Griffin, W. S., Sheng, J. G., Royston, M. C., Gentleman, S. M., McKenzie, J. E., Graham, D. I., Roberts, G. W., & Mrak, R. E. (1998). Glial-neuronal interactions in Alzheimer's disease: The potential role of a ''cytokine cycle'' in disease progression. *Brain Pathology, 8,* 65–72.

Grohr, P., Solomon, G. F., & Benton, D. (1994). Immunological and psychological correlates of perceived place in lifespan in elderly women. *Research perspectives in psychoneuroimmunology,* Key Biscayne, FL, November 16–20.

Guidi, L., Bartoloni, C., Frasca, D., Antico, L., Pili, R., Cursi, F., Tempesta, E., Rumi, C., Menini, E., Carbonin, P., Doria, G., & Gambassi, G. (1991). Impairment of lymphocyte activities in depressed aged subjects. *Mechanisms of Aging and Development, 60,* 13–24.

Hadden, J. W. (1998). Thymic endocrinology. *Annals of the New York Academy of Science, 840,* 352–358.

Hankinson, S. E., Willett, W. C., Colditz, G. A., Hunter, D. J., Michaud, D. S., Deroo, B., Rosner, B., Speizer, F. E., & Pollak, M. (1998). Circulating concentrations of insulin-like growth factor-I and risk of breast cancer. *Lancet, 351,* 1393–1396.

Hansen, M. K., Taishi, P., Chen, Z., & Krueger, J. M. (1998). Vagotomy blocks the induction of interleukin-1beta (IL-1beta) mRNA in the brain of rats in response to systemic IL-1beta. *Journal of Neuroscience, 18,* 2247–2253.

Herbert, T. B., & Cohen, S. (1993). Depression and immunity: A meta-analytic review. *Psychological Bulletin, 113,* 472–486.

Hollenbeck, C. B., Haskell, W., Rosentha, M., & Reaven, G. M. (1985). Effect of habitual physical activity on regulation of insulin-stimulated glucose disposal in older males. *Journal of the American Gerontological Society, 33,* 273–277.

Hu, J., Akama, K. T., Krafft, G. A., Chromy, B. A., & Van Eldik, L. J, (1998). Amyloid-beta peptide activates cultured astrocytes: Morphological alterations, cytokine induction and nitric oxide release. *Brain Research, 785,* 195–206.

Ironson, G., Solomon, G. F., Cruess, D., Barroso, J., & Stivers M. (1995). Psychosocial factors related to long survival with HIV/AIDS. *Journal of Clinical Psychology and Psychotherapy, 2,* 249–266.

Irwin, M., Daniels, M., Risch, S. D., Bloom, E., & Weiner, H. (1988). Plasma cortisol and natural killer cell activity during bereavement. *Biological Psychiatry, 24,* 173–178.

Irwin, M., Lecher, U., & Caldwell, D. (1991). Depression and reduced natural killer cytotoxity: A longitudinal study of depressed patients and control subjects. *Psychological Medicine, 22,* 1045–1050.

Irwin, M., Mascovich, A., Gillin, C., Willoughby, R., Pike, J., & Smith, T. L (1994). Partial sleep deprivation reduces natural killer cell activity in humans. *Psychosomatic Medicine, 56,* 493–498.

Jerrels, T. R., Marietta, C. A., Eckhardt, M. J., Majchrowicz, E., & Wright, R. F. G. (1986). Effects of ethanol administration on parameters of immunocompetence in rats. *Journal of Leukocyte Biology, 29,* 499–510.

Kalman, J., Juhasz, A., Laird, G., Dickens, P., Jardanhazy, T., Rimanoczy, A., Boncz, I., Parry-Jones, W. L., & Janka, Z. (1997). Serum interleukin-6 levels correlate with the severity of dementia in Down syndrome and in Alzheimer's disease. *Acta Neurologica Scandinavica, 96,* 236–240.

Kaplan, J. R., Pettersson, K., & Manuck, S. B. (1991). Role of sympathoadrenal activation in the initiation and progression of atherosclerosis. *Circulation, 84* (supplement VI), 23–31.

Katila, H., Apelberg, B., Hurme, M., & Rimon, R. (1994). Plasma levels of interleukin-1$\beta$ and interleukin-6 in schizophrenia, other psychoses, and affective disorders. *Schizophrenia Research, 12,* 29–34.

Keast, D. (1996). Immune responses to overtraining and fatigue. In L. Hoffman-Goetz (Ed.), *Exercise and immune function* (pp. 121–141). Boca Raton, FL: CRC Press.

Kelley, K. W., Meier, W. A., Minshall, C., Schacher, D. H., Liu, Q., Van Hoy, R., Burgess, W., & Dantzer, R. (1998). Insulin growth factor-I inhibits apoptosis in hematopoietic progenitor cells. Implications in thymic aging. *Annals of the New York Academy of Science, 840,* 518–524.

Kemeney, M. E., Fahey, J. L., Schneider, S., Taylor, S. E., Weiner, H., & Visscher, B. (1989). Psychosocial co-factors in HIV infection: Associations among bereavement, depression and immunity. *Psychosomatic Medicine, 51,* 244–266.

Kennedy, G. J. (1991). Persistence and remission of depressive symptoms in late life. *American Journal of Psychiatry, 148,* 174–178.

Kiecolt-Glaser, J. K., Dura, J. R., Speicher, C. E., Trask, J., & Glaser, R. (1991). Spousal caregivers of dementia victims. Longitudinal changes in immunity and health. *Psychosomatic Medicine, 53,* 345–362.

Kiecolt-Glaser, J. K., Glaser, R., Shuttleworth, E., Dyer, C., Ogrocki, P., & Speicher, C. E. (1987). Chronic stress and immunity in family caregivers of Alzheimer's disease victims. *Psychosomatic Medicine, 49,* 523–535.

Kiecolt-Glaser, J. K., Glaser, R., Williger, D., Stout, J., Messick, G., Sheppard, S., Ricker, D., Romisher, S. C., Briner, W., Bonnell, G., & Donnerberg, R. (1985). Psychosocial enhancement of immunocompetence in a geriatric population. *Health Psychology, 4,* 25–41.

King, A. C., & Brassington, G. (1997). Enhancing physical and psychological functioning in older family caregivers: The role of regular physical activity. *Annals of Behavioral Medicine, 19,* 91–100.

Kitamura, Y., Shimohama, S., Ota, T., Matsuoka, Y., Nomura, Y., & Taniguchi, T., (1997). Alteration of transcription factors NF-kappaB and STAT1 in Alzheimer's disease brains. *Neuroscience Letters, 237,* 17–20.

Koenig, H. G., Cohen, H. J., George, L. K., Hays, J. C., Larson, D. B., & Blazer, D. G. (1997). Attendance of religious services, interleukin-6, and other biological parameters of immune function in older adults. *International Journal of Psychiatry in Medicine, 27,* 233–250.

Kouzis, A., Eaton, W. W., & Leaf, P. J. (1995). Psychopathology and mortality in the general population. *Social Psychiatry and Psychiatric Epidemiology 30,* 165–170.

Laman, J. D., de Smet, B. J. G. L. Schoneveld, A., & van Meurs, M. (1997). CD40–CD40L interactions in atherosclerosis. *Immunology Today, 18,* 231–239.

Lewis, S. L., Kroening, C. E., Bonner, P. N., & Cooper, C. L. (1999). *Relaxation therapy improves immune function in caregivers of Alzheimer's patients.* Vancouver, BC: American Psychosomatic Society.

Li, Z. G., Davis, V. A., & Brooks, P. M. (1993). Effect of gonadal steroids on the production of IL-1 and IL-6 by blood mononuclear cells in vitro. *Clinical Experimental Rheumatology, 11,* 157–162.

Licinio, J., Kling, M. A., & Hauser, P. (1998). Cytokines and brain function: Relevance to interferon-alpha-induced mood and cognitive changes. *Seminars in Oncology, 25*(1), 30–38.

Lissoni, P., Brivio, O., Brivio, F., Barni, S., Tancini, G., Crippa, D., & Meregalli, S. (1996). Adjuvant therapy with the pineal hormone melatonin in patients with lympho node relapse due to malignant melanoma. *Journal of Pineal Research, 21,* 239–242.

Lissoni, P., Paolorossi, F., Ardizzoia, A., Barni, S., Chilelli, M., Mancuso, M., Tancini, G., Conti, A., & Maestroni, G. J. (1997). A randomized study of chemotherapy with cisplatin plus etoposide versus chemoendocrine therapy with cisplatin, etoposide and the pineal hormone melatonin as a first-line treatment of advanced non-small cell lung cancer patients in a poor clinical state. *Journal of Pineal Research, 23,* 15–19.

Lutgendorf, S. K., Garand, L., Buckwalter, K. E., Reimer, T. T., Hong, S.-Y., & U Lubaroff, D. M. (1999). Life stress and elevated IL-6 in healthy elderly women. *Journals of Gerontology: Medical Sciences, 54A,* M1–M6.

Lutgendorf, S. K., Vitaliano, P. P., Tripp-Reimer, T. T., Harvey, J. H., & Luberoff, D. M. (1999). Sense of coherence buffers effects of life stress on NK activity in healthy older adults. *Psychology and Aging, 14,* 552–563.

Maes, M., Stevens, W. J., Declerck, L. S., Bridts, C. H., Peeters, D., Schotte, C., & Cosyns, P. (1993). Significantly increased expression of T-cell activation markers (interleukin-2 and HLA-DR) in depression: Further evidence for an inflammatory process during that illness. *Progress in NeuroPsychopharmacology and Biological Psychiatry, 17,* 241–255.

Maes, M., Vandoolaeghe, E., Ranjan, R., Bosmans, E., Berghmans, R., & Desnyder, R. (1995). Increased serum interleukin-1-receptor-antagonist concentrations in major depression. *Journal of Affective Disorders, 36,* 29–36. .

Maison, P., Balkau, B., Simon, D., Chanson, P., Rosselin, G., & Eschwege, E. (1998). Growth hormone as a risk for premature mortality in healthy subjects—Data from the Paris prospective study. *British Medical Journal, 316,* 1132–1133.

Malaise, M. G., Hazee-Hagelstein, M. T., Reuter, A. M., Vrinds-Gavaert, Y., Goldstein, G., & Franchimont, P. (1987). Thymopoetin and thymopentin enhance the levels of ACTH, BE, and beta-lipoprotein from rat pituitary cells *in vitro. Acta Endocrinologica, 114,* 455–560.

Mantovani, A., Bussolini, F., & Introna, M. (1997). Cytokine regulation of endothelial cell function from molecular level to the bedside. *Immunology Today, 18,* 231–239.

Mariotti, S., Barbesino, G., Caturegli, P., Bartalena, L., Sansoni, P., Fagnoni, F., Monti, D., Fagiolo, U., Franceschi, C., & Pinchera, A. (1993). Complex alteration of thyroid function in healthy centenarians. *Journal of Clinical Endocrinolology and Metabolism, 77,* 1130–1134.

Mariotti, S., Sansoni, P., Barbesino, G., Caturegli, P., Monti, D., Cossarizza, A., Giacomelli, T., Passeri, G., Fagiolo, U., & Pinchera, A. (1992). Thyroid and other organ-specific autoantibodies in healthy centenarians. *Lancet, 339,* 1506–1508.

McNaughton, M. E., Smith, L. W., Patterson, T. L., & Grant, I. (1990). Stress, social support, coping resources, and immune status in elderly women. *Journal of Nervous and Mental Disease, 38,* 460–461.

Miller, R. A. (1996). Aging and the immune response. In E. L. Schneider & J. E. Rowe (Eds.), *Handbook of the biology of aging* (4th ed.) (pp. 335–392). San Diego: Academic Press.

Moldofsky, H., Lue, F. A., Davidson, J. R., & Gorczynski, R. (1989). Effects of sleep deprivation on human immune functions. *Federation of American Societies of Experimental Biology Journal, 3,* 192–897.

Moos, R. H., & Solomon, G. F. (1964). Personality correlates of the rapidity of progression of rheumatoid arthritis. *Annals of Rheumatic Diseases, 23,* 145–151.

Moos, R. H., & Solomon, G. F. (1965). Personality correlates of the degree of functional incapacity of patients with physical diseases. *Journal of Chronic Disease, 18,* 1019–1038.

Morley, J. E. (1999, in press). Immunosenescence. In J. E. Morley, J. Armbrecht, & R. M. Coe (Eds.). *Geriatric Science.* Baltimore: Johns Hopkins Press.

Morley, J. E., Flood, J. F., Silver, A. J., & Kaiser, F. E. (1994). Effects of peripherally secreted hormones on behavior. *Neurobiology of Aging, 15,* 573–577.

Morley, J. E., & Perry, H. M. (1991). The management of diabetes mellitus in older individuals. *Drugs, 41,* 548–565.

Muller, K., & Bendtzen, K. (1996). 1,25-Dihydroxyvitamin D3 as a natural regulator of human immune functions. *Journal of Investigative Dermatology, 1,* 68–71.

Naliboff, B. D., Benton, D., Solomon, G. F., Morley, J. E., Fahey, J. L., Bloom, E. T., Makinodan, T., & Gilmore, S. L. (1991). Immunological changes in young and old adults during brief laboratory stress. *Psychosomatic Medicine, 53,* 121–132.

Neri, B., de Leonardis, V., Gemelli, M. T., di Loro, F., Mottola, A., Ponchietti, R., Raugei, A., & Cini, G. (1998). Melatonin as biological response modifier in cancer patients. *Anticancer Research, 18,* 1329–1332.

Nieman, D. C., Henson, D. A., Gusewitch, G., Warren, B. J., Dotson, R. C., Butterworth, D. E., & Nehlsen-Camarella, S. L. (1993). Physical activity and immune function in elderly women. *Medical Science of Sports and Exercise, 25,* 823–826.

Norman, D. C., Morley, J. E., & Chang, M-P. (1988). Aging decreases β-endorphin enhancement of T-cell mitogenesis in mice. *Mechanisms of Aging and Development. 44,* 185–191.

Papadakis, M. A., Grady, D., Black, D., Tierney, M. J., Gooding, G. A., Schambelan, M., & Grunfeld, C. (1996). Growth hormone replacement in healthy older men improves body composition but not functional ability. *Annals of Internal Medicine, 124,* 708–716.

Pennix, B. W. J. H., Guralnik, J. M., Ferrucci, L., Simonsick, E. M., Deeg, P. J. H., & Wallace, R. B. (1998). Depressive symptoms and physical decline in community-dwelling older persons. *Journal of the American Medical Association, 279,* 1720–1726.

Rada, P., Mark, G. P., Vitek, M. P., Mangano, R. M., Blume, A. J., Beer, B., & Hoebel, B. G., (1991). Interleukin-1 beta decreases acetylcholine measured by microdialysis in the hippocampus of freely moving rats. *Brain Research, 550,* 287–290.

Reed, K. M., Kemeny, M. E., Taylor, S. E., Wang, H. Y., & Fisher, E. R. (1994). Realistic acceptance as a predictor of decreased survival time in gay men with HIV/AIDS. *Health Psychology, 13,* 299–307.

Ridker, P. M., Cushman, M., Stampfer, M. J., Tracy, R. P., & Henekens, C. H. (1997). Inflammation, aspirin, and the risk of cardiovascular disease in apparently healthy men. *New England Journal of Medicine, 336,* 973–979.

Rincón, H. G., Solomon, G. F., Benton, D., & Rubenstein, L. Z. (1996). Exercise in frail elderly men decreases natural killer cell activity. *Aging: Clinical and Experimental Research, 8,* 109–112.

Roberts, G. W., Gentleman, S. M., Lynch, A., & Graham, D. I. (1991). Beta A4 amyloid protein deposition in brain after head trauma. *Lancet, 338,* 1422–1423.

Rodin, J. (1986). Aging and health: effects of sense of control *Science, 233,* 1271–1276.

Rosenthal, M. J., Fajardo, M., Gilmore, S., Morley, J. E., & Naliboff, B. D., (1998). Hospitalization and mortality of diabetes in older adults. A 3-year prospective study. *Diabetes Care, 21,* 231–235.

Saikku, P., Keinonen, M., Tankeneh, L., Kinanmake, E., Ekman, M., Mahninen, V., Mantarri, M., Frick, M., & Huttunen, J. (1992). Chronic Chlamydia pneumoniae infection as a risk factor for coronary artery disease in the Helsinki Heart Study. *Annals of Internal Medicine, 116,* 273–278.

Scanlon, J. M., Vitaliano, P. P., Ochs, H., Savage, M. V., & Borson, S. (1998). CD4 and CD8 counts are associated with interaction of gender and psychosocial stress. *Psychosomatic Medicine, 60,* 644–653.

Schleifer, S. J., Keller, S. E., Bond, R. N., Cohen, J., & Stein, M. (1989). Major depressive disorder and immunity: Role of age, sex, severity, and hospitalization. *Archives of General Psychiatry, 45,* 81–89.

Schleifer, S. J., Keller, S. E., Camerino, M., Thornton, J., & Stein, M. (1983). Suppression of lymphocyte stimulation following bereavement. *Journal of the American Medical Association, 250,* 374–377.

Shinkai, S., Konishi, M., & Sheppard, R. J. (1996). Aging, exercise, and the immune system. *Exercise Immunology Review, 3,* 68–95.

Sidney, K. H., & Shephard, R. J. (1987). Frequency and intensity of exercise training for elderly subjects. *Medical Science of Sports and Exercise, 10,* 125–131.

Sieber, W. J., Rodin, J., Larson, L., Ortega, S., & Cummings, N. (1992). Modulation of human natural killer cell activity by exposure to uncontrollable stress. *Brain, Behavior, and Immunity, 6,* 141–156.

Simonsick, E. M., Lafferty, M. E., Phillips, C. L., de Leon, C. F. M., Kasl, S. V., Seeman, T. E., Fillenbaum, G., Herbert, P., & Lemke, J. H. (1993). Risk due to inactivity in physically capable older adults. *American Journal of Public Health, 83,* 1443–1450.

Sluzewska, A., Rybakowski, J., Bosmans, E., Sobieska, M., Berghmans, R., Maes, M., & Witorowicz, K. (1996). Indicators of immune activation in major depression. *Psychiatric Research, 64,* 161–167

Solomon, G. F. (1991). Psychosocial factors, exercise, and immunity: Athletes, elderly persons, and AIDS patients. *International Journal of Sports Medicine, 15,* S50–S52.

Solomon, G. F., Fiatarone, M. A., Benton, D., Morley, J. E., Bloom, E., & Makinodan, T. (1988). Psychoimmunologic and endorphin function in the aged. *Annals of the New York Academy of Sciences, 521,* 43–58.

Solomon, G. F., & Moos, R. H. (1965a). Psychologic aspects of response to treatment in rheumatoid arthritis. *GP, 32,* 113–119.

Solomon, G. F., & Moos, R. H. (1965b). The relationship of personality to the presence of rheumatoid factor in symptomatic relatives of patients with rheumatoid arthritis. *Psychosomatic Medicine, 27,* 350–360.

Solomon, G. F., Temoshok, L., O'Leary, A., & Zich, J. (1987). An intensive pilot study of long-surviving persons with AIDS. *Annals of the New York Academy of Sciences, 496,* 628–636.

Song, H., Price, P. W., & Cerny, J. (1997). Age-related changes in antibody repertoire: Contribution from T cells. *Immunological Review, 160,* 55–62.

Spangelo, B. L., & MacLeod, R. M. (1988). Thymic stromal elements contain prolactin and growth hormone releasing activities. *Progress in NeuroEndocrinImmunology, 1,* 9–10.

Spurrell, M., & Creed, F. H. (1993) Lymphocyte response in depressed patients and subjects anticipating bereavement. *British Journal of Psychiatry, 162,* 60–64.

Sternberg, E. M., Wilder, R. L., Chrousos, G. P., & Gold, P. W. (1991). The stress response and the pathogenesis of arthritis. In J. A. McCubbin, P. G. Kaufman, & C. B. Nemeroff (Eds.), *Stress, neuropeptides, and systemic disease* (pp. 287–300). San Diego: Academic Press.

Travis, J. (1993). Army targets a potential vaccine against cholesterol (Article reporting work of C. Ahring and other investigators). *Science, 262,* 1974–1975.

Unützer, J., Patrick, D. L., Simon, G., Grembowski, D., Walker, E., Rutter, C., & Katoni, W. (1997). Depressive symptoms and the cost of health services in HMO patients aged 65 years and older. *Journal of the American Medical Association, 277,* 1618–1623.

Uthgennant, D., Schoolmann, D., Pietrowsky, R., Fehm, Y., & Born, J. (1995). Effects of sleep on the production of cytokines in humans. *Psychosomatic Medicine, 57,* 97–104.

Waterhouse, J., Reilly, T., & Atkinson, G. (1998). Melatonin & jet lag. *British Journal of Sports Medicine, 32,* 98–99.

Watson, R. (Ed.) (1995). *Alcohol, drugs of abuse and immune functions.* Boca Raton, FL: CRC Press.

Weitzman, R., Laor, N., Podliszewski, E., Notti, I., Djaldetti, M., & Bessler, H. (1994). Cytokine production in major depressed patients before and after clomipramine treatment. *Biological Psychiatry, 35,* 42–47.

Whooley, M. A., & Browner, W. S. (1998). Depression is associated with increased mortality in elderly women. *Archives of Internal Medicine, 158,* 2129–2135.

Wick, G., Schett, G., & Amberger, A. (1995). Is atherosclerosis an immunologically-mediated disease? *Immunology Today, 16,* 27–33.

Wittert, G. A., & Morley, J. E. (1997). Effects of aging on the hormonal response to stress. In K. P. Ober (Ed.), *Endocrinology of critical disease* (pp. 299–309). Totowa NJ: Humana Press.

Yen, S. S., Morales, A. J., & Khorram, O. (1995). Replacement of DHEA in aging men and women. Potential remedial effects. *Annals of the New York Academy of Sciences, 774,* 128–142.

Yirmiya, R., & Taylor, A. N. (Eds.) (1993). *Alcohol, immunity and cancer.* Boca Raton, FL: CRC Press.

# Author Index

## C

# Subject Index

## A

Abortion, recurrent, **2:**425

Acetylcholine, **2:**113

Acetylcholinesterase, **1:**63–66, 78, 79, 241–242

AchE, *see* acetylcholinesterase

Acquired immune deficiency syndrome, **1:**97–98, 100–101
  opportunistic infections, **2:**585
  antiretroviral medications, **2:**586

Acquired immune response
  cellular activation, **2:**125–126
  immunoglobulin A, **2:**126
  lymphocyte proliferation, **2:**125

ACTH, *see* adrenocorticotropic hormone

Acute coronary syndromes, **2:**526–527, 529, 531, 536–537

Acute phase proteins, **1:**564, **2:**529–530, 538

Adaptor proteins, **1:**12

Adenosine, **1:**677–678

Adenosine 3′,5′-cyclic monophosphate, **1:**117–121, 140–141

Adenosine triphosphate (ATP), **1:**198

Adenylyl cyclase, **1:**117–118, 120–121

Adhesion molecules, **1:**223, 235, 555–556, **2:**116, 351, 354, 434, 440–441

Adjuvant-induced arthritis, **1:**92–95, 98–99, 207–208

Adrenergic activity
  Beta-adrenoceptor activation, **2:**552–553
  corticosteroids, **2:**553
  ex-vivo suppression, **2:**552
  human natural killer cell activity, **2:**553–554
  intracellular mechanisms, **2:**553
  in vitro suppression, **2:**552–553
  natural killer cells and, **2:**551–554
  tumor increases, **2:**552

Adrenergic receptors, **1:**161–179, 198 **2:**113

Adrenocorticotropic hormone, **2:**486, 650, 665

Affect, **2:**87–88, 90–95

Aggression, **1:**707, **2:**38–43, 80–82, 95–96, 98, 175–177, 252

Aging
  disease susceptibility and, **2:**636
  hippocampal degeneration and, **2:**636–637
  hypothalamic-pituitary-adrenal hyperactivity, **2:**637
  immunity and, **2:**702–704, 709–710
    hormones, **2:**702–704
  lymphoid tissue and, **1:**86–87
  mental health and, **2:**708–709
  psychosocial influences on immunity, **2:**704–707
  thymic function and, **2:**704

AIDS, *see* Acquired immune deficiency syndrome

Alcohol, **2:**656–658, 687–695

Alcoholism, **2:**706–707

Alexithymia, **2:**94

Allergy, **2:**136, 138–146

Alpha adrenergic receptors, **1:**118, 146

α-MSH, *see* Alpha-melanocyte stimulating hormone

Alpha-melanocyte stimulating hormone, **1:**574, 577

Alternative medicine, **2:**161–169

Alzheimer's disease, **1:**550–551, **2:**354–356, 358–359, 710–711
  amyloid precursor protein, **1:**551
  beta-amyloid protein **1:**551
  nitric oxide, **1:**551
  pro-inflammatory cytokines, **1:**550

Amygdala, **2:**323

Analgesia, **2:**115–117
  peripheral, **1:**399

Angina, **2:**527

Animal
  models, advantages and disadvantages, **2:**484
  welfare, **2:**44

Antibiotics, **2:**540

Antibody secretion, **1:**417

Anti-thymocyte serum, **2:**42–43

Anxiety, **1:**;706, **2:**206–207
  dental **2:**646–649

Apoptosis, **1:**134–136, 247, **2:**55, 255–256, 353, 587, 694

L-arginine, **2:**255–257

Arthritis, **1:**263, 639, 641
  adjuvant-induced, **2:**234,-235

Asthma, **2:**136–137, 140, 215

Astrocytes, **2:**349–350

Atherosclerosis, **2:**407, 711–712

ATP, *see* Adenosine triphosphate

Attention, **2:**135

Autoimmunity, **1:**92–99, **2:**399–414
  handedness and, **2:**412
  organ-specific, **2**, 401
  non-specific, **2:**401
  pregnancy and, **2:**412

Autoimmune disease, **1:**262–263
  animal models of, **2:**423
  diabetes, **2:**183
  experimental allergic encephalomyelitis, **2:**183
  penetrance, **2:**184
  stress and, **2:**214–215
  sympathetic regulation of, **1:**24–30
  systemic lupus erythematosus, **2:**183–184

Autonomic nervous system, *see also* sympathetic nervous system; parasympathetic nervous system, **2:**435–436

## B

BBB, *see* Blood-brain barrier

B-cells, **1:**251, 254
  cyclic adenosine monophosphate, **1:**174–175
  effects of marijuana on, **1:**424
  immunoglobulin secretion, **1:**172–174
  isotype switching, **2:**56
  proliferation, **1:**170–174, 257–258, 276–277
  radioligand binding, **1:**174

B lymphocytes, *see* B-cells

Baseline, measurement of, **2:**267–268

Bereavement, **2:**704–705

Tonsil, **1:**78–79
Toxic shock syndrome toxin, **2:**258
Transcription factors, **1:**556–557
 AP-1, **1:**557
 NFφB, **1:**556–557
Transforming growth factor beta, **1:**553–555,
 **2:**661
 physiological effects of, **1:**554–555
 receptors, **1:**553–554
 signaling, **1:**554
Traumatic stress, **2:**335–342
 neuroendocrine changes and, **2:**340–
 341
*Trichinella spiralis*, **2:**492
Triple response, **2:**472–473
Trichotillomania, **2:**412
Tuberculin skin test, **2:**143–144, 147, 155
Tuberculosis, **1:**290–291, **2:**491
 stress and, **1:**290–291
Tumors, growth and metastases, **1:**209–210
Tumor necrosis factor alpha (TNFα), **1:**205–
 207, 551–553, **2:**59–60, 662
 catecholamine regulation of, **1:**205
 effects on brain cells, **1:**552–553
 receptors, **1:**552
 signaling, **1:**552

Type A behavior pattern, **2:**533–534
Tyrosine hydroxylase, Innervation of
 lymphoid tissue, **1:**60–61, 80, 84–85

# U

U69, 593, **2:**257–259
Urticaria, **2:**135, 140

# V

Viral infection
 influenza virus, **1:**652
 neurochemical responses to, **1:**652–
 653
 Newcastle disease virus, **1:**652
Varicella zoster, **2:**147, 155
Vascular endothelial growth factor, **2:**662
Vasoactive intestinal peptide (VIP), **1:**72–74,
 76–77, 79–81, 248–250, **2:**113
 receptors, **2:**113
Vasopressin, **1:**719–720
Vital exhaustion, *see* exhaustion
Vagotomy, **1:**568–573, 710

Vagus nerve, **1:**568–573, 678–679
*Valerianae radix*, **2:**168

# W

Warts, **2:**136
West Nile virus, **2:**490
 encephalitis, **2:**490
Worry, **2:**92–93
Wound
 contraction, **2:**615, 618
 healing, **2:**215–216, 614–620, 659–662
 fibroblasts, **2:**617–618
 growth factors, **2:**618–619
 macrophages, **2:**617
 models of, **2:**614–615
 neutrophils
 pro-inflammatory cytokines, **2:**619–620
 remodeling, **2:**618
 strength, **2:**615

# Y

*Yersinia (pasteurella) pestis*, **2:**492

ISBN 0-12-044316-3

9 780120 443161

90114